FITZPATRICK'S

COLOR ATLAS AND SYNOPSIS OF CLINICAL DERMATOLOGY

SIXTH EDITION

Available Translations of Fitzpatrick's *Color Atlas and Synopsis of Clinical Dermatology,*
Fifth Edition

Chinese (Short Form)	McGraw-Hill Education (Asia), Jurong, Singapore
Chinese (Long Form)	McGraw-Hill International Enterprises, Inc., Taipei, Taiwan
Greek	Paschalidis Medical Publications, Athens, Greece
Indonesian	Penerbit Salemba Medika, Jakarta, Indonesia
Italian	McGraw-Hill, s.r.l., Milan, Italy
Portuguese	McGraw-Hill Interamericana Editores, S.A. de C.V., Mexico City
Spanish	McGraw-Hill Interamericana de Espana. S.A., Madrid

FITZPATRICK'S
COLOR ATLAS AND SYNOPSIS OF CLINICAL DERMATOLOGY
SIXTH EDITION

Klaus Wolff
Professor and Chairman Emeritus
Department of Dermatology
Medical University of Vienna
Chief Emeritus, Dermatology Service
General Hospital of Vienna
Vienna, Austria

Richard Allen Johnson
Clinical Instructor and Associate in Dermatology
Massachusetts General Hospital
Harvard Medical School
Boston, Massachusetts

mcgraw-hillmedical.com

New York   Chicago   San Francisco   Lisbon   London   Madrid   Mexico City
Milan   New Delhi   San Juan   Seoul   Singapore   Sydney   Toronto

Fitzpatrick's Color Atlas And Synopsis Of Clinical Dermatology, Sixth Edition

1234567890 DOC DOC 12 11 10 9

ISBN 978-0-07-159975-7
MHID 0-07-159975-4

This book was set in Times Roman by Aptara, Inc. The editors were Anne M. Sydor and Mariapaz Ramos Englis. The production supervisor was Phil Galea. The text designers were Alan Barnett and Alicia Fox of Alan Barnett Design. The line art was prepared by Susan Gilbert. The index was prepared by Jerry Ralya.

R R Donnelley was printer and binder.

This book is printed on acid-free paper.

Library of Congress Cataloging-in-Publication Data
Fitzpatrick's color atlas and synopsis of clinical dermatology.—6th ed. /
Klaus Wolff,
    Richard Allen Johnson.
        p. ; cm.
    Includes bibliographical references and index.
    ISBN-13: 978-0-07-159975-7 (softcover : alk. paper)
    ISBN-10: 0-07-159975-4 (softcover : alk. paper)   1. Dermatology—Atlases.
    I. Wolff, Klaus, 1935- II.
Johnson, Richard Allen, 1940- III. Fitzpatrick, Thomas B. (Thomas Bernard),
1919-2003.   IV. Title: Color atlas and synopsis of clinical dermatology.
    [DNLM: 1. Skin Diseases—Atlases. WR 17 F5591 2009]
    RL81.C65 2009
    616.5—dc22
                                                        2008052749

THOMAS BERNARD FITZPATRICK
19 December 1919 – 16 August 2003

This Sixth Edition of *Fitzpatrick's Color Atlas and Synopsis of Clinical Dermatology* is dedicated to Thomas B. Fitzpatrick, the founding Author who was part of the Atlas for the first four editions. On August 16, 2003, Thomas B. Fitzpatrick succumbed to a disease he had fought patiently and courageously. One of the giants of dermatology had gone—a man who had moved the world of dermatology had left the scene.

The name Thomas B. Fitzpatrick is associated with many milestones: the melanosome and tyrosinase, the epidermal melanin unit, skin phototypes, melanoma, PUVA photochemotherapy, sun protection factors, vitiligo, and many others; the landmark books *Fitzpatrick's Dermatology in General Medicine* and this *Color Atlas and Synopsis of Clinical Dermatology* are milestones in themselves. Thomas B. Fitzpatrick was a towering personality—what he created in the twentieth century is a challenge for the dermatosciences of the future.

This Sixth Edition of *Fitzpatrick's Color Atlas and Synopsis of Clinical Dermatology* is dedicated to **Mariapaz Ramos Englis**, who has been Production Editor for the *Atlas* on the last five editions. She has worked tirelessly and precisely to ensure the quality of the book, often using her personal time to see to the myriad details involved in producing the book. She has adapted and evolved with the book and with publishing as it has transitioned from working with paper and slides to floppy disks, e-mail submission, and online publication. Her dedication, patience, and passion have made her the soul of the *Atlas* for the last two decades.

NOTICE

Medicine is an ever-changing science. As new research and clinical experience broaden our knowledge, changes in treatment and drug therapy are required. The authors and the publisher of this work have checked with sources believed to be reliable in their efforts to provide information that is complete and generally in accord with the standards accepted at the time of publication. However, in view of the possibility of human error or changes in medical sciences, neither the authors nor the publisher nor any other party who has been involved in the preparation or publication of this work warrants that the information contained herein is in every respect accurate or complete, and they disclaim all responsibility for any errors or omissions or for the results obtained from use of the information contained in this work. Readers are encouraged to confirm the information contained herein with other sources. For example and in particular, readers are advised to check the product information sheet included in the package of each drug they plan to administer to be certain that the information contained in this work is accurate and that changes have not been made in the recommended dose or in the contraindications for administration. This recommendation is of particular importance in connection with new or infrequently used drugs.

CONTENTS

PART I
DISORDERS PRESENTING IN THE SKIN AND MUCOUS MEMBRANES

SECTION 1
DISORDERS OF SEBACEOUS AND APOCRINE GLANDS   2

SECTION 2
ECZEMA/DERMATITIS   20

SECTION 3
PSORIASIS   53

SECTION 10

PHOTOSENSITIVITY, PHOTO-INDUCED DISORDERS, AND DISORDERS BY IONIZING RADIATION — 232

SECTION 11

PRECANCEROUS LESIONS AND CUTANEOUS CARCINOMAS — 274

SECTION 12

MELANOMA PRECURSORS AND PRIMARY CUTANEOUS MELANOMA   300

SECTION 13

PIGMENTARY DISORDERS   334

PART II

DERMATOLOGY AND INTERNAL MEDICINE

SECTION 14

THE SKIN SIGNS IN IMMUNE, AUTOIMMUNE, AND RHEUMATIC DISORDERS   354

SECTION 15

ENDOCRINE, METABOLIC, NUTRITIONAL, AND GENETIC DISEASES   420

SECTION 16

SKIN SIGNS OF VASCULAR INSUFFICIENCY   **458**

SECTION 17

SKIN SIGNS OF RENAL INSUFFICIENCY   **480**

SECTION 18

SKIN SIGNS OF SYSTEMIC CANCERS   **486**

PART III
DISEASES DUE TO MICROBIAL AGENTS

SECTION 31

HUMAN RETROVIRAL INFECTIONS AND MUCOCUTANEOUS MANIFESTATIONS OF HIV/AIDS DISEASE — 942

PART IV
SKIN SIGNS OF HAIR, NAIL, AND MUCOSAL DISORDERS

SECTION 32

DISORDERS OF HAIR FOLLICLES AND RELATED DISORDERS — 961

SECTION 33

DISORDERS OF THE NAIL APPARATUS — 1000

SECTION 34

DISORDERS OF THE MOUTH   1028

SECTION 35

DISORDERS OF THE GENITALIA, PERINEUM, AND ANUS **1046**

PREFACE

The *First Edition* of this book appeared 26 years ago (1983) and has been expanded pari passu with the major developments that have occurred in dermatology over the past two and a half decades. Dermatology is now one of the most sought after medical specialties because the burden of skin disease has become enormous and the many new innovative therapies available today attract large patient populations.

The *Color Atlas and Synopsis of Clinical Dermatology* has been used by thousands of primary care physicians, dermatologists, internists, and other health care providers principally because it facilitates dermatologic diagnosis by providing color photographs of skin lesions and, juxtaposed, a succinct summary outline of skin disorders as well as the skin signs of systemic diseases.

The Sixth Edition has been extensively revised, rewritten, and expanded by the addition of new sections. Roughly 80% of the old images have been replaced by new ones and additional images have been added. There is a complete update of etiology, pathogenesis, management and therapy and there is now an online version. The previous edition of the *Atlas* has been translated into seven languages.

ACKNOWLEDGMENT

Our secretary, Renate Kosma, worked hard to meet the demands of the authors. In the present McGraw-Hill team, we appreciated the counsel of Scott Grillo, Vice President and Publisher; Anne M. Sydor, Executive Editor; Mariapaz Ramos Englis, Senior Managing Editor; Phil Galea, Senior Production Manager, who expertly managed the production process; Lindsey Zahuranec and M. Lorraine Andrews, the editorial assistants, for their invaluble help;. Alan Barnett and Alicia Fox, of Alan Barnett Design; and Susan Gilbert, for her lovely line illustrations.

But the major force behind this edition and previous editions was Mariapaz Ramos Englis whose good nature, good judgment, loyalty to the authors, and, most of all, patience, guided the authors to make an even better book.

INTRODUCTION

The *Color Atlas and Synopsis of Clinical Dermatology* is proposed as a "field guide" to the recognition of skin disorders and their management. The skin is a treasury of important lesions that can usually be recognized clinically. Gross morphology in the form of skin lesions remains the hard core of dermatologic diagnosis, and therefore this text is accompanied by over 900 color photographs illustrating skin diseases, skin manifestations of internal diseases, infections, tumors, and incidental skin findings in otherwise well individuals. We have endeavored to include information relevant to gender dermatology and a large number of images showing skin disease in different ethnic populations. This *Atlas* covers the entire field of clinical dermatology but does not include very rare syndromes or conditions. With respect to these the reader is referred to another McGraw-Hill Publication: *Fitzpatrick's Dermatology in General Medicine*, 7th ed., 2008, edited by Klaus Wolff, Lowell A. Goldsmith, Stephen I. Katz, Barbara A. Gilchrest, Amy S. Paller, and David J. Leffell.

This text is intended for all physicians and other health care providers, including medical students, dermatology residents, internists, oncologists, and infectious disease specialists dealing with diseases with skin manifestations. For non-dermatologists, it is advisable to start with "Approach to Dermatologic Diagnosis" and "Outline of Dermatologic Diagnosis," below, to familiarize themselves with the principles of dermatologic nomenclature and lines of thought.

The *Atlas* is organized in 4 Parts, subdivided into 36 Sections, and there are 4 short Appendices. Each section has a color label that is reflected by the bar on the top of each page. This is to help the reader to find his or her bearings rapidly when leafing through the book. Also, the first page of each section carries an "icon," i.e., a small photograph of a condition that is representative for that particular section.

Each disease is labeled with little symbols to provide first-glance information on incidence (squares) and morbidity (circles).

☐ rare   ○ low morbidity
◨ not so common   ◑ considerable morbidity
■ common   ● serious

For instance, the symbols ■ ● for melanoma are meant to indicate that melanoma is common and serious. There are also some variations in this symbology. For instance, ☐→■ means that the disease is rare but may be common in specific populations or in endemic regions or in epidemics. Another example ◑→● indicates that the disease causes considerable morbidity and may become serious. In addition, each disease is labeled with the respective ICD9/10 codes.

Since, for reasons of space, not all manifestations of skin diseases and variations thereof can be shown in this printed version of *Color Atlas and Synopsis of Clinical Dermatology*, there is an online version of the book that contains "picture galleries" of most of the conditions discussed here. The symbol ⬲ in the text refers to such a picture gallery in the online version. So, for instance, if reading about psoriasis and finding this symbol ⬲, look up the psoriasis picture gallery in the online version for additional clinical images.

APPROACH TO DERMATOLOGIC DIAGNOSIS

There are two distinct clinical situations regarding the nature of skin changes:

I. The skin changes are *incidental* findings in *well* and *ill* individuals noted during the routine general physical examination
   - *"Bumps and blemishes"*: many asymptomatic lesions that are medically inconsequential may be present in well and ill persons and are not the reason for the visit to the physician; every general physician should be able to recognize these lesions to differentiate them from asymptomatic but important, e.g., malignant, lesions.
   - *Important skin lesions not* noted by the patient but that must not be overlooked by the physician: e.g., atypical nevi, melanoma, basal cell carcinoma, squamous cell carcinoma, café-au-lait macules in von Recklinghausen disease, xanthomas.

II. The skin changes are the *chief complaint* of the patient
   - "Minor" problems: e.g., localized itchy rash, "rash," rash in groin, nodules such as common moles, seborrheic keratoses.
   - "4-S": *s*erious *s*kin *s*igns in *s*ick patients

SERIOUS SKIN SIGNS IN SICK PATIENTS

- **Generalized red rash with fever**
  - Viral exanthems
  - Rickettsial exanthems
  - Drug eruptions
  - Bacterial infections with toxin production.
- **Generalized red rash with blisters and prominent mouth lesions**
  - Erythema multiforme (major)
  - Toxic epidermal necrolysis
  - Pemphigus

- Bullous pemphigoid
- Drug eruptions
- **Generalized red rash with pustules**
  - Pustular psoriasis (von Zumbusch)
  - Drug eruptions
- **Generalized rash with vesicles**
  - Disseminated herpes simplex
  - Generalized herpes zoster
  - Varicella
  - Drug eruptions
- **Generalized red rash with scaling over whole body**
  - Exfoliative erythroderma
- **Generalized wheals and soft tissue swelling**
  - Urticaria and angioedema
- **Generalized purpura**
  - Thrombocytopenia
  - Purpura fulminans
  - Drug eruptions
- **Generalized purpura that can be palpated**
  - Vasculitis
  - Bacterial endocarditis
- **Multiple skin infarcts**
  - Meningococcemia
  - Gonococcemia
  - Disseminated intravascular coagulopathy
- **Localized skin infarcts**
  - Calciphylaxis
  - Atherosclerosis obliterans
  - Atheroembolization
  - Warfarin necrosis
  - Antiphospholipid antibody syndrome
- **Facial inflammatory edema with fever**
  - Erysipelas
  - Lupus erythematosus

OUTLINE OF DERMATOLOGIC DIAGNOSIS

In contrast to other fields of clinical medicine, patients should be examined before a detailed history is taken because patients can see their lesions and thus often present with a history that is flawed with their own interpretation of the origin or causes of the skin eruption. Also, diagnostic accuracy is higher when objective examination is approached without preconceived ideas. However, a history should always be obtained but if taken during or after the visual and physical examination, it can be streamlined and more focused following the objective findings.

Thus, recognizing, analysing, and properly interpreting skin lesions are the sine qua non of dermatologic diagnosis.

PHYSICAL EXAMINATION

Appearance   Uncomfortable, "toxic," well
Vital Signs   Pulse, respiration, temperature
Skin: "Learning to Read"   The entire skin should be inspected and this should include mucous membranes, genital and anal regions, as well as hair and nails and peripheral lymph nodes. Reading the skin is like reading a text. The basic skin lesions are like the letters of the alphabet: their shape, color, margination, and other features combined will lead to words, and their localization and distribution to a sentence or paragraph. The prerequisite of dermatologic diagnosis is thus the recognition of (1) the type of skin lesion, (2) the color, (3) margination, (4) consistency, (5) shape, (6) arrangement, and (7) distribution of lesions.

Recognizing Letters: Types of Skin Lesions

• *Macule* (Latin: *macula,* "spot") A macule is a circumscribed area of change in skin color without elevation or depression. It is thus not palpable. Macules can be well- and ill-defined. Macules may be of any size or color (Image I-1). White, as in vitiligo; brown, as in café-au-lait spots; blue, as in Mongolian spots; or red, as in permanent vascular abnormalities such as port-wine stains or capillary dilatation due to inflammation (erythema). Pressure of a glass slide (*diascopy*) on the border of a red lesion detects the extravasation of red blood cells. If the redness remains under pressure from the slide, the lesion is purpuric, that is, results from extravasated red blood cells; if the redness disappears, the lesion is due to vascular dilatation. A rash consisting of macules is called a *macular exanthem.*

IMAGE I-1   Macule

• *Papule* (Latin: *papula,* "pimple") A papule is a superficial, elevated, solid lesion, generally considered <0.5 cm in diameter. Most of it is elevated above, rather than deep within, the plane of the surrounding skin (Image I-2). A papule is palpable. It may be well- or ill-defined. In papules the elevation is caused by metabolic or locally produced deposits, by localized cellular infiltrates, inflammatory or noninflammatory, or by hyperplasia of local cellular elements. Superficial papules are sharply defined. Deeper dermal papules have indistinct borders. Papules may be dome-shaped, cone-shaped or flat-topped (as in lichen planus) or consist of multiple, small, closely packed, projected elevations that are known as a *vegetation* (Image I-2). A rash consisting of papules is called a *papular exanthem.* Papular exanthems may be grouped ("lichenoid") or disseminated (dispersed). Confluence of papules leads to the development of larger, usually flat-topped, circumscribed, plateau-like elevations known as plaques (French: *plaque,* "plate"). See below.

IMAGE I-2   Papule

- *Plaque* A plaque is a plateau-like elevation above the skin surface that occupies a relatively large surface area in comparison with its height above the skin (Image I-3). It is usually well defined. Frequently it is formed by a confluence of papules, as in psoriasis. *Lichenification* is a less well-defined, large plaque where the skin appears thickened and the skin markings are accentuated. Lichenification occurs in atopic dermatitis, eczematous dermatitis, psoriasis, lichen simplex chronicus and mycosis fungoides. A *patch* is a barely elevated plaque—a lesion fitting between a macule and a plaque—as in parapsoriasis or Kaposi sarcoma.

IMAGE I-3   Plaque

- *Nodule* (Latin: *nodulus,* "small knot") A nodule is a palpable, solid, round or ellipsoidal lesion that is larger than a papule (Image I-4) and may involve the epidermis, dermis, or subcutaneous tissue. The depth of involvement and the size differentiate a nodule from a papule. Nodules result from inflammatory infiltrates, neoplasms, or metabolic deposits in the dermis or subcutaneous tissue. Nodules may be well defined (superficial) or ill defined (deep); if localized in the subcutaneous tissue, they can often be better felt than seen. Nodules can be hard or soft upon palpation. They may be dome-shaped and smooth or may have a warty surface or crater-like central depression.
- *Wheal* A wheal is a rounded or flat-topped, pale red papule or plaque that is characteristically evanescent, disappearing within 24–48 h (Image I-5). It is due to edema in the papillary body of the dermis. Wheals may be round, gyrate, or irregular with pseudopods—changing rapidly in size and shape due to shifting papillary edema. A rash consisting of wheals is called an *urticarial exanthem* or *urticaria.*

IMAGE I-4   Nodule

IMAGE I-5   Wheal

- *Vesicle-Bulla* (*Blister*) (Latin: *vesicula*, "little bladder"; *bulla*, "bubble")   A vesicle (<0.5 cm) or a bulla (>0.5 cm) is a circumscribed, elevated, superficial cavity containing fluid (Image I-6). Vesicles are dome-shaped (as in contact dermatitis, dermatitis herpetiformis), umbilicated (as in herpes simplex), or flaccid (as in pemphigus). Often the roof of a vesicle/bulla is so thin that it is transparent, and the serum or blood in the cavity can be seen. Vesicles containing serum are yellowish; those

containing blood from red to black. Vesicles and bullae arise from a cleavage at various levels of the superficial skin; the cleavage may be subcorneal or within the visible epidermis (i.e., intraepidermal vesication) or at the epidermal-dermal interface (i.e., subepidermal), as in Image I-6. Since vesicles/bullae are always superficial they are always well defined. A rash consisting of vesicles is called a *vesicular exanthem*; a rash consisting of bullae a *bullous exanthem*.

IMAGE I-6   Vesicle

• *Pustule* (Latin: *pustula*, "pustule") A pustule is a circumscribed, superficial cavity of the skin that contains a purulent exudate (Image I-7), which may be white, yellow, greenish-yellow, or hemorrhagic. Pustules thus differ from vesicles in that they are not clear but have a turbid content. This process may arise in a hair follicle or independently.

Pustules may vary in size and shape. Pustules are usually dome-shaped, but follicular pustules are conical and usually contain a hair in the center. The vesicular lesions of herpes simplex and varicella zoster virus infections may become pustular. A rash consisting of pustules is called a *pustular exanthem*.

IMAGE I-7   Pustule

• *Crusts* (Latin: *crusta*, "rind, bark, shell") Crusts develop when serum, blood, or purulent exudate dries on the skin surface (Image I-8). Crusts may be thin, delicate, and friable (*A*) or thick and adherent. Crusts are yellow when formed from dried serum; green or yellow-green when formed from purulent exudate; or brown, dark red, or black when

formed from blood. Superficial crusts occur as honey-colored, delicate, glistening particulates on the surface and are typically found in impetigo. When the exudate involves the entire epidermis, the crusts may be thick and adherent, and if it is accompanied by necrosis of the deeper tissues (e.g., the dermis), the condition is known as *ecthyma*.

IMAGE I-8   Crust

• *Scales (squames)* (Latin: *squama*, "scale") Scales are flakes of stratum corneum (Image I-9). They may be large (like membranes, tiny (like dust), pityriasiform (Greek: *pityron*,

"bran"), adherent, or loose. A rash consisting of papules with scales is called a *papulosquamous exanthem*.

IMAGE I-9   Scale

- *Erosion*   An erosion is a defect only of the epidermis, not involving the dermis (Image I-10); in contrast to an ulcer, which always heals with scar formation (see below), an erosion heals without a scar. An erosion is sharply defined and is red and oozes. There are superficial erosions, which are subcorneal or run through the epidermis, and deep erosions, the base of which is the papillary body (Image I-10). Except for physical abrasions, erosions are always the result of intraepidermal or subepidermal cleavage and thus of vesicles or bullae.

IMAGE I-10   Erosion

- *Ulcer* (Latin: *ulcus*, "sore")   An ulcer is a skin defect that extends into the dermis or deeper (Image I-11) into the subcutis and always occurs within pathologically altered tissue. An ulcer is therefore always a secondary phenomenon. The pathologically altered tissue giving rise to an ulcer is usually seen at the border or the base of the ulcer and is helpful in determining its cause. Other features helpful in this respect are whether borders are elevated, undermined, hard, or soggy; location of the ulcer; discharge; and any associated topographic features, such as nodules, exoriations, varicosities, hair distribution, presence or absence of sweating, and arterial pulses. Ulcers always heal with scar formation.

- *Scar*   A scar is the fibrous tissue replacement of the tissue defect by previous ulcer or a wound. Scars can be hypertrophic and hard (Image I-12) or atrophic and soft with a thinning or loss of all tissue compartments of the skin (Image I-12).
- *Atrophy*   This refers to a diminution of some or all layers of the skin (Image I-13). Epidermal atrophy is manifested by a thinning of the epidermis, which becomes transparent, revealing the papillary and subpapillary vessels; there are loss of skin texture and cigarette paper–like wrinkling. In dermal atrophy there are loss of connective tissue of the dermis and depression of the lesion (Image I-13).

IMAGE I-11   Ulcer

IMAGE I-12   Scar

IMAGE I-13   Atrophy

- *Cyst* A cyst is a cavity containing liquid or solid or semisolid (Image I-14) materials and may be superficial or deep. Visually it appears like a spherical, most often dome-shaped papule or nodule, but upon palpation it is resilient. It is lined by an epithelium and often has a fibrous capsule; depending on its contents it may be skin colored, yellow, red, or blue. An epidermal cyst producing kerati-naceous material and a pilar cyst that is lined by a multilayered epithelium are shown in Image I-14.

IMAGE I-14   Cyst

Shaping Letters into Words: Further Characterization of Identified Lesions

- *Color*   Pink, red, purple [purpuric lesions do not blanch with pressure with a glass slide (diascopy)], white, tan, brown, black, blue, grey, yellow. The color can be uniform or variegated.
- *Margination*   Well defined (can be traced with the tip of a pencil), ill defined.
- *Shape*   Round, oval, polygonal, polycyclic, annular (ring-shaped), iris, serpiginous (snakelike), umbilicated.
- *Palpation*   Consider (1) *consistency* (soft, firm, hard, fluctuant, boardlike); (2) *deviation in temperature* (hot, cold); and (3) *mobility*. Note presence of *tenderness*, and estimate the *depth* of the lesion (i.e., dermal or subcutaneous).

Forming Sentences and Understanding the Text: Evaluation of Arrangement, Patterns, and Distribution

- *Number*   Single or multiple lesions.
- *Arrangement*   Multiple lesions may be (1) *grouped*: herpetiform, arciform, annular, reticulated (net-shaped), linear, serpiginous (snakelike); or (2) *disseminated*: scattered discrete lesions.
- *Confluence*   Yes or no.
- *Distribution*   Consider (1) *extent*: isolated (single lesions), localized, regional, generalized, universal, and (2) *pattern*: symmetric, exposed areas, sites of pressure, intertriginous area, follicular localization, random, following dermatomes or Blaschko lines.

Table I-1 provides an algorithm showing how to proceed.

HISTORY

Demographics   Age, race, sex, occupation.
History

1. **Constitutional symptoms**
   - "Acute illness" syndrome: headaches, chills, feverishness, weakness
   - "Chronic illness" syndrome: fatigue, weakness, anorexia, weight loss, malaise

2. **History of skin lesions. Seven key questions:**
   - When? Onset
   - Where? Site of onset
   - Does it itch or hurt? Symptoms
   - How has it spread (pattern of spread)? Evolution
   - How have individual lesions changed? Evolution
   - Provocative factors? Heat, cold, sun, exercise, travel history, drug ingestion, pregnancy, season
   - Previous treatment(s)? Topical and systemic,

3. **General history of present illness as indicated by clinical situation, with particular attention to constitutional and prodromal symptoms**

4. **Past medical history**
   - Operations
   - Illnesses (hospitalized?)
   - Allergies, especially drug allergies
   - Medications (present and past)
   - Habits (smoking, alcohol intake, drug abuse)
   - Atopic history (asthma, hay fever, eczema)

TABLE I-1   Algorithm for Evaluating Skin Lesions

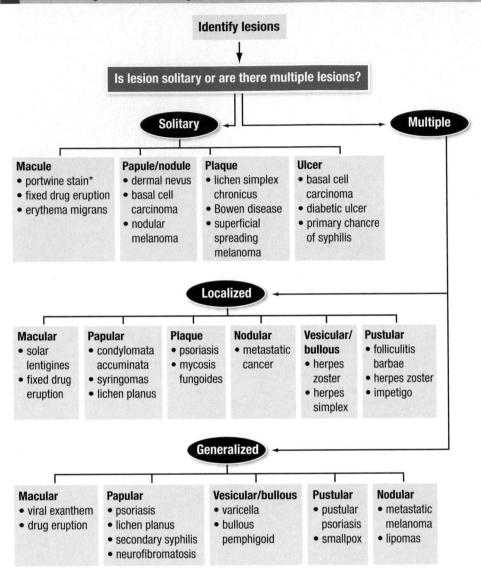

*Bulleted conditions are examples

5. **Family medical history (particularly of psoriasis, atopy, melanoma, xanthomas, tuberous sclerosis)**
6. **Social history, with particular reference to occupation, hobbies, exposures, travel, injecting drug use**
7. **Sexual history: history of risk factors of HIV: blood transfusions, IV drugs, sexually active, multiple partners, sexually transmitted disease?**

REVIEW OF SYMPTOMS

This should be done as indicated by the clinical situation, with particular attention to possible connections between signs and disease of other organ systems (e.g., rheumatic complaints, myalgias, arthralgias, Raynaud phenomenon, sicca symptoms).

SPECIAL CLINICAL AND LABORATORY AIDS TO DERMATOLOGIC DIAGNOSIS

SPECIAL TECHNIQUES USED IN CLINICAL EXAMINATION

Magnification with hand lens. To examine lesions for fine morphologic detail, it is necessary to use a magnifying glass (hand lens) (7×) or a binocular microscope (5× to 40×). Magnification is especially helpful in the diagnosis of lupus erythematosus (follicular plugging), lichen planus (Wickham striae), basal cell carcinomas (translucence and telangiectasia), and melanoma (subtle changes in color, especially gray or blue); this is best visualized after application of a drop of mineral oil. Use of the dermatoscope is discussed below (see "Dermoscopy").

Oblique lighting of the skin lesion, done in a darkened room, is often required to detect slight degrees of elevation or depression, and it is useful in the visualization of the surface configuration of lesions and in estimating the extent of the eruption.

Subdued lighting in the examining room enhances the contrast between circumscribed hypopigmented or hyperpigmented lesions and normal skin.

Wood lamp (ultraviolet long-wave light, "black" light) is valuable in the diagnosis of certain skin and hair diseases and of porphyria. With the Wood lamp (365 nm), fluorescent pigments and subtle color differences of melanin pigmentation can be visualized; the Wood lamp also helps to estimate variation in the lightness of lesions in relation to the normal skin color in both dark-skinned and fair-skinned persons; e.g., the lesions seen in tuberous sclerosis and tinea versicolor are hypomelanotic and are not as white as the lesions seen in vitiligo, which are amelanotic. Circumscribed hypermelanosis, such as a freckle and melasma, is much more evident (darker) under the Wood lamp. By contrast, dermal melanin, as in a Mongolian sacral spot, does not become accentuated under the Wood lamp. Therefore, it is possible to localize the site of melanin by use of the Wood lamp; *however, this is more difficult or not possible in patients with brown or black skin.*

Wood lamp is particularly useful in the detection of the fluorescence of dermatophytosis in the hair shaft (green to yellow) and of erythrasma (coral red). A presumptive diagnosis of porphyria can be made if a pinkish-red fluorescence is demonstrated in urine examined with the Wood lamp; addition of dilute hydrochloric acid intensifies the fluorescence.

Diascopy consists of firmly pressing a microscopic slide or a glass spatula over a skin lesion. The examiner will find this procedure of special value in determining whether the red color of a macule or papule is due to capillary dilatation (erythema) or to extravasation of blood (purpura) that does not blanch. Diascopy is also useful for the detection of the glassy yellow-brown appearance of papules in sarcoidosis, tuberculosis of the skin, lymphoma, and granuloma annulare.

Dermoscopy (also called *epiluminescence microscopy*). A hand lens with built-in lighting and a magnification of 10× to 30× is called a *dermatoscope* and permits the noninvasive inspection of deeper layers of the epidermis and beyond. This is particularly useful in the distinction of benign and malignant growth patterns in pigmented lesions. *Digital dermoscopy* is particularly useful in the monitoring of pigmented skin lesions because images are stored electronically and can be retrieved and examined at a later date to permit comparison quantitatively and qualitatively and to detect changes over time. Digital dermoscopy uses computer image analysis programs that provide (1) objective measurements of changes; (2) rapid storage, retrieval, and transmission of images to experts for further discussion (teledermatology); and (3) extraction of morphologic features for numerical analysis. Dermoscopy and digital dermoscopy require special training.

CLINICAL SIGNS

Darier sign is "positive" when a brown macular or a slightly papular lesion of urticaria pigmentosa (mastocytosis) becomes a palpable wheal after being vigorously rubbed with an instrument such as the blunt end of a pen. The wheal may not appear for 5–10 min.

Auspitz sign is "positive" when slight scratching or curetting of a scaly lesion reveals punctate bleeding points within the lesion. This suggests psoriasis, but it is not specific.

The *Nikolsky phenomenon* is positive when the epidermis is dislodged from the dermis by lateral, shearing pressure with a finger, resulting in an erosion. It is an important diagnostic sign in acantholytic disorders such as pemphigus or the staphylococcal scalded skin (SSS) syndrome or other blistering or epidermonecrotic disorders, such as toxic epidermal necrolysis.

CLINICAL TESTS

Patch testing is used to document and validate a diagnosis of allergic contact sensitization and identify the causative agent. Substances to be tested are applied to the skin in shallow cups (Finn chambers), affixed with a tape and left in place for 24–48 h. Contact hypersensitivity will show as a papular vesicular reaction that develops within 48–72 h when the test is read. It is a unique means of in vivo reproduction of disease in diminutive proportions, for sensitization affects all the skin and may therefore be elicited at any cutaneous site. The patch test is easier and safer than a "use test" with a questionable allergen, for test items can be applied in low concentrations in small areas of skin for short periods of time (see Section 2).

Photopatch testing is a combination of patch testing and UV irradiation of the test site and is used to document photoallergy (see Section 10).

Prick testing is used to determine type I allergies. A drop of a solution containing a minute concentration of the allergen is placed on the skin and the skin is pierced through this drop with a needle. Piercing should not go beyond the papillary body. A positive reaction will appear as a wheal within 20 min. The patient has to be under observation for possible anaphylaxis.

Acetowhitening facilitates detection of subclinical penile or vulvar warts. Gauze saturated with 5% acetic acid (white vinegar) is wrapped around the glans penis or used on the cervix and anus. After 5–10 min, the penis or vulva is inspected with a 10× hand lens. Warts appear as small white papules.

LABORATORY TESTS

Microscopic Examination of Scales, Crusts, Serum, and Hair

Gram stains of smears and *cultures of exudates and of tissue minces* should be made in lesions suspected of being bacterial or yeast (*Candida albicans*) infections. Ulcers and nodules require a scalpel biopsy in which a wedge of tissue consisting of all three layers of skin is obtained; the biopsy specimen is divided into one-half for histopathology and one-half for culture. This is minced in a sterile mortar and then cultured for bacteria (including typical and atypical mycobacteria) and fungi.

Microscopic examination for mycelia should be made of the roofs of vesicles or of scales (the advancing borders are preferable) or of the hair in dermatophytoses. The tissue is cleared with 10–30% KOH and warmed gently. Hyphae and spores will light up by their birefringence (Fig. 25-1). Fungal cultures with Sabouraud medium should be made (see Section 25).

Microscopic examination of cells obtained from the base of vesicles (Tzanck preparation) may reveal the presence of acantholytic cells in the acantholytic diseases (e.g., pemphigus or SSS syndrome) or of giant epithelial cells and multinucleated giant cells (containing 10–12 nuclei) in herpes simplex, herpes zoster, and varicella. Material from the base of a vesicle obtained by *gentle* curettage with a scalpel is smeared on a glass slide, stained with either Giemsa or Wright stain or methylene blue, and examined to determine whether there are acantholytic or giant epithelial cells, which are diagnostic (Fig. 27-27). In addition, culture, immunofluorescence tests, or polymerase chain reaction for herpes have to be ordered.

Laboratory diagnosis of scabies. The diagnosis is established by identification of the mite, or ova or feces, in skin scrapings removed from the papules or burrows (see Section 28). Using a sterile scalpel blade on which a drop of sterile mineral oil has been placed, apply oil to the surface of the burrow or papule. Scrape the papule or burrow vigorously to remove the entire top of the papule; tiny flecks of blood will appear in the oil. Transfer the oil to a microscopic slide and examine for mites, ova, and feces. The mites are 0.2–0.4 mm in size and have four pairs of legs (see Section 28).

Biopsy of the Skin

Biopsy of the skin is one of the simplest, most rewarding diagnostic techniques because of the easy accessibility of the skin and the variety of techniques for study of the excised specimen (e.g., histopathology, immunopathology, polymerase chain reaction, electron microscopy).

Selection of the site of the biopsy is based primarily on the stage of the eruption, and early lesions are usually more typical; this is especially important in vesiculobullous eruptions (e.g., pemphigus, herpes simplex), in which the lesion should be no more than 24 h old. However, older lesions (2–6 weeks) are often more characteristic in discoid lupus erythematosus.

A common technique for diagnostic biopsy is the use of a 3- to 4-mm punch, a small tubular knife much like a corkscrew, which by rotating movements between the thumb and index finger cuts through the epidermis, dermis, and subcutaneous tissue; the base is cut off with scissors. If immunofluorescence is indicated (e.g., as in bullous diseases or lupus erythematosus), a special medium for transport to the laboratory is required.

For nodules, however, a large wedge should be removed by excision including subcutaneous tissue. Furthermore, when indicated, lesions should be bisected, one-half for histology and the other half sent in a sterile container for bacterial and fungal cultures or in special fixatives or cell culture media, or frozen for immunopathologic examination.

Specimens for light microscopy should be fixed immediately in buffered neutral formalin. A brief but detailed summary of the clinical history and description of the lesions should accompany the specimen. Biopsy is indicated in *all* skin lesions that are suspected of being neoplasms, in all bullous disorders with immunofluoresence used simultaneously, and in all dermatologic disorders in which a specific diagnosis is not possible by clinical examination alone.

PART I

DISORDERS PRESENTING IN THE SKIN AND MUCOUS MEMBRANES

DISORDERS OF SEBACEOUS AND APOCRINE GLANDS

ACNE VULGARIS (COMMON ACNE) AND CYSTIC ACNE ■ ○→◑

- An inflammation of pilosebaceous units, very common
- Appears in certain body areas (face, trunk, rarely buttocks)
- Most frequently in adolescents

- Manifests as comedones, papulopustules, nodules, and cysts
- Results in pitted, depressed, or hypertrophic scars

ICD-9: 706.1 ∘ ICD-10: L70.0

EPIDEMIOLOGY

Occurrence   Very common, affecting approximately 85% of young people.
Age of Onset   Puberty—10 to 17 years in females, 14 to 19 in males; however, may appear first at 25 years or older.
Sex   More severe in males than in females.
Race   Lower incidence in Asians and Africans.
Genetic Aspects   Multifactorial genetic background. Familial predisposition: majority of individuals with cystic acne have parent(s) with a history of severe acne. Severe acne may be associated with XYY syndrome.

PATHOGENESIS

Key factors are follicular keratinization, androgens, and *Propionibacterium acnes* (Image 1-1).
  Acne results from a change in the keratinization pattern in the pilosebaceous unit, with the keratinous material becoming more dense and blocking secretion of sebum. These keratin plugs are called *comedones* and represent the "time bombs" of acne. Linoleic acid, which regulates keratinocyte proliferation, is decreased in acne. Comedonal plugging and a complex interaction between androgens and bacteria (*P. acnes*) in the plugged pilosebaceous units lead to inflammation. Androgens (qualitatively and quantitatively normal in the serum) stimulate sebaceous glands to produce larger amounts of sebum. Bacteria contain lipase, which converts lipid into fatty acids, and

produce proinflammatory mediators, [interleukin 1, tumor necrosis factor TNF α]. Fatty acids and proinflammatory mediators cause a sterile inflammatory response to the pilosebaceous unit. The distended follicle walls break, and the contents (sebum, lipids, fatty acids, keratin, bacteria) enter the dermis, provoking an inflammatory and foreign-body response (papule, pustule, nodule). Rupture plus intense inflammation lead to scars.
Contributory Factors   Acnegenic mineral oils, rarely dioxin and others.
Drugs   Lithium, hydantoin, isoniazid, glucocorticoids, oral contraceptives, iodides, bromides and androgens (e.g., testosterone), danazol.
Others   *Emotional stress* can definitely cause exacerbations. *Occlusion* and *pressure* on the skin, such as by leaning face on hands, *very important* and often unrecognized exacerbating factor (*acne mechanica*). Acne is not caused by chocolate or fatty foods or, in fact, by any kind of food.

CLINICAL MANIFESTATION

Duration of Lesions   Weeks to months.
Season   Often worse in fall and winter.
Symptoms   Pain in lesions (especially nodulocystic type).
Skin Lesions   *Comedones*—open (blackheads) or closed (whiteheads); *comedonal acne* (Fig. 1-1). *Papules* and *papulopustules*—i.e., a papule topped by a pustule; *papulopustular acne* (Fig. 1-2). *Nodules* or *cysts*—1–4 cm in

FIGURE 1-1   Acne vulgaris: comedones   Comedones are keratin plugs that form within follicular ostia, frequently associated with surrounding erythema and pustule formation. Comedones associated with small ostia are referred to as closed comedones or "white heads"; those associated with large ostia are referred to as open comedones or "black heads." Comedones are best treated with topical retinoids.

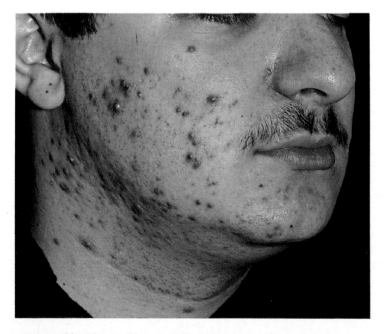

FIGURE 1-2   20-year-old male   In this case of papulopustular acne, some inflammatory papules become nodular and thus represent early stages of nodulocystic acne.

diameter (Fig. 1-3); *nodulocystic acne.* Soft nodules result from repeated follicular ruptures and reencapsulations with inflammation, abscess formation, and foreign-body reaction. Cysts are actually pseudocysts as they are not lined by epithelium but represent fluctuating abscesses (Image 1-1). Round isolated single nodules and cysts coalesce to linear mounds and sinus tracts (Fig. 1-4). *Sinuses*: draining epithelial-lined tracts, usually with nodular acne. *Scars*: atrophic depressed (often pitted) or hypertrophic (at times, keloidal). *Seborrhea* of the face and scalp often present and sometimes severe. For more clinical pictures, see acne picture gallery on online version. ⏎
Sites of Predilection Face, neck, trunk, upper arms, buttocks.

Special Forms
Acne Conglobata   Severe cystic acne (Figs. 1-4 and 1-5) with more involvement of the trunk than the face. Coalescing nodules, cysts, abscesses, and ulceration; occurs also on buttocks. Spontaneous remission is long delayed. Rarely, acne conglobata seen in XYY genotype (tall males, slightly mentally retarded, with aggressive behavior) or in the polycystic ovary syndrome. ⏎

Acne Fulminans   Teenage boys (ages 13 to 17). *Acute onset*, severe cystic acne with concomitant suppuration and always *ulceration*; also present are malaise, fatigue, fever, generalized arthralgias, leukocytosis, and elevated erythrocyte sedimentation rate. ⏎

SAPHO Syndrome   Synovitis, *a*cne, acne fulminans, *p*almoplantar pustulosis, *h*idradenitis suppurativa, hyperostosis, and *o*steitis. Rare.

PAPA Syndrome   Sterile *p*yogenic *a*rthritis, *p*yoderma gangrenosum *a*cne. An inherited autoinflammatory disorder; very rare.

Tropical Acne   Flare of acne, usually with severe folliculitis, inflammatory nodules, and draining cysts on trunk and buttocks in tropical climates; secondary infection with *Staphylococcus aureus.*

Acne with Facial Edema   Associated with recalcitrant, disfiguring midline facial edema. Woody induration with and without erythema.

Acne in the Adult Woman   Persistent acne in an (often) hirsute female with or without *irregular* menses needs an evaluation for hypersecretion of adrenal and ovarian androgens:

A

Microcomedone
- hyperkeratotic infundibulum
- cohesive corneocytes
- sebum secretion

B

Comedone
- accumulation of shed corneocytes and sebum
- dilation of follicular ostium

C

Inflammatory papule/ pustule
- further expansion of follicular unit
- proliferation of *Propionibacterium acnes* perifollicular inflammation

D

Nodule
- rupture of follicular wall
- marked perifollicular inflammation
- scarring

IMAGE 1-1   A–D. Acne pathogenesis   [From Zaenglein AL et al. Acne vulgaris and acneiform eruptions, in Wolff K et al (eds): *Fitzpatrick's Dermatology in General Medicine,* 7th ed. New York, McGraw-Hill, 2008.]

FIGURE 1-3 Nodulocystic acne A symmetric distribution in the face of a teenage boy. This image clearly shows that even nodulocystic acne starts with comedones—both open and closed comedones can be seen in this face—that then transform into papulopustular lesions, which enlarge and coalesce eventually to lead to nodulocystic acne. It is not surprising that these lesions are very painful, and it is understandable that nodulocystic acne also severely impacts the social life of these adolescents.

total testosterone, free testosterone, and/or dehydroepiandrosterone sulfate (DHEAS) (e.g., in the polycystic ovary syndrome).

Recalcitrant Acne Can be related to congenital adrenal hyperplasia (11β- or 21β- hydroxylase deficiencies).

Acne Excoriée Mild acne, usually in young women, associated with extensive excoriations and scarring due to emotional and psychological problems (obsessive compulsive disorder).

Neonatal Acne On nose and cheeks in newborns or infants, related to glandular development; transient.

Occupational Acne Due to exposure to tar derivatives, cutting oils, chlorinated hydrocarbons (see "Chloracne," below). Large comedones, inflammatory papules and cysts; not restricted to predilection sites of acne but can appear on other (covered) body sites.

Chloracne Due to exposure to chlorinated aromatic hydrocarbons in electrical conductors, insecticides, and herbicides. Sometimes very severe due to industrial accidents or intended poisoning (e.g., dioxin).

Acne Cosmetica Due to comedogenic cosmetics.

Pomade Acne   On the forehead, usually in Africans applying pomade to hair.

Acne Mechanica   Flares of preexisting acne in face, because of leaning face on hands, or on forehead, from pressure of football helmet. 📷

Acne-Like Conditions

Steroid Acne   Following systemic or topical glucocorticoids. Monomorphous folliculitis—small erythematous papules and pustules *without* comedones. 📷

Drug-Induced Acne   Monomorphous acne-like eruption due to phenytoin, lithium, isoniazid, high-dose vitamin B complex, epidermal growth factor inhibitors (see Section 22), halogenated compounds. No comedones. 📷

Acne Aestivalis   Papular eruption after sun exposure ("Mallorca acne"). Usually on forehead, shoulders, arms, neck, and chest. No comedones. Pathogenesis unknown.

Gram-Negative Folliculitis   Multiple tiny yellow pustules develop on top of acne vulgaris as a result of long-term antibiotic administration.

DIAGNOSIS AND DIFFERENTIAL DIAGNOSIS

Note: Comedones are required for diagnosis of any type of acne. Comedones are not a feature of acne-like conditions (above) and of the conditions listed below.

Face   *S. aureus* folliculitis, pseudofolliculitis barbae, rosacea, perioral dermatitis.

Trunk   *Malassezia* folliculitis, "hot-tub" pseudomonas folliculitis, *S. aureus* folliculitis, and acne-like conditions (see above).

LABORATORY EXAMINATION

No laboratory examinations required. If there is suspicion of an endocrine disorder, free testosterone, follicle-stimulating hormone, luteinizing hormone, and DHEAS should be determined to exclude hyperandrogenism and polycystic ovary syndrome. *Note*: In the overwhelming majority of acne patients, hormone levels are normal.

Laboratory examinations [transaminases (ALT, AST), triglycerides, and cholesterol levels] may be required if systemic isotretinoin treatment is planned (see below).

COURSE

Acne most often clears spontaneously by the early twenties but can persist to the fourth decade or older. Flares occur in the winter and with the onset of menses. The sequela is scarring (for clinical examples see 📷, which should be avoided by proper treatment, *especially with oral isotretinoin early in the course of the disease* (see below).

MANAGEMENT

The psychological impact of acne (perceived cosmetic disfigurement) should be assessed individually in each patient and therapy modified accordingly. The goal of therapy is to remove the plugging of the pilar drainage, reduce sebum production, and treat bacterial colonization.

Mild Acne

Topical antibiotics (clindamycin and erythromycin)

Benzoyl peroxide gels (2%, 5%, or 10%)

Topical retinoids (tretinoin, adapalene) require detailed instructions regarding gradual increases in concentration from 0.01% to 0.025% to 0.05% cream/gel or liquid. After improvement, medication is reduced to the lowest effective maintenance.

Improvement occurs over a period of months (2–5) but may take even longer for noninflamed comedones. Topical retinoids are applied in the evening; topical antibiotics and benzoyl peroxide gels are applied during the day.

Combination therapy is best, using benzoyl peroxide–erythromycin gels *plus* topical retinoids (tretinoin *or* tazarotene gel, adapalene). *Note:* acne surgery (extractions of comedones) is helpful only when properly done and after pretreatment with topical retinoids.

Moderate Acne   Oral antibiotics are added to the above regimen. Most effective antibiotic is minocycline, 50–100 mg twice daily, or doxycycline, 50–100 mg twice daily, and this is tapered to 50- mg/d as acne lessens. In females, moderate acne can be controlled with high doses of oral estrogens combined with progesterone or antiandrogens, but recurrences are the rule after cessation of treatment. Cerebrovascular accidents are a serious risk. *Note:* for inflammatory cysts and nodules, intralesional triamcinolone (0.05 mL of a 3- to 5-mg/mL suspension) is indicated.

Severe Acne   In addition to the topical treatment outlined above, systemic treatment with isotretinoin is indicated for cystic or conglobate acne or for acne refractory to treatment. This retinoid inhibits sebaceous gland function and keratinization and is very effective.

FIGURE 1-4 Acne conglobata In this severe nodulocystic acne, there are large confluent nodules and cysts forming linear mounds that correspond to interconnecting channels. There is postulation, scarring and lesions are very painful.

Oral isotretinoin leads to complete remission in almost all cases, which last for months to years in the majority of patients.

Indications for Oral Isotretinoin For moderate and severe, recalcitrant, nodular acne. The patient must have been resistant to other acne therapies, including systemic antibiotics.

Contraindications Isotretinoin is teratogenic. Therefore, pregnancy must be prevented and effective contraception is necessary, i.e., oral. Both tetracycline and isotretinoin may cause pseudotumor cerebri (benign intracranial swelling); therefore, the two medications should *never* be used together.

Warnings Blood lipids and transaminases (ALT, AST) should be determined before therapy. About 25% of patients can develop *increased plasma triglycerides*; 15% of patients a decrease in *high-density lipoproteins*, and about 7% an *increase in cholesterol levels*. This may increase the cardiovascular risk. When levels of serum triglycerides rise above 800 mg/μL, the patient may develop acute pancreatitis. Patients should not take vitamin supplements containing vitamin A. *Hepatotoxicity* has been very rarely reported in the form of clinical hepatitis, but patients may develop mild to moderate elevation of transaminase levels that normalize

FIGURE 1-5   Acne conglobata Inflammatory nodules and cysts have coalesced, forming abscesses and even leading to ulceration. There are multiple comedones and many recent red scars following resolution of inflammatory lesions on the upper chest, neck, and arms.

with reduction of the dose of the drug. *Eyes: night blindness* has been reported, and patients should be warned about driving at night. Also, patients may have *decreased tolerance to contact lenses* during and after therapy. *Skin:* an eczema-like rash due to drug-induced dryness often appears, and this responds dramatically to low potency (class III) topical glucocorticoids. Dry lips and cheilitis occur in practically all patients and must be treated. Reversible thinning of hair may occur very rarely, as may paronychia. *Nose:* dryness of nasal mucosa and nose bleeds (rare). *Other systems:* rarely, depression, headaches, arthritis, and muscular pain. For additional rare possible complications, consult the package insert.

Dosage Isotretinoin, 0.5 to 1 mg/kg given in divided doses with food. Most patients improve and clear within 20 weeks with 1 mg/kg. For severe disease, especially on the trunk, 2 mg/kg and longer treatment may be required. As many as three or more courses of isotretinoin have been given in refractory cases, but in most cases a single course is sufficient to induce lasting remission.

Other Systemic Treatments for Severe Acne Systemic glucocorticoids may be required in severe acne conglobata, acne fulminans, and the SAPHO and PAPA syndromes. The TNF-α inhibitor infliximab and anakinra are investigational drugs in these severe forms and show promising effects. *Note:* For inflammatory cysts and nodules, intralesional triamcinolone (0.05 mL of a 3 to 5 mg/mL solution) is indicated. Website: *http://www.aad.org/pamphlets/acnepamp.html*

ROSACEA   ICD-9: 695.3 ∘ ICD-10: L71

- A common chronic inflammatory acneiform disorder of the facial pilosebaceous units.
- It is coupled with an increased reactivity of capillaries leading to flushing and telangiectasia.
- May result in rubbery thickening of nose, cheeks, forehead, or chin due to sebaceous hyperplasia, edema, and fibrosis

EPIDEMIOLOGY

Occurrence   Common, affecting approximately 10% of fair-skinned people.

Age of Onset   30 to 50 years; peak incidence between 40 and 50 years.

Sex   Females predominantly, but rhinophyma occurs mostly in males.

Race   Celtic persons (skin phototypes I and II) but also southern Mediterraneans; less frequent or rare in pigmented persons (skin phototypes V and VI, i.e., brown and black)

STAGING (PLEWIG AND KLIGMAN CLASSIFICATION)

The rosacea diathesis: episodic erythema, "flushing and blushing"

Stage I: Persistent erythema with telangiectases

Stage II: Persistent erythema, telangiectases, papules, tiny pustules.

Stage III: Persistent deep erythema, dense telangiectases, papules, pustules, nodules; rarely persistent "solid" edema of the central part of the face

Note: progression from one stage to another does not always occur. Rosacea may start with stage II or III and stages may overlap.

CLINICAL MANIFESTATION

Usually a history of episodic reddening of the face (flushing) with increases in skin temperature in response to heat stimuli in the mouth (hot liquids); spicy foods; alcohol,. Exposure to sun—rosacea is often associated with solar elastosis—and heat (such as chefs working near a hot stove) may cause exacerbations. Acne may have preceded the onset of rosacea by years; nevertheless, rosacea may and usually does arise

de novo without any preceding history of acne or seborrhea.

Duration of Lesions   Days, weeks, months.

Skin Symptoms   Concern about cosmetic facial appearance; patients are often perceived as being alcoholic—which, of course, is not true.

Skin Lesions   *Early* Pathognomonic flushing— "red face" (Fig. 1-6); tiny papules and papulopustules (2–3 mm), pustule often small (≤1 mm) and on the apex of the papule (Figs. 1-7 and 1-8). *No comedones*.

Late Red facies and dusky-red papules and nodules (Figs. 1-6 to 1-9) Scattered, discrete lesions. Telangiectases. Marked sebaceous hyperplasia and lymphedema in chronic rosacea, causing disfigurement of the nose, forehead, eyelids, ears, and chin. 🕮

Distribution Characteristic is the symmetric localization on the face (Fig. 1-7). Rarely, neck, chest (V-shaped area), back, and scalp.

Special Lesions

Rhinophyma (enlarged nose), *metophyma* (enlarged cushion-like swelling of the forehead), *blepharophyma* (swelling of the eyelids), *otophyma* (cauliflower-like swelling of the earlobes), and *gnathophyma* (swelling of the chin) result from marked sebaceous gland hyperplasia (Fig. 1-11) and fibrosis. Upon palpation: soft, rubber-like. 🕮

Eye Involvement

"Red" eyes as a result of chronic blepharitis, conjunctivitis, and episcleritis. Rosacea keratitis, albeit rare, is a serious problem because corneal ulcers may develop. 🕮

LABORATORY EXAMINATIONS

Bacterial Culture   Rule out *S. aureus* infection. Scrapings may reveal massive concurrent *Demodex folliculorum* infestation.

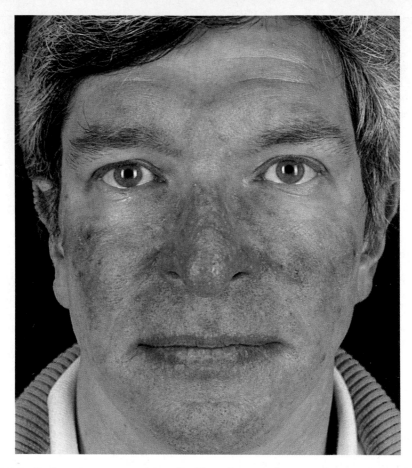

FIGURE 1-6 Erythematous rosacea (stage I)   The early stages of rosacea often present by episodic erythema, "flushing and blushing," which is followed by persistent erythema, which is due to multiple tiny telangiectasias, resulting in a red face.

Dermatopathology Nonspecific perifollicular and pericapillary inflammation with occasional foci of "tuberculoid" granulomatous areas; dilated capillaries. Foci of neutrophils high and within the follicle. *Later stages*: diffuse hypertrophy of the connective tissue, sebaceous gland hyperplasia, epithelioid granuloma without caseation, and foreign-body giant cells.

Rhinophyma Very marked lobular sebaceous hyperplasia (*glandular type*) and/or marked increase in connective tissue (*fibrous type*) with large ectatic veins (*fibroangiomatous type*).

DIFFERENTIAL DIAGNOSIS

Facial Papules/Pustules Acne (in rosacea there are no comedones), perioral dermatitis,

S. aureus folliculitis, gram-negative folliculitis, *D. folliculorum* infestation.

Facial Flushing/Erythema Seborrheic dermatitis, prolonged use of topical glucocorticoids, systemic lupus erythematosus; dermatomyositis.

COURSE

Prolonged Recurrences are common. After a few years, the disease may disappear spontaneously; usually it is for life time. Men and very rarely women may develop rhinophyma.

MANAGEMENT

Prevention Marked reduction or elimination of alcohol may be helpful in some patients.

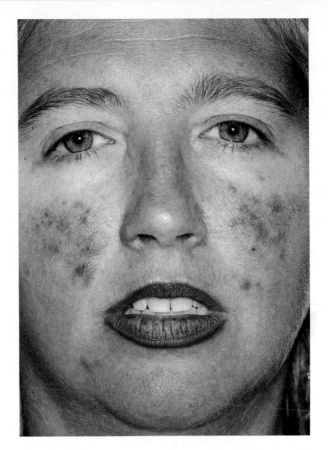

FIGURE 1-7 Rosacea Moderately severe rosacea in a 29-year-old female with persistent erythema, telangiectasia, red papules (stage II), and tiny pustules.

Topical

Metronidazole gel or *cream*, 0.75%, twice daily

Metronidazole cream, 1%, once daily

Sodium sulfacetamide, sulfur lotions 10% and 5%

Topical antibiotics (e.g., erythromycin gel) are less effective.

Systemic Oral antibiotics are more effective than topical treatment.

Minocycline or doxycycline, 50–100 mg twice daily, first-line antibiotics; very effective (doxycycline is a phototoxic drug and its use limits exposure to sunlight in summer).

Tetracycline, 1–1.5 g/d in divided doses until clear; then gradually reduce to once-daily doses of 250–500 mg, most effective is oral metronidazole 500 mg BID.

A dose of 50 mg minocycline or doxycycline or 250–500 g tetracycline is given as maintenance.

Oral Isotretinoin For individuals with severe disease (especially stage III) not responding to antibiotics and topical treatments. A low-dose regimen of 0.1–0.5 mg/kg body weight per day is effective in most patients, but occasionally 1 mg/kg may be required.

Ivermectin 12 mg PO in case of massive demodex infestation.

Rhinophyma and Telangiectasia Treated by surgery or laser surgery with excellent cosmetic results. Website *http://www.aad.org/pamphlets/rosacea.html*

FIGURE 1-8   Rosacea, stages II-III   Telangiectasia, papules and pustules, and some swelling in a 50-year-old woman. There are no comedones.

FIGURE 1-9   Papulopustular rosacea (transition of stage II to stage III)   In this 65-year-old female, rosacea involves almost the entire face, sparing only the upper lip and chin. Papules and pustules have coalesced—again no comedones—and have already led to some swelling of the cheeks, which present "solid" edema.

FIGURE 1-10   Rosacea, transition of stage II to III   Multiple bright red papules and pustules and some swelling of the right cheek of a 52-year-old woman. Note that in this case lesions are clustered, the forehead is free of telangiectasia, and the lesions are not absolutely symmetric.

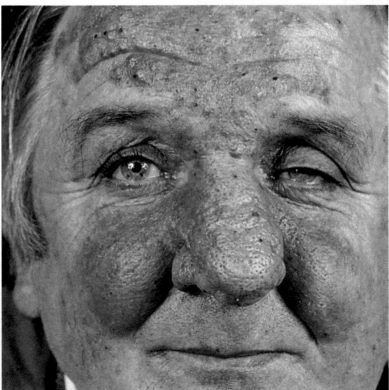

FIGURE 1-11   Rosacea (stage III)   Here the persistent "solid" edema of the nose, forehead, and parts of the cheeks is the leading symptom. Papules, pustules, and crusted pustules are superimposed on this persistent edema. The enlarged nose feels rubbery and already represents rhinophyma.

PERIORAL DERMATITIS   ICD-9: 695.3 ∘ ICD-10: L71.0 ■ ○➔◑*

- ■ Discrete erythematous micropapules and microvesicles,
- ■ Often confluent in the perioral and periorbital skin

- ■ Occurs mainly in young women; can occur in children and the old
- * Rarely

EPIDEMIOLOGY AND ETIOLOGY

Age of Onset   16–45 years; can occur in children and the old.
Sex   Females predominantly.
Etiology   Unknown but may be markedly aggravated by potent topical (fluorinated) glucocorticoids.

CLINICAL MANIFESTATION

Duration of Lesions   Weeks to months. Skin symptoms perceived as cosmetic disfigurement; occasional itching or burning, feeling of tightness.
Skin Lesions   1- to 2-mm erythematous papulopustules on an erythematous background (Fig. 1-12) irregularly grouped, symmetric. Lesions increase in number with central

confluence and satellites; confluent plaques may appear eczematous with tiny scales. There are no comedones.
Distribution   Initially perioral. Rim of sparing around the vermilion border of lips (Fig. 1-12). At times, in the periorbital area (Figs. 1-13, 1-14). Uncommonly, only periorbital involvement; occasionally, glabella and forehead. Commonly on the moustache area and lateral chin. ✑

LABORATORY EXAMINATIONS

Culture   Rule out *S. aureus* infection.

DIFFERENTIAL DIAGNOSIS

Allergic contact dermatitis, atopic dermatitis, seborrheic dermatitis, rosacea, acne vulgaris, steroid acne.

FIGURE 1-12   Perioral dermatitis   Moderate involvement with early confluence of tiny papules and a few pustules in a perioral distribution in a young woman. Note typical sparing of the vermilion border (mucocutaneous junction).

COURSE

Appearance of lesions usually subacute over weeks to months. At times, misdiagnosed as an eczematous or a seborrheic dermatitis and treated with a potent topical glucocorticoid preparation, aggravating perioral dermatitis or inducing steroid acne. Untreated, perioral dermatitis fluctuates in activity over months to years but is not nearly as chronic as rosacea.

MANAGEMENT

Topical
Avoid topical glucocorticoids!

> *Metronidazole*, 0.75% gel two times daily or 1% once daily
> *Erythromycin*, 2% gel applied twice daily

Systemic

> *Minocycline* or *doxycycline*, 100 mg daily until clear, then 50 mg daily for another 2 months (caution, doxycycline is a photosensitizing drug) or
> *Tetracycline*, 500 mg twice daily until clear, then 500 mg daily for 1 month, then 250 mg daily for an additional month.

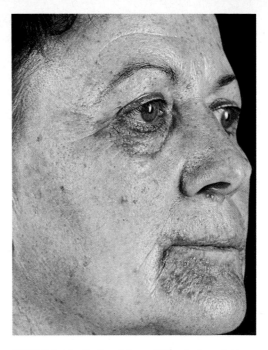

FIGURE 1-13   Perioral dermatitis   Preferential location on the chin but also on the lower eyelids in a 64-year-old woman. At this age, differential diagnosis includes rosacea, but it would be unusual for rosacea to involve the perioral region and eyelids but sparing the cheeks and nose.

FIGURE 1-14   Periorbital dermatitis   Note presence of tiny papules and a few pustules around the eye. This is a much less common site than the lesions around the mouth.

HIDRADENITIS SUPPURATIVA   ICD-9: 705.83 ○ ICD-10: L73.2   ▯ ◐

- A chronic, suppurative, often cicatricial disease of apocrine gland–bearing skin.
- Involves the axillae, the anogenital region, and, rarely, the scalp (called *cicatrizing perifolliculitis*).
- May be associated with severe nodulocystic acne and pilonidal sinuses (termed *follicular occlusion syndrome*).

Synonyms: Apocrinitis, hidradenitis axillaris, abscess of the apocrine sweat glands.

EPIDEMIOLOGY

Age of Onset   From puberty to climacteric.
Sex   Affects more females than males; estimated to be 4% of female population. Males more often have anogenital and females axillary involvement.
Race   All races.
Heredity   Mother-daughter transmission has been observed. Families give a history of nodulocystic acne and hidradenitis suppurativa occurring separately or together in blood relatives.

ETIOLOGY AND PATHOGENESIS

Unknown. Predisposing factors: obesity, genetic predisposition to acne, follicular plugging of apocrine regions, secondary bacterial infection.

PATHOGENESIS

The following sequence may be the mechanism of the development of the lesions: keratinous plugging of the hair follicle → dilatation hair follicle and secondarily of the apocrine duct → inflammatory changes limited to a single apocrine gland → bacterial growth in dilated follicle and duct → rupture resulting in extension of inflammation/infection → extension of suppuration/tissue destruction → ulceration and fibrosis, sinus tract formation.

CLINICAL MANIFESTATION

Symptoms: Intermittent pain and marked point tenderness related to abscess.
Skin Lesions   Initial lesion: *very tender*, red inflammatory nodule/abscess (Fig. 1-15) that may resolve or drain purulent/seropurulent material. The same lesion may appear repeatedly in the same location. Open comedones, and at times unique *double* comedones, are highly characteristic (Fig. 1-15), may be present even when active nodules are absent. Eventually, moderately to exquisitely tender sinus tracts may form. Pus drains from opening of abscess and sinus tracts; fibrosis, "bridge" scars, hypertrophic and keloidal scars, contractures form (Figs. 1-16, 1-17). Rarely, lymphedema of the associated limb may develop.
Distribution   Axillae, breasts, anogenital area, groin. Often bilateral in axillae and/or anogenital area; may extend over entire back, buttocks, perineum involving scrotum or vulva (Fig. 1-18), and scalp. ☑
Associated Findings   Cystic acne, pilonidal sinus. Often obesity.

LABORATORY EXAMINATIONS

Bacteriology   Various pathogens may secondarily colonize or "infect" lesions. These include *S. aureus*, streptococci, *Escherichia coli*, *Proteus mirabilis*, and *Pseudomonas aeruginosa*.
Dermatopathology   *Early*: keratin occlusion of hair follicle, ductal/tubular dilatation, inflammatory changes limited to follicular apparatus. *Late*: destruction of apocrine/eccrine/pilosebaceous apparatus, fibrosis, pseudoepitheliomatous hyperplasia in sinuses.

DIFFERENTIAL DIAGNOSIS

Painful papule, nodule, abscess in groin and axilla. *Early*: furuncle, carbuncle, lymphadenitis, ruptured inclusion cyst, painful lymphadenopathy in lymphogranuloma venereum or cat-scratch disease. *Late*: lymphogranuloma venereum, donovanosis, scrofuloderma, actinomycosis, sinus tracts and fistulas associated with ulcerative colitis and regional enteritis.

FIGURE 1-15 Hidradenitis suppurativa Many black comedones, some of which are paired, are a characteristic finding, associated with deep, exquisitely painful abscesses and old scars in the axilla.

FIGURE 1-16 Hidradenitis suppurativa Multiple bulging and depressed scars puckering the surrounding skin and draining sinuses in the axilla of a 22-year-old female.

COURSE AND PROGNOSIS

The severity of the disease varies considerably. Many patients have only mild involvement with recurrent, self-healing, tender red nodules and do not seek therapy. The disease usually undergoes a spontaneous remission with age (>35 years). In some individuals, the course can be relentlessly progressive, with marked morbidity related to chronic pain, draining sinuses, and scarring, with restricted mobility (Fig. 1-18) ☑. Complications (rare): fistulas to urethra, bladder, and/or rectum; anemia, amyloidosis.

MANAGEMENT

Hidradenitis suppurativa is *not* simply an infection, and systemic antibiotics are only part of the treatment program. Combinations of (1) intralesional glucocorticoids, (2) surgery, (3) oral antibiotics, and (4) isotretinoin are used.

Medical Management
Acute Painful Lesions   *Nodule* Intralesional triamcinolone (3–5 mg/mL).
Abscess   Intralesional triamcinolone (3–5 mg/mL) into the wall followed by incision and drainage of abscess fluid.
Chronic Low-Grade Disease   Oral antibiotics: erythromycin (250 – 500 mg qid), tetracycline (250–500 mg qid), or minocycline (100 mg twice daily) until lesions resolve, or a combination of clindamycin twice daily 300 mg bid with rifampin (300 mg twice daily); may take weeks.
Prednisone   May be given concurrently if pain and inflammation are severe: 70 mg daily for 2 to 3 days, tapered over 14 days.
Oral Isotretinoin   Not useful in severe disease, but useful in early disease to prevent follicular plugging and when combined with surgical excision of individual lesions.

Surgical Management
- Incise and drain acute abscesses.
- Excise chronic recurrent, fibrotic nodules or sinus tracts. If one or two nodules can be pinpointed with recurrent disease, they can be excised with a good result.
- With extensive, chronic disease, complete excision of axilla or involved anogenital area may be required. Excision should extend down to fascia and requires split skin grafting. ☑

Psychological Management
These patients need constant reassurance, as they become very depressed because of the nature of the illness, e.g., pain, soiling of clothing by draining pus, odor, and the site of occurrence (anogenital area). Therefore, every effort should be made to deal with the disease, using every modality possible.

FIGURE 1-17 Hidradenitis suppurativa Severe scarring on the buttocks, inflammatory painful nodules with fistulas and draining sinuses. When the patient sits down, pus will squirt from the sinus openings.

FIGURE 1-18 Hidradenitis suppurativa The entire perigenital and perianal skin as well as the buttocks and inner aspects of the thighs are involved in this 50-year-old male. There is considerable inflammation, and pressure releases purulent exudate from multiple sinuses. The patient had to wear a large diaper, because whenever he was seated, secretions would squirt from the sinuses.

ECZEMA/DERMATITIS

The terms *eczema* and *dermatitis* are used interchangeably, denoting a polymorphic inflammatory reaction pattern involving the epidermis and dermis. There are many etiologies and a wide range of clinical findings. Acute eczema/dermatitis is characterized by pruritus, erythema, and vesiculation; chronic eczema/dermatitis, by pruritus, xerosis, lichenification, hyperkeratosis, ± fissuring.

CONTACT DERMATITIS   ICD-9:692-9 ○ ICD-10:L25

Contact dermatitis is a generic term applied to acute or chronic inflammatory reactions to substances that come in contact with the skin. Irritant contact dermatitis (ICD) is caused by a chemical irritant; allergic contact dermatitis (ACD) by an antigen (allergen) that elicits a type IV (cell-mediated or delayed) hypersensitivity reaction.

    The acute form of ICD occurs after a single exposure to the offending agent that is toxic to the skin (e.g., croton oil, phenols, kerosene, organic solvents, sodium and potassium hydroxide, lime acids) and in severe cases may lead to necrosis. It is dependent on concentration of the offending agent and occurs in everyone, depending on the penetrability and thickness of the stratum corneum. There is a threshold concentration for these substances above which they cause acute dermatitis and below which they do not. This sets acute ICD apart from acute ACD, which is dependent on sensitization and thus occurs only in sensitized individuals. Depending on the degree of sensitization, minute amounts of the offending agents may elicit a reaction. Since ICD is a toxic phenomenon, it is confined to the area of exposure and is therefore always sharply marginated and never spreads. ACD is an immunologic reaction that tends to involve the surrounding skin (spreading phenomenon) and may even spread beyond affected sites. Generalization may occur.

IRRITANT CONTACT DERMATITIS (ICD)
ICD-9:692.9 ○ ICD-10:L24

- ICD is a localized disease confined to areas exposed to irritants.
- It is caused by exposure of the skin to chemical or other physical agents that are capable of irritating the skin, acutely or chronically.
- Severe irritants cause toxic reactions even after a short exposure.
- Most cases are caused by chronic cumulative exposure to one or more irritants.
- The hands are the most commonly affected area.

- In addition to dermatitis, irritant contact responses of the skin include: subjective irritancy, transient irritant reactions, persistent irritant reactions, toxic (caustic) burn.
- Irritant contact responses of skin appendages and pigmentary system include: follicular and acneiform eruptions, miliaria, pigmentary changes (hypo- and hyperpigmentation), granulomatous reactions, and alopecia.

TABLE 2-1 Most Common Irritant/Toxic Agents

- Soaps, detergents, waterless hand cleaners
- Acids and alkalis*: hydrofluoric acid, cement, chromic acid, phosphorus, ethylene oxide, phenol, metal salts.
- Industrial solvents: coal tar solvents, petroleum, chlorinated hydrocarbons, alcohol solvents, ethylene glycol ether, turpentine, ethyl ether, acetone, carbon dioxide, DMSO, dioxane, styrene.
- Plants: Euphorbiaceae (spurges, crotons, poinsettias, machneel tree). Racunculaceae (buttercup), Cruciferae (black mustard), Urticaceae (nettles), Solanaceae (pepper, capsaicin), Opuntia (prickly pear).
- Others: fiberglass, wool, rough synthetic clothing, fire-retardant fabrics, "NCR" paper.

*Lead to chemical burns and necrosis, if concentrated.

EPIDEMIOLOGY

ICD is the most common form of occupational skin disease, accounting for up to 80% of all occupational skin disorders. However, ICD need not be occupational and can occur in anyone being exposed to a substance irritant or toxic to the skin.

Occupational Exposure Individuals engaged in the following occupations/activities are at risk for ICD: housekeeping; hairdressing; medical, dental, and veterinary services; cleaning; floral arranging; agriculture; horticulture; forestry; food preparation and catering; printing; painting; metal work; mechanical engineering; car maintenance; construction; fishing.

ETIOLOGY

Etiologic Agents (Table 2-1) Abrasives, cleaning agents, oxidizing agents (e.g., sodium hypochlorite); reducing agents, plants and animal enzymes, secretions; dessicant powders, dust, soils; excessive exposure to water.

Predisposing Factors Atopics with a history of atopic dermatitis are at highest risk for ICD; the majority of workers with significant occupational ICD are atopics. Others: white skin, temperature (low), climate (low humidity), occlusion, mechanical irritation. Cement ICD tends to flare in summer in hot humid climates.

PATHOGENESIS

Irritants (both chemical and physical), cause cell damage if applied for sufficient time and in adequate concentration. ICD occurs when defense or repair capacity of the skin is unable to maintain normal skin integrity and function or when penetration of chemical(s) induces an inflammatory response. Lesser irritants cause reaction only after prolonged exposure. The initial reaction is usually limited to the site of contact with the irritant; the concentration of irritant diffusing outside the area of contact almost always falls below the critical threshold necessary to provoke a reaction.

Mechanisms involved in acute and chronic phases of ICD are fundamentally different. Acute reactions involve direct cytotoxic damage to keratinocytes. Chronic ICD results from repeated exposures that cause slow damage to cell membranes, disrupting the skin barrier and leading to protein denaturation and cellular toxicity.

ACUTE IRRITANT CONTACT DERMATITIS

CLINICAL MANIFESTATION

Symptoms In some individuals, subjective symptoms (burning, stinging, smarting) may be the only manifestations. Painful sensations can occur within seconds after exposure (immediate-type stinging), e.g., to acids, chloroform, and methanol. Delayed-type stinging occurs within 1 to 2 min, peaking at 5 to 10 min, fading by 30 min, and is caused by agents such as aluminum chloride, phenol, propylene glycol, and others. In acute delayed ICD, objective skin symptoms do not start until 8–24 h after exposure (e.g., anthralin, ethylene oxide, benzalkonium chloride) and are accompanied by burning rather then itching.

Skin Findings May occur minutes after exposure or may be delayed up to ≥ 24 h. The spectrum of changes ranges from erythema to vesiculation (Figs. 2-1 and 2-2) and caustic burn with necrosis. Acute ICD represents sharply demarcated erythema and superficial edema, corresponding to the application site of the toxic substance (Fig. 2-1). Lesions do not spread beyond the site of contact. In more severe reactions vesicles and blisters arise within the erythematous lesions (Figs. 2-1 and 2-2), followed by erosions and/or even frank necrosis, as with acids or alkaline solutions. No papules. Configuration often bizarre or linear ("outside job" or dripping effect) (Fig. 2-1).

Evolution of Lesions   Erythema with a dull, nonglistening surface (Fig. 2-1) → vesiculation (or blister formation) (Figs. 2-1 and 2-2) → erosion → crusting → shedding of crusts and scaling or (in chemical burn) erythema → necrosis → shedding of necrotic tissue → ulceration → healing. ☑

Distribution   Isolated, localized to one region or generalized (plant dermatitis), depending on contact with toxic agent.

Duration   Days, weeks depending on tissue damage.

Constitutional Symptoms

Usually none, but in widespread acute ICD "acute illness" syndrome, fever may occur.

CHRONIC IRRITANT CONTACT DERMATITIS

TYPES

Cumulative ICD   Most common; develops slowly after repeated additive exposure to mild irritants (water, soap, detergents, etc.), usually on hands. Repeated exposures to toxic or subtoxic concentrations of offending agents usually associated with a chronic disturbance of the barrier function that allows even subtoxic concentrations of offending agents to penetrate into the skin and elicit a chronic inflammatory response; e.g., after repeated exposure to alkaline detergents and organic solvents, which, if applied only once to normal skin, do not elicit a reaction. Injury (e.g., repeated rubbing of the skin), prolonged soaking in water, or chronic contact after repeated, cumulative physical trauma—friction, pressure, abrasions in individuals engaged in manual work (*traumatic ICD*).

Irritant Reaction ICD   Early, subclinical dermatitis on hands of individuals exposed to wet work. Usually during first months of training of hair dressers or of metal workers, smarting and burning sensations.

CLINICAL MANIFESTATION

Symptoms   Stinging, smarting, burning, *and* itching; pain as fissures develop.

Skin Findings   Dryness → chapping → erythema (Fig. 2-3) → hyperkeratosis and scaling → fissures and crusting (Fig. 2-4). Sharp margination gives way to ill-defined borders, lichenification. In *irritant reaction ICD* also vesicles, pustules, and erosions. ☑

Distribution   Usually on hands (Figs. 2-3 and 2-4). In *cumulative ICD* usually starting at finger webspaces, spreading to sides and dorsal surface of hands and then to palms. In housewives often starting on fingertips (*pulpitis*) (Fig. 2-3). Rarely in other locations exposed to irritants and/or trauma, e.g., in violinists on mandible or neck, or on exposed sites as in *airborne ICD* (see below).

Duration   Chronic, months to years.

Constitutional Symptoms

None, except when infection occurs. Chronic ICD (e.g., hand dermatitis; see below) can become a severe occupational and emotional problem.

LABORATORY EXAMINATION

Histopathology   In acute ICD, epidermal cell necrosis, neutrophils, vesiculation, and necrosis. In chronic ICD, acanthosis, hyperkeratosis, lymphocytic infiltrate.

Patch Tests   These are negative in ICD unless allergic contact dermatitis is also present (see below).

SPECIAL FORMS OF ICD

Hand Dermatitis

Most cases of chronic ICD occur on the hands and are occupational. Often sensitization to allergens (such as nickel or chromate salts) occurs, and then ACD (acute and/or chronic) is superimposed on ICD. A typical example is hand dermatitis in construction and cement workers. Cement is alkaline and corrosive, leading to chronic ICD; chromates in cement sensitize and lead to ACD (see Fig. 2-6). In such cases the eruption may spread beyond the hands and may even generalize. ☑

FIGURE 2-1 Acute irritant contact dermatitis following application of a cream containing nonylva-nillamid and nicotinic acid-butoxyethylester prescribed for lower back pain The "streaky pattern" indicates an outside job. The eruption is characterized by a massive erythema with vesiculation and blister formation and is confined to the sites exposed to the toxic agent.

FIGURE 2-2 Acute irritant contact dermatitis on the hand due to an industrial solvent There is massive blistering on the palm.

Airborne ICD

Characteristically face, neck, anterior chest, and arms are involved. Most frequent causes are irritating dust and volatile chemicals (ammonia, solvents, formaldehyde, epoxy resins, cement, fiberglass, sawdust from toxic woods). This has to be distinguished from photoallergic contact dermatitis (see Section 10).

Pustular and Acneiform ICD

ICD may target follicles and become pustular and papulopustular. It may result from metals, mineral oils, greases, cutting fluids, naphthalenes.

DIAGNOSIS AND DIFFERENTIAL DIAGNOSIS

Diagnosis is by history and clinical examination (lesions, pattern, site). Most important differential diagnosis is ACD (see Table 2-3, p. 32). On palms and soles: palmoplantar psoriasis; in exposed sites: photoallergic contact dermatitis.

COURSE AND PROGNOSIS

Healing usually occurs within 2 weeks of removal of noxious stimuli; in more chronic cases, 6 weeks or longer may be required. In the setting of occupational ICD, only one-third of individuals have complete remission and two-thirds may require allocation to another job; atopic individuals have a worse prognosis. In cases of chronic subcritical levels of irritant, some workers develop tolerance, or "hardening."

MANAGEMENT

Prevention

- Avoid irritant or caustic chemical(s) by wearing protective clothing (i.e., goggles, shields, gloves).
- If contact does occur, wash with water or weak neutralizing solution.
- Barrier creams.
- In occupational ICD that persists in spite of adherence to the above measures, change of job may be necessary.

TREATMENT

Acute   Identify and remove the etiologic agent. Wet dressings with gauze soaked in Burow's solution, changed every 2–3 h. Larger vesicles may be drained, but tops should *not* be removed. Topical class I glucocorticoid preparations. In severe cases, systemic glucocorticoids may be indicated. Prednisone: 2-week course, 60 mg initially, tapering by steps of 10 mg.

Subacute and Chronic   Identify and remove etiologic/pathogenic agent. Employ a potent topical glucocorticoid preparation, betamethasone dipropionate or clobetasol propionate, and provide adequate lubrication. As healing occurs, continue with lubricating/protective creams or ointments. The topical calcineurin inhibitors pimecrolimus and tacrolimus are usually not potent enough to suppress the chronic inflammation and its sequelae sufficiently.

In chronic ICD of hands a "hardening effect" can be achieved in most cases with topical (soak or bath)-PUVA therapy (see page 68).

FIGURE 2-3   Early chronic irritant contact dermatitis in a housewife   This has resulted from repeated exposure to soaps and detergents. Note glistening fingertips (pulpitis).

FIGURE 2-4 ***A*. Chronic irritant dermatitis with acute exacerbation in a housewife** The patient used turpentine to clean her hands after painting. Erythema, fissuring, and scaling. Differential diagnosis is allergic contact dermatitis and palmar psoriasis. Patch tests to turpentine were negative. ***B*. Irritant contact dermatitis** in a construction worker who works with cement. Note the hyperkeratoses, scaling and fissuring. There is also minimal pustulation.

ALLERGIC CONTACT DERMATITIS   ICD-9 : 692.9 ∘ ICD-10 : L24   ■ ◑

- ACD is a systemic disease defined by hapten-specific T cell–mediated inflammation.
- One of the most frequent, vexing, and costly skin problems.

- An eczematous (papules, vesicles, pruritic) dermatitis
- Due to reexposure to a substance to which the individual is sensitized.

EPIDEMIOLOGY

Frequent. Accounts for 7% of occupationally related illnesses in the United States. However, there are data suggesting that the actual indicence rate is 10 to 50 times greater than reported in the U.S. Bureau of Labor Statistics data. Nonoccupational ACD is estimated to be three times greater than occupational ACD.

Age of Onset   No influence on capacity for sensitization; however, allergic contact dermatitis is uncommon in young children and in individuals older than 70 years.

Occupation   One of the most important causes of disability in industry.

PATHOGENESIS

ACD is a classic, delayed, cell-mediated hypersensitivity reaction. Exposure to a strong sensitizer such as poison ivy resin results in sensitization in a week or so, while exposure to a weak allergen may take months to years for sensitization. The antigen is taken up by Langerhans cells, which process the antigen and migrate from the epidermis to the draining lymph nodes, where they present the processed antigen in association with MHC class II molecules to T cells that then proliferate. Sensitized T cells leave the lymph node, enter the blood circulation, home to the skin, and, after being presented by Langerhans cells with the same specific antigen, produce and mediate the release by other cells of a variety of cytokines. Thus, all the skin becomes hypersensitive to the contact allergen and will react wherever the specific allergen is presented.

ALLERGENS

Contact allergens are diverse and range from metal salts to antibiotics, dyes to plant products.

Thus, allergens are found in jewelry, personal care products, topical medications, plants, house remedies, and chemicals the individual may come in contact with at work. The most common allergens in the United States are listed in Table 2-2.

CLINICAL MANIFESTATION

The eruption starts in a sensitized individual 48 h or days after contact with the allergen; repeated exposures lead to a crescendo reaction, i.e., the eruption worsens. Site of the eruption is confined to site of exposure. With phytoallergic (poison ivy), exposure sites may not be apparent to the patient. Haptens can be blotted on to face or penis without direct contact.

Symptoms   Subjective symptoms are intense pruritus; in severe reactions also stinging and pain.

Constitutional Symptoms   "Acute illness" syndrome, including fever, but only in severe allergic contact dermatitis (e.g., poison ivy).

Skin Lesions   The appearance of ACD depends on severity, location, and duration.

Type   *Acute*   Well-demarcated erythema and edema on which are superimposed closely spaced, nonumbilicated vesicles, and/or papules (Fig. 2-5); in severe reactions, bullae, confluent erosions exuding serum, and crusts. The same reaction can occur after several weeks at sites not exposed.

Subacute   Plaques of mild erythema showing small, dry scales, sometimes associated with small, red, pointed or rounded (Figs. 2-6, 2-7), firm papules.

Chronic   Plaques of lichenification (thickening of the epidermis with deepening of the skin lines in parallel or rhomboidal pattern), scaling with satellite, small, firm, rounded or flat-topped papules, excoriations, erythema, and pigmentation. ⌇

FIGURE 2-5   Acute allergic contact dermatitis on the lips due to lipstick   The patient was hypersensitive to eosin. Note bright erythema, microvesiculation. At close inspection a papular component can be discerned. At this stage there is still sharp margination.

FIGURE 2-6   Allergic contact dermatitis of hands: chromates   Confluent papules, vesicles, erosions and crusts on the dorsum of the left hand in a construction worker who was allergic to chromates.

TABLE 2-2   Top Ten Contact Allergens (North American Contact Dermatitis Group) and Other Common Contact Allergens*

Allergen	Principal Sources of Contact
Nickel sulfate	Metals, metals in clothing, jewelry, catalyzing agents
Neomycin sulfate	Usually contained in creams, ointments
Balsam of Peru	Topical medications
Fragrance mix	Fragrances, cosmetics
Thimerosal	Antiseptics
Sodium gold thiosulfate	Medication
Formaldehyde	Disinfectant, curing agents, plastics
Quaternium-15	Disinfectant
Bacitracin	Ointments, powder
Cobalt chloride	Cement, galvanization, industrial oils, cooling agents, eyeshades
Methyldibromoglutaronitrile, phenoxylethanol	Preservatives, cosmetics
Carba mix	Rubber, latex
Para-phenylendiamine	Black or dark dyes of textiles, printer's ink
Thiuram	Rubber
Parahydroxybenzoic acid ester	Conserving agent in foodstuffs
Propylene glycol	Preservatives, cosmetics
Procaine, benzocaine	Local anesthetics
Sulfonamides	Medication
Turpentine	Solvents, shoe polish, printer's ink
Mercury salts	Disinfectant, impregnation
Chromates	Cement, antioxidants, industrial oils, matches, leather
Parabenes	Biocides, preservatives
Cinnamic aldehyde	Fragrance, perfume
Pentadecylcatechols	Plants, e.g., poison ivy

* Over 3700 chemicals have been reported to cause ACD.

Arrangement   Initially, confined to area of contact with allergen [e.g., earlobe (earrings), dorsum of foot (shoes), wrist (watch or watchband), collar-like (necklace), lips (lipstick)]. Often linear, with artificial patterns, an "outside job." Plant contact often results in linear lesions (e.g., *Rhus* dermatitis). Initially confined to site of contact, later spreading beyond.

Distribution   *Extent*   Isolated, localized to one region (e.g., shoe dermatitis), or generalized (e.g., plant dermatitis).

Pattern   Random or on exposed areas (as in airborne ACD).

COURSE

Evolution of ACD   The duration of ACD varies among individuals, resolving in some in 1–2 weeks. ACD continues to get worse as long as allergen continues to come into contact with the skin.

Acute   Erythema → papules → vesicles → erosions → crusts → scaling.

Note: In the acute forms of contact dermatitis, papules occur only in ACD, not in ICD.

Chronic   Papules → scaling → lichenification → excoriations. Chronic inflammation with thickening, fissuring, scaling, and crusting results.

Note: Contact dermatitis is always confined to the site of exposure to the allergen. Margination is originally sharp in ACD; however, it spreads in the periphery beyond the actual site of exposure. If strong sensitization has occurred, spreading to other parts of the body and generalization occur. The main differences between toxic irritant and allergic contact dermatitis are summarized in Table 2-3.

FIGURE 2-7 Allergic contact dermatitis due to nickel, subacute Note a mix of papular, vesicular, and crusted lesions and loss of sharp margination. The patient was a retired watchmaker who used a metal clasp on the dorsum of the left hand while repairing watches. He was known to be allergic to nickel.

LABORATORY EXAMINATIONS

Dermatopathology *Acute* Prototype of spongiotic dermatitis. Inflammation with intraepidermal intercellular edema (*spongiosis*), lymphocytes and eosinophils in the epidermis, and monocyte and histiocyte infiltration in the dermis.
Chronic In chronic ACD there are also spongiosis plus acanthosis, elongation of rete ridges, and elongation and broadening of papillae; hyperkeratosis; and a lymphocytic infiltrate.
Patch Tests In ACD sensitization is present on every part of the skin; therefore, application of the allergen to any area of normal skin provokes an eczematous reaction. A positive patch test shows erythema and papules, as well as possibly vesicles confined to the test site. Patch tests should be delayed until the dermatitis has subsided for at least 2 weeks and should be performed on a previously uninvolved site. (See "Clinical Tests," Introduction.)

DIAGNOSIS AND DIFFERENTIAL DIAGNOSIS

By history and clinical findings, including evaluation of site and distribution. Histopathology may be helpful; verification of offending agent (allergen) by patch test. Exclude ICD (Table 2-3), atopic dermatitis, seborrheic dermatitis (face), psoriasis (palms and soles), epidermal dermatophytosis (KOH), fixed drug eruption, erysipelas phytophotodermatitis.

SPECIAL FORMS OF ACD

ALLERGIC CONTACT DERMATITIS DUE TO PLANTS

- Termed *allergic phytodermatitis* (APD)
- Occurs in sensitized individuals after exposure to a wide variety of plant allergens
- Characterized by an acute, very pruritic, eczematous dermatitis, often in a linear arrangement
- In the United States, poison ivy/oak are by far the most common plants implicated

Note: Phytophotodermatitis is a different entity; it is a photosensitivity reaction occurring in any individual with a photosensitizing plant–derived chemical on the skin and subsequent sun exposure (see Section 10)

EPIDEMIOLOGY AND ETIOLOGY

Age of Onset   Occurs in individuals of all ages. Very young and very old are less likely to be sensitized to plants. Sensitization is lifelong.

Etiology   Pentadecylcatechols, present in the Anacardiaceae plant family, are the most common sensitizers in the United States. They cross-react with other phenolic compounds such as resorcinol, hexylresorcinol, and hydroxyquinones.

Plants   *Anacardiaceae Family* Poison ivy (*Toxicodendron radicans*) and poison oak (*T. querifolium, T. diversilobum*) 🔲. Also poison sumac (*T. vernix*). Plants related to poison ivy group: Brazilian pepper, cashew nut tree, ginkgo tree, Indian marker nut tree, lacquer tree, mango tree, rengas tree.

Geography   Poison ivy occurs throughout the United States (except extreme southwest) and southern Canada; poison oak on the west coast. Poison sumac and poison dogwood grow only in woody, swampy areas.

Exposure   Telephone and electrical workers working outdoors. Leaves, stems, seeds, flowers, berries, and roots contain milky sap that turns to a black resin on exposure to air. Cashew oil: unroasted cashew nuts (heat destroys hapten); cashew oil in wood (Haitian voodoo dolls, swizzle sticks), resins, printer's ink. Mango rind. Marking nut tree of India: laundry marker (dhobi itch). Furniture lacquer from Japanese lacquer tree.

Season   APD usually occurs in the spring, summer, and fall; can occur year-round if exposed to stems or roots. In southwest of the United States, occurs year-round.

PATHOGENESIS

All *Toxicodendron* plants contain identical allergens. Hapten is present in milky sap in leaves, stems, seeds, flowers, berries, and roots. The oleoresins are referred to as *urushiol*. The haptens are the pentadecylcatechols (1, 2-hydroxybenzenes with a 15-carbon side chain in position three). Washing with soap and water removes oleoresins.

More than 70% of individuals can be sensitized to *Toxicodendron* haptens. Dark-skinned individuals are less susceptible to APD. After first exposure (sensitization) dermatitis occurs 7–12 days later. In a previously sensitized person (may be many decades before), dermatitis occurs (especially on face or genitalia) in <12 h after reexposure. Difference in clinical course varies with individual reactivity, inoculum of hapten on skin, and regional variation.

Note: Blister fluid does not contain hapten and cannot spread the dermatitis; exposure to smoke from the burning plant is harmless, but dermatitis can occur from particulate matter in the smoke.

CLINICAL MANIFESTATION

Exposure   *Poison Ivy/Oak Dermatitis*   Direct plant exposure: plant brushes against exposed skin giving rise to linear lesions (Fig. 2-8); resin usually is not able to penetrate the thick stratum corneum of palms/soles. Clothing: wearing clothing previously contaminated with resin can reexpose the skin.

Food Containing Urushiol   Eating unpeeled mango or unroasted cashew nuts can expose lips to oleoresin. Mucous membranes uncommonly experience APD, but ingestion of urushiol can produce allergic contact dermatitis of the anus and perineum.

Skin Symptoms   Pruritus mild to severe. Often sensed before any detectable skin changes. Pain in some cases. Secondary infection associated with local tenderness.

Constitutional Symptoms   Sleep deprivation due to pruritus.

Skin Lesions   Initially, well-demarcated patches of erythema, characteristic linear lesions (Fig. 2-8); rapidly evolve into papules and edematous plaques; may be severe especially on face and/or genitals, resembling cellulitis (Figs. 2-9, 35-16) Microvesiculation may evolve to vesicles and/or bullae (Figs. 2-8 and 2-10). Erosions, crusts. With resolution, erythematous plaques ± scale, ± erosion, ± crusting. Postinflammatory hyperpigmentation common in darker skinned individuals.

Distribution   Most commonly on exposed extremities, where contact with the plant occurs; blotting can transfer to any exposed site; palms/soles are usually spared; however, lateral fingers can be involved.

Clothing-Protected Sites   Oleoresin can penetrate damp clothing onto covered skin.

Nonexposed Sites   "Id"-like reaction or some systemic absorption can be associated with disseminated urticarial, erythema multiforme–like, or scarlatiniform lesions away from sites of exposure in some individuals with well-established APD.

FIGURE 2-8   Allergic phytodermatitis of leg: poison ivy   Linear vesicular lesions with erythema and edema on the calf at sites of direct contact of the skin 5 days after exposure with the poison ivy leaf.

FIGURE 2-9   Allergic phytodermatitis of face: poison ivy   Very pruritic erythema, edema, microvesiculation of the cheeks and periorbital area in a previously sensitized 7-year-old boy, occurring 3 days after exposure.

LABORATORY EXAMINATIONS

Dermatopathology   See ACD, above.
Patch Tests with Pentadecylcatechols   Con-traindicated. Can sensitize the individual to hapten.

TABLE 2-3   Differences Between Irritant and Allergic Contact Dermatitis*

		Irritant CD	Allergic CD
Symptoms	Acute	**Stinging, smarting → itching**	**Itching → pain**
	Chronic	Itching/pain	Itching/pain
Lesions	Acute	Erythema → vesicles → erosions → crusts → scaling	Erythema → **papules** → vesicles → erosions → crust → scaling
	Chronic	Papules, plaques, fissures, scaling, crusts	Papules, plaques, scaling, crusts
Margination and site	Acute	**Sharp, strictly confined to site of exposure**	Sharp, confined to site of exposure **but spreading in the periphery; usually tiny papules; may become generalized**
	Chronic	Ill-defined	Ill-defined, **spreads**
Evolution	Acute	**Rapid** (few hours after exposure)	**Not so rapid** (12–72 h after exposure)
	Chronic	Months to years of repeated exposure	Months or longer; exacerbation after every reexposure
Causative agents		**Dependent on concentration of agent and state of skin barrier; occurs only above threshold level**	**Relatively independent of amount applied, usually very low concentrations sufficient but depends on degree of sensitization**
Incidence		**May occur in practically everyone**	**Occurs only in the sensitized**

*Differences are printed in bold.

DIAGNOSIS

By history and clinical findings.

DIFFERENTIAL DIAGNOSIS

ACD to other allergens, phytophotodermatitis (see Section 10), soft-tissue infection (cellulitis, erysipelas), atopic dermatitis, inflammatory dermatophytosis, early herpes zoster, fixed drug eruption.

SYSTEMIC ACD (SACD)

- After systemic exposure to an allergen to which the individual had prior ACD.
- A delayed T cell–mediated reaction.
- Examples: ACD to ethylenediamine → subsequent reaction to aminophylline (which contains ethylene diamine); poison ivy dermatitis → subsequent reaction to ingestion of cashew nuts; also antibiotics, sulfonamides, propylene glycol, metal ions, sorbic acid, fragrances.

AIRBORNE ACD

- Contact with airborne allergens in exposed body sites, notably the face (Fig. 2-11); also including eyelids, "V" of the neck, arms, and legs.
- In contrast to airborne ICD, papular from the beginning, extremely itchy.
- Prolonged repetitive exposure leads to dry, lichenified ACD with erosions and crusting (Fig. 2-11).
- Due to plant allergens, especially from compositae, natural resins, woods, essential oils volatizing from aroma therapy.

MANAGEMENT OF ACD

Termination of Exposure   Identify and remove the etiologic agent.

FIGURE 2-10   Acute allergic phytodermatitis, bullous   This eruption occurred in a patient who had walked bare-foot through a forest. It later spread as a papular eruption to the rest of the body. Similar lesions were present on the other foot and lower leg. Differential diagnosis included acute bullous contact dermatitis to caterpillars. Phytophotodermatitis was excluded because at the time of exposure there was a heavily clouded sky and a papular eruption occurred later on. Caterpillar dermatitis was excluded because of the multiplicity of the lesions and because upon patch testing the patient was positive to toxicodendron haptens. Note, patch testing to urushiol is no longer done to avoid sensitization of patients.

Topical Therapy   Topical glucocorticoid ointments/gels (classes I to III) are effective for early nonbullous lesions. Larger vesicles may be drained, but tops should not be removed. Wet dressings with cloths soaked in Burow solution changed every 2–3 h. Since treatment with glucocorticoids is usually short-term in ACD, there is usually no danger of glucocorticoid side effects. An exception is airborne ACD, which may require systemic treatment. The topical calcineurin inhibitors pimecrolimus and tacrolimus are effective in ACD but to a lesser degree than glucocorticoids.

Systemic Therapy   Glucocorticoids are indicated if severe (i.e., if patient cannot perform usual daily functions, cannot sleep). Prednisone beginning at 70 mg (adults), tapering by 5–10 mg/d over a 1- to 2-week period.

In airborne ACD where complete avoidance of allergen may be impossible, immunosuppression with oral cyclosporine may become necessary.

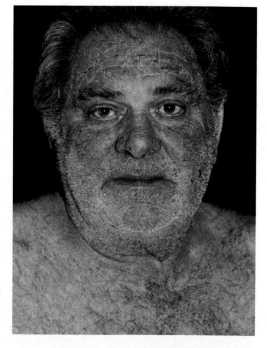

FIGURE 2-11   Airborne allergic contact dermatitis on the face   Extremely itchy, confluent papular, erosive, and crusted/scaly lesions with lichenification on the forehead, following exposure to pinewood dust.

ATOPIC DERMATITIS   ICD-9 : 691.8 ○ ICD-10 : L20   ■ ◑

- An acute, subacute, or chronic relapsing skin disorder
- Usually begins in infancy
- Prevalance peak of 15–20% in early childhood
- Characterized principally by dry skin and pruritus; consequent rubbing leads to incrased inflammation and lichenification and to further itching and scratching: *itch-scratch cycle*
- Diagnosis is based on clinical findings
- Often associated with a personal or family history of AD, allergic rhinitis, and asthma; 35% of infants with AD develop asthma later in life

- Associated with skin barrier dysfunction, IgE reactivity
- Genetic basis influenced by environmental factors; alterations in immunologic responses in T cells, antigen processing, inflammatory cytokine release, allergen sensitivity, infection

Synonyms: IgE dermatitis, "eczema," atopic eczema.

EPIDEMIOLOGY

Age of Onset   First 2 months of life and by the first years in 60% of patients. 30% are seen for the first time by age 5, and only 10% develop AD between 6 and 20 years of age. Rarely AD has an adult onset.

Gender   Slightly more common in males than females.

Prevalence   Between 7 and 15% reported in population studies in Scandinavia and Germany.

Genetic Aspects   The inheritance pattern has not been ascertained. However, in one series, 60% of adults with AD had children with AD. The prevalence in children was higher (81%) when both parents had AD.

Eliciting Factors   *Inhalants*   Specific aeroallergens, especially dust mites and pollens, have been shown to cause exacerbations of AD.

Microbial Agents   Exotoxins of *Staphylococcus aureus* may act as superantigens and stimulate activation of T cells and macrophages.

Autoallergens   Sera of patients with AD contain IgE antibodies directed at human proteins. The release of these autoallergens from damaged tissue could trigger IgE or T cell responses, suggesting maintenance of allergic inflammation by endogenous antigens.

Foods   *Subset* of infants and children have flares of AD with eggs, milk, peanuts, soybeans, fish, and wheat.

Other Exacerbating Factors

Skin Barrier Disruption: decrease of barrier function associated with impaired filaggrin production, reduced ceramide levels, and increased transepidermal water loss by frequent bathing and hand washing; dehydration is an important exacerbating factor.

Infections: S. aureus is almost always present in severe cases; group A streptococcus; rarely fungus (dermatophytosis, candidiasis).

Season: in temperate climates, AD usually improves in summer, flares in winter.

Clothing: pruritus flares *after* taking off clothing. Wool is an important trigger; wool clothing or blankets directly in contact with skin (also wool clothing of parents, fur of pets, carpets).

Emotional Stress: results from the disease or is itself an exacerbating factor in flares of the disease.

PATHOGENESIS

Complex interaction of skin barrier, genetic, environmental, pharmacologic, and immunologic factors. Type I (IgE-mediated) hypersensitivity reaction occurring as a result of the release of vasoactive substances from both mast cells and basophils that have been sensitized by the interaction of the antigen with IgE (reaginic or skin-sensitizing antibody). The role of IgE in AD is still not fully clarified, but epidermal Langerhans cells possess high-affinity IgE receptors through which an eczema-like reaction can be mediated. T_H2 and T_H1 both contribute to skin inflammation in AD. Actute T cell infiltration in AD is associated with a predominance of interleukin (IL) 4 and IL-13 expression, and chronic inflammation in AD

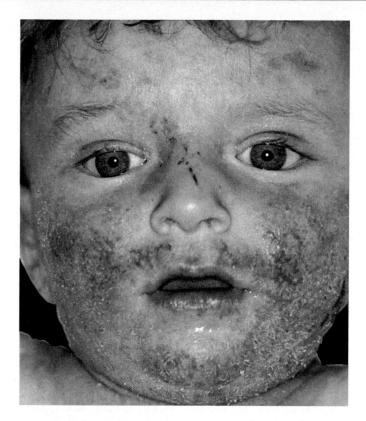

FIGURE 2-12 Atopic dermatitis: infantile Puffy face, confluent erythema, papules, microvesiculation, scaling, and crusting

FIGURE 2-13 Atopic dermatitis: infantile-type Skin of forehead is dry, cracked and scaly. In addition, there are oozing erosions.

with increased IL-5, granulocyte-macrophage colony-stimulating factor (GM-CSF), IL-12, and interferon (IFN) γ. Thus, skin inflammation in AD shows a biphasic pattern of T cell activation.

CLINICAL MANIFESTATION

Skin Symptoms   Patients have dry skin. Pruritus is the sine qua non of atopic dermatitis— "eczema is the itch that rashes." The constant scratching leads to a vicious cycle of itch → scratch → rash → itch → scratch.

Other Symptoms of Atopy   Allergic rhinitis, characterized by sneezing, rhinorrhea, obstruction of nasal passages, conjuctival and pharyngeal itching, and lacrimation; seasonal when associated with pollen.

Skin Lesions   *Acute*   Poorly defined erythematous patches, papules, and plaques with or without scale. Edema with widespread involvement; skin appears "puffy" and edematous (Fig. 2-12). Erosions: moist, crusted. Linear or punctate, resulting from scratching. Secondarily infected sites: *S. aureus*. Oozing erosions (Figs. 2-12 and 2-13) and/or pustules (usually follicular). Skin may be extremely dry and cracked and scaly (Fig. 2-13).

Chronic   Lichenification (thickening of the skin with accentuation of skin markings): results from repeated rubbing or scratching (Figs. 2-14 and 2-15); follicular lichenification (especially in brown and black persons) (Fig. 2-16). Fissures: painful, especially in flexures (Fig. 2-15), on palms, fingers, and soles. Alopecia: lateral one-third of the eyebrows as a result of rubbing. Periorbital pigmentation: also as a result of compulsive rubbing 🔊. Characteristic infraorbital fold below eyelids (Dennie-Morgan sign).

Distribution   Predilection for the flexures, front and sides of the neck, eyelids, forehead, face, wrists, and dorsa of the feet and hands (Image 2-1). Generalized in severe disease (Fig. 2-17).

Special Features Related to Age

Infantile AD   The lesions present as red skin, tiny vesicles on "puffy" surface. Scaling, exudation with wet crusts and cracks (fissures) (Figs. 2-12 to 2-14). Skin lesions seem to be a reaction to itching and rubbing. 🔊

Childhood-type AD   The lesions are papular, lichenified plaques, erosions, crusts, especially on the antecubital and popliteal fossae (Figs. 2-15, to 2-17), the neck and face; may be generalized. 🔊

Adult-type AD   There is a similar distribution, mostly flexural but also face and neck, with lichenification and exoriations being the most conspicuous symptoms (Figs. 2-18, 2-19). May be generalized. 🔊

Special Features Related to Ethnicity

In blacks but also dark-brown skin, so-called follicular eczema is common; characterized by discrete follicular papules (Figs. 2-16, 2-19, 2-20) involving hair follicles of the involved site. 🔊

Associated Findings

"White" dermatographism is a special and unique feature of involved skin: stroking will not lead to redness as in normal skin but to blanching 🔊; delayed blanch to cholinergic agents. *Ichthyosis vulgaris* and *keratosis pilaris* (see page 75) occur in 10% of patients. Vernal conjunctivitis with papillary hypertrophy or cobblestoning of upper eyelid conjuctiva. Atopic keratoconjunctivitis is disabling, may result in corneal scarring. Keratoconus rare. Cataracts in a small percentage.

DIAGNOSIS

History in infancy, clinical findings (typical distribution sites, morphology of lesions, white dermatographism).

DIFFERENTIAL DIAGNOSIS

Seborrheic dermatitis, ICD, ACD, psoriasis, nummular eczema, dermatophytosis, early stages of mycosis fungoides. Rarely, acrodermatitis enteropathica, glucagonoma syndrome, histidinemia, phenylketonuria; also, some immunologic disorders including Wiskott-Aldrich syndrome, X-linked agammaglobulinemia, hyper-IgE syndrome, and selective IgA deficiency; Langerhans cell histiocytosis, Letterer-Siwe type.

LABORATORY EXAMINATIONS

Bacterial Culture   Colonization with *S. aureus* very common in the nares and in the involved skin; almost 90% of patients with severe AD are secondarily colonized/infected. Look out for methicillin-resistant *S. aureus* (MRSA).

Viral Culture   Rule out herpes simplex virus (HSV) infection in crusted lesions (eczema herpeticum; see Section 27).

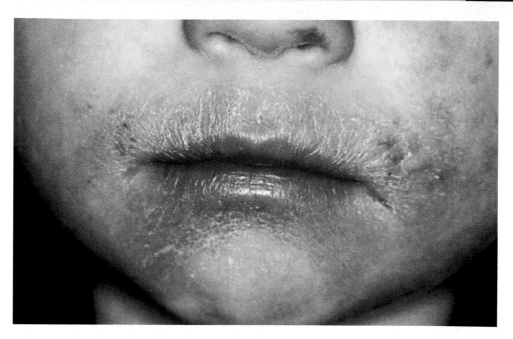

FIGURE 2-14   Childhood atopic dermatitis   A typical localization of atopic dermatitis in children is the region around the mouth. In this child there is lichenification and fissuring and crusting.

FIGURE 2-15   Childhood atopic dermatitis   One of the hallmarks of atopic dermatitis is lichenification in the flexural regions as shown in this picture. Note the thickening of the skin with exaggerated skin lines and erosions.

Blood Studies   Increased IgE in serum, eosinophilia. HSV antigen detection for diagnosis of acute HSV infection.

Dermatopathology   Various degrees of acanthosis with rare intraepidermal intercellular edema (spongiosis). The dermal infiltrate is composed of lymphocytes, monocytes, and mast cells with few or no eosinophils.

SPECIAL FORMS OF AD

Hand Dermatitis   Aggravated by wetting and washing with detergents, harsh soaps, and *disinfectants;* leads to ICD in the atopic. Clinically indistinguishable from "normal" ICD (see p. 22).

Exfoliative Dermatitis (See Section 8)   Erythroderma in patients with extensive skin involvement. Generalized redness, scaling, weeping, crusting, lymphadenopathy, fever, and systemic toxicity.

COMPLICATIONS

Secondary infection with *S. aureus* 🔁 and herpes simplex virus (eczema herpeticum, see Section 27). Rarely keratoconus, cataracts and keratoconjunctivitis with secondary herpetic infection 🔁 and corneal ulcers.

COURSE AND PROGNOSIS

Untreated involved sites persist for months or years. Spontaneous, more or less complete remission during childhood occurs in >40% with occasional, more severe recurrences during adolescence. In many patients, the disease persists for 15–20 years, but is less severe. From 30 to 50% of patients develop asthma and/or hay fever. Adult-onset AD often runs a severe course. *S. aureus* infection leads to extensive erosions and crusting, and herpes simplex infection to eczema herpeticum, which may be life-threatening (see Section 27).

MANAGEMENT

Education of the patient to avoid rubbing and scratching is most important. Topical antipruritic (menthol/camphor) lotions are helpful in controlling the pruritus but are useless if emollients are not used and the patient continues to scratch and rub the plaques.

An allergic workup is rarely helpful in uncovering an allergen; however, in patients who are hypersensitive to house dust mites, various pollens, and animal hair proteins, exposure to the appropriate allergen may cause flares. Atopic dermatitis is considered by many to be related, at least in part, to emotional stress. It may exacerbate with sweating.

Patients should be warned of their special problems with herpes simplex and the frequency of superimposed staphylococcal infection, for which oral antibiotics are indicated. Antiviral drugs for herpes simplex are indicated if HSV infection is suspected.

IMAGE 2-1   Predilection sites of atopic dermatitis.

FIGURE 2-16 Atopic dermatitis in black child: follicular   Pruritic follicular papules on the posterior leg. Follicular eczema is a reaction pattern that occurs more commonly in African and Asian children.

Acute

1. Wet dressings and topical glucocorticoids; topical antibiotics (mupirocin ointment) when indicated.
2. Hydroxyzine, 10–100 mg four times daily for pruritus.
3. Oral antibiotics (dicloxacillin, erythromycin) to eliminate *S. aureus* and treat MRSA according to sensitivity as shown by culture.

Subacute and Chronic

1. Hydration (oilated baths or baths with oatmeal powder) followed by application of unscented emollients (e.g., hydrated petrolatum) form the basic daily treatment needed to prevent xerosis. Soap showers are permissible to wash the body folds, but soap should seldom be used on the other parts of the skin surface. 12% ammonium lactate or 10% α-hydroxy acid lotion is very effective for the xerosis seen in AD.
2. Topical anti-inflammatory agents such as glucocorticoids, hydroxyquinoline preparations, and tar are the mainstays of treatment. Of these, glucocorticoids are the most effective. However, topical glucocorticoids may lead to skin atrophy if used for prolonged periods of time and if used excessively will lead to suppression of the pituitary-adrenal axis, osteoporosis, growth retardation. Another problem is "glucocorticoidophobia." Patients or their parents are increasingly aware of glucocorticoid side effects and refuse their use, no matter how beneficial they may be.
3. New topical nonsteroidal anti-inflammatory agents, the calcineurin inhibitors tacrolimus and pimecrolimus, are gradually replacing glucocorticoids in most patients. They potently suppress itching and inflammation and do not lead to skin atrophy. They are usually not effective enough to suppress acute flares but work very well in minor flares and subacute atopic dermatitis.
4. Oral H_1 antihistamines are useful in reducing itching.

5. Systemic glucocorticoids should be avoided, except in rare instances in adults for only short courses (rescue treatment). They are widely overused. Osteopenia and cataracts are complications. For severe intractable disease, prednisone, 60–80 mg daily for 2 days, then halving the dose each 2 days for the next 6 days. Patients with AD tend to become dependent on oral glucocorticoids. Often, small doses (5–10 mg) make the difference in control and can be reduced gradually to even 2.5 mg/d, as is often used for the control of asthma. Intramuscular glucocorticoids are risky and should be avoided.

6. UVA-UVB phototherapy (combination of UVA plus UVB and increasing the radiation dose each treatment, with a frequency of two to three times weekly). Narrow band UV (311 nm), PUVA photochemotherapy also effective.

7. In severe cases of adult AD and in normotensive healthy persons without renal disease cyclosporine treatment (starting dose 5 mg/kg per day) is indicated when all other treatments fail, but should be monitored closely. Treatment is limited to 3–6 months because of potential side effects, including hypertension and reduced renal function. Blood pressure should be checked weekly and chemistry panels biweekly. Nifedipine can be used for moderate increases in blood pressure.

8. Patients should learn and use stress management techniques.

9. A suggested algorithm of AD management is as follows (see Image 2-2):

   • Baseline therapy of dryness with emollients
   • Suppression of mild to moderate AD by prolonged topical pimecrolimus or tacrolimus and continued emollients
   • Supression of severe flares with topical glucocorticoids followed by pimecrolimus or tacrolimus and emollients
   • Oral and topical antibiotics to eliminate *S. aureus*
   • Hydroxyzine to suppress pruritus

Website: *http://www.aad.org/pamphlets/eczema.html.*

FIGURE 2-17   Childood atopic dermatitis   This is a generalized eruption consisting of confluent, inflammatory papules that are erosive, excoriated, and crusted.

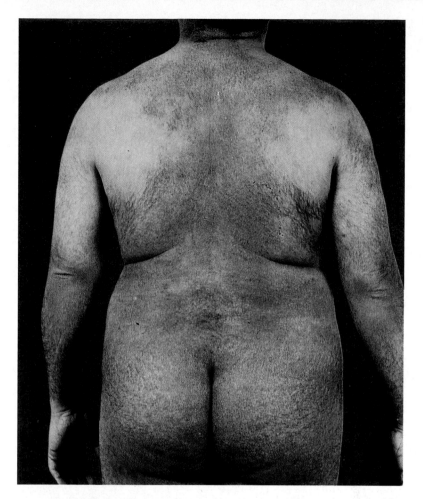

FIGURE 2-18 **Adult atopic dermatitis in dark skin** Generalized eruption of follicular papules that are more heavily pigmented than normal skin in a 53-year-old woman of African extraction.

Strategy for treatment with topical calcineurin inhibitors

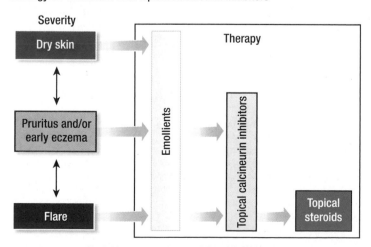

IMAGE 2-2 **Treatment algorithm of AD.**

FIGURE 2-19   Adult atopic dermatitis   Lichenification does not only occur in the big flexural folds but may also affect the face in this 53-year-old woman of Indonesian extraction.

FIGURE 2-20   Adult atopic dermatitis in heavily pigmented Asian skin   There are multiple pruritic follicular papules that are a typical reaction pattern in African and Asian skin.

LICHEN SIMPLEX CHRONICUS   (LSC) ICD-9:698.3 ∘ ICD-10:L28

- A special localized form of lichenification, occurring in circumscribed plaques.
- Results from repetitive rubbing and scratching.
- Lichenification is a characteristic feature of atopic dermatitis, whether generalized or localized.

- LSC can last for decades unless the rubbing and scratching are stopped by treatment.
- Occurs in individuals older than 20 years, is more frequent in women, and possibly more frequent in Asians.

PATHOGENESIS

A special predilection of the skin to respond to physical trauma by epidermal hyperplasia; skin becomes highly sensitive to touch. The very abnormal itching hyperexcitability of lichenified skin arises in response to minimal external stimuli that would not elicit an itch response in normal skin. Emotional stress in some cases. It becomes a habit and may persist for months to years, with resulting marked lichenification.

Many patients have AD or an atopic background.

Skin symptoms consist of pruritus, often in paroxysms. The lichenified skin is like an erogenous zone—it becomes a pleasure (orgiastic) to scratch. Often the areas on the feet are rubbed at night with the heel and the toes. The rubbing becomes automatic and reflexive and an unconscious habit. Most patients with LSC give a history of itch attacks starting from minor stimuli: putting on clothes, removing

FIGURE 2-21 Lichen simplex chronicus Confluent, papular, follicular eczema, creating a plaque of lichen simplex chronicus of the posterior neck and occipital scalp. Condition had been present for many years as a result of chronic rubbing of the area.

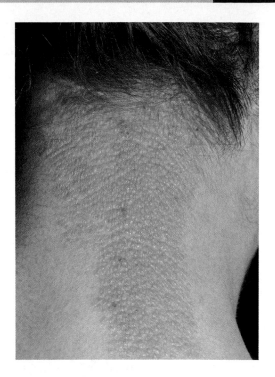

ointments, clothes rubbing the skin; in bed, the skin becomes warmer and the warmth precipitates itching.

CLINICAL MANIFESTATION

Skin Lesions A solid plaque of lichenification, arising from the confluence of small papules; scaling is minimal except on lower extremities (Fig. 2-21). Lichenified skin is palpably thickened; skin markings (barely visible in normal skin) are accentuated and can be seen readily. Excoriations are often present. Usually dull red, later brown or black hyperpigmentation, especially in skin phototypes IV, V, and VI. Round, oval, linear (following path of scratching). Usually sharply defined. Isolated single lesion or several randomly scattered plaques. Nuchal area (female) (Fig. 2-21), scalp, ankles, lower legs, upper thighs, exterior forearms, vulva, pubis, anal area, scrotum (See Fig. 35-18), and groin.

In black skin, lichenification may assume a special type of pattern—there is not a solid plaque, but the lichenification consists instead of a multitude of small (2- to 3-mm) closely set papules—i.e., a "follicular" pattern (as in Fig. 2-16).

DIFFERENTIAL DIAGNOSIS

Includes a chronic pruritic plaque of psoriasis vulgaris, early stages of mycosis fungoides, ICD, ACD, epidermal dermatophytosis.

LABORATORY EXAMINATION

Dermatopathology Hyperplasia of all components of epidermis: hyperkeratosis, acanthosis, and elongated and broad rete ridges. Spongiosis is infrequent. In the dermis there is a chronic inflammatory infiltrate.

MANAGEMENT

Difficult. Repeatedly explain to the patient that the rubbing and scratching must be stopped. It is important to apply occlusive bandages at night to prevent rubbing. Topical glucocorticoid preparations or tar preparations such as combinations of 5% crude coal tar in zinc oxide paste plus class II glucocorticoids all covered by occlusive dressings are effective for body areas where this approach is feasible (e.g., legs, arms). Occlusive dressings: topical glucocorticoids are applied to lesion and covered by an occlusive (plastic) dressing (like saran wrap). Glucocorticoids incorporated in adhesive plastic tape are also very effective, left for 24 hours. Unna Boot: a gauze roll dressing impregnated with zinc oxide paste is wrapped around a large lichenified area such as the calf. The dressing can be left on for up to 1 week.

Intralesional triamcinolone is often highly effective in smaller lesions (3 mg/mL; higher concentrations may cause atrophy). Oral hydroxyzine, 25–50 g at night, may be helpful.

PRURIGO NODULARIS (PN)   ICD-9 698.3 ∘ ICD-10 : L28.1

- Is often associated with AD or occurs without AD.
- PN patients with AD are younger and have reactivity to environmental allergens; nonatopic PN patients are older and lack hypersensitivities to environmental allergens.
- PN starts with piercing pruritus that leads to picking and scratching.
- Dome-shaped nodules—several millimeters to 2 cm—develop on sites in which persistent itching and scratching occur (Fig. 2-22). 🔁
- Nodules are often eroded, excoriated, and sometimes even ulcerated as patients dig into them with their nails.

- Usually multiple on the extremities.
- PN usually occurs in younger or middle-age females, who often exhibit signs of neurotic stigmatization.
- Lesions persist for months after the trauma has been discontinued.
- Treatment: intralesional triamcinolone, occlusive dressings with high-potency glucocorticoids. In severe cases, thalidomide 50–100 mg. Watch out for contraindications! PO neurontin 300 mg TID may be helpful.

FIGURE 2-22   Prurigo nodularis   Multiple, firm, excoriated nodules arising at sites of chronically picked or excoriated skin. Often occurring in patients with atopy but also without it. This is a 36-year-old male with HIV disease. He had MRSA secondary infection of prurigo nodules. Cellulitis originated in prurigo nodules requiring multiple hospitalizations.

DYSHIDROTIC ECZEMATOUS DERMATITIS (DED)

- Dyshidrotic eczema is a special vesicular type of hand and foot dermatitis.
- An acute, chronic, or recurrent dermatosis of the fingers, palms, and soles.
- Sudden onset of many deep-seated pruritic, clear "tapioca-like" vesicles (Fig. 2-23). ⚡

- Large bullae and bacterial infection can occur.
- Later, scaling fissures and lichenification.

Synonyms: Pompholyx, vesicular palmar eczema.

ICD-9 : 705.81 ○ ICD-10 : L30.1

LABORATORY EXAMINATIONS

Bacterial Culture Vesicles of DED are sterile. But rule out *S. aureus* infection.
KOH Preparation Rule out epidermal dermatophytosis.
Dermatopathology Eczematous inflammation (spongiosis and intraepidermal edema) with intraepidermal vesicles.

COURSE AND PROGNOSIS

Recurrent attacks are the rule. Spontaneous remissions in 2–3 weeks. Interval between attacks is weeks to months. Secondary infection may complicate the course: pustules, crusts, cellulitis, lymphangitis, and painful lymphadenopathy. Disabling because of severe, frequently recurring outbreaks.

MANAGEMENT

Wet Dressing For vesicular stage: Burow wet dressings. Large bullae drained with a puncture but not unroofed.
Fissures Topical application of flexible collodion.

Glucocorticoids
Topical High-potency glucocorticoids with plastic occlusive dressings for 1 to maximum of 2 weeks.
Intralesional Injection Triamcinolone, 3 mg/mL. Very effective for small areas of involvement.
Systemic In severe cases, a short, tapered course of prednisone can be given: 70 mg/d, tapering by 10 or 5 mg/d over 7 or 14 days.
Systemic Antibiotic For suspected (localized pain) or documented secondarily infected lesions (usually *S. aureus;* less commonly group A streptococcus).
PUVA (See page 68) Oral or topical as "soaks." Successful in many patients if given over prolonged periods of time and worth trying, especially in severe cases.

FIGURE 2-23 Dyshidrotic eczematous dermatitis Confluent tapioca-like vesicles and crusted (excoriated) erosions on the dorsum of fingers and finger webs.

NUMMULAR ECZEMA (NE)   ◧ ◑

- Nummular eczema is a chronic, pruritic, inflammatory dermatitis occurring in the form of coin-shaped plaques composed of grouped small papules and vesicles on an erythematous base.

- It is especially common on the extremities during winter months; often seen in atopic individuals;

Synonym: Discoid eczema, microbial eczema.

ICD-9:692.9 ∘ ICD-10:L30.9

EPIDEMIOLOGY

Two peaks in incidence: young adulthood and old age. Fall and winter.

PATHOGENESIS

Unknown. Unrelated to atopic diathesis; IgE levels normal. Incidence peaks in winter, when xerosis is maximal. *S. aureus* often present but pathogenic significance not proven.

CLINICAL MANIFESTATION

Skin Symptoms   Pruritus, often intense.
Skin Lesions   Closely grouped, small vesicles and papules that coalesce into plaques (Fig. 2-24A), often more than 4 to 5 cm in diameter, with an erythematous base with distinct borders. Plaques may become exudative and crust (Fig. 2-24B). Excoriations secondary to scratching. Dry scaly plaques that may be lichenified. Round or *coin-shaped* (Fig. 2-24A), hence the adjective *nummular* (Latin: *nummularis,* "like a coin"). Margins often more pronounced than center. 🔎
Distribution   Regional clusters of lesions (e.g., on legs or trunk) or generalized, scattered. Lower legs (older men), trunk, hands and fingers (younger females).

DIFFERENTIAL DIAGNOSIS

Scaling Plaques   Epidermal dermatophytosis, ICD or ACD, psoriasis, early stages of mycosis fungoides, impetigo, familial pemphigus.

LABORATORY EXAMINATIONS

Bacterial Culture   Rule out *S. aureus* infection.
Dermatopathology   Subacute inflammation with acanthosis and spongiosis.

COURSE AND PROGNOSIS

Chronic. Lesions last from weeks to months. Often difficult to control even with potent topical glucocorticoid preparations.

MANAGEMENT

Skin Hydration   "Moisturize" involved skin after bath or shower with hydrated petrolatum or other moisturizing cream.
Glucocorticoids *Topical Preparations* Classes I and II applied twice daily until lesions have resolved. Steroid impregnated tape. *Intralesional* triamcinolone, 3 mg/mL.
Crude Coal Tar   2–5% crude coal tar ointment daily. May be combined with glucocorticoid preparation. Tar baths are useful in patients with refractory lesions.
Systemic Therapy   Systemic antibiotics if *S. aureus* is present.
PUVA or UVB 311-nm Therapy   Very effective.

FIGURE 2-24   Nummular eczema   A. Pruritic, round, nummular (coin-shaped) plaques with erythema, scales, and crusts on the forearm. **B.** A close-up of a lesion in another patient reveals that this inflammatory plaque consists of confluent papulovesicular lesions that ooze a serous fluid and lead to crusting and are usually yellow.

AUTOSENSITIZATION DERMATITIS   ICD-9:692.9 ∘ ICD-10:L30.9 ▪ ◑

- An often unrecognized generalized pruritic dermatitis directly related to a primary dermatitis elsewhere.

- For example, a patient with venous stasis dermatitis on the lower legs may develop pruritic, symmetric, scattered, erythematous, maculopapular, or papulovesicular lesions on the trunk, forearms, thighs, or legs.

- These persist and spread until the basic underlying primary dermatitis is controlled.

- Similarly, autosensitization may occur as an "id" reaction in inflammatory tinea pedis and manifests as a dyshidrosiform, vesicular eruption on

the feet and hands (Fig. 2-25) and papulovesicular eczematoid lesions on the trunk.

- The phenomenon results from the release of cytokines in the primary dermatitis, as a result of sensitization. These cytokines circulate in the blood and heighten the sensitivity of the distant skin areas.

- The diagnosis of autosensitization dermatitis is often *post hoc*, i.e., the distant eruption disappears when the primary dermatitis is controlled.

- Oral glucocorticoids hasten the disappearance of the lesions.

SEBORRHEIC DERMATITIS (SD)   ICD-9:609.1 ∘ ICD-10:L21.9 ▪ ○ → ◑

- A very common chronic dermatosis characterized by redness and scaling and occurring in regions where the sebaceous glands are most active, such as the face and scalp, the presternal area, and in the body folds. Mild scalp SD causes flaking, i.e., dandruff.

- Generalized SD, failure to thrive, and diarrhea in an infant should bring to mind Leiner disease with a variety of immunodeficiency disorders.

Synonyms: "Cradle cap" (infants), pityriasis sicca (dandruff).

EPIDEMIOLOGY AND ETIOLOGY

Age of Onset   Infancy (within the first months), puberty, most between 20 and 50 years or older.
Sex   More common in males.
Incidence   2 to 5% of the population.
Predisposing and Exacerbating Factors   In immunocompetent patients there is often a hereditary diathesis, the so-called seborrheic state, with marked seborrhea and marginal blepharitis. May be associated with psoriasis as a prepsoriasis state in which the patient later develops psoriasis; in some patients a mix of lesions (superficial scales on the scalp and eyebrows and polycyclic scaling patches on the trunk) suggests the use of the term *seborrhiasis*. There is reputedly an increased incidence in Parkinson disease and facial paralysis. Also, some neuroleptic drugs are possibly a factor, but the disease is so common that this has not been proved. Emotional stress is a putative factor in flares. HIV-infected individuals have an increased incidence, and severe intractable SD

should be a clue to the existence of HIV disease (see also Section 31).

PATHOGENESIS

Malassezia furfur is said to play a role in the pathogenesis, and the response to topical ketoconazole and selenium sulfide is some indication that this yeast may be pathogenic; also the frequency of SD in immunosuppressed patients (HIV/AIDS, cardiac transplants). SD-like lesions are seen in nutritional deficiencies such as zinc deficiency (as a result of IV alimentation) and experimental niacin deficiency and in Parkinson disease (including drug-induced). SD develops in experimental pyridoxine deficiency in humans.

CLINICAL MANIFESTATION

Duration of Lesions   Gradual onset.
Seasonal Variations   Some patients are worse in winter in a dry, indoor environment. Sunlight exposure causes SD to flare in a few

FIGURE 2-25 Autosensitization dermatitis ("id" reaction): dermatophytid Vesicles and bullae on the finger and the lateral foot of a 21-year-old female. Bullous (inflammatory) tinea pedis was present and was associated with dermatophytid reaction. Prednisone was given for 2 weeks; pruritus and vesiculation resolved.

patients and promotes improvement of the condition in others.

Skin Symptoms Pruritus is variable, often increased by perspiration.

Skin Lesions Orange-red or gray-white skin, often with "greasy" or white dry scaling macules, papules of varying size (5–20 mm), or patches, rather sharply marginated (Fig. 2-26). Sticky crusts and fissures are common in the folds behind the external ear. On the scalp there is mostly marked scaling ("dandruff"), diffuse involvement of scalp. Scattered, discrete on the face and trunk. Nummular, polycyclic, and even annular on the trunk 🔁.

Distribution and Major Types of Lesions (Based on Localization and Age) *Hairy Areas of Head* Scalp, eyebrows, eyelashes (blepharitis), beard (follicular orifices); cradle cap: erythema and yellow-orange scales and crusts on the scalp in infants 🔁.

Face The flush ("butterfly") areas, on forehead ("corona seborrhoica"), nasolabial folds, eyebrows, glabella (Fig. 2-26). The erythema of SD is often overlooked and thought to be the flushing of rosacea. SD does not respond to treatment of rosacea. Ears: retroauricular, meatus.

Trunk Simulating lesions of pityriasis rosea or pityriasis versicolor; yellowish-brown patches over the sternum common.

Body Folds Axillae, groins, anogenital area, submammary areas, umbilicus, and diaper area

in infants (Fig. 2-27)—presents as a diffuse, exudative, sharply marginated, brightly erythematous eruption; erosions and fissures common.

Genitalia Often with yellow crusts and psoriasiform lesions. 🔁

DIAGNOSIS/DIFFERENTIAL DIAGNOSIS

Usually made on clinical criteria.

Red Scaly Plaques *Common* Mild psoriasis vulgaris (sometimes may be indistinguishable), impetigo (rule out by smears for bacteria), dermatophytosis (tinea capitis, tinea facialis, tinea corporis), pityriasis versicolor, intertriginous candidiasis (KOH: rule out dermatophytes and yeasts), subacute lupus erythematosus (rule out by biopsy), "seborrheic" papules in secondary syphilis (darkfield: rule out *Treponema pallidum*).

Rare Langerhans cell histiocytosis (occurs in infants, often associated with purpura), acrodermatitis enteropathica, zinc deficiency, pemphigus foliaceus, glucagonoma syndrome.

LABORATORY STUDIES

Dermatopathology Focal parakeratosis, with few neutrophils, moderate acanthosis, spongiosis (intercellular edema), nonspecific inflammation of the dermis. A characteristic feature is neutrophils at the tips of the dilated follicular openings, which appear as crusts/scales.

COURSE AND PROGNOSIS

SD is very common, affecting the majority of individuals at some time during life. The condition improves in the summer and flares in the fall. Recurrences and remissions, especially on the scalp, may be associated with alopecia in severe cases. Infantile and adolescent SD disappears with age. Seborrheic erythroderma may occur. *Seborrheic erythroderma with diarrhea and failure to thrive (Leiner disease) in infants is associated with a variety of immunodeficiency disorders including defective yeast opsonization, C3 deficiency, severe combined immunodeficiency, hypogammaglobulinemia, and hyperimmunoglobulinemia.*

MANAGEMENT

Requires initial therapy followed by chronic maintenance therapy. Topical glucocorticoid preparations are effective but can cause atrophy and erythema and telangiectasia, especially on the face, or initiation/exacerbation of perioral dermatitis or rosacea. UV radiation is beneficial for many individuals. Topical calcineurin inhibitors are highly effective.

Initial Topical Therapy
Scalp   *Adults*   Effective over-the-counter (OTC) *shampoos* containing selenium sulfide, zinc pyrithione, are helpful. By prescription (U.S.), 2% ketoconazole shampoo, used initially to treat and subsequently to control the symptoms; lather can be used on face and chest during shower. Tar shampoos (OTC) are equally effective in many patients. Low-potency *glucocorticoid* solution, lotion, or gels following

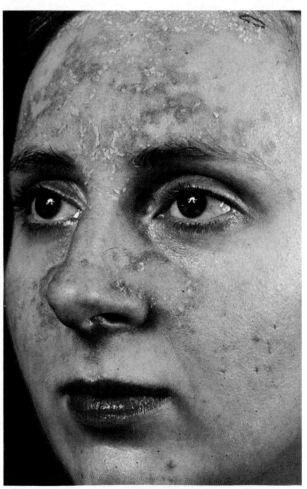

FIGURE 2-26   Seborrheic dermatitis of face: adult-type   Erythema and yellow-orange scaling annular of the forehead, cheeks, nasolabial folds, and chin. Scalp and retroauricular areas were also involved.

FIGURE 2-27 Seborrheic dermatitis: infantile-type Erythema and orange scales and crusting in the diaper region of an infant. This is difficult to distinguish in the diaper region from psoriasis and *Candida* has to be ruled out by KOH.

a medicated shampoo (ketoconazole or tar) for more severe cases. Pimecrolimus, 1% cream, is very beneficial.

Infants For cradle cap, removal of crusts with warm olive oil compresses, followed by baby shampoo, 2% ketoconazole shampoo, and application of 1–2.5% hydrocortisone cream, 2% ketoconazole cream, 1% pimecrolimus cream.

Face and Trunk *Ketoconazole shampoo, 2%*. Glucocorticoid cream and lotions: initially 1 or 2.5% hydrocortisone cream, 2% ketoconazole cream, 1% pimecrolimus cream, 0.03 or 0.1% tacrolimus ointment.

More potent glucocorticoid lotions (e.g., clobetasol propionate) may be used for *initial* control and are used along with the medicated shampoos.

Eyelids Gentle removal of the crusts in the morning with a cotton ball dipped in diluted baby shampoo. Apply 10% sodium sulfacetamide in a suspension containing 0.2% prednisolone and 0.12% phenylephrine (use cautiously because it contains glucocorticoids). Sodium sulfacetamide ointment alone is also effective, as is 2% ketoconazole cream, 1%

pimecrolimus cream, or 0.03% tacrolimus ointment.

Intertriginous Areas *Ketoconazole, 2%*; if uncontrolled with these treatments, Castellani paint for dermatitis of the body folds is often very effective, but staining is a problem. Pimecrolimus cream, 1%; tacrolimus ointment, 0.03 or 0.1%.

Systemic Therapy

In severe cases, 13-*cis* retinoic acid orally, 1 mg/kg, is highly effective. Contraception should be used in females of child-bearing age. In milder cases, itraconazole 100 twice daily for 2 weeks is also effective.

Maintenance Therapy

Ketoconazole 2% shampoo; tar shampoos may be equally effective; ketoconazole cream. If these do not work, then the old "standard," 3% sulfur precipitate and 2% salicylic acid in an oil-in-water base is effective; this must be properly compounded. Also, 1–2.5% hydrocortisone cream daily will work, but patients should be monitored for signs of atrophy. 1% pimecrolimus cream and 0.03% tacrolimus ointment are safe and effective.

ASTEATOTIC DERMATITIS   ICD-9:692.89 ∘ ICD-10:L30.9   ■ ○→◑

- A common pruritic dermatitis that occurs especially in older persons, in the winter in temperate climates—related to the low humidity of heated houses.

- The sites of predilection are the legs (Fig. 2-28), arms, and hands but also the trunk.

- Dry, "cracked," superficially fissured skin with slight scaling. 🔲

- The incessant pruritus can lead to lichenification, which can even persist when the environmental conditions have been corrected.

- The disorder results from too frequent bathing in hot soapy baths or showers and/or in older persons living in rooms with a high environmental temperature and low relative humidity.

- Management: avoiding overbathing with soap, especially tub baths, and increasing the ambient humidity to >50%, by using room humidifiers; also using tepid water baths containing bath oils for hydration, followed by immediate liberal application of emollient ointments, such as hydrated petrolatum. If skin is inflamed, use medium-potency glucocorticoid ointments, applied twice daily until the eczematous component has resolved.

Synonym: Eczema *craquelé* (French *craquelé*, "marred with cracks," such as in old china and ceramic tile).

FIGURE 2-28   Asteatotic dermatitis   In this 65-year-old man lesions have coalesced to involve the entire skin of the lower leg. The erythematous, scaling lesions are extremely pruritic.

PSORIASIS

- Psoriasis affects 1.5–2% of the population in western countries. World wide occurrence.
- A chronic disorder with polygenic predisposition and triggering environmental factors such as bacterial infection, trauma, or drugs.
- Several clinical expressions. Typical lesions are chronic, recurring, scaly papules and plaques. Pustular eruptions and erythroderma occur.
- Clinical presentation varies among individuals, from those with only a few localized plaques to those with generalized skin involvement.
- Psoriatic arthritis occurs in 10–25% of the patients.
- The pathogenesis is determined by a polygenic trait with an ongoing T cell–driven autoreactive immune response.

CLASSIFICATION

Psoriasis vulgaris
  Acute guttate
  Chronic stable plaque
  Palmoplantar
  Inverse

Psoriatic erythroderma
Pustular psoriasis
  Pustular psoriasis of von Zumbusch
  Palmoplantar pustulosis
  Acrodermatitis continua

PSORIASIS VULGARIS   ICD-9 : 696.1 ○ ICD-10 : L 40.0

EPIDEMIOLOGY

Age of Onset   *Early*: Peak incidence occurs at 22.5 years of age (in children, the mean age of onset is 8 years). *Late*: Presents about age 55. *Early onset* predicts a more severe and long-lasting disease, and there is usually a positive family history of psoriasis.

Incidence   Psoriasis affects 1.5–2% of the population in western countries. In the United States, there are 3 to 5 million persons with psoriasis. Most have localized psoriasis, but approximately 300,000 persons have generalized psoriasis.

Sex   Equal incidence in males and females.

Race   Low incidence in West Africans, Japanese, and Inuits; very low incidence or absence in North and South American Indians.

Heredity   Polygenic trait. When one parent has psoriasis, 8% of offspring develop psoriasis; when both parents have psoriasis, 41% of children develop psoriasis. HLA types most frequently associated with psoriasis are HLA- B13, -B17,-Bw57, and, most importantly, HLA-Cw6, which presents antigens to CD8+ T cells and is thus a candidate for functional involvement.

Trigger Factors   *Physical trauma* (Koebner phenomenon) is a major factor in eliciting lesions; rubbing and scratching stimulate the psoriatic proliferative process. *Infections*: acute streptococcal infection precipitates guttate psoriasis. *Stress*: a factor in flares of psoriasis is said to be as high as 40% in adults and higher in children. *Drugs*: systemic glucocorticoids, oral lithium, antimalarial drugs, interferon, and β-adrenergic blockers can cause flares in existing psoriasis and cause a psoriasiform drug eruption. *Alcohol ingestion* is a putative trigger factor.

PATHOGENESIS

The most obvious abnormalities in psoriasis are (1) an alteration of the cell kinetics of keratinocytes with a shortening of the cell cycle from 311 to 36 h, resulting in 28 times the normal production of epidermal cells, and (2) CD8+ T cells, which are the overwhelming T cell population in lesions. The epidermis and dermis react as an integrated system: the described changes in the germinative layer of the epidermis and inflammatory changes in the dermis, which trigger the epidermal changes. Psoriasis is a T cell–driven disease. There are many CD8+ T cells present in psoriatic lesions surrounding the upper dermal blood vessels, and the cytokine spectrum is that of a T_H1 response. Maintenance of psoriatic lesions is considered an ongoing autoreactive immune response.

CLINICAL MANIFESTATION

There are two major types:

1. *Eruptive, inflammatory type* with multiple small (guttate or nummular) lesions and a greater tendency toward spontaneous resolution (Figs. 3-1 and 3-2); relatively rare (<2.0% of all psoriasis); similar to an exanthem: a shower of lesions appears rather rapidly and in young adults, often but not always following streptococcal pharyngitis.
2. *Chronic stable (plaque) psoriasis* (Figs. 3-3; 3-4): Majority of patients, with chronic indolent lesions present for months and years, changing only slowly.

Skin Symptoms   Pruritus is reasonably common, especially in scalp and anogenital psoriasis.

Skin Lesions   The classic lesion of psoriasis is a sharply marginated erythematous papule with a silvery-white scale (Fig. 3-1). Scales are lamellar, loose, and easily removed by scratching. Removal of scale results in the appearance of minute blood droplets (*Auspitz sign*). Papules grow to sharply marginated plaques with lamellar scaling (Fig. 3-3) that coalesce to form polycyclic or serpiginous patterns (Fig. 3-4). May occur anywhere on the body but there are classic predilection sites (see Image 3-1).

Acute Guttate Type   Salmon-pink papules (guttate: Latin *gutta*, "drop"), 2.0 mm to 1.0 cm with or without scales (Figs. 3-1; 3-2) scales may not be visible but become apparent upon scraping. Scattered discrete lesions, like a rash; generally concentrated on the trunk (Fig. 3-2), less on the face and scalp, and usually sparing palms and soles. Guttate lesions may resolve spontaneously within a few weeks but usually become recurrent and may evolve into chronic, stable psoriasis. 🗗

Chronic Stable Type   Sharply marginated, dull-red plaques with loosely adherent, lamellar, silvery-white scales (Fig. 3-3). Plaques coalesce to form polycyclic, geographic lesions (Fig. 3-4) and may partially regress, resulting in annular, serpiginous, and arciform patterns. Lamellar scaling can easily be removed, or, when the lesion is extremely chronic, it adheres tightly to the underlying inflammatory and infiltrated skin, resulting in hyperkeratosis that looks like the shell of an oyster (Fig. 3-5). 🗗

Distribution and Predilection Sites

Acute Guttate   Disseminated, generalized, mainly trunk (Fig. 3-2).

Chronic Stable   Single lesion or lesions localized to one or more predilection sites: elbows, knees, sacralgluteal region, scalp, palm/soles (Image 3-1). Sometimes only regional involvement (scalp), often generalized.

Pattern   Bilateral, often symmetric (predilection sites); often spares exposed areas.

Special Sites

Palms and Soles   May be the only areas involved. There is massive silvery white or yellowish hyperkeratosis and scaling, which in contrast to lesions on the trunk, is not easily removed (Fig. 3-6). Desquamation of hyperkeratosis will, however, reveal an inflammatory plaque at the base that is always sharply demarcated (Fig. 3-7). There may be cracking and painful fissures and bleeding. 🗗

Scalp   Plaques, sharply marginated, with thick adherent scales (Fig. 3-8). Scattered discrete or diffuse involvement of entire scalp. Often very pruritic. *Note:* psoriasis of the scalp does not lead to hair loss, even after years of thick plaque-type involvement. Scalp psoriasis may be part of generalized psoriasis or coexist with isolated plaques, or the scalp may be only site involved. 🗗

Face   Uncommonly involved, and when involved, usually associated with a refractory type of psoriasis (Fig. 3-9).

FIGURE 3-1 **Psoriasis vulgaris** Primary lesions are well-defined, reddish or salmon-pink papules, droplike, with a loosely adherent silvery-white lamellar scale.

FIGURE 3-2 **Psoriasis vulgaris: buttocks (guttate type)** Discrete, erythematous, scaling, small papules that tend to coalesce, appearing after a group A streptococcal pharyngitis. There was a family history of psoriasis.

Chronic Psoriasis of the Perianal and Genital Regions and of the Body Folds—Inverse Psoriasis   Due to the warm and moist environment in these regions psoriatic plaques are usually not scaly but are macerated, often bright red and fissured (Figs. 3-10, 35-7, 35-8). The sharp demarcation permits distinction from intertrigo, candidiasis, contact dermatitis, tinea cruris. ✐

Nails   Fingernails and toenails frequently (25%) involved, especially with concomitant arthritis (Fig. 3-11A). Nail changes include pitting, subungual hyperkeratosis, onycholysis, and yellowish-brown spots under the nail plate—the *oil spot* (pathognomonic) (See Figs. 33-8, 33-9). ✐

LABORATORY EXAMINATIONS

Dermatopathology

- Marked overall thickening of the epidermis (acanthosis) and thinning of epidermis over elongated dermal papillae
- Increased mitosis of keratinocytes, fibroblasts, and endothelial cells
- Parakeratotic hyperkeratosis (nuclei retained in the stratum corneum)

- Inflammatory cells in the dermis (lymphocytes and monocytes) and in the epidermis (lymphocytes and polymorphonuclear cells), forming microabscesses of Munro in the stratum corneum.

Serology   Increased antistreptolysin titer in acute guttate psoriasis with antecedent streptococcal infection. Sudden onset of psoriasis may be associated with HIV infection. Determination of HIV serostatus is indicated in at-risk individuals. Serum uric acid is increased in 50% of patients, usually correlated with the extent of the disease; there is an increased risk of gouty arthritis. The levels of uric acid decrease as therapy is effective.

Culture   Throat culture for group A β-hemolytic streptococcus infection.

DIAGNOSIS AND DIFFERENTIAL DIAGNOSIS

Diagnosis is made on clinical grounds.

Acute Guttate Psoriasis   Any maculopapular drug eruption, secondary syphilis, pityriasis rosea.

Nails

IMAGE 3-1   Predilection sites of psoriasis.

FIGURE 3-3   Psoriasis vulgaris: elbow   Chronic stable plaque psoriasis on the elbow. In this location scales can either accumulate to oyster shelllike hyperkeratosis, or are shed in large sheets revealing a beefy-red base. This plaque has arisen from the coalescence of smaller, papular lesions.

Small Scaling Plaques   *Seborrheic dermatitis*—may be indistinguishable in sites involved and morphology; sometimes termed *seborrhiasis*. *Lichen simplex chronicus*—may complicate psoriasis as a result of pruritus. *Psoriasiform drug eruptions*—especially beta blockers, gold, and methyldopa. *Tinea corporis*—KOH examination is mandatory, particularly in single lesions. *Mycosis fungoides*—scaling plaques can be an initial stage of mycosis fungoides. Biopsy.
Large Geographic Plaques   Tinea corporis, mycosis fungoides.
Scalp Psoriasis   Seborrheic dermatitis, tinea capitis.
Inverse Psoriasis   Tinea, candidiasis, intertrigo, extramammary Paget disease. *Glucagonoma syndrome*—an important differential because this is a serious disease; the lesions look like inverse psoriasis. Langerhans cell histiocytosis (see page 516), Hailey-Hailey disease (see page 105).
Nails   Onychomycosis. KOH is mandatory.

COURSE AND PROGNOSIS

Acute guttate psoriasis appears rapidly, a generalized "rash." Sometimes this type of psoriasis disappears spontaneously in a few weeks without any treatment. More often, guttate psoriasis evolves into chronic plaque psoriasis. This is stable and may undergo remission after months or years, recur, and be a lifelong companion. Chronic generalized psoriasis is one of the "miseries that beset mankind," causing shame and embarrassment and a compromised lifestyle. The "heartbreak of psoriasis" is no joke. As the writer John Updike (who himself has psoriasis) so poignantly said about being a person with psoriasis, "I am silvery, scaly. Puddles of flakes form wherever I rest my flesh. Lusty, though we are loathsome to love. Keen-sighted, though we hate to look upon ourselves. The name of the disease, spiritually speaking, is Humiliation."

FIGURE 3-4   Psoriasis vulgaris: chronic stable type   Multiple large scaling plaques on the trunk, buttock, and legs. Lesions are round or polycyclic and confluent forming geographic patterns. Although this is the classical manifestation of chronic stable plaque psoriasis, the eruption is still ongoing, as evidenced by the small guttate lesions in the lumbar and lower back area. This patient was cleared by acitretin/PUVA combination treatment within 4 weeks.

FIGURE 3-5   Chronic plaquelike psoriasis in a 30-year-old man of Arabian descent   The hyper-keratotic horny plaque covering the underlying inflammatory tissue obscures all erythema; and due to the high melanin content, the scales appear dirty-gray. The irregular, sharply defined brown areas are postinflammatory hyperpigmentation in previous psoriatic plaques.

FIGURE 3-6   Psoriasis vulgaris: soles   Erythematous plaques with thick, yellowish, lamellar scale
and desquamation on sites of pressure arising on the
plantar feet. Note sharp demarcation of the inflammatory lesion on the arch of the foot. Similar lesions
were present on the palms.

FIGURE 3-7   Psoriasis, palmar involvement
Psoriatic plaque on the palm of a 45-year-old woman,
which on first sight suggests chronic irritative dermatitis. The sparing in the center of the palm and
the sharp delineation of the lesion suggest psoriasis,
which was also present on other parts of the body.

FIGURE 3-8   Psoriasis of the scalp   There is massive compaction of horny material on the entire scalp.
Desquamation has occurred on the forehead, which is also involved with psoriasis.

FIGURE 3-9   Psoriasis, facial involvement   Classic psoriatic plaque on the forehead of a 21-year-old male who also had massive scalp involvement.

FIGURE 3-10   Psoriasis vulgaris: inverse pattern   This picture shows the difference between plaque psoriasis on nonfrictional regions, such as the sacrum, and intertriginous region, such as the gluteal fold. Here the environment is moist and warm, which facilitates shedding of the scaly material. In the intergluteal fold the lesion is macerated and grayish on an erythematous base.

FIGURE 3-11 **A. Psoriasis of the fingernails** Pits have progressed to elkonyxis (holes in the nail plates) and there is transverse and longitudinal ridging. This patient also has perionychial psoriasis and psoriatic arthritis. **B. Psoriatic arthritis**, late stage leading to arthritis mutilans. Destruction of the interphalangeal joints has lead to the phenomenon of telescope fingers and to a severe mutilation of the hands with considerable functional impairment. For further images of nail involvement see Section 33 and 🔁.

PUSTULAR PSORIASIS   ICD-9:696.1

- Characterized by pustules, not papules, arising on normal or inflamed, erythematous skin. Two types.

PALMOPLANTAR PUSTULOSIS   ICD-9:696.1 ∘ ICD-10:L40.3

- A chronic, relapsing eruption limited to the palms and soles.
- Numerous very typical sterile, yellow, deep-seated pustules that evolve into dusky-red crusts.

- Considered by some as a localized form of pustular psoriasis (barber-type) and by others as a separate entity.

EPIDEMIOLOGY

Incidence   Low as compared to psoriasis vulgaris.
Age of Onset   50 to 60 years. More common in females (4:1).

CLINICAL MANIFESTATION

Symptoms   Stinging, burning → itching. Eruptions come and go, in waves.
Skin Lesions   Pustules in stages of evolution, 2–5 mm, deep-seated, yellow, develop into dusky-red macules and crusts; present in areas of erythema and scaling or normal skin (Fig. 3-12). Limited to palms and soles, may be only a localized patch on the sole or hand, or involve both hands and feet with a predilection of thenar and hypothenar, flexor aspects of fingers, heels, and insteps; acral portions of the fingers and toes usually spared.

DIFFERENTIAL DIAGNOSIS

Conditions confined to palms and soles. Epidermal dermatophytosis (tinea manus, tinea pedis), dyshidrotic eczematous dermatitis, irritant or allergic contact dermatitis, herpes simplex virus (HSV) infection (if localized to one site).

LABORATORY EXAMINATIONS

KOH Preparations   To exclude dermatophytosis.
Bacterial or Viral Culture   To exclude *Staphylococcus aureus* infection and HSV infection.
Dermatopathology   Edema and exocytosis of mononuclear cells that appear first to form a vesicle, and later myriads of neutrophils, which form a unilocular spongiform pustule. Acanthosis.

COURSE AND PROGNOSIS

Persistent for years and characterized by unexplained remissions and exacerbations; rarely psoriasis vulgaris may develop elsewhere.

FIGURE 3-12 **Palmar pustulosis** Creamy-yellow pustules that are partially confluent on the palm of a 28-year-old female. Pustules are sterile and pruritic, and when they get larger, become painful. At the time of this eruption there was no other evidence of psoriasis anywhere else on the body, but 2 years later the patient developed chronic stable plaque psoriasis on the trunk.

GENERALIZED ACUTE PUSTULAR PSORIASIS (VON ZUMBUSCH)   ICD-9:696.1 ∘ ICD-10:L40.1   ☐ ●

- A life-threatening medical problem with an abrupt onset.
- Skin involvement starts with a burning fiery-red erythema that spreads in hours with pinpoint sterile pustules appearing in clusters.

- Fever, generalized weakness, severe malaise, and leukocytosis are features in almost every patient.

EPIDEMIOLOGY

Rare, occurs in adults, rarely in children.

PATHOGENESIS

Unknown. The fever and leukocytosis result from the release of cytokines and chemokines from the skin into the circulation. There are no known precipitating factors, and the patient may or may not have had a stable plaque-type psoriasis in the past.

CLINICAL MANIFESTATION

Onset of Lesions   The constellation of fiery-red erythema followed by formation of pustules occurs over a period of less than 1 day. Waves of pustules may follow each other; as one set dries, another appears.
Skin Symptoms   Marked burning, tenderness.
Constitutional Symptoms   Headache, chills, feverishness, marked fatigue, severe malaise.
Appearance of Patient   Frightened, "toxic."
Vital Signs   Fast pulse, rapid breathing, fever that may be high.
Skin Lesions   There is a sequence of burning, diffuse erythema followed by the appearance of clusters of tiny, nonfollicular, and very superficial yellowish to whitish pustules that usually become confluent, forming circinate lesions and "lakes" of pus (Figs. 3-13 and 3-14), Nikolsky phenomenon is positive. Removal of the tops of pustules yields superficial, oozing erosions. Crusting. Once crusts are shed, new crops of pustules may appear in the same site. Pustules are sterile. The eruption is generalized. 🖉

Hair and Nails   Nails become thickened, and there is onycholysis; subungual "lakes" of pus lead to shedding of nails; hair loss of the telogen defluvium type (see Section 33) may develop in 2 or 3 months.
Mucous Membranes   Circinate desquamation of the tongue. This is the only form of psoriasis that involves mucous membranes.

DIFFERENTIAL DIAGNOSIS

Widespread Erythema with Pustules   The abrupt onset and the typical evolution of erythema followed by pustulation are highly characteristic. Nevertheless, blood cultures should always be obtained because of possible superinfection and bacteremia, especially with *S. aureus*. Generalized HSV infection has umbilicated pustules, and the Tzanck tests and viral cultures establish the diagnosis. Generalized pustular drug eruptions [e.g., after furosemide, amoxicillin/clavulanic acid, and other drugs (acute generalized exanthematous pustulosis, see Section 22)] may be clinically indistinguishable, but patients are less toxic. Psoriasis cum pustulatione (see below) has lesions of classic psoriasis with pustulation.

LABORATORY EXAMINATIONS

Dermatopathology   Large spongiform pustules resulting from the migration of neutrophils to the upper stratum malpighi, where they aggregate within the interstices between the degenerated and thinned keratinocytes.
Bacterial Culture of Tissue   Pustules are sterile. Rule out *S. aureus* infection.
Hematologic   Polymorphonuclear leukocytosis—white blood cell count as high as 20,000/μL.

FIGURE 3-13 Generalized acute pustular psoriasis (von Zumbusch) Multiple pustules on highly erythematous skin. Close-up of lesions shows that they are very superficial, creamy white, and coalesce, forming lakes of pus.

FIGURE 3-14 Generalized acute pustular psoriasis (von Zumbusch) This female patient was toxic and had fever and peripheral leukocytosis. The entire body was covered with showers of creamy-white coalescing pustules on a fiery-red base. Since these pustules are very superficial, they can be literally wiped off, which results in red oozing erosions.

COURSE AND PROGNOSIS

These patients are often brought to the emergency rooms of hospitals, and there is the question of overwhelming bacteremia until a dermatologist is consulted and the blood cultures are shown to be negative. Relapses and remissions may occur over a period of years. In the elderly prognosis is guarded if not treated. May follow, evolve into, or be followed by psoriasis vulgaris.

SPECIAL TYPES

Impetigo Herpetiformis   This is von Zumbusch pustular psoriasis in a pregnant woman with hypocalcemia, leading to tetanic seizures.

Annular Type   This type of pustular psoriasis occurs in children, with less consitutional symptoms. 🖉

Psoriasis cum Pustulatione (psoriasis with postulation)   This is maltreated stable plaque psoriasis where pustulation of psoriatic lesions and the surrounding normal skin occurs 🖉, usually after irritating topical treatment (e.g., anthralin) or systemic glucocorticoids; may become generalized but patients are usually nontoxic. 🖉

Acrodermatitis Continua of Hallopeau   This is a chronic recurrent pustulation of nail folds, nail bed, and distal fingers leading to loss of nails. It can occur alone or in association with pustular psoriasis of von Zumbusch. 🖉

FIGURE 3-15   Acrodermatitis continua   of Hallopeau with acral pustule formation, subungual lakes of pus, and destruction of nail plates. This may lead to permanent loss of nails and scarring.

PSORIATIC ERYTHRODERMA   ICD-9:696.1 ○ ICD-10:L40

This is a condition in which psoriasis involves practically the entire skin and leads to constitutional symptoms. It is a serious condition and is discussed in Section 8.

PSORIATIC ARTHRITIS   ICD-9:696.0 ○ ICD-10:L40.5

- Psoriatic arthritis is included among the seronegative spondyloarthropathies, which include ankylosing spondylitis, enteropathic arthritis, and reactive arthritis.
- Asymmetric peripheral joint involvement of upper extremities and especially smaller joints.
- Axial form involves vertebral column, sacroiliitis.

- Associated with MHC class I antigens, while rheumatoid arthritis is associated with MHC class II antigens.
- Incidence is 5–8%. Rare before age 20.
- *May be present (in 10% of individuals) without any visible psoriasis; if so, search for a family history.*

TYPES

1. "Distal"—seronegative, without subcutaneous nodules, and involving, asymmetrically, a few distal interphalangeal joints of the hands and feet: an asymmetric oligoarthritis. **℮**
2. Enthesitis—inflammation of ligament insertion into bone.
3. Multilating psoriatic arthritis with bone erosion and ultimately leading to osteolysis or ankylosis.
4. "Axial"—especially involving the sacroiliac, hip, and cervical areas with ankylosing spondylitis.

SKIN SYMPTOMS AND SIGNS

Swelling, redness, tenderness of involved joints or site of enthesitis (e.g., insertion of Achilles tendon in calcaneus). Dactylitis—sausage fingers. May or may not be associated with psoriasis elsewhere. Often psoriatic involvement of fingertips and periungual skin. **℮** Massive nail involvement by psoriasis is frequent (Fig. 3-11A).**℮**
Arthritis may lead to arthritis mutilans: destruction of interphalangeal joints results in telescope fingers with mutilation of hand and considerable functional impairment (Fig. 3-11B).

MANAGEMENT OF PSORIASIS

Factors Influencing Selection of Treatment

1. Age: childhood, adolescence, young adulthood, middle age, >60 years.
2. Type of psoriasis: guttate, plaque, palmar and palmopustular, generalized pustular psoriasis, erythrodermic psoriasis.
3. Site and extent of involvement: *localized* to palms and soles, scalp, anogenital area, scattered plaques but <5% involvement; *generalized* and >30% involvement.
4. Previous treatment: ionizing radiation, systemic glucocorticoids, photochemotherapy

(PUVA), cyclosporine (CS), methotrexate (MTX).
5. Associated medical disorders (e.g., HIV disease).

Ideally all patients with suspected psoriasis should be seen at least once by a dermatologist to establish the diagnosis and select the best available treatment regimen. Localized psoriasis (covering <5% of the body surface) can be managed by the primary care physician if a proper regimen is selected. Psoriasis of all other types, especially generalized psoriasis, should be managed by a dermatologist who has access to and knowledge of all therapies, as combinations and "rotational" therapy shifting from ultraviolet to PUVA to MTX or the "biologicals."

In the following pages management of psoriasis is discussed in the context of types of psoriasis, sites, and extent of involvement.

LOCALIZED PSORIASIS

This consists of a limited number of chronic stable psoriasis plaques (see Fig. 3-3) on the predilection sites or elsewhere. Here, first-line therapies are topical treatments.

Trunk and Extremities

- Topical fluorinated glucocorticoids (betamethasone valerate, fluocinolone acetonide, betamethasone propionate, clobetasol propionate) in ointment base applied after the scales are removed by soaking in water. *Ointment* applied to wet skin, covered with plastic wrap, left on overnight. Glucocorticoid-impregnated tape useful for small plaques.
- Hydrocolloid dressing, left on for 24–48 h, is effective and prevents scratching. During the day, classes I and II fluorinated glucocorticoid creams can be used without occlusion. Patients develop tolerance (tachyphylaxis) after long periods. *Caveat*: Prolonged application of the fluorinated glucocorticoids leads to atrophy of the skin, permanent striae, and unsightly telangiectasia. Clobetasol-17-propionate is stronger and active even without occlusion. To avoid systemic effects of this class I glucocorticoid: maximum of 50 g ointment per week.
- For small plaques (≤4 cm), triamcinolone acetonide aqueous suspension 3 mg/mL diluted with normal saline is injected into the lesion. Must be *intradermal*. *Warning*: Hypopigmentation at the injection site can result; this is more apparent in brown and black skin but is reversible.
- Topical anthralin preparations are excellent when used properly. Can be very irritant; therefore follow directions on the package insert with attention to details.
- Vitamin D analogues (calcipotriene, 0.005%, ointment and cream) are good nonsteroidal antipsoriatic topical agents and are not associated with cutaneous atrophy. Not as potent as class I glucocorticoids (e.g., clobetasol propionate) but can be combined with them. Calcipotriene should not be applied to more than 40% of the body surface and not more

than 100 g per week to avoid hypercalcemia. Topical tacrolimus, 0.1%, has efficacy similar to that of vitamin D analogues.
- Topical pimecrolimus, 1%, is effective in inverse psoriasis and seborrheic dermatitis–like psoriasis of the face and ear canals.
- Tazarotene (a topical retinoid, 0.05 and 0.1% gel) has similar efficacy but can best be combined with class II (medium strength) topical glucocorticoids, as it can cause irritation.
- When there is >10% (palm of the hand = 1%) involvement with psoriatic plaques, it is preferable to combine these topical treatments with 311-nm UVB phototherapy or PUVA photochemotherapy.

Scalp   *Mild*   Superficial scaling and lacking thick plaques: Tar or ketoconazole shampoos *followed by* betamethasone valerate, 1% lotion; if refractory, clobetasol propionate, 0.05% scalp application.

Severe   Thick, adherent plaques (Fig. 3-8): Removal of scales from plaques before active treatment by 10% salicylic acid in mineral oil, covered with a plastic cap and left on overnight. After shedding of scales, fluocinolone cream or lotion with the scalp covered with plastic or a shower cap, left on overnight or for 6 h. When the thickness of the plaques is reduced, clobetasol propionate, 0.05% lotion, or calcipotriene lotion can be used for maintenance. If unsuccessful or rapid recurrence or if associated with generalized psoriasis, consider systemic treatment (see below).

Palms and Soles (Figs. 3-6 and 3-7)   Occlusive dressings with class I topical *glucocorticoids* in petrolatum. If ineffective, *PUVA photochemotherapy*, administered in specially designed hand-and-foot lighting cabinets that deliver UVA. *PUVA "soaks"*: In this treatment the hands and feet are immersed in a solution of 8-methoxypsoralen (10 mg/L of warm water) for 15 min and then exposed to hand and foot UVA phototherapy units. Retinoids (acitretin > isotretinoin) given orally are effective in removing the thick hyperkeratosis of the palms and soles; however, combination with topical glucocorticoids or PUVA (Re-PUVA) is much more efficacious. Systemic treatments should be considered.

Palmoplantar Pustulosis (Fig. 3-12)   The condition is recalcitrant to treatment, but persistence in treatment can be rewarding.

PUVA "Soaks" of Hands and Feet (See above) Ideal for this condition. Re-PUVA (see below) is highly efficacious.

Topical Glucocorticoids, Dithranol, and Coal Tar   Ineffective. Strong glucocorticoids under plastic occlusion (e.g., for the night) may be effective but do not prevent recurrences. MTX or CS for recalcitrant cases.

Inverse Psoriasis (Fig. 3-10)   Initiate therapy with *topical glucocorticoids* (caution: these are atrophy-prone regions, steroids should be applied for only limited periods of time); switch to topical vitamin D derivatives or tazarotene or topical tacrolimus or pimecrolimus. Tar baths or Castellani paint sometimes useful. If resistant or recurrent, consider systemic therapy.

Nails (Fig. 3-11; See also Section 33 🔁)   Topical treatments of the fingernails are unsatisfactory. Note also that nail psoriasis may disappear spontaneously or pari passu with successful treatment of psoriasis. Injection of the nail fold with intradermal triamcinolone acetonide (3 mg/mL) effective but painful and impractical when all nails are involved. PUVA photochemotherapy somewhat effective when administered in special hand-and-foot lighting units providing high-intensity UVA. Long-term systemic retinoids (acitretin, 0.5 mg/kg) are also effective, as are systemic MTX and CS therapy. Since a diseased nail (plate) cannot be cured, therapy of nails aims at securing *regrowth* of a normal nail plate. It therefore depends on the speed of nail growth, which is slow and thus requires a long time; this should be taken into account when considering treatment that may cause side effects when administered over a prolonged period of time.

GENERALIZED PSORIASIS

Acute, Guttate Psoriasis (Fig. 3-2)   Treat streptococcal infection with antibiotics. Topical treatment as for localized psoriasis. Narrowband UVB irradiation most effective. If it fails, oral PUVA photochemotherapy (see below).

Generalized Plaque-Type Psoriasis (Fig. 3-4) Performed either by office-based dermatologist or in a psoriasis center where all major options are available: phototherapy, PUVA, or systemic treatments which are given as either mono– or combined or rotational therapy. Combination therapy denotes the combination of two or more modalities (as in chemotherapy); rotational therapy denotes switching the patient after clearing and a subsequent relapse to another different treatment. This is done to prevent cumulative long-term side effects.

Narrow-Band UVB Phototherapy (311 nm) Effective only in psoriasis with very thin plaques; effectiveness is increased by combination with topical glucocorticoids, vitamin D analogues, tazarotene, or topical tacrolimus/pimecrolimus.

Oral PUVA Photochemotherapy   Treatment consists of oral ingestion of 8-methoxypsoralen (8-MOP) (0.6 mg 8-MOP per kilogram body weight) or, in some European countries, 5-MOP (1.2 mg/kg body weight) and exposure to doses of UVA that are adjusted to the sensitivity of the patient. UVA is given 1 h (8-MOP) or 2 h (5-MOP) after ingestion of the psoralen, starting at a dose of 0.5 to 1 J/cm^2, adjusted upward for skin phototype. Alternatively, phototoxicity testing is done prior to treatment, which permits a better adjustment of the UVA dose to the individual's sensitivity to PUVA. The UVA dose is increased at successive treatment sessions. Treatments are performed two or three times a week or, with a more aggresive protocol, four times a week. Most patients clear after 19 to 25 treatments, and the amount of UVA needed ranges from 100 to 245 J/cm^2.

Long-term side effects: PUVA keratoses and squamous cell carcinomas in some patients who receive an excessive number of treatments. Re-PUVA (see below) reduces the total number of treatments.

In patients with recalcitrant plaque-type psoriasis, acitretin (in males) or isotretinoin (in females) may be combined with other antipsoriatic therapy, e.g., PUVA, UVB (311 nm), topical glucocorticoids, or anthralin. These combination modalities reduce the length of treatments as well as the total amount of antipsoriatic drug necessary for clearing. Topical glucocorticoids, calcipotriene ointments, anthralin, oral MTX, and oral acitretin, combined with either PUVA or 311-nm UVB, are all effective in reducing the dose of one another.

Oral Retinoids   Acitretin, and isotretinoin are very effective in inducing desquamation but only moderately effective in suppressing psoriatic plaques (an exception is pustular psoriasis—see below). They are highly effective when combined according to established protocols with 311-nm UVB or PUVA (called Re-PUVA). *The latter is in fact the most effective therapy to date for generalized plaque psoriasis.* A combination of PUVA with acitretin (0,75 mg/kg body weight) is used for males; for females, PUVA is combined with isotretinoin (1 mg/kg body weight). Contraception is mandatory during treatment and for 2 months after it is completed. Combinations of oral retinoids and PUVA improve the efficacy of each and permit a reduction of the dose and duration of each if refractory to treatment. For side effects of retinoids, see page 80 and package insert.

Methotrexate Therapy   Oral MTX is one of the most effective treatments and certainly the most convenient treatment for generalized plaque type psoriasis. Nevertheless, MTX is a potentially dangerous drug, principally because of liver toxicity that can occur after prolonged use. Also, response is slow and long-term treatment is required. Hepatic toxicity may occur after cumulative doses in normal persons ($\geq$1.5 g), but additional risk factors include a history of or actual alcohol intake, abnormal liver chemistries, IV drug use, and obesity. Inasmuch as hepatic toxicity is related to total life dose, this therapy should, in general, not be given to young patients who may face many years of therapy.

Schedule of Methotrexate Therapy with the Triple-Dose (Weinstein) Regimen   Preferred by most over the single-dose MTX once weekly. Begin with a test dose of 5 mg (2.5-mg tablet followed 24 h later with a second 2.5-mg tablet); this dose will ascertain whether there is a special sensitivity to MTX. A complete blood count (CBC), liver function tests, and serum creatinine levels are obtained before start of treatment, after 1 week, and 2 weeks thereafter as the dose of MTX is increased. One tablet (2.5 mg) is given every 12 h for a total of three doses, i.e., 7.5 mg/week (1/1/1 tablet schedule). Some patients respond to this dose; if not, the dose is increased after 2 weeks to 2/2/2, or 15 mg/week total dose, to which most patients respond. This regimen achieves an 80% improvement but total clearing only in some, and higher doses increase the risk of toxicity. Higher doses may be needed in overweight patients. As patients respond the dose of MTX can be reduced by one or two tablets periodically.

CBC, Liver Function, and Creatinine   These have to be monitored every 3 months. In patients with normal liver chemistries and no risk factors present, a liver biopsy should be done after a cumulative dose of approximately 1500 mg MTX; if the post-MTX liver biopsy is normal, repeat liver biopsy should be done after further therapy with an additional 1000 to 1500 mg MTX. Be aware of the various drug interactions with MTX.

Cyclosporine[1]   CS treatment is highly effective at a dose of 3–5 mg/kg per day. As the patient responds, the dose is tapered to the lowest effective maintenance dose. Monitoring blood pressure and serum creatinine is mandatory because of the known nephrotoxicity of the drug. *CS should be employed only in patients without risk factors.*

Monoclonal Antibodies and Fusion Proteins[2] (so-called biologicals)   Some of these proteins, specifically targeted to pathogenically relevant receptors on T cells or to cytokines, have been approved and more are being developed. They should be employed only by specifically trained dermatologists who are familiar with the dosage schedules, drug interactions, and short- or long-term side effects.

Alefacept   is a human lymphocyte function–associated antigen (LFA)-3-IgG1 fusion protein that prevents interaction of LFA-3 and CD2. CD2 is upregulated in memory effector T cells (CD45Ro$^+$), which explains the preferential depletion of these cells by Alefacept. It is given intramuscularly once weekly, but more than one-third of patients do not respond for unknown reasons. Repeated administration leads to improved response and there may be long periods of remissions.

Efalizumab   is a humanized anti-CD11a monoclonal antibody that blocks the interaction of LFI-1 with its ligand intercellular adhesion molecule 1. It is given subcutaneously once a week and is usually highly effective, but some patients show exacerbation of disease and there are rebounds.

Tumor necrosis factor (TNF) α *antagonists* that are effective in psoriasis are infliximab, adalimumab, and etanercept. *Infliximab* is a chimeric monoclonal antibody with a high specificity, affinity, and avidity for TNF-α. It is administered as intravenous infusion at weeks 0, 2 and 6 and is highly effective in psoriasis (although currently only FDA approved for psoriatic arthritis). *Adalimumab* is also very effective. It is a fully human recombinant monoclonal antibody that specifically targets TNF-α. It is administered subcutaneously every other week and is similarly as effective as infliximab. *Etanercept* is a human recombinant, soluble TNF-α receptor that binds TNF-α and neutralizes its activity. It is administered as subcutaneous injections twice weekly and is less effective than infliximab and adalimumab but is highly effective in psoriatic arthritis.

---

[1]For details and drug interactions, see MJ Mihatsch, K Wolff: Consensus Conference on Cyclosporin A for Psoriasis. Br J Dermatol 126:621, 1992.

[2]For details and drug interaction, see S Richardson, J Gelfand, in K Wolff et al (eds): *Fitzpatrick's Dermatology, in General Medicine*, 7th ed, New York, McGraw-Hill, pp 2223–2236, 2008.

Anti-interleukin(IL) 12/interleukin 23 p40 is a newer agent developed for chronic plaque psoriasis and has shown promising efficacy in phase I trials. It is a human IgG1κ monoclonal antibody that binds to the common p40 subunit of human IL-12 and IL-23, preventing its interaction with its receptor.

All these biologicals and others currently developed and in clinical trials have side effects, and there are long-term safety concerns. Also, they are currently extremely expensive which limits their use in clinical practice. For doses, warnings, and side effects see[2] and package inserts.

GENERALIZED PUSTULAR PSORIASIS (SEE FIGS. 3-13, 3-14)

These ill patients with generalized rash should be hospitalized and treated in the same manner as patients with extensive burns, toxic epidermal necrolysis, or exfoliative erythroderma—in a specialized unit: isolation, fluid replacement, and repeated blood cultures are necessary. Rapid suppression and resolution of lesions is achieved by oral retinoids (acitretin, 50 mg/d). Supportive measures should include fluid intake, IV antibiotics to prevent septicemia, cardiac support, temperature control, topical lubricants, and antiseptic baths. Systemic glucocorticoids to be used only as rescue intervention as rapid tachyphylaxis occurs. Oral PUVA photochemotherapy is effective, but logistics are usually prohibitive in a toxic patient with fever.

ACRODERMATITIS CONTINUA HALLOPEAU

(Figure 3-15) Oral retinoids as in von Zumbusch pustular psoriasis; MTX, once-a-week schedule, is the second-line choice.

PSORIATIC ARTHRITIS

Should be recognized early in order to prevent bony destruction. MTX, once-a-week schedule as outlined above; infliximab or etanercept are highly effective.

ICHTHYOSES

- A group of hereditary disorders characterized by an excess accumulation of cutaneous scale, varying from very mild and asymptomatic to life-threatening.
- A relatively large number of types of hereditary ichthyoses exist; most are extremely rare and often part of multiorgan syndromes. The four most common and important types are discussed here plus a brief discussion of two types affecting newborns.
- Selected rare, but important, hereditary ichthyoses are discussed in the online version. 🔁

- Acquired ichthyosis can be a manifestation of systemic disease, malignancy, drugs, endocrine disease, autoimmune disease, and HIV and other infections.
- Support groups such as Foundation for Ichthyosis and Related Skin Types (FIRST) exist.

For an in-depth discussion of ichthyoses, see P Fleckman, JJ DiGiovanna, in K Wolff et al (eds): *Fitzpatrick's Dermatology in General Medicine*, 7th ed. New York, McGraw-Hill, pp 401–424, 2008.

CLASSIFICATION

Dominant ichthyosis vulgaris (DIV)
X-linked recessive ichthyosis (XLI)
Lamellar ichthyosis (LI)
Epidermolytic hyperkeratosis (EH)

ETIOLOGY AND PATHOGENESIS

Individual keratin genes may not be expressed or may result in the formation of abnormal keratins. In DIV and XLI, formation of thickened stratum corneum is caused by increased adhesiveness of the stratum corneum cells and/or failure of normal cell separation. Abnormal stratum corneum formation results in variable increases in transepidermal water loss. The etiology of the most common ichthyosis, DIV, is unknown, but there are mutations in the gene encoding profilaggrin; in XLI, there is a steroid sulfatase deficiency. LI shows increased germinative cell hyperplasia and increased transit rate through the epidermis, and there is a transglutaminase deficiency. In EH, there are mutations in the genes encoding keratins 1 or 10; here the disturbance of epidermal differentiation and the expression of abnormal keratin genes result in vacuolization of the upper epidermal layers, blistering, and hyperkeratosis.

CLINICAL MANIFESTATION

All four types of ichthyosis tend to be worse during the dry, cold winter months and improve during the hot, humid summer. Patients living in tropical climates may remain symptom-free but may experience appearance or worsening of symptoms on moving to a temperate climate.

DOMINANT ICHTHYOSIS VULGARIS (DIV)

- Characterized by usually mild generalized xerosis with scaling, most pronounced on lower legs; in severe cases large, tessellated scales occur.
- Hyperlinear palms and soles.

- Perifollicular hyperkeratosis (keratosis pilaris) usually on arms and legs.
- Frequently associated with atopy.

ICD-9 : 757.1 ∘ ICD-10 : Q 80.0

EPIDEMIOLOGY

Age of Onset   3 to 12 months.

Sex   Equal incidence in males and females. Autosomal dominant inheritance.
Incidence   Common (1 in 250).

FIGURE 4-1 Ichthyosis vulgaris: chest Fine fish scalelike hyperkeratosis of the pectoral area. This is a mild form of ichthyosis vulgaris.

FIGURE 4-2 Ichthyosis vulgaris: legs
Grayish tessellated (tilelike), firmly bound down scales. The similarity to fish skin or the skin of an amphibian is quite obvious. Note sparing of popliteal fossae. This is a more severe form of ichthyosis vulgaris.

PATHOGENESIS

Etiology unknown. There is reduced or absent filaggrin. Epidermis proliferates normally, but keratin is retained with a resultant thickened stratum corneum.

CLINICAL MANIFESTATION

Very commonly associated with atopy. Xerosis and pruritus worse in winter months. Cosmetic concern to many patients, particularly when hyperkeratosis is severe.

Skin Lesions Xerosis (dry skin) with fine, powdery scaling but also larger, firmly adherent tacked-down scales in a fish-scale pattern (Figs. 4-1 and 4-2). Diffuse general involvement, accentuated on the shins, arms, and back but also on the buttocks and lateral thighs; axillae and the antecubital and popliteal fossae spared (Fig. 4-2; Image 4-1); face usually also spared but cheeks and forehead may be involved. *Keratosis pilaris* is perifollicular hyperkeratosis with little, spiny hyperkeratotic follicular papules of normal skin color, either grouped or disseminated, mostly on the extensor surfaces of the extremities (Fig. 4-3); in childhood, also on cheeks. Hands and feet usually spared, but palmoplantar markings are more accentuated (hyperlinear). ✐

Associated Diseases More than 50% of individuals with DIV also have atopic dermatitis; rarely, keratopathy can occur.

DIFFERENTIAL DIAGNOSIS

Xerosis/Hyperkeratosis Xerosis; acquired ichthyoses, all other forms of ichthyosis.

LABORATORY EXAMINATION

Dermatopathology Compact hyperkeratosis; reduced or absent granular layer; germinative layer flattened. Electron microscopy: small, poorly formed keratohyalin granules.

DIAGNOSIS

Usually by clinical findings; abnormal keratohyalin granules in electron microscopy.

COURSE AND PROGNOSIS

Improvement in the summer, in humid climates, and in adulthood. Keratosis pilaris occurring on the cheeks during childhood usually improves during adulthood.

MANAGEMENT

Hydration of Stratum Corneum Pliability of stratum corneum is a function of its water content. Hydration best accomplished by immersion in a bath followed by the application of petrolatum. Urea-containing creams bind water in the stratum corneum.

Keratolytic Agents Propylene glycol–glycerin–lactic acid mixtures. Propylene glycol (44–60% in water); 6% salicylic acid in propylene glycol and alcohol, which is used under plastic occlusion (beware of hypersalicism). α-Hydroxy acids (lactic acid or glycolic acid) control scaling. Urea-containing preparations (2–10%) are effective.

Systemic Retinoids Isotretinoin and acitretin are very effective, but careful monitoring for toxicity is required. Only severe cases may require intermittent therapy.

Keratosis pilaris

IMAGE 4-1 Distribution of ichthyosis vulgaris
Dots indicate keratosis pilaris

FIGURE 4-3 Ichthyosis vulgaris. Keratosis pilaris: arm Small, follicular, horny spines occur as a manifestation of mild ichthyosis vulgaris; arising mostly on the shoulders, upper arms, and thighs. Desquamation of the nonfollicular skin results in hypomelanotic (less pigmented) spots similar to pityriasis alba (compare with Fig. 13-16).

X-LINKED ICHTHYOSIS (XLI)   ICD-9:757.1 ∘ ICD-10:Q 80.1   ▮ ◑

- Occurs in males.
- Onset soon after birth.
- Prominent, dirty brown scales on the neck, extremities, trunk, and buttocks.
- Involvement of flexural regions.
- Absence of palm and sole involvement.
- Corneal opacities in 50% of adult males.

EPIDEMIOLOGY

Age of Onset Birth or infancy. Males.
Incidence 1:2000 to 1:6000.

ETIOLOGY AND PATHOGENESIS

X-linked recessive; gene locus Xp22.32.
Genetic Defect Steroid sulfatase deficiency—abnormal cholesterol metabolism, accumulation of cholesterol sulfate; is associated with failure to shed senescent keratinocytes normally, resulting clinically in retention hyperkeratosis associated with normal epidermal proliferation.

CLINICAL MANIFESTATION

Onset of skin abnormality at 2–6 weeks of age; corneal opacities develop during the second to third week. Usually asymptomatic; may also be present in female carriers of XLI. Discomfort due to xerosis. Cosmetic disfigurement due to the dirty brown scales.

Skin Lesions Large adherent scales that appear brown or dirty (Fig. 4-4); most pronounced on posterior neck, extensor arms, antecubital and popliteal fossae, and trunk. ✎ Absence of palm/sole and face involvement (Image 4-2).

Eye Lesions   Comma-shaped stromal corneal opacities in 50% of adult males, asymptomatic. Present in some female carriers.

Genitourinary Abnormality   Cryptorchidism in 20% of individuals.

DIFFERENTIAL DIAGNOSIS

All forms of ichthyosis, syndromic ichthyoses.

LABORATORY EXAMINATIONS

Chemistry   Cholesterol sulfate level elevated. Increased mobility of β-lipoproteins in electrophoresis. Steroid sulfatase decreased or absent.

Dermatopathology   Hyperkeratosis; granular layer present, sometimes hypergranulosis.

DIAGNOSIS

By family history and clinical findings.

Prenatal Diagnosis   Via amniocentesis and chorionic villus sampling; steroid sulfatase assay detects enzyme deficiency.

COURSE AND PROGNOSIS

No improvement with age. Usually worse in temperate climates and in winter season. With placental sulfatase deficiency, failure of labor to begin or progress in mother carrying affected fetus.

MANAGEMENT

Topical Therapy

Hydration of Stratum Corneum   Pliability of stratum corneum is a function of its water content. Hydration best accomplished by immersion in a bath followed by the application of petrolatum. Urea-containing creams bind water in the stratum corneum.

Keratolytic Agents   Propylene glycol–glycerin–lactic acid mixtures. Propylene glycol (44–60% in water); 6% salicylic acid in propylene glycol and alcohol, which is used under plastic occlusion. α-Hydroxy acids (lactic acid or glycolic acid) (beware of hypersalicism) control scaling. Urea-containing preparations (2–10%) are effective.

Systemic Retinoids   Isotretinoin and acitretin are very effective, but careful monitoring for toxicity is required. Only severe cases may require intermittent therapy.

Systemic Treatment

Acitretin, 0.5–1 mg/kg orally until marked improvement, then taper dose to maintenance level. Continuous laboratory monitoring and, in long-term regimens, x-rays for calcifications and diffuse idiopathic skeletal hyperostosis (DISH) syndrome mandatory.

IMAGE 4-2   Distribution of X-linked ichthyosis.

FIGURE 4-4 X-linked ichthyosis: trunk, buttocks and arms Dark hyperkeratosis with tessellated scales gives a dirty appearance in this 12-year-old boy of African ethnicity.

LAMELLAR ICHTHYOSIS (LI)   ICD-9:757.1 ○ ICD-10:Q 80.2   ☐ ◑

- Often presents at birth as collodion baby (see page 78)
- Collodion-like membrane soon shed with subsequent large, coarse scales involving entire body.
- Flexural areas involved.

- Palmoplantar involvement varies.
- Extropium, eclabium, alopecia may occur.
- Heat intolerance.

EPIDEMIOLOGY

Age of Onset At birth, usually as collodion baby.
Sex Presents equally in both sexes.
Incidence ≤1:300,000.

ETIOLOGY AND PATHOGENESIS

Mode of Inheritance Autosomal recessive; gene locus varies. In one subset there is mutation in the gene encoding transglutaminase 1, an enzyme that catalyzes the cross-linking of proteins during the formation of cornified envelopes of corneocytes. In another, a mutation in the gene encoding ATP-binding cassette, subfamily A, member 12—controlling membrane transport/lipid metabolism. In a third subset, there is a mutation in the gene encoding arachidonate lipoxygenase, controlling hydroperoxidase isomerase.[1]

CLINICAL MANIFESTATION

Heat intolerance, usually during exercise and hot weather, because of inability to sweat. Water loss (excess)/dehydration due to fissuring of stratum corneum. Increased nutritional requirements for young children due to rapid growth and shedding of stratum corneum. Painful palmar/plantar fissures.

Skin Lesions *Newborn* Collodion baby, encased in a translucent collodion-like membrane (see Fig. 4-8); shed in a few weeks. Ectropion; eclabion. Generalized erythroderma.

Child/Adult Large parchment–like hyperkeratosis (Fig. 4-5) over entire body; fracturing of the hyperkeratotic plate results in a tessellated (tilelike) pattern (Fig. 4-6). Scales are large and very thick and brown, over most of the body (Fig. 4-6), accentuated on lower extremities, and involving the flexural areas. Hyperkeratosis around joints may be verrucous. 🖉. Hands/feet: keratoderma; accentuation of palmar/plantar creases (Image 4-3) but may vary. Erythroderma may develop.
Hair Bound down by scales; frequent infections may result in scarring alopecia (Fig. 4-5).
Nails Dystrophy secondary to nail fold inflammation.
Mucous Membranes Usually spared.
Eye Lesions Ectropion (Fig. 4-5).
Lips Eclabium.
🖉

DIFFERENTIAL DIAGNOSIS

X-linked ichthyosis, epidermolytic hyperkeratosis, congenital ichthyosiform erythroderma, syndromic ichthyoses.

LABORATORY EXAMINATIONS

Culture Rule out secondary infection and sepsis, especially in newborns.
Dermatopathology Hyperkeratosis; granular layer present; acanthosis. Epidermal transglutaminase decreased in transglutaminase-deficient subtype.

COURSE AND PROGNOSIS

Collodion membrane present at birth is shed within first few days to weeks (see Fig. 4-8). Newborns are at risk for hypernatremic dehydration, secondary infection, and sepsis. Disorder persists throughout life. No improvement with age.

---

[1]For details on genes identified in autosomal recessive ichthyoses, see P Fleckman, JJ DiGiovanna, in K Wolff et al: *Fitzpatrick's Dermatology in General Medicine*, 7th ed. New York, McGraw-Hill, pp 401–424, 2008.

FIGURE 4-5   Lamellar ichthyosis   Parchment-like hyperkeratosis gives the impression of the skin being too tight on the face of this 6-year-old Arab boy. There is pronounced ectropium and beginning alopecia.

Hair loss

IMAGE 4-3   Distribution of lamellar ichthyosis.

Obstruction of eccrine sweat glands with resultant impairment of sweating.

MANAGEMENT

Newborn   Care in neonatal intensive care unit. High-humidity chamber. Emolliation. Monitor electrolytes, fluids. Follow for signs of local or systemic infection.

Child/Adult   *Emollients*   Hydrated petrolatum.

Keratolytics   As in DIV and XLI.

Overheating   Parents and affected individuals should be instructed about overheating and heat prostration that can follow exercise, high environmental temperatures, and fever. Repeated application of water to skin can somewhat replace function of sweating, cooling the body.

Retinoids   Acitretin and, to a lesser degree, isotretinoin (0.5–1 mg/kg) are effective. Monitor continuously for serum triglycerides, transaminases, and bony toxicities if given over prolonged period of time. Teratogenicity requires effective contraception.

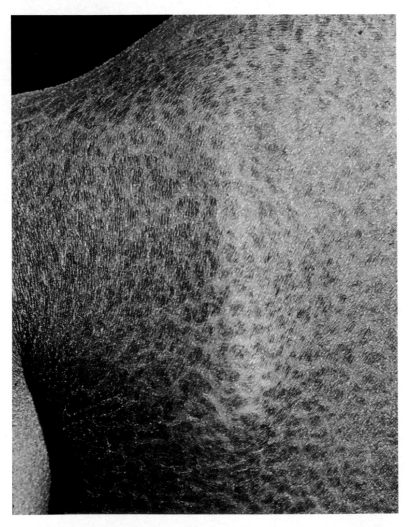

FIGURE 4-6   Lamellar ichthyosis: Shoulder   Tesselated (tilelike) hyperkeratosis gives the appearance of reptilian scales on the shoulder and back. The entire body was involved and there was ectropium.

EPIDERMOLYTIC HYPERKERATOSIS (EH)
ICD-9 : 757.1 ∘ ICD-10 : Q 80.8

- Presents at or shortly after birth with blistering.
- With time skin becomes keratotic, verrucous.
- Shedding of hyperkeratotic masses results in circumscribed islands of normal-appearing skin.

- Involvement of flexural areas.
- Palmar and plantar involvement.
- Secondary pyogenic infections.

EPIDEMIOLOGY

Age of Onset   Birth or shortly thereafter.
Sex   Equal incidence in males and females.
Incidence   Very rare.

ETIOLOGY AND PATHOGENESIS

Mode of Inheritance   Autosomal dominant. Mutations of genes that encode the epidermal differentiation keratins, keratin 1 and 10.[2] Structural protein abnormality → keratin intermediate filament dysfunction → epidermal fragility.

CLINICAL MANIFESTATION

Blistering may recur periodically, leading to denuded areas, secondary infection, and sepsis. Hyperkeratotic lesions become verrucous, particularly in the flexural areas, and are associated with an unpleasant odor.

Skin Lesions   Blistering at birth or shortly thereafter. Generalized or localized. Denuded areas heal with normal-appearing skin. With time, the skin becomes keratotic and verrucous (Fig. 4-7), particularly in the flexural areas, knees, and elbows. Hyperkeratotic scales adhere to underlying skin, often in a mountain range–like appearance; may be quite dark in color and associated with an unpleasant odor (like rancid butter). Recurrent blisters in hyperkeratotic areas (Fig. 4-7) and also shedding of hyperkeratotic masses result in circumscribed areas of skin that are relatively normal in appearance. A valuable diagnostic sign. Secondary pyogenic infections, especially impetigo. ⊿

Generalized distribution with prominent involvement of flexural areas (Image 4-4). Palmar and plantar involvement (hyperkeratosis). (*Note*: A variant of epidermolytic hyperkeratosis is localized to palms and soles and is genetically distinct from the generalized form.)

Hair and Nails   Hair normal, but involvement of the nails may produce abnormal nail plates.
Mucous Membranes   Spared.

LABORATORY EXAMINATION

Dermatopathology   Giant, coarse keratohyalin granules and vacuolization of the granular layer, resulting in cell lysis and subcorneal multiloculated blisters. Papillomatosis, acanthosis, and hyperkeratosis.

COURSE AND PROGNOSIS

Blister formation and massive hyperkeratosis are prone to bacterial superinfection, which is probably also responsible for the unpleasant odor. Palmar involvement can adversely affect manual dexterity.

MANAGEMENT

Topical application of α-hydroxy acids. Antimicrobial therapy. Systemic retinoids (isotretinoin and acitretin) may transiently lead to a worsening of the condition because of increased blister formation but later improve the skin dramatically owing to a relative normalization of epidermal differentiation. Predisposes to impetigo. Determine dose carefully, and monitor for side effects.

[2]For other subtypes and genes involved, see P Fleckman, JJ DiGiovanna, in K Wolff et al (eds): *Fitzpatrick's Dermatology in General Medicine*, 7th ed. New York, McGraw-Hill, pp 401–424, 2008.

FIGURE 4-7   Epidermolytic hyperkeratosis: arms and hands   Mountain rangelike hyperkeratosis of the dorsum of hands with blistering that results in erosions and shedding of large sheets of keratin.

IMAGE 4-4   Distribution of epidermolytic hyperkeratosis.

ICHTHYOSIS IN THE NEWBORN

COLLODION BABY   ICD-9 : 757.1 ∘ ICD-10 : Q 80.2

- Encasement of entire baby in a transparent parchment-like membrane (Fig. 4-8A) impairs respiration and sucking.
- Breaking and shedding of the collodion membrane initially leads to difficulties in thermoregulation and increased risk of infection.
- Skin is bright red and moist. After healing, skin appears normal for some time until signs of ichthyosis develop.

- Collodion baby may be the initial presentation of lamellar ichthyosis or some less common forms of ichthyosis not discussed here.
- Collodion baby also may be a condition which, after the collodion membrane is shed and the resultant erythema has cleared, will progress to normal skin for the rest of the child's life (Fig. 4-8B).

MANAGEMENT

Newborns should be kept in an incubator in which the air is saturated with water. Careful monitoring of temperature and parenteral fluids and nutrient replacement may be necessary for some time. Infection of the skin and lungs is an important problem, and aggressive antibiotic therapy may be indicated.

A

B

FIGURE 4-8   Ichthyosis in the newborn
A. "Collodion baby" shortly after birth with a parchment-like membrane covering the entire skin. The membrane has ruptured and is being shed leaving oozing, raw-looking skin.
B. At 8 months of age, the same infant is a beautiful baby with minimal residual scale and erythema.

HARLEQUIN FETUS   ICD-9 : 757.1 ∘ ICD-10 : Q 80.4

- Harlequin fetus is an extremely rare condition in which the child is born with very thick plates of stratum corneum separated by deep cracks and fissures.
- Eclabium, ectropion, and absence of or rudimentary ears result in a grotesque appearance.

- These babies usually die shortly after birth, but there are reports of survival for weeks to several months.
- This condition is different from collodion baby and the other forms of ichthyosis, with an unusual fibrous protein within the epidermis.

SYNDROMIC ICHTHYOSES   ICD-9 : 757.1 ∘ ICD-10 : Q 80.9

- These are a number of rare syndromic ichthyoses where ichthyotic skin changes are associated with metabolic and/or functional and structural abnormalities.
- For *erythroderma variabilis, keratitis-ichthyosis and deafness (KID) syndrome, Child syndrome,*

and *Netherton syndrome* see Ichthyosis picture gallery in the online version. 🖳
- For others see P Fleckman, JJ DiGiovanna, in K Wolff et al: *Fitzpatrick's Dermatology in General Medicine,* 7th ed. New York, McGraw-Hill, pp 401–424, 2008.

ACQUIRED ICHTHYOSES   ICD-9 : 701.1 ∘ ICD-10 : L 85.0

- Development in adulthood.
- Associated with malignancies (Hodgkin disease but also non-Hodgkin lymphomas and other malignancies).
- Associated with AIDS.
- Associated with sarcoidosis.
- Associated with systemic lupus erythematosus, dermatomyositis, mixed connective tissue disease, eosinophilic fasciitis.

- Associated with graft-versus-host disease.
- Associated with drugs (nicotinic acid, tripanarol, butyrophenol, dixyrazine, nafoxidine.
- Occurs in Kava drinkers: *Kava dermopathy.*

INHERITED KERATODERMAS OF PALMS AND SOLES

- Palmoplantar keratodermas (PPK) are a rare and diverse group of keratinization disorders.
- PPK may be found alone or concomitant with (related) lesions elsewhere on the body or may be part of complex syndromes.
- Clinical classification distinguishes between diffuse, focal (striate), and punctate PPK.

- Symptoms include pain, associated with manual labor and walking, and secondary infections.
- The genetic basis of most PKK involves mutations in keratin genes or genes encoding connexin and desmosomal proteins.
- Treatment consist of keratolytics and systemic retinoids.

CLASSIFICATION

There exist more than twenty different PKK either confined to palms and soles (simple) or in combination with lesions elsewhere (complex) or as part of a multiorgan syndrome (syndromic). The underlying gene defects for almost everyone of these are

FIGURE 4-9   Plantar keratoderma, diffuse type   Yellow waxy diffuse hyperkeratosis on both soles.

unknown.[3] In this book only three simple PKK phenotypes will be discussed:

Diffuse PKK
Punctate PKK
Focal PKK

DIFFUSE PALMOPLANTAR KERATODERMA

Two main types exist. Epidermolytic and nonepidermolytic. Nonepidermolytic PKK is autosomal dominant, presenting in infancy; it

[3]For additional discussion, including genetics and pathogenesis, the reader is reffered to DP Kelsell, IM Leigh, in K Wolff et al: *Fitzpatrick's Dermatology in General Medicine*, 7th ed. New York, McGraw-Hill, pp 424–431, 2008.

consists of symmetric well-demarcated diffuse waxy thickening of the stratum corneum of palms and soles (Fig. 4-9). Spread to dorsum of hands and wrists occurs. Epidermolytic diffuse PKK is also autosomal dominant; the keratoderma is also well-defined, diffuse, and symmetric but is not waxy but has fine fissuring on the surface. 🔌

Symptoms, if at all, consist of pain with manual work and walking.

PUNCTATE PALMOPLANTAR KERATODERMA

An autosomal dominant PKK arising in adolescence and consisting of multiple punctate keratoses symmetrically on palms and soles (Fig. 4-10). Lesions may resemble palmar/plantar warts and get worse by physical trauma. Tenderness and pain.

FIGURE 4-10   Punctate plantar keratoderma   Multiple, discrete droplike keratoses resembling plantar warts. Lesions had been present since late childhood and have become worse, particularly in the pressure areas.

FOCAL PALMOPLANTAR KERATODERMA

Mostly striate in appearance, autosomal dominant. Linear hyperkeratotic calluses usually extending from the palm to the tips of the fingers (Fig. 4-11). Arises in childhood and gets worse with manual labor. 🖉

LABORATORY EXAMINATION

Histopathology nondiagnostic in nonepidermolytic PKK. Hyperkeratosis, acanthosis, papillomatosis. In epidermolytic PKK, epidermolytic hyperkeratosis.

DIFFERENTIAL DIAGNOSIS

Hyperkeratotic chronic irritant dermatitis, psoriasis, calluses, palmar/plantar warts.

FIGURE 4-11 **Striate (focal) palmar keratoderma** There are linear verrucous hyperkeratoses extending from the palm onto the fingers. Manual work aggravates these lesions, which can become fissured and painful.

COURSE AND PROGNOSIS

Does not improve with age, life-long companion. Gets worse with physical trauma (manual labor, walking); complications are bacterial and fungal infections.

MANAGEMENT

Topical Physical examination débridement (chiropody) reduces keratotic masses. Topical keratolytic agents: 10–20% salicylic acid ointment, corn plasters (20–40% salicylic acid). 40–60% propylene glycol under overnight occlusion.

Systemic Acitretin or, in women of childbearing age, isotretinoin, 0.5 mg/kg body weight very beneficial, but shedding of hyperkeratosis is often associated with increased sensitivity, which may interfere with manual work and walking. Blistering may occur in epidermolytic PKK. Beware of teratogenicity and long-term complications.

MISCELLANEOUS EPIDERMAL DISORDERS

ACANTHOSIS NIGRICANS (AN)
ICD-9 : 701.2 ∘ ICD-10 : L 83

- Asymmetric velvety thickening and hyperpigmentation of the skin, chiefly on the neck, axilla, groins, and other body folds.
- May be hyperkeratotic and associated with skin tags.

- A cutaneous marker related to heredity, obesity, endocrine disorders (particularly diabetes), drug administration, and malignancy.
- Insidious onset; in malignancy, rapid.

CLASSIFICATION

Type 1: Hereditary Benign AN   No associated endocrine disorder.

Type 2: Benign AN   Endocrine disorders associated with insulin resistance: insulin-resistant type II diabetes mellitus, hyperandrogenic states, acromegaly/gigantism, Cushing disease, hypogonadal syndromes with insulin resistance, Addison disease, hypothyroidism.

Type 3: Pseudo-AN   Associated with obesity; more common in patients with darker pigmentation. Common in metabolic syndrome. Obesity produces insulin resistance.

Type 4: Drug-induced AN   Nicotinic acid in high dosage, stilbestrol in young males, glucocorticoid therapy, diethylstilbestrol/oral contraceptive, growth hormone therapy.

Type 5: Malignant AN   Paraneoplastic, usually adenocarcinoma of gastrointestinal or genitourinary tract; less commonly, lymphoma (see Section 18).

EPIDEMIOLOGY

Age of Onset   Type 1: during childhood or puberty; other types dependent on associated conditions.

ETIOLOGY AND PATHOGENESIS

Dependent on associated disorder. In a subset of women with hyperandrogenism and insulin intolerance and AN, loss-of-function mutation in the insulin receptor or anti-insulin receptor antibodies can be found (types A and B). It is postulated that excess growth factor stimulation in the skin leads to proliferation of keratinocytes and fibroblasts. In hyperinsulinemia AN, excess insulin binding to insulin–like growth factor 1 receptor and fibroblast growth factor receptor has also been implicated. In malignancy-associated AN, transforming growth factor β released from tumor cells may stimulate keratinocyte proliferation via epidermal growth factor receptors.

CLINICAL MANIFESTATION

Insidious onset; first visible change is darkening of pigmentation.

Skin Lesions   All types of AN: Darkening of pigmentation, skin appears dirty (Fig. 5-1). As skin thickens, appears velvety; skin lines accentuated; surface becomes rugose, mammillated. Type 3: velvety patch on inner, upper thigh at site of chafing; often has many skin tags in body folds and neck. Type 5: hyperkeratosis and hyperpigmentation more pronounced (see Fig. 18-16). Hyperkeratosis of palms/soles, with accentuation of papillary markings: "Tripe hands" (see Fig. 18-18), involvement of oral mucosa and vermilion border of lips (see Fig. 18-17).

FIGURE 5-1 Acanthosis nigricans Velvety, dark-brown to gray thickening of the skin of the armpit with prominent skin folds and feathered edges in a 30-year-old obese woman from the Middle East. There were similar changes on the neck, the antecubital fossae, and on the knuckles.

Distribution Most commonly, axillae; (Fig. 5-1), neck (back, sides) also, groins, anogenitalia, antecubital fossae, knuckles, submammary, umbilicus.

Mucous Membranes Oral mucosa: velvety texture with delicate furrows. Type 5: Mucous membranes and mucocutaneous junctions commonly involved; warty papillomatous thickenings periorally (see Fig. 18-17). 🔲

General Examination
Examine for underlying endocrine disorders in overweight to morbidly obese persons and malignancy.

DIAGNOSIS AND DIFFERENTIAL DIAGNOSIS

Clinical Findings Dark thickened flexural skin: Confluent and reticulated papillomatosis (Gougerot-Carteaud syndrome), pityriasis versicolor, X-linked ichthyosis, retention hyperkeratosis, nicotinic acid ingestion.

LABORATORY EXAMINATIONS

Chemistry Rule out diabetes mellitus; metabolic syndrome

Dermatopathology Papillomatosis, hyperkeratosis; epidermis thrown into irregular folds, showing various degrees of acanthosis.

Imaging and Endoscopy Rule out associated malignancy.

COURSE AND PROGNOSIS

Type 1: Accentuated at puberty and, at times, regresses when older. Type 2: Depends on underlying disturbance. Type 3: May regress after significant weight loss. Type 4: Resolves when causative drug is discontinued. Type 5: AN may precede other symptoms of malignancy by 5 years; removal of malignancy may be followed by regression of AN.

MANAGEMENT

Symptomatic. Treat associated disorder. Topical keratolytic and/or topical or systemic retinoids may improve AN.

DARIER DISEASE (DD) ICD-9 : 701.1 ∘ ICD-10 : L 87

- A rare autosomal dominant inherited disease with late onset.
- Multiple discrete scaling, crusted and pruritic papules mainly in seborrheic and flexural areas.
- Malodorous and disfiguring, also involving nails and mucous membranes.
- Itching and/or painful.

- Histologically characterized by suprabasal acantholysis and dyskeratosis.
- Caused by loss-of-function mutation in the *ATP2A2* gene.
- Synonym: Darier-White disease, keratosis follicularis.

EPIDEMIOLOGY AND ETIOLOGY

Rare.

Age of Onset Usually in the first or second decade, males and females equally affected.

Genetics Autosomal dominant trait, new mutations common, penetrance >95%. Loss-of-function mutations in the *ATP2A2* gene encoding sarco/endoplasmic reticulum calcium adenosine triphosphatase isoform 2 (SERCA 2), which impair intracellular Ca^{2+} signaling.

Precipitating Factors Frequently worse in summer with heat and humidity as major factors; can be exacerbated by UVB, mechanical trauma, bacterial infections. Often associated with affective disorders and rarely with decreased intelligence.

CLINICAL MANIFESTATION

Usually insidious; onset is abrupt after precipitating factors; associated with severe pruritus and often pain.

Skin Lesions Multiple discrete scaling of crusted, pruritic papules (Fig. 5-2); when scaling crust is removed, a slitlike opening becomes visible (Fig. 5-3). Confluence to large plaques covered by hypertrophic warty masses that are foul smelling, particularly in intertriginous areas.

Distribution Corresponding to the "seborrheic areas": chest (Fig. 5-2), back, ears, nasolabial folds, forehead (Fig. 5-3), scalp; axilla, neck, groin.

FIGURE 5-2 Darier disease: chest Primary lesions are reddish-brown, scaling and crusted papules that feel warty when stroked. Where crusts have been removed there are slitlike erosions that are later covered by hemorrhagic crusts.

FIGURE 5-3   Darier disease: forehead Partly coalescing, hyperkeratotic papules that are eroded and crusted. The main concern of this young female was disfigurement.

Palms and Soles Multiple, flat, cobblestone-like papules.

Appendages Hair not involved, but permanent alopecia may result from extensive scalp involvement. Nails thin, splitting distally and showing characteristic V-shaped scalloping (see Fig. 33-31).

Mucous Membranes White, centrally depressed papules on mucosa of cheeks, hard and soft palate, and gums, "cobblestone" lesions.

🖉

DISEASE ASSOCIATION

Associated with *acrokeratosis verruciformis*, allelic with DD. Multiple, small flat-topped papules predominantly on dorsa of hands and feet.

LABORATORY EXAMINATION

Dermatopathology Dyskeratotic cells in the spinous layer (corps ronds) and stratum corneum (grains), suprabasal acantholysis and clefts (lacunae), papillary overgrowth of the epidermis and hyperkeratosis.

DIAGNOSIS AND DIFFERENTIAL DIAGNOSIS

Diagnosis based on history of familial involvement, clinical appearance, and histopathology. May be confused with seborrheic dermatitis, Grover disease, benign familial pemphigus (Hailey-Hailey disease), and pemphigus foliaceus. Acrokeratosis verruciformis: flat warts (verrucae planae juveniles).

COURSE AND PROGNOSIS

Persisting throughout life, not associated with cutaneous malignancies.

MANAGEMENT

Sunscreens to avoid UV-induced exacerbations, avoidance of friction and rubbing (turtle neck sweaters), antibiotic therapy (systemic and topical) to suppress bacterial infection, topical retinoids (tazarotene and adapalene) or systemic retinoids (isotretinoin or acitretin). Systemic therapy can be modified according to seasonal variation of the disease.

GROVER DISEASE (GD)   ICD-9 : 702.8 ○ ICD-10 : L 11.1   □ ◑

- A pruritic dermatosis located principally on the trunk, occurring as crops of discrete papular or papulovesicular lesions, sparse to numerous.
- Occurs in adults.
- Pruritus is main symptom.
- Usually transient but a persistent form is recognized.

- Principal histopathologic feature: variable focal acantholysis and dyskeratosis.
- No evidence of genetic predisposition.
- Synonym: transient acantholytic dermatosis.

EPIDEMIOLOGY

Age of Onset   Middle age and older, mean age 50 years.
Sex   Males > females.
Precipitating Factors   Heavy, sweat-inducing exercise, excessive solar exposure, exposure to heat, and persistent fever; may also occur in bedridden patients, with heat and sweating as factors.

CLINICAL MANIFESTATION

Usually abrupt onset of pruritus and simultaneous appearance of crops of lesions.

Skin Lesions   Skin-colored, pink or reddish papules (small, 3 to 5 mm, some with slight scale or smooth) (Fig. 5-4), papulovesicles, and erosions. Very similar to Darier disease. Upon palpation, smooth or warty. Scattered, discrete on central trunk (Fig. 5-4) and proximal extremities.

LABORATORY EXAMINATION

Dermatopathology   Acantholysis and spongiosis, focal acantholytic dyskeratosis occurring at the same time and simulating Darier disease, pemphigus foliaceus, and Hailey-Hailey disease; in the dermis there is a superficial infiltrate of eosinophils, lymphocytes, and histiocytes.

DIAGNOSIS AND DIFFERENTIAL DIAGNOSIS

Often difficult.
Small Discrete Pruritic Papules on Chest   Darier disease, heat rash (miliaria rubra), papular urticaria, scabies, dermatitis herpetiformis (here there is grouping and the lesions are symmetric), Pityrosporum or eosinophilic folliculitis, insect bites, and drug eruptions.

COURSE AND PROGNOSIS

The disease is by no means always transient, and there appear to be two types: acute ("transient") and chronic relapsing. The mean duration in one series was 47 weeks.

MANAGEMENT

Topical   Class I topical glucocorticoids under plastic (e.g., dry-cleaning plastic suit bags with holes cut for arms) are used for 4 h.
Systemic   Oral glucocorticoids and dapsone have been used with success, but relapses occur after withdrawal.
Phototherapy   UVB or PUVA photochemotherapy may be useful for patients who do not respond to topical glucocorticoids under occlusion. Isotretinoin has been used in refractory cases.

FIGURE 5-4   **Grover disease**   A rash consisting of reddish, hyperkeratotic scaling and/or crusted papules with a sandpaper feel upon palpation. Papules are discrete, scattered on the central trunk and very pruritic.

PITYRIASIS RUBRA PILARIS (PRP)
ICD-9 : 696.4 ∘ ICD-10 : L 44.4

- Rare, chronic, papulosquamous disorder often progressing to erythroderma.
- Six types exist.
- Follicular hyperkeratotic papules, reddish-orange progressing to generalized erythroderma. Sharply demarcated islands of unaffected (normal) skin.
- Waxy, diffuse, orange keratoderma of palms and soles; nails may be affected.
- Most effective therapy is methotrexate, retinoids.

CLASSIFICATION[1]

Type 1: Classic Adult   Generalized, beginning on head and neck.

Type 2: Atypical Adult   Generalized, sparse hair.

Type 3: Classic Juvenile   Appears within the first two years of life, generalized.

Type 4: Circumscribed Juvenile   In prepubertal children, localized.

Type 5: Atypical Juvenile   Onset in first few years of life, familial, generalized.

[1] W.A.D. Griffiths Pityriasis rubra pilaris. Clin Exp Dermatol 5:105, 1980; and A. Gonzáles-López et al: Br J Dermatol 140:931, 1999.

Type 6: HIV-Associated   Generalized, associated with acne conglobata, hidradenitis suppurativa, and lichen spinulosus.

EPIDEMIOLOGY

Estimated incidence 1: 5000 and in 1 in 15,000 dermatology patients. Bimodal distribution with a peak incidence in the first and fifth decades of life. Affects both sexes and occurs in all races.

ETIOLOGY AND PATHOGENESIS

Unknown. A dysfunction in vitamin A metabolism has been suggested but not proven. Genetic factors are believed to play a critical role in the induction of PRP.

CLINICAL MANIFESTATION

Both insidious and rapid onset occur.

Skin Lesions   All types of PRP. An eruption of follicular hyperkeratotic papules of reddish-orange color usually spreading in a cephalocaudal direction (Fig. 5-5). Confluence to a reddish-orange psoriasiform, scaling dermatitis with sharply demarcated islands of unaffected skin (Fig. 5-6). Progression to erythroderma (except for type 2 and type 4) (Fig. 5-7).
Distribution   Types 1, 2, 3, 5, and 6: Generalized, classically beginning on the head and neck, then spreading caudally.
Scalp and Hair   Scalp affected, as in psoriasis, often leading to asbestos-like accumulation of scale. Hair not affected except in type 2 where sparse scalp hair is observed.
Mucous Membranes   Spared.
Nails   Common but not diagnostic. Distal yellow-brown discoloration, nail plate thickening, subungual hyperkeratosis, and splinter hemorrhages. See section 33.
Associated Conditions   Ichthyosiform lesions on legs in type 2. Scleroderma-like appearance of hands and feet in type 5. Acne conglobata, hidradenitis suppurativa, and lichen spinulosus in type 6. 🕮

DIAGNOSIS AND DIFFERENTIAL DIAGNOSIS

The diagnosis is made on clinical grounds. The differential diagnosis includes psoriasis, follicular ichthyosis, erythrokeratoderma variabilis, nonbullous ichthyosiform erythroderma.

LABORATORY EXAMINATIONS

Chemistry   No diagnostic features.
Histopathology   Not diagnostic. Suggestive: Hyperkeratosis, acanthosis with broad short rete ridges, alternating autokeratosis and parakeratosis. Keratinous plugs of follicular infundibula and perifollicular areas of parakeratosis may be present. Prominent granular layer may distinguish PRP from psoriasis. Superficial perivascular lymphocytic infiltrate.

COURSE AND PROGNOSIS

A socially and psychologically disabling condition. Long duration; type 3 often resolves after 2 years; type 4 may clear. Type 5 has a very chronic course. Type 6 may respond to highly active antiretroviral therapy (HAART).

MANAGEMENT

Topical therapies consist of emollients, keratolytic agents, vitamin D_3 (calciproptriol),

FIGURE 5-5   Pityriasis rubra pilaris (type 1, classic adult)   Initial lesions are discrete, disseminated follicular hyperkeratotic papules of reddish-orange color.

FIGURE 5-6   Darier disease (type 1, classic adult)   Generalized papules beginning on the head and neck have coalesced on the chest of a 57-year-old male who had taken estrogens. There are sharply demarcated islands of unaffected normal skin.

FIGURE 5-7   Pityriasis rubra pilaris (type 1, classic adult)   Orange-reddish papules have coalesced to near erythroderma, sparing isolated islands of normal skin. Also note erythroderma, involvement of the hands in this 55-year-old woman.

glucocorticoids, and vitamin A analogues (tazaroten). All not very effective. Phototherapy [ultraviolet A phototherapy, narrowband ultraviolet B phototherapy, and photochemotherapy (PUVA)] are effective in some cases.

Most effective treatment consists of systemic administration of methotrexate or retinoids (both as in psoriasis). In type 6 HAART. The anti-TNF agents, e.g., remicade and enbrel, are effective.

DISSEMINATED SUPERFICIAL ACTINIC POROKERATOSIS (DSAP) ■ ◑

- DSAP is the most common form of the porokeratoses (for classification see porokeratosis picture gallery in the online version.)🔗

- Uniformly small, annular flat papules ranging from 2 to 5 mm in diameter.

- Distributed symmetrically on the extremities and located predominantly in sun-exposed sites.

- Typically spare palms, soles, and mucous membranes.

- Characteristic feature: well-demarcated hyperkeratotic border of individual lesions, usually < 1 mm in height with a characteristic longitudinal furrow encircling the entire lesion (Figs. 5-8 and 5-9).

- As lesions progress, the central area becomes atrophic and unhidrotic.

- Symptoms: asymptomatic or mildly pruritic cosmetically disfiguring.

- Tends to be inherited as an autosomal dominant disorder.

- Pathogenesis unknown.

- A benign condition, but rarely a precursor for in situ or invasive squamous cell carcinoma.

- Treatment: topical 5-fluorouracil, retinoids, and imiquimod. Topical retinoids may improve lesions.

- Patients should be monitored for SCC.

ICD-9 : 692.75 ○ ICD-10 : Q 82.8

FIGURE 5-8   Disseminated superficial actinic porokeratosis   Very flat annular papules with a very characteristic hyperkeratotic border surrounding the lesion. Individual lesions have coalesced to irregular patches, which are also surrounded by the porokeratotic border. This is on the lower arm of a 55-year-old female who had been chronically sun-exposed for decades. The eruption was distributed symmetrically on arms and legs but only in sun-exposed sites.

FIGURE 5-9   Disseminated superficial actinic porokeratosis   Small annular flat papules up to 4 mm in diameter surrounded by a well-demarcated hyperkeratotic border. With a hand lens the longitudinal furrow encircling the entire lesion can be seen.

BULLOUS DISEASES

HEREDITARY EPIDERMOLYSIS BULLOSA (EB)

- A spectrum of rare genodermatoses in which a disturbed coherence of the epidermis and/or dermis leads to blister formation following trauma. Hence, the designation *mechano-bullous dermatoses*.

- Disease manifestations range from very mild to severely mutilating and even lethal forms that differ in mode of inheritance, clinical manifestations, and associated findings.

- Classification based on the site of blister formation distinguishes three main groups: epidermolytic or EB simplex (EBS), junctional EB (JEB), and dermolytic, or dystrophic, EB (DEB).

- In each of these groups there are several distinct types of EB based on clinical, genetic, histologic, and biochemical evaluation.

ICD-9 : 757.39 ∘ ICD-10 : Q 81

CLASSIFICATION

Based on level of cleavage and blister formation there are three main types:

- Epidermolytic. Cleavage occurs in keratinocytes: EB simplex (EBS)
- Junctional. Cleavage occurs in basal lamina: junctional EB (JEB)
- Dermatolytic. Cleavage occurs in most superficial papillary dermis: dermolytic, or dystrophic, EB (DEB)

In each of these groups there are several distinct types of EB based on clinical, genetic, histologic/electronmicroscopic, and biochemical evaluation (Table 6-1). Only the most important are discussed here.

EPIDEMIOLOGY

The overall incidence of hereditary EB is placed at 19.6 live births per 1 million births in the United States. Stratified by subtype, the incidences are 11 for EBS, 2 for JEB, and 5 for DEB. The estimated prevalence in the United States is 8.2 per million, but this figure represents only the most severe cases as it does not include the majority of very mild disease going unreported.

ETIOLOGY AND PATHOGENESIS

Genetic Defects   Molecules involved are listed in Table 6-1 and localization in the tissue and sites of cleavage are shown in Image 6-1.

CLINICAL PHENOTYPES

EB Simplex (EBS)

A trauma-induced, intraepidermal blistering, based in most cases on mutations of the genes for keratins 5 and 14 resulting in a disturbance of the stability of the keratin filament network (Table 6-1). This causes cytolysis of basal keratinocytes and a cleft in the basal cell layer (Image 6-1). Different subgroups have considerable phenotypic variations (Table 6-1), and there are eight distinct forms, most of which are dominantly inherited. The two most common are described below.

Generalized EBS (Table 6-1)   The so-called Koebner variant is dominantly inherited, with onset at birth to early infancy. There is generalized blistering following trauma with a predilection for traumatized body sites such as feet, hands, elbows, and knees. Blisters are tense or flaccid at first and lead to erosions (Fig. 6-1). There is rapid healing and only minimal scarring at sites of repeated blistering. Palmoplantar

FIGURE 6-1 **Generalized EBS** This 4-year- old girl has had blistering since very early infancy with predilection for traumatized body sites such as palms and soles but also elbows and knees. Blistering also occurs in other areas such as the forearm, as shown here, and on the trunk. Note that despite multiple blistering episodes there is hardly any evidence of scarring on the palms of this child.

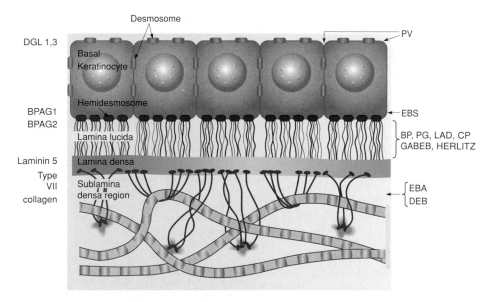

IMAGE 6-1 Localization of target adhesion sites and cleft formation in selected hereditary and autoimmune bullous diseases. (Modified from Fig. 30-5 in JL Bolognia et al: *Dermatology*; Mosby, London, Philadelphia, 2003; with permission.)

TABLE 6-1 Classification of Epidermolysis Bullosa

Level of Separation	Disease	Defect
Simplex	Generalized/Koebner	KRT5/KRT14
Simplex	Herpetiformis/Dowling-Meara	KRT5/KRT14
Simplex	Localized/Weber-Cockayne	KRT5/KRT14
Simplex	Ogna	KRT5/KRT14
Simplex	Superficialis	KRT5/KRT14
Simplex	Mottled pigmentation	KRT5
Hemidesmosomal[a]	EB with muscular dystrophy	PLEC1
Hemidesmosomal[b]	EB with pyloric atresia	ITGB4/ITGA6
Junctional	Gravis/Herlitz	LAMB3/LAMA3/LAMG2
Junctional	Mitis	LAMB3/LAMA3/LAMG2
Junctional[c]	Generalized atrophic benign	COL17A1/LAMB3
Junctional	Localized	COL17A1
Dystrophic	Pasini	COL7A1
Dystrophic	Cockayne-Touraine	COL7A1
Dystrophic	Localized RDEB	COL7A1
Dystrophic	Hallopeau-Siemens	COL7A1
Variable	Kindler syndrome	KIND1
Desmosomal	Ectodermal dysplasia-skin fragility	PKP1

COL7A1, collagen, type VII, α_1; EB, epidermolysis bullosa; ITGB, integrin β; KRT, keratin; LAMA, laminin α; LAMB, laminin β; PKP, plakophilin; PLEC, plectin; RDEB, recessive dystrophic epidermolysis bullosa.
[a]Alternatively classified as simplex.
[b]Alternatively classified as junctional.
[c]Case with type XVII collagen cytoplasmic deletion showed both junctional and hemidesmosomal levels of skin separation.

Source: From M.P. Marinkovich, EA Bauer: Inherited epidermolysis bullosa, in K Wolff et al. (eds.): *Fitzpatrick's Dermatology in General Medicine* 7th edition. New York, McGraw-Hill, 2008

hyperkeratoses may be present. Nails, teeth, and oral mucosa are usually spared.

Localized EBS Weber-Cockayne subtype (Table 6-1). This is the most common form of EBS. Onset in childhood or later. The disease may not present itself until adulthood, when thick-walled blisters on the feet and hands occur after excessive exercise, manual work, or military training (Fig. 6-2). Increased ambient temperature facilitates lesions. Hyperhidrosis of palms and soles is associated, and secondary infection of blistered lesions often occurs.

Junctional EB (JEB)

All forms of JEB share the pathologic feature of blister formation within the lamina lucida of the basement membrane (Image 6-1). Mutations are in the gene for collagen XVII and laminin (Table 6-1). This trait is autosomal recessive and comprises clinical phenotypes depending on the type of genetic lesion and environmental factors. The three principal subtypes (see Table 6-1) are described below.

JEB Gravis (Herlitz EB) Patients often do not survive infancy; the mortality rate is 40% during the first year of life. There is generalized blistering at birth (Fig. 6-3) or clinically distinctive and severe periorificial granulation, loss of nails, and involvement of most mucosal surfaces. The skin of these children may be completely denuded, representing oozing painful erosion. Associated findings include all symptoms resulting from generalized epithelial blistering with respiratory, gastrointestinal, and genitourinary organ systems involved.

JEB Mitis These children may have moderate or severe JEB at birth but survive infancy and clinically improve with age. Periorificial nonhealing erosions during childhood.

Generalized Atrophic Benign Epidermolysis Bullosa (GABEB) GABEB is a separate JEB that presents at birth with generalized cutaneous

FIGURE 6-2 Localized EBS Thick-walled blisters on the soles. The disease presented itself for the first time during military training when this 19-year-old man had to march over a long distance.

FIGURE 6-3 Junctional epidermolysis bullosa (Herlitz variant) There are large eroded, oozing and bleeding areas that occurred intrapartum. When this newborn is lifted up, dislodgment of epidermis as well as erosions occur with manual handling.

blistering (Fig. 6-4) and erosions not only on the extremities but also on the trunk, face, and scalp. Survival to adulthood is the rule, but blistering on traumatized areas continues (Fig. 6-5). It is particularly pronounced with increased ambient temperature, and there is atrophic healing of the lesions. Nail dystrophy, nonscarring or scarring alopecia, mild oral mucous membrane involvement; enamel defects may occur. Mutations are in the genes for collagen type XVII and laminin (Table 6-1).

Dystrophic Epidermolysis Bullosa (DEB)

A spectrum of dermolytic diseases where blistering occurs below the basal lamina (Image 6-1); healing is therefore usually accompanied by scarring and milia formation—hence, the name *dystrophic*. There are four principal subtypes, and all are due to mutations in anchoring fibril type VII collagen (Table 6-1). Anchoring fibrils are therefore only rudimentary or absent. Of the four main types of DEB, only two are described below.

Dominant DEB   Cockayne-Touraine disease. Onset in infancy or early childhood with acral blistering and nail dystrophy; milia and scar formation, which may be hypertrophic or hyperplastic. Oral lesions are uncommon, and teeth are usually normal.

Recessive DEB (RDEB)   Comprises a larger spectrum of clinical phenotypes. The localized, less severe form (RDEB mitis) occurs at birth, shows acral blistering, atrophic scarring, and little or no mucosal involvement. Generalized, severe RDEB, the Hallopeau-Siemens variant, is mutilating. There is generalized blistering at birth, and progression and repeated blistering at the same sites (Fig. 6-6) result in remarkable scarring and ulcerations, syndactyly with loss of nails (Fig. 6-7) and even mitten-like deformities of hands and feet, flexion contractures. There are enamel defects with caries and parodontitis, strictures and scarring in the oral mucous membrane and esophagus, urethral and anal stenosis, and ocular surface scarring; also malnutrition, growth retardation, and anemia.

The most serious complication is squamous cell carcinoma in chronic recurrent erosions.

DIAGNOSIS

Based on clinical appearance and history. Histopathology determines the level of cleavage, which is further defined by electron microscopy and/or immunohistochemical mapping. Western blot, Northern blot, restriction fragment length polymorphism (RFLP) analysis, and DNA sequences may then identify the mutated gene.

MANAGEMENT

There is as yet no causal therapy for EB, but gene therapy is being investigated. Management is tailored to the severity and extent of skin involvement and consists of supportive skin care, supportive care for other organ systems, and systemic therapies for complications. Wound management, nutritional support, and infection control are key to the management of all EB patients.

In EBS, maintenance of a cool environment and use of soft, well-ventilated shoes, are important. Blistered skin is treated by saline compresses and topical antibiotics or, in the case of inflammation, with topical steroids. More severely affected JEB and DEB patients are treated like patients in a burn unit. Gentle bathing and cleansing are followed by protective emollients and nonadherent dressings.

Management of cutaneous infection is important, and surgical treatment is often required in DEB for the release of fused digits and correction of limb contractures.

Although rare, EB and, in particular, JEB and DEB pose a major health and socioeconomic problem. Organizations such as the Dystrophic Epidermolysis Bullosa Research Association (DEBRA) offer assistance that includes patient education and support.

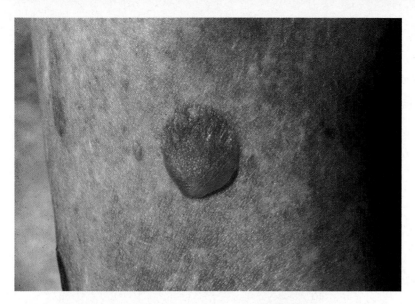

FIGURE 6-4   Generalized atrophic benign epidermolysis bullosa (GABEB)   This 19-year-old man has had cutaneous blistering since birth, with blisters and erosions arising on the elbows and knees but also on the trunk and arms following trauma. Note: ill-defined erythemas at sites of previous blistering. There is no scarring but some spotty atrophy.

FIGURE 6-5   Generalized atrophic benign epidermolysis bullosa (GABEB)   This 20-year-old man has had generalized cutaneous blistering since birth. Note: erosions on the left lower back and hemorrhagic crusts on the lower arms. Erythema on the back indicates sites of previous blistering.

FIGURE 6-6   Generalized recessive dystrophic epidermolysis bullosa (RDEB)   In this severe disease blistering occurs often at the same sites, as in this 10-year-old girl. Blisters lead to erosions and these become ulcers that have a low tendency to heal. When healing occurs it results in scarring. This girl also has enamel defects with caries, strictures of the esophagus, severe anemia, and considerable growth retardation. It is obvious that these large wounds are portal entries for systemic infection.

FIGURE 6-7   Generalized recessive dystrophic epidermolysis bullosa (RDEB)   Loss of all fingernails, syndactyly, and severe atrophic scarring on the dorsa of the hand.

FAMILIAL BENIGN PEMPHIGUS

- Familial benign pemphigus, or Hailey-Hailey disease, is a rare genodermatosis with dominant inheritance that is classically described as a blistering disorder but actually presents as an erythematous, erosive, oozing condition with cracks and fissures localized to the nape of the neck, axillae (Fig. 6-8).

- Submammary regions, inguinal folds, and scrotum *are major sites of involvement.*

- The underlying pathologic process is acantholysis whereby the fragility of the epidermis is due to a defect in the adhesion complex between desmosomal proteins and tonofilaments.

- The genetic abnormality lies in *ATP2CI*, which encodes an ATP-powered calcium pump.

- Onset is usually between the third and fourth decades.

- Often mistaken for intertrigo, candidiasis, or frictional or contact dermatitis.

- Individual lesions consist of microscopically small flaccid vesicles on an erythematous background that soon turn into eroded plaques with the described, highly characteristic, fissured appearance (Fig. 6-8).

- Crusting, scaling, and hypertrophic vegetative growths may occur.

- Histology explains the clinical appearance as epidermal cells lose their coherence with acantholysis throughout the epithelium, giving the appearance of a dilapidated brick wall.

- Colonization of the lesions, particularly by *Staphylococcus aureus,* is a trigger for further acantholysis and maintenance of the pathologic process. Secondary colonization by *Candida* has a similar effect.

- Treatment rests on antimicrobial therapy, administered both topically and systemically; systemically, the tetracyclines seem to work better than most. Mupirocin topically. Topical glucocorticoids depress the anti-inflammatory response and accelerate healing. In severe cases, dermabrasion or carbon dioxide laser vaporization leads to healing with scars, which are resistant to recurrences. The condition becomes less troublesome with age.

ICD-9 : 694.5 ○ ICD-10 : Q 82.8

FIGURE 6-8   Familial benign pemphigus   This 46-year-old male has had oozing lesions in both axillae, occasionally in the groins and sometimes also on the nape of the neck, for several years. Eruptions worsen during the summer months. The father and sister have similar lesions that wax and wane. Lesions are painful and show typical cracks and fissures within an erosive erythematous plaque. Although classified among the blistering diseases, familial benign pemphigus hardly ever shows intact vesicles and is often mistaken for intertrigo.

PEMPHIGUS   ICD-9:694.4 ∘ ICD-10:L10   □ ●

- A serious, acute or chronic, bullous autoimmune disease of skin and mucous membranes based on acantholysis.
- Two major types: pemphigus vulgaris (PV) and pemphigus foliaceus (PF)
- PV: flaccid blisters on skin and erosions on mucous membranes. PF: scaly and crusted skin lesions.

- PV: suprabasal acantholysis. PF: subcorneal acantholysis
- IgG autoantibodies to desmogleins, transmembrane desmosomal adhesion molecules.
- Serious and often fatal unless treated with immunosuppressive agents.

CLASSIFICATION

Two major types: pemphigus vulgaris (PV) and pemphigus foliaceus (PF). In addition, paraneoplastic pemphigus (PP) associated with malignancy and IgA pemphigus (Table 6-2).

EPIDEMIOLOGY

PV: Rare, more common in Jews and people of Mediterranean descent. In Jerusalem the incidence is estimated at 16 per million, whereas in France and Germany it is 1.3 per million.

PF: Also rare but endemic in rural areas in Brazil (fogo selvagem), where the prevalence can be as high as 3.4%.
Age of Onset 40 to 60 years; fogo selvagem also in children and young adults.
Sex Equal incidence in males and females, but predominance of females with PF in Tunisia and Colombia.

ETIOLOGY AND PATHOGENESIS

An autoimmune disorder. Loss of the normal cell-to-cell adhesion in the epidermis (*acantholysis*) occurs as a result of circulating antibodies of the IgG class; these antibodies bind to desmogleins, transmembrane glycoproteins in the desmosomes, members of the cadherin superfamily. In PV, desmoglein 3 (in some, also desmoglein 1). All patients with PV have autoantibodies to desmoglein 3. Those with mucocutaneous PV also have antibodies to desmoglein 1; those with only mucosal involvement, only to desmoglein 3. In contrast, PF patients have autoantibodies only to desmoglein 1. These autoantibodies interfere with calcium-sensitive adhesion function and thus induce acantholysis (Image 6-2).

CLINICAL MANIFESTATION

PV usually starts in the oral mucosa, and months may elapse before skin lesions occur; lesions may be localized for months, after which generalized bullae occur. Less frequently there may be a generalized, acute eruption of bullae from the beginning. No pruritus (as occurs in pemphigoid but burning and pain in erosions or eroded bullae). Painful and tender mouth lesions may prevent adequate food intake. Epistaxis, hoarseness, dysphagia. Weakness, malaise, weight loss. PF has no mucosal lesion and starts with scaly, crusted lesion on an erythematous base, initially in seborrheic areas.

Skin Lesions of PV Round or oval vesicles and bullae with serous content, flaccid (flabby) (Fig. 6-9), easily ruptured, and weeping (Fig. 6-10), arising on *normal* skin, randomly scattered, discrete. Localized (e.g., to mouth or circumscribed skin area), or generalized with a random pattern. Extensive erosions that bleed easily (Fig. 6-11), crusts particularly on scalp.

TABLE 6-2   Classification of Pemphigus

Pemphigus vulgaris
  Pemphigus vulgaris: localized and generalized
  Pemphigus vegetans: localized
  Drug-induced
Pemphigus foliaceus
  Pemphigus foliaceus: generalized
  Pemphigus erythematosus: localized
  Fogo selvagem: endemic
  Drug-induced
Paraneoplastic pemphigus: associated with malignancy
IgA pemphigus: subcorneal pustular dermatosis and
  intraepidermal neutrophilic IgA dermatitis

FIGURE 6-9   Pemphigus vulgaris   This is the classic initial lesion: flaccid, easily ruptured vesicle or bulla on normal-appearing skin. Ruptured vesicles lead to erosions that subsequently crust.

IMAGE 6-2   Desmoglein compensation   Triangles represent the distribution of Dsg 1 and 3 in skin and mucous membranes. Anti-Dsg 1 antibodies in pemphigus foliaceus cause acantholysis only in the superficial epidermis of skin. In the deep epidermis and in mucous membranes, Dsg 3 compensates for antibody-induced loss of function of Dsg 1. In early pemphigus vulgaris, antibodies are present only against Dsg 3, which cause blisters only in the deep mucous membrane where Dsg 3 is present without compensatory Dsg 1. However, in mucocutaneous pemphigus, antibodies against both Dsg 1 and Dsg 3 are present, and blisters form in both mucous membrane and skin. The blister is deep probably because antibodies diffuse from the dermis and interfere first with the function of desmosomes at the base of the epidermis. [From J Stanley, in K Wolff et al (eds): *Fitzpatrick's Dermatology in General Medicine*, 7th ed. New York, McGraw-Hill, 2008, p 463.]

Since blisters rupture so easily, only erosions are seen in many patients. These are very painful (Fig. 6-11).

Nikolsky Sign Dislodging of epidermis by lateral finger pressure in the vicinity of lesions, which leads to an erosion. Pressure on bulla leads to lateral extension of blister.

Sites of Predilection Scalp, face, chest, axillae, groin, umbilicus. In bedridden patients, there is extensive involvement of back (Fig. 6-11).

Mucous Membranes Bullae rarely seen, erosions of mouth and nose, pharynx and larynx, vagina. ✎

Skin Lesions of PF Most commonly on face, scalp, upper chest, and abdomen. Scaly, crusted erosions on an erythematous base. In early or localized disease, sharply demarcated in seborrheic areas; may stay localized for a long time or progress to generalized disease and exfoliative erythroderma. ✎ Initial lesion also a flaccid bulla but this is rarely seen because of superficial location (see histopathology below). ✎

VARIANTS (SEE TABLE 6-2)

Pemphigus Vegetans (PVeg) Usually confined to intertriginous regions, perioral area, neck, and scalp. Granulomatous vegetating purulent plaques that extend centrifugally. In these patients there is a granulomatous response to the autoimmune damage of PV. ✎

Drug-Induced PV Clinically identical to sporadic PV. Several different drugs implicated, most significantly, captopril and D-penicillamine.

Brazilian Pemphigus (Fogo Selvagem) A distinctive form of PF endemic to south central Brazil. Clinically, histologically, and immunopathologically identical to PF. Patients improve when moved to urban areas but relapse after returning to endemic regions. It is speculated that the disease is somehow related to an arthropod-borne infectious agent, with clustering similar to that of the *black fly—Similium incrimanum*. More than 1000 new cases per year are estimated to occur in the endemic regions.

Pemphigus Erythematosus (PE) Synonym: Senear-Usher syndrome. A localized variety of PF largely confined to seborrheic sites. Erythematous, crusted, and erosive lesions in the "butterfly" area of the face, forehead, and presternal and interscapular regions. These patients have immunoglobulin and complement deposits at the dermal-epidermal junction, in addition to intercellular pemphigus antibody in the epidermis, and may have antinuclear antibodies, as is the case in lupus erythematosus. ✎

Drug-Induced Pemphigus PF As in PV, associated with D-penicillamine and less frequently by captopril and other drugs. In most, but not all, instances the eruption resolves after termination of therapy with the offending drug.

PARANEOPLASTIC PEMPHIGUS (PNP)

This is a disease sui generis (see Section 18). Mucous membranes primarily and most severely involved. Lesions combine features of pemphigus vulgaris and erythema multiforme, clinically and histologically.

LABORATORY EXAMINATIONS

Dermatopathology PV: Light microscopy (select early small bulla or, if not present, margin of larger bulla or erosion): Separation of keratinocytes, suprabasally, leading to split just *above* the basal cell layer and vesicles containing separated, rounded-up (acantholytic) keratinocytes. PF: Superficial form with acantholysis in the granular layer of the epidermis.

Immunopathology Direct immunofluorescence (IF) staining reveals IgG and often C3 deposited in lesional and paralesional skin in *the intercellular substance of the epidermis*.

Serum Autoantibodies (IgG) detected by indirect IF (IIF) or enzyme-linked immunosorbent assay (ELISA). Titer usually correlates with activity of disease process. In PV autoantibodies are directed against a 130-kDa glycoprotein designated desmoglein 3 and located in desmosomes. In PF circulating autoantibodies to a 160-kDa intercellular (cell surface) antigen, desmoglein 1, in the desmosomes of keratinocytes. PV (130 kDa) and PF (160 kDa) antigens differ (Image 6-2). This explains the different sites of acantholysis and thus the different clinical appearance of the two conditions.

DIAGNOSIS AND DIFFERENTIAL DIAGNOSIS

Can be a difficult problem if only mouth lesions are present. Aphthae, mucosal lichen planus, erythema multiforme. Differential diagnosis includes all forms of acquired bullous diseases (see Table 6-3). Biopsy of the skin and mucous membrane, direct IF, and demonstration of circulating autoantibodies confirm a high index of suspicion.

COURSE

In most cases the disease inexorably progresses to death unless treated aggressively with

FIGURE 6-10   Pemphigus vulgaris   Widespread confluent flaccid blisters on the lower back of a 40-year-old male who had a generalized eruption including scalp and mucous membranes. The eroded lesions are extremely painful.

FIGURE 6-11   Pemphigus vulgaris   Widespread confluent erosions that are very painful and bleed easily in a 53-year-old male. There are hardly any intact blisters because they are so fragile and break easily. The blood tracts go sideways because the patient had been lying on his right side before the photograph was taken.

immunosuppressive agents. The mortality rate has been markedly reduced since treatment has become available. Currently, morbidity related to glucocorticoids and immunosuppresive therapies.

MANAGEMENT

Glucocorticoids   2 to 3 mg/kg body weight of prednisone until cessation of new blister formation and disappearance of Nikolsky sign. Then rapid reduction to about half the initial dose until patient is almost clear, followed by very slow tapering of dose to minimal effective maintenance dose.

Concomitant Immunosuppressive Therapy
Immunosuppressive agents are given concomitantly for their glucocorticoid-sparing effect:

Azathioprine, 2–3 mg/kg body weight until complete clearing; tapering of dose to 1 mg/kg. Azathioprine alone is continued even after cessation of glucocorticoid treatment and may have to be continued for many months or years.

Methotrexate, either orally (PO) or IM at doses of 25 to 35 mg/week. Dose adjustments are made as with azathioprine.

Cyclophosphamide, 100–200 mg daily, with reduction to maintenance doses of 50–100 mg/d. Alternatively, cyclophosphamide "bolus" therapy with 1000 mg IV once a week or every 2 weeks in the initial phases, followed by 50–100 mg/d PO as maintenance.

Plasmapheresis, in conjunction with glucocorticoids and immunosuppressive agents in poorly controlled patients, in the initial phases of treatment to reduce antibody titers.

Gold therapy, for milder cases. After an initial test dose of 10 mg IM, 25–50 mg of gold sodium thiomalate is given IM at weekly intervals to a maximum cumulative dose of 1 g.

Mycophenolate mofetil (1 g twice daily) has been reported to be beneficial, and clinical studies are ongoing.

High-dose intravenous immunoglobulin (HIVIg) (2 g/kg body weight every 3–4 weeks) has been reported to have a glucocorticoid-sparing effect. Expensive.

Rituximab (monoclonal antibody to CD20) presumably targets B cells, the precursors of (auto) antibody-producing plasma cells. Given as intravenous therapy once a week for 4 weeks, shows dramatic effects in some and at least partial remission in other patients. Serious infections may be seen.

Other Measures   Cleansing baths, wet dressings, topical and intralesional glucocorticoids, antimicrobial therapy per documented bacterial infections. Correction of fluid and electrolyte imbalance.

Monitoring   Clinical, for improvement of skin lesions and development of drug-related side effects. Laboratory monitoring of pemphigus antibody titers and for hematologic and metabolic indicators of glucocorticoid- and/or immunosuppressive-induced adverse effects.

TABLE 6-3   Differential Diagnosis of Important Acquired Bullous Diseases

Disease	Skin Lesions	Mucous Membranes	Distribution
PV	Flaccid bullae on normal skin, erosions	Almost always involved, erosions	Anywhere, localized or generalized
PF	Crusted erosions, occasionally flaccid vesicles	Rarely involved	Exposed, seborrheic regions or generalized
PVeg	Granulating plaques, occasionally vesicles at margin	As in PV	Intertriginous regions, scalp
Bullous pemphigoid	Tense bullae on normal and erythematous skin; urticarial plaques and papules	Mouth involved in 10–35%	Anywhere, localized or generalized
EBA	Tense bullae and erosions, noninflammatory or BP-, DH- or LAD-like presentation	May be severely involved (oral esophagus, vagina)	Traumatized regions or random
Dermatitis herpetiformis	Grouped papules, vesicles, urticarial plaques, crusted	None	Predilection sites: elbows, knees, gluteal, sacral, and scapular areas
Linear IgA dermatosis	Annular, grouped papules, vesicles, and bullae	Oral erosions and ulcers, conjunctival erosions and scarring	Anywhere

Disease	Histopathology	Immunopathology/Skin	Serum
PV	Suprabasal acantholysis	IgG intercellular pattern	IgG AB to intercellular substance of epidermis (IIF) ELISA: AB to desmoglein 3 >> desmoglein 1
PF	Acantholysis in granular layer	IgG, intracellular pattern	IgG AB to intercellular substance of epidermis (IIF) ELISA: AB to desmoglein 1 only
PVeg	Acantholysis ± intraepidermal neutrophilic abscesses, epidermal hyperplasia	As in PV	As in PV
Bullous pemphigoid	Subepidermal blister	IgG and C3 linear at BMZ	IgG AB to BMZ (IIF); directed to BPAG1 and BPAG2
EBA	Subepidermal blister	Linear IgG at BMZ	IgG AB to BMZ (IIF) directed to type VII collagen (ELISA, Western blot)
Dermatitis herpetiformis	Papillary microabscesses, subepidermal vesicle	Granular IgA in tips of papillae	Antiendomysial antibodies
Linear IgA dermatosis	Subepidermal blister with neutrophils	Linear IgA at BMZ	Low titers of IgA AB against BMZ

Note: AB, antibody; BMZ, basement membrane zone; BP, bullous pemphigoid; DH, dermatitis herpetiformis; EB, epidermolysis bullosa acquisita; ELISA, enzyme-linked immunosorbent assay; IIF, indirect immunofluorescence; LAD, linear IgA dermatosis; PF, pemphigus foliaceus; PV, pemphigus vulgaris; PVeg, pemphigus vegetans.

BULLOUS PEMPHIGOID (BP)   ICD-9 : 694.5 ∘ ICD-10 : L12.0 ▯ ◐ → ●

- A bullous autoimmune disease usually in elderly patients.
- Pruritic papular and/or urticarial lesions with large tense bullae.
- Subepidermal blisters with eosinophils.
- C3 and IgG at epidermal basement membrane, antibasement membrane IgG autoantibodies in serum.

- Autoantigens are keratinocyte hemidesmosome proteins.
- Therapy includes topical and systemic glucocorticoids and other immunosuppressives.

EPIDEMIOLOGY

Age of Onset   60 to 80 years.

Sex   Equal incidence in males and females. No known racial predilection.

Incidence   The most common bullous autoimmune disease. Seven per million in Germany and France. Far more common in authors' experience in very old people.

ETIOLOGY AND PATHOGENESIS

Interaction of autoantibody with bullous pemphigoid antigen [BPAG1 and BPAG2 (collagen type XVII)] in hemidesmosomes of basal keratinocytes (Image 6-1) is followed by complement activation and attraction of neutrophils and eosinophils. Bullous lesion results from interaction of multiple bioactive molecules released from inflammatory cells. Not yet completely clarified.

CLINICAL MANIFESTATION

Often starts with a prodromal eruption (urticarial, papular lesions) and evolves in weeks to months to bullae that may appear suddenly as a generalized eruption. Initially no symptoms except moderate or severe pruritus; later, tenderness of eroded lesions. No constitutional symptoms, except in widespread, severe disease.

Skin Lesions   Erythematous, papular or urticarial-type lesions (Fig. 6-12) may precede bullae formation by months. Bullae: large, tense, firm-topped, oval or round (Fig. 6-13); may arise in normal, erythematous, or urticarial skin and contain serous or hemorrhagic fluid. The eruption may be localized or generalized, usually scattered but also grouped in arciform and serpiginous patterns. Bullae rupture less easily than in pemphigus, but sometimes large, bright red, oozing, and bleeding erosions become a

major problem. Usually, however, the originally tense bullae collapse and transform into crusts.

Sites of Predilection   Axillae; medial aspects of thighs, groins, abdomen; flexor aspects of forearms; lower legs (often first manifestation).

Mucous Membranes   Practically only in the mouth (10–35%); less severe and painful and less easily ruptured than in pemphigus. ▨

LABORATORY EXAMINATIONS

Dermatopathology   *Light Microscopy*   Neutrophils in "Indian-file" alignment at dermal-epidermal junction; neutrophils, eosinophils, and lymphocytes in papillary dermis; *subepidermal* bulla.

Electron Microscopy   Junctional cleavage, i.e., split occurs in lamina lucida of basement membrane.

Immunopathology   Linear IgG deposits along the basement membrane zone. Also, C3, which may occur in the absence of IgG.

Serum   Circulating antibasement membrane IgG antibodies detected by IIF in 70% of patients. Titers do not correlate with course of disease. Autoantibodies in bullous pemphigoid recognize two types of antigens. BPAG1 is a 230-kDa glycoprotein that has high homology with desmoplakin I and is part of hemidesmosomes. BPAG2 is a transmembranous 180-kDa polypeptide (type XVII collagen).

Hematology   Eosinophilia (not always).

DIAGNOSIS AND DIFFERENTIAL DIAGNOSIS

Clinical appearance, histopathology, and immunology permit a differentiation from other bullous diseases (see Table 6-3 on p 111).

MANAGEMENT

Systemic prednisone with starting doses of 50–100 mg/d continued until clear, either alone

FIGURE 6-12 Bullous pemphigoid Early lesions in a 75-year-old female. Note urticarial plaques and a small, tense blister with a clear serous content.

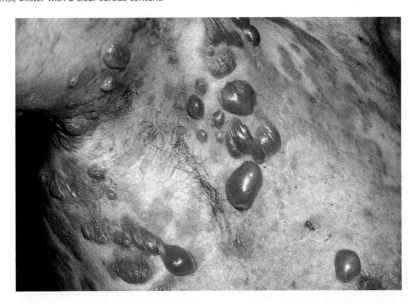

FIGURE 6-13 Bullous pemphigoid This 77-year-old male has a generalized eruption with confluent urticarial plaques and multiple tense blisters. The condition is severely pruritic.

or combined with azathioprine, 150 mg daily, for remission induction and 50–100 mg for maintenance; in refractory cases IVIG: plasmapheresis in milder cases, sulfones (dapsone), 100–150 mg/d. Low-dose MTX 2.5 to 10 mg weekly PO is effective and safe in elderly. In very mild cases and for local recurrences, topical glucocorticoid or topical tacrolimus therapy may be beneficial. Tetracycline ± nicotinamide has been reported to be effective in some cases.

COURSE AND PROGNOSIS

Patients often go into a permanent remission after therapy and do not require further therapy; local recurrences can sometimes be controlled with topical glucocorticoids; clobetasol with occlusion to urticarial areas. Also, intralesional triamcinolone for localized disease. Some cases go into spontaneous remission without therapy.

CICATRICIAL PEMPHIGOID (CP)   ICD-9 : 694.6 ∘ ICD-10 : L12.1   ☐ ●

- A rare disease, largely of the elderly.
- Blisters that rupture easily and also erosions resulting from epithelial fragility in the mouth; oropharynx; and, more rarely, the nasopharyngeal, esophageal, genital, and rectal mucosae.
- Ocular involvement may initially manifest as unilateral or bilateral conjunctivitis with burning, dryness, and foreign-body sensation.
- Chronic involvement results in scarring, symblepharon (Fig. 6-14), and, in severe disease, fusion of the bulbar and palpebral conjunctiva.
- Entropion and trichiasis result in corneal irritation, superficial punctate keratinopathy, corneal neovascularization, ulceration, and blindness.
- Scarring also in the larynx; esophageal involvement results in stricture formation leading to dysphagia or dynophagia.

- The skin is involved in roughly 30% of patients.
- Antigens to which autoantibodies may be directed include BPAG2, laminin 5, integrin subunits β_4 and α_6, type VII collagen, and BPAG1.
- *Brunsting-Perry pemphigoid* describes a subset of patients whose skin lesions recur at the same sites, mainly on the head and neck, and also lead to scarring.
- *Management*: Most patients respond to dapsone in combination with low-dose prednisone. Some patients may require more aggressive immunosuppressive treatment with cyclophosphamide or azathioprine, in combination with glucocorticoids. In addition, surgical intervention for scarring and supportive measures. ✍
- *Synonym*: Mucous membrane pemphigoid.

FIGURE 6-14   Cicatricial pemphigoid   This scarring condition in a 78-year-old female started with bilateral conjunctival pain and foreign body sensation as the first symptoms. The conjunctiva then became erosive with scarring and fibrous tracts between eyelids and the eye.

PEMPHIGOID GESTATIONIS (PG)   ICD-9 : 646.8 ○ ICD-10 : L12.8 □ ◑

- A rare pruritic and polymorphic inflammatory bullous dermatosis of pregnancy and the postpartum period.

- The estimated incidence is from 1 in 1700 to 1 in 10,000 deliveries.

- Extremely pruritic vesicular eruption mainly on the abdomen but also on other areas, with sparing of the mucous membranes. Lesions vary from erythematous, edematous papules to urticarial plaques to vesicles and tense bullae (Fig. 6-15).

- PG usually begins from the fourth to the seventh month of pregnancy but can also occur in the first trimester and in the immediate postpartum period.

- It may recur in subsequent pregnancies; if it does, it is likely to begin earlier.

- PG can be exacerbated by the use of estrogen- and progesterone-containing medications.

- Histopathologically it is a subepidermal blistering condition, and there is a heavy linear deposition of C3 along the basement membrane zone with concomitant IgG deposition in roughly 30% of patients.

- Serum contains IgG antibasal membrane antibodies, but these are detected in only 20% of patients by IIF. ELISA and immunoblotting assays detect autoantibodies in >70%, directed to BP180 (type XVII collagen), a 180-kDa transmembrane protein in hemidesmosomes. They are avid complement-fixing IgG1 antibodies that bind to amniotic epithelial basement membrane. They can also be detected in the blood of some infants.

- Some 5% of babies born to mothers with PG have urticarial, vesicular, or bullous lesions, which resolve spontaneously during the first several weeks. No significant maternal morbidity (pruritus) and mortality. There is a slight increase in premature and small-for-gestational-age births. Some reports of fetal prognosis have revealed significant fetal death and premature deliveries, whereas others have suggested no increase in fetal mortality.

- *Management* is geared to suppressing blister formation and relieving the intense pruritus. Prednisone, 20–40 mg/d, is given but sometimes higher doses are required. Prednisone is tapered gradually during the postpartum period. Only a few patients do not require systemic prednisone and can be managed with antihistamines and topical glucocorticoids. ⧉

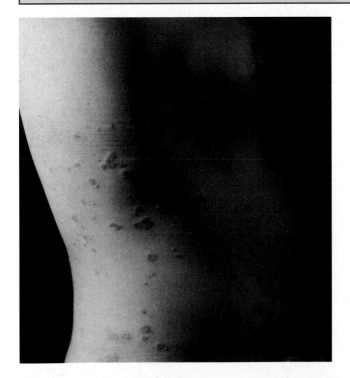

FIGURE 6-15   Pemphigoid gestationis   A. Erythematous papules that were highly pruritic and had appeared on the trunk and abdomen of this 33-year-old pregnant female (third trimester) and were a cause of great concern. At this time there were no blisters and diagnosis was established by biopsy and immunopathology.

FIGURE 6-15   (Continued)
B. Urticarial plaques and small vescicles and blisters in another patient who had similar eruptions in previous pregnancies. She responded rapidly to systemic glucocorticolds. The delivery was uneventful, and the baby was healthy.

DERMATITIS HERPETIFORMIS (DH)   ICD-9:694.0 ∘ ICD-10:L13.0

- A chronic, recurrent, intensely pruritic eruption occurring symmetrically on the extremities and the trunk.
- Consists of tiny vesicles, papules, and urticarial plaques that are arranged in groups.
- Associated with gluten-sensitive enteropathy (GSE).

- Characterized histologically by papillary collection of neutrophils.
- Granular IgA deposits in paralesional or normal skin are diagnostic.
- Responds to sulfa drugs and, to a lesser extent, to a gluten-free diet.

EPIDEMIOLOGY

Prevalence in Caucasians varies from 10 to 39 per 100,000 persons.
Age of Onset   20 to 60 years, but most common at 30 to 40 years; may occur in children.
Sex   Male:female ratio is 2:1.

ETIOLOGY AND PATHOGENESIS

The GSE probably relates to IgA deposits in the skin. Patients have antibodies to transglutaminases (TGs) that may be the major autoantigens in this disease. Epidermal TG autoantibody probably binds to TG in the gut and circulates either alone or as immune complexes and deposits in skin. With additional factors IgA activates complement via the alternative pathway, with subsequent chemotaxis of neutrophils releasing their enzymes and producing tissue injury.

CLINICAL MANIFESTATION

Pruritus, intense, episodic; burning or stinging of the skin; rarely, pruritus may be absent.

Symptoms often precede the appearance of skin lesions by 8 to 12 h. Ingestion of iodides and overload of gluten are exacerbating factors.

Systems Review Laboratory evidence of small-bowel malabsorption is detected in 10–20%. GSE occurs in nearly all patients and is demonstrated by small-bowel biopsy. There are usually no systemic symptoms.

Skin Lesions Lesions consist of erythematous papules or wheal-like plaques; tiny firm-topped vesicles, sometimes hemorrhagic (Fig. 6-16); occasionally bullae. Lesions are arranged in groups (hence the name *herpertiformis*); the distribution is strikingly symmetric. Scratching results in excoriations, crusts (Fig. 6-17). Postinflammatory hyper-and hypopigmentation at sites of healed lesions.

Sites of Predilection Typical and almost diagnostic: extensor areas—elbows, knees. Buttocks, scapular and sacral areas (Image 6-3 and Figs. 6-16 and 6-17). Here, often in a "butterfly" fashion. Scalp, face, and hairline. ✐

LABORATORY EXAMINATIONS

Immunogenetics Association with HLA-B8, HLA-DR, and HLA-DQ.

Dermatopathology Biopsy is best from early erythematous papule. Microabscesses (polymorphonuclear cells and eosinophils) at the tips of the dermal papillae. Dermal infiltration of neutrophils and eosinophils. *Subepidermal vesicle.*

Immunofluorescence Of *perilesional* skin, best on the buttocks. Granular IgA deposits in tips of papillae that correlate well with small-bowel disease. Granular IgA is found in almost-normal skin in most patients and is diagnostic. Also found are C3 and C5and alternative complement pathway components.

Circulating Autoantibodies Antireticulin antibodies of the IgA and IgG types, thyroid antimicrosomal antibodies, and antinuclear antibodies can be present. Putative immune complexes in 20–40% of patients. IgA antibodies binding to the intermyofibril substance of smooth muscles (*antiendomysial antibodies*) are present in most patients and have specificity for TGs.

Other Studies Steatorrhea (20–30%) and abnormal D-xylose absorption (10–73%). Anemia secondary to iron or folate deficiency. *Endoscopy of small bowel*: blunting and flattening of the villi (80–90%) in the small bowel as in celiac disease. Lesions are focal; verification is by small-bowel biopsy.

DIAGNOSIS AND DIFFERENTIAL DIAGNOSIS

Grouped papulovesicles at predilection sites accompanied by severe pruritus are highly suggestive. Biopsy of early lesions usually diagnostic, but IgA deposits in perilesional skin detected by IF are the best confirming evidence. Differential

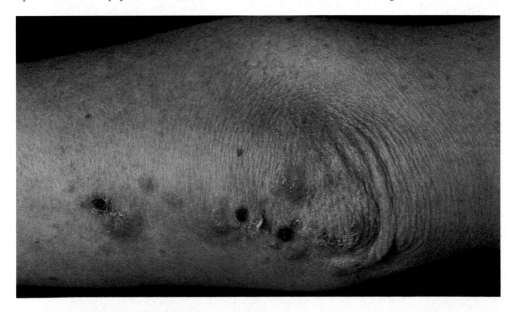

FIGURE 6-16 Dermatitis herpetiformis These are the classic early lesions. Papules, urticarial plaques, small grouped vesicles, and crusts on the elbow of a 23-year-old male.

FIGURE 6-17 **Dermatitis herpetiformis**
In this 56-year-old male patient with a generalized highly pruritic eruption, the diagnosis can be made upon first sight by the distribution of the lesions. Most heavily involved are the elbows; the scapular, sacral, and gluteal areas; and (not seen in this picture) the knees. Upon close inspection there are grouped papules, small vesicles, crusts, and erosions on an erythematous base and there is postinflammatory hypo- and hyperpigmentation. Because of pruritus the patient had previously been diagnosed as having atopic dermatitis, scabies, and allergic contact dermatitis and had responded only poorly to topical glucocorticoids. This particular eruption occurred after he had spent a vacation on the Dalmation coast (having been told that sunbathing would be good for his condition) where his meals consisted of seafood (iodides) and white bread (gluten).

diagnosis is to allergic contact dermatitis, atopic dermatitis, scabies, neurotic excoriations, papular urticaria, bullous pemphigoid, pemphigoid gestationis (see Table 6-3).

COURSE

Prolonged, for many years, with a third of the patients eventually having a spontaneous remission.

MANAGEMENT

Systemic Therapy *Dapsone* 100–150 mg daily, with gradual reduction to 50–25 mg and often as low as 50 mg twice a week. There is a dramatic response, often within hours. Obtain a glucose-6-phosphate dehydrogenase level before starting sulfones; obtain methemoglobin levels in the initial 2 weeks, and follow blood counts carefully for the first few months.

Sulfapyridine 1–1.5 g/d, with plenty of fluids, if dapsone contraindicated or not tolerated. Monitor for casts in urine and kidney function.
Diet A gluten-free diet *may* suppress the disease or allow reduction of the dosage of dapsone or sulfapyridine, but response is very slow.

IMAGE 6-3 Dermatitis herpetiformis. Pattern of distribution.

LINEAR IgA DERMATOSIS (LAD) ICD-9:702.8 □ ◑

- A rare, immune-mediated, subepidermal blistering skin disease defined by the presence of homogeneous linear deposits of IgA at the cutaneous basement membrane zone (Image 6-1).

- It is clearly separate from dermatitis herpetiformis (DH) on the basis of immunopathology, immunogenetics, and lack of association with GSE.

- LAD most often occurs after puberty.

- Clinical manifestations are very similar to those of DH, but there is more blistering. Patients present with combinations of annular or grouped papules, vesicles, and bullae (Fig. 6-18) that are distributed symmetrically on trunk and extremities including elbows, knees, and buttocks. The lesions are very pruritic but less severe than those of DH.

- Mucosal involvement is important and ranges from large asymptomatic oral erosions and ulceration to severe oral disease alone, or severe generalized cutaneous involvement and oral disease similar to that in cicatricial pemphigoid.

- It is identical with chronic bullous disease of childhood (CBDC), which is a rare blistering disease that occurs predominantly in children <5 years (Fig. 6-19).

- Circulating autoantibodies against various epidermal basement membrane antigens have been found.

- LAD has been associated with drugs: vancomycin, lithium, phenytoin, sulfamethoxazole/trimethoprim, furosemide, captopril, diclofenac, and others.

- There is a small risk of lymphoid malignancies, and associated ulcerative colitis has been reported.

- *Management*: Patients respond to dapsone or sulfapyridine but in addition, most may require low-dose prednisone. Patients do not respond to a gluten-free diet. ℮

FIGURE 6-18 Linear IgA dermatosis There are multiple grouped, confluent vesicles, bullae, and crusts on an urticarial and erythematous base. There were similar lesions on the trunk and the upper extremities.

FIGURE 6-19 Linear IgA dermatosis (chronic, bullous disease of childhood) Extensive blistering on the upper extremities and trunk in a 7-year-old child. Note: blisters are both tense and flaccid. They are grouped and there is no notable inflammation.

EPIDERMOLYSIS BULLOSA ACQUISITA (EBA)

- A chronic subepidermal bullous disease associated with autoimmunity to the type VII collagen within the anchoring fibrils in the basement membrane zone.

- Four types: the *classic mechano-bullous presentation* is a noninflammatory, blistering eruption with acral distribution that heals with scarring and milia formation. It is a mechano-bullous disease marked by skin fragility, and patients have tense blisters within noninflamed skin, erosions, and scars in traumatized regions such as the dorsa of the hands, knuckles, elbows, knees, sacral area, and toes. This presentation thus resembles porphyria cutanea tarda (see Section 10) or hereditary epidermolysis bullosa.

- The *bullous pemphigoid–like presentation* is a widespread inflammatory vesiculo-bullous eruption where erythematous or even urticarial skin lesions are associated with tense bullae involving the trunk, central body, and skin folds in addition to the extremities (Fig. 6-20).

- *Cicatricial pemphigoid–like presentation* has prominent mucosal involvement—erosions and scarring in the mouth, esophagus, conjunctiva, anus, and vagina.

- The *IgA bullous dermatosis–like presentation* shows vesicles arranged in an annular fashion that are reminiscent of linear IgA bullous dermatosis, DH, or CBDC.

- Histopathology of lesional skin: subepidermal blisters with a clean separation between the epidermis and dermis.

- Immunopathology reveals linear IgG (plus IgA, IgM, factor B, and properdin) at the dermal-epidermal junction. If salt split-skin IIF is performed, circulating antibasement membrane zone antibodies bind the floor of the blister, in contrast to bullous pemphigoid where antibodies are bound to the roof.

- Antibodies in EBA sera will bind to a 290-kDa band in Western blots containing type VII collagen. An ELISA that is very specific for antibodies to type VII collagen is now available.

- *Treatment* of EBA is difficult, particularly in patients with the classic mechano-bullous presentation. Patients are refractory to high doses of systemic glucocorticoids, azathioprine, methotrexate, and cyclophosphamide, which are somewhat helpful in the inflammatory BP-like form of the disease. Some EBA patients improve on dapsone and high doses of colchicine. Supportive therapy is warranted in all patients with EBA. �

ICD-9 : 694.8 ○ ICD-10 : L12.3

FIGURE 6-20 **Epidermolysis bullosa acquisita**   This is a the bullous pemphigoid-like presentation with tense bullae, erosions, and crusts on an erythematous base. There is extensive postinflammatory pigmentation due to previous blistering.

MISCELLANEOUS INFLAMMATORY DISORDERS

PITYRIASIS ROSEA (PR)   ICD-9: 696.4 ○ ICD-10: L42

- Pityriasis rosea (PR) is an acute exanthematous eruption with a distinctive morphology and often with a characteristic self-limited course.

- Initially, a single (primary, or "herald") plaque lesion develops, usually on the trunk; 1 or 2 weeks later a generalized secondary eruption develops in a typical distribution pattern.

- The entire process remits spontaneously in 6 weeks.

- Reactivation of human herpesvirus (HHV) 7 and HHV-6 is the most probable cause.

EPIDEMIOLOGY AND ETIOLOGY

Age of Onset   10–43 years, but can occur rarely in infants and old persons.
Season   Spring and fall.
Etiology   There is good evidence that PR is associated with reactivation of HHV-7 or HHV-6, two closely related β-herpesviruses.

CLINICAL MANIFESTATION

Duration of Lesions   A single herald patch precedes the exanthematous phase; which develops over a period of 1–2 weeks. Pruritus—absent (25%), mild (50%), or severe (25%).

Skin Lesions   *Herald Patch*   80% of patients. Oval, slightly raised plaque or patch 2–5 cm, salmon-red, fine collarette scale at periphery; may be multiple (Fig. 7-1*B*).
Exanthem   Fine scaling papules and plaques with marginal collarette (Fig. 7-1*A*). Dull pink or tawny. Oval, scattered, with characteristic distribution with the long axes of the oval lesions following the lines of cleavage in a "Christmas tree" pattern (Image 7-1). Lesions usually confined to trunk and proximal aspects of the arms and legs. Rarely on face.

Atypical Pityriasis Rosea   Lesions may be present only on the face and neck. The primary plaque may be absent, may be the sole manifestation of the disease, or may be multiple. Most confusing are the examples of pityriasis rosea with vesicles or simulating erythema multiforme. This usually results from irritation and sweating, often as a consequence of inadequate treatment (*pityriasis rosea irritata*).

DIFFERENTIAL DIAGNOSIS

Multiple Small Scaling Plaques   *Drug eruptions* (e.g., captopril, barbiturates); *secondary syphilis* (obtain serology); *guttate psoriasis* (no marginal collarette); *small plaque parapsoriasis*; *erythema migrans* with secondary lesions; *erythema multiforme; tinea corporis.*

LABORATORY EXAMINATION

Dermatopathology   Patchy or diffuse parakeratosis, absence of granular layer, slight acanthosis, focal spongiosis, microscopic vesicles. Occasional dyskeratotic cells with an eosinophilic homogeneous appearance. Edema of dermis, homogenization of the collagen. Perivascular infiltrate mononuclear cells.

FIGURE 7-1 Pityriasis rosea *A.* Overview of exanthem of pityriasis rosea with the herald patch shown in B. There are papules and small plaques with oval configurations that follow the lines of cleavage. The fine scaling of the salmon-red papules cannot be seen at this magnification, while the collarette of the herald patch is quite obvious. *B.* Herald patch. An erythematous (salmon-red) plaque with a collarette scale on the trailing edge of the advancing border. Collarette means that scale is attached at periphery and loose toward the center of the lesion.

COURSE

Spontaneous remission in 6–12 weeks or less. Recurrences are uncommon.

MANAGEMENT

Symptomatic Oral antihistamines and/or topical antipruritic lotions for relief of pruritus. Topical glucocorticoids. May be improved by UVB phototherapy or natural sunlight exposure if treatment is begun in the first week of eruption. Short course of systemic glucocorticoids.

Herald patch

IMAGE 7–1   Pityriasis rosea: Distribution "Christmas tree" pattern on the back.

PARAPSORIASIS EN PLAQUES (PP)

- Rare eruptions with worldwide occurrence.
- Two types are recognized: small-plaque PP and large-plaque PP.
- Lesions are only slightly infiltrated, yellowish or fawn-colored patches. In small-plaque PP (SPP) lesions are small (<5 cm) round to oval or linear mostly on the trunk. Large-plaque PP (LPP) also oval or irregularly shaped and >5 cm. May be poikilodermatous.
- SPP does not progress to mycosis fungoides (MF). LPP, by contrast, exists on a continuum with patch-stage MF and can progress to overt MF.
- Treatment consists of topical glucocorticoids, phototherapy, or photochemotherapy (PUVA).

SMALL-PLAQUE PARAPSORIASIS (DIGITATE DERMATOSIS), SPP   ☐ ○
ICD-9:696.2 ∘ ICD-10:L41.3

CLINICAL MANIFESTATION

Gradual development over months. Rare pruritus. Middle age.

Skin Lesions   Round, oval, erythematous, yellowish or fawn-colored, only minimally elevated patches, <5 cm in diameter (Fig. 7-2*B*).

Slight scale and wrinkled surface with cigarette-paper appearance. Linear finger-like (digitate) shapes on trunk, proximal extremities, and buttocks, following lines of cleavage, giving appearance of a hug that left fingerprints (hence, *digital dermatosis*) (Fig. 7-2*A*). 🖉

DIFFERENTIAL DIAGNOSIS

Pityriasis rosea, large-plaque parapsoriasis, drug eruptions, nummular eczema, tinea corporis, mycosis fungoides.

FIGURE 7-2   Digitate dermatosis (small-plaque parapsoriasis)   *A.* The lesions are asymptomatic, yellowish or fawn-colored, very thin, well-defined, slightly scaly patches. They are oval and follow the lines of cleavage of the skin, giving the appearance of a "hug" that left fingerprints on the trunk. The long axis of these lesions often reaches more than 5 cm. ***B.*** Close up of smaller lesions showing wrinkling of surface.

LABORATORY EXAMINATION

Dermatopathology Spongiform dermatitis with focal areas of hyperkeratosis, parakeratosis, and exocytosis. In the dermis there are a mild superficial vascular lymphohistiocytic infiltrate (predominantly CD4+ T cells) and dermal edema.

MANAGEMENT

No treatment necessary, but patients should be reassured. Disease may be treated with lubricant or topical steroids. Broad-band phototherapy; UVB (311 nm) and PUVA are highly effective.

LARGE-PLAQUE PARAPSORIASIS (LPP)

☐ ◑   ICD-9:692.2 ∘ ICD-10:L41.4

CLINICAL MANIFESTATION

Gradual development over months and years, starting with one or two plaques. Pruritus is rare; the lesions may disappear after exposure to sun in the summer to recur in the fall and winter. Middle age.

Skin Lesions Barely elevated, erythematous, dusky-red, sometimes yellowish plaques that are actually patches (Fig. 7-3*A*), with or without slight atrophy and smooth or slightly scaling surface (Fig. 7-3*B*). Circular, >10 cm in diameter, or irregular and well defined; and randomly scattered on trunk, buttocks, breasts, or extremities.

DIFFERENTIAL DIAGNOSIS

Scaling Plaques "Early" stages of mycosis fungoides. The development of *infiltration* in the lesions, *atrophy*, and *poikilodermatous changes* are clues to early mycosis fungoides.

LABORATORY EXAMINATIONS

Dermatopathology Nonspecific or, later, a bandlike mononuclear cell infiltrate (CD4+) with atrophy of the epidermis, vacuolization of the basal cell layer, capillary dilatation. There are no atypical lymphocytes. Mild exocytosis. Predominance of CD4+ T cells, frequent CD7 antigen deficiency, and, in the epidermis, expression of class II HLA antigens.
Peripheral Blood Monoclonal T helper cells with skin-homing specificity can be detected.

COURSE AND PROGNOSIS

The lesions persist for life and can progress to mycosis fungoides (see Section 20).

MANAGEMENT

Topical Temporary remission with topical glucocorticoids.
Phototherapy Good responses to narrow-band 311-nm UVB or PUVA photochemotherapy.

FIGURE 7-3   Large-plaque parapsoriasis (parapsoriasis en plaques)   *A.* The lesions are asymptomatic, well-defined, rounded, slightly scaly, thin plaques or patches. The lesions can be larger than 10 cm and are light red-brown or salmon-pink. There may be atrophy in some areas. The lesions here are located on the extremities but they are more commonly noted on the trunk. These lesions must be carefully followed and repeated biopsies are necessary to detect mycosis fungoides. This entity may be considered as a prestage of mycosis fungoides. ***B.*** Close up of lesions showing minimal scaling and wrinkled surface.

A

B

LICHEN PLANUS (LP)   ICD-9 : 697.0 ∘ ICD-10 : L43

- Worldwide occurrence; incidence less than one percent, all races.

- LP is an acute or chronic inflammatory dermatosis involving skin and/or mucous membranes.

- Characterized by flat-topped (Latin *planus*, "flat"), pink to violaceous, shiny, pruritic polygonal papules. The features of the lesions have been designated as the four P's—papule, purple, polygonal, pruritic.

- Distribution: predilection for flexural aspects of arms and legs, can become generalized.

- In the mouth milky-white reticulated papules; may become erosive and even ulcerate.

- Main symptom: pruritus; in the mouth, pain.

- Therapy: topical and systemic glucocorticoids, cyclosporine.

EPIDEMIOLOGY AND ETIOLOGY

Age of Onset   30–60 years.
Sex   Females > males.
Race   Hypertrophic LP more common in blacks.
Etiology   Idiopathic in most cases but cell-mediated immunity plays a major role. Majority of lymphocytes in the infiltrate are CD8+ and CD45Ro+ (memory) cells. Drugs, metals (gold, mercury), or infection [hepatitis C virus (HCV)] result in alteration in cell-mediated immunity. There could be HLA-associated genetic susceptibility that would explain a predisposition in certain persons. Lichenoid lesions of chronic graft-versus-host disease (GVHD) of skin are indistinguishable from those of LP (see Section 21).

CLINICAL MANIFESTATION

Onset   Acute (days) or insidious (over weeks). Lesions last months to years, asymptomatic or pruritic; sometimes severe pruritus. Mucous membrane lesions are painful, especially when ulcerated.

Skin Lesions   Papules, flat-topped, 1 to 10 mm, sharply defined, shiny (Fig. 7-4). Violaceous, with white lines (Wickham striae) (Fig. 7-4A), seen best with hand lens after application of mineral oil. Polygonal or oval (Fig. 7-4B). Grouped (Figs. 7-4 and 7-5), annular, or disseminated scattered discrete lesions when generalized (Fig. 7-6). In dark-skinned individuals, postinflammatory hyperpigmentation is common. May present on lips (Fig. 7-7A) and in a linear arrangement after trauma (Koebner

or isomorphic phenomenon (Fig. 7-7B).
Sites of Predilection   Wrists [flexor (Fig. 7-4A)], lumbar region, shins [thicker, hyperkeratotic lesions (Fig. 7-5B)], scalp, glans penis (See Figs. 35-9, 35-10), mouth (Image 7-2). ✑

Variants
Hypertrophic   Large thick plaques arise on the foot, dorsum of hands (Fig. 7-5A), and shins (Fig. 7-5B); more common in black males. Although typical LP papule is smooth, hypertrophic lesions may become hyperkeratotic.
Atrophic   White-bluish, well-demarcated papules and plaques with central atrophy.
Follicular   Individual keratotic-follicular papules and plaques that lead to cicatricial alopecia. Spinous follicular lesions, typical skin and mucous membrane LP, and cicatricial alopecia of the scalp (See Figs. 32-19, 32-20) are called *Graham Little syndrome.* (See Section 32.)
Vesicular   Vesicular or bullous lesions may develop within LP patches or independent of them within normal-appearing skin. There are direct immunofluorescence findings consistent with bullous pemphigoid, and the sera of these patients contain bullous pemphigoid IgG autoantibodies (see Section 6). ✑
Pigmentosus   Hyperpigmented, dark-brown macules in sun-exposed areas and flexural folds. In Latin Americans and other dark-skinned populations. Significant similarity with ashy dermatosis (see Section 13).
Actinicus   Papular LP lesions arise in sun-exposed sites, especially the dorsa of hands and arms.
Ulcerative   LP may lead to therapy-resistant ulcers, particularly on the soles, requiring skin grafting. ✑

A

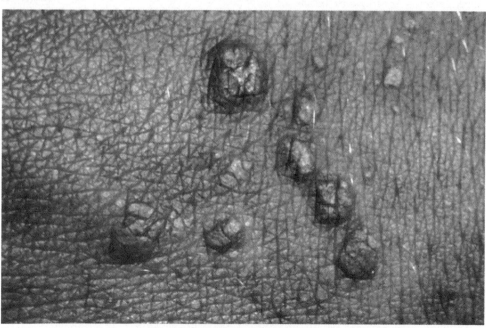

B

FIGURE 7-4   Lichen planus   *A.* Flat-topped, polygonal, sharply defined papules of violaceous color, grouped and confluent. Surface is shiny and, upon close inspection with a hand lens, fine white lines are revealed (Wickham striae, arrow). ***B.*** Close up of flat-topped shiny violaceous papules that are polygonal.

Mucous Membranes   Some 40–60% of individuals with LP have oropharyngeal involvement (see Section 34).

Reticular LP   Reticulate (netlike) pattern of lacy white hyperkeratosis on buccal mucosa (see Fig. 34-3), lips (Fig. 7-7*A*), tongue, gingiva; the most common pattern of oral LP.

Erosive or Ulcerative LP   Superficial erosion with/without overlying fibrin clot; occurs on tongue and buccal mucosa (see Fig. 34-3); shiny red painful erosion of gingiva (desquamative gingivitis) (see Fig. 34-5) or lips (Fig. 7-7*A*). Carcinoma may very rarely develop in mouth lesions. 🔎

Genitalia   Papular (see Figs. 35-9, 35-10) agminated, annular, or erosive lesions arise on penis (especially glans), scrotum, labia majora, labia minora, vagina.

Hair and Nails   *Scalp*   Follicular LP, atrophic scalp skin with scarring alopecia (See Figs. 32-19, 32-20). (See Section 32.)

Nails   Destruction of nail fold and nail bed with longitudinal splintering (see Fig. 33-10). 🔎

LICHEN PLANUS–LIKE ERUPTIONS

Lichen planus–like eruptions closely mimic typical LP, both clinically and histologically. They occur as a clinical manifestation of chronic GVHD, in dermatomyositis, and as cutaneous manifestations of malignant lymphoma but may also develop as the result of therapy with certain drugs and after industrial use of certain compounds (Table 7-1).

DIAGNOSIS AND DIFFERENTIAL DIAGNOSIS

Clinical findings confirmed by histopathology.

Skin Lesions   *Papular LP*   Chronic cutaneous lupus erythematosus, psoriasis, pityriasis rosea, eczematous dermatitis, lichenoid GVHD; single lesions: superficial basal cell carcinoma, Bowen disease (in situ squamous cell carcinoma).

Hypertrophic LP   Psoriasis vulgaris, lichen simplex chronicus, prurigo nodularis, stasis dermatitis, Kaposi sarcoma.

Drug-Induced LP   See Table 7-1.

Mucous Membranes   Leukoplakia, pseudomembranous candidiasis (thrush), HIV-associated hairy leukoplakia, lupus erythematosus, bite trauma, mucous patches of secondary syphilis, pemphigus vulgaris, bullous pemphigoid (see Section 34).

LABORATORY EXAMINATION

Dermatopathology   Inflammation with hyperkeratosis, increased granular layer, irregular acanthosis, liquefaction degeneration of the basal cell layer, and bandlike mononuclear infiltrate that hugs the epidermis. Keratinocyte apoptosis (colloid, Civatte bodies) is found at the dermal-epidermal junction. Direct immunofluorescence reveals heavy deposits of fibrin at the junction and IgM and, less frequently, IgA, IgG, and C3 in the colloid bodies.

COURSE

Cutaneous LP usually persists for months, but in some cases, for years; hypertrophic LP on the shins and oral LP often for decades. The incidence of oral squamous cell carcinoma in individuals with oral LP is increased (5%); patients should be followed at regular intervals.

MANAGEMENT

Local Therapy
Glucocorticoids Topical glucocorticoids with occlusion for cutaneous lesions. Intralesional triamcinolone (3 mg/mL) is helpful for symptomatic cutaneous or oral mucosal lesions and lips.

Cyclosporine and Tacrolimus Solutions   Retention "mouthwash" for severely symptomatic oral LP.

Systemic Therapy
Cyclosporine   In very resistant and generalized cases, 5 mg/kg per day will induce rapid remission, quite often not followed by recurrence.

Glucocorticoids   Oral prednisone is effective for individuals with symptomatic pruritus, painful erosions, dysphagia, or cosmetic disfigurement. A short, tapered course is preferred: 70 mg initially, tapered by 5 mg/day.

Systemic Retinoids (Acitretin)   1 mg/kg per day is helpful as adjunctive measure in severe (oral, hypertrophic) cases, but usually additional topical treatment is required.

PUVA Photochemotherapy
In individuals with generalized LP or cases resistant to topical therapy.

Other Treatments
Mycophenolate mofetil, heparin analogues (enoxaparin) in low doses have antiproliferative and immunomodulatory properties; azathioprine.

A B

FIGURE 7-5 Hypertrophic lichen planus **A.** Confluent hyperkeratotic papules and plaques on the dorsum of the hand of a light-colored man of African descent. Hyperkeratosis covers Wickham striae, and the characteristic violaceous color of the lesions can be seen only at the very margins. **B.** Hypertrophic lichen planus on the lower leg of a 50-year-old man of Arabian descent. Lesions form thick plaques of a dark brown violaceous color and have a hyperkeratotic surface.

TABLE 7-1   Agents Inducing Lichen Planus and Lichenoid Reactions

Common inducers
- Gold salts
- β blockers
- Antimalarials
- Thiazide diuretics
- Furosemide
- Spironolactone
- Penicillamine

Less common
- ACE inhibitors
- Calcium channel blockers
- Sulfonylurea
- Nonsteroidal anti-inflammatory drugs
- Ketoconazole
- Tetracycline
- Phenothiazine
- Sulfasalazine
- Carbamazepine
- Lithium

Less common
- Antituberculosis drugs
- Iodides
- Radiocontrast media
- Methyldopa
- Heavy metals

Inducers of lichen planus by contact
- Color film developers
- Dental restorative materials
- Musk ambrette
- Nickle
- Gold

Inducers of photodistributed lichenoid eruption
- 5-Fluorouracil
- Carbamazepine
- Chlorpromazine
- Diazoxide
- Ethambutol

Inducers of photodistributed lichenoid eruption (*continued*)
- Pyritinol
- Quinine
- Quinidine
- Tetracycline
- Thiazide
- Furosemide

Inducers of oral lichen planus and lichenoid eruption
- Allopurinol
- ACE inhibitors
- Cyanamide
- Dental restorative materials
- Gold salts
- Ketoconazole
- Nonsteroidal anti-inflammatory drugs
- Penicillamines
- Sulfonylurea

ACE, angiotensin-converting enzyme.

FIGURE 7-6   Disseminated lichen planus   A shower of disseminated papules on the trunk and the extremities (not shown) in a 45-year-old Filipino. Due to the ethnic color of the skin, the papules are not as violaceous as in Caucasians but have a brownish hue.

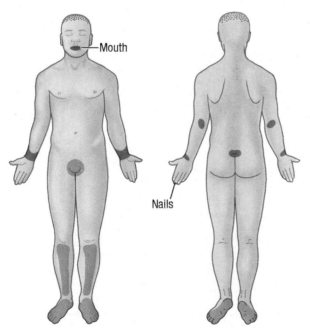

IMAGE 7–2   Lichen planus: predilection sites.

A

B

FIGURE 7-7   Lichen planus   *A.* Silvery-white, confluent, flat-topped papules on the lips. Note: Wickham striae (arrow). B. Lichen planus, Koebner phenomenon. Linear arrangement of flat-topped, shiny papules that erupted after scratching.

GRANULOMA ANNULARE (GA)   ICD-9:695.89 ∘ ICD-10:L92.0   ■ ○→◑

- A common self-limited, asymptomatic, chronic dermatosis of the dermis.
- Usually occurs in children and young adults.
- Consists of papules in an annular arrangement, commonly arising on the dorsa of the hands and feet, elbows, and knees.
- Sometimes becomes generalized in distribution.
- Unless disfiguring, no treatment is an option.

EPIDEMIOLOGY

Common.
Age of Onset   Children and young adults.
Sex   Female:male ratio 2:1.

ETIOLOGY AND PATHOGENESIS

Unknown. An immunologically mediated necrotizing inflammation that surrounds blood vessels, altering collagen and elastic tissue. Generalized GA may be associated with diabetes mellitus.

CLINICAL MANIFESTATION

Duration months to years. Usually asymptomatic and only cosmetic disfigurement.

Skin Lesions   Firm, smooth, shiny, beaded, dermal papules and plaques, 1–5 cm annular, arciform plaques with central depression (see Fig. 7-8A, B), skin-colored, violaceous, erythematous. *Subcutaneous GA* (rare): painless, skin-colored, deep dermal or subcutaneous, solitary or multiple nodules.
Distribution   Isolated lesion, particularly on dorsum of hand, finger, or lower arm (Fig. 7-8A), multiple lesions on extremities and trunk (Fig. 7-8B), or generalized (papular; older patients) (Fig. 7-8C). Subcutaneous lesions are located near joints, palms and soles, buttocks.

Variants

- *Perforating* lesions are very rare and mostly on the hands; central umbilication followed by crusting and ulceration; this type was associated with diabetes in one series.
- May rarely involve fascia and tendons, causing sclerosis.
- Generalized GA: in this form a search for diabetes mellitus should be made.

DIFFERENTIAL DIAGNOSIS

GA is important because of its similarity to more serious conditions.
Papular Lesions and Plaques   Necrobiosis lipoidica, papular sarcoid, lichen planus, lymphocytic infiltrate of Jessner.
Subcutaneous Nodules   Rheumatoid nodules: confusion can occur because of the similar pathology of GA and rheumatic nodule or rheumatoid nodules. Also subcutaneous fungal infections such as sporotrichosis and NTM (*M. marinum*).
Annular Lesions   Tinea, erythema migrans, sarcoid, lichen planus.

LABORATORY EXAMINATION

Dermatopathology   Foci of chronic inflammatory and histiocytic infiltrations in superficial and mid-dermis, with necrobiosis of connective tissue surrounded by a wall of palisading histiocytes and multinucleated giant cells.

COURSE

The disease disappears in 75% of patients in 2 years. Recurrences are common (40%), but they also disappear.

MANAGEMENT

GA is a local skin disorder and not a marker for internal disease, and spontaneous remission is the rule. *No treatment is an option if the lesions are not disfiguring.* Lesions may resolve after biopsy.
Topical Therapy   *Topical Glucocorticoids* - Applied under plastic occlusion or hydrocolloid.
Intralesional Triamcinolone   3 mg/mL into lesions is very effective.
Cryospray   Superficial lesions respond to liquid nitrogen, but atrophy may occur.
PUVA Photochemotherapy   Effective in generalized GA.
Systemic Glucocorticoids   Effective in generalized GA, but recurrences common.

A

B

C

FIGURE 7-8 Granuloma annulare ***A.*** Confluent, pearly-white papules forming a well-demarcated ring with central regression. ***B.*** Multiple granulomata forming annular and semicircular plaques with central regression on the arm of a 45-year-old man of African extraction. ***C.*** Disseminated granuloma annulare in a Caucasian. Multiple, well-defined, pearly-white papules, some of which show a central depression.

MORPHEA   ICD-9 : 701.0 ∘ ICD-10 : L94.0

- A localized and circumscribed cutaneous sclerosis characterized by early violaceous, later ivory-colored, hardened skin.
- May be solitary, linear, generalized, and, rarely, accompanied by atrophy of underlying structures.
- It is unrelated to systemic scleroderma.

- *Synonyms:* Localized scleroderma, circumscribed scleroderma.

EPIDEMIOLOGY AND ETIOLOGY

Incidence   Rare between the ages of 20 and 50; in linear morphea, earlier. Pansclerotic Morphea, a disabling disorder, usually starts before age 14.

Sex   Females are affected about three times as often as males, including children. Linear scleroderma is the same in males and females.

Etiology   Unknown. At least some patients (predominantly in Europe) with classic morphea have sclerosis due to *Borrelia burgdorferi* infection, and, if not too sclerotic, the lesions can disappear with prolonged courses of oral antibiotics. Pigmentation, however, persists. Morphea has been noted after x-irradiation for breast cancer. Morphea is not related to systemic scleroderma.

CLASSIFICATION OF VARIOUS TYPES OF LOCALIZED SCLERODERMA

- *Circumscribed:* plaques or bands
- *Macular:* small, confluent patches
- *Linear scleroderma:* upper or lower extremity
- *Frontoparietal (en coup de sabre)*
- *Generalized morphea*
- *Pansclerotic:* involvement of dermis, fat, fascia, muscle, bone.

CLINICAL MANIFESTATION

Symptoms   Usually none. No history of Raynaud phenomenon. Linear and pansclerotic morphea can result in major facial or limb asymmetry, flexion contractures, and disability. Can cause severe disfigurement.

Skin Findings   *Plaques*—circumscribed, indurated, hard, but poorly defined areas of skin; 2–15 cm in diameter, round or oval, often better felt than seen. Initially, purplish or mauve.

In time, surface becomes smooth and shiny after months to years, ivory with lilac-colored edge "lilac ring" (Fig. 7-9). May have hyper- and hypopigmentation in involved sclerotic areas (Fig. 7-10). Rarely, lesions become atrophic and hyperpigmented without going through a sclerotic stage (atrophoderma of Pasini and Pierini) (see Fig. 7-13*B*).

Distribution

Circumscribed: Trunk (Fig. 7-9), limbs, face, genitalia; less commonly, axillae, perineum, areolae.

Generalized: Initially on trunk (upper, breasts, abdomen) (Fig. 7-10) thighs.

Linear: Usually on extremity (Fig. 7-11) or *frontoparietal*—scalp and face (Fig. 7-12); here it may resemble a scar from a strike with a saber (*en coup de sabre*).

Macular: Small (<3 mm) macular patches, confluent (Fig. 7-13*A*); clinically indistinguishable from lichen sclerosus et atrophicus (see p. 142).

Atrophic: Atrophoderma of Pasini and Pierini (Fig. 7-13*B*).

Pansclerotic: On trunk (Fig. 7-14) or extremities.

Mouth   With linear morphea of head, may have associated hemiatrophy of tongue.

Hair and Nails   Scarring alopecia with scalp plaque. Particularly with linear morphea of the head. Nail dystrophy in linear lesions of extremity or in pansclerotic morphea.

General Examination
Morphea around joints and linear morphea may lead to flexion contractures. Pansclerotic morphea is associated with atrophy and fibrosis of muscle (Fig. 7-14). Extensive involvement of trunk may result in restricted respiration. With linear morphea of the head (Fig. 7-12), there may be associated atrophy of ocular structures and atrophy of bone. *Note:* morphea may be associated with lichen sclerosus et atrophicus.

FIGURE 7-9 Morphea This is an indurated ivory-colored, shiny plaque with a lilac-colored, ill-defined border (arrows). Most lesions are better felt than seen because they are indurated.

DIAGNOSIS AND DIFFERENTIAL DIAGNOSIS

Clinical, confirmed by biopsy. Sclerotic plaque associated with *B. burgdorferi* infection, acrodermatitis chronica atrophicans, progressive systemic sclerosis, lichen sclerosus et atrophicus, eosinophilic fasciitis, toxic oil syndrome, eosinophilia-myalgia syndrome associated with L-tryptophan ingestion, scleredema, Parry-Romberg syndrome (hemiatrophy).

LABORATORY EXAMINATIONS

Serology Appropriate serologic testing to rule out *B. burgdorferi* infection.

Dermatopathology Epidermis appears normal to atrophic with loss of rete ridges. Dermis edematous with homogeneous and eosinophilic collagen. Slight infiltrate, perivascular or diffuse; lymphocytes, plasma cells, macrophages. Later, dermis thickened with few fibroblasts

FIGURE 7-10   Morphea   Irregular, brownish, indurated lesions with focal ivory-colored macular lesions on the left hip. Similar lesions were also found on the chest and on the back.

and dense collagen; inflammatory infiltrate at dermal-subcutis junction; dermal appendages disappear progressively. Pansclerotic lesions show fibrosis and disappearance of subcutaneous tissue, with fibrosis involving fascia. Silver stains should be performed to rule out *B. burgdorferi* infection. Histopathology distinct from that of lichen sclerosus et atrophicus.

DIAGNOSIS

Clinical diagnosis, usually confirmed by skin biopsy.

COURSE

May be slowly progressive; "burn out" and spontaneous remissions can rarely occur.

MANAGEMENT

There is no effective treatment for morphea, but some reports of treatment are as follows:

Morphea-Like Lesions Associated with Lyme Borreliosis   In patients with early involvement, there may be a reversal of sclerosis with high-dose parenteral penicillin or ceftriaxone; treatment given in several courses over a time span of several months. Best response if combined with oral glucocorticoids.

Phototherapy with UVA-1 (340–400 nm)   In our experience, the treatment is not easy or very successful because of the prolonged irradiation times and the disfiguring hyperpigmentation of the irradiated areas.

FIGURE 7-11 Linear Morphea
Indurated, ivory-white lesion extending from upper thigh to the dorsum of the foot. Induration is pronounced, and in the region above the knee it extends to the fascia (pan-sclerotic morphea). If progressive, it will limit the movement of the joint.

FIGURE 7-12 Linear morphea, "en coup de sabre" Two linear, partially ivory-white (on the scalp) and hyperpigmented (on the forehead) depressed lesions extending from the crown of the head, where they have led to alopecia, over the forehead to the orbita. They look like scars after strikes with a saber, hence the French designation. These lesions can extend to the bone and rarely to the dura mater.

A

B

FIGURE 7-13   Macular form of morphea   *A.* There are multiple, shining, ivory-white macules with conflu-ence leading to a reticulated pattern. These lesions are rather superficial and therefore less indurated. An impor-tant differential diagnosis is lichen sclerosus et atrophicus. ***B.*** Atrophic, hyperpigmented form of morphea (called atrophoderma of Pasini and Pierini). There is a diffuse brown and sharply defined hyperpigmentation with a less pigmented follicular pattern. These lesions are atrophic and not indurated.

FIGURE 7-14   Pansclerotic morphea   This type affects all layers of the skin including the fascia and even muscle. The skin is glistening, hyperpigmented, and hard as wood. It is obvious that pansclerotic morphea leads to considerable functional impairment. If these lesions occur on the upper trunk, they can impair excursion of the chest and thus breathing.

LICHEN SCLEROSUS et ATROPHICUS (LSA)
ICD-9 : 701.0 ◦ ICD-10 : L90.0

- LSA is a chronic atrophic disorder mainly of the anogenital skin of females but also of males and of the general skin.

- A disease of adults, but also occurring in children 1–13 years of age. Females ten times more often affected than males.

- Whitish, ivory or porcelain-white, sharply demarcated, individual papules may become confluent, forming *plaques* (Fig. 7-15). Surface of lesions may be elevated or in the same plane as normal skin; older lesions may be depressed. Dilated pilosebaceous or sweat duct orifices filled with keratin plugs (dells); if plugging is marked, surface appears hyperkeratotic (Fig. 7-15C).

- *Bullae* and *erosions* occur and *purpura* is often a characteristic and identifying feature (Fig. 7-15B); *telangiectasia*.

- Lesions occur on general skin or on the genitalia. On vulva, hyperkeratotic plaques may become erosive, macerated; vulva may become atrophic, shrunken, especially clitoris and labia minora, with vaginal introitus reduced in size (see Fig. 35-16). Fusion of labia minora and majora.

- In uncircumcised males, prepuce first shows ivory white confluent papules (see Figs. 35-12, 35-14) but then becomes sclerotic and cannot be retracted (*phimosis*). Glans appears ivory or porcelain-white, semitransparent, resembling mother-of-pearl with admixed purpuric hemorrhages.

- Nongenital LSA usually asymptomatic; genital symptomatic. In females, vulvar lesions may be sensitive, especially while walking; pruritus; painful, especially if erosions are present; dysuria; dyspareunia. In males, recurrent balanitis, acquired phimosis.

- The histopathology is diagnostic with a dense lymphocytic infiltrate hugging the initially hypertrophic and later, atrophic epidermis and then sinking down into the dermis, being separated from the epidermis by an edematous, structureless subepidermal zone.

- The etiology of LSA is unknown, but reports from Europe have documented an association of DNA of *Borrelia* spp. with LSA in cases from Germany and Japan; DNA of the spirochetes detected in these patients was not found in any of the American samples.

- The course of LSA waxes and wanes. In girls it may undergo spontaneous resolution; in women it leads to atrophy of the vulva and in men to phimosis. Patients should be checked for the occurrence of squamous cell carcinoma of the vulva and penis.

- Management is very important, as this disease can cause a devastating atrophy of the labia minora and clitoral hood. Potent topical *glucocorticoid preparations* (clobetasol propionate) have proved effective for genital LSA and should be used for 6–8 weeks only. Patients should be monitored for signs of glucocorticoid-induced atrophy. *Pimecrolimus* and *tacrolimus* are almost as effective. *Topical androgens* are less used now because they can sometimes cause a clitoral hypertrophy. *Systemic therapy*: hydrochloroquine, 125–150 mg/d, for weeks to a few months (monitor for ocular side effects).

- In males, *circumcision* relieves symptoms of phimosis and in some cases can result in remission.

FIGURE 7-15 Lichen sclerosus et atrophicus **A.** Multiple, ivory-white, indurated and slightly hyper-keratotic papules on the chest of a 42-year-old woman. **B.** The ivory-white papules of lichen sclerosus here have merged to form a superficially indurated and also atrophic plaque of sharp margination. Hemorrhage in the center of this plaque is an important differential diagnostic sign to the macular form of morphea. **C.** Lichen sclerosus in the groin region of a 60-year-old female. Here the papules have merged to form a large hyper-keratotic plaque with sharp definition. There are also crusts resulting from erosions.

PIGMENTED PURPURIC DERMATOSES (PPD)   □ ○

- PPD are distinguished by their clinical characteristics, having identical dermatopathologic findings, and include:
  - *Schamberg disease*, also known as progressive pigmented purpuric dermatosis or progressive pigmentary purpura
  - *Majocchi disease*, also known as purpura annularis telangiectodes
  - *Gougerot-Blum disease*, also known as pigmented purpuric lichenoid dermatitis or purpura pigmentosa chronica
  - *Lichen aureus*, also known as lichen purpuricus.

- Clinically, each entity shows recent pinpoint cayenne pepper–colored hemorrhages associated with older hemorrhages and hemosiderin deposition. Capillaritis histologically.

- PPD are significant only if they are a cosmetic concern to the patient; they are important because they are often mistaken as manifestations of vasculitis or thrombocytopenia.

- *Synonym*: Capillaritis of unknown cause.

ICD-9: 709.1 ○ ICD-10: L81.7

EPIDEMIOLOGY AND ETIOLOGY

Age of Onset   30–60 years; uncommon in children.
Sex   More common in males.
Etiology   Unknown. Primary process believed to be cell-mediated immune injury with subsequent vascular damage and erythrocyte extravasation. Other etiologic factors: pressure, trauma, drugs (acetaminophen, ampicillin-carbromal, diuretics, meprobamate, nonsteroidal anti-inflammatory drugs, zomepirac sodium).
Onset and Duration   Insidious, slow to evolve except drug-induced variant, which may develop rapidly and be more generalized in distribution. Persists for months to years. Most drug-induced purpuras resolve more quickly after discontinuation of the drug. Usually asymptomatic but may be mildly pruritic. It can be quite cosmetically disfiguring. Any pruritus probably related to dermatitis (asteatotic, atopic, or stasis) on lower legs.

CLINICAL MANIFESTATION

Schamberg Disease   Discrete clusters of pinhead-sized red macules and barely palpable papules become confluent, coalescing into patches (Fig. 7-16). Diascopy reveals pinpoint hemorrhages (hence the term *purpura*). New lesions are red; older lesions tan to brown, representing degradation of extravasated erythrocytes with the formation of hemosiderin. Overall color impression: reddish brown, "cayenne pepper" (Fig. 7-16). Lower extremities (especially pretibial and on ankles) but may extend proximally to lower trunk and to upper extremities. Usually bilateral but may be unilateral. Uncommonly, generalized.

Majocchi Disease   Essentially an annular form of Schamberg disease with telangiectasias (Fig. 7-17). An arciform variant has also been described.
Gougerot-Blum Disease   Lichenoid papules, plaques, macules in association with lesions of Schamberg disease.
Lichen Aureus   Solitary or few patches or plaques, rust-colored, purple, or golden, arising on the extremities or trunk.

LABORATORY EXAMINATIONS

Dermatopathology   Epidermal involvement varies, but dermal pathology (capillaritis) with extravasation of erythrocytes, hemosiderin pigment–laden macrophages (more extensive in lichen aureus), mild perivascular and interstitial lymphohistiocytic infiltrate in reticular dermis is common to all. Immunofluorescence is variable and nonspecific.

DIAGNOSIS AND DIFFERENTIAL DIAGNOSIS

Nonpalpable Purpura   Chronic venous insufficiency with clotting abnormalities, glucocorticoid usage, cutaneous T cell lymphoma; dysproteinemias, nummular eczema, old fixed drug eruption, parapsoriasis, poikiloderma vasculare atrophicans, primary amyloidosis, scurvy, senile purpura, stasis dermatitis, thrombocytopenia, trauma.
Palpable Purpura   Leukocytoclastic vasculitis. Thrombocytopenic purpura.

FIGURE 7-16   Pigmented purpuric dermatosis: Schamberg disease   Multiple discrete and confluent nonpalpable, nonblanching purpuric lesions on the leg. Acute microhemorrhages resolve with deposition of hemosiderin, creating a brown peppered stain.

COURSE

Chronic (months to years), slow to evolve and resolve; spontaneous resolution has occurred. In lesions of long standing, hemosiderin deposits resolve very slowly (months to years). Almost all cases due to drugs clear within months after discontinuation of the offending agent.

MANAGEMENT

Symptomatic   Long-standing lesions are cosmetically disfiguring, and patients may choose to treat these lesions. Topical low- and middle-potency glucocorticoid preparations may inhibit new purpuric lesions. Systemic tetracycline or minocycline (50 mg twice daily) are effective. PUVA is effective in severe forms. *Supportive stockings required in all forms.*

FIGURE 7-17   Pigmented purpuric dermatosis: Majocchi disease   Multiple nonpalpable, nonblanching purpuric lesions arranged in annular configurations. Note: disfiguring dark brown discoloration of old lesions.

PITYRIASIS LICHENOIDES (ACUTE AND CHRONIC) (PL)
ICD-9:696.2 ∘ ICD-10:L41.0/L41.1   ☐ ○

- PL is an eruption of unknown etiology, characterized clinically by successive crops of a wide range of morphologic lesions.
- Classified into an acute form, pityriasis lichenoides et varioliformis acuta (PLEVA, Mucha-Habermann disease), and a chronic form, pityriasis lichenoides chronica (PLC, guttate parapsoriasis of Juliusberg).

- However, most patients have lesions of PLEVA and PLC simultaneously.
- PLEVA is important because it can be mistaken for lymphomatoid papulosis (see Section 20).
- *Synonym:* Guttate parapsoriasis.

EPIDEMIOLOGY AND ETIOLOGY

Age of Onset   Adolescents and young adults.
Sex   More common in males than females.
Etiology   Unknown.

CLINICAL MANIFESTATION

Lesions tend to appear in crops over a period of weeks or months. Uncommonly, patients with an acute onset of the disorder may have symptoms of an acute infection with fever, malaise, and headache. Cutaneous lesions are usually asymptomatic but may be pruritic or sensitive to touch. Lesions may heal with significant scarring and postinflammatory pigmentation. Especially in that it occurs in adolescents and young adults.

Skin Lesions   Initially, randomly distributed, bright-red edematous papules (i.e., lichenoides), less commonly vesicles, which undergo central necrosis with hemorrhagic crusting (i.e., varioliformis, hence the designation *PLEVA*) (Fig. 7-18*A* and *B*). In the chronic form (PLC), scaling papules of reddish-brown color and a central mica-like scale are seen (Fig. 7-18*C*). Postinflammatory hypo- or hyperpigmentation often present after lesions resolve. PLEVA may heal with depressed or elevated scars.
Distribution Randomly arranged, most commonly on trunk, proximal extremities but also generalized, including palms and soles. ✌
Oral and Genital Mucosa   Inflammatory papules and necrotic lesions may occur.

LABORATORY EXAMINATION

Dermatopathology   *Epidermis*: spongiosis, keratinocyte necrosis, vesiculation, ulceration; exocytosis or erythrocytes within epidermis. *Dermis*: Edema, chronic inflammatory cell infiltrate in wedge shape extending to deep reticular dermis; hemorrhage; vessels congested with blood; endothelial cells swollen.

DIAGNOSIS AND DIFFERENTIAL DIAGNOSIS

Clinical diagnosis is confirmed by skin biopsy. Differential diagnosis: varicella, guttate psoriasis, lymphomatoid papulosis.

COURSE AND PROGNOSIS

New lesions appear in successive crops. PLC tends to resolve spontaneously after 6–12 months. In some cases, relapses after many months or years.

MANAGEMENT

Most patients do not require any therapeutic intervention. Oral erythromycin and tetracycline are reported to be effective in some cases. Ultraviolet radiation (whether natural sunlight or broad-band UVB), 311-nm UVB, and PUVA are the treatments of choice if oral antibiotics fail after a 2-week trial.

FIGURE 7-18   Pityriasis lichenoides et varioliformis acuta (PLEVA)   A. Randomly distributed red papules of different size, some of which show hemorrhagic crusting. In this 5-year-old child the eruption appeared in
crops over a period of 10 days. **B. PLEVA** lesions in a 38-year-old Indonesian man. Lesions are more hyperpigmented and there is considerable scaling and crusting. **C. Pityriasis lichenoids chronica (PLC)** Discrete papules
with fine mica-like scales which become more visible after slight scraping. In contrast to PLEVA (Fig. 7-18A and B),
there is no hemorrhagic crusting.

ERYTHEMA MULTIFORME SYNDROME (EM)   ■ ◐

- A common reaction pattern of blood vessels in the dermis with secondary epidermal changes.
- Manifests clinically as characteristic erythematous iris-shaped papular and vesiculobullous lesions.
- Typically involving the extremities (especially the palms and soles) and the mucous membranes.

- Benign course with frequent recurrences.
- Most cases related to herpes simplex virus (HSV) infection
- Recurrences can be prevented by long-term anti-HSV medication.

ICD-9:695.1 ○ ICD-10:L51

EPIDEMIOLOGY

Age of Onset   50% under 20 years.
Sex   More frequent in males than in females.

ETIOLOGY

A cutaneous reaction to a variety of antigenic stimuli, most commonly to herpes simplex.
Infection   Especially following herpes simplex, *Mycoplasma*.
Drugs   Sulfonamides, phenytoin, barbiturates, phenylbutazone, penicillin, allopurinol.
Idiopathic   Probably also due to undetected herpes simplex or *Mycoplasma*.

CLINICAL MANIFESTATION

Evolution of lesions over several days. May have history of prior EM. May be pruritic or painful, particularly mouth lesions. In severe forms constitutional symptoms such as fever, weakness, malaise.

Skin Lesions   Lesions may develop over ≥10 days. Macule → papule (1–2 cm) → vesicles and bullae in the center of the papule; (Fig. 7-19). Dull red. *Iris* or *targetlike lesions* result and are typical (Figs. 7-19 and 7-20). Localized to hands and face or generalized (Figs. 7-21 and 7-22). Bilateral and often symmetric.
Sites of Predilection   Dorsa of hands, palms, and soles; forearms; feet; face (Figs. 7-20 and 7-21); elbows and knees; penis (50%) and vulva (Image 7-3).
Mucous Membranes   Erosions with fibrin membranes; occasionally ulcerations: lips (Fig. 7-20), oropharynx, nasal, conjunctival (Fig. 7-21), vulvar, anal.
Other Organs   Eyes, with corneal ulcers, anterior uveitis. ✏

COURSE

Mild Forms (EM Minor)   Little or no mucous membrane involvement; vesicles but no bullae or systemic symptoms. Eruption usually confined to extremities, face, classic target lesions (Figs. 7-19 and 7-20). Recurrent EM minor is usually associated with an outbreak of herpes simplex preceding it by several days.
Severe Forms (EM Major)   Most often occurs as a drug reaction, always with mucous membrane involvement; severe, extensive, tendency to become confluent and bullous, positive Nikolsky sign in erythematous lesions (Fig. 7-21). Systemic symptoms: fever, prostration. Cheilitis and stomatitis interfere with eating; vulvitis and balanitis with micturition. Conjunctivitis can lead to keratitis and ulceration; lesions also in pharynx and larynx.

LABORATORY EXAMINATION

Dermatopathology   Inflammation characterized by perivascular mononuclear infiltrate, edema of the upper dermis; apoptosis of keratinocytes with focal epidermal necrosis and subepidermal bulla formation. In severe cases, complete necrosis of epidermis as in toxic epidermal necrolysis. (See Section 8.)

DIAGNOSIS AND DIFFERENTIAL DIAGNOSIS

The target-like lesion and the symmetry are quite typical, and the diagnosis is not difficult.
Acute Exanthematic Eruptions   Drug eruption, psoriasis, secondary syphilis, urticaria, generalized Sweet syndrome. Mucous membrane lesions may present a difficult differential diagnosis: bullous diseases, fixed drug eruption, acute lupus erythematosus, primary herpetic gingivostomatitis.

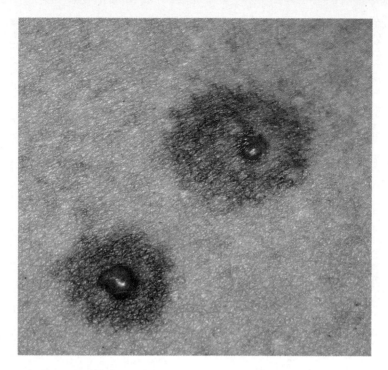

FIGURE 7-19 Erythema multiforme Iris or target lesions on the lower arm of a 15-year-old. These are sharply defined flat papules with a central vesicle.

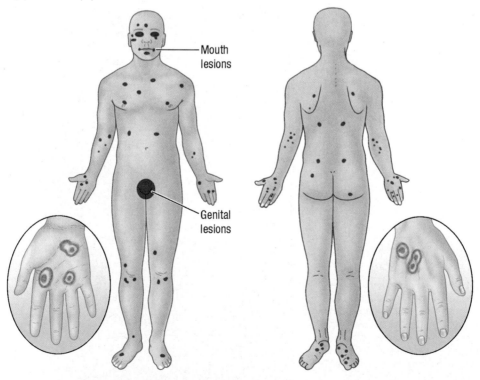

IMAGE 7-3 Erythema multiforme predilection sites and distribution.

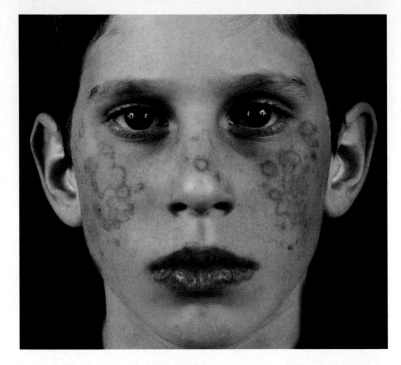

FIGURE 7-20   Erythema multiforme: minor   Multiple, confluent, target-like papules on the face of a 12-year-old boy. The target morphology of the lesions is best seen on the lips.

FIGURE 7-21   Erythema multiforme: major   Erythematous, confluent, target-like papules, plaques, and erosions on the trunk, the arms, and the face. Facial lesions are erosive and crusted. There is erosive cheilitis indicating mucosal involvement, and there is conjunctivitis.

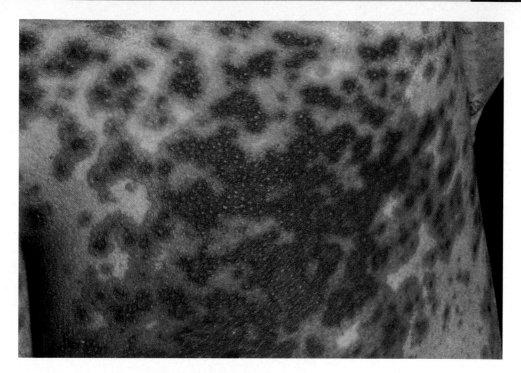

FIGURE 7-22 Erythema multiforme: major   Multiple, target lesions have coalesced, and erosions will develop. This patient had fever and mucosal involvement of mouth, conjunctiva, and genitalia.

MANAGEMENT

Prevention   Control of herpes simplex using oral valacyclovir or famciclovir may prevent development of recurrent EM.

Glucocorticoids   In severely ill patients, systemic glucocorticoids are usually given (prednisone, 50–80 mg/d in divided doses, quickly tapered), but their effectiveness has not been established by controlled studies.

ERYTHEMA NODOSUM (EN) SYNDROME
ICD-9:695.2 ∘ ICD-10:L52

- EN is an important and common acute inflammatory/immunologic reaction pattern of the subcutaneous fat.
- Characterized by the appearance of painful nodules on the lower legs.

- Lesions are bright red and flat but nodular upon palpation.
- Often fever and arthritis.
- Multiple and diverse etiologies.

EPIDEMIOLOGY AND ETIOLOGY

The most common type of panniculitis, with a peak incidence at 20–30 years, but any age may be affected. Three to six times more common on females than males.

Etiology   EN is not a disease but a cutaneous reaction pattern to various etiologic agents. Etiologic associations include infections, drugs, and other inflammatory/granulomatous diseases, notably sarcoidosis (Table 7-2).

CLINICAL MANIFESTATION

Painful, tender lesions, usually of a few days' duration, are accompanied by fever, malaise, and arthralgia (50%), most frequently of ankle joints. Other symptoms, depending on etiology.

Skin Lesions   Indurated, very tender nodules (3–20 cm), not sharply marginated (Fig. 7-23), deep seated in the subcutaneous fat, mostly on the anterior lower legs, bilateral but not symmetric. Nodules are bright to deep red and are appreciated as such only upon palpation. The term *erythema nodosum* best describes the skin lesions: *they look like erythema but feel like nodules* (Fig. 7-23). Lesions are oval, round, arciform; as they age, they become violaceous, brownish, yellowish, green, like resolving hematomas. Lesions may also occur on knees and arms but only rarely on the face and on the neck. 🕮

LABORATORY EXAMINATIONS

Hematology   Elevated erythrocyte sedimentation rate (ESR), C-reactive protein elevated, leukocytosis.

Bacterial Culture   Culture throat for group A β-hemolytic streptococcus, stool for *Yersinia*.

Imaging   Radiologic examination of the chest and gallium scan are important to rule out or prove sarcoidosis.

Dermatopathology   Acute (polymorphonuclear) and chronic (granulomatous) inflammation in the panniculus and around blood vessels in the septum and adjacent fat. It is a septal panniculitis.

COURSE

Spontaneous resolution occurs in 6 weeks, with new lesions erupting during that time. Course depends on the etiology. Lesions never break down or ulcerate and heal without scarring.

DIAGNOSIS AND DIFFERENTIAL DIAGNOSIS

Diagnosis rests on clinical criteria, may be supported by histopathology. Differential diagnosis includes all other forms of panniculitis, panarteritis nodosa, nodular vasculitis, pretibial myxedema, nonulcerated gumma, and lymphoma.

MANAGEMENT

Symptomatic   Bed rest or compressive bandages (lower legs), wet dressings.

Anti-Inflammatory Treatment   Salicylates, nonsteroidal anti-inflammatory drugs. Systemic glucocorticoids—response is rapid, but their use is indicated only when the etiology is known (and infectious agents are excluded).

TABLE 7-2   Causes of Erythema Nodosum[a]

Infections	Other
Bacterial	**Drugs**
Streptococcal infections; tuberculosis, yersiniosis Other: *Salmonella, Campylobacter, Shigella,* brucellosis, psittacosis, *Mycoplasma*	Sulfonamides; bromides and iodides; Oral contraceptives Other: minocycline, gold salts, penicillin, salicylates
Fungal	**Malignancies**
Coccidioidomycosis, blastomycosis, histoplasmosis, sporotrichosis, dermatophytosis	Hodgkin and non-Hodgkin lymphoma, leukemia, renal cell carcinoma
Viral	**Other**
Infectious mononucleosis, hepatitis B, orf, herpes simplex	Sarcoidosis Inflammatory bowel disease: ulcerative colitis, Crohn disease
Other	
Amebiasis, giardiasis, ascariasis	Behçet disease

[a]for a more complete list of etiologic factors in EN, see L Requena et al, in K, Wolff et al (eds,): *Fitzpatrick's Dermatology in General Medicine,* 7th ed, New York, McGraw-Hill, 2008, p 569–585

FIGURE 7-23   Erythema nodosum   Indurated, very tender, inflammatory nodules mostly in the pretibial region. Lesions are seen as red, ill-defined erythemas but palpated as deep-seated nodules, hence the designation. In this 49-year-old female there was also fever and arthritis of the ankle joints following an upper respiratory tract infection. The throat cultures yielded β-hemolytic streptococci.

OTHER PANNICULITIDES   ICD-9 : 729.3 ∘ ICD-10 : M79.3   □ ◑ → ●

- Panniculitis is the term used to describe diseases where the major focus of inflammation is in the subcutaneous tissue. In general, panniculitis presents as an erythematous or violaceous nodule in the subcutaneous fat that may be tender or not, that may ulcerate or heal without scarring, and that may be soft or hard on palpation. Thus, the term *panniculitis* describes a wide spectrum of disease manifestations, although diagnostic clues can be derived from the history, distribution, or characteristics of the lesions.

- An accurate diagnosis requires an ample deep skin biopsy that should reach down to or even beyond the fascia. The panniculitides are classified histologically as lobular or septal, depending on where the disease process begins. However, a sharp distinction between septal and lobular is often not possible. Panniculitis may also be associated with vasculitis, but in most cases there is no vasculitis. A simplified classification of panniculitis is given in Table 7-3.

- Only idiopathic lobular panniculitis (Pfeiffer-Weber-Christian disease), pancreatic panniculitis, and α^1 antitrypsin-deficiency panniculitis are briefly discussed here. Other diseases in which panniculitis occurs are referred to in the table.[1]

- *Idiopathic lobular panniculitis* (ILP), which occurs predominantly in females 30–60 years of age, but can also occur in childhood, manifests as crops of subcutaneous inflammatory and tender nodules, primarily on the lower extremities but also on the trunk and elsewhere (Fig. 7-24). Occasionally, lesions can break down, discharging an oily yellow-brown liquid; generally accompanied by malaise, fatigue, fever, arthralgia, and myalgia. There may be focal necrosis in the intravisceral and perivisceral fat of internal organs, including the mesenteric and omental fat, pericardium, and pleura. Organ involvement may present as hepatomegaly, abdominal pain, nausea, and vomiting.

- The etiology is unknown. *Note:* many cases of ILP have been reclassified as other manifestations of lobular panniculitis and there is a now growing doubt that ILP exists as an entity.

- *Pancreatic panniculitis* is characterized clinically by painful erythematous nodules and plaques that may fluctuate and occur at any site, with a predilection for abdomen, buttocks, legs (Fig. 7-25). Frequently accompanied by arthritis and polyserositis. Associated with either pancreatitis or pancreatic carcinoma. It affects middle-aged to elderly individuals, males more often than females. History: alcoholism, abdominal pain, weight loss, or recent-onset diabetes mellitus. Skin biopsy reveals lobular panniculitis, and after biopsy liquefied fat drains from the biopsy site. General examination may reveal pleural effusion, ascites, and arthritis, particularly of the ankles.

- Laboratory: eosinophilia, hyperlipasemia, hyperamylasemia, and increased excretion of amylase and/or lipase in the urine. The pathophysiology is probably a breakdown of subcutaneous fat caused by enzymes (amylase, trypsin, lipase) released into the circulation from a diseased pancreas. The course and prognosis depend on the type of pancreatic disease. Treatment is directed at the underlying pancreatic disorder.

- α_1 *Antitrypsin-deficiency panniculitis* is also characterized by recurrent tender, erythematous, subcutaneous nodules ranging from 1 to 5 cm and located predominantly on the trunk and the proximal extremities, very much like those shown in Fig. 7-25. Nodules break down and discharge a clear serous or oily fluid. Diagnosis is substantiated by a decrease in the level of serum α_1 antitrypsin, and treatment consists of oral dapsone in doses up to 200 mg/d. The intravenous infusion of human α_1-proteinase inhibitor concentrate has been shown to be very effective.

[1]The reader is also referred to L.Requena et al, in K Wolff et al (eds): *Fitzpatrick's Dermatology in General Medicine,* 7th ed. New York, McGraw-Hill, 2008, p 569.

TABLE 7-3 Simplified Classification of Panniculitis

	Lobular Panniculitis	Septal Panniculitis
Neonatal	Sclerema neonatorum, neonatal subcutaneous fat necrosis	
Physical	Cold, trauma	
Drugs	Poststeroid panniculitis	Erythema nodosum
Idiopathic	Idiopathic lobular panniculitis (Pfeiffer-Weber-Christian) syndrome	Eosinophilic fasciitis
		Eosinophilia myalgia syndrome
Pancreatic	With pancreatitis or carcinoma of the pancreas	
Panniculitis with other systemic disease	Lupus erythematosus; sarcoidosis, lymphoma, histiocytic cytophagic panniculitis	Scleroderma
With vasculitis	Nodular vasculitis	Thrombophlebitis, panarteritis nodosa
Metabolic deficiency	α_1-antitrypsin deficiency	

FIGURE 7-24 Idiopathic lobular panniculitis in a 5-year-old boy   Although lesions usually arise on the lower extremities, they may manifest as crops of subcutaneous inflammatory and tender nodules also on the trunk and on the face. Usually occurring in females 30 to 60 years old, it can also appear in children, as is the case with this boy. No etiologic agent was found. There was hepatomegaly, and abdominal pain. The patient responded to glucocorticoids but had recurrences.

FIGURE 7-25   Pancreatic panniculitis There are multiple, painful, erythematous nodules and plaques that fluctuate on the lower extremities, but similar lesions were also found on the trunk and on the buttocks.

PYODERMA GANGRENOSUM (PG)   ICD-9:686.01 ○ ICD-10:L88   ☐ ●

- PG is a rapidly evolving, idiopathic, chronic, and severely debilitating skin disease.
- It is characterized by neutrophilic infiltration and destruction of tissue.
- It occurs most commonly in association with a systemic disease, especially chronic ulcerative colitis.
- It also occurs with arthritis, hematologic dyscrasias, and malignancy but may occur also alone.

- It is characterized by the presence of irregular, boggy, blue-red ulcers with undermined borders surrounding purulent necrotic bases.
- There is no laboratory test that establishes the diagnosis.
- The mainstays of treatment are immunosuppressive or modulating agents.

EPIDEMIOLOGY

Rare, prevalence unknown. All age groups affected with a peak between 40 and 60 years. Slight preponderance of females.

ETIOLOGY AND PATHOGENESIS

Unknown. Although called pyoderma, it does not have a microbial etiology. PG is counted among the neutrophilic dermatoses because of the massive neutrophilic infiltrates within the skin.

CLINICAL MANIFESTATION

Two Types *Acute:* acute onset with painful hemorrhagic pustule or painful nodule either de novo or after minimal trauma. *Chronic:* slow progression with granulation and hyperkeratosis. Less painful.

Skin Lesions *Acute:* Superficial hemorrhagic pustule surrounded by erythematous halo; very painful (Fig. 7-26*A*). Breakdown occurs with ulcer formation, whereby ulcer borders are dusky-red or purple, irregular and raised, undermined, boggy with perforations that drain pus (Fig. 7-26*B*). The base of the ulcer is purulent with hemorrhagic exudate, partially covered by necrotic eschar (Fig. 7-27), with or without granulation tissue. Pustules both at the advancing border and in the ulcer base; a halo of erythema spreads centrifugally at the advancing edge of the ulcer (Figs. 7-26*B* and 7-27). *Chronic:* lesions may slowly progress, grazing over large areas of the body and exhibiting massive granulation within the ulcer from the outset (Fig. 7-28) and crusting and even hyperkeratosis on the margins (Fig. 7-29, page 160). Lesions are usually solitary but may be multiple and form clusters that coalesce. Most common sites: lower extremities (Figs. 7-26*B* and 7-29) > buttocks > abdomen (Fig. 7-27) > face (Fig. 7-28). Healing of ulcers results in thin atrophic cribriform scars.
Mucous Membranes Rarely, aphthous stomatitis–like lesions; massive ulceration of oral mucosa and conjuctivae.
🖉

General Examination
Patient may appear ill.

Associated Systemic Diseases
Up to 50% of cases occur without associated disease. Remainder of cases associated with large- and small-bowel disease (Crohn disease, ulcerative colitis), diverticulosis (diverticulitis), arthritis, paraproteinemia and myeloma, leukemia, active chronic hepatitis, Behçet syndrome.

LABORATORY EXAMINATIONS

There is no single diagnostic test.
ESR Variably elevated.
Dermatopathology Not diagnostic. Neutrophilic inflammation with abscess formation and necrosis.

DIAGNOSIS AND DIFFERENTIAL DIAGNOSIS

Clinical findings plus history and course; confirmed by nonspecific dermatopathology showing neutrophilic inflammation with abscesses and necrosis. Differential diagnosis: ecthyma and ecthyma gangrenosum, atypical mycobacterial infection, clostridial infection, deep mycoses, amebiasis, leishmaniasis, bromoderma, pemphigus vegetans, stasis ulcers, Wegener granulomatosis.

COURSE AND PROGNOSIS

Untreated, course may last months to years, but spontaneous healing can occur. Ulceration may extend rapidly within a few days or slowly. Healing may occur centrally with peripheral extension. New ulcers may appear as older lesions resolve. Pathergy, i.e., slight trauma initiating new PG lesion, noted at sites of minor trauma, biopsy, or needle sticks.

MANAGEMENT

With Associated Underlying Disease Treat underlying disease.
For PG High doses of oral glucocorticoids or IV glucocorticoid pulse therapy (1–2 g/d prednisolone) may be required. Sulfasalazine (particularly in cases associated with Crohn disease), sulfones, cyclosporine, and, more recently, infliximab, etanercept, adalimumab have been shown to be effective in uncontrolled studies.
Topical In singular lesion, topical tacrolimus ointment or intralesional triamcinolone.

FIGURE 7-26   Pyoderma gangrenosum   A. The initial lesion is a hemorrhagic nonfollicular pustule surrounded by an erythematous halo and is very painful. **B.** Lesions rapidly enlarge and break down centrally as shown here. Note: erythematous halo around the individual lesions. There is accompanying edema of the right foot. Lesions are extremely painful.

FIGURE 7-27 Pyoderma gangrenosum A very large ulcer with raised bullous undermined borders covered with hemorrhagic and fibrinous exudate. When the bullae are opened, pus is drained. This lesion arose acutely and spread rapidly following laparatomy for an ovarian carcinoma.

FIGURE 7-28 Pyoderma gangrenosum: chronic type The lesion involves the upper eyelid and represents an ulcer with elevated granulating base with multiple abscesses. The lesion later spread slowly to involve the temporal and zygomatic regions and eventually healed under systemic glucocorticoid treatment, leaving a thin cribriform scar that did not impair the function of the eyelid.

FIGURE 7-29 **Pyoderma gangrenosum: chronic type** This lesion, which appears like a plaque, spread only slowly but was also surrounded by an erythematous border. The lesion is crusted and hyperkeratotic and is less painful than the lesions in acute pyoderma gangrenosum.

SWEET SYNDROME (SS) ICD-9:695.89 ∘ ICD-10:L98.2

- An uncommon, acute and recurrent, cytokine-induced skin reaction associated with various etiologies.
- Painful plaque-forming inflammatory papules, often with massive exudations giving the appearance of vesiculation (pseudovesiculation).
- Associated with fever, arthralgia, and peripheral leukocytosis.
- Associated with infection, malignancy, or drugs.
- Treatment: systemic glucocorticoids, potassium iodide, dapsone, or colchicine.
- *Synonym:* Acute febrile neutrophilic dermatosis.

EPIDEMIOLOGY AND ETIOLOGY

Age of Onset Most 30–60 years.
Sex Women > men.
Etiology Unknown, possibly hypersensitivity reaction. Inflammatory bowel disease. SS is counted among the neutrophilic dermatoses.
Associated Disorders Febrile upper respiratory tract infection. In some cases associated with *Yersinia* infection. Hematologic malignancy; drugs: granulocyte colony-stimulating factor (G-GSF).

CLINICAL MANIFESTATION

Prodromes are febrile upper respiratory tract infections. Gastrointestinal symptoms (diarrhea), tonsillitis, influenza-like illness, 1–3 weeks before skin lesions. Lesions tender/painful. Fever (not always present), headache, arthralgia, general malaise.

Skin Lesions Bright red, smooth, tender papules (2–4 mm in diameter) that coalesce to form irregular, sharply bordered, inflammatory plaques (Fig. 7-30A). Pseudovesiculation: intense edema gives the appearance of vesiculation (Figs. 7-30A and 7-31A). Lesions

A   B

FIGURE 7-30   Sweet syndrome   A. An erythematous, edematous plaque that has formed from coalescing papules on the right cheek. The border of the plaque looks as if composed of vesicles, but palpation reveals that it is solid (pseudovesiculation). This lesion occurred in a 26-year-old female following an upper respiratory infection, and the patient also had fever and leukocytosis. **B.** A similar eruption in a 52-year-old female. Note: multiple, coalescing, inflammatory and very exudative papules on the neck. This patient also had leukocytosis and fever. In addition, there is vitiligo.

A   B

FIGURE 7-31   Sweet syndrome   A. Coalescing exudative papules that look like vesicles. Upon palpation lesions were solid. **B.** Bullous type of Sweet syndrome. These are true bullae and pustules. The patient had myelomonocytic leukemia.

arise rapidly, and as they evolve, central clearing may lead to annular or arcuate patterns. Tiny, superficial pustules may occur. If associated with leukemia, bullous lesions may occur (Fig. 7-31*B*) and lesions may mimic pyoderma gangrenosum. May present as a single lesion or multiple lesions, asymmetrically distributed. Most common on face (Fig. 7-30*A*), neck (Fig. 7-30*B*), and upper extremities but also on lower extremities, where lesions may be deep in the fat and thus mimic panniculitis or erythema nodosum. Truncal lesions are uncommon but widespread, and generalized forms occur.
Mucous Membranes   ± Conjunctivitis, episcleritis.

General Examination
Patient may appear ill. There may be involvement of cardiovascular, central nervous system, gastrointestinal, hepatic, musculoskeletal, ocular, pulmonary, renal, and splenic organs.

LABORATORY EXAMINATIONS

Complete Blood Count   Leukocytosis with neutrophilia (not always persistent).
ESR   Elevated.
Dermatopathology   Diagnostic. Epidermis usually normal but may show subcorneal pustulation. Massive edema of papillary body, dense leukocytic infiltrate with starburst pattern in mid-dermis, consisting of neutrophils with occasional eosinophils/lymphoid cells. Leukocytoclasia, nuclear dust, but other signs of vasculitis absent. ± Neutrophilic infiltrates in subcutaneous tissue.

DIAGNOSIS AND DIFFERENTIAL DIAGNOSIS

Clinical impression plus skin biopsy confirmation.
Very Edematous Acute Plaques   Erythema multiforme, erythema nodosum, prevesicular herpes simplex infection, preulcerative pyoderma gangrenosum.

COURSE AND PROGNOSIS

Untreated, lesions enlarge over a period of days or weeks and eventually resolve without scarring. With oral prednisone, lesions resolve within a few days. Recurrences occur in 50% of patients, often in previously involved sites. Some cases follow *Yersinia* infection or are associated with acute myelocytic leukemia, transient myeloid proliferation, various malignant tumors, ulcerative colitis, benign monoclonal gammopathy; some follow drug administration, most commonly by GSF.

MANAGEMENT

Rule out sepsis.
Prednisone   30–50 mg/d, tapering in 2–3 weeks; some, but not all, patients respond to dapsone, 100 mg/d, or to potassium iodide. Some to colchicine.
Antibiotic Therapy   Clears eruption in *Yersinia*–associated cases; in all other cases antibiotics are ineffective.

GRANULOMA FACIALE (GF) ICD-9:686.1 ○ ICD-10:L92.2 □ ○

- A rare, localized inflammatory disease of unknown etiology, clinically characterized by reddish-brown papules or small plaques primarily in the face.
- Single or multiple lesions with characteristic orange peel-like surface (Fig. 7-32).

- Histologically, chronic leukocytoclastic vasculitis with eosinophils, fibrin deposition, and fibrosis.
- Therapy: topical glucocorticoids; dapsone.

FIGURE 7-32 Granuloma faciale: classic presentation A single, sharply defined, brown plaque with a characteristic orange peel-like surface.

SEVERE AND LIFE-THREATENING SKIN ERUPTIONS IN THE ACUTELY ILL PATIENT

EXFOLIATIVE ERYTHRODERMA SYNDROME (EES) □→□ ◑→●

- EES is a serious, at times life-threatening, reaction pattern of the skin characterized by generalized and uniform redness and scaling involving practically the entire skin.
- It is associated with fever, malaise, shivers, and generalized lymphadenopathy, and fever.
- Two stages, acute and chronic, merge one into the other. In the acute and subacute phases, there is rapid onset of generalized vivid red erythema and fine branny scales; the patient feels hot and cold, shivers, and has fever. In chronic EES, the skin thickens, and scaling continues and becomes lamellar.

- There is a loss of scalp and body hair, and the nails become thickened and separated from the nail bed (onycholysis).
- There may be hyperpigmentation or patchy loss of pigment in patients whose normal skin color is brown or black.
- The most frequent preexisting skin disorders are (in order of frequency) psoriasis, atopic dermatitis, adverse cutaneous drug reaction, lymphoma, allergic contact dermatitis, and pityriasis rubra pilaris.

ICD-9: 695.9

[See "Sézary Syndrome" (Section 20) for a special consideration of this form of EES.]

EPIDEMIOLOGY

Age of Onset Usually >50 years; in children, EES usually results from pityriasis rubra pilaris or atopic dermatitis.

Sex Males > females.

ETIOLOGY

Some 50% of patients have history of preexisting dermatosis, which is recognizable only in the acute or subacute stage. Most frequent preexisting skin disorders are (in the order of frequency) psoriasis, atopic dermatitis, adverse cutaneous drug reactions, cutaneous T cell lymphoma, allergic contact dermatitis, and pityriasis rubra pilaris (Table 8-1). Drugs most commonly implicated in EES are shown in Table 8-2. In 20% of patients it is not possible to identify the cause by history or histology.

TABLE 8-1 Etiology of Exfoliative Dermatitis in Adults

Cause[a]	Average Percent[b]
Undetermined or unclassified	23
Psoriasis	23
Atopic dermatitis, eczema	16
Drug allergy	15
Lymphoma, leukemia	11
Allergic contact dermatitis	5
Seborrheic dermatitis	5
Stasis dermatitis with "id" reaction	3
Pityriasis rubra pilaris	2
Pemphigus foliaceus	1

[a]For a complete list of diseases associated with EES, see exfoliative dermatitis picture gallery in the online version. ◪
[b]As collated from the literature.

Source: Abbreviated from MH Jih et al, in IM Freedberg et al (eds): *Fitzpatrick's Dermatology in General Medicine,* 6th ed. New York, McGraw-Hill, 2003.

PATHOGENESIS

The metabolic response to exfoliative dermatitis may be profound. Large amounts of warm blood are present in the skin due to the dilation of capillaries, and there is considerable heat dissipation through insensible fluid loss and by convection. Also, there may be high-output cardiac failure; the loss of scales through exfoliation can be considerable, up to 9 g/m^2 of body surface per day, and this may contribute to the reduction in serum albumin and the edema of the lower extremities so often noted in these patients.

CLINICAL MANIFESTATION

Depending on the etiology, the acute phase may develop rapidly, as in a drug reaction, lymphoma, eczema, or psoriasis. At this early acute stage it is still possible to identify the preexisting dermatosis. There is fever, pruritus, fatigue, weakness, anorexia, weight loss, malaise, feeling cold, shivers.

Appearance of Patient   Frightened, red, "toxic," may be malodorous.

Skin Lesions   Skin is red, thickened, scaly. Dermatitis is uniform involving the entire body surface (Figs. 8-1 to 8-3), except for pityriasis

---

TABLE 8-2   Drugs that Cause Exfoliative Dermatitis[a]

Allopurinol[b]	Codeine	Mercurials	Sulfasalazine
Aminoglycosides	Cyanamide	Mesna	Sulfonamides
Aminophylline	Dapsone	Methylprednisolone	Sulfonylureas
Amiodarone	Dideoxyinosine	Minocycline	
Amonafide	Diflunisal	Mitomycin C	Tar preparations
Ampicillin	Diphenylhydantoin	Omeprazole	Terbinafine
Antimalarials	Ephedrine	Penicillin	Terbutaline
Arsenicals	Ethambutol	Pentostatin	Thalidomide
Aspirin	Ethylenediamine	Peritrate and	Thiacetazone
		glyceryl trinitrate	
Aztreonam	Etretinate	Pheneturide	Thiazide diuretics
Bactrim	Fluorouracil	Phenolphthalein	Ticlopidine
Barbiturates	GM-CSF	Phenothiazines	Timolol maleate
Bromodeoxyuridine	**Gold**	Phenylbutazone	eyedrops
Budenoside	Herbal medications	Phenytoin	Tobramycin
Calcium channel	Indeloxazine	Phototherapy	Tocainide
blockers	hydrochloride		
Captopril	Indinavir	Plaquenil	Trimetrexate
Carbamazepine	Interleukin 2	Practolol	Trovafloxacin
Carboplatin	Iodine	**Quinidine**	Tumor necrosis
Cefoxitin	Isoniazid	Ranitidine	factor α
Cephalosporins	Isosorbide dinitrate	Retinoids	Vancomycin
Cimetidine	Lansoprazole	Ribostamycin	Yohimbine
Cisplatin	Lidocaine	Rifampicin	Zidovudine
Clodronate	**Lithium**	St. John's wort	
Clofazamine	Mefloquine	Streptomycin	

[a]For a more extensive list of drugs implicated in EES, see exfoliative dermatitis syndrome picture gallery in the online version. 🔲
[b]The more commonly implicated agents are listed in bold.

Source: MH Jih, A Kimyai-Asadi, and IM Freedberg, in IM Freedberg et al. (eds): *Fitzpatrick's Dermatology in General Medicine*, 6th ed. New York. McGraw-Hill, 2003. p.487.

rubra pilaris, where EES spares sharply defined areas of normal skin (see Fig. 5-7). Thickening leads to exaggerated skin folds (Figs. 8-2 and 8-3); scaling may be fine and branny and may be barely perceptible (Fig. 8-2) or large, up to 0.5 cm, and lamellar (Fig. 8-1).

Palms and Soles Usually involved, with massive hyperkeratosis and deep fissures in pityriasis rubra pilaris, Sézary syndrome, and psoriasis.

Hair Telogen effluvium, even alopecia, except for EES arising in eczema or psoriasis.

Nails Thickening of nail plates, onycholysis, shedding of nails.

Pigmentation In chronic EES there may be hyperpigmentation or patchy loss of pigment in patients whose normal skin is brown or black.

General Examination
Lymph nodes generalized, rubbery, and usually small; enlarged in Sézary syndrome. Edema of lower legs and ankles.

LABORATORY EXAMINATIONS

Chemistry Low serum albumin and increase in gammaglobulins; electrolyte imbalance; acute-phase proteins increased.

Hematology Leukocytosis.

Bacterial Culture *Skin*: rule out secondary *Staphylococcus aureus* infection. *Blood*: rule out sepsis.

Dermatopathology Depends on type of underlying disease. Parakeratosis, inter- and intracellular edema, acanthosis with elongation of the rete ridges, and exocytosis of cells. There is edema of the dermis and a chronic inflammatory infiltrate.

Imaging CT scans or MRI should be used to find evidence of lymphoma.

Lymph Node Biopsy When there is suspicion of lymphoma.

DIAGNOSIS

Diagnosis is not easy, and the history of the preexisting dermatosis may be the only clue.

Also, pathognomonic signs and symptoms of the preexisting dermatosis may help, e.g., dusky-red color in psoriasis and yellowish-red in pityriasis rubra pilaris; typical nail changes of psoriasis; lichenification, erosions, and excoriations in atopic dermatitis and eczema; diffuse, relatively nonscaling palmar hyperkeratoses with fissures in cutaneous T cell lymphoma (CTCL) and pityriasis rubra pilaris; sharply demarcated patches of noninvolved skin within the erythroderma in pityriasis rubra pilaris; massive hyperkeratotic scale of scalp, usually without hair loss in psoriasis and with hair loss in CTCL and pityriasis rubra pilaris; in the latter and in CTCL, ectropion may occur.

COURSE AND PROGNOSIS

Guarded, depends on underlying etiology. Despite the best attention to all details, patients may succumb to infections or, if they have cardiac problems, to cardiac failure ("high-output" failure) or, as was often the case in the past, to the effects of prolonged glucocorticoid therapy.

MANAGEMENT

This is an important medical problem that should be dealt with in a modern inpatient dermatology facility with experienced personnel. The patient should be hospitalized in a single room, at least for the beginning workup and during the development of a therapeutic program. The hospital room conditions (heat and cold) should be adjusted to the patient's needs; most often these patients need a warm room with many blankets.

Topical Water baths with added bath oils, followed by application of bland emollients.

Systemic Oral glucocorticoids for remission induction but not for maintenance; *systemic and topical therapy as required by underlying condition.*

Supportive Supportive cardiac, fluid, electrolyte, protein replacement therapy as required.

FIGURE 8-1 **Exfoliative dermatitis: psoriasis** There is universal erythema, thickening of the skin, and heavy scaling. This patient had psoriasis as suggested by the large silvery white scales and the scalp and nail involvement not seen in this illustration. The patient had fatigue, weakness, malaise, and was shivering. It is quite obvious that such massive scaling can lead to protein loss and the maximal dilatation of skin capillaries to considerable heat dissipation and high-output cardiac failure

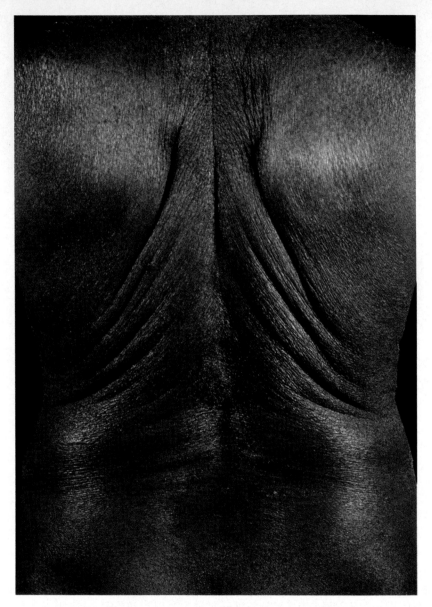

FIGURE 8-2 **Exfoliative dermatitis: drug-induced** This is generalized erythroderma with thickening of skin resulting in increased skin folds, universal redness, a fine brawny scaling. This patient had developed erythroderma following the injection of gold salts for rheumatoid arthritis.

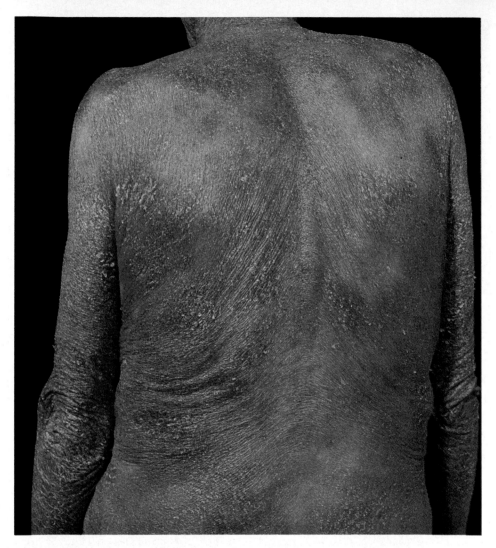

FIGURE 8-3   Exfoliative dermatitis: cutaneous T cell lymphoma   There is universal erythema, thickening, and scaling. Note that in contrast to erythroderma shown in Figs. 8-1 and 8-2 the degree of erythema and thickness is not uniform and the redness has a brownish hue. In addition, this elderly patient had hair loss, massive involvement of palms and soles with diffuse hyperkeratoses, cracks, and fissures. Generalized lymphadenopathy was also present.

RASHES IN THE ACUTELY ILL FEBRILE PATIENT   □ ●

- The sudden appearance of a rash and fever cause anxiety for the patient. Medical advice is sought immediately and often in the emergency units of hospitals; about 10% of all patients seeking emergency medical care have a dermatologic problem.

- The diagnosis of an acute rash with a fever is a clinical challenge (Figs. 8-4 and 8-5) If a diagnosis is not established promptly in certain patients [e.g., those having septicemia (Fig. 8-6)], lifesaving treatment may be delayed.

- The cutaneous findings alone are often diagnostic before confirmatory laboratory data are available. As in problems of the acute abdomen, the results of some laboratory tests, such as microbiologic cultures, may not be available immediately. On the basis of a differential diagnosis, appropriate therapy—whether antibiotics or glucocorticoids—may be started. Furthermore, prompt diagnosis and isolation of the patient with a contagious disease, which may have serious consequences, prevent spread to other persons. For example, varicella in adults (see Figs. 27-39 and 27-40) rarely can be fatal. Contagious diseases presenting with rash and fever as the major findings include *viral infections* (Fig. 8-5), enterovirus, and parvovirus infections (see Fig. 27-24*A, B*) and *bacterial infections* [streptococcal (see Fig. 24-48),

staphylococcal (see Fig. 24-40), meningococcal (see Figs. 24-50, 24-51), typhoid, and syphilis (see Fig. 30-21)].

- The physical diagnosis of skin eruptions is a discipline based mainly on precise identification of the type of skin lesion. The physician must not only identify and classify the *type* of skin lesion but also look for additional morphologic clues such as the *configuration* (annular? iris?) of the individual lesion, the *arrangement* (zosteriform? linear?) of the lesions, the *distribution pattern* (exposed areas? centripetal or centrifugal? mucous membranes?).

- In the *differential diagnosis* of exanthems it is important to determine, by history, the *site of first appearance* [the rash of Rocky Mountain spotted fever characteristically appears first on the wrists and ankles (see Figs. 26-1, 26-2)], and very important is the *temporal evolution* of the rash. [Measles (see Figs. 8-5 and 27-22) spreads from head to toes in a period of 3 days, while the rash of rubella (see Fig. 27-21) spreads rapidly in 24 to 48 h from head to toes and then sequentially clears—first face, then trunk, and then limbs.]

- Although there may be some overlap, the differential diagnostic possibilities may be grouped into five main categories according to the type of lesion (Table 8-3).

LABORATORY TESTS AVAILABLE FOR QUICK DIAGNOSIS

The physician should make use of the following laboratory tests immediately or within 8 h:

1 *Direct smear from the base of a vesicle.* This procedure, known as the *Tzanck test*, is described in the Introduction. Smears are examined for acantholytic cells, giant acanthocytes, and/or multinucleated giant cells (see Fig. 27-27).

2 *Viral culture*, negative stain (electron microscopy), polymerase chain reaction for infections with herpes viruses, direct fluorescence (DIF) technique.

3 *Gram stain of aspirates or scraping.* This is essential for proper diagnosis of pustules. Organisms can be seen in the lesions of acute meningococcemia, rarely in the skin lesions of gonococcemia and ecthyma gangrenosum.

4 *Touch preparation.* This is especially helpful in deep fungal infections and leishmaniasis. The dermal part of a skin biopsy specimen is touched repeatedly to a glass slide; the touch preparation is *immediately* fixed in 95% ethyl alcohol. Special stains are then performed, and the slide examined for organisms in the cytology laboratory.

5 *Biopsy of the skin lesion.* All purpuric lesions should be biopsied. Inflammatory dermal nodules and most ulcers should be biopsied (at base and margin) and a portion of tissue minced and cultured for bacteria and fungi. A 3- to 4-mm trephine and local anesthesia are used. In many laboratories the biopsy specimen can be processed within 8 h if necessary. In gangrenous cellulitis (see Section 24) frozen sections of a deep biopsy will verify the diagnosis in minutes.

FIGURE 8-4   Generalized fixed drug eruption: tetracycline.   Prostrated, 59-year-old woman with fever. Multiple confluent violaceous red erythematous areas, some of which later became bullous.

FIGURE 8-5   Generalized rash with fever: measles   Young woman with high fever, cough, conjunctivitis, and a confluent maculopapular eruption in the edematous face. The rash also involves the trunk and the extremities. The patient has measles.

TABLE 8-3   Generalized Eruptions in the Acutely Ill Patient: Diagnosis According to Type of Lesion[a]

Generalized Eruptions Manifested by Macules, Papules	Generalized Eruptions Manifested by Wheals, Plaques	Generalized Eruptions Manifested by Vesicles, Bullae, or Pustules	Generalized Eruptions Manifested by Purpuric Macules, Purpuric Papules, or Purpuric Vesicles	Diseases Manifested by Widespread Erythema ± Papules Followed by Desquamation
Drug hypersensitivities	Serum sickness	Drug	Drug hypersensitivities	Drug hypersensitivities
Acute HIV syndrome	Sweet syndrome	hypersensitivities	Meningococcemia[b]	Staphylococcal
Erythema infectiosum	Acute urticaria	Allergic contact	(acute or chronic)	scalded-skin
(parvovirus B19)	Erythema	dermatitis from	Gonococcemia[b]	syndrome
Cytomegalovirus,	marginatum	plants	Staphylococcemia	Toxic shock syndrome
primary infection		Rickettsialpox	*Pseudomonas*	Kawasaki syndrome
Epstein-Barr virus,		Gonococcemia	bacteremia	Graft-versus-host
primary infection		Varicella	Subacute bacterial	reaction
Exanthem subitum		(chickenpox)[c]	endocarditis	Erythroderma
(HHV 6)		Eczema herpeticum[c]	Enterovirus infections	(exfoliative
		Enterovirus infections	(echovirus, Coxsackie)	dermatitis)
Measles (rubeola)		(Coxsackie),	Rickettsial diseases:	
German measles (rubella)[d]		including hand-foot-	Rocky Mountain	
Enterovirus infections		and-mouth disease	spotted fever	
(echovirus and Coxsackie)		Toxic epidermal	Typhus, louse-borne	
Adenovirus infections		necrolysis	(epidemic)	
Scarlet fever		Smallpox or variola	"Allergic" vasculitis[b]	
Ehrlichiosis		Staphylococcal	Disseminated	
Typhoid fever		scalded-skin	intravascular	
Secondary syphilis		syndrome	coagulation (purpura	
Typhus, murine (endemic)		Erythema multiforme	fulminans[b])	
Rocky Mountain spotted		Kawasaki disease	*Vibrio* infections	
fever (early lesions)[d]		von Zumbusch		
Other spotted fevers		pustular psoriasis		
Disseminated deep fungal		Acute graft-versus-		
infection in immuno-		host reaction		
compromised patients				
Erythema multiforme				
Systemic lupus erythematosus				
Acute graft-versus-host reaction				

[a]With regard to the detailed morphologies, the reader is
referred to the
respective sections.
[b]Often present as infarcts.

[c]Umbilicated vesicles.
[d]May have arthralgia or musculoskeletal pain.
[e]Leading to large areas of black necrosis.

6 *Blood and urine examinations.* Blood culture, rapid serologic tests for syphilis, and serology for lupus erythematosus require 24 h. Examination of urine sediment may reveal red cell casts in allergic vasculitis.

7 *Dark-field examination.* In the skin lesions of secondary syphilis, repeated examination of papules may show *Treponema pallidum.* The dark-field examination is not reliable in the mouth because nonpathogenic organisms are almost impossible to differentiate from *T. pallidum*, but a lymph node aspirate can be subjected to dark-field examination.

FIGURE 8-6 Generalized purpura necrosis and fever: DIC 54-year-old woman with fever, prostration, and extensive geographic infarctions on the face, the trunk, and the extremities. This is disseminated intravascular coagulation: purpura fulminans following sepsis after abdominal surgery.

STEVENS-JOHNSON SYNDROME (SJS) AND TOXIC EPIDERMAL NECROLYSIS (TEN) ICD-9:695.1 ∘ ICD-10:L51.1/51.2 ☐ ●

- SJS and TEN are acute life-threatening muco-cutaneous reaction characterized by extensive necrosis and detachment of the epidermis.

- They are severe variants of an identical pathologic process and differ only in the percentage of body surface involved.

- Either idiopathic or drug-induced.

- Pathomechanism is widespread apoptosis of keratinocytes induced by a cell-mediated cytotoxic reaction.

- Confluent erythematous purpuric and target-like macules evolve into flaccid blisters and epidermal detachment mostly on the trunk and extremities, and there is associated mucous membrane involvement.

- Histopathologically: full-thickness necrosis of the epidermis and a sparse lymphocytic infiltrate.

- Treatment is symptomatic. Systemic treatment with glucocorticoids and high-dose intravenous immunoglobulin is controversial.

DEFINITION

TEN is a maximal variant of SJS differing only in the extent of body surface involvement. Both can start with macular and target-like like lesions; however, about 50% of TEN cases do not, and in these the condition evolves from diffuse erythema to immediate necrosis and epidermal detachment.

There is now consensus that SJS and TEN are different from erythema multiforme(EM).

SJS: <10% epidermal detachment
SJS/TEN overlap: 10–30% epidermal detachment.
TEN: >30% epidermal detachment.

EPIDEMIOLOGY

Age of Onset Any age, but most common in adults >40 years. Equal sex incidence.
Overall Incidence *TEN*: 0.4–1.2 per million person-years. *SJS*: 1.2–6 per million person-years.
Risk Factors Systemic lupus erythematosus, HLA-B12, HIV/AIDS.

ETIOLOGY AND PATHOGENESIS

Polyetiologic reaction pattern, but drugs are clearly the leading causative factor. *TEN*: 80% of cases have strong association with specific medication (Table 8-4); <5% of patients report no drug use. Also: chemicals, *Mycoplasma pneumoniae*, viral infections, immunization. *SJS*: 50% are associated with drug exposure; etiology often not clear-cut.

Pathogenesis of SJS-TEN is only partially understood. It is viewed as a cytotoxic immune reaction aimed at the destruction of keratinocytes expressing foreign (drug-related) antigens. Epidermal injury is based on the induction of apoptosis. Drug-specific activation of T cells has been shown in vitro on peripheral blood mononuclear cells of patients with drug eruptions. The nature of the antigens that drive the cytotoxic cellular immune reaction is not well understood. Drugs or their metabolites act as haptens and render keratinocytes antigenic by binding to their surfaces. Cutaneous drug eruptions have been linked to a defect of the detoxification systems of liver and skin, which results in direct toxicity or alteration of antigenic properties of keratinocytes. Cytokines produced by activated mononuclear cells and keratinocytes probably contribute to local cell death, fever, and malaise.

CLINICAL MANIFESTATION

Time from first drug exposure to onset of symptoms: 1–3 weeks. Occurs more rapidly with rechallenge. Often after days of ingestion of the drug; newly added drug is most suspect. Prodromes: fever, malaise, arthralgias 1–3 days prior to mucocutaneous lesions. Mild to moderate skin tenderness, conjunctival burning

TABLE 8-4 Medications and the Risk of Toxic Epidermal Necrolysis

High Risk	Lower Risk	Doubtful Risk	No Evidence of Risk
Allopurinol	Acetic acid NSAIDs (e.g., diclofenac)	Paracetamol (acetaminophen)	Aspirin
Sulfamethoxazole	Aminopenicillins	Pyrazolone analgesics	Sulfonylurea
Sulfadiazine	Cephalosporins	Corticosteroids	Thiazide diuretics
Sulfapyridine	Quinolones	Other NSAIDs (except aspirin)	Furosemide
Sulfadoxine	Cyclins	Sertraline	Aldactone
Sulfasalazine	Macrolides		Calcium channel blockers
Carbamazepine			β Blockers
Lamotrigine			Angiotensin-converting enzyme inhibitors
Phenobarbital			Angiotensin II receptor antagonists
Phenytoin			Statins
Phenylbutazone			Hormones
Nevirapine			Vitamins
Oxicam NSAIDs			
Thiacetazone			

NSAIDs, nonsteroidal anti-inflammatory drugs.

Source: L. Valeyrie-Allanore, J-C Roujeau: Epidermal necrolysis, in *Fitzpatrick's Dermatology in General Medicine*, 7e, K Wolff et al (eds). New York , McGraw-Hill, 2008, Chap. 39.

or itching, then skin pain, burning sensation, tenderness, paresthesia. Mouth lesions are painful, tender. Impaired alimentation, photophobia, painful micturition, anxiety.

Skin Lesions *Prodromal Rash* Is morbilliform, can be target lesion–like, with/without purpura (Fig. 8-7); rapid confluence of individual lesions (Fig. 8-8); alternatively, can start with diffuse erythema (Fig. 8-9).
Early Necrotic epidermis first appears as macular areas with crinkled surface that enlarge and coalesce (Fig. 8-7). Sheetlike loss of epidermis (Figs. 8-7 to 8-9). Raised flaccid blisters that spread with lateral pressure (Nikolsky sign) on erythematous areas. With trauma, full-thickness epidermal detachment yields exposed, red, oozing dermis (Figs.8-8 and 8-9) resembling a second-degree thermal burn.
Recovery Regrowth of epidermis begins within days; completed in >3 weeks. Pressure points and periorificial sites exhibit delayed healing. Skin that is not denuded acutely is shed in sheets, especially palms/soles. Nails and eyelashes may be shed.
Distribution Initial erythema on face, extremities, becoming confluent over a few hours or days. Epidermal sloughing may be general-

ized, resulting in large denuded areas (Figs. 8-8 and 8-9). Scalp, palms, soles may be less severely involved or spared. *SJS*: widely distributed with prominent involvement of trunk and face. *TEN*: generalized, universal.
Mucous Membranes Invariably involved, i.e., erythema, painful erosions: lips, buccal mucosa, conjunctiva, genital and anal skin.
Eyes 85% have conjunctival lesions: hyperemia, pseudomembrane formation; keratitis, corneal erosions; later synechiae between eyelids and bulbar conjunctiva.
Hair and Nails Eyelashes and nails may be shed in TEN.

GENERAL FINDINGS

- Fever usually higher in TEN than in SJS.
- Usually mentally alert. Distress due to severe pain.
- Cardiovascular: pulse may be >120 beats/min. Blood pressure.
- Renal: tubular necrosis may occur. Acute renal failure.
- Respiratory and GI tracts: sloughing of epithelium with erosions.

FIGURE 8-7   TEN, exanthematic presentation   There is a widespread confluent macular rash with crinkling of the epidermis in some areas and detachment of the epidermis in others, leaving oozing red erosions. This eruption was due to allopurinol.

LABORATORY EXAMINATIONS

Hematology Anemia, lymphopenia; eosinophilia uncommon. Neutropenia correlates with poor prognosis. Serum urea increased, serum bicarbonate decreased.

Dermatopathology *Early* Vacuolization/ necrosis of basal keratinocytes and individual cell necrosis (apoptosis) throughout the epidermis.

Late Full-thickness epidermal necrosis and detachment with formation of subepidermal split above basement membrane. Sparse lymphocytic infiltrate in dermis. Immunofluorescence studies unremarkable, ruling out other blistering disorders.

TABLE 8-5   SCORTEN: A Prognostic Scoring System for Patients with Epidermal Necrolysis [a]

SCORTEN Prognostic Factors	Points
• Age > 40 yr	1
• Heart rate > 120 beats/min	1
• Cancer or hematologic malignancy	1
• Body surface area involved > 10 percent	1
• Serum urea level > 10 mM	1
• Serum bicarbonate level < 20 mM	1
• Serum glucose level > 14 mM	1

SCORTEN	Mortality Rate (%)
0–1	3.2
2	12.1
3	35.8
4	58.3
> 5	90

[a]*Note by authors:* Although it is highly appreciated that we now have a scoring system, we do have a reservation with SCORTEN. Only one point is assigned to body surface area involvement (>10%). There is definitely a prognostic difference between, e.g., 20% and 70% body surface area involvement and this should be reflected in the total score.

Source: Data from S Bastuji-Garin et al: SCORTEN: A severity-of-illness score for toxic epidermal necrolysis. *J Invest Dermatol* **115**: 149, 2000; from L Valeyrie-Allanore, J-C Roujeau: Epidermal necrolysis, in *Fitzpatrick's Dermatology in General Medicine*, 7th ed, K Wolff et al (eds). New York, McGraw-Hill, 2008, Chap. 39.

DIAGNOSIS AND DIFFERENTIAL DIAGNOSIS

Early Exanthematous drug eruptions, EM major, scarlet fever, phototoxic eruptions, toxic shock syndrome, graft-versus-host disease (GVHD).

Fully Evolved EM major (typical target lesions, predominantly on extremities), GVHD (may mimic TEN; less mucosal involvement), thermal burns, phototoxic reactions, staphylococcal scalded-skin syndrome (in young children, rare in adults), generalized bullous fixed drug eruption, exfoliative dermatitis.

COURSE AND PROGNOSIS

Average duration of progression is <4 days. A prognostic scoring system is shown in Table 8-5. Course similar to that of extensive thermal burns. Prognosis related to extent of skin necrosis. Transcutaneous fluid loss is large and varies with area of denudation; associated electrolyte abnormalities. Prerenal azotemia common. Bacterial colonization common and associated with sepsis. Other complications include hypermetabolic state and diffuse interstitial pneumonitis. Mortality rate for TEN is 30%, mainly in elderly; for SJS, 5–12%. Mortality related to sepsis, GI hemorrhage, fluid/electrolyte imbalance. If the patient survives the first episode of SJS/TEN, reexposure to the causative drug may be followed by recurrence within hours to days, more severe than the initial episode.

SEQUELAE

Skin Scarring, hypo- and hyperpigmentation, eruptive nevomelanocytic nevi, abnormal regrowth of nails.

Eyes Common, including Sjögren-like sicca syndrome with deficiency of mucin in tears; entropion, trichiasis, squamous metaplasia, neovascularization of conjunctiva and cornea; synblepharon, punctate keratitis, corneal scarring; persistent photophobia, burning eyes, visual impairment, blindness.

Anogenitalia: Phimosis, vaginal synechiae.

MANAGEMENT

Acute SJS/TEN

- Early diagnosis and withdrawal of suspected drug(s) are very important.
- Patients are best cared for in an intermediate or intensive care unit.

FIGURE 8-8 TEN, exanthematic presentation
A macular rash that is still visible on the lower flank has coalesced, and dislodgment and shedding of the necrotic epidermis has led to large, oozing, extremely painful erosions. This resembles scalding. The eruption was due to a sulfonamide.

FIGURE 8-9 TEN, non-exanthematic diffuse presentation This 60-year-old man developed diffuse erythema over almost the entire body, which then resulted in epidermal crinkling, detachment, and shedding of epidermis leaving large erosions. This is reminiscent of scalding.

- Manage replacement of IV fluids and electrolytes as for patient with a third-degree thermal burn. However, less fluid usually required as for thermal burn of similar extent.
- Systemic glucocorticoids early in the disease and in high doses are reported helpful in reducing morbidity or mortality (as is also the experience of the authors), but this has been questioned. Late in the disease they are contraindicated.
- High-dose IV immunoglobulins halt progression of TEN if administered early. This is questioned by some authors; the discrepancy may be explained by the different products and batches used.

- Pentoxifylline IV by continuous drip early on in the eruption has been anecdotally reported to be beneficial.
- With oropharyngeal involvement, suction frequently to prevent aspiration pneumonitis.
- Surgical debridement not recommended.
- Diagnose and treat complicating infections, including sepsis (fever, hypotension, change in mental status).
- Treat eye lesions early with erythromycin ointment.

Prevention The patient must be aware of the likely offending drug and that other drugs of the same class can cross-react. These drugs must never be readministered. Patient should wear a medical alert bracelet.

BENIGN NEOPLASMS AND HYPERPLASIAS

DISORDERS OF MELANOCYTES

ACQUIRED NEVOMELANOCYTIC NEVI ■ ○

- Nevomelanocytic nevi (NMN), commonly called *moles*, are very common, small (<1 cm), circumscribed, acquired pigmented macules, papules, or nodules.
- Composed of groups of melanocytic nevus cells located in the epidermis, dermis, and, rarely, subcutaneous tissue.

- They are benign, acquired tumors arising as nevus cell clusters at the dermal-epidermal junction (*junctional NMN*), invading the papillary dermis (*compound NMN*), and ending their life cycle as *dermal NMN* with nevus cells located exclusively in the dermis where, with progressive age, there will be fibrosis.

EPIDEMIOLOGY AND ETIOLOGY

One of the most common acquired new growths in Caucasians (most adults have about 20 nevi), less common in blacks or pigmented persons, and sometimes absent in persons with red hair and marked freckling (skin phototype I).

Race   Blacks and Asians have more nevi on the palms, soles, nail beds.

Heredity   Common acquired NMN occur in family clusters. Dysplastic melanocytic nevi (DN) (see Section 12), which are putative precursor lesions of malignant melanoma, occur in virtually every patient with familial cutaneous melanoma and in 30–50% of patients with sporadic nonfamilial primary melanoma.

Sun Exposure   A factor in the induction of nevi on the exposed areas.

Significance   Risk of melanoma is related to the numbers of NMN and to DN. In the latter, even if only a few lesions are present.

CLINICAL MANIFESTATION

Duration and Evolution of Lesions   NMN appear in early childhood and reach a maximum in young adulthood even though some NMN may arise in adulthood. Later on there is a gradual involution and fibrosis of lesions, and most disappear after the age of 60. In contrast, DN continue to appear throughout life and are believed not to involute (see Section 12).

Skin Symptoms   NMN are asymptomatic. However, NMN initially grow and growth is often accompanied by itching. If a lesion *persistently* itches or is tender, it should be followed carefully or excised, since *persistent* pruritus may be an early indication of malignant change.

CLASSIFICATION

NMN are multiple (Fig. 9-1) and can be classified according to their state of evolution and thus according to the site of the clusters of nevus cells.

1. *Junctional melanocytic NMN*: These arise at the dermal-epidermal junction, on the epidermal side of the basement membrane; in other words, they are intraepidermal (Fig. 9-2).
2. *Compound melanocytic NMN*: Nevus cells invade the papillary dermis, and nevus cell nests are now found both intraepidermally and dermally (Fig. 9-3).

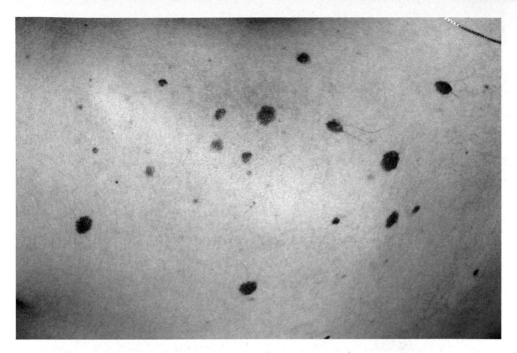

FIGURE 9-1 Multiple NMN on the shoulder of a 32-year-old female. Most of these nevi are junctional NMN, some are slightly elevated and thus compound NMN. Note relatively uniform shape and color of the lesions. Due to different developmental stages they are of varying size ranging from 1 to 4 mm in diameter and they are regular and have a relatively uniform shape.

3. *Dermal melanocytic NMN*: These represent the last stage of the evolution of NMN. "Dropping off" into the dermis is now completed, and the nevus grows or remains intradermal. With progressive age, there will be gradual fibrosis (Fig. 9-4).

Thus, melanocytic NMN undergo the evolution from junctional → compound → dermal NMN. Since the capacity of NMN cells to form melanin is greatest when they are located at the dermal-epidermal junction (intraepidermally) and since NMN cells lose their capacity for melanization, the further they penetrate into the dermis, the lesser is the intensity of pigmentation with the increase in the dermal proportion of the nevus. Purely dermal NMN are therefore almost always without pigment. In a simplified manner, the clinical appearance of NMN along this evolutionary path can be characterized as follows: junctional NMN is flat and dark, compound NMN is raised and dark, and dermal NMN is raised and light. This evolution also reflects the age at which the different types of NMN are found. Junctional and compound NMN are usually seen in childhood and through the teens, whereas dermal NMN start manifesting in the third and fourth decade.

Junctional Melanocytic Nevocellular Nevi
Lesions Macule, or only very slightly raised (Figs. 9-2, 33-13). Uniform tan, brown, dark brown, or even black. Round or oval with smooth, regular borders. Scattered discrete lesions. Never >1 cm in diameter; if >1 cm, the "mole" is a congenital nevomelanocytic nevus, an atypical nevus, or a melanoma (see Section 12).

Compound Melanocytic Nevocellular Nevi
Lesions Papules or small nodules (Fig. 9-3). Dark brown, sometimes even black; dome-shaped, smooth or cobblestone-like surface, regular and sharply defined border, sometimes papillomatous or hyperkeratotic. Never >1 cm in diameter; if >1 cm, the mole is a congenital nevomelanocytic nevus, an atypical nevus, a melanoma. Consistency either firm or soft. Color may become mottled as progressive conversion into dermal NMN occurs. May have hairs.

FIGURE 9-2   A–D Junctional NMN   Lesions are completely flat (**A, B**) or minimally elevated as in **C.** and **D.** They are symmetric with a regular border and, depending on the skin type of the individuals, have different shades of brown to black (**D**).

Dermal Melanocytic Nevocellular Nevi

Lesions   Sharply defined papule or nodule. Skin-colored, tan or flecks of brown, often with telangiectasia. Round, dome-shaped (Fig. 9-4), smooth surface, diameter <1 cm. Usually not present before the second or third decade. Older lesions, mostly on the trunk, may become pedunculated and do not disappear spontaneously. May be hairy.

Distribution   Face, trunk, extremities, scalp. Random, but some predilection for sun-exposed areas. Occasionally palmar and plantar, in which case these NMN usually have the appearance of junctional NMN. 🗎

DIAGNOSIS AND DIFFERENTIAL DIAGNOSIS

Diagnosis   Made clinically. As for all pigmented lesions the ABCDE rule applies (see page 310). In cases of doubt apply dermoscopy (epiluminescence microscopy), and if malignancy cannot be excluded even by this procedure, excise lesions with a narrow margin.

Differential Diagnosis   *Junctional NMN:* all flat, deeply pigmented lesions. Solar lentigo, flat atypical nevus, lentigo maligna. *Compound NMN:* all raised pigmented lesions. Seborrheic keratosis, DN, small superficial spreading melanoma, early nodular melanoma, pigmented

A

B

FIGURE 9-3   Compound NMN   Uniformly pigmented papules and small domed nodules. **A.** The lesion to the left is flatter and tan with a more elevated darker center; the larger lesion (on the right) is older and chocolate-brown; the left lesion is younger and has a predominantly junctional component at the periphery. **B.** A heavily pigmented dome-shaped lesion in the eyebrow. It is sharply defined, uniformly black, smooth and slightly cobblestone-like surface, sharply and regularly defined. It measures less than 5 mm.

basal cell carcinoma, dermatofibroma, Spitz nevus, blue nevus. *Dermal NMN*: all light tan or skin-colored papules. Basal cell carcinoma, neurofibroma, trichoepithelioma, dermatofibroma, sebaceous hyperplasia.

MANAGEMENT

Indications for removal of acquired melanocytic NMN are the following:

Site: Lesions on the scalp (only if difficult to follow and not a classic dermal NMN); mucous membranes, anogenital area.
Growth: If there is rapid change in size.
Color: If color becomes variegated.
Border: If irregular borders are present or develop.
Erosions: If lesion becomes eroded without major trauma.
Symptoms: If lesion begins to *persistently* itch, hurt, or bleed.

Dermoscopy: If criteria for melanoma or an dysplastic nevus are present or appear de novo.

Melanocytic NMN *never* become malignant because of manipulation or trauma. In those cases where this was claimed, the lesion was initially a melanoma. If there is an indication for the removal of an NMN, the nevus should always be excised for histologic diagnosis and for definite treatment (particularly applicable to and decisive in ruling out congenital, dysplastic, or blue nevi). Removal of papillomatous, compound, or dermal NMN for cosmetic reasons by electrocautery requires that a nevus be unequivocally diagnosed as benign NMN and histology be performed. If an early melanoma cannot be excluded with certainty, an excision for histologic examination is obligatory but can be performed with narrow margins.

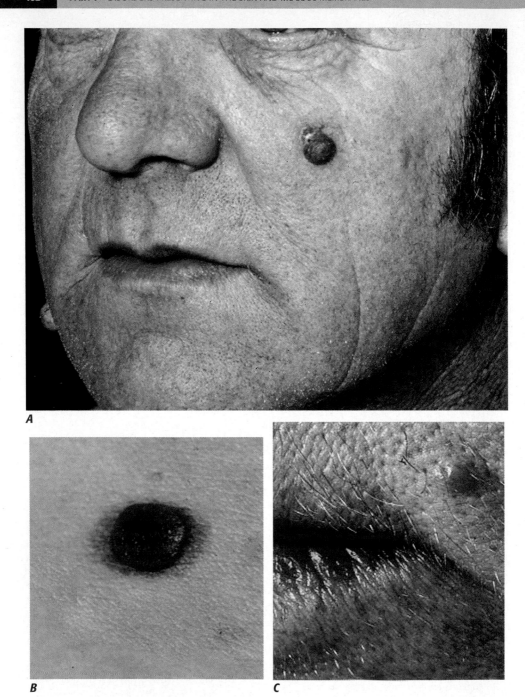

A

B   *C*

FIGURE 9-4   Dermal melanocytic NMN   *A.* Two dome-shaped, sharply defined relatively soft tan nodules on the left cheek and right lateral mandibular region in a 60-year-old male. These lesions were previously much darker and less elevated. ***B.*** A larger magnification of a dermal NMN. This lesion is sharply defined, has a reddish color with a central regular pigmented spot where the nevus obviously is still compound in nature. ***C.*** Old dermal nevus on the upper lip of a 65-year-old woman. This lesion is relatively hard, has a smooth surface and a pinkish color. This lesion is in regression.

HALO NEVOMELANOCYTIC NEVUS ICD-9:216.9 ∘ ICD-10:D22-M8723/0 ■ ○

- An NMN that is encircled by a halo of leukoderma or depigmentation. The leukoderma is based on a decrease of melanin in melanocytes and/or disappearance of melanocytes at the dermal-epidermal junction.
- A white halo around a NMN indicates regression

- Halo nevi most often undergo spontaneous involution, often with regression of the centrally located pigmented nevus.
- Halo NMN may indicate incipient vitiligo.

Synonym: Sutton leukoderma acquisitum centrifugum.

EPIDEMIOLOGY

Overall prevalence 1%. Onset in the first three decades. Occurs spontaneously and in patients with vitiligo (18–26%). Also in patients with metastatic melanoma (around metastatic lesions and around primary melanoma). May herald vitiligo. All races, both sexes. Halo nevi occur in siblings and in those with a family history of vitiligo.

PATHOGENESIS

Immunologic phenomena, both humoral and cellular, are responsible for the dynamic changes that eventually lead to nevus involution.

CLINICAL MANIFESTATION

There are three stages: (1) Development (in months) of white halo around preexisting NMN; halo may be preceded by faint erythema; (2) disappearance (months to years) of NMN; and (3) repigmentation (months to years) of halo.

PHYSICAL EXAMINATION

Skin Lesions Papular brown NMN (<5 mm) with oval or round halo of sharply marginated hypomelanosis (Figs. 9-5 and 9-6*A*). The NMN is *centrally* located. These usually show depigmentation with wood lamp examination. Scattered discrete lesions (1 to >30) mostly on the trunk, but in general the same distribution as of NMN (Fig. 9-5). May begin with erythema around NMN (Fig. 9-6*B*).

Special Forms
Congenital halo NMN occur rarely. ✐

DIAGNOSIS AND DIFFERENTIAL DIAGNOSIS

If clinical findings atypical: the nevus has variegation of color and/or irregular borders, confirm histologically and exclude melanoma.
"Halo" Depigmentation around Other Lesions Can occur around blue nevus, congenital NMN, Spitz juvenile nevus, verruca plana, primary melanoma, melanoma metastases, dermatofibroma, neurofibroma.

FIGURE 9-5 Halo melanocytic NMN on the back of a 22-year-old female There are five halo nevi, all with a pigmented dot-like central junctional or compound NMN surrounded by a hypo- or amelanotic halo. The arrow indicates one lesion where the central nevus has completely regressed, the reddish color indicates telangiectasia.

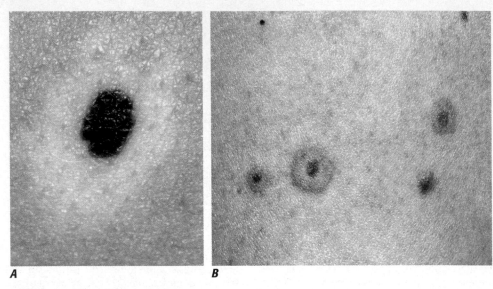

A   *B*

FIGURE 9-6   Halo melanocytic NMN   *A.* Larger magnification of a halo NMN. The nevus is a junctional NMN (compare with Fig. 9-2) that is surrounded by a hypomelanotic (almost white) halo. ***B.*** Several tan junctional NMN that are surrounded by an erythematous halo. This is the early stage of halo development. The erythematous rim will later be replaced by a hypomelanotic halo.

LABORATORY EXAMINATION

Dermatopathology   Junctional dermal or compound nevus surrounded by lymphocytic infiltrate (lymphocytes and histiocytes) around and between nevus cells. Nevus cells develop evidence of cell damage undergo apoptosis, and disappear. Halo shows decrease or total absence of melanin and melanocytes.

MANAGEMENT

Reassurance. Excision if the features of the nevus are atypical: variegation of color, irregular borders.

BLUE NEVUS   ICD-9:216.9 ∘ ICD-10:D22. M8780   ▮ ○

- A blue nevus is an acquired, firm, dark-blue to gray-to-black, sharply defined papule or nodule representing a localized proliferation of melanin-producing *dermal* melanocytes.

- A blue nevus is benign. So-called cellular blue nevi are larger and have very rare tendency to become malignant.

  Synonyms: Blue neuronevus, dermal melanocytoma.

EPIDEMIOLOGY

Onset   In childhood and late adolescence. Equal sex distribution.
Variants   Three types: common blue nevus, cellular blue nevus, combined blue nevus–nevomelanocytic nevus.

PATHOGENESIS

Ectopic accumulations of melanin-producing melanocytes (not nevus cells) in the dermis derived from melanoblasts that became arrested during their migration from neural crest to sites in the skin.

CLINICAL MANIFESTATION

Nearly always asymptomatic, occasionally of cosmetic concern; often feared to be melanoma.

PHYSICAL EXAMINATION

Skin Lesions Papules to nodules, blue, blue-gray, blue-black, usually <10 mm in diameter (Figs. 9-7 and 9-8*A*). *Cellular blue nevi* are larger (1–3 cm) (Fig. 9-8*B*). Occasionally have target-like pattern of pigmentation. Usually round to oval. *Combined blue nevus–NMN*: blue-brown or blue-black with a lighter rim.
Sites of Predilection Most commonly located on the dorsa of hands (Fig. 9-8*A*) or feet (50%), but many occur in the face (Fig. 9-7); cellular blue nevi occur on the buttocks, lower back, scalp (Fig. 9-8*B*), and face. ☒

LABORATORY EXAMINATION

Dermatopathology Melanin-containing wavy dermal melanocytes with long thin dendrites grouped in irregular bundles admixed with melanin-containing macrophages in the upper or middle dermis: excessive fibrous tissue production in upper reticular dermis. *Cellular blue nevus*: in addition to spindle-shaped melanocytes, epithelioid nevus cells in dermis and subcutaneous fat in nests and neuroid forms. *Combined blue nevus–NMN*: combination of blue nevus and compound NMN.

DIAGNOSIS AND DIFFERENTIAL DIAGNOSIS

Usually made on clinical findings, at times confirmed by excision and dermatopathologic examination to rule out nodular melanoma.
Blue/Gray Papule Dermatofibroma, glomus tumor, primary (nodular) or metastatic melanoma, pigmented spindle cell (Spitz) nevus, traumatic tattoo, angiokeratoma, pigmented basal cell carcinoma.

COURSE AND PROGNOSIS

Most remain unchanged. Malignant melanoma rarely develops in *cellular* blue nevi.

MANAGEMENT

Blue nevi <10 mm in diameter and stable for many years usually do not need excision. Sudden appearance or change of an apparent blue nevus warrants surgical excision and dermatopathologic examination. Cellular blue nevi (≥1–3 cm; Fig. 9-8*B*) are usually excised to rule out melanoma.

FIGURE 9-7   Blue nevus There are four tan junctional NMN and one bluish-black round lesion on the cheek of a 17-year-old girl. In contrast to the junctional NMNs the blue nevus is palpable with a relatively high consistency and upon dermoscopy will appear as an ill-defined uniformly bluish lesion deep in the dermis.

A   *B*

FIGURE 9-8   Blue nevus and cellular blue nevus   *A.* This blue nevus has regular borders but is not circular and is solidly blue-black in color. The epidermis is smooth, indicating that the lesion is in the dermis. The consistency is increased and the margins are well defined. Differential diagnosis must include nodular melanoma. If the lesion has been present for years, a biopsy is not necessary. If the lesion was noted only a few months ago, excision biopsies are required to rule out nodular melanoma. However, dermoscopy greatly facilitates the clinical differential diagnosis showing none of the features of nodular melanoma and will therefore render an excisional biopsy unnecessary. ***B.*** This cellular blue nevus appeared as two large, bluish-black nodules on the scalp. After excision, histology showed that they were contiguous and thus represented one single lesion. Cellular blue nevi are much larger and should always be excised to rule out melanoma, which, albeit rarely, can develop in these lesions.

NEVUS SPILUS   ICD-9:216.9 ∘ ICD-10:D22   ■ ○

- A rather common melanocytic lesion that consists of a light brown pigmented macule varying from a few centimeters to a very large area (>15 cm), and many dark brown small macules (2–3 mm) or papules scattered throughout the pigmented background (Fig. 9-9*A*). The pigment in the macular background may be so faint that it can be recognized only under Wood light (Fig. 9-9*B*).

- The pathology of the background of the macular pigmented lesion is the same as lentigo simplex, i.e., increased numbers of melanocytes, while the flat or raised lesions scattered throughout are either junctional or compound; rarely, these are DN.

- The lesions are not as common as junctional or compound NMN but are not at all rare. In one series, the nevus spilus was present in 3% of white patients.

- Malignant melanoma very rarely arises in these lesions. ∅

FIGURE 9-9 Nevus spilus A. This dark brown pigmented macule measuring about 10 cm along the long axis is peppered with many small, dark brown to black macules and papules. **B.** This is also nevus spilus but the macular background is only slightly pigmented so that it will be revealed only under Wood light. The lesion is peppered with many small dark brown macules and flat papules.

SPITZ NEVUS   ICD-9:216.9 ∘ ICD-10:D22-M8772

- Spitz nevus is a benign, dome-shaped, hairless, small (<1 cm in diameter) nodule, most often pink or tan (Fig. 9-10A). There is often a history of recent rapid growth.
- Incidence is 1.4:100,000 (Australia). It occurs at all ages. A third of the patients are children <10 years, a third are 10–20 years old, and a third are >20; rarely seen in persons ≥40 years. *Lesions* arise within months. They are papules or dome-shaped or relatively flat nodules, round, well-cirumscribed, smooth-topped, and hairless. They are a uniform pink (Fig. 9-10A), tan, brown, dark brown, or even black (Fig. 9-10B); are firm; and usually distributed on the head and neck.
- *Differential diagnosis* includes all pink, tan, or darkly pigmented papules: pyogenic granuloma, hemangioma, molluscum contagiosum, juvenile xanthogranuloma, mastocytoma, dermatofibroma, NMN, DN, nodular melanoma.
- *Dermatopathology* consists of hyperplasia of the epidermis and of melanocytes, dilatation of capillaries. There are admixed large epithelioid cells, large spindle cells with abundant cytoplasm, and occasional mitotic figures. There are sometimes bizarre cytologic patterns: nests of large cells extend from the epidermis ("raining down") into the reticular dermis as fascicles of cells form an "inverted triangle," with the base lying at the dermal-epidermal junction and the apex in the reticular dermis.
- Histologic examination must be done to confirm the clinical diagnosis. Excision in its entirety is important because the condition recurs in 10–15% of all cases in lesions that have not been excised completely. Spitz nevi are benign, but there can be a histologic similarity to melanoma and the histopathologic diagnosis requires the help of an experienced dermatopathologist.
- Spitz tumors probably do not usually involute, as do common acquired NMN nevi. However, some lesions have been observed to transform into common compound NMN, and some undergo fibrosis and in late stages may resemble dermatofibromas.
- *Synonyms*: Pigmented and epithelioid spindle cell nevus. Years ago these were called "juvenile melanoma." ◢

FIGURE 9-10   Spitz nevus   *A.* Pink dome-shaped nodule on the cheek of a young woman, developing abruptly within the previous 12 months; the lesion can be mistaken for a hemangioma. ***B.*** Pigmented Spitz nevus. A black papule surrounded by a tan macular region (lentiginous) developed within a few months on the back of a young female; as such a lesion cannot be distinguished from a nodular melanoma, the lesion was excised and the diagnosis confirmed histologically.

MONGOLIAN SPOT   ICD-9 : 757.33   □ ■* ○

- These congenital gray-blue macular lesions are characteristically located on the lumbosacral area (Fig. 9-11) but can also occur on the back, scalp, or anywhere on the skin. There is usually a single lesion, but rarely, several truncal lesions can be present at birth (Fig. 9-12).

- The underlying pathology is dispersed spindle-shaped melanocytes within the dermis (dermal melanocytosis). Melanocytes are not normally present in the dermis, and it is believed that these ectopic melanocytes represent pigment cells that have been interrupted in their migration from the neural crest to the epidermis.

- Mongolian spots may disappear in early childhood, in contrast to nevus of Ota (see Fig. 9-13A).

- As the term *Mongolian* implies, these lesions are found almost always (99–100%) in infants of Asiatic and Native American origin; however, they have been reported in black and, rarely, in white infants.

- No melanomas have been reported to occur in these lesions.

* In Asians.

FIGURE 9-11   Mongolian spot   A large gray-blue macular lesion involving the entire lumbosacral and gluteal area and the left thigh in a baby from Sri Lanka. Although Mongolian spots are common in Asians, the parents of this baby were alarmed because the lesion was so large.

FIGURE 9-12   Mongolian spots   Multiple, ill-defined, bluish lesions are scattered on the back of this child of Japanese descent. They were present at birth. Most of these lesions disappeared later in childhood.

NEVUS OF OTA   ICD-9:216.9 ∘ ICD-10:D22   ■* ○

- This pigmentary disorder is very common in Asian populations and is said to occur in 1% of dermatologic outpatients in Japan. It has been reported in East Indians, blacks, and, rarely, whites.

- The pigmentation, which can be quite subtle or markedly disfiguring, consists of a mottled, dusky admixture of blue and brown hyperpigmentation of the skin. The pigmentation mostly involves the skin and mucous membranes innervated by the first and second branches of the trigeminal nerve (Fig. 9-13).

- The blue hue results from the presence of ectopic melanocytes in the dermis. It can occur in the hard palate and in the conjunctivae (Fig. 9-13*B*), sclerae, and tympanic membranes.

- Nevus of Ota may be bilateral (Fig. 9-13*C*). It may be congenital but is not hereditary; more often it appears in early childhood or during puberty and remains for life, in contrast to the Mongolian spot, which may disappear in early childhood.

- Treatment with lasers is an effective modality for this disfiguring disorder.

- Malignant melanoma can occur but is rare. ⬈

*In Asians.

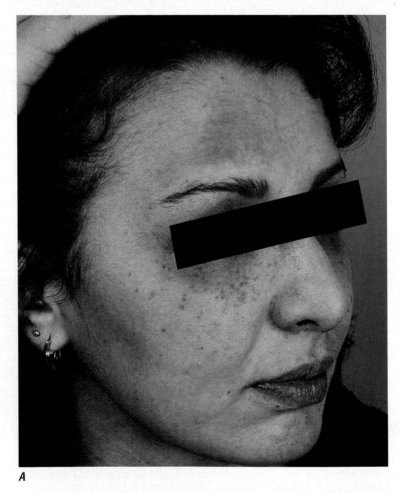

A

FIGURE 9-13   Nevus of Ota   *A.* There is an ill-defined, mottled, dusky, gray to bluish hyperpigmentation in the regions supplied by the first and second branches of the trigeminal nerve. The lesion was unilateral and there was also hyperpigmentation of the sclera.

B

C

FIGURE 9-13 Nevus of Ota (Continued) ***B.*** Brownish to gray hyperpigmentation on the upper and lower lids and a speckled hyperpigmentation of the sclera in a Pakistani boy. The lesion is unilateral. ***C.*** Bilateral nevus of Ota with involvement of the sclerae in a Japanese child.

VASCULAR TUMORS AND MALFORMATIONS

- The present binary biologic classification distinguishes between vascular tumors and vascular malformations. The latter are subclassified according to the structural components into capillary, venous, lymphatic, arterial, or combined forms.

- *Vascular tumors* (e.g., hemangiomas) show endothelial hyperplasia, whereas *malformations* have a normal endothelial turnover.

- Hemangiomas of infancy are not present at birth but appear postnatally; grow rapidly during the first year (proliferating phase), undergo slow spontaneous regression during childhood (involution phase), and remain stable thereafter.

- Vascular malformations are errors of morphogenesis and are presumed to occur during intrauterine life. Most are present at birth, though some do not appear until years later. Once manifest they grow proportionally, but enlargement can occur as a result of various factors.

- Both vascular tumors and malformations can be separated into slow-flow or fast-flow types.

- Classification of vascular tumors and malformations is shown in Table 9-1 and the distinguishing features of vascular tumors and vascular malformations are shown in Table 9-2.

TABLE 9-1   Classification of Vascular Anomalies

Vascular Tumors	Vascular Malformations

■ Hemangioma
  • Hemangioma of infancy
  • Congenital
    ◦ Rapidly involuting congenital hemangioma
    ◦ Noninvoluting congenital hemangioma
■ Hemangioendotheliomas
  • Kaposiform hemangioendothelioma
  • Tufted angioma
■ Angiosarcoma
	■ Capillary
	  • Capillary malformation (port-wine stain)
	  • Telangiectasia (hereditary benign telangiectasia; essential telangiectasia)
	  • Hereditary hemorrhagic telangiectasia
	  • Capillary malformation-arteriovenous malformation
	  • Sturge-Weber syndrome
	■ Venous
	  • Venous malformation
	  • Familial form: Cutaneomucosal venous malformation
	  • Glomuvenous malformation
	  • Blue rubber bleb nevus or Bean syndromes
	■ Lymphatic
	  • Lymphatic malformation
	  • Primary lymphoedemas
	■ Arterial
	  • Arteriovenous malformation
	  • Capillary malformation-arteriovenous malformation
	  • Arteriovenous fistula
	■ Syndromic malformations
	  • Slow-flow
	    ◦ Klippel-Trénaunay syndrome (capillary-lymphaticovenous malformation)
	    ◦ Marffucci syndrome
	  • Fast-flow
	    ◦ Parkes Weber syndrome

Source: LM Boon, and M Vikkulla, in K Wolff et al (eds): *Fitzpatrick's Dermatology in General Medicine*, 7th ed. New York, McGraw-Hill, 2008, pp 1651–1666.

TABLE 9-2 Distinguishing Features of Vascular Tumors (Hemangiomas) and Vascular Malformations

	Tumors	Malformations
Presence at birth	Usually postnatal, 30% nascent, rarely full grown	100% (presumably), not always obvious
Male:female ratio	1:3–1:5	1:1
Incidence	1–12.6% at birth; 10–12% at 1 year	0.3–0.5% port-wine stain
Natural history	Phases: proliferating, involuting, and involuted	Proportionate growth; can expand
Cellular	Endothelial hyperplasia	Normal endothelial turnover
Skeletal changes	Occasional mass effect on adjacent bone; rare hypertrophy	Slow-flow: distortion, hypertrophy, or hyperplasia
		Fast-flow: destruction, distortion, or hypertrophy

Source: S Virnelli-Grevelink, JB Mulliken, in IM Freedberg et al (eds): *Fitzpatrick's Dermatology in General Medicine*, 6th ed. New York, McGraw-Hill, 2003, pp 1002–1019.

VASCULAR TUMORS

HEMANGIOMA OF INFANCY (HI)
ICD-9 : 757.32 ∘ ICD-10 : D18.0-M9131 ■ ○ → ◑

(Formerly strawberry, cherry, capillary hemangioma.)

EPIDEMIOLOGY

HI is the most common tumor of infancy. The incidence in newborns is between 1 and 2.5%; in white children by 1 year of age it is 10%. Females more affected than males by a 3 to 1 ratio.

ETIOLOGY AND PATHOGENESIS

HI is a localized proliferative process of angioblastic mesenchyme. It represents a clonal expansion of endothelial cells that may result from somatic mutations of genes regulating endothelial cell proliferation.

CLINICAL MANIFESTATION

The initial proliferative phase lasts from 3 to 9 months, sometimes more. HIs usually enlarge rapidly during the first year. In a subsequent phase of involution the HI regresses, and this occurs gradually over 2 to 6 years and is usually complete by the age of 10. Involution varies greatly between individuals and is not correlated with size, location, or appearance of the lesion.

Skin Lesions Soft, bright red to deep purple, compressible. On diascopy, does not blanch completely. Nodule or plaque, 1–8 cm (Figs. 9-14*A*, 9-15*A*). With the onset of spontaneous regression, a white-to-gray area appears on the surface of the central part of the lesion (Fig. 9-15*A*). Ulceration may occur.

Distribution Lesions are usually solitary and localized or extend over an entire region (Fig. 9-16). Head and neck 50%, trunk 25%. Face, trunk, legs, oral mucous membrane.

SPECIAL PRESENTATIONS

Deep Hemangioma (Formerly, cavernous hemangioma.) In the lower dermis and subcutaneous fat. Localized, firm rubbery mass of bluish or normal skin color with telangiectases in overlying skin (Fig. 9-17). Can be combined with superficial hemangioma (Fig. 9-15*A*). Does not involute as well as superficial type.

Multiple HIs   Multiple small (<2 cm), cherry-red papular lesions involving skin alone (*benign cutaneous hemangiomatosis*) or skin and internal organs (*diffuse neonatal hemangiomatosis*).

Congenital Hemangiomas   These develop in utero and are subdivided into rapidly involuting congenital hemangiomas (RICH) and noninvoluting congenital hemangiomas (NICH). They present as violaceous tumors with overlying telangiectasia with large veins in periphery or as red-violaceous plaques invading deeper tissues. NICH are fast-flow hemangiomas requiring surgery. ☐

LABORATORY EXAMINATION

Dermatopathology   Proliferation of endothelial cells in various amounts in the dermis and/or subcutaneous tissue; there is usually more endothelial proliferation in the superficial type and little in the deep angiomas. GLUT-1 immunoreactivity is found in all hemangiomas but not in vascular malformations.

DIAGNOSIS

Made on clinical findings and MRI; Doppler and arteriography to demonstrate fast flow. Determine GLUT-1 immunoreactivity to rule out vascular malformation.

COURSE AND PROGNOSIS

HIs spontaneously involute by the fifth year, with some few percent disappearing only by age 10 (Figs. 9-14*B* and 9-15*B*). There is virtually no residual skin change at the site in most lesions (80%); in the rest there is atrophy, depigmentation, telangiectasia, and scarring. HIs may, however, pose a considerable problem during the growth phase when they interfere with vital functions, such as obstruction of vision (Fig. 9-16) or of larynx, nose, or mouth. Deeper lesions, especially those involving mucous membranes, may not involute completely. Synovial involvement may be associated with hemophilia-like arthropathy. Special forms of HI, *tufted angiomas* and *Kaposiform hemangioendothelioma* may have platelet entrapment, thrombocytopenia (Kasabach-Merritt syndrome), and even disseminated intravascular coagulation. Rarely, morbidity associated with HI occurs secondary to hemorrhage or high-output heart failure.

MANAGEMENT

Each lesion must be judged individually regarding the decision to treat or not to treat and the selection of a treatment mode. Systemic treatment is difficult, requires experience, and should be performed by an expert. Surgical and medical interventions include continuous wave or pulsed dye laser, cryosurgery, intralesional and systemic high-dose glucocorticoids, interferon α (IFN-α), and propanolol. For the majority of HIs active nonintervention is the best approach because spontaneous resolution gives the best cosmetic results (Figs. 9-14*B*, 9-15*B*). Treatment is indicated in about a quarter of HIs (5% that ulcerate; 20% that obstruct vital structures, i.e., eyes, ears, larynx) and in the <1% that are life threatening.

A   B

FIGURE 9-14   Hemangioma of infancy   A. This bright red nodular plaque in an infant of African extraction is frightening to the parents, and caution is needed to prevent scarring from the treatment itself. Since most of these lesions disappear spontaneously with only 20% showing residual atrophy or depigmentation, a wait-and-see strategy is recommended. **B.** The same lesion after 3 years. The hemangioma has faded spontaneously, and there is only slight residual atrophy.

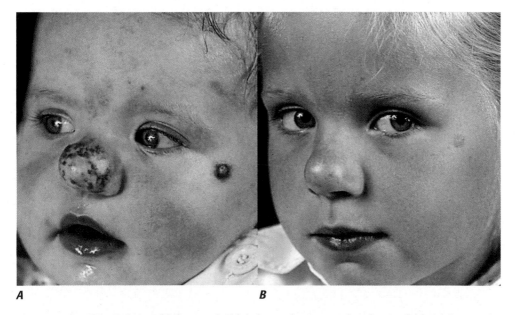

A   B

FIGURE 9-15   Hemangioma of infancy   A. This lesion on the nose consists of a superficial and deep portion and incipient involution is already apparent for the superficial compartment. Note an additional small hemangioma of infancy on the left zygomalic region. **B.** By the fifth year the hemangioma on the nose has almost disappeared and so has the lesion on the zygomatic region, that, however, has left a small scar.

FIGURE 9-16 **Hemangioma of infancy** Here it involves a large segment of skin. While involution is already apparent on the forehead, the lesion on the upper eyelid and the medial canthus is impairing proper function of the lid, and this indicates that vision might be impaired in the future. In this patient, treatment was indicated.

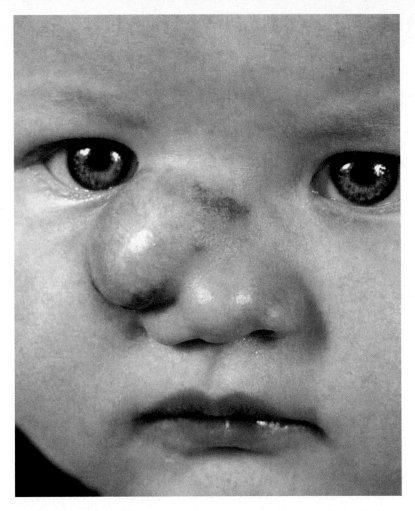

FIGURE 9-17 Hemangioma of infancy, deep lesion There is a rubbery mass in the subcutis associated with a superficial (red) portion. These lesions hardly regress. The hemangioma was removed by surgery.

PYOGENIC GRANULOMA   ICD-9:686.1 ∘ ICD-10:L98.0   ■ ◑

- Pyogenic granuloma is a rapidly developing vascular lesion usually following minor trauma.

- This is a very common solitary eroded vascular nodule that bleeds spontaneously or after minor trauma. The lesion has a smooth surface, with or without crusts, with or without erosion (Fig. 9-18*A*). It appears as a bright red, dusky red, violaceous, or brown-black papule with a collar of hyperplastic epidermis at the base (Fig. 9-18*B*) and occurs on the fingers, lips, mouth, trunk, and toes.

- Histopathologically there are lobular aggregates of proliferating capillaries with edema and numerous neutrophils. Thus, pyogenic granuloma is neither pyogenic (associated with bacterial infection of the skin) nor a granuloma.

- Treatment is surgical excision or curettage with electrodesiccation at the base.

- The importance of pyogenic granuloma is that it can be mistaken for amelanotic nodular melanoma, and vice versa. ⊵

A

B

FIGURE 9-18   Pyogenic granuloma   *A.* This is a solitary eroded vascular nodule that bleeds spontaneously or after minor trauma. The lesions usually have a smooth surface, with or without crusts, with or without erosion. ***B.*** On palms and soles they have a typical collar of thickened stratum corneum at the base. This collar can best be seen when viewed from the side, as is the case here.

GLOMUS TUMOR   ICD-9:228.0 ∘ ICD-10:M8711/0

- This is a tumor of the glomus body. The *glomus body* is an anatomic and functional unit composed of specialized smooth muscle, the *glomus cells* that surround thin-walled endothelial spaces; this anatomic unit functions as an arteriovenous shunt linking arterioles and venules. The glomus cells surround the narrow lumen of the Sucquet-Hoyer canal that branches from the arteriole and leads to the collecting venule segment that acts as a reservoir. Glomus bodies are present on the pads and nail beds of the fingers and toes and also on the volar aspect of hands and feet, in the skin of the ears, and in the center of the face.

- The glomus tumor presents as an exquisitely tender subungual or subcutaneous papule or nodule. Glomus tumors are characterized by paroxysmal painful attacks, especially elicited by exposure to cold. They are most often present as solitary subungual tumors (Fig. 9-19A) but may rarely occur as multiple papules or nodules. These are noted, especially in children, as discrete papules or sometimes plaques anywhere on the skin surface (Fig. 9-19B).

- Therapy is by excision. ₴

A   B

FIGURE 9-19   Glomus tumor   A. This is an exquisitely painful subungual nodule of reddish color; pain becomes paroxysmal upon exposure to cold. **B.** Glomus tumor on the palm of a 16-year-old boy.

ANGIOSARCOMA* ICD-10:M9120/3 ☐ ●

- This is a rare, highly malignant proliferation of endothelial cells manifesting as purpuric macules (Fig. 9-20*A*) and/or papules and nodules of bright red or violaceous and even black color (Fig. 9-20*B*). Nodules are solid, bleed easily, and ulcerate (Fig. 9-20*C*).
- They occur in normal skin, usually on the scalp and upper forehead or in localized lymphedema, for instance in postmastectomy lymphedema

(*Stuart-Treves syndrome*) or postirradiation lymphedema (Fig. 9-20*B*).
- Histologically: channels lined by pleomorphic endothelial cells with a high number of mitoses.
- Treatment is by surgery and/or chemotherapy (liposomal doxorubicin). The 5-year survival is just above 10%. ☑

*Angiosarcoma, although not a beign neoplasm, is discussed here because it fits with other vascular tumors.

FIGURE 9-20   Angiosarcoma   *A.* Early lesions appear as dusky erythematous macules. ***B.*** More advanced lesions are red to black papules and nodules that bleed easily. ***C.*** Advanced angiosarcoma with bleeding purple to black nodules, ulceration, and concomitant edema.

VASCULAR MALFORMATIONS

- These are malformations that do not undergo spontaneous involution.
- *Capillary malformations* (CMs) (e.g., nevus flammeus, or port-wine stain, according to the old nomenclature), *lymphatic malformation, capillary-lymphatic malformation* (CLM), *venous malformation* (VM), and *arteriovenous malformation* (AVM) are distinguished.
- Histologically they consist of enlarged, tortuous vessels of various types.
- Only the most common and important are being dealt with here.

CAPILLARY MALFORMATIONS

PORT-WINE STAIN   ICD-9 : 757.32 ∘ ICD-10 : Q82.5

- A port-wine stain (PWS) is an irregularly shaped, red or violaceous, macular CM that is present at birth and never disappears spontaneously.
- It is common (0.3% of newborns); the malformation is usually confined to the skin.
- May be associated with vascular malformations in the eye and leptomeninges (Sturge-Weber syndrome).
- *Synonym*: Nevus flammeus.

Skin Lesions   These are macular (Fig. 9-21) with varying hues of pink to purple. Large lesions follow a dermatomal distribution and are usually unilateral (85%) though not always. Most commonly involve the face where the CM occurs in the distribution of the trigeminal nerve (Fig. 9-21), usually the superior and middle branches; mucosal involvement of conjunctiva and mouth may occur. CM may also involve other sites. With increasing age of the patient, papules or rubbery nodules (Fig. 9-22) often develop, leading to significant disfigurement. ⊠

Clinical Variant
Nevus flammeus nuchae ("stork bite," erythema nuchae, salmon patch) occurs in approximately one-third of infants on the nape of the neck and tends to regress spontaneously. Similar lesions may occur on eyelids and glabella. It is not really a CM but rather a transitory vasodilatation phenomenon.

HISTOPATHOLOGY

Reveals ectasia of capillaries and no proliferation of endothelial cells. GLUT-1 immunoreactivity is negative.

FIGURE 9-21   Port-wine stain   Sharply marginated, port-wine red macule occurring in a distribution of the second branch of the trigeminal nerve in a child.

COURSE AND PROGNOSIS

PWSs are CMs that do not regress spontaneously. The area of involvement tends to increase in proportion to the size of the child. In adulthood, PWSs usually become raised with papular and nodular areas and are the cause of significant progressive cosmetic disfigurement (Fig. 9-22).

MANAGEMENT

During the macular phase, PWS can be covered with makeup. Treatment with tunable dye or copper vapor lasers is highly effective.

SYNDROMIC CM

Sturge-Weber syndrome (SWS) is the association of PWS in the trigeminal distribution with vascular malformations in the eye and leptomeninges and superficial calcifications of the brain. SWS may be associated with contralateral hemiparesis, muscular hemiatrophy, epilepsy, and mental retardation; glaucoma and ocular palsy may occur. Skull x-rays show characteristic calcifications of vascular malformations or localized linear calcification along cerebral convolutions. CT scan should be done. It should, however, be noted that PWS with trigeminal distribution is common and does not necessarily indicate the presence of SWS. *Klippel-Trénaunay-Weber syndrome* may have an associated PWS overlying the deeper vascular malformation of soft tissue and bone. *PWS on the midline back* may be associated with an underlying arteriovenous malformation of the spinal cord.

FIGURE 9-22   Port-wine stain   With increasing age, the color deepens and papular and nodular vascular lesions develop within the previously macular lesion, causing progressively increasing disfigurement.

SPIDER ANGIOMA   ICD-9:448.1 ○ ICD-10:I78.1

- Spider angioma is a very common red focal telangiectatic network of dilated capillaries radiating from a central arteriole (punctum) (Fig. 9-23A). The central papular punctum is the site of the feeding arteriole with macular radiating telangiectatic vessels. Up to 1.5 cm in diameter. Usually solitary.

- On diascopy, the radiating telangiectasia blanches and the central arteriole may pulsate.

- Most commonly occurs on the face, forearms, and hands.

- It frequently occurs in normal persons and is more common in females; occurs in children.

- It may be associated with hyperestrogenic states, such as pregnancy (one or more in two-thirds of pregnant women), or occurs in patients receiving estrogen therapy, e.g., oral contraceptives, or in those with hepatocellular disease such as subacute and chronic viral hepatitis and alcoholic cirrhosis (Fig. 9-23B).

- Spider angioma arising in childhood and pregnancy may regress spontaneously.

- The lesion may be confused with *hereditary hemorrhagic telangiectasia, ataxia-telangiectasia,* or *telangiectasia* in systemic scleroderma.

- Lesions may be treated easily with electro- or laser surgery.

- *Synonyms*: Nevus araneus, spider nevus, arterial spider, spider telangiectasia, vascular spider.

A

B

FIGURE 9-23   Spider nevus   A. Two small papules from which telangiectasias radiate. Upon compression the lesion blanches completely. **B.** Spider nevi on the chest of a patient with cirrhosis.

VENOUS LAKE   ICD-9 : 528.5 ∘ ICD-10 : K13.0   ■ ○

- A venous lake is a dark blue to violaceous, asymptomatic, soft papule resulting from a dilated venule, occurring on the face, lips, and ears of patients >50 years of age (Fig. 9-24A, B).

- The etiology is unknown, but it has been related to solar exposure.

- These lesions are few in number and remain for years. The lesion results from a dilated cavity lined with a single layer of flattened endothelial cells and a thin wall of fibrous tissue filled with red blood cells.

- Due to its dark blue or sometimes even black color, the lesion may be confused with nodular melanoma or pyogenic granuloma.

- The lesion can be partially compressed and lightened up by diascopy, and the use of dermoscopy permits its easy diagnosis as a vascular lesion.

- Management is for cosmetic reasons and can be accomplished with electrosurgery, laser, or, rarely, with surgical excision.

A   B

FIGURE 9-24   Venous lake   A. On the cheek of a 70-year-old male. The lesion was almost black and became a matter of concern to the patient, who feared he might have melanoma. However, it blanched completely after compression. **B.** Venous lake on the cheek of an 82-year-old female. This bluish-black nodule blanched completely after compression.

CHERRY ANGIOMA   ICD-9:228.0 ∘ ICD-10:I78.8   ■ ○

- Cherry angiomas are exceedingly common, asymptomatic, bright red to violaceous or even black, domed vascular lesions (~3 mm) (Fig. 9-25) or occurring as myriads of tiny red papular spots simulating petechiae.

- They are found principally on the trunk. The lesions appear first at about age 30 and increase in number over the years.

- There are hardly any elderly people who do not have at least a few lesions.

- The histology consists of numerous moderately dilated capillaries lined by flattened endothelial cells; stroma is edematous with homogenization of collagen.

- They are of no consequence other than their cosmetic appearance. Management is electro- or laser coagulation if indicated cosmetically. Cryosurgery is not effective.

- *Synonyms*: Campbell de Morgan spots, senile (hem)angioma.

FIGURE 9-25   Cherry angiomas   These bright red, violaceous or even black lesions appear progressively on the trunk with advancing age.

ANGIOKERATOMA   ICD-9 : 448.9 ∘ ICD-10 : M9141/0

- The term *angio* ("blood vessel") *keratoma* would imply a vascular tumor with keratotic elements. But, in fact, capillaries and postcapillary venules are packed into the papillary body just beneath and bulging into the epidermis, leading to hyperkeratosis. This and the fact that the lumina are usually at least partially thrombosed impart a firm consistency to the lesions.

- Angiokeratomas are dark violaceous to black, often keratotic papules or small plaques that are hard upon palpation and cannot be compressed by diascopy (Fig. 9-26).

- Angiokeratoma can appear as a solitary lesion (*solitary angiokeratoma*), and then the most important differential diagnosis is a small nodular or superficial spreading melanoma (Fig. 9-26).

- The most common is *angiokeratoma of Fordyce*; this disease involves the scrotum and vulva; the lesions are multiple papules (≤4 mm) that are dark red in color and present in quite large numbers (Fig. 9-27).

- *Angiokeratoma of Mibelli* comprises pink to dark red and even black papules that occur on the elbows, knees, and dorsa of the hands. This autosomal dominant disease is rare and occurs in young females.

- *Angiokeratoma corporis diffusum (Fabry disease)*, an X-linked recessive disease, is an inborn error of metabolism in which there is a deficiency of α-galactosidase A leading to an accumulation of neutral glycosphingolipid ceramide trihexoside in endothelial cells, fibrocytes, and pericytes in the dermis, heart, kidneys, and autonomic nervous system. Lesions are numerous dark red, punctate, and tiny (<1 mm) (Fig. 9-28), located on the lower half of the body: lower abdomen, genitalia, and buttocks, although lesions may also occur on the lips. The homozygous males have not only the skin lesions but also symptoms related to involvement of other organ systems: acroparesthesias, excruciating pain, transient ischemic attacks, and myocardial infarction. Heterozygous females may have corneal opacities. Fabry disease is rare. ∎

FIGURE 9-26   Angiokeratoma: solitary   This black, firm lesion with a pebbled surface immediately sparks the suspicion of superficial spreading melanoma. It is noncompressible, but dermoscopy reveals the typical lacunae of thrombosed vascular spaces. Nonetheless, such lesions should be excised.

FIGURE 9-27 Angiokeratoma of Fordyce Reddish, violaceous and black papules on the scrotum. They blanch upon diascopy and this verifies the diagnosis. Note: Thrombosed angiokeratomas do not blanch.

FIGURE 9-28 Angiokeratoma corporis diffusum (Fabry disease) Numerous red, punctate lesions on the lower flank.

LYMPHATIC MALFORMATION (LM)

LYMPHANGIOMA   ICD-9 : 228.1 ◦ ICD-10 : D18.1-M9170/0   □ ○

- The term *lymphatic malformation* is the terminology for what was formerly called "lymphangioma."

- These typical lesions comprise multiple, grouped, small macroscopic vesicles filled with clear or serosanguineous fluid ("frog-spawn") (Fig. 9-29). However, these are not true vesicles but microcystic lesions (lymphangioma) as opposed to a macrocystic lesion (cystic hygroma), which is located deep in the dermis and subcutis and appears as a large soft subcutaneous tumor often distorting the face or an extremity.

- The microcystic LM is present at birth or appears in infancy or childhood. It may disappear spontaneously, but this is extremely rare. Bacterial infection may occur.

- LM may occur as an isolated solitary lesion, as in Fig. 9-29, or cover large areas (up to 10 × 20 cm); it may be associated with a capillary venous lymphatic (CVL) malformation.

- The lesion can be excised, if feasible, or treated with sclerotherapy.

FIGURE 9-29   Lymphatic malformation (lymphangioma)   Frog-spawnlike confluent grouped "vesicles" filled with a serosanguineous fluid.

CAPILLARY/VENOUS MALFORMATIONS (CVMs)   □ ○➔◑➔●

- CVMs are deep vascular malformations characterized by soft, compressible deep-tissue swelling. Lesions are not apparent at birth but become so during childhood.

- They manifest as soft tissue swelling, dome-shaped or multinodular (Fig. 9-30), and are slow-flow lesions. When vascular malformation extends to the epidermis, the surface may be verrucous. The borders are poorly defined, and there is considerable variation in size. Often, CVMs are normal skin color, with the nodular portion blue to purple. They are easily compressed and fill promptly when pressure is released. Some types may be tender, and they may be associated with CMs.

- CVMs may be complicated by ulceration and bleeding, scarring, and secondary infection; and, with large lesions, by high-output heart failure.

- CVMs may interfere with food intake or breathing and, if located on the eyelids or in the vicinity of the eyes, will obstruct vision and may lead to blindness.

- There is no satisfactory treatment except compression. In larger lesions—if organ function is compromised—surgical procedures and intravascular coagulation should be performed. High-dose systemic glucocorticoids or IFN-α may be effective.

ICD-9 : 757.32

VARIANTS

Vascular Hamartomas CVLs with deep soft tissue involvement and resultant swelling or diffuse enlargement of an extremity. May involve skeletal muscle with muscle atrophy. Cutaneous changes include dilated tortuous veins and arteriovenous fistulas.

Klippel-Trénaunay Syndrome A CVM or CVL malformation, slow-flow lesion. Local overgrowth of soft tissue and bone results in enlargement of an extremity. Associated cutaneous changes include phlebectasia, nevus flammeus–like cutaneous CM (Fig. 9-31), lymphatic hypoplasia, and lymphedema.

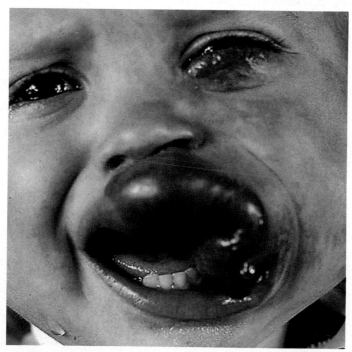

FIGURE 9-30 Capillary-venous malformation In an infant. There is a soft, compressible, bluish-red tissue swelling distorting the upper lip and lower eyelid. It is a slow-flow lesion but requires therapeutic intervention.

Blue Rubber Bleb Nevus A venous malformation that is spontaneously painful and/or tender. It is a compressible, soft, blue swelling in the dermis and subcutaneous tissue. Size ranges from a few millimeters to several centimeters (Fig. 9-32). The lesion may exhibit localized hyperhidrosis over CVL malformations and occurs, often multiply, on the trunk and upper arms. Similar vascular lesions can occur in the gastrointestinal tract and may be a source of hemorrhage.

Marfucci Syndrome A slow-flow venous or lymphatic/venous malformation associated with enchondromas and manifested as hard nodules on fingers or toes and as bony deformities. Patients may develop chondrosarcoma.

Parkes-Weber Syndrome A fast-flow capillary arteriovenous malformation (CAVM) or CM, with soft tissue and skeletal hypertrophy. 🖉

FIGURE 9-31   Capillary-venous malformation   In a 31-year-old woman. This nevus flammeus–like lesion was associated with phlebectasia, lymphedema, and an enlarged right lower extremity (Klippel-Trénaunay syndrome).

FIGURE 9-32   Blue rubber bleb nevus   A spontaneously painful and tender venous malformation. There are a number of compressible bluish-violaceous papules and nodules on the upper arm.

MISCELLANEOUS CYSTS AND PSEUDOCYSTS

EPIDERMOID CYST   ICD-9 : 706.2 ∘ ICD-10 : L72.0   ■ ○

- An epidermoid cyst is the most common cutaneous cyst, derived from epidermis or the epithelium of the hair follicle, and is formed by cystic enclosure of epithelium within the dermis that becomes filled with keratin and lipid-rich debris.

- It occurs in young to middle-aged adults on the face, neck, upper trunk, and scrotum.

- The lesion, which is usually solitary but may be multiple, is a dermal-to-subcutaneous nodule, 0.5–5 cm, which often connects with the surface by keratin-filled pores (Fig. 9-33*A*).

- The cyst has an epidermal-like wall (stratified squamous epithelium with well-formed granular layer); the content of the cyst is keratinaceous material–cream-colored with a pasty consistency and the odor of rancid cheese. Scrotal lesions may calcify.

- The cyst wall is relatively thin. Following rupture of the wall, the irritating cyst contents initiate an inflammatory reaction, enlarging the lesion manyfold; the lesion is now associated with a great deal of pain. Ruptured cysts (Fig. 9-33*B*) are often misdiagnosed as being infected rather than ruptured.

- *Synonyms:* Wen, sebaceous cyst, infundibular cyst, epidermal cyst. ▣

A   *B*

FIGURE 9-33   Epidermoid cyst   *A.* A rounded nodule within the dermis. Not always is there an opening through which caseous keratinous material can be expressed. ***B.*** Ruptured epidermoid cyst. These inflammatory lesions are often misdiagnosed as being infected.

TRICHILEMMAL CYST ICD-9 : 706.2 ∘ ICD-10 : L72.0 ■ ○

- A trichilemmal cyst is the second most common type of cutaneous cyst and is seen most often in middle age, more frequently in females. It is often familial and occurs frequently as multiple lesions.

- These are smooth, firm, dome-shaped, 0.5- to 5-cm nodules or tumors; they lack the central punctum seen in epidermoid cysts. They are not connected to the epidermis.

- Over 90% occur on the scalp, and the overlying scalp hair is usually normal but may be thinned if the cyst is large (Fig. 9-34).

- The cyst wall is usually thick, and the cyst can be removed intact. The wall is a stratified squamous epithelium with a palisaded outer layer resembling that of the outer root sheath of hair follicles. The inner layer is corrugated without a granular layer.

- The cyst contains keratin—very dense, homogeneous; it is often calcified, with cholesterol clefts. If cyst ruptures, it may be inflamed and very painful.

- *Synonyms:* Pilar cyst, isthmus catagen cyst. *Archaic* terms: Wen, sebaceous cyst. ⊠

EPIDERMAL INCLUSION CYST ◫ ○

- An epidermal inclusion cyst occurs secondary to traumatic implantation of epidermis into the dermis. Traumatically grafted epidermis grows in the dermis, with accumulation of keratin within the cyst cavity, enclosed in a stratified squamous epithelium with a well-formed granular layer.

- The lesion appears as a dermal nodule (Fig. 9-35) and most commonly occurs on the palms, soles, and fingers.

- It should be excised.

- *Synonym*: Traumatic epidermoid cyst.

FIGURE 9-34 Trichilemmal cyst A firm, dome-shaped nodule on the scalp. Pressure by the cyst has caused atrophy of hair bulbs and it thus appears without hairs.

FIGURE 9-35 Epidermal inclusion cyst A small dermal nodule on the knee at the site of the laceration.

MILIUM ■ ○

- A milium is a 1- to 2-mm, superficial, white to yellow, keratin-containing epidermal cyst, occurring multiply, located on the eyelids, cheeks, and forehead in pilosebaceous follicles (Fig. 9-36*A*, *B*).

- The lesions can occur at any age, even in infants.

- Milia arise either de novo, especially around the eye, or in association with various dermatoses with subepidermal bullae or vesicles (pemphigoid, porphyria cutanea tarda, bullous lichen planus, epidermolysis bullosa) (Fig. 9-36*C*) and skin trauma (abrasion, burns, dermabrasion, radiation therapy).

- Incision and expression of contents are the method of treatment. ☒

A

B

C

FIGURE 9-36 Milium *A.* A small chalk-white or yellowish papule on the cheek, it can be slit with a scalpel, releasing a little ball of horny material. ***B.*** A slightly larger lesion on the lower lid of an African woman. ***C.*** Multiple milia on the trunk of a child with hereditary dystrophic epidermolysis bullosa (see Section 6).

DIGITAL MYXOID CYST   ICD-9 : 727.41 ∘ ICD-10 : M25.8

- A digital myxoid cyst is a pseudocyst occurring over the distal interphalangeal joint and the base of the nail of the finger (Fig: 9-37*A*) or toe, often associated with Heberden's (osteophytic) node.

- The lesion occurs in older patients, usually >60 years of age.

- It is usually a solitary cyst, rubbery, translucent. A clear gelatinous viscous fluid may be extruded (Fig. 9-37*B*).

- When the myxoid cyst is over the nail matrix, a nail plate dystrophy occurs in the form of a 1- to 2-mm groove that extends to the length of the nail (Figs.9-37*A*, 33-12). (See Section 33.)

- Various methods of management have been advocated, including surgical excision, incision and drainage, injection of sclerosing material, and injection of a triamcinolone suspension. A simple and most effective method is to make a small incision, express the gelatinous contents, and use a firm compression bandage over the lesion over a period of weeks.

- *Synonyms*: Mucous cyst, synovial cyst, myxoid pseudocyst. ⊵

A   *B*

FIGURE 9-37   Digital myxoid cyst   A. The cyst has led to a 3- to 4-mm groove of the nail plate. **B.** Slitting it with a scalpel and pressure releases a gelatinous viscous fluid.

MISCELLANEOUS BENIGN NEOPLASMS AND HYPERPLASIAS

SEBORRHEIC KERATOSIS ICD-9:702.1 ○ ICD-10:L82 ■ ○

- The seborrheic keratosis is the most common of the benign epithelial tumors.
- These lesions, which are hereditary, do not appear until age 30 and continue to occur over a lifetime, varying in extent from a few scattered lesions to literally hundreds in some very elderly patients.
- Lesions range from small, barely elevated papules to plaques with a warty surface and a "stuck on" appearance.

- Lesions are benign and do not require treatment except for cosmetic reasons. They can become irritated or traumatized, with pain and bleeding. SCC should be ruled out.
- *Synonym: verruca seborrhoica.*

EPIDEMIOLOGY

Onset Rarely before 30 years.
Sex Slightly more common and more extensive involvement in males.

CLINICAL MANIFESTATION

Evolve over months to years. Rarely pruritic; tender if secondarily infected.
Skin Lesions *Early* Small, 1- to 3-mm, barely elevated papule, later a larger plaque (Figs. 9-38

FIGURE 9-38 Seborrheic keratosis, solitary A slightly raised, keratotic, brown, flat plaque on the zygomatic region in an older female. The differential diagnosis includes lentigo maligna and lentigo maligna melanoma.

and 9-39) with or without pigment. The surface has a greasy feel and often shows, with a hand lens, fine stippling like the surface of a thimble. Elevation can be demonstrated by lightly freezing the lesion with LN2. Lesions such as lentigo (benigna or maligna) are macules; SKs have a sharply marginated elevated edge in comparison. *Late* Plaque with warty surface and "stuck on" appearance (Fig. 9-40), "greasy." With a hand lens horn cysts can often be seen; with dermoscopy they can always be seen and are diagnostic. Size from 1 to 6 cm. Flat nodule. Brown, gray, black, skin-colored, round or oval (Figs. 9-39 and 9-40*A, B*).

Distribution Isolated lesion or generalized. Face, trunk (Fig. 9-41), upper extremities. In dark skinned people, multiple, small black lesions in the face are called *dermatosis papulosa nigra* (Fig. 9-39). SKs are most dense in sun-exposed site with dermatoheliosis. When numerous and dense, SKs may become confluent. In females, commonly occur in submammary intertriginous skin.

🖉

LABORATORY EXAMINATION

Dermatopathology Proliferation of monomorphous keratinocytes (with marked papillomatosis) and melanocytes, formation of horn cysts. Some lesions can exhibit atypia of keratinocytes, mimicking Bowen disease (SCCIS), flat or squamous cell carcinoma (SCC), and these should be excised.

DIAGNOSIS AND DIFFERENTIAL DIAGNOSIS

Clinically, the diagnosis is made easily. Curettage may be helpful: seborrheic keratosis comes off easily after slight freezing and permits histopathologic examination.

"Tan Macules" Early "flat" lesions may be confused with solar lentigo or spreading pigmented actinic keratosis (see Fig. 10-28).

Skin-Colored/Tan/Black Verrucous Papules/Plaques Larger pigmented lesions are easily mistaken for pigmented basal cell carcinoma (BCC) or malignant melanoma (only biopsy will settle this, or dermoscopy will be of assistance); verruca vulgaris may be similar in clinical appearance, but thrombosed capillaries are present in verrucae.

COURSE AND PROGNOSIS

Lesions develop with increasing age; they are benign and do not become malignant.

MANAGEMENT

Light electrocautery permits the whole lesion to be easily rubbed off. Then the base can be lightly cauterized to prevent recurrence. This, however, precludes histopathologic verification of diagnosis and should be done only by an experienced diagnostician. Cryosurgery with liquid nitrogen spray works only in flat lesions, and recurrences are possibly more frequent. The best approach is curettage after slight freezing with cryospray, which also permits histopathologic examination. In a solid black lesion without horn cysts, a punch biopsy is mandatory to rule out malignant melanoma; in this case a shave biopsy should not be performed as, in the case of melanoma, it will not permit evaluation of the level of invasion.

FIGURE 9-39   Seborrheic keratosis (dermatosis papulosa nigra) · This consists of a myriad of tiny black lesions, some enlarging to more than a centimeter. This is seen in Black Africans, African Americans, and deeply pigmented South East Asians. Treatment is a problem because hypopigmented spots can arise at sites where these seborrheic keratoses have been removed.

A *B*

FIGURE 9-40 **Seborrheic keratosis** *A.* Small, heavily pigmented seborrheic keratoses can have a smooth surface and present a differential diagnostic challenge: pigmented basal cell carcinoma and nodular melanoma have to be excluded. *B.* Large seborrheic keratoses have a "stuck on" appearance, can be very dark and irregular. Due to their multiplicity they usually do not present a diagnostic problem. As shown here, they can be disfiguring.

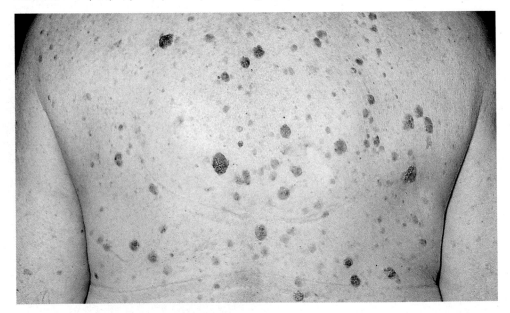

FIGURE 9-41 **Seborrheic keratoses, multiple** Multiple brown, warty papules and nodules on the back, having a "greasy" feel and "stuck on" appearance. This picture also shows the evolution of the lesions: from small only slightly tan, very thin papules or plaques to larger, darker nodular lesions with a verrucous surface. Practically all lesions on the back of this elderly patient are seborrheic keratoses; what they have in common is that they give the impression that they could be scraped off easily, which, in fact, they can.

BECKER NEVUS ICD-9:216 ∘ ICD-10:M8720/0

- Becker nevus (BN) is a distinctive asymptomatic clinical lesion that is a pigmented hamartoma—i. e., a developmental anomaly consisting of changes in pigmentation, hair growth, and a slightly elevated smooth verrucous surface (Fig. 9-42*A* and *B*).

- It occurs mostly in males and in all races. It appears not at birth but usually before 15 years of age and sometimes after this age.

- The lesion is predominantly a macule but with a papular verrucous surface not unlike the lesion of acanthosis nigricans. It is light brown in color and has a geographic pattern with sharply demarcated borders (Fig. 9-42*A*).

- Commonest locations are the shoulders and the back. The increased hair growth follows the onset of the pigmentation and is localized to the areas that are pigmented. The pigmentation is related to increased melanin in basal cells and not to an increased number of melanocytes.

- It is differentiated from a hairy congenital melanocytic nevus, because BN is not usually present at birth, and from café au lait macules because these are not hairy.

- The lesion extends for a year or two and then remains stable, only rarely fading.

- There is very rarely hypoplasia of underlying structures, e.g., shortening of the arm or reduced breast development in areas under the lesion.

- Management: the hypertrichosis can be of cosmetic concern to some individuals. ✎

A   *B*

FIGURE 9-42 Becker nevus *A.* A slightly raised light-tan plaque with sharply defined and highly irregular border and barely visible hypertrichosis on the chest of a 16-year-old male patient. *B.* In this case of Becker nevus the massive hypertrichosis conceals the tan background plaque.

TRICHOEPITHELIOMA   ICD-9:M8100/0 ICD-10:D23

- Trichoepitheliomas are benign appendage tumors with hair bulb differentiation.
- The lesions, which appear at puberty, occur on the face and less often on the scalp, neck, and upper trunk (Fig. 9-43A).
- Lesions may be only a few small pink or skin-colored papules at first gradually increase in

number and may become quite large and be confused with BCC (Fig. 9-43A).
- Trichoepitheliomas can also appear as solitary tumors, which may be nodular, or appear as ill-defined plaques like sclerosing BCC (Fig. 9-43B).

SYRINGOMA   ICD-9:216.0 -216.9 ◦ ICD-10:D23- M8407/0

- Syringomas are benign adenomas of the eccrine ducts. They are 1- to 2-mm, skin-colored or yellow, firm papules that occur mostly in women, beginning at puberty; they may be familial.
- Most often multiple rather than solitary, they occur most frequently on lower periorbital area, usually symmetrically but also on the eyelids

(Fig. 9-44) and on the face, axillae, umbilicus, upper chest, and vulva.
- The lesions have a specific histologic pattern: many small ducts in the dermis with comma-like tails with the appearance of "tadpoles."
- The lesions can be disfiguring, and most patients want them removed; this can be done easily with electrosurgery.

A

FIGURE 9-43   Trichoepitheliomas   A. Multiple, small, sharply defined smooth papules that look like early BCCs.

B

FIGURE 9-43   Trichoepitheliomas (Continued)   *B.* Trichoepithelioma, solitary type. A nodular tumor on the upper lip that can be confused with a basal carcinoma or squamous cell carcinoma.

FIGURE 9-44   Syringomas   Symmetric eruption of 1- to 2-mm skin-colored, smooth papules on the upper and lower eyelids.

SEBACEOUS HYPERPLASIA   ICD-9 : 706.9   ■ ○

- These are very common lesions in older persons and are confused with small BCCs. Also occurs in solid organ transplant recipients treated with cyclosporine. The lesions are 1 to 3 mm in diameter and have both telangiectasia and central umbilication (Fig. 9-45).

- Two features distinguish sebaceous hyperplasia from nodular BCC: (1) sebaceous hyperplasia is

soft to palpation, not firm as in nodular BCC (not superficial); and (2) with firm lateral compression it is often possible to elicit a very small globule of sebum in the valley of the umbilicated portion of the lesion.

- Sebaceous hyperplasias can be destroyed with light electrocautery. ⚡

NEVUS SEBACEOUS   ICD-9 : 216.3   □ ◑

- This congenital malformation of sebaceous differentiation occurs on the scalp or, rarely, on the face (Fig. 9-46).

- A hairless, thin, elevated, 1- to 2-cm plaque, sometimes larger, with a characteristic orange color and a pebbly or warty surface.

- About 10% of patients can be expected to develop BCC in the lesion.

- Excision is recommended at around puberty for cosmetic reasons and to prevent the occurrence of BCC.

- *Synonym*: Organoid nevus. ⚡

EPIDERMAL NEVUS   ICD-9 : 216   □ ○→◑

- As the name *nevus* implies this is a developmental (hamartomatous) disorder characterized by hyperplasia of epidermal structures (epidermis and adnexa). There are no nevomelanocytic nevus cells.

- Epidermal nevus is usually present at birth or occurs in infancy; rarely, it develops in puberty. All epidermal nevi on the head/neck region are present at birth.

- There are several variants of epidermal nevi. The *verrucous epidermal nevus* may be localized or multiple. The lesions are skin-colored, brown, or grayish-brown (Fig. 9-47) and are composed of closely set verrucous papules, well circumscribed; they are often in a linear arrangement—especially on the leg—or they may appear in Blaschko lines on the trunk. Excision is the best treatment, if feasible. Biopsy of the lesions should be considered to rule out BCC.

- When the lesions are extensive they are termed *systematized epidermal nevus*, and when they

are located on half the body they are termed *nevus unius lateris*.

- The lesions can exhibit erythema, scaling, and crusting and are then called *inflammatory linear verrucous epidermal nevus* (ILVEN). The lesions gradually enlarge and become stable in adolescence.

- There is also a *noninflammatory linear verrucous epidermal nevus* (NILVEN).

- Extensive epidermal nevi (*epidermal nevus syndrome*) may be multisystem disorders and may be associated with developmental abnormalities (bone cysts, hyperplasia of bone, scoliosis, spina bifida, kyphosis), vitamin D–resistant rickets, and neurologic problems (mental retardation, seizures, cortical atrophy, hydrocephalus). These patients require a complete examination, including the eyes (cataracts, optic nerve hypoplasia), and cardiac studies to rule out aneurysms, patent ductus arteriosus. ⚡

FIGURE 9-45 **Sebaceous hyperplasia** 1- to 4-mm smooth papules with central umbilication on the forehead.

FIGURE 9-46 **Nevus sebaceous** An elevated plaque of orange color and pebbly surface. Note that the lesion is hairless on the scalp.

FIGURE 9-47 **Epidermal nevus** A grayish irregular plaque with a verrucous surface on the ear extending linearly down to the neck.

BENIGN DERMAL AND SUBCUTANEOUS NEOPLASMS AND HYPERPLASIAS

LIPOMA   ICD-9:214 ○ ICD-10:D17- M8850/0   ■ ○

- Lipomas are single or multiple, benign subcutaneous tumors that are easily recognized because they are soft, rounded, or lobulated and movable against the overlying skin (Fig. 9-48 *A, B*).
- Many lipomas are small but may also enlarge to > 6 cm.
- They occur especially on the neck, trunk, and on the extremities (Fig. 9-48) but can occur anywhere on the body.
- Lipomas are composed of fat cells that have the same morphology as normal fat cells within a connective tissue framework. Angiolipomas have a vascular component and may be tender in cold ambient temperature and with compression.
- Angiolipomas often require excision, whereas other lipomas should be excised only when

considered disfiguring. Liposuction can also be performed when liposomas are soft and thus have only a minor connective tissue component.
- *Familial lipoma syndrome*, an autosomal dominant trait appearing in early adulthood, consists of hundreds of slowly growing nontender lesions.
- *Adipositas dolorosa*, or *Dercum disease*, occurs in women in middle age; there are multiple tender, not circumscribed but rather diffuse fatty deposits.
- *Benign symmetric lipomatosis*, which affects middle-aged men, consists of many large nontender, coalescing poorly circumscribed lipomas, mostly on the trunk and upper extremities; they coalesce on the neck and may lead to a "horse-collar" appearance. ⊠

DERMATOFIBROMA   ICD-9:216 ○ ICD-10:D23- M8832/0   ■ ○

- A dermatofibroma is a very common, button-like dermal nodule, usually occurring on the extremities.
- Important only because of its cosmetic appearance or its being mistaken for other lesions,

such as malignant melanoma when it is pigmented.
- Rarely, the lesion may be tender.
- *Synonyms*: Solitary histiocytoma, sclerosing hemangioma.

EPIDEMIOLOGY AND ETIOLOGY

Very common, occurs mostly in adults. Females > males.

Etiology   Unknown. It is considered by many to represent a late histiocytic reaction to an arthropod bite.

Skin Lesions   Usually asymptomatic papule or nodule (Fig. 9-49*A*), 3 to 10 mm in diameter. Surface variably domed but may be depressed below plane of surrounding skin. Texture of

surface may be dull, shiny, or scaling. Top may be crusted or scarred secondary to excoriation or shaving. Borders ill defined, fading to normal skin. *Color*: variable—skin-colored, pink, brown, tan, dark chocolate brown (Fig. 9-49*B*). Usually darker at center, fading to normal skin color at margin. Firm. *Dimple sign*: lateral compression with thumb and index finger produces a depression or "dimple" (Fig. 9-49*C*).

Distribution   Legs > arms > trunk. Hardly ever occurs on head, palms, soles. Usually solitary; may be multiple, randomly scattered.

A   **B**

FIGURE 9-48   Lipoma   A. Well-defined, soft, rounded tumors in the subcutis, movable both against the overlying skin and the underlying structures, in a 56-year-old male patient. In this patient lesions were symmetric and were also found on the trunk and upper extremities. **B.** Multiple lipomas on the lower arm of a 50-year-old patient. These lesions were also symmetric.

LABORATORY EXAMINATION

Dermatopathology   Whorling fascicles of spindle cells with small amounts of pale blue cytoplasm and elongated nuclei. Some tumors extend to the panniculus. Pigmented dermatofibromas (Fig. 9-49B) contain lipids or hemosiderin pigment in the histiocytes in addition to hyperpigmentation of the epidermis. Overlying epidermis frequently hyperplastic.

DIAGNOSIS AND DIFFERENTIAL DIAGNOSIS

Clinical findings—"dimple" sign (Fig. 9-49C), but there are other lesions that can result in depression with lateral pressure, e.g., papulonodular lesions containing mucin, scar, blue nevus, pilar cyst, metastatic carcinoma, Kaposi sarcoma, dermatofibrosarcoma protuberans.

COURSE AND PROGNOSIS

Lesions appear gradually over several months, may persist without increase in size for years to decades, and may regress spontaneously.

MANAGEMENT

Surgical removal is not usually indicated, as the resulting scar is often less cosmetically acceptable. Cryosurgery with a cotton-tip applicator is often effective and produces a cosmetically acceptable scar in most patients.

A

B   *C*

FIGURE 9-49   Dermatofibroma   *A.* A dome-shaped, slightly erythematous and tan nodule with a button-like, firm consistency. ***B.*** This lesion is pigmented. Can be confused with blue nevus or even nodular melanoma. The pigment is melanin and hemosiderin. ***C.*** "Dimple sign." Dimpling of the lesion is seen when pinched between two fingers.

HYPERTROPHIC SCARS AND KELOIDS ICD-9:701.4 ◦ ICD-10:L91.0 ■ ◐

- Hypertrophic scars and keloids are exuberant fibrous repair tissues after a cutaneous injury.
- A *hypertrophic scar* remains confined to the site of original injury.
- A *keloid*, however, extends beyond this site, often with clawlike extensions.

- May be cosmetically very unsightly and pose a serious problem for the patient if the lesion is large and on the ear or face or over a joint.

EPIDEMIOLOGY AND ETIOLOGY

Age of Onset Third decade, but all ages.
Sex Equal incidence in males and females.
Race Much more common in blacks and in persons with blood group A.
Etiology Unknown. They usually follow injury to skin, i.e., surgical scar, laceration, abrasion, cryosurgery, and electrocoagulation as well as vaccination, acne, etc. *Keloid may also arise spontaneously, without history of injury, usually in presternal site.*

CLINICAL MANIFESTATION

Skin Symptoms Usually asymptomatic. May be pruritic or painful if touched.

Skin Lesions Papules to nodules (Fig. 9-50A, B) to large tuberous lesions. Most often the color of the normal skin but also bright red or bluish. May be linear after traumatic or surgical injury (Fig. 9-50A). Hypertrophic scars tend to be elevated and are confined to approximately the site of the original injury (Fig. 9-50). Keloids, however, may extend in a clawlike fashion far beyond any slight original injury (Figs. 9-51, 9-52A) or may be nodular; tumor-like. Firm to hard; may be tender, surface smooth. Spontaneous keloids arise de novo without trauma or surgery, and usually occur on the chest (Fig. 9-52B).
Distribution Earlobes, shoulders, upper back, chest. ▨

B

A

FIGURE 9-50 Hypertrophic scar *A.* A broad, raised scar developing at the site of surgical incision with telangiectatic blood vessels and a shiny atrophic epidermis. *B.* Multiple hypertrophic scars on the chest of a 22-year-old male with a history of severe acne conglobata.

LABORATORY EXAMINATION

Dermatopathology *Hypertrophic Scar* Whorls of young fibrous tissue and fibroblasts in haphazard arrangement.

Keloid Features of hypertrophic scar with added feature of thick, eosinophilic, acellular bands of collagen.

DIAGNOSIS AND DIFFERENTIAL DIAGNOSIS

Clinical diagnosis; biopsy not warranted unless there is clinical doubt, because this may induce new hypertrophic scarring. Differential diagnosis includes dermatofibroma, dermatofibrosarcoma protuberans, desmoid tumor, scar with sarcoidosis, foreign-body granuloma.

COURSE AND PROGNOSIS

Hypertrophic scars tend to regress, in time becoming flatter and softer. Keloids, however, may continue to expand in size for decades.

MANAGEMENT

This is a real challenge, as no treatment is highly effective.

Intralesional Glucocorticoids Intralesional injection of triamcinolone (10–40 mg/mL) every month may reduce pruritus or sensitivity of lesion, as well as reduce its volume and flatten it. This works quite well in small hypertrophic scars but less well in keloids. Can be combined with cryotherapy whereby the lesion is initially frozen with liquid nitrogen, allowed to thaw, and then injected with triamcinolone (10–40 mg/mL). After freezing, the lesion becomes edematous and is much easier to inject.

Surgical Excision Lesions that are excised surgically often recur larger than the original lesion. Excision with immediate postsurgical radiotherapy is beneficial.

Silicone Cream and Silicone Gel Sheet Reported to be beneficial in keloids and is painless and noninvasive. Not very effective in authors' experience.

Prevention Individuals prone to hypertrophic scars or keloids should be advised to avoid cosmetic procedures such as ear piercing. Scars from burns tend to become hypertrophic. Can be prevented by compression garments.

FIGURE 9-51   Keloids   Well-defined irregular nodules, very hard on palpation, in the auricular region and cheek of a 30-year-old man. The lesions on the earlobe arose after piercing, the lesion on the mandibular region after incision of an inflamed cyst.

A

B

FIGURE 9-52 Keloids *A.* Keloid after a deep burn. Note sausage- and clawlike extensions of the keloid into normal skin. *B.* Spontaneous keloids that arose without apparent cause on the chest of a 19-year-old man.

INFANTILE DIGITAL FIBROMATOSIS   ICD-9 : 757.3 ∘ ICD-10 : M72   □ ○

- A rare form of superficial juvenile fibromatosis.
- Presenting as asymptomatic flesh-colored or pink firm nodule on fingers and toes (Fig. 9-53).
- Appears in the first year of life, less commonly in childhood.

- Histologically interlacing bundles of myofibroblasts with eosinophilic inclusions.
- Benign. Spontaneous regression is rare. Treatment is surgical
- *Synonym*: Rye tumor.

FIGURE 9-53   Infantile digital fibromatosis
A well-defined pink nodule on the finger of an infant. Usually the third to fifth digits are affected. Here, the tumor is found on the second digit.

SKIN TAG ICD-9:701.9 ○ ICD-10:L91.8 ■ ○

- A skin tag is a very common, soft, skin-colored or tan or brown, round or oval, pedunculated papilloma (polyp) (Fig. 9-54); it is usually constricted at the base and may vary in size from >1 mm to as large as 10 mm.

- Histologic findings include a thinned epidermis and a loose fibrous tissue stroma.

- Usually asymptomatic but occasionally may become tender following trauma or torsion and may become crusted or hemorrhagic.

- It occurs more often in the middle aged and in the elderly.

- More common in females and in obese patients and most often noted in intertriginous areas (axillae, inframammary, groin) and on the neck and eyelids.

- It occurs in acanthosis nigricans and metabolic syndrome.

- May be confused with a pedunculated seborrheic keratosis, dermal or compound melanocytic nevus, solitary neurofibroma, or molluscum contagiosum.

- Lesions tend to become larger and more numerous over time, especially during pregnancy. Following spontaneous torsion, autoamputation can occur.

- Management is accomplished with simple snipping with scissors, electrodesiccation, or cryosurgery.

- *Synonyms:* Acrochordon, cutaneous papilloma, soft fibroma.

FIGURE 9-54 Skin tags Soft skin-colored and tan pedunculated papillomas. These are very common in the elderly obese and are obligatory lesions in acanthosis nigricans, as in this patient.

PHOTOSENSITIVITY, PHOTO-INDUCED DISORDERS, AND DISORDERS BY IONIZING RADIATION

SKIN REACTIONS TO SUNLIGHT   ICD-9 : 692.70 ∘ ICD-10 : L56.8

The term *photosensitivity* describes an abnormal response to light, usually sunlight, occurring within minutes, hours, or days of exposure and lasting up to weeks, months, and even longer. Cutaneous photosensitivity reactions require absorption of photon energy by appropriately shaped molecules leading to molecular deformity. Energy is either dispersed harmlessly or is directed to chemical reactions that lead to molecular, cellular, and tissue damage resulting in clinical disease. Absorbing molecules can be (1) exogenous agents applied topically or systemically, (2) endogenous molecules either usually present in skin or produced by an abnormal metabolism, or (3) a combination of exogenous and endogenous molecules that have acquired antigenic properties and thus elicit a photoradiation-driven immune reaction. *Photosensitivity disorders occur only in body regions exposed to solar radiation* (Image 10-1).

There are three broad types of *acute photosensitivity*:

1. A *sunburn*-type response with the development of morphologic skin changes simulating a normal sunburn with erythema, edema, and bullae, such as in phototoxic reactions to drugs or phytophotodermatitis.

2. A *rash* response to light exposure with development of varied morphologic expressions: macules, papules, or plaques, as in eczematous dermatitis. These are usually photoallergic in nature or belong to the so-called idiopathic photodermatoses such as polymorphous light eruption.

3. *Urticarial* responses are typical for solar urticaria; urticarial lesions can also occur in erythropoietic porphyria.

   Chronic photosensitivity: chronic repeated sun exposures over time result in polymorphic skin changes that have been termed *dermatoheliosis*, or photoaging. A classification of skin reactions to sunlight is shown in Table 10-1.

BASICS OF CLINICAL PHOTOMEDICINE

The main culprit of solar radiation–induced skin pathology is the ultraviolet portion of the solar spectrum. Ultraviolet radiation (UVR) in photomedicine is divided into two principal types: UVB (290–320 nm), the "sunburn spectrum," and UVA (320–400 nm). UVA is subdivided into UVA-1 (340–400 nm) and UVA-2 (320–340 nm). The unit of measurement of sunburn is the *minimum erythema dose* (MED), which is the minimum ultraviolet exposure that produces a clearly marginated erythema in the irradiated site 24 h after a single exposure. The MED is expressed as the amount of energy delivered per unit area: mJ/cm^2 (UVB) or J/cm^2 (UVA). The MED for UVB in Caucasians is 20–40 mJ/cm^2 (for a skin phototype I or II, about 20 min in northern latitudes at noon in June) and for UVA is 15–20 J/cm^2 (about 120 min in northern latitudes at noon in June). UVB erythema develops in 6–24 h and fades within 72–120 h. UVA erythema develops in 4–16 h and fades within 48–120 h.

Variations in Sun Reactivity in Normal Persons: Fitzpatrick Skin Phototypes (Table 10-2)

Sunburn is seen most frequently in individuals who have pale white or white skin and a limited capacity to develop *facultative*, or inducible, melanin pigmentation (tanning) after exposure to UVR. Basic skin color (*constitutive* melanin pigmentation) is divided into white, brown, and black. Not all persons with white skin have the same capacity to develop tanning, and this

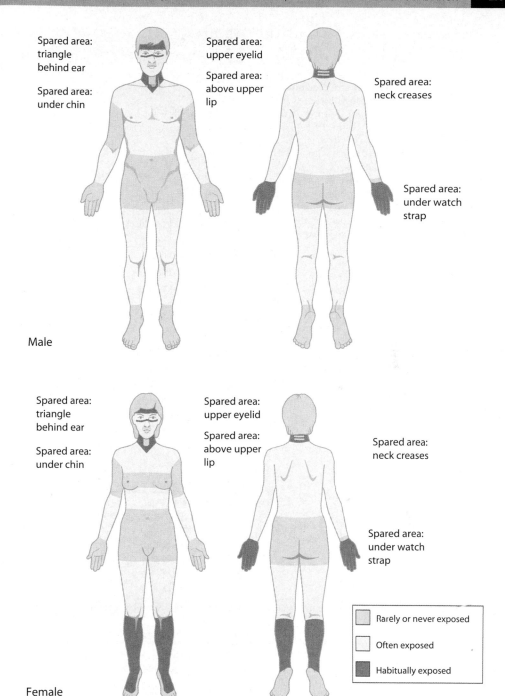

IMAGE 10-1 Variations in solar exposure on different body areas.

fact is the principal basis for the classification of "white" persons into four *skin phototypes* (SPT). The SPT is based on the basic skin color (Table 10-2) and on a *person's own estimate* of sunburning and tanning. One question permits the identification of the SPT: "Do you tan easily?" Persons with SPT I or II will say immediately, "No," and those with SPT III or IV will say, "Yes." Persons with SPT I or II are regarded as "melanocompromised," and those with SPT III or IV as "melanocompetent."

SPT I persons usually have pale white skin color, blond or red hair, and blue eyes; but, in fact, they may have dark brown hair and brown eyes, while their skin color is pale white. SPT I persons sunburn easily with short exposures and do not tan.

SPT II persons are a subgroup of SPT I and sunburn easily but *tan with difficulty,* whereas SPT III persons may have some sunburn with short exposures but can develop marked tanning. It is estimated that about 25% of white-skinned persons in the United States are SPT I and II. SPT IV persons tan with ease and do not sunburn with short exposures. SPT IV persons may have blond hair and blue eyes but more often have brown hair and brown eyes and light tan (beige) constitutive skin color. Persons with constitutive brown skin are termed SPT V and with black skin SPT VI. Note that sunburn depends on the amount of UVR energy absorbed. Thus, with excessive sun exposure, even SPT VI person can have a sunburn.

TABLE 10-1   Simplified Classification of Skin Reactions to Sunlight

Phototoxicity
  Sunburn
  Drug-/chemical-induced
  Plant-induced (phytophotodermatitis)
Photoallergy
  Drug-/chemical-induced
  Chronic actinic dermatitis
  Solar urticaria
Idiopathic
  Polymorphous light eruption
  Actinic prurigo[a]
  Hydroa vacciniforme[a]
Metabolic and nutritional
  Porphyria cutanea tarda
  Variegate porphyria
  Erythropoietic protoporphyria
  Pellagra[a]
DNA-deficient photodermatoses
  Xeroderma pigmentosum[a]
  Other rare syndromes[a]
Photoexacerbated dermatoses
Chronic photodamage
  Dermatoheliosis (photoaging)
  Solar lentigo
  Actinic keratoses
  Skin cancer[b]

[a]Conditions not dealt with here and the reader is referred to K Wolff et al (eds): *Fitzpatrick's Dermatology in General Medicine,* 7th ed. New York, McGraw-Hill, 2008.
[b]For coverage of skin cancer, see Sections 11 and 12.

TABLE 10-2   Classification of Fitzpatrick's Skin Phototypes (SPT)

SPT	Basic Skin Color	Response to Sun Exposure
I	Pale white	Do not tan, burn easily
II	White	Tan with difficulty, burn easily
III	White	Tan easily but may burn initially
IV	Light brown/olive	Tan easily, hardly burn
V	Brown	Tan easily, usually do not burn
VI	Black	Become darker, do not burn

> **ACUTE SUN DAMAGE (SUNBURN)**   ICD-9:692.71 ○ ICD-10:L55   ■ ○→○
>
> - Sunburn is an acute, delayed, and transient inflammatory response of normal skin after exposure to UVR from sunlight or artificial sources.
> - By nature it is a phototoxic reaction.
>
> - Sunburn is characterized by erythema (Fig. 10-1*A*) and, if severe, by vesicles and bullae, edema, tenderness, and pain (Fig. 10-1*B*).

EPIDEMIOLOGY

Sunburn depends on the amount of UVR energy delivered and the susceptibility of the individual (SPT). It will therefore occur more often around midday, with decreasing latitude, increasing altitude, and decreasing SPT. Thus, the "ideal" setting for a sunburn to occur would be an SPT I individual (highest susceptibility) on Mt. Kenya (high altitude, close to the equator) at noon (UVR is highest). Of course, sunburn can occur at any latitude, but the probability for it to occur decreases with increasing distance from the equator. Sunburn is seen more often in those who frequent beaches or travel to sunny vacation areas. Sunburn also increases with respect to other ambient conditions, such as UVR reflectance from snow, water, or a glacier.

Age Very young children and elderly persons are said to have a reduced capacity to sunburn, although this has not been thoroughly documented.

PATHOGENESIS

The chromophores (molecules that absorb UVR) for UVB sunburn erythema are not known, but damage to DNA may be the initiating event. The damage to DNA results in excision of pyrimidine dimers, and that itself initiates a protective tanning response. The mediators that cause the erythema include histamine for both UVA and UVB. In UVB erythema, other mediators include tumor necrosis factor α (TNF-α), serotonin, prostaglandins, nitric oxide, lysosomal enzymes, and kinins. The cytokine TNF-α can be detected as early as 1 h after exposure. The resolution of erythema is associated with interleukin (IL) 10, IL-4, and transforming growth factor β_1.

CLINICAL MANIFESTATION

Exposure to the sun or an artificial UV source. Onset of symptoms depends on intensity of exposure; erythema develops after 6 h and peaks after 24 h.

Skin Symptoms Pruritus may be severe even in mild sunburn; pain and tenderness occur with severe sunburn.

Constitutional Symptoms Headache, chills, feverishness, and weakness are not infrequent in severe sunburn; some SPT I and II persons develop headache and malaise even after short exposures.

General Appearance In severe sunburn, the patient is "toxic"—with fever, weakness, lassitude, and a rapid pulse rate.

Skin Lesions Confluent bright erythema always confined to sun-exposed areas and thus sharply marginated at the border between exposed and covered skin (Fig. 10-1*A*). Edema, vesicles, and even bullae; always uniform erythema and no "rash," as occurs in most photoallergic reactions. Edematous areas are raised and tender. As edema and erythema fade vesicles and blisters dry to crusts, which are then shed (Fig. 10-1*B*).

Distribution Strictly confined to areas of exposure; sunburn can occur in areas covered with clothing, depending on the degree of UV transmission through clothing, the level of exposure, and the SPT of the person.

Mucous Membranes Sunburn of the tongue can occur rarely in mountain climbers who hold their mouth open "panting"; it is frequent on the vermilion border of the lips.

LABORATORY EXAMINATIONS

Dermatopathology "Sunburn" cells in the epidermis (apoptotic keratinocytes); also, exocytosis of lymphocytes, vacuolization of melanocytes and Langerhans cells. *Dermis*: endothelial cell swelling of superficial blood vessels. More prominent with UVA erythema, with a denser mononuclear infiltrate and more severe vascular changes.

Serology and Hematology   To rule out systemic lupus erythematosus (SLE) obtain antinuclear antibody (ANA) level. Leukopenia may be present in SLE.

DIAGNOSIS AND DIFFERENTIAL DIAGNOSIS

History of UVR exposure and sites of reaction on exposed areas. *Phototoxic erythema*: obtain history of medications that can induce phototoxic erythema. *SLE* can cause a sunburn-type erythema. *Erythropoietic protoporphyria* causes erythema, vesicles, edema, purpura, and, only rarely, urticarial wheals.

COURSE AND PROGNOSIS

Sunburn, unlike thermal burns, cannot be classified on the basis of depth, i.e., first-, second-, and third-degree. Third-degree burns after UVR do not occur, and none of the features of third-degree thermal burns are seen: scarring, loss of sensation, loss of sweating, hair loss. A perma-

nent reaction from severe ultraviolet burns is mottled depigmentation, probably related to the destruction of melanocytes, and eruptive solar lentigines (see Fig. 10-22).

MANAGEMENT

Prevention   Persons with SPT I or II should avoid sunbathing, especially between 11 A.M. and 2 P.M. Clothing: UV-screening cloth garments. There are now many highly effective topical chemical filters (sunscreens) in lotion, gel, and cream formulations. It is still not clear whether regular use of topical sunscreens can prevent melanoma of the skin, but there is reasonable proof that topical sunscreens reduce the induction of solar keratoses and, probably, squamous cell carcinoma.

Moderate Sunburn   *Topical*   Cool wet dressings, topical glucocorticoids.

Systemic   Acetylsalicylic acid, indomethacin, NSAIDs.

Severe Sunburn   Bed rest. If very severe, a "toxic" patient may require hospitalization for fluid replacement, prophylaxis of infection, etc. *Topical*   Cool wet dressings, topical glucocorticoids.

Systemic   Oral glucocorticoids are often given, but their efficacy has not been established by controlled studies. Indomethacin.

DRUG-/CHEMICAL-INDUCED PHOTOSENSITIVITY   ICD-9:692.79 ∘ ICD-10:L56.0

- This describes the interaction of UVR with a chemical/drug within the skin.
- Two mechanisms are recognized: *phototoxic reactions,* which are photochemical reactions leading to skin pathology, and
- *photoallergic reactions,* where a photoallergen is formed that initiates an immunologic response

and manifests in skin as a type IV immunologic reaction.
- The main clinical difference between phototoxic and photoallergic eruptions is that the former manifests like an irritant (toxic) contact dermatitis or sunburn and the latter like an allergic eczematous contact dermatitis (Table 10-3).

A

B

FIGURE 10-1   Acute sunburn   A. Painful, tender, bright erythema with mild edema of the upper back with sharp demarcation between the sun-exposed and sun-protected white areas. **B.** 48 hours after acute sunburn. Erythema is fading and blisters have dried to crusts.

TABLE 10-3 Characteristics of Phototoxicity and Photoallergy

	Phototoxicity	Photoallergy
Clinical presentation	Sunburn reaction: erythema, edema, vesicles and bullae; frequently resolves with hyperpigmentation; burning, smarting	Eczematous lesions, papules, vesicles, scaling, crusting; usually pruritic
Histology	Apoptotic keratinocytes, sparse dermal infiltrate of lymphocytes, macrophages, and neutrophils	Spongiotic dermatitis, dense, dermal lymphohistiocytic infiltrate
Pathophysiology	Direct tissue injury	Type IV delayed hypersensitivity reponse
Occurrence after first exposure	Yes	No
Onset of eruption after exposure	Minutes to hours	24–48 h
Dosage of agent needed for eruption	Large	Small
Cross-reactivity with other agents	Rare	Common
Diagnosis	Clinical + phototests	Clinical + phototests + photopatch tests

Adapted from H Lim, in K Wolff et al (eds): *Fitzpatrick's Dermatology in General Medicine,* 7th ed. New York, McGraw-Hill, 2008.

PHOTOTOXIC DRUG-/CHEMICAL-INDUCED PHOTOSENSITIVITY   ICD-9:692.79 ∘ ICD-10:L56.0

- This describes an adverse reaction of the skin that results from simultaneous exposure to certain drugs (via ingestion, injection, or topical application) and to UVR or visible light.
- The chemicals may be therapeutic, cosmetic, industrial, or agricultural.
- There are two types of reaction: (1) systemic phototoxic dermatitis, occurring in individuals systemically exposed to a photosensitizing agent

(drug) and subsequent UVR; and (2) local phototoxic dermatitis, occurring in individuals topically exposed to the photosensitizing agent and subsequent UVR.
- Both are *exaggerated sunburn responses* (erythema, edema, vesicles, and/or bullae).
- Systemic phototoxic dermatitis occurs in all *UVR-exposed sites;* local phototoxic dermatitis only in the *topical application sites.*

TABLE 10-4 Systemic Phototoxic Agents[a]

Property	Generic Name	Property	Generic Name
Antianxiety drugs	Alprazolam	Diuretics	Hydrochlorothiazide
	Chlordiazepoxide		**Dyazide**
Anticancer drugs	Adriamycin	Dyes	Fluorescein
	Dacarbazine		Methylene blue
	Fluorouracil	Furocoumarins	Psoralens
	Methotrexate		**5-Methoxypsoralen**
	Vinblastine		**8-Methoxypsoralen**
Antidepressants	Tricyclics		**4, 5', 8-Trimethylpsoralen**
	Amitriptyline	Hypoglycemics	Sulfonylureas:
	Desipramine		Acetohexamide
	Imipramine		Chlorpropamide
Antifungals	Griseofulvin		Glipizide
Antimalarials	Chloroquine		Glyburide
	Quinine		Tolazamide
Antimicrobials	Quinolones		**Tolbutamide**
	Ciprofloxacin	NSAIDs	Acetic acid derivative
	Enoxacin		Diclofenac
	Gemifloxacin		Anthranilic acid derivative
	Lomefloxacin		Mefenamic acid
	Moxifloxacin		Enolic acid derivative:
	Nalidixic acid		**Piroxicam**
	Norfloxacin		Propionic acid derivatives
	Ofloxacin		Ibuprofen
	Sparfloxacin		Ketoprofen
	Sulfonamides		**Naproxen**
	Tetracyclines		Oxaprozin
	Demeclocycline		Tiaprofenic acid
	Doxycycline		Salicylic acid derivative
	Minocycline		Diflunisal
	Tetracycline		Others
	Trimethoprim		Celecoxib
	Voriconazole		**Nabumetone**
Antipsychotic	Phenothiazines	Photodynamic	**Porfimer**
drugs	**Chlorpromazine**	therapy agents	**Verteporfin**
	Perphenazine	Retinoids	Acitretin
	Prochlorperazine		Isotretinoin
	Thioridazine	Other	Flutamide
	Trifluoperazine		Hypericin
Cardiac	**Amiodarone**		Pyridoxine (vitamin B$_6$)
medications	Quinidine		Ranitidine
Diuretics	**Furosemide**		
	Thiazides		
	Bendroflumethiazide		
	Chlorothiazide		

[a]Commonly reported drugs are printed in bold.
Source: Adapted from H Lim, in K Wolff et al (eds): *Fitzpatrick's Dermatology in General Medicine,* 7th ed. New York, McGraw-Hill, 2008.

SYSTEMIC PHOTOTOXIC DERMATITIS   ICD-9:692.79 ∘ ICD-10:656.0

EPIDEMIOLOGY

Occurs in everyone after ingestion of a sufficient dose of a photosensitizing drug and subsequent UVR. Therefore all ages, both sexes, all races, and all types of skin color. Phototoxic drug reactions are more frequent than photoallergic drug sensitivity.

ETIOLOGY AND PATHOGENESIS

Formation of toxic photoproducts such as free radicals or reactive oxygen species such as singlet oxygen. The principal sites of damage are nuclear DNA or cell membranes (plasma, lysosomal, mitochondrial). The action spectrum is UVA. Drugs eliciting systemic phototoxic dermatitis are listed in Table 10-4. Some drugs causing phototoxic reactions can also elicit photoallergic reactions (see below).

CLINICAL MANIFESTATION

An "exaggerated sunburn" after solar or UVR exposure that *normally would not elicit a sunburn in that particular individual.* Occurs usually within hours after exposure, with some agents such as psoralens after 24 h, and peaking at 48 h. Skin symptoms: burning, stinging, pruritus.

Skin Lesions   *Early:* The skin lesions are those of an "exaggerated sunburn." Erythema, edema (Fig. 10-2*A*), and vesicle and bulla formation (Fig. 10-2*B*) confined exclusively to areas exposed to light. An eczematous reaction is *not* seen in phototoxic reactions.
Special Presentations: Pseudoporphyria   With some drugs there is little erythema but pronounced blistering and skin fragility with erosions (see Fig. 22-13) and, upon repeated exposures, healing milia formation, particularly on the dorsa of hands and lower arms. Clinically indistinguishable from porphyria cutanea tarda (see Fig. 10-11)—hence the term *pseudoporphyria* (see Section 22).
Nails   Subungual hemorrhage and photo-onycholysis can occur with certain drugs (psoralens, demethylchlortetracycline, benoxaprofen).
Pigmentation   Marked brown epidermal melanin pigmentation may occur in the course of some eruptions. With certain drugs especially

(chlorpromazine and amiodarone), a slate gray dermal melanin pigmentation develops (see Section 22). ☒

LABORATORY EXAMINATIONS

Dermatopathology   Inflammation, "sunburn cells" (apoptotic keratinocytes) in the epidermis, epidermal necrobiosis, intraepidermal and subepidermal vesiculation. Absence of eczematous changes.
Phototesting   For verification of the incriminating agent, template test sites are exposed to increasing doses of UVA (*phototoxic reactions are almost always due to UVA*) while patient is on the drug. The UVA MED will be much lower than that for normal individuals of the same skin phototype. After drug is excreted and then eliminated from the skin, a repeat UVA phototest will reveal an *increase* in the UVA MED. This test may be important if patient is on multiple potentially phototoxic drugs.

DIAGNOSIS AND DIFFERENTIAL DIAGNOSIS

History of exposure to drugs is most important, as are the types of morphologic changes in the skin characteristic of phototoxic drug eruptions: confluent erythema, edema, vesicles, bullae. Differential diagnosis includes regular sunburn, phototoxic reactions due to excess of endogenous porphyrins, and photosensitivity due to other diseases, e.g., SLE.

COURSE AND PROGNOSIS

Phototoxic drug sensitivity is a major problem, since the abnormal reactions seriously limit or exclude the use of important drugs: diuretics, antihypertensive agents, drugs used in psychiatry. Whereas, as a rule, phototoxicity occurs in practically anyone who is on a phototoxic drug—in contrast to photoallergy, which occurs only in the sensitized—some individuals nonetheless show phototoxic reactions to a particular drug and others do not. It is not known why. Phototoxic drug reactions disappear after cessation of drug.

MANAGEMENT

As for sunburn.

FIGURE 10-2   Phototoxic drug-induced photosensitivity   A. Massive edema and erythema in the face of a 17-year-old girl who was treated with demethylchlortetracycline for acne. Note absence of erythema from neck, which was shaded. **B.** Dusky erythema with blistering on the dorsa of both hands in a patient treated with piroxicam.

TOPICAL PHOTOTOXIC DEMATITIS   ICD-9 : 692.79 ∘ ICD-10 : L56.0 ▯ ◑

- Here there is inadvertent contact with or therapeutic application of a photosensitizer, followed by UVA irradiation (practically all topical photosensitizers have an action spectrum in the UVA range).

- The most common topical phototoxic agents are listed in Table 10-5, and the most common route of contact is either therapeutic or occupational exposure.

- Clinical presentation is like acute irritant contact dermatitis (see Section 2), with erythema,

swelling, vesiculation, and blistering confined to the sites of contact with the phototoxic agent.

- Symptoms are smarting, stinging, and burning rather than itching.

- Healing usually results in pronounced pigmentation. The most common and thus important topical phototoxic dermatitis is phytophotodermatitis, described below.

PHYTOPHOTODERMATITIS (PPD)   ICD-9:692.72 ∘ ICD-10:L56.2 ■ ◐

- Phytophotodermatitis (plant + light = dermatitis) is an inflammation of the skin caused by contact with certain plants during recreational or occupational exposure to sunlight.
- The inflammatory response is a phototoxic re-action to photosensitizing chemicals in several plant families.
- Common types of PPD are due to exposure to limes, celery, and meadow grass.

Synonyms: Berloque dermatitis, lime dermatitis.

EPIDEMIOLOGY AND ETIOLOGY

Common. Usually in spring and summer or all year in tropical climates. PPD can occur at any age.

Race   All skin colors; brown- and black-skinned persons may develop only marked spotty dark pigmentation without erythema or bullous lesions.

Occupation   Celery pickers, carrot processors, gardeners [exposed to carrot greens or to "gas plant" (*Dictamnus albus*)], and bartenders (lime juice) who are exposed to sun in outside bars. Nonoccupational: housewives and users of perfumes containing oil of bergamot; persons in holiday drinking time drinks or eating oranges in the sun.

Etiology   Phototoxic reaction caused by photoactive furocoumarins (psoralens) contained in the plants (Table 10-5).

CLINICAL MANIFESTATION

The patient gives a history of exposure to certain plants (lime, lemon, wild parsley, celery, giant hogweed, parsnips, carrot greens, figs). Lime juice is a frequent cause: making lime drinks, hair rinses with lime juice. Women who use perfumes containing oil of bergamot (which contains bergapten, 5-methoxypsoralen) may develop streaks of pigmentation only in areas where the perfume was applied, especially the sides of the neck. This is called *berloque derma-titis* (French: *berloque*, "pendant"). Persons walk-ing on beaches containing meadow grass and children playing in grassy meadows develop PPD on the legs; meadow grass contains agrimony.

Skin Symptoms   Smarting, sensation of sunburn, pain, later pruritus.

Skin Lesions   Acute: erythema, edema, vesicles, and bullae (Fig. 10-3). Lesions may appear pseudopapular before vesicles are evident. Often bizarre streaks, artificial patterns that indicate an "outside job" (Fig. 10-4). Scattered areas on the sites of contact, especially the arms, legs, and face. Residual hyperpigmentation in bizarre streaks (berloque dermatitis) (Fig. 10-5). ▨

DIAGNOSIS AND DIFFERENTIAL DIAGNOSIS

Easily made if the pattern is recognized and a careful history is taken. Differential diagnosis is primarily acute irritant contact dermatitis, with streaky pattern poison ivy dermatitis (see Figs. 2-8, 2-10), but this is eczematous.

COURSE

May be an important occupational problem, as in celery pickers. The acute eruption has a short life and fades spontaneously, but the pigmentation may last for many weeks.

MANAGEMENT

Wet dressings may be indicated in the acute vesicular stage. Topical glucocorticoids.

■ TABLE 10-5   Common Topical Phototoxic Agents

Agent	Exposure
Rose Bengal	Ophthalmologic examination
Fluorescein	Dye
Furocoumarins	Occur naturally in plants (mostly *Compositae* spp.; *Umbiliferae* spp.; fruits and vegetables (lime, lemon, celery, fig, parsley, parsnip); used in perfumes and cosmetics (e.g., oil of bergamot); and used for topical photochemotherapy
Tar	Topical therapeutic agent, roofing materials, road tarring

FIGURE 10-3   Phytophotodermatitis (plant + light): acute with blisters   These bullae were the result of exposure to umbiliferae and the sun. This 50-year-old housewife was weeding her garden on a sunny day. Umbiliferae contain bergapten (5-methoxypsoralen), which is a potent topical phototoxic chemical.

FIGURE 10-5   Berloque dermatitis   The patient had applied a fragrant bath oil to her shoulders and chest but showered only the front of her body before going into the sun. The bath oil contained oil of bergamot, and pigmentation is now noted where it trickled down from the shoulders to the buttocks. (Courtesy of Dr. Thomas Schwarz.)

FIGURE 10-4   Phytophotodermatitis   In a 48-year-old man who was sunbathing in a meadow. Immediately before vesicles and blisters arise erythematous lesions may appear raised, giving the false impression of being papular. Note streaky pattern.

PHOTOALLERGIC DRUG-/CHEMICAL-INDUCED PHOTOSENSITIVITY ICD-9:692.72 ∘ ICD-10:L56.1 ■ ◑

- This results from interaction of a photoallergen and UVA radiation.
- In sensitized individuals exposure to a photoallergen and sunlight results in a pruritic eczematous eruption confined to exposed sites and clinically indistinguishable from allergic contact dermatitis.
- In most patients the eliciting drug/chemical has been applied topically, but systemic elicitation also occurs.

EPIDEMIOLOGY

Age of Onset   More common in adults.
Race   All skin phototypes and colors.
Incidence   Photoallergic drug reactions occur much less frequently than do phototoxic drug reactions.

ETIOLOGY AND PATHOGENESIS

Topically applied chemical/drug plus UVA radiation. The chemicals are disinfectants, antimicrobials, agents in sunscreens, perfumes in aftershaves, or whiteners (Table 10-6). The chemical agent present in the skin absorbs photons and forms a photoproduct; this then binds to a soluble or membrane-bound protein to form an antigen to which a type IV immune response is elicited. Since photoallergy depends on individual immunologic reactivity, it develops in only a small percentage of persons exposed to drugs and light and is elicited only in those who have been sensitized. Photoallergy can also be induced by systemic administration of a drug and elicited by topical administration of the same drug, and vice versa. UVA is always required.

CLINICAL MANIFESTATION

May be unclear in that the initial exposure induces sensitization to delayed-type hypersensitivity reactions, and the eruption occurs only on subsequent exposure. Topically applied photosensitizers are the most frequent cause of photoallergic eruptions (Table 10-6). Eruption is highly pruritic.

Skin Lesions   The morphology of the skin reaction is much different from that in phototoxic drug sensitivity. Acute photoallergic reaction patterns are clinically indistinguishable from allergic contact dermatitis (Fig. 10-6): papular, vesicular, scaling, and crusted. Occasionally there can also be a lichenoid eruption similar to lichen planus. In chronic drug photoallergy, there is scaling, lichenification, and marked

TABLE 10-6   Topical Photoallergens[a]

Group	Chemical Name
Sunscreens	UVB absorbers:
	para-Aminobenzoic acid (PABA)
	Cinnamates
	Salicylates
	UVA absorbers:
	Anthranilate
	Benzophenones
Fragrances	**6-Methylcoumarin**
	Musk ambrette
	Sandalwood oil
Antibacterials	**Dibromosalicylanilide**
	Tetrachlorosalicylanilide
	Tribromosalicylanilide
	Chlorhexidine
	Dimethylol-dimethyl hydantoin
	Hexachlorophene
	Bithionol
	Dichlorophene
	Triclosan
	Sulfonamides
Antifungals	Thiobischlorophenol
	Buclosamide
	Bromochlorosalicylanilide
Others	**Chlorpromazine**
	Clioquinol
	Ketoprofen
	Olaquindox
	Promethazine
	Quinidine
	Thiourea

[a]Commonly reported drugs are printed in bold.

Source: Adapted from H Lim, in K Wolff et al (eds): *Fitzpatrick's Dermatology in General Medicine,* 7th ed. New York, McGraw-Hill, 2008.

pruritus mimicking atopic dermatitis or, again, chronic allergic contact dermatitis (Fig. 10-6; see also "Eczema/Dermatitis," Section 2.)

Distribution   Confined primarily to areas exposed to light (distribution pattern of photosensitivity), but there may be spreading onto adjacent nonexposed skin; therefore, it is not so well circumscribed as in phototoxic reactions. Of diagnostic help is the fact that in the face the upper eyelids, the area under the nose, and a thin strip of skin between the lower lip and the chin are often spared (shaded areas) (Fig. 10-6). ✐

LABORATORY EXAMINATION

Dermatopathology   Acute and chronic delayed-type hypersensitivity reaction: epidermal spongiosis with lymphocytic infiltration.

DIAGNOSIS

History of exposure to drug is most important, as well as the types of morphologic changes in the skin: this is essentially an allergic contact dermatitis pattern. In essence, the differential diagnosis between this and phototoxic eruptions is identical to that described for toxic/irritant and allergic contact dermatitis (see Section 2).

Diagnosis requires the use of patch and photopatch tests. Photopatch tests are done in duplicate because photoallergens can also cause contact hypersensitivity. Photoallergens are applied to the skin and covered. After 24 h, one set of the duplicate test sites is exposed to UVA while the other set remains covered; test sites are read for reactions after 48–96 h. An eczematous reaction in the irradiated site but not in the

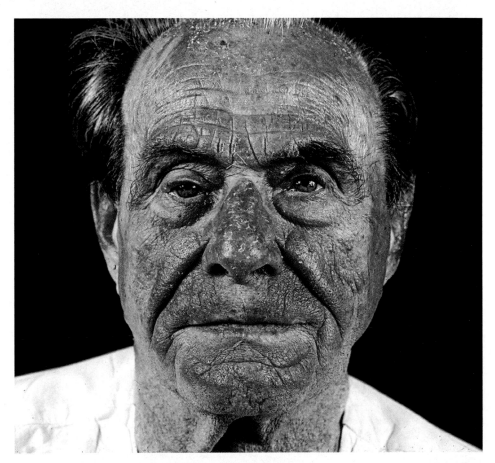

FIGURE 10-6   Photoallergic drug-induced photosensitivity   This 60-year-old male shows an eczematous dermatitis in the face. He was taking trimethoprim-sulfamethoxazole. Note sparing of eyelids (protected by sunglasses), under the nose, and the area under the lower lip (shaded areas).

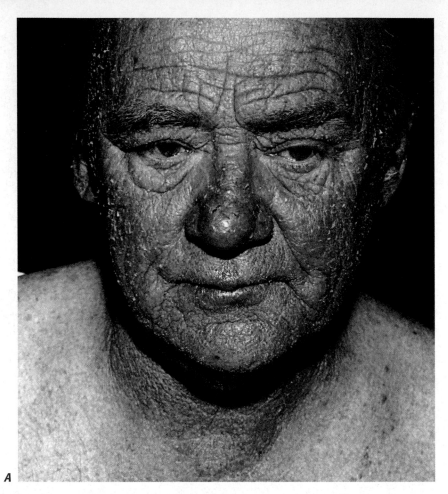

A

FIGURE 10-7   Drug-induced photosensitivity: persistent light eruption   *A.* Erythematous plaques confined to the face and neck, sparing the shoulders. This male has excruciating pruritus.

nonirradiated site confirms photoallergy to the particular agent tested.

COURSE AND PROGNOSIS

Photoallergic dermatitis can persist for months to years. This is known as *persistent light reaction,* or *chronic actinic dermatitis* (Fig. 10-7*A, B*), The classic generalized persistent light reactions were caused by exposure to soaps containing salicylanilides (Table 10-6). In *persistent light reaction,* the action spectrum usually broadens to involve UVB, and the condition persists despite discontinuation of the causative photoallergen, with each new UV exposure aggravating the condition. Chronic

eczema-like lichenified and extremely itchy confluent plaques result (Fig. 10-7*A, B*), which lead to gross disfigurement and a distressing situation for the patient. As the condition is now independent of the original photoallergen and is aggravated by each new solar exposure, avoidance of photoallergen does not cure the disease. In contrast to earlier belief, chronic actinic dermatitis does not progress to lymphoma.

MANAGEMENT

In severe cases, immunosuppression (azathioprine plus glucocorticoids or oral cyclosporine) is required.

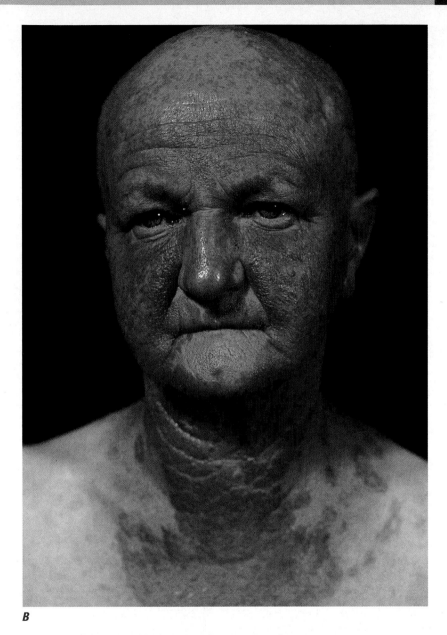

B

FIGURE 10-7 **Drug-induced photosensitivity: persistent light eruption (Continued)** *B.* Persistent light eruption with infiltrated eczematous eruption in the face and the neck.

POLYMORPHOUS LIGHT ERUPTION   ICD-9:692.72 ∘ ICD-10:L56.4 ■ ◑

- Polymorphous light eruption (PMLE) is a term that describes a group of heterogeneous, idiopathic, acquired, acute recurrent eruptions characterized by delayed abnormal reactions to UVR.
- Manifested by varied lesions, including erythematous macules, papules, plaques, and vesicles.

However, in each patient the eruption is consistently monomorphous.
- By far the most frequent morphologic types are the papular and papulovesicular eruptions.

EPIDEMIOLOGY

Incidence Most common photodermatosis. Prevalence from 10% in Boston, 14% in London, to 21% in Sweden. Average age is 23 years, much more common in females. All races, but most common in SPT I, II, III, and IV. In American Indians (North and South America) there is a *hereditary* type of PMLE that is called *actinic prurigo*.

Geography PMLE is less frequently observed in areas that have high solar intensity throughout the year and in persons who have adapted to persistent sun exposures. In fact, PMLE often occurs for the first time in persons traveling for short vacations to tropical areas in winter from northern latitudes.

PATHOGENESIS

Possibly a delayed-type hypersensitivity reaction to an (auto-) antigen induced by UVR; suggested by the morphology of the lesions and the histologic pattern, which shows an infiltration of T cells. More commonly, UVA is the action spectrum, but PMLE lesions have been evoked with UVB and with both UVA and UVB. Since UVA is transmitted through window glass, PMLE can be precipitated while riding in a car. Areas of the skin habitually exposed (face and neck) are often spared, despite severe involvement of the arms, trunk, and legs.

CLINICAL MANIFESTATION

Onset and Duration of Lesions PMLE appears in spring or early summer, and not infrequently the eruption does not recur by the end of summer, suggesting a "hardening." PMLE most often appears within hours of exposure and, once established, persists for 7 to 10 days, thereby limiting the vacationer's subsequent time in the

sun. Symptoms are pruritus (may precede the onset of the rash) and paresthesia (tingling).

Skin Lesions The papular (Fig. 10-8) and papulovesicular types are the most frequent. Less common are plaques or urticarial plaques (Fig. 10-9). The lesions are pink to red. In the individual patient, lesions are quite monomorphous, i.e., either papular or papulovesicular or urticarial plaques. Recurrences follow the original pattern.

Distribution The eruption often spares the face and appears most frequently on the forearms, V area of the neck, arms, and chest (Fig. 10-8). The lesions may also occur on the face (Fig. 10-9), if there has not been previous exposure. ◪

LABORATORY EXAMINATIONS

Dermatopathology Edema of the epidermis, spongiosis, vesicle formation, and mild liquefaction degeneration of the basal layer. A dense lymphocytic infiltrate is present in the dermis, with occasional neutrophils. There is edema of the papillary dermis and endothelial swelling.

Immunofluorescence (Direct) Negative. ANA negative. There is no leukopenia.

DIAGNOSIS

The diagnosis is not difficult: delayed onset of eruption, characteristic morphology, histopathologic changes that rule out lupus erythematosus, and the history of disappearance of the eruption in days. In plaque-type PMLE, a biopsy and immunofluorescence studies are mandatory to rule out SLE (Fig. 10-9). *Phototesting* is done with both UVB and UVA. Test sites are exposed daily, starting with 2 MEDs of UVB and UVA, respectively, for 1 week to 10 days, using increments of the UV dose. In 50% of patients, a PMLE-like eruption will occur

FIGURE 10-8 Polymorphic light eruption Clusters of confluent, extremely pruritic papules on the exposed chest, occurred in an Arabian man the day following the first sun exposure of the season. The eruption also involved the arms, but spared the face and dorsal hands.

FIGURE 10-9 Polymorphic light eruption Erythematous plaques in the face following first sun exposure of the season. The butterfly distribution is very similar to that of lupus erythematosus.

in the test sites, confirming the diagnosis. The eruption in the test site mimics the type of PMLE in that particular patient. This also helps to determine whether the action spectrum is UVB, UVA, or both.

COURSE AND PROGNOSIS

The course is chronic and recurrent and may, in fact, become worse each season. Although some patients may develop "tolerance" by the end of the summer, the eruption usually recurs the following spring and/or when the person travels to tropical areas in the winter. However, spontaneous improvement or even cessation of eruptions occurs after years.

MANAGEMENT

Prevention   Sunblocks, even the potent UVA-UVB sunscreens, are not always effective but should be tried first in every patient.

Systemic   β-Carotene, 60 mg three times a day for 2 weeks, before going in the sun. Oral prednisone 20 mg/day given 2 days before and 2 days during exposure is a good prophylaxis. Also, intramuscular triamcinolone acetonide, 40 mg, will suppress an eruption when administered a few days before a trip to a sunny region.

PUVA Photochemotherapy   This is very effective when given in early spring by inducing "tolerance" for the summer. PUVA treatments have to be given before the sunny season, have to be repeated each spring, but are usually not necessary for more than 3 or 4 years. *Narrow-band UVB* (311 nm) is used with equal success.

SOLAR URTICARIA   ICD-9 : 708.9 ∘ ICD-10 : L56.3   ☐ ◑

- Uncommon sunlight-induced whealing confined to exposed body sites.
- Eruption occurs within minutes of exposure and resolves in a few hours. Very disabling and sometimes life threatening.
- Action spectrum is UVB, UVA, and visible light or any combination thereof. Most commonly UVA (Fig. 10-10).

- Is an immediate type I hypersensitivity response to cutaneous and/or circulating photoallergens.
- Therapy: multiple phototherapy sessions in low but increasing doses on the same day ("rush hardening"); oral immunosuppressive agents or plasmapheresis.
- Prevention: sun avoidance, sunscreens with high protection factors against action spectrum. ⏎

PHOTOEXACERBATED DERMATOSES

- Various wavelengths of UVR and/or visible light can elicit or aggravate a number of dermatoses.
- In these cases the eruption is invariably similar to that of the primary condition.

- An abbreviated list is given in alphabetical order in Table 10-7, but it should be emphasized that among these disorders SLE is by far the most important.

FIGURE 10-10   Solar urticaria, test sites   The upper row of the template test sites were exposed to increasing doses of UVB and revealed only erythema (figures indicate mJ/cm^2 applied). 24 hours later the template test sites in the lower row were exposed to 0.5 and 1 J/cm^2 UVA (which are extremely low doses) and immediately after the exposure this picture was taken. Note massive urticarial reaction in the UVA-exposed test sites.

TABLE 10-7   Diseases Exacerbated by Ultraviolet Irradiation

Acne	Pellagra
Atopic eczema	Pemphigus foliaceus (erythematosus)
Carcinoid syndrome	Pityriasis rubra pilaris
Cutaneous T cell lymphoma	Psoriasis
Darier disease	Reticulate erythematous mucinosis syndrome
Dermatomyositis	Rosacea
Disseminated superficial actinic porokeratosis	Seborrheic dermatitis
Erythema multiforme	**Lupus erythematosus**
Familial benign chronic pemphigus	Transient acantholytic dermatosis
(Hailey-Hailey disease)	(Grover disease)
Keratosis follicularis (Darier disease)	Herpes labialis
Lichen planus	

METABOLIC PHOTOSENSITIVITY—THE PORPHYRIAS

PORPHYRIA CUTANEA TARDA   ICD-9:277.1 ∘ ICD-10:E80.1   ▮ ◑

- Porphyria cutanea tarda (PCT) occurs mostly in adults.
- Patients do not present with characteristic photosensitivity but with complaints of "fragile skin," vesicles, and bullae, particularly on the dorsa of the hands, after minor trauma.
- The diagnosis is confirmed by the presence of a pinkish-red fluorescence in the urine when examined with a Wood lamp.

- PCT is distinct from variegate porphyria (VP) and acute intermittent porphyria (AIP) in that patients with PCT do not have acute life-threatening attacks.
- Furthermore, the drugs that induce PCT are fewer than the drugs that induce VP and AIP.
- For classification of the porphyrias, see Table 10-8.

TABLE 10-8   Classification and Differential Diagnosis of Porphyrias

	Congenital Erythropoietic Porphyrias	Erythropoietic Protoporphyria	Porphyria Cutanea Tarda	Variegate Porphyria	Intermittent Acute Porphyria
Inheritance	Autosomal recessive	Autosomal dominant	Autosomal dominant (familial form)	Autosomal dominant	Autosomal dominant
Signs and symptoms					
Photosensitivity	Yes	Yes	Yes	Yes	No
Cutaneous lesions	Yes	Yes	Yes	Yes	No
Attacks of abdominal pain	No	No	No	Yes	Yes
Neuropsychiatric syndrome	No	No	No	Yes	Yes
Laboratory abnormalities	+	+	+	+	+
Red blood cells					
Fluorescence	+	+	−	−	−
Uroporphyrin	+++	N	N	N	N
Coproporphyrin	++	+	N	N	N
Protoporphyrin	(+)	+++	N	N	N
Plasma					
Fluorescence	+	+	−	+	−
Urine					
Fluorescence	−	−	+	±	−
Porphobilinogen	N	N	N	(+++)	(+++)
Uroporphyrin	+++	N	+++	+++	+++
Feces					
Protoporphyrin	+	++	N	+++	N

Note: N, normal; +, above normal; ++, moderately increased; +++, markedly increased; (+++), frequently increased (depends on whether patient has an attack, or is in remission); (+), increased in some patients.

EPIDEMIOLOGY

Onset 30 to 50 years, rarely in children; females on oral contraceptives; males on estrogen therapy for prostate cancer. Equal in males and in females.

Heredity Most PCT patients have *type I* (*acquired*) induced by drugs or chemicals. *Type II* (*hereditary*), autosomal dominant; possibly these patients actually have VP, but this is not yet resolved. There is also a "dual" type with VP and PCT in the same family.

ETIOLOGY AND PATHOGENESIS

PCT is caused by either an inherited or acquired deficiency of UROGEN decarboxylase. In type I (sporadic, acquired PCT-symptomatic) the enzyme is deficient only in the liver; in type II (PCT-hereditary) it is also deficient in red blood cells (RBCs) and fibroblasts. *Chemicals and drugs that induce PCT:* Ethanol, estrogen, hexachlorobenzene (fungicide), chlorinated phenols, iron, tetrachlorodibenzo-*p*-dioxin. High doses of chloroquine lead to clinical manifestations in "latent" cases (low doses are used as treatment). *Other predisposing factors:* Diabetes mellitus (25%), hepatitis C virus, also, hemochromatosis.

CLINICAL MANIFESTATION

Duration of Lesions No acute skin changes but gradual onset. Patients may present with fragility of skin and bullae on the hands and feet based on a photosensitivity reaction to sun and yet will have a suntan. Pain from erosions in easily traumatized skin ("fragile skin").

Skin Lesions Tense bullae and erosions on normal-appearing skin (Fig. 10-11); slowly heal to form pink atrophic scars, milia (1–2 mm) on dorsa of hands and feet, nose, forehead, or (bald) scalp. Purple-red suffusion ("heliotrope") of central facial skin (Fig. 10-12A), especially periorbital areas. Brown hypermelanosis, diffuse, on exposed areas. Hypertrichosis of face (Fig. 10-13). Scleroderma-like changes, diffuse or circumscribed, waxy yellowish-white areas on exposed areas of face (Fig. 10-12B), neck, and trunk, sparing the doubly clothed area of the breast in females. ◪

FIGURE 10-11 Porphyria cutanea tarda Bullae and atrophic depigmented scars on the dorsum of both hands. This is not an acute reaction to initial sun exposure but develops over time with repeated sun exposure and occurs after minor trauma. The patient presents with a history of "fragile" skin and bullae.

LABORATORY EXAMINATIONS

Dermatopathology Bullae, subepidermal with "festooned" (undulating) base. PAS staining reveals thickened vascular walls. Paucity of an inflammatory infiltrate.

Immunofluorescence IgG and other immunoglobulins at the dermal-epidermal junction and in and around blood vessels, in the sun-exposed areas of the skin.

Chemistry Plasma iron and liver enzymes may be increased. High level of iron stores in the liver. The patient may have hemochromatosis. *Blood glucose* is increased in those patients with diabetes mellitus (25% of patients).

Porphyrin Studies in Stool and Urine (Table 10-8) Increased uroporphyrin (I isomer, 60%) in urine and plasma. Increased isocoproporphyrin (type III) and 7-carboxyl-porphyrin in the feces. In contrast, VP has markedly elevated fecal protoporphyrin as the diagnostic hallmark. No increase in δ-aminolevulinic acid or porphobilinogen in the urine.

Simple Test Wood lamp examination of the urine shows orange-red fluorescence (Fig. 10-14); to enhance, add a few drops of 10% hydrochloric acid.

Liver Biopsy Reveals porphyrin fluorescence and often fatty liver. May also show cirrhosis, hemochromatosis.

DIAGNOSIS AND DIFFERENTIAL DIAGNOSIS

By clinical features, pink-red fluorescence of urine and elevated urinary porphyrins. Bullae on dorsa of hands and feet can occur in *pseudo-PCT* (see Section 22). Phototoxic reactions occur in chronic renal failure with hemodialysis. Tanning salon radiation (visible and UVA). May occasionally resemble dyshidrotic eczema but bullae are on the dorsa. *Epidermolysis bullosa acquisita* (see Section 6) has the same clinical picture (increased skin fragility, easy bruising, and light- and trauma-provoked bullae) and some of the histology (subepidermal bullae with little or no dermal inflammation).

MANAGEMENT

1. Avoid ethanol, stop drugs that could be inducing PCT (such as estrogen), and eliminate exposure to chemicals (chlorinated phenols, tetrachlorodibenzo-*p*-dioxin). In some patients, complete avoidance of ethanol ingestion will result in a clinical and biochemical remission and in depletion of the high level of iron stores in the liver.
2. Phlebotomy is done by removing 500 mL of blood at weekly or biweekly intervals until the hemoglobin is decreased to 10 g. Clinical

FIGURE 10-12 Porphyria cutanea tarda *A.* Very subtle periorbital violaceous coloration.

and biochemical remission occurs within 5 to 12 months after regular phlebotomy. Relapse within a year is uncommon (5–10%).

3. Low-dose chloroquine is used to induce remission of PCT in patients in whom phlebotomy is contraindicated because of anemia. Since chloroquine can exacerbate the disease and, in higher doses, may even induce hepatic failure in these patients, this treatment requires considerable experience. However, long-lasting remissions and, in a portion of patients, clinical and biochemical "cure" can be achieved.

The best approach currently used by one of us (K.W.) is to start with a course of three consecutive phlebotomies every other day followed by 150 mg/d, of chloroquine PO. Close clinical and laboratory monitoring (transaminases, porphyrin excretion in urine), are required to adjust the chloroquine dose, which is eventually tapered to 150 mg twice a week and continued for several months.

FIGURE 10-12   Porphyria cutanea tarda (Continued)   **B.** Sclerodermoid thickening, scars, and erosions on the forehead.

FIGURE 10-13   Porphyria cutanea tarda   Hypertrichosis in a woman who had been on a prolonged regimen with estrogens. Under Wood light her urine showed a bright coral-red fluorescence, as shown in Fig. 10-14.

FIGURE 10-14   Porphyria cutanea tarda: Wood light   Coral-red fluorescence of the urine of a patient with PCT as compared to that of a normal control.

VARIEGATE PORPHYRIA ICD-9:277. 1 ∘ ICD-10:E80.2 □ (■*) ◐→●

- Variegate porphyria (VP) is a serious autosomal dominant disorder of heme biosynthesis.
- Skin lesions that are identical to those of PCT (vesicles and bullae, skin fragility, milia, and scarring of the dorsa of the hands and fingers).
- Acute attacks of abdominal pain, neuropsychiatric manifestations.
- Increased excretion of porphyrins; especially characteristic are high levels of protoporphyrin in the feces.

Synonym: Porphyria variegata.

*In South Africa

EPIDEMIOLOGY

Age of Onset At puberty; peak, second to fourth decades.
Race All races; especially common in white South Africans (3:1000) (a large proportion of the present white population was descended from an early Dutch settler who emigrated to South Africa from Holland in 1680 to where VP can be traced).
Incidence It is increasingly recognized in Europe (Finland) and the United States.
Heredity Autosomal dominant.

ETIOLOGY AND PATHOGENESIS

PROTOGEN oxidase defect resulting in an accumulation of protophyrinogen in the liver, which is excreted in the bile and is nonenzymatically converted to protoporphyrin; this accounts for the high fecal protoporphyrin. The basic metabolic defect is accentuated by ingestion of certain drugs (Table 10-9), with the resultant precipitation of acute attacks of abdominal pain and neuropsychiatric disorders (delirium, seizures, personality changes).

CLINICAL MANIFESTATION

Change with Seasons Skin lesions occur during the summer season but may persist throughout the winter; lesions result from exposure to sunlight. Painful erosions, skin fragility.
Systems Review Acute attacks of abdominal pain, constipation, nausea and vomiting, muscle weakness, seizures, confusional state, psychiatric symptoms (depression, coma); rarely, cranial nerve involvement, bulbar paralysis, sensory loss, and paresthesias.
Drug Exposure See Table 10-9.

Skin Lesions PCT-like vesicles or, more commonly, bullae (Fig. 10-15); erosions, milia; sclerosis (scleroderma-like changes); scars (pink, atrophic). Periorbital heliotrope hue, diffuse melanoderma and hypertrichosis on exposed areas. Localization to dorsa of hands, fingers, and feet, as in PCT.
Miscellaneous Findings Neurologic, especially peripheral neuropathy.

LABORATORY EXAMINATIONS

Dermatopathology As for PCT

TABLE 10-9 Drugs Hazardous to Patients with Variegate Porphyria

Anesthetics: barbiturates and halothane	Imipramine
Anticonvulsants: hydantoins,	Methyldopa
carbamazepine, ethosuximide,	Minor tranquilizers: chlordiazepoxide,
methsuximide, phensuximide, primidone	diazepam, oxazepam, flurazepam,
	meprobamate
Antimicrobial agents: chloramphenicol griseofulvin,	
novobiocin, pyrazinamide,	Pentazocine
sulfonamides	Phenylbutazone
	Sulfonylureas: chlorpropamide,
Ergot preparations	tolbutamide
Ethyl alcohol	Theophylline
Hormones: estrogens, progestin, oral contraceptive	
preparations	

General Laboratory Examination   *Porphyrins*
See Table 10-8.
Plasma   Distinctive plasma fluorescence with emission maximum at 626 nm.
Urine   Increased porphobilinogen during acute attacks.
Stool   High protoporphyrin.

COURSE AND PROGNOSIS

Lifetime disease. Prognosis good, if exacerbating factors are avoided. Rarely, death can occur after ingestion or injection of drugs (e.g., barbiturates, general anesthesia) that induce increased amounts of cytochrome P450 and create a demand for increased synthesis of heme.

DIFFERENTIAL DIAGNOSIS

Pseudoporphyria, scleroderma, acquired epidermolysis bullosa, hereditary coproporphyria, PCT.

MANAGEMENT

None; oral β-carotene may or may not control the skin manifestations but has no effect on porphyrin metabolism or the important systemic manifestations.

FIGURE 10-15   Variegate porphyria   Bullae on the dorsum of the foot and toes, a common site of sun exposure in patients wearing open footwear. This 42-year-old female was diagnosed with porphyria cutanea tarda. The lesions in porphyria cutanea tarda are identical to the lesions in variegate porphyria. This patient, however, gave a history of recurrent attacks of abdominal pain, which was a clue to the diagnosis of variegate porphyria; this diagnosis was established by the detection of elevated stool protoporphyrins. Variegate porphyria (or South African porphyria) is akin to acute intermittent porphyria, in which there are no skin lesions but a fatal outcome may occur with ingestion of certain drugs (see Table 10-9). In South Africa every white patient who is scheduled for major surgery must have laboratory tests for porphyrins since variegate porphyria is common in that country.

ERYTHROPOIETIC PROTOPORPHYRIA   ICD-9:277.1 ∘ ICD-10:F80.0   ☐ ◑

- This hereditary metabolic disorder of porphyrin metabolism is unique among the porphyrias in that porphyrins or porphyrin precursors are usually not excreted in the urine.
- Erythropoietic protoporphyria (EPP) is characterized by an acute sunburn-like photosensitivity, in contrast to the other common porphyrias (PCT or VP), in which obvious acute photosensitivity is *not* a presenting complaint.

- Symptoms occur rapidly within minutes of sun exposure and consist of stinging and burning.
- Skin signs are erythema, edema, and purpura.
- Rarely there may be cirrhosis of the liver and liver failure.
- (Preventive) treatment consists of β-carotene PO.

Synonym: Erythrohepatic protoporphyria.

EPIDEMIOLOGY

Incidence Uncommon; series reported from Europe (in The Netherlands, 1:100,000; Austria, United Kingdom) and the United States.
Age of Onset Acute photosensitivity begins early in childhood; rarely, late onset in early adulthood.
Sex Equal in males and females.
Race All ethnic groups, including blacks.
Heredity Autosomal dominant with variable penetrance.

PATHOGENESIS

The defective enzyme is ferrochelatase. This defect occurs at the step in porphyrin metabolism in which protoporphyrin is converted to heme by ferrochelatase. This leads to an accumulation of protoporphyrin that is highly photosensitizing.

CLINICAL MANIFESTATION

Important sequence of symptoms: stinging, burning, and itching occur *within a few minutes* of sunlight exposure; erythema and edema appear only after 1 to 8 h. Children may choose not to go out in the direct sunlight after a few painful episodes, which may cause serious sociopsychologic problems. Symptoms occur when exposed to sunlight through window glass. Photosensitivity is less common in the winter months in temperate areas.
Systems Review Biliary colic, even in children.

Skin Changes in Acute Reactions to Sunlight
Exposure Bright red erythema, later edema (swelling of hands especially), purpura [especially on the nose, cheeks (Fig. 10-16),

backs of hands (Fig. 10-17), and tips of ears]. Urticaria uncommon; vesicles or bullae rarely occur. These changes appear within 1–8 h after subjective symptoms and subside after several hours or days.

Skin Changes After Chronic Recurrent Exposures
Shallow, often linear scars, on the nose and dorsa of the hands ("aged knuckles"). Diffuse wrinkling of the skin of the nose, around the lips, and the cheeks, with obvious thickening and a waxy color (Fig. 10-18). Crusted, erosive lesions may occur on the nose and lips. In contrast to PCT, absence of sclerodermoid changes, hypertrichosis, and hyperpigmentation. ▨

General Medical Findings
Hemolytic anemia with hypersplenism (rare). Cholelithiasis (12%), even in children; stones contain large amounts of protoporphyrin. Liver disease from massive deposition of protoporphyrin in hepatocytes occurs; fatal hepatic cirrhosis is rare, but occurs.

LABORATORY EXAMINATIONS

Porphyrin Studies (See Table 10-8) Increased protoporphyrin in red blood cells, plasma, and stools, but no excretion in the urine except in the rare cases with fatal hepatic cirrhosis. Decreased activity of the enzyme ferrochelatase in the bone marrow, liver, and skin fibroblasts.
Liver Function Tests for liver function indicated. Liver biopsy: portal and periportal fibrosis and deposits of brown pigment and birefringent granules in hepatocytes and Kupffer cells. Cirrhosis and portal hypertension may develop.
Radiography Gallstones may be present.
Special Examination for Fluorescent Erythrocytes RBCs in a blood smear exhibit a characteristic

transient fluorescence when examined with a fluorescence microscope with a mercury or tungsten-iodide lamp that emits 400-nm radiation (Fig. 10-19).

Dermatopathology   Marked eosinophilic homogenization and thickening of the blood vessels in the papillary dermis; there is an accumulation of an amorphous, hyaline-like eosinophilic substance in and around blood vessels.

DIAGNOSIS

In EPP there is photosensitivity with an exaggerated sunburn response without blisters that appears much earlier than ordinary sunburn erythema. Also, the skin changes occur behind window glass. *There is no other photosensitivity disorder in which the symptoms appear so rapidly (minutes after exposure to sunlight).* Porphyrin examination establishes the diagnosis with elevated free protoporphyrin levels in the RBCs and in the stool. The fecal protoporphyrin is most consistently elevated, but urinary porphyrins are not. In chronic cases, the waxy thickening and wrinkling of facial skin is diagnostic.

Differential Diagnosis   Hyalinosis cutis et mucosae.

COURSE AND PROGNOSIS

EPP persists throughout life, but the photosensitivity may become less apparent in late adulthood. Liver cirrhosis may become manifest in adults. Rarely, fatal outcome due to hepatic failure.

MANAGEMENT

There is no treatment for the basic metabolic abnormality, but symptomatic relief of the photosensitivity can be achieved in most patients with oral β-carotene in divided doses of 180 mg/d. Therapeutic levels of carotenoids are achieved in 1–2 months. Patients on β-carotene can remain outdoors longer by a factor of 8 to 10 but will still burn if exposures are too long. Nevertheless, many patients can participate in outdoor activities for the first time. There is no toxicity with prolonged treatment with β-carotene. Protection by β-carotene can be considerably enhanced by PUVA-induced tanning.

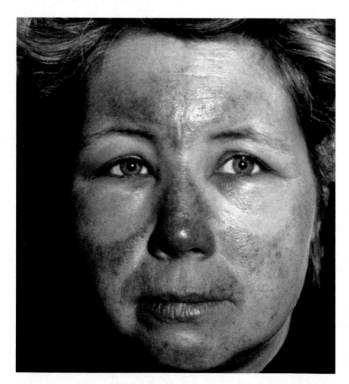

FIGURE 10-16   Erythropoietic protoporphyria   Diffuse erythematous swelling of the nose, forehead, and cheeks with petechial hemorrhage and telangiectasia. There are no porphyrins in the urine. A clue to the diagnosis is the history of tingling and burning within 4 to 5 min of sun exposure. The face of this woman appears yellow-orange because she was on β-carotene, which obviously did not protect her sufficiently.

FIGURE 10-17 Erythropoietic protoporphyria Massive petechial, confluent hemorrhage on the dorsa of the hands of a 16-year-old 24 h after exposure to the sun.

FIGURE 10-18 Erythropoietic protoporphyria
Erythema, edema, erosion, crusting of the nose with less severe changes on the chin of a 15-year-old female. Deep wrinkling and a peculiar waxy thickening on the upper lip and cheeks make the patient look much older as they are similar to dermatoheliosis in photoaged skin.

FIGURE 10-19 Erythropoietic protoporphyria
Fluorescent red blood cells. The left panel shows the blood cell smear viewed with visible light. The right panel was the same smear examined with a tungsten-iodide lamp that emits only 400-nm radiation. Note red fluorescence of erythrocytes. Note also that only a minority of red blood cells fluoresce and that to different degrees.

CHRONIC PHOTODAMAGE

DERMATOHELIOSIS ("PHOTOAGING") ICD-9:692.74 ∘ ICD-10:L57.9   ■ ○

- Repeated solar injuries over many years ultimately can result in the development of a skin syndrome, *dermatoheliosis* (DHe).
- It occurs in persons with SPT I to III and in persons with SPT IV who have had heavy cumulative exposure to sunlight, such as lifeguards and outdoor workers, over a lifetime.
- DHe describes a polymorphic response of various components of the skin (especially cells in the epidermis, the vascular system, and the dermal

connective tissue) to prolonged and/or excessive sun exposure.
- Its severity depends principally on the duration and intensity of sun exposure and on the indigenous (constitutive) skin color and the capacity to tan (facultative melanin pigmentation).

Note: If you want to demonstrate to an older patient the role of UVR in photoaging just have him/her undress and compare the quality of his/her facial skin to that of the suprapubic skin.

EPIDEMIOLOGY

Age of Onset Most often in persons >40 years.
Sex Higher incidence in males.
Skin Phototype Persons with SPT I and II are most susceptible, but persons with SPT III and IV and even V (brown skin color) can develop DHe.
Incidence Very common. The most susceptible persons with SPT I and II comprise about 25% of the white population in the United States.
Occupation Farmers ("farmer's skin"), telephone linemen; sea workers ("sailor's skin"), construction workers, and lifeguards; tennis, swimming, and ski instructors; mountain guides, sportspersons, and "beach bums"; persons who spend considerable time in mountain or sea resorts.
Geography DHe is more severe in white populations living in areas with high solar UVR (at high altitudes or in low latitudes). Young white children (age 10) living in southern Borneo (cool climate with high UVR) have been observed to have DHe, including solar keratoses.

PATHOGENESIS

While UVB is the most obvious damaging UVR, UVA in high doses can produce connective tissue changes in mice. In addition, visible (400–700 nm) and infrared (1000–1,000,000 nm) radiations have been implicated. The action spectrum for DHe is not known for certain; there is some experimental evidence in mice that infrared radiation is implicated, in addition to UVB and UVA.

CLINICAL MANIFESTATION

Personal History There is a history of intensive exposure to sun in youth (<20 years), even though sun exposure may have been quite limited in later adult life, and/or significant sun exposure in adulthood. Because skin phototypes are genetically determined, there is often a family history of DHe.

Skin Lesions A combination of atrophy (of epidermis), hypertrophy (of papillary dermis due to elastosis), telangiectases, spotty depigmentation and hyperpigmentation, and spotty hyperkeratosis in light-exposed areas. Skin appears wrinkled, wizened, leathery, "prematurely aged" (Fig. 10-20). Both fine, cigarette paper–like and deep furrow-like wrinkling; skin is waxy, papular with a yellowish hue, and both glistening and rough (Fig. 10-21). There may be telangiectasia and bruising, Bateman or senile purpura due to fragility of small vessels. Macular hyperpigmentations: *solar lentigines* (see below); macular hypopigmentations; *guttate hypomelanosis*, <3 mm in diameter, on the extremities. Comedones, particularly periorbital (termed *Favre-Racouchet disease*), particularly in cigarette smokers. Individuals with DHe invariably have actinic keratoses. Also, seborrheic keratoses that are misdiagnosed as lentigos.
Distribution Exposed areas, particularly face, periorbital and perioral areas, scalp (bald males). Nuchal area: cutis rhomboidalis ("red neck") with rhomboidal furrows; lower arms, dorsa of hands. Pattern hair loss in both sexes, although much less so in females. ∎

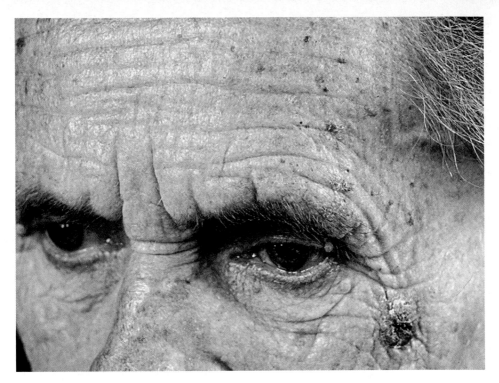

FIGURE 10-20   Dermatoheliosis   Severe deep wrinkling. The skin appears waxy, papular with a yellowish hue (actinic elastosis). This 68-year-old female mountain farmer lived at an altitude of 1000 m and had been working outdoors all her life. There is basal cell carcinoma in the left zygomatic region.

FIGURE 10-21   Severe dermatoheliosis on the forearm of a 70-year-old female farmhand   The skin is waxy, deeply wrinkled, and dry. Multiple solar keratoses have been removed from this arm by cryotherapy.

LABORATORY EXAMINATION

Dermatopathology   Acanthosis of epidermis, increased horny layer. Flattening of the dermal-epidermal junction. Atypia of the keratinocytes. Loss of small vessels in the papillary dermis.

Elastosis: Degraded elastic tissue with accumulation of coarse amorphous masses and increase in glycosaminoglycans in the upper dermis. Decrease in collagen.

COURSE AND PROGNOSIS

The appearance of DHe marks a relatively young person as "old," a state that everyone tries to delay. DHe is inexorably progressive and irreversible, but some repair of connective tissue effects can occur if the skin is protected. Some processes leading to DHe continue to progress, however, even when sun exposures are severely restricted in later life; solar keratoses and lentigines develop in the sun-damaged skin that is now being protected by avoidance and sunblocks. Yet there are documented examples of spontaneous reversal of solar keratoses.

MANAGEMENT

Current management is to prevent skin cancers and the development of DHe with the use of protective sunblocks, a change of behavior in the sun, and the use of topical chemotherapy (tretinoin) that reverses some of the changes of DHe.

Topical Treatment   *Tretinoin* in lotions, gels, and creams in varying concentrations reverses some aspects of DHe, especially in the connective tissue and vascular changes. Topical *tazarotene* has also been shown to reduce the effects of photoaging in short-term studies. Topical tretinoin can alter the progression of incipient epithelial skin cancers. *5-Fluorouracil* in lotions and creams and imiquimod are highly effective in causing a disappearance of solar keratoses. Topical imiquimod improves cosmetic appearance of photoaged skin: histology shows repair of photodamage.

Prevention   Persons of SPT I and II should be identified early in life and advised that they are susceptible to the development of DHe and skin cancers, including melanoma. These persons should never sunbathe and should, from an early age, adopt a daily program of self-protection using sun-filtering clothing and substantive and effective topical sun-protective solutions, gels, or lotions that can filter DNA-damaging UVB; effective UVA filters are now available. SPT I and II persons should avoid the peak hours of UVB intensity, which are the 2 h before and after solar noon.

Caution: There is some experimental evidence that while sunscreens protect from sunburn, they do not protect from UV-induced local immunosuppression. Prevention of sunburn may lure individuals into exposing themselves to the sun for prolonged periods, which may abrogate immunosurveillance mechanisms in the skin. This has been linked to the rising incidence of melanoma but is not proven.

SOLAR LENTIGO   ICD-9 : 709.09

- Solar lentigo is a circumscribed 1- to 3-cm brown macule resulting from a localized proliferation of melanocytes due to acute or chronic exposure to sunlight.

- Multiple lesions usually arise in sun-exposed sites.

EPIDEMIOLOGY AND ETIOLOGY

Age of Onset   Usually >40 years but may be 30 years in sunny climates and in susceptible persons.

Race   Most common in Caucasians but seen also in Asians.

Skin Phototype   Generally correlated with skin phototypes I to III and duration and intensity of solar exposure.

Etiology   Solar lentigines may arise acutely after sunburns and after overdosage of PUVA (*PUVA lentigines*).

CLINICAL MANIFESTATION

Skin Lesions Strictly macular, 1 to 3 cm, and as large as 5 cm. Light yellow, light brown, or dark brown; variegated mix of brown and not uniform color (Figs. 10-22 and 10-23), as in café au lait macules. Round, oval, with slightly irregular border, ill defined (Fig. 10-23). Scattered, discrete lesions, stellate and sharply defined after acute sunburn (Fig. 10-22).

Distribution Exclusively exposed areas: forehead, cheeks, nose, dorsa of hands and forearms, upper back, chest, shins.

🖉

FIGURE 10-22   Dermatoheliosis: solar lentigines   Multiple stellate brown macules on the shoulder occurred after a sunburn. They are all of about the same size and sharply marginated, which is characteristic of sunburn-induced solar lentigines.

FIGURE 10-23   Dermatoheliosis: solar lentigines   Multiple, variegated, tan-to-dark-brown macules on the malar and frontal areas in the face. Solar lentigines are not the same as ephelides (freckles)—they do not fade in the winter as freckles do. In contrast to the sharply marginated solar lentigines shown in Fig. 10-22, which are due to an acute sunburn, the solar lentigines shown here are of different sizes and partially ill defined and confluent, which is characteristic of chronic cumulative solar damage.

LABORATORY EXAMINATION

Dermatopathology Club-shaped elongated rete ridges that show hypermelanosis and an increased number of melanocytes in the basal layer.

DIFFERENTIAL DIAGNOSIS

Brown Macules "Flat," acquired, brown lesions on the exposed skin of the face, which may on cursory examination appear to be similar, have distinctive features: solar lentigo, freckles, seborrheic keratosis, spreading pigmented actinic keratosis (SPAK), lentigo maligna.

MANAGEMENT

Cryosurgery or laser surgery are effective. No more than 10 s of liquid nitrogen should be administered; otherwise depigmentation of normal skin will occur.

CHONDRODERMATITIS NODULARIS HELICIS ICD-9:380.0 ∘ ICD-10:H61.0

- Usually occurs as a single elongated, exquisitely tender nodule or a "beading" of the free border of helix of the ear. Common, probably due to constant mechanical trauma and most probably to UV radiation.
- Appears spontaneously, enlarges quickly, measuring less than 1 cm (Fig. 10-24), firm, well-defined, round to oval with sloping margins.
- Either embedded in the skin or elevated several millimeters and with dome-shaped surface, white-waxy and translucent, and often ulcerated (Fig. 10-24).
- More common in males than in females.

- Spontaneous pain or tenderness is the initial presenting complaint. Can be intense and stabbing, paroxysmal or continuous.
- Differential diagnosis includes basal cell and squamous cell carcinoma, actinic keratosis, in situ or invasive SCC, hypertrophic solar keratosis, and keratoacanthoma. One also has to think of gouty tophus, rheumatoid and rheumatic nodules, and discoid lupus erythematosus.
- Management includes intralesional injection of triamcinolone acetonide, carbon dioxide laser, surgery. The definitive treatment is excisional surgery including the underlying cartilage.

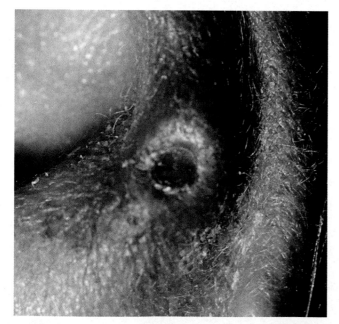

FIGURE 10-24 Chondrodermatitis nodularis helicis An extremely painful nodule with central ulceration on the anthelix of a 60-year-old female. The central ulcer is covered with a crust and can be mistaken for a basal cell carcinoma.

ACTINIC KERATOSIS   ICD-9:702.0 ∘ ICD-10:L57.0   ■ ◑

- These single or multiple, discrete, dry, rough, adherent scaly lesions occur on the habitually sun-exposed skin of adults, usually on a background of dermatoheliosis.

- Actinic keratoses can progress to squamous cell carcinoma.

  Synonym: Solar keratosis.

EPIDEMIOLOGY

Age of Onset Middle age, although in Australia and southwestern United States solar keratoses may occur in persons <30 years.
Sex More common in males.
Race SPT I, II, and III; rare in SPT IV; almost never in blacks or South Indians.
Occupation Outdoor workers (especially farmers, ranchers, sailors) and outdoor sportspersons (tennis, golf, mountain climbing, deep-sea fishing).

PATHOGENESIS

Prolonged and repeated solar exposure in susceptible persons (SPT I, II, and III) leads to cumulative damage to keratinocytes by the action of UVR, principally, if not exclusively, UVB (290–320 nm).

CLINICAL MANIFESTATION

Duration of Lesions (Fig. 10-25) Months to years.
Skin Symptoms Lesions may be tender. On examination, painful if excoriated with a fingernail; patient winces.

FIGURE 10-25 Solar keratoses Erythematous macules and papules with coarse, adherent scale become confluent on this bald scalp with dermatoheliosis. These hyperkeratoses are yellowish-grey. They are better felt than seen; gently abrading lesions with a fingernail usually induces pain, even in early subtle lesions, a helpful diagnostic finding.

Skin Lesions Adherent hyperkeratotic scale, which is removed with difficulty and pain (Figs. 10-25 and 10-26). May be papular. Skin-colored, yellow-brown, or brown—"dirty" (Fig. 10-26); often there is a reddish tinge (Fig. 10-25). Rough, like coarse sandpaper, "better felt than seen" on palpation with a finger. Most commonly <1 cm, oval or round (Fig. 10-27A, B).

Special Presentation: SPAK (spreading pigmented actinic keratosis). This lesion is best described as "looks like lentigo maligna but feels like actinic keratosis" (Fig. 10-28). It is a rather uncommon variant of solar keratosis. The distinctive features of SPAK include size (>1.5 cm), pigmentation (brown to black and variegated), and history of sopur spreading, especially the verrucous surface. The lesion is important because it can mimic lentigo maligna (LM). Keratotic nature of the lesion can best be evaluated when the lesion is slightly frozen with LN2. Sharply marginated scale is seen with solar and seborrheic keratoses. Lentigos are completely flat. It is, however, easily distinguished from LM because LM is completely flat without evidence of verrucous change. Biopsy is necessary to confirm the clinical diagnosis.

Distribution Isolated single lesion or scattered discrete lesions. Face [forehead, nose, cheeks (Figs. 10-25 and 10-26), temples, vermilion border of lower lip], ears (in males), neck (sides), forearms, and hands (dorsa), shins, and the scalp in bald males (Fig. 10-25). Males with early pattern alopecia are especially prone to severe dermatoheliosis and solar keratosis on the exposed scalp. ▨

LABORATORY EXAMINATION

Dermatopathology Large bright-staining keratinocytes, with mild to moderate pleomorphism in the basal layer extending into follicles, atypical (dyskeratotic) keratinocytes, parakeratosis.

DIAGNOSIS AND DIFFERENTIAL DIAGNOSIS

Usually made on clinical findings. Differential: Chronic cutaneous lupus erythematosus; seborrheic keratosis, flat warts, squamous cell carcinoma (SCC) in situ, superficial basal cell carcinoma. Highly hyperkeratotic lesions and SPAK may require biopsy to rule out SCC (in situ or invasive) or LM.

COURSE AND PROGNOSIS

Solar keratoses may disappear spontaneously, but in general remain for years. The actual incidence of SCC arising in preexisting solar keratoses is unknown but has been estimated at one SCC developing annually in 1000 solar keratoses.

MANAGEMENT

Prevention Avoided by use of highly effective UVB/UVA sunscreens, which should be applied daily to the face, neck, and ears during the summer in northern latitudes for SPT I and SPT II persons and for those SPT III persons who sustain prolonged sunlight exposures.

Topical Therapy *Cryosurgery* Light spray or with cotton-tipped applicator is effective in most cases.

5-Fluorouracil (5-FU) Cream 5% Effective, but difficult for many individuals. Treatment of facial lesions causes significant erythema and erosions, resulting in temporary cosmetic disfigurement. Apply twice daily for 2 to 4 weeks on face; may require longer period of therapy on dorsum of hands or lower legs. Efficacy can be increased and duration of treatment can be shortened if applied under occlusion and/or combined with topical tretinoin. This, however, leads to confluent erosions and may require hospitalization. Reepithelialization occurs after treatment is discontinued. Pretreatment with light cryosurgery to hyperkeratotic lesions may improve efficacy of 5-FU cream.

Imiquimod (twice weekly for 16 weeks) Causes cytokine dermatitis, also leads to irritation and erosions but is highly effective.

Topical Retinoids Used chronically, is effective for treatment of dermatoheliosis and superficial solar keratoses.

Diclofenac Gel Used chronically, is effective in superficial acting keratoses; also irritating.

Facial Peels Trichloroacetic acid (5–10%) effective for widespread lesions.

Laser Surgery Erbium or carbon dioxide lasers. Usually effective for individual lesions. For extensive facial lesions, facial resurfacing is effective.

Photodynamic Therapy Effective but painful and cumbersome.

Systemic Therapy Acitretin or isotretinoin are effective in reducing the number of solar keratoses and SCC in situ in patients with advanced dermatoheliosis, especially in immunocompromised patients. Lesions recur once therapy is discontinued.

FIGURE 10-26 Actinic keratoses, close up Yellow-greyish tightly adherent scales on the forehead of an 80-year-old man. Abrading these hyperkeratoses is painful. There is a small basal cell carcinoma at the border of the hairy scalp.

A *B*

FIGURE 10-27 Solar keratoses, higher magnification *A.* A sharply defined yellow-brownish tightly adherent, rough hyperkeratosis. *B.* This lesion is even more elevated and has a "stuck-on" appearance like a seborrheic keratosis. However, it is not greasy and soft but rather hard, rough, and painful when scraped.

FIGURE 10-28   Spreading pigmented actinic keratosis (SPAK)   "Looks like lentigo maligna" (see Fig. 12-7) but is rough and therefore "feels like actinic keratosis." A nonpigmented actinic keratosis is seen in the preauricular region.

SKIN REACTIONS TO IONIZING RADIATION

RADIATION DERMATITIS   ICD-9:692.82 ∘ ICD-10:L58

- Radiation dermatitis is defined as skin changes resulting from exposure to ionizing radiation.
- *Reversible effects* are pain, erythema, epilation, suppression of sebaceous glands, and pigmentation (lasting for weeks to months to years).

- *Irreversible effects* are atrophy, sclerosis, telangiectasias, ulceration, and radiation-induced cancers.

Type of Exposure

Result of therapy (for cancer, formerly also used for acne and psoriasis, and fungal infections of the scalp in children), accidental, or occupational (e.g., formerly, in dentists who held the film in the mouth with their fingers). The radiation causing radiodermatitis includes superficial and deep x-ray radiation, electron-beam therapy, and grenz-ray therapy. It is a prevailing myth among some dermatologists that grenz rays are "soft" and not carcinogenic; it has been estimated that SCC can appear from >5000 cGy of grenz rays.

Types of Reactions

Acute   Temporary erythema that lasts 3 days and then persistent erythema, which reaches a peak in 2 weeks and is painful; pigmentation appears about day 20; a late erythema can also occur beginning on day 35–40, and this lasts 2–3 weeks. Massive reactions lead to blistering erosions (Fig. 10-29) and ulceration, also painful; may occur as recall phenomenon. Permanent scarring may result.

Chronic   After *fractional* but relatively intensive therapy with total doses of 3000–6000 rad, there develops an epidermolytic reaction in 3 weeks. This is repaired in 3–6 weeks, and scars and hypopigmentation develop; there is loss of all skin appendages and atrophy of the epidermis and dermis. During the next 2–5 years, the atrophy increases (Fig. 10-30); there is hyper- and hypopigmentation (poikiloderma), telangiectasia (Figs. 10-30 and 10-31), and superficial venules

FIGURE 10-29   Radiation dermatitis: acute, recall phenomenon   This patient had breast cancer. She had a lumpectomy, methotrexate, and x-ray therapy and developed painful erythema and erosions at the irradiated site.

become ectatic. There are hyperkeratoses (x-ray keratoses) (Fig. 10-34A). Necrosis and painful ulceration (Fig. 10-32) are rare but occur in accidental exposure or error in dose: either one or a few accidentally high doses or multiple small doses at frequent intervals (monthly or weekly). When necrosis occurs, it is leathery, yellow, and adherent and the base and surrounding skin are extremely painful (Fig. 10-32). Ulcerations have a very poor tendency to heal and usually require surgical intervention. Accidental exposure occurs mostly in occupational exposure and affects the hands, feet, and face. There is a destruction of the fingerprint pattern, xerosis, scanty hair, atrophy of sebaceous and sweat glands, and development of keratoses (Fig. 10-34A).

Nails Longitudinal striations (Fig. 10-34B) show thickening, dystrophy. Diclofenac used chronically is effective in keratoses. 🔲

COURSE, PROGNOSIS, AND MANAGEMENT

Chronic radiation dermatitis is permanent, progressive, and irreversible. SCC may develop in 4–40 years (Figs. 10-33 and 10-34A, B), with a median of 7–12 years, almost exclusively from the chronic repeated types of exposures. SCC always develops within the area of radiodermatitis, (Fig. 10-34A, B). Tumors metastasize in about 25%; despite extensive surgery (excision, grafts, etc.), the prognosis is poor, and recurrences are common. Basal cell carcinoma (BCC) may also occur in chronic radiation dermatitis and appears mostly in patients formerly treated with x-rays for acne vulgaris and acne cystica or epilation (tinea capitis) (Fig. 10-31). The tumors may appear 40–50 years after exposure. Excision and grafting are often possible before the cancer develops.

FIGURE 10-30 **Radiation dermatitis: chronic** There is sclerosis combined with atrophy and telangiectasia. This is the result of the irradiation of an infantile hemangioma in infancy.

FIGURE 10-31 **Radiation dermatitis: chronic** There is poikiloderma (brown: hyperpigmentation; white: hypopigmentation; red: telangiectasia) combined with atrophy and sclerosis. Hairs are absent. These massive skin changes are the result of overdosed irradiation the patient received as a child for fungal infection of the scalp. He is a candidate for SCC in the future.

FIGURE 10-33 Radiation dermatitis: chronic with squamous cell carcinoma A large slightly elevated ulcer in an area of atrophy, fibrosis, poikiloderma, and telangiectasia on the chest wall. This occurred 20 years after radical mastectomy, axillary lymph node dissection, and radiotherapy. The ulceration was primarily due to radionecrosis. Now the border of the ulcer is elevated and firm: this is SCC arising in this radiation dermatitis.

FIGURE 10-32 Radiation dermatitis: chronic An area of severe telangiectasia with a central necrosis that is leathery, yellowish-white, and tightly adherent. Surgical removal will reveal a deep ulcer. The lesion is extremely painful.

A

B

FIGURE 10-34 Radiation-induced squamous cell carcinoma ***A.*** These are the hands of an elderly radiologist who decades ago had disregarded precautionary measures and hardly wore gloves doing fluoroscopic work. There are multiple x-ray keratoses; the hyperkeratotic lesion on the right thumb has destroyed the nail and represents x-ray-induced SCC. ***B.*** Nail changes in site of radiation exposure. Note the linear striations resulting from damage to the nail matrix. At the nailfold and extending proximally on the thumb, there is an irregular erythematous plaque that represents mostly SCC in situ but, focally, also invasive SCC.

PRECANCEROUS LESIONS AND CUTANEOUS CARCINOMAS

EPIDERMAL PRECANCERS AND CANCERS

Cutaneous epithelial cancers [nonmelanoma skin cancer (NMSC)] are the easiest of all cancers to diagnose and treat. They originate most commonly in the epidermal germinative keratinocytes or adnexal structures (e.g., sweat apparatus, hair follicle). The two principal NMSCs are basal cell carcinoma (BCC) and squamous cell carcinoma (SCC). SCC often has its origin in an identifiable dysplastic in situ lesion that can be treated before frank invasion occurs. In contrast, in situ BCC is not known, but minimally invasive "superficial" BCCs are common.

The most common etiology of NMSC in fair-skinned individuals is sunlight, ultraviolet radiation (UVR), and human papillomavirus (HPV). Solar keratoses are the most common precursor lesions of SCC in situ (SCCIS) and invasive SCC occurring at sites of chronic sun exposure in individuals of northern European heritage (see Section 10). UVR and HPV cause the spectrum of changes ranging from epithelial dysplasia to SCCIS to invasive SCC. Much less commonly, NMSC can be caused by ionizing radiation (arising in sites of chronic radiation damage), chronic inflammation, hydrocarbons (tar), and chronic ingestion of inorganic arsenic; these tumors can be much more aggressive than those associated with UVR or HPV. In the increasing population of immunosuppressed individuals (those with HIV/AIDS disease, solid organ transplant recipients, etc.), UVR- and HPV-induced SCCs are much more common and can be more aggressive.

EPITHELIAL PRECANCEROUS LESIONS AND SCCIS

Dysplasia of epidermal keratinocytes in epidermis and squamous mucosa can involve the lower portion of the epidermis or the full thickness. Basal cells mature into dysplastic keratinocytes resulting in a hyperkeratotic papule, or plaque, clinically identified as "keratosis." A continuum exists from dysplasia to SCCIS to invasive SCC. These lesions have various associated eponyms such as Bowen disease or erythroplasia of Queyrat, which as descriptive morphologic terms are helpful; terms such as UVR- or HPV-associated SCCIS, however, will be more meaningful but can be used only for those lesions with known etiology.

Epithelial precancerous lesions and SCCIS can be classified as follows:

- UVR-induced
  - Solar (actinic) keratoses
  - Spreading pigmented actinic keratoses (SPAK)
  - Lichenoid actinic keratoses
  - Bowenoid actinic keratoses
  - SCCIS (Bowen disease)
- HPV-induced
  - Low-grade squamous intraepithelial lesion (LSIL)
  - High-grade squamous intraepithelial lesion (HSIL)
  - SCCIS (Bowenoid papulosis)
- Arsenical keratoses
  - Palmoplantar keratoses
  - Bowenoid arsenical keratoses
- Hydrocarbon (tar) keratoses
- Thermal keratoses
- Keratoses in chronic radiation dermatitis
- Chronic cicatrix (scar) keratoses

SOLAR OR ACTINIC KERATOSIS

These single or multiple, discrete, dry, rough, adherent scaly lesions occur on the habitually sun-exposed skin of adults. They can progress to SCCIS, which can then progress to invasive SCC. (Fig. 11-1).

Synonym: Solar and actinic keratosis are synonymous.

For a full discussion of this condition, see Section 10, p. 267.

FIGURE 11-1   Solar keratoses and invasive squamous cell carcinoma   Multiple, tightly adherent dirty-looking solar keratoses (see also Figs. 10-25 to 10-27). The large nodule shown here is covered by hyperkeratoses and hemorrhagic crusts; it is partially eroded and firm. This nodule is invasive squamous cell carcinoma. The image is shown to demonstrate the transition from precancerous lesions to frank carcinoma.

CUTANEOUS HORN   ICD-9 : 702.2 ∘ ICD-10 : L85.8

- A cutaneous horn (CH) is a *clinical* entity having the appearance of an animal horn with a papular or nodular base and a keratotic cap of various shapes and lengths (Fig. 11-2).

- CHs most commonly represent hypertrophic solar keratoses. However, in situ or invasive SCC is often present at the base of a CH.

- CHs usually arise within areas of dermatoheliosis on the face, ear, dorsum of hands, or forearms, and shins.

- Nonprecancerous CH formation can also occur in seborrheic keratoses, warts, and keratoacanthomas.

- Clinically, CHs vary in size from a few millimeters to several centimeters (Fig. 11-2). The horn may be white, black, or yellowish in color and straight, curved, or spiral in shape.

- Histologically there is usually hypertrophic actinic keratosis, SCCIS or invasive SCC at the base. Because of the possibility of invasive SCC, a CH should always be excised.

FIGURE 11-2   Cutaneous horn: hypertrophic actinic keratosis   A hornlike projection of keratin on a slightly raised base in the setting of advanced dermatoheliosis on the upper eyelid in an 85-year-old female. Excision showed invasive SCC at the base of the lesion.

ARSENICAL KERATOSES   ICD-9:692.4 ∘ ICD-10:L85.8   ☐ ◑

- Appear decades after chronic arsenic ingestion (medicinal, occupational, or environmental exposure).
- Arsenical keratoses have the potential to become SCCIS or invasive SCC. These are currently being seen in West Bengal and Bangladesh.
- Two types: punctate, yellow papules on palms and soles (Fig. 11-3A); keratoses indistinguishable

from actinic keratoses on the trunk and elsewhere. These are often associated with small SCCIS of the Bowen-type and hypopigmented slightly depressed macules ("raindrops in the dust") (Fig. 11-3B).
- Treatment—as for solar keratoses.

SQUAMOUS CELL CARCINOMA IN SITU   ICD-9:173.0 ∘
ICD-10:M8070/2   ■ ◑

- Presents as solitary or multiple macules, papules, or plaques, which may be hyperkeratotic or scaling.
- SCCIS is most often caused by UVR or HPV infection.
- Commonly arises in epithelial dysplastic lesions such as solar keratoses or HPV-induced squamous epithelial lesions (SIL) (see Sections 27 and 30).
- Pink or red, sharply defined scaly plaques on the skin are called *Bowen disease*; similar but usually

nonscaly lesions on the glans and vulva are called *erythroplasia*.
- Anogenital HPV-induced SCCIS is referred to as *bowenoid papulosis*.
- Untreated SSCIS may progress to invasive SCC. With HPV-induced SCCIS in HIV/AIDS, lesions often resolve completely with successful ART and immune reconstitution.
- Treatment is topical 5-fluorouracil, imiquimod, cryosurgery, CO_2 laser evaporation, or excision, including Mohs micrographic surgery.

FIGURE 11-3   Arsenical keratoses   A. Multiple punctate, tightly adherent and very hard keratoses on the palm. **B.** Arsenical keratoses on the back. Multiple lesions are seen here ranging from red to tan, dark brown, and white. The brown lesions are a mix of arsenical keratoses (hard, rough) and small seborrheic keratoses (soft and smooth). The difference can be better felt than seen. The red lesions are small Bowenoid keratoses and Bowen disease (see Fig. 11-4). The white macular areas are slightly depressed and represent superficial atrophic scars from spontaneously shed or treated arsenical keratoses. The entire picture gives the impression of "rain drops in the dust."

ETIOLOGY

UVR, HPV, arsenic, tar, chronic heat exposure, chronic radiation dermatitis.

CLINICAL MANIFESTATION

Lesions are most often asymptomatic but may bleed. Nodule formation or onset of pain or tenderness within SCCIS suggests progression to invasive SCC.

Skin Findings Appears as a sharply demarcated, scaling, or hyperkeratotic macule, papule, or plaque (Fig. 11-4). Solitary or multiple lesions are pink or red in color and have a slightly scaling surface, small erosions, and can be crusted. Such lesions are always well-defined and are called *Bowen disease* (Fig. 11-4).

Red, sharply demarcated, glistening macular or plaque-like SCCIS on the glans penis or labia minora are called *erythroplasia of Queyrat* (see Section 35). Anogenital HPV-induced SCCIS may be red, tan, brown, or black in color and are referred to as *bowenoid papulosis* (see Section 35). Eroded lesions may have areas of crusting. SCCIS may be mistaken for a patch of eczema or psoriasis and go undiagnosed for years, resulting in large lesions with annular or polycyclic borders (Fig. 11-5). Once invasion occurs, nodular lesions appear within the plaque and the lesion is then commonly called *Bowen carcinoma* (Fig. 11-5).

Distribution UVR-induced SCCIS commonly arises within a solar keratosis in the setting of photoaging (dermatoheliosis). HPV-induced SCCIS arises within an area of low-grade or high-grade SIL, mostly in the genital area but also periungually, most commonly on the thumb or in the nail bed (see Fig. 33-15) (Image 11-1).

LABORATORY EXAMINATION

Dermatopathology Carcinoma in situ with loss of epidermal architecture and regular differentiation; keratinocyte polymorphism, single cell dyskeratosis, increased mitotic rate, multinuclear cells. Epidermis may be thickened but basement membrane intact.

DIAGNOSIS AND DIFFERENTIAL DIAGNOSIS

Clinical diagnosis confirmed by dermatopathologic findings. Differential diagnosis includes all well-demarcated pink-red plaque(s): Nummular eczema, psoriasis, seborrheic keratosis, solar keratoses, verruca vulgaris, verruca plana, condyloma acuminatum, superficial BCC; amelanotic melanoma, Paget disease.

COURSE AND PROGNOSIS

Untreated SCCIS will progress to invasive SCC (Fig. 11-5). In HIV/AIDS, resolves with successful ART. Lymph node metastasis can occur without demonstrable invasion. Metastatic dissemination from lymph nodes.

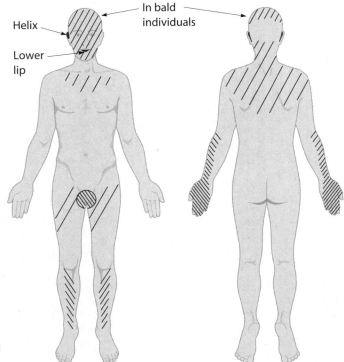

IMAGE 11-1   Squamous cell carcinoma: predilection sites.

MANAGEMENT

Topical Chemotherapy   *5-Fluorouracil* cream applied every day or twice daily, with or without tape occlusion, is effective. So is *imiquimod*, but both require considerable time.

Cryosurgery   Highly effective. Lesions are usu-ally treated more aggressively than solar kera-toses, and superficial scarring will result.

Photodynamic Therapy   Effective but still cum-bersome and painful.

Surgical Excision   Has the highest cure rate but the greatest chance of causing cosmetically disfiguring scars. It should be done in all lesions where invasion cannot be excluded by biopsy.

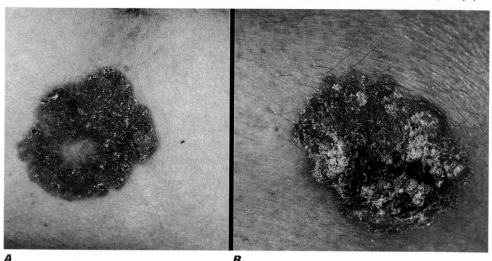

A   *B*

FIGURE 11-4   Squamous cell carcinoma in situ: Bowen disease   *A.* A large, sharply demarcated, scaly, erythematous plaque simulating a psoriatic lesion. ***B.*** A similar psoriasiform plaque with a mix of scales, hyper-keratosis, and hemorrhagic crusts on the surface.

FIGURE 11-5   Squamous cell carcinoma in situ: Bowen disease and invasive SCC: Bowen carcinoma
A large variegated orange, brown to gray plaque on the back, sharply defined, with irregular outlines represents SCCIS, or Bowen disease. The red nodule on this plaque indicates that here the lesion is not any more an in situ lesion but that invasive carcinoma has developed. It is an undifferentiated carcinoma.

INVASIVE SQUAMOUS CELL CARCINOMA (SCC) ■ ●

- SCC of the skin is a malignant tumor of keratinocytes, arising in the epidermis.

- SCC usually arises in epidermal precancerous lesions (see above) and, depending on etiology and level of differentiation, varies in its aggressiveness.

- The lesion is a plaque or a nodule with varying degrees of keratinization in the nodule and/or on the surface. Thumb rule: undifferentiated SCC is soft and has no hyperkeratosis; differentiated SCC is hard on palpation and has hyperkeratosis.

- The majority of UVR-induced lesions have a low rate of distant metastasis in otherwise healthy individuals. More aggressive SCCs occur in immunosuppressed individuals with a greater incidence of metastasis.

- Treatment is by surgery.

ICD-9 : 173.0 ○ ICD-10 : M8076/2-3

EPIDEMIOLOGY AND ETIOLOGY

Ultraviolet Radiation

Age of Onset Older than 55 years of age in the United States; in Australia, New Zealand, in Florida, Southwest and Southern California persons in their twenties and thirties.

Incidence Continental United States: 12 per 100,000 white males; 7 per 100,000 white females. Hawaii: 62 per 100,000 whites.

Sex Males > females, but SCC can occur more frequently on the legs of females.

Exposure Sunlight. Phototherapy, PUVA (oral psoralen + UVA). Excessive photochemotherapy can lead to promotion of SCC, particularly in patients with skin phototypes I and II or in patients with history of previous exposure to ionizing radiation or methotrexate treatment for psoriasis.

Race Persons with white skin and poor tanning capacity (skin phototypes I and II) (see Section 10). Brown- or black-skinned persons can develop SCC from numerous etiologic agents other than UVR.

Geography Most common in areas that have many days of sunshine annually, i.e., in Australia and southwestern United States.

Occupation Persons working outdoors—farmers, sailors, lifeguards, telephone line installers, construction workers, dock workers.

Human Papillomavirus

Oncogenic HPV type-16, -18, -31 most commonly, -33, -35, -39, -40, and -51 to -60 are associated with epithelial dysplasia, SCCIS, and invasive SCC. HPV-5, -8, -9 have also been isolated from SCCs.

Other Etiologic Factors

Immunosuppression Solid organ transplant recipients, individuals with chronic immunosuppression of inflammatory disorders, and those with HIV disease are associated with an increased incidence of UVR- and HPV-induced SCCIS and invasive SCCs. SCCs in these individuals are more aggressive than in nonimmunosuppressed individuals.

Chronic Inflammation Chronic cutaneous lupus erythematosus, chronic ulcers, burn scars, chronic radiation dermatitis, lichen planus of oral mucosa.

Industrial Carcinogens Pitch, tar, crude paraffin oil, fuel oil, creosote, lubricating oil, nitrosoureas.

Inorganic Arsenic Trivalent arsenic had been used in the past in medications such as Asiatic pills, Donovan pills, Fowler solution (used as a treatment for psoriasis). Historically trivalent arsenic was used for treatment of psoriasis. Arsenic is still present in drinking water in some geographic regions (West Bengal and Bangladesh).

CLINICAL MANIFESTATION

Slowly evolving—any isolated keratotic or eroded papule or plaque in a suspect patient that persists for over a month is considered a carcinoma until proved otherwise. Also, a nodule evolving in a plaque that meets the clinical criteria of SCCIS (Bowen disease), a chronically eroded lesion on the lower lip or on the penis, or nodular lesions evolving in or at the margin of a chronic venous ulcer or within chronic radiation dermatitis. Note that SCC is always asymptomatic. Potential carcinogens often can be detected only after detailed interrogation of the patient.

Rapidly evolving—invasive SCC can erupt within a few weeks and is often painful and/or tender.

For didactic reasons, two types can be distinguished:

1. Highly differentiated SCCs, which practically always show signs of keratinization either within or on the surface (hyperkeratosis) of the tumor. These are firm or hard upon palpation (Figs. 11-6 to 11-8 and Figs. 11-10 to 11-12).

2. Poorly differentiated SCCs, which do not show signs of keratinization and clinically appear fleshy, granulomatous, amd consequently are soft upon palpation (Figs. 11-5 and 11-9).

A   *B*

FIGURE 11-6 **Squamous cell carcinoma: invasive on the lip, two stages of development** **A.** A large but subtle nodule, which is better felt than seen, on the vermilion border of the lower lip with areas of hyperkeratosis and erosion, arising in the setting of dermatoheliosis of the lip (cheilitis actinica). **B.** This nodule is larger and can be felt to infiltrate the entire lip.

FIGURE 11-7 **Squamous cell carcinoma** A round nodule, firm and indolent with a central black eschar. Note yellowish color in the periphery of the tumor indicating the presence of keratin. All three SCC shown in Fig. 11-6 and here are hard and occur on the lower lip. SCC hardly occurs on the upper lip because this is shaded from the sun. SCC on the lip is easily distinguished from nodular BCC because BCC does not develop hyperkeratosis or keratosis inside the tumor and does not occur on the vermilion lip.

Differentiated SCC

Lesions   Indurated papule, plaque, or nodule (Figs. 11-1, 11-6 to 11-8); adherent thick keratotic scale or hyperkeratosis (Figs. 11-1, 11-6, 11-7, 11-8, 11-11); when eroded or ulcerated, the lesion may have a crust in the center and a firm, hyperkeratotic, elevated margin (Figs. 11-7 and 11-8). Horny material may be expressed from the margin or the center of the lesion (Figs. 11-7, 11-8, and 11-10). Erythematous, yellowish, skin color. Hard. Polygonal, oval, round (Figs. 11-6 and 11-10), or umbilicated and ulcerated. ◪

Distribution   Usually isolated but may be multiple. Usually exposed areas. Sun-induced keratotic and/or ulcerated lesions especially on the bald scalp (Fig. 11-1), cheeks, nose, lower lips (Fig. 11-6), ears (Fig. 11-11), preauricular area, dorsa of the hands (Fig. 11-10), forearms, trunk, and shins (females) (Fig. 11-12).

Other Physical Findings   Regional lymphadenopathy due to metastases.

Special Features   In UV-related SCC evidence of *dermatoheliosis* and *solar keratoses*. SCCs of the lips develop from leukoplasia or actinic cheilitis; in 90% of cases they are found on the lower lip (Fig. 11-6). In chronic radiodermatitis they arise from radiation-induced keratoses (see Fig. 10-34); in individuals with a history of chronic intake of arsenic, from arsenical keratoses. Differentiated (i.e., hyperkeratotic) SCC due to HPV on genitalia; SCC due to excessive PUVA therapy on lower extremities (pretibial) or on genitalia. SCCs in scars from burns, in chronic stasis ulcers of long duration, and in sites of chronic inflammation are often difficult to identify. Suspicion is indicated when nodular lesions are hard and show signs of keratinization (Figs. 11-8, 11-10, and 11-11).

Special form: carcinoma cuniculatum, usually on the soles, highly differentiated, HPV-related but can also occur in other settings (Fig. 11-13). ◪

Histopathology   SCCs with various grades of anaplasia and keratinization.

Undifferentiated SCC

Lesions   Fleshy, granulating, easily vulnerable, erosive papules and nodules and papillomatous vegetations (Fig. 11-9). Ulceration with a necrotic base and soft, fleshy margin. Bleeds easily, crusting. Red. Soft. Polygonal, irregular, often cauliflower-like.

Distribution   Isolated but also multiple, particularly on the genitalia, where they arise from erythroplasia (see Fig. 35-24) and on the trunk (Fig. 11-5), lower extremities, or face, where they arise from Bowen disease. ◪

Miscellaneous Other Skin Changes   Lymphadenopathy as evidence of regional metastases is far more common than with differentiated, hyperkeratotic SCCs.

Histopathology   Anaplastic SCC with multiple mitoses and little evidence of differentiation and keratinization.

DIFFERENTIAL DIAGNOSIS

As stated previously, any persistent nodule, plaque, or ulcer, but especially when these occur in sun-damaged skin, on the lower lips, in areas of radiodermatitis, in old burn scars, or on the genitalia, must be examined for SCC. Keratoacanthoma may be clinically indistinguishable from differentiated SCC (Fig. 11-8*A*).

MANAGEMENT

Surgery   Depending on localization and extent of lesion, excision with primary closure, skin flaps, or grafting. Microscopically controlled surgery in difficult sites. Radiotherapy should be performed only if surgery is not feasible.

COURSE AND PROGNOSIS

Recurrence and Metastases   SCC causes local tissue destruction but it has a significant potential for metastases. Metastases are directed to regional lymph nodes and appear 1 to 3 years after initial diagnosis. In-transit metastases occur. In solid organ transplant recipients, can be present when SCC is diagnosed/detected or shortly after. SCC in the skin has an overall metastatic rate of 3–4% and tends to occur with tumors that are large, recurrent, and involve deep structures of cutaneous nerves. High-risk SCCs are defined as having a diameter >2 cm, a level of invasion > 4 mm, and Clark levels IV or V[*]; tumor involvement of bone, muscle, and nerve (so-called neurotropic SCC, occurs frequently on the forehead and scalp); location on ear, lip, and genitalia; tumors arising in a scar or following ionizing radiation are usually highly dedifferentiated tumors. Cancers arising in chronic osteomyelitis sinus tracts, in burn scars, and in sites

---

[*]Clark level I, intraepidermal; level II, invades papillary dermis; level III fills papillary dermis; level IV, invades reticular dermis; level V, invades subcutaneous fat.

A   **B**

FIGURE 11-8 Squamous cell carcinoma, well differentiated   A. A nodule on the lower arm covered with a dome-shaped dark hyperkeratosis. **B.** A large, round, hard nodule on the nose with central hyperkeratosis. Neither lesion can be distinguished from keratoacanthoma (see Fig. 11-15).

FIGURE 11-9 Squamous cell carcinoma, undifferentiated There is a circular, dome-shaped reddish nodule with partly eroded surface on the temple of a 78-year-old male. The lesion shows no hyperkeratoses and is soft and friable. When scraped it bleeds easily.

of radiation dermatitis have a metastatic rate of 31, 20, and 18%, respectively. On the other hand, SCC arising in solar keratoses have the lowest potential for metastasis. A special group of high-risk SCCs are those in patients who are immunosuppressed (Fig. 11-14).

SCCs in Immunosuppression Organ transplant recipients have a markedly increased incidence of NMSCs, primarily SCC, which is 40 to 50 times greater than in the general population. Risk factors include skin type, cumulative sun exposure, age at transplantation, male sex, HPV infections, the degree and length of immunosuppression, and the type of immunosuppressant. Lesions are often multiple, usually in sun-exposed sites but also in the genital, anal, and perigenital regions (Fig. 11-14).

These tumors grow rapidly and are aggressive; in one series of heart-transplant patients from Australia, 27% died of skin cancer.

Patients with AIDS have only a slight increased risk of NMSC. In one series a fourfold increase in their risk of developing lip SCC was noted. However, SCC of the anus is significantly increased in this population (see also Section 21).

FIGURE 11-10   Squamous cell carcinoma, advanced, well differentiated, on the hand of a 65-year-old farmer   The big nodule is smooth, very hard upon palpation, and shows a yellowish color, focally indicating keratin in the body of the nodule. If the lesion were incised in the yellowish areas, a yellowish-white material (keratin) could be expressed.

FIGURE 11-11   Squamous cell carcinoma, highly differentiated, on the ear   There is a relatively large plaque covered by adherent hard hyperkeratoses. Although SCCs are in general not painful, lesions on the helix or anthelix usually are, as was the case in this 69-year-old man.

FIGURE 11-12   Squamous cell carcinoma in the setting of chronic statis dermatitis and long-standing, nonhealing venous ulcer   There was a venous ulcer of more than 10 years' duration at the site, which was unsuccessfully treated with topical remedies. Gradually the center of the ulcer became harder and elevated and now represents a firm elevated, easily bleeding mass with yellow necroses. Long-standing ulcers of the leg should always be biopsied to rule out squamous cell carcinoma.

FIGURE 11-14   Squamous cell carcinoma in a renal transplant recipient on the base of the scrotum   In addition to this ulcerating firm nodule of the base of the scrotum, the patient had smaller, similar lesions elsewhere on the body. Since he had psoriasis and had therefore spent considerable time in the sun, the lesions in the sun-exposed sides were probably due to UVR. The lesion shown here was probably initiated by HPV as he had a similar lesion perianally and on the glans.

FIGURE 11-13   Squamous cell carcinoma (carcinoma cuniculatum) in a patient with peripheral neuropathy due to leprosy   A large fungating, partially necrotic and hyperkeratotic tumor on the sole of the foot. The lesion had been considered a neuropathic ulcer, ascribed to leprosy, but continued growing and became elevated and ulcerated.

KERATOACANTHOMA (KA)   ICD-9 : 238.2 ∘ ICD-10 : L58.8

- KA is a special lesion; formerly considered a pseudocancer it is now regarded by most as a variant of squamous cell carcinoma.
- A relatively common, rapidly growing epithelial tumor with potential for tissue destruction and (rare) metastasis; however, in most cases spontaneous regression.

- A dome-shaped nodule with central keratotic plug (Fig. 11-15A).
- Predilection for sun-exposed sites.
- Multiple KAs occur.
- Treatment is by excision.

EPIDEMIOLOGY

Age of Onset   Over 50 years; rare below 20 years. Male:female ratio 2:1.

PATHOGENESIS

Human papillomavirus (HPV) -9, -16, -19, -25, and -37 have been identified in KAs. Other possible etiologic factors include UV radiation and chemical carcinogens (industrial: pitch and tar).

CLINICAL MANIFESTATION

Rapid growth, achieving a size of 2.5 cm within a few weeks. No symptoms, but there are occasional tenderness and cosmetic disfigurement.

Skin Lesions   Nodule, dome-shaped, often with a central keratotic plug (Fig. 11-15). Skin-colored or slightly red, tan/brown. Firm but not hard. 2.5 cm (range, 1–10 cm), round. Keratotic plug may appear like a cutaneous horn. Removal of plug results in a crater.
Distribution   Isolated single lesion. Uncommonly, may be multiple, eruptive. On exposed skin: cheeks, nose, ears, hands (dorsa).

LABORATORY EXAMINATION

Dermatopathology   A representative biopsy that extends through the entire lesion to preserve the architecture of the nodule or primary excision is required. Central, large, irregularly shaped crater filled with keratin. The surrounding epidermis extends in a liplike manner over the sides of the crater. The keratinocytes are atypical and many are dyskeratotic. Differentiation of KA from highly differentiated SCC is difficult and may not always be possible.

DIAGNOSIS AND DIFFERENTIAL DIAGNOSIS

Clinical findings confirmed by representative biopsy. SCC, hypertrophic solar keratosis, verruca vulgaris.

COURSE AND PROGNOSIS

Spontaneous regression in 2–6 months or sometimes >1 year in most cases. There is progressive keratinization with expansion of the central keratotic plug until all epithelial tumor tissue is converted into horny material and shed (Figs. 11-15B and 11-15C) which leads to a scar. However, KA is locally destructive; lymph node and visceral metastases have been observed in some cases.

MANAGEMENT

Surgery   Surgical excision is recommended in that KA cannot be distinguished from SCC on clinical findings.
Multiple KAs   Systemic retinoids and methotrexate have been used.

A   *B*   *C*

FIGURE 11-15 Keratoacanthoma showing different stages of evolution ***A.*** Initially there is a round dome-shaped, very firm nodule, reddish with a central hyperkeratotic plug. This has been partially shed leaving a central crater. ***B.*** Hyperkeratosis has progressed and has now replaced most of the nodule, leaving only a thin rim of tumor tissue in the periphery. ***C.*** Further progression of hyperkeratoses and keratinization has now replaced all of the tumor and will be later shed, leaving a scar. Since this evolution is not always predictable, keratoacanthoma should always be excised in the early stages.

BASAL CELL CARCINOMA (BCC)   ICD-9:173.0 ○ ICD-10:C33.M8090/3 ■ ◑ → ●

- BCC is the most common cancer in humans.
- Caused by UVR; *PTCH* gene mutation in most cases.
- Clinically different types: nodular, ulcerating, pigmented, sclerosing, and superficial.

- BCC is locally invasive, aggressive, and destructive but slow growing, and there is very limited (literally no) tendency to metastasize.
- Treatment is by surgical excision, Mohs micrographic surgery, electrodesiccation, and curettage. Also cryosurgery and imiquimod cream.

EPIDEMIOLOGY

Age of Onset Older than 40 years.
Sex Males > females.
Incidence United States: 500–1000 per 100,000, higher in the sunbelt; >400,000 new patients annually.
Race Rare in brown- and black-skinned persons.

ETIOLOGY

UVR, mostly of the UVB spectrum (290–320 nm) that induces mutations in suppressor genes. The propensity for multiple BCC may be inherited. Associated with mutations in the *PTCH* gene in many cases.
Predisposing Factors Skin phototypes I and II and albinos are highly susceptible to develop BCC with prolonged sun exposure. Also a history of heavy sun exposure in youth predisposes the skin to the development of BCC later in life. Previous therapy with x-rays for facial acne greatly increases the risk of BCC, even in those persons with a good ability to tan (skin phototypes III and IV). Superficial multicentric BCC occurs 30–40 years after ingestion of arsenic but also without apparent cause.

CLINICAL MANIFESTATION

Slowly evolving, usually asymptomatic. Erosion or bleeding with minimal trauma may be first symptom.

Skin Lesions There are five *clinical* types: nodular, ulcerating, sclerosing (cicatricial), superficial, and pigmented.

- *Nodular BCC:* Papule or nodule, translucent or "pearly." Skin-colored or reddish, smooth surface with telangiectasia, well defined, firm (Figs. 11-16 and 11-17). Portions of nodular BCC may have erosions or stipples of melanin pigmentation.

- *Ulcerating BCC:* Ulcer (often covered with a crust) with a rolled border (rodent ulcer), which again is translucent, pearly, smooth with telangiectasia, and firm (Figs. 11-18 and 11-19).
- *Sclerosing BCC:* Appears as a small patch of morphea or a superficial scar, often ill-defined, skin-colored, whitish but also with peppery pigmentation (Fig. 11-20). In this infiltrating type of BCC there is an excessive amount of fibrous stroma. Histologically, finger-like strands of tumor extend far into the surrounding tissue, and excision therefore requires wide margins. Sclerosing BCC can progress to nodular or ulcerating BCC (Figs. 11-20*B* and 11-21).
- *Superficial multicentric BCCs:* Appear as thin plaques (Figs. 11-22 and 11-23). Pink or red; characteristic fine threadlike border and telangiectasia can be seen with the aid of a hand lens. This is the only form of BCC that can exhibit a considerable amount of scaling. This can also give rise to nodular and ulcerating BCC (Fig. 11-23). BCC often bleeds with minimal excoriation by fingernail. Solar keratosis, in comparison, does not bleed but is somewhat painful with excoriation.
- *Pigmented BCC:* May be brown to blue or black (Fig. 11-24). Smooth, glistening surface; hard, firm; may be indistinguishable from superficial spreading or nodular melanoma but is usually harder. *Cystic* lesions may occur: round, oval shape, depressed center ("umbilicated"). Stippled pigmentation can be seen in any of BCC types.

Distribution   (Image 11-2) Isolated single lesion; multiple lesions are not infrequent; > 90% occur in the face. Search carefully for "danger sites": medial and lateral canthi (Fig. 11-17*A, B, C*), nasolabial fold (Fig. 11-16*B*), behind the ears (Figs. 11-18*B* and 11-19). Superficial multicentric BCCs occur on the trunk (Figs. 11-22 and 11-23). BCC usually arises only from epidermis that has a capacity to develop (hair) follicles. Therefore, BCCs rarely occur on the vermilion border of the lips or on the genital mucous membranes. ⊠

LABORATORY EXAMINATION

Dermatopathology   Solid tumor consisting of proliferating atypical basal cells, large, oval, deep-blue staining on H&E, but with little anaplasia and infrequent mitoses; palisading arrangement at periphery; variable amounts of mucinous stroma.

DIAGNOSIS AND DIFFERENTIAL DIAGNOSIS

Serious BCCs occurring in the danger sites (central part of the face, behind the ears) are readily detectable by careful examination with good lighting, a hand lens, and careful palpation and dermoscopy. Diagnosis is made clinically and confirmed microscopically. Differential

A

B

FIGURE 11-16   Basal cell carcinoma: nodular type   *A.* A small pearly papule (arrow) on the nostril and an even smaller one (small arrow) in the nasolabial fold. These are very early stages of BCC. The gray arrow denotes a dermal NMN. ***B.*** This is a further advanced nodular BCC. A solitary, shiny, nodule with large telangiectatic vessels on the ala nasi, arising on skin with dermatoheliosis.

FIGURE 11-17 Basal cell carcinoma: nodular type A. A glistening, smooth plaque on the lower eyelid with multiple telangiectasias. **B.** An oval, pearly nodule on the nose close to the inner canthus. **C.** A smooth, pearly tumor with telangiectasia below the lower eyelid. Tumor feels hard, is well defined, and is asymptomatic. **D.** A large, firm reddish glistening nodule with small ulcerations on the nose.

diagnosis includes all smooth papules such as dermal nevomelanocytic nevi, trichoepithelioma, dermatofibroma, and others; if pigmented, superficial spreading and nodular melanoma; if ulcerated, all nonpainful firm ulcers including SCC and a (extragenital) primary chancre of syphilis.

MANAGEMENT

Excision with primary closure, skin flaps, or grafts. Cryosurgery and electrosurgery are options, but only for very small lesions and not in the danger sites or on the scalp.

FIGURE 11-18   Basal cell carcinoma, ulcerated: Rodent ulcer   A. A large circular ulcer on the tip of the nose with a wall-like border. **B.** A similar lesion in the retroauricular region. There is a rolled pearly border surrounding the ulcer. **C.** Rodent ulcer in the preauricular region. A rolled pearly border surrounds an ulcer with yellow necroses and a tiny black crust. **D.** A deep ulcer with a surrounding rolled border, smooth, glistening and partly covered with crusts in the mandibular region. All these lesions are hard upon palpation.

For lesions in the danger sites (nasolabial area, around the eyes, in the ear canal, in the posterior auricular sulcus, and on the scalp) and sclerosing BCC, microscopically controlled surgery (Mohs surgery) is the best approach. Radiation therapy is an alternative only when disfigurement may be a problem with surgical excision (e.g., eyelids or large lesions in the nasolabial area) or in very old age.

There are a variety of topical treatments that can be used for superficial BCCs but only for those tumors below the neck; *cryosurgery* is effective but leaves a white scar that remains for life. Electrocautery with curettage is also simple and effective, but it leaves scars and should be used only in small lesions. Topical 5-fluorouracil ointment and imiquimod cream for superficial BCC, 5 times a week, for 6 weeks, are effective, do not cause scars, but require considerable time and may not radically remove all tumor tissue. Imiquimod requires compliance by patient or caregiver. Imiquimod is especially

FIGURE 11-19   A large rodent ulcer in the nuchal and retroauricular area extending to the temple
The entire lesion consists of a firm granulating tissue, partially covered by hemorrhagic crusts. The diagnosis can be made only by examining the border, which is rolled, elevated, firm, and smooth.

A   *B*

FIGURE 11-20   Basal cell carcinoma: sclerosing type   *A.* A small inconspicuous area resembling superficial morphea, ill defined, yellowish with telangiectasia. Upon palpation, however, a platelike induration can be felt and this extends beyond the visible margins of the lesion. After verification of the diagnosis by biopsy, it will require excision with wide margins. ***B.*** A large depressed area resembling a scar on the nose; on the right (lateral) and medial margins of this "scar" there is the typical rolled border of a nodular BCC. This lesion is shown to demonstrate that sclerosing and nodular BCC are simply two different growth patterns.

FIGURE 11-21 Basal cell carcinoma, sclerosing, nodular, and ulcerating A large lesion, which looks like morphea and is whitish and firm upon palpation but within the level of the skin, is found on the temple and in the supraciliar region. Within lesion and at the margins there are small nodules of BCCs. On the lateral canthus of the eye there is a large ulcer with rolled borders representing rodent ulcer. Again this figure is shown to demonstrate that the different types of basal cell carcinoma are just different growth patterns.

A   *B*

FIGURE 11-22 Superficial basal cell carcinoma: solitary lesion and multiple lesions **A.** This bright red lesion has a slightly elevated rolled border that can be detected with "side lighting"; although this lesion is typical enough to be diagnosed clinically, a biopsy is necessary to verify the diagnosis. **B.** Many superficial basal cell carcinomas on the trunk. They appear as brightly erythematous, often scaling, flat lesions, often without a rolled border. The hypopigmented areas represent superficial scars after cryotherapy of superficial BCCs.

FIGURE 11-23 Superficial basal cell carcinoma, invasive There are two irregular red areas with rolled borders and central telangiectasia. In the larger lesion the BCC is elevated with an irregular surface and now assumes the morphology and growth behavior of a nodular BCC, on the right the lesion is erosive and will progress to an ulcer.

good for young persons who do not want scars. Photodynamic therapy is effective only in very superficial lesions and radiation sessions (photodynamic dye + visible light) are painful.

COURSE AND PROGNOSIS

BCC does not metastasize. The reason for this is the tumor's growth dependency on its stroma, which on invasion of tumor cells into the vessels is not disseminated with the tumor cells. When tumor cells lodge at distant sites, they do not multiply and grow because of the absence of growth factors derived from their stroma. Exceptions occur when a BCC shows signs of dedifferentiation, for instance, after inadequate radiotherapy. Most lesions are readily controlled by various surgical techniques. Serious problems, however, may occur with BCC arising in the danger sites of the head. In these sites the tumor may invade deeply, cause extensive destruction of muscle and bone, and even invade to the dura mater. In such cases, death may result from hemorrhage of eroded large vessels or infection.

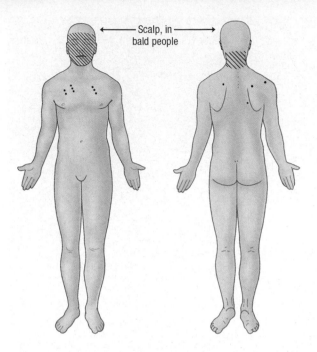

Scalp, in bald people

IMAGE 11-2   Basal cell carcinoma: predilection sites   Dots indicate superficial multicentric BCCs.

BASAL CELL NEVUS SYNDROME (BCNS)   ICD-9 : 173.0

- This autosomal dominant disorder is caused by mutations in the patched gene that resides on chromosome 9q (9q22).

- It affects skin with multiple BCCs and so-called palmoplantar pits and has a variable expression of abnormalities in a number of systems, including skeletal malformations, soft tissue, eyes, CNS, and endocrine organs.

- The syndrome occurs mostly in whites but also in brown- and black-skinned people, and there is an equal sex incidence.

- BCCs begin singly in childhood or early adolescence and continue throughout life.

- There are more BCCs on the sun-exposed areas of the skin, but they also occur in covered areas and there may be hundreds of lesions.

- Characteristic general features are frontal bossing, a broad nasal root, and hypertelorism. A systems review may reveal congenital anomalies including undescended testes and hydrocephalus. Other *extracutaneous lesions* are mandibular jaw odontogenic keratocysts, which may be multiple and may be unilateral or bilateral. There may be defective dentition, bifid or splayed ribs, pectus excavatum, short fourth metacarpals, scoliosis,

and kyphosis. Eye lesions include strabismus, hypertelorism, dystopia canthorum, cataracts, glaucoma, and coloboma with blindness. There may be agenesis of the corpus callosum, medulloblastoma, and calcification of the falx. Mental retardation is rare, however. Fibrosarcoma of the jaw, ovarian fibromas, teratomas, and cystadenomas have been reported.

- *Skin lesions* are small, pinpoint to larger nodular BCCs (Fig. 11-25), but "regular," nodular, ulcerating, and sclerosing BCCs also occur. Tumors on the eyelids, axillae, and neck tend to be pedunculated and are often symmetric on the face. There are characteristic palmoplantar lesions, which are present in 50% and are small pits that are pinpoint to several millimeters in size and 1 mm deep (Fig. 11-26).

- The significance of the syndrome is that a large number of skin cancers create a lifetime problem of vigilance. The multiple excisions can cause a considerable amount of scarring (Fig. 11-25). The tumors continue throughout life, and the patient must be followed carefully.

- *Synonyms*: Gorlin syndrome, nevoid basal cell carcinoma syndrome.

FIGURE 11-24 Basal cell carcinoma, pigmented ***A.*** A nodule with irregular borders and variegation of melanin hues, easily confused with a malignant melanoma. Features indicating BCC are the areas of translucency and surface telangiectasia. ***B.*** An irregular pitch-black plaque with a central area of regression. This pigmented BCC is clinically indistinguishable from superficial spreading melanoma. Compare with Fig. 12-10C.

FIGURE 11-26 Basal cell nevus syndrome: palmar pits Palmar surface of hand showing 1- to 2-mm, sharply marginated, depressed lesions, i.e., palmar pits.

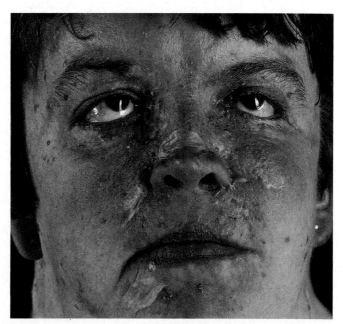

FIGURE 11-25 Basal cell nevus syndrome: small basal cell carcinomas Small reddish papular lesions are dispersed over the entire face. All of these represent small BCCs. Note considerable scarring from removal of previous lesions. Note also frontal bossing and strabismus.

MALIGNANT APPENDAGE TUMORS   ICD-9:173.0

- Carcinomas of the eccrine sweat gland are rare and include eccrine porocarcinoma, syringoid eccrine carcinoma, mucinous carcinoma, and clear cell eccrine carcinoma.
- Carcinomas of the apocrine glands are also rare, arising in axillae, nipples, vulva, and eyelids.

- Carcinomas of the sebaceous glands are equally rare, most commonly arising on the eyelids.
- These lesions are clinically indistinguishable from other carcinomas and are usually more aggressive than other invasive cutaneous SCCs.

MERKEL CELL CARCINOMA   ICD-9:173.0 ◦ ICD-10:C44.M8247/3

- Merkel cell carcinoma (MCC) (cutaneous neuroendocrine tumor) is a rare malignant solid tumor thought to be derived from a specialized epithelial cell, the Merkel cell. It is a nonkeratizing, "clear" cell present in the basal cell layer of the epidermis, free in the dermis, and around hair follicles as the hair disk of Pinkus.
- MCC occurs almost exclusively in white people.
- MCC is 10 to 30 times as common in immunosuppressed patients as in nonimmunosuppressed patients.
- The etiology is unknown but may be related to chronic UVR damage. Polyoma virus has been found in 80% of MCC.
- The tumor may be solitary or multiple and occurs on the head and on the extremities.
- There is a high rate of recurrence following excision, but, more important, it spreads to the regional lymph nodes in > 50% of patients and is disseminated to the viscera and CNS.
- MCC presents as a cutaneous to subcutaneous papule, nodule, or tumor (0.5–5 cm) (Figs. 11-27, 11-28, 36-23), which is pink, red to violet or reddish-brown, dome-shaped, and usually solitary. The overlying skin is intact, but larger lesions may ulcerate.

- They grow rapidly and usually occur in persons > 50 years.
- Dermatopathology shows nodular or diffuse patterns of aggregated, deeply blue staining, small basaloid or lymphoma-like-looking cells that can also be arranged in sheets forming nests, cords, and trabeculae.
- Immunocytochemistry shows cytokeratin and neurofilament markers, chromogranin A, and neuron-specific enolase; electron microscopy reveals the characteristic organelles.
- Treatment is by excision or Moh surgery, and sentinel node biopsy or prophylactic regional node dissection is advocated because of the high rate of regional metastases. Radiation therapy to site of MCC and regional LN is given in most cases except for very small lesions.
- Recurrence rates are high; in one series, even without a local recurrence, about 60% of patients developed regional node metastases, as did 86% of those patients with a local recurrence. Prognosis is guarded.

FIGURE 11-27 Merkel cell carcinoma A small violaceous nodule above the pinna that had been present for about 2 weeks. Sentinel lymph node biopsy revealed metastasis of neuroendocrine carcinoma. Also note actinic keratoses on the helix and concha.

A

B

FIGURE 11-28 Merkel cell carcinoma *A.* A barely noticeable 6-mm slightly dermal nodule below the hairline that had been present for about 6 weeks. Preauricular lymph node metastasis was also present. *B.* A violaceous dermal nodule, 3 cm in diameter on the forearm of a 60-year-old man. There was metastasis to the axillary lymph nodes.

DERMATOFIBROSARCOMA PROTUBERANS (DFSP) ICD-10:M8833/3 ☐ ◑

- A rare, locally aggressive tumor, slow growing, initially often misinterpreted as a scar.
- DFSP is a firm indurated plaque, skin-colored to red-brown with exophytic nodules (Fig. 11-29).
- An atrophic variant may resemble slcerosing BCC, morphea, or scar.
- Occurs on the trunk, followed by the extremities, and only 15% in the head and neck region.

- Locally aggressive with a high rate of recurrence and rare metastases.
- Diagnosis is made by histopathology, and therapy is wide surgical excision. Recurrences respond to Gleevec.

✐

FIGURE 11-29   Dermatofibrosarcoma protuberans   An irregular sclerotic skin-colored to reddish plaque of increased consistency on the back of a 40-year-old male. On the lower margin there is a reddish nodule representing exophytic growth. This lesion needs to be excised with large margins to prevent a recurrence.

ATYPICAL FIBROSARCOMA (AFX)   ICD-9 : 173.0

- A not so rare rapidly growing tumor of intermediate malignant potential.
- AFX is an asymptomatic, solitary papule, nodule, or plaque often resembling an SCC or BCC initially.

- Occurs in sun-damaged skin of older patients especially on forehead, scalp. nose, and ears (Fig. 11-30).
- Treatment is surgical.

FIGURE 11-30   Atypical fibroxanthoma   This is a 57-year-old male with dermatoheliosis and a history of solar keratoses, invasive and in situ squamous carcinoma, and basal cell carcinoma. This nodule on the vertex was clinically atypical for either basal cell carcinoma or squamous cell carcinoma; histopathology revealed atypical fibroxanthoma.

MELANOMA PRECURSORS AND PRIMARY CUTANEOUS MELANOMA

PRECURSORS OF CUTANEOUS MELANOMA

Precursors of melanoma are lesions that are benign per se but have the potential of turning malignant and thus giving rise to melanoma.

Two such entities are recognized: (1) dysplastic nevomelanocytic nevi, and (2) congenital nevomelanocytic nevi.

DYSPLASTIC MELANOCYTIC NEVUS   ICD-9 : 238.2 ∘ ICD-10 : D48-5   ■ ◑

- Dysplastic melanocytic nevi (DN) are a special type of acquired, circumscribed, pigmented lesions that represent disordered proliferations of variably atypical melanocytes.
- DN arise de novo or as part of a compound melanocytic nevus.
- DN are clinically distinctive from common acquired nevi: larger and more variegated in color, asymmetric in outline, irregular borders; they also have characteristic histologic features.

- DN are regarded as potential precursors of superficial spreading melanoma and also as markers of persons at risk for developing primary malignant melanoma of the skin, either within the DN or on "normal" skin.
- DN occur either sporadically or in the context of the *familial DN syndrome*: kindreds with familial multiple DN and melanomas (formerly FAMMM, or B-K mole syndrome).
- Synonyms: atypical melanocytic nevus, dark nevus

EPIDEMIOLOGY

Age of Onset   Children and adults.
Prevalence   DN are present in 5% of the general white population. They occur in almost every patient with familial cutaneous melanoma and in 30–50% of patients with sporadic nonfamilial primary melanomas of the skin.
Sex   Equal in males and females.
Race   White persons. Data on persons with brown or black skin are not available; DN are rarely seen in the Japanese population.
Transmission   Autosomal dominant.

PATHOGENESIS

Multiple loci have been implicated in familial melanoma/DN syndrome. It is assumed than an abnormal clone of melanocytes can be activated by exposure to sunlight. Immunosuppressed

patients (renal transplantation) with DN have a higher incidence of melanoma. DN favor the exposed areas of the skin, and this may be related to the degree of sun exposure.

CLINICAL MANIFESTATION

Duration of Lesions   DN usually arise later in childhood than common acquired nevomelanocytic nevi (NMN), appearing first in late childhood, just before puberty. New lesions continue to develop over many years in affected persons; in contrast, common acquired NMN do not appear after middle age and disappear entirely in older persons. Also, whereas common NMN are usually in a roughly comparable stage of development in a given body region (e.g., junctional, compound, dermal), DN appear "out of step," e.g., a mix of large and small, flat and raised, tan and very dark lesions (Fig. 12-1A).

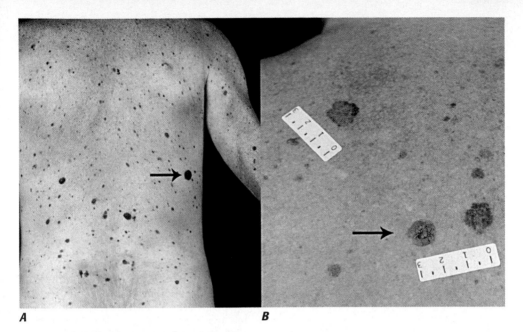

A   **B**

FIGURE 12-1 Dysplastic nevi A. Overview of the back of a patient with common and dysplastic nevi. Note a number of lesions are of different size and color, "out of step". The lesion marked by an arrow was an SSM. **B.** Larger magnification of two DNs. Note irregularity, variegation of color which are different in the two lesions ("out of step"). Also, the lesions are 1 cm or larger in diameter. The arrow denotes a seborrheic keratosis. The smaller lesions are common NMN.

TABLE 12-1   Comparative Features of Common Nevomelanocytic Nevi (NMN), Dysplastic Nevi (DN), and Superficial Spreading Melanoma (SSM)

Lesion	NMN Figs. 9–1 to 9–4)	DN (Figs. 12–1 and 12–2)	SSM (Figs. 12–10 and 12–11)
Number	Several or many	One or many	Single (1–2% have multiple)
Distribution	Mostly trunk, extremities	Mostly trunk, extremities	Anywhere but predominant upper back, legs
Onset	Childhood, adolescence	Early adolescence	Any age, most in adulthood
Type	Macules (junctional) Papules (compound, dermal)	Macules with raised portions (asymmetrically, maculopapular)	Plaque, irregular
A Asymmetry	Symmetry	Asymmetry	Greater asymmetry
B Border	Regular, well-defined	Irregular, ill- and well-defined	Irregular, well-defined
C Color	Tan, brown, dark brown, uniform, orderly pattern	Tan, brown, dark brown, pink, red, not uniform, variegated pattern, "fried egg," "targetoid"	Tan, brown, dark brown, black, pink, red, blue, white, usually a mix, highly variegated, spotted, speckled pattern
D Diameter	<5 mm, rarely <10 mm	Up to 15 mm	Most >5 mm (but, of course, starts smaller)
E Enlargement	Stops in adolescence	Continues in adulthood but limited	Growth in size at any age, unlimited

DN are thought not to undergo spontaneous regression at all or at least much less than common acquired NMN.

Precipitating Factors   Exposure to sunlight is regarded by some as an inducing agent for DN; nevertheless, DN are not infrequently observed in completely covered areas such as the scalp and anogenital areas.

Skin Symptoms   Asymptomatic.

Family History   In the familial setting, family members can develop melanoma without the presence of DN.

Clinical Features   DN show some of the features of common NMN and some of superficial spreading melanoma, so that they occupy an intermediary position between these two morphologies (Table 12-1). No single feature is diagnostic; rather, there is a constellation of findings. They are more irregular, lighter than common NMN, usually maculopapular (DN have a macular component); have distinct *and* indistinct borders (Figs. 12-1 and 12-2), and a greater complexity of color than common nevi (Figs. 12-1 and 12-2) but less than melanoma. "Fried-egg" and "targeted" types (see Fig. 12-2*E* and Table 12-1). Melanoma arising in an DN appears initially as a small papule (often of a different color) or change in color pattern and massive color change within the precursor lesion (Fig. 12-3). ▨

Dermoscopy   This noninvasive technique allows for clinical improvement of diagnostic accuracy in DN by >50%. *Digital dermoscopy* permits computerized follow-up of lesions and immediate detection of any change over time, indicating developing malignancy.

LABORATORY EXAMINATION

Dermatopathology   Hyperplasia and proliferation of melanocytes in a single-file, "lentiginous" pattern in the basal cell layer either as spindle cells or as epithelioid cells and as irregular and dyshesive nests. "Atypical" melanocytes, "bridging" between rete ridges by melanocytic nests; spindle-shaped melanocytes oriented parallel to skin surface. Lamellar fibroplasia and concentric eosinophilic fibrosis (not a constant feature). Histologic atypia do not always correlate with clinical atypia. DN may arise in contiguity with a compound NMN (rarely, a junctional nevus) that is centrally located, i.e., DN often have extension of intraepidermal melanocytic hyperplasia beyond the shoulder of the dermal nevus component; some DN may not have a dermal nevus component.

DIAGNOSIS AND DIFFERENTIAL DIAGNOSIS

The diagnosis of DN is made by clinical recognition of typical distinctive lesions (see Table 12-1), and diagnostic accuracy is considerably improved by dermoscopy. The clinicopathologic correlations are now well documented. Siblings, children, and parents should also be examined for DN once the diagnosis is established in a family member.

Differential Diagnosis   Congenital NMN, common acquired NMN, superficial spreading malignant melanoma, melanoma in situ, lentigo maligna, Spitz nevus, pigmented basal cell carcinoma.

Association with Melanoma   DN are regarded as markers for persons at risk for melanoma and as precursors of superficial spreading melanoma. Anatomic association (in contiguity) of DN has been observed in 36% of sporadic primary melanomas, in about 70% of familial primary melanomas, and in 94% of melanomas with familial melanoma and DN.

Lifetime Risks of Developing Primary Malignant Melanoma

- General population: 1.2%
- Familial DN syndrome with *two* blood relatives with melanoma: 100%
- All other patients with DN: 18%
- The presence of *one* DN doubles the risk for development of melanoma; with ≥10 DN, the risk increases 12-fold.

MANAGEMENT

Surgical excision of lesions with narrow margins. Laser or other types of physical destruction should *never* be used because they do not permit histopathologic verification of diagnosis. The following guidelines for selection of lesions to be excised are suggested:

- Lesions that are changing (increase in size, change in pigmentation pattern, changes in shape and/or border); decision is best and most reliably made by digital dermoscopy.
- Lesions that cannot be closely followed by the patient by self-examination (on the scalp, genitalia, upper back).

Patients with DN in the familial melanoma setting need to be followed carefully: in familial DN, every 3 months; in sporadic DN, every 6 months to 1 year. Search for changes in existing DN and development of new nevi. Photographic follow-up is important, with the trunk

FIGURE 12-2 Dysplastic nevi *A.* A large, uniformly tan, very flat macular oval lesion. The notched border on the left and the size (>1 cm) are the only criteria making this suspicious of a DN. ***B.*** Though relatively symmetric this lesion is macular and papular with a variegated color and measures 1.5 cm in diameter. The smaller lesions are common NMN. ***C.*** A highly asymmetric, both ill- and sharply defined margin, a notched border, and variegated brown to black color. It is clinically indistinguishable from an SSM (see Figs. 12-10A, B) but was histologically a DN. ***D*** This lesion is asymmetric with an irregular, notched border; it has a macular component and a pebbly surface in the papular portion. ***E.*** A relatively symmetric sharply defined lesion with an eccentric, more heavily pigmented area (targetoid lesion).

and extremities; also (1:1) of larger lesions (>6 mm) and all lesions that have some variegation. Most reliable method is digitalized dermoscopy, which should be available in every pigmented lesion and melanoma center. Patients should be given color-illustrated pamphlets that depict the clinical appearance of DN, malignant melanoma, and common acquired NMN. Patients with DN (familial and nonfamilial) should not sunbathe and should use sunscreens when outdoors. They should not use tanning parlors. Family members of the patient should also be examined regularly.

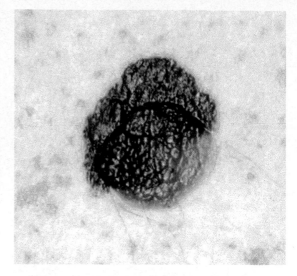

FIGURE 12-3   Superficial spreading melanoma: arising within a dysplastic nevus   The upper dark brown portion with a pinkish rim of this lesion is a dysplastic nevus; the variegated blue-black and pink plaque in the lower half of the lesion is the superficial spreading melanoma (0.9-mm thickness) arising within the dysplastic nevus.

CONGENITAL NEVOMELANOCYTIC NEVUS (CNMN)   ICD-9 : 757.33 ∘ ICD-10 : D22

- CNMN are pigmented lesions of the skin usually present at birth; rare varieties of CNMN can develop and become clinically apparent during infancy.
- CNMN may be any size from very small to very large.

- CNMN are benign nevomelanocytic neoplasms.
- However, all CNMN, regardless of size, may be precursors of malignant melanoma.

*Giant CNMC are very rare.

EPIDEMIOLOGY

Prevalence   Present in 1% of white newborns; the majority <3 cm in diameter. Larger CNMN are present in 1:2000 to 1:20,000 newborns. Lesions ≥9.9 cm in diameter have a prevalence of 1:20,000, and giant CNMN (occupying a major portion of a major anatomic site) occur in 1:500,000 newborns.

Age of Onset   Present at birth (congenital). Some CNMN become visible only after birth (*tardive*), "fading in" as a relatively large lesion over a period of weeks.

Sex   Equal prevalence in males and females.

Race   All races.

PATHOGENESIS

Congenital and acquired nevomelanocytic nevi are presumed to occur as the result of a developmental defect in neural crest–derived melanoblasts. This defect probably occurs after 10 weeks in utero but before the sixth uterine month; the occurrence of the "split" nevus of the eyelid, i.e., half of the nevus on the upper and half on the lower eyelid, is an indication that nevomelanocytes migrating from the neural crest were in place in this site before the eyelids split (24 weeks).

Small and Large CNMN   CNMN have a rather wide range of clinical features, but the following are typical (Figs. 12-4 and 12-5): CNMN usually distort the skin surface to some degree and are therefore a plaque with or without coarse terminal dark brown or black hairs (hair growth has a delayed onset) (Figs. 12-4B, 12-5B). Sharply demarcated (Fig. 12-4) or merging imperceptibly with surrounding skin; regular or irregular contours. Large lesions may be "wormy" or soft (Fig. 12-5*A*), rarely firm (desmoplastic type). Skin surface smooth or "pebbly," mamillated, rugose, cerebriform, bulbous, tuberous, or lobular (Fig. 12-5*A*). These surface changes are observed more frequently in lesions that extend deep into the reticular dermis.
Color   Light or dark brown. With dermoscopy a fine speckling of a darker hue with a lighter surrounding brown hue is seen; often the pigmentation is follicular. "Halo" CNMN are rare.
Size   Small (Fig. 12-4), large (>20 cm), or giant (Fig. 12-5). "Acquired" nevomelanocytic nevi > 1.5 cm in diameter should be regarded as probably tardive CNMN or they represent DN.
Shape   Oval or round.
Distribution of Lesions   Isolated, discrete lesion in any site. Fewer than 5% of CNMN are multiple. Multiple lesions are more common in association with large CNMN. Numerous small CNMN occur in patients with giant CNMN, in whom there may be numerous small CNMN on the trunk and extremities away from the site of the giant CNMN (Fig. 12-5*A*). ⊠

Very Large ("Giant") CNMN
Giant CNMN of the head and neck may be associated with involvement of the leptomeninges with the same pathologic process; this presentation may be asymptomatic or manifested by seizures, focal neurologic defects, or obstructive hydrocephalus. Giant CNMN is usually a plaque with surface distortion, covering entire segments of the trunk, extremities, head, or neck (Fig. 12-5). ⊠

Melanoma in CNMN
A papule or nodule arises within CNMN (Fig. 12-6). Often melanoma arises in dermal or subcutaneous nevomelanocytes and can be far advanced when detected.

DIFFERENTIAL DIAGNOSIS

Common acquired NMN, DN, congenital blue nevus, nevus spilus, Becker nevus, pigmented epidermal nevi, and café-au-lait macules should be considered in the differential diagnosis of CNMN. Small CNMN are virtually indistinguishable clinically from common acquired NMN except for size, and lesions >1.5 cm may be presumed to be either tardive CNMN or DN.

A   *B*

FIGURE 12-4   Congenital nevomelanocytic nevus   A. Small, variegated brown plaque on the nose. The lesion was present at birth. Note that lesion is hairy. **B.** Congenital nevomelanocytic nevus, intermediate size. Sharply demarcated chocolate-brown plaque with sharply defined borders in an infant. With increasing age, lesions may become elevated and hairy and very discrete hairiness is also noted in this lesion.

LABORATORY EXAMINATION

Histopathology Nevomelanocytes occur as well-ordered clusters (*theques*) in the epidermis and in the dermis as sheets, nests, or cords. *A diffuse infiltration of strands of nevomelanocytes in the lower one-third of the reticular dermis and subcutis is, when present, quite specific for CNMN.* In large and giant CNMN, the nevomelanocytes may extend into the muscle, bone, dura mater, and cranium.

COURSE AND PROGNOSIS

By definition, CNMN appear at birth, but CNMN may arise during infancy (*tardive CNMN*). The life history of CNMN is not documented, but CNMN have been observed in elderly persons, an age when the common acquired NMN have disappeared.

Large or giant CNMN: The lifetime risk for development of melanoma in large CNMN has been estimated to be at least 6.3%. In 50% of patients who develop melanoma in large CNMN, the diagnosis is made between the ages of 3 and 5 years. Melanoma that develops in a large CNMN has a poor prognosis because it is detected late.

Small CNMN: The lifetime risk of developing malignant melanoma is 1–5%. Based on the detection of congenital nevi in association with melanoma by means of histology and a careful history, a significantly increased risk is apparent for developing melanoma in persons with small CNMN. This risk is as high as 21-fold based on history and 3- to 10-fold based on histology. The expected association of small CNMN and melanoma is <1:171,000 based on chance alone. Nonetheless, small CNMN should be considered for prophylactic excision at puberty if there are no atypical features (variegated color and irregular borders); small CNMN with atypical features should be excised immediately.

MANAGEMENT

Surgical Excision The only acceptable method. *Small and large CNMN:* Excision, with full-thickness skin graft, if required; swing flaps, tissue expanders for large lesions. *Giant CNMN:* Risk of development of melanoma is significant even in the first 3 to 5 years of age, and thus giant CNMN should be removed as soon as possible. Individual considerations are necessary (size, location, degree of loss of function, or amount of mutilation). New surgical techniques utilizing the patient's own normal skin grown in tissue culture can now be used to facilitate removal of very large CNMN. Also, tissue expanders can be used.

FIGURE 12-5   Giant congenital nevomelanocytic nevus   *A*. In this baby the lesion involves the majority of the skin, with complete replacement of normal skin on the back and multiple smaller CNMN on the buttocks and thighs. There is hypertrichosis in the upper portion. Melanoma developing in a giant CNMN is difficult to diagnose early in a setting of such highly abnormal tissue.

**FIGURE 12-5   Giant congenital nevomelanocytic nevus (Continued)   *B.* Giant CNMN in a 52-year-old male. The massive hypertrichosis adds to the difficulty of diagnosing melanoma in this lesion at this stage.

FIGURE 12-6   Melanoma: arising in small CNMN   A black plaque on the thigh of a 36-year-old female, which has been present since birth. Recently a slightly less pigmented excentric nodule had appeared in this lesion. This is a melanoma.

CUTANEOUS MELANOMA ICD-9 : 172 ∘ ICD-10 : C43 ■ ●

Cutaneous melanoma is the most malignant tumor of the skin. Melanoma arises from the malignant transformation of melanocytes at the dermal-epidermal junction or from the nevomelanocytes of dysplastic melanocytic nevi or CNMN that become invasive and metastasize after various time intervals.

CLASSIFICATION OF MELANOMA

I   De novo melanoma
  A. Melanoma in situ (MIS)
  B. Lentigo maligna melanoma (LMM)
  C. Superficial spreading melanoma (SSM)
  D. Nodular melanoma (NM)
  E. Acral-lentiginous melanoma (ALM)
  F. Melanoma of the mucous membranes
  G. Desmoplastic melanoma

II   Melanoma arising from precursors
  A. Melanoma arising in dysplastic nevomelanocytic nevi
  B. Melanoma arising in congenital nevomelanocytic nevi
  C. Melanoma arising in common NMN

FOUR IMPORTANT MESSAGES CONCERNING CUTANEOUS MELANOMA

1. Melanoma of the Skin Is Approaching Epidemic Proportions

Melanoma is a common malignancy and its incidence is on the rise. In the United States the lifetime risk of invasive melanoma developing was only 1 in 1500 in 1935; in 1992 it was 1 in 105, in 2002 it was 1 in 75, and in 2010 it is estimated that it will be 1 in 50. In 2008, 60,000 cases of melanoma were recorded and there were 8000 deaths from melanoma in the United States; the number of melanomas in the United States continues to increase by 7% per year. Cutaneous melanoma currently represents 5% of newly diagnosed cancer in men and 6% in women. It is the leading fatal illness arising in the skin and is responsible for 80% of deaths from skin cancer. U.S. cancer statistics show that melanoma had the second highest mortality rate increase among men ≥65 years old. On the other hand, deaths from melanoma occur at a younger age than deaths from most other cancers, and melanoma is among the most common types of cancer in young adults.

2. Early Recognition and Excision of Primary Melanoma Result in Virtual Cure

Current cutaneous melanoma education stresses the detection of early melanoma, with high cure rates after surgical excision. Of all the cancers, melanoma of the skin is the most rewarding for detection of early curable primary tumors, thereby preventing metastatic disease and death. Early accessability to physicians is especially important because curability is directly related to size and depth of invasion of the tumor. At the present time, the most critical tool for conquering this disease is, therefore, the identification of early "thin" melanomas by clinical examination. Total skin examination for melanoma and its precursors should be done routinely.

About 30% of melanomas arise in a preexisting melanocytic lesion; 70% arise in normal skin. Almost all melanomas show an initial radial growth phase followed by a subsequent vertical growth phase. Since metastasis occurs only infrequently during the radial growth phase, detection of early melanomas (i.e., "thin" melanomas) during this phase is essential.

There is the paradox that even with a rising mortality rate, there has been an encouraging improvement in the overall prognosis of melanoma with very high 5-year survival rates (approaching 98%) for thin (<0.75 mm) primary melanoma and an 83% rate for all stages. The favorable prognosis is entirely attributable to early detection.

3. All Physicians and Nurses Have the Responsibility of Detecting Early Melanoma

Early detection of primary melanoma assures increased survival; advanced primary melanoma has a poor prognosis and survival. The survival rate plummets when there is regional metastasis to lymph nodes. The seriousness of this disease thus places the responsibility on the health care provider in the pivotal role: not to overlook pigmented lesions. This is especially true for the primary care physician, the nurse, the physical therapist, or a health care provider who sees the total skin of the body. Therefore, it is recommended that in clinical practice, no matter what is the presenting complaint, total examination of the body should be requested of all nonpigmented (i.e., white) patients at the time of the first encounter and that all

TABLE 12-2 Fitzpatrick MMRISK

A mnemonic device for promoting melanoma risk awareness among physicians and patients. Each letter represents one of the major risk factors for melanoma of the skin.

M	Moles: atypical (dysplastic nevus) (>5)
M	Moles: common moles (numerous, >50)
R	Red hair and freckling (often these persons have few or no moles)
I	Inability to tan: skin phototypes I and II
S	Sunburn: severe sunburn especially before age 14
K	Kindred: family history of melanoma

body regions, including the scalp, toewebs, and orifices (mouth, anus, vulva), be examined. It is helpful to question patients according to a mnemonic list of melanoma risk (Table 12-2).

4. Examination of All Acquired Pigmented Lesions According to the ABCDE Rule

This rule analyzes pigmented lesions according to symmetry, border, color, diameter, growth and elevation (see page 310). While it does not apply to all types of melanoma it permits differential diagnostic separation of most melanomas from common nevi and other pigmented lesions.

ETIOLOGY AND PATHOGENESIS

The etiology and pathogenesis of cutaneous melanoma are unknown. Epidemiologic studies demonstrate a role for genetic predisposition and sun exposure in melanoma development. The major genes involved in melanoma development reside on chromosome 9p21. 25 to 40% of members of melanoma-prone families have mutations in cyclin-dependent kinase inhibitor 2A (*CDKN2A*) and a few families in cyclin-dependent kinase 4 (*CDK4*). These are tumor suppressor genes that provide a rational basis for the link to susceptibility to melanoma.

There is convincing evidence from epidemiologic studies that exposure to solar radiation is the major cause of cutaneous melanoma. Cutaneous melanoma is a greater problem in light-skinned whites (skin types I and II), and sunburns during childhood and intermittent burning exposure in fair skin seem to have a higher impact than cumulative UV exposure over time. Other predisposing and risk factors are the presence of precursor lesions (dysplastic melanocytic nevi and congenital nevomelanocytic nevi) and a family history of melanoma in parents, children or siblings. Risk factors for melanoma are listed in Table 12-3.

MELANOMA GROWTH PATTERNS

Almost all melanomas show an initial radial growth phase followed by a subsequent vertical growth phase. *Radial growth phase* refers to a mostly intraepidermal, preinvasive, or minimally invasive growth pattern; *vertical growth* refers to growth into the dermis and thus into the vicinity of vessels that serve as avenues for metastasis. Since most melanomas produce melanin

TABLE 12-3 Risk Factors for the Development of Melanoma

- Genetic markers (*CDKN2a* mutation)
- Skin type I/II
- Family history of dysplastic nevi or melanoma
- Personal history of melanoma
- Ultraviolet irradiation, particularly sunburns during childhood and intermittent burning exposures
- Number (>50) and size (>5 mm) of melanocytic nevi
- Congenital nevi
- Number of dysplastic nevi (>5)
- Dysplastic melanocytic nevus syndrome

pigment, even preinvasive melanomas in their radial growth phase are clinically detectable by their color patterns. The prognostic difference among the clinical types of melanoma relates mainly to the duration of the radial growth phase, which may last from years to decades in lentigo maligna melanoma, from months to 2 years in superficial spreading melanoma, and 6 months or less in nodular melanoma.

DATA AND FACTS

- Melanoma represents 5% of all cancers by incidence in males and 6% in females.
- Number of new cases in the United States in 2008: 62,000.
- U.S. lifetime risk of developing invasive melanoma in 2010: 1/50.
- New melanoma deaths in United States, 2008: 8400.
- Most frequent sites
- Whites
  Male: back, upper extremities.
  Female: back, lower legs.
- Blacks and Asians: soles, mucous membranes, palms, nail beds.
- Frequency of melanoma by type of tumor: superficial spreading melanoma: 70%; nodular melanoma: 15%; lentigo maligna melanoma: 5%; acral and unclassified melanoma: 10%.

MELANOMA RECOGNITION

Six Signs of Malignant Melanoma (ABCDE Rule)

A *Asymmetry* in shape—one-half unlike the other half.

B *Border* is irregular—edges irregularly scalloped, notched, sharply defined.

C *Color* is not uniform; mottled—haphazard display of colors; all shades of brown, black, gray, red, and white.

D *Diameter* is usually large—greater than the tip of a pencil eraser (6.0 mm); others use D for "ugly duckling" sign: lesion is different with respect to change in size, shape, color.

E *Elevation* is almost always present and is irregular—surface distortion is assessed by side-lighting. Melanoma in situ and acral lentiginous lesions initially macular; others use E for *Enlargement*—a history of an increase in the size of lesion is one of the most important signs of malignant melanoma.

CLINICAL PRESENTATIONS OF MELANOMA

The clinical characteristics of the four major types of melanoma are summarized in Table 12-4. Also discussed in this section are melanoma in situ and desmoplastic melanoma.

TABLE 12-4 Four Major Types of Melanoma

Type	Frequency, %	Site	Radial Growth	Vertical Growth
Superficial spreading	70	Any site, lower extremities, trunk	Months to 2 years	Delayed
Nodular	15	Any site, trunk, head, neck	No clinically perceptible radial growth	Immediate
Lentigo maligna melanoma	5	Face, neck, dorsa of hands	Years	Much delayed
Acral lentiginous melanoma	5–10	Palms, soles, subungual	Months to years	Early but recognition delayed

MELANOMA IN SITU (MIS)   ICD-9:232 ∘ ICD-10:D02   ■ ◑

The clinical features of MIS are not always clearly presented. MIS is primarily a histopathologic definition, and the term is used when melanoma cells are confined to the epidermis, above the basement membrane; basilar melanocytic atypia, hyperplasia, and spread either occur in single-file alignment along the basal membrane or are distributed throughout the epidermis (pagetoid spread). Every melanoma starts as an in situ lesion, but MIS is clinically diagnosable only when the radial growth phase is long enough for it to become visually detectable. Such lesions are flat, within the level of the skin, and thus a *macule* (Fig. 12-7) or a macule with barely perceptible

elevation (Fig. 12-8), with irregular borders and marked variegation of color: brown, dark brown, and black or reddish tones but without gray or blue, as this occurs only when melanin (within macrophages) or melanocytes or melanoma cells are located in the dermis. The clinical distinction between melanoma in situ and severely atypical dysplastic nevi may not be possible. Most life insurance companies at the present time do not regard this lesion as a malignancy, but it definitely is.

The clinical correlations of MIS are *lentigo maligna* (Fig. 12-7) and flat *superficial spreading melanoma* (Fig. 12-8) and these are discussed in the respective sections below.

FIGURE 12-7   Melanoma in situ: lentigo maligna   A large, very irregular and asymmetric macule on the preauricular region of a 78-year-old male. There is striking variegation of pigmentation (tan, brown, dark brown, black).

LENTIGO MALIGNA MELANOMA (LMM)   ICD-9:232 ○ ICD-10:D02   ◼ ●

- The least common (<5%) of the four principal melanoma types of white persons [the others are superficial spreading melanoma (SSM), nodular melanoma (NM), and acral lentiginous melanoma (ALM)].

- It occurs in older persons on the most sun-exposed areas—the face and forearms.

- Sunlight is the most important pathogenic factor in LMM.

- LMM always starts as *lentigo maligna* (LM), which represents a macular intraepidermal neoplasm and is an MIS (Fig. 12-7). LM is thus not a precursor but an evolving lesion of melanoma.

- Focal papular and nodular areas signal a switch from the radial to the vertical growth phase and thus invasion into the dermis; the lesion is now called LMM (Image 12-1).

- For the most important clinical characteristics, see Table 12-4.

EPIDEMIOLOGY

Age of Onset   Median age 65.
Sex   Equal incidence in males and females.
Race   Rare in brown- (e.g., Asians, East Indians) and extremely rare in black-skinned (African Americans and Africans) persons. Highest incidence in whites and skin phototypes I, II, and III.
Incidence   5% of primary cutaneous melanomas.
Predisposing Factors   Same factors as in sun-induced nonmelanoma skin cancer: older population, outdoor occupations (farmers, sailors, construction workers).

PATHOGENESIS

In contrast to SSM and NM, which appear to be related to intermittent high-intensity sun exposure and occur on the intermittently exposed areas (back and legs) of young or middle-aged adults, LM and LMM occur on the face, neck, and dorsa of the forearms or hands (Table 12-4); furthermore, LM and LMM occur almost always in older persons with evidence of heavily sundamaged skin (dermatoheliosis). The evolution of the lesion most clearly reveals the transition from the radial to the vertical growth phase and from a clinically recognizable MIS to invasive melanoma (Image 12-1).

CLINICAL MANIFESTATION

LMM very slowly evolves from LM over a period of several years, sometimes up to 20 years. There is practically always a background of dermatoheliosis.

Skin Lesions   *Lentigo Maligna*   Uniformly *flat*, macule (Fig. 12-7); 0.5 cm or larger, up to 20 cm (Fig. 12-9A). Usually well defined, in some areas also blurred borders or highly irregular

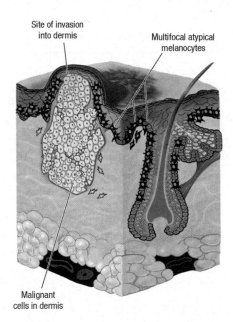

Site of invasion into dermis

Multifocal atypical melanocytes

Malignant cells in dermis

IMAGE 12-1   Lentigo maligna melanoma.
Illustrated on the right is a large, variegated, freckle-like macule (not elevated above the plane of the skin) with irregular borders; the ten areas show increased numbers of melanocytes, usually atypical and bizarre, and are distributed single file along the basal layer; at certain places in the dermis, malignant melanocytes have invaded and formed prominent nests. At the left is a large nodule that is composed of epithelioid cells in this illustration; the nodules of all four main subtypes of melanoma are indistinguishable from each other.

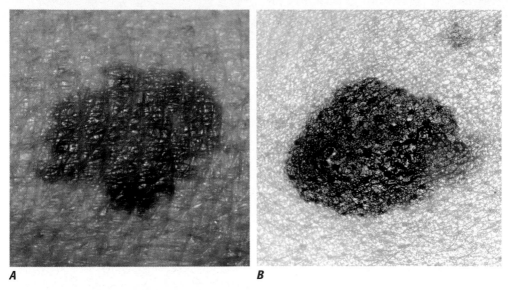

A   *B*

FIGURE 12-8 Melanoma in situ, superficial spreading type *A.* Barely elevated plaque on the arm of a 75-year-old white male was first noted 5 years previously, gradually increasing in size. The lesion is asymmetric and there is also asymmetry in the distribution of color that is variegated and shows dark-brown specks against a tan background. Dermatopathology of the lesion showed a superficial spreading melanoma in situ. *B.* An almost oval, barely elevated small plaque that has a relatively regular border but is striking with regard to the variegation in color: tan, dark brown, and even black with an orange portion on the right. Dermatopathology again showed MIS with a pagetoid growth pattern of intraepidermal melanoma cells.

A   *B*

FIGURE 12-9 Lentigo maligna *A.* A very large lentigo maligna on the right cheek with the typical variega-tion in color (tan, brown, black) and highly irregular shape. The lesion is flat, macular, and thus represents in situ melanoma. *B.* The classically macular lentigo maligna is highly irregular in shape and variegated in color. How-ever, there is a bluish component and a large pink nodule in the infraorbital region, indicating a switch from the radial to the vertical growth phase and thus invasiveness: the lesion is now called lentigo maligna melanoma.

borders, often with a notch; "geographic" shape with inlets and peninsulas (Fig. 12-9B). Early lesions tan, advanced lesions: striking variations in hues of brown and black (speckled), appears like a "stain" (Fig. 12-7); haphazard network of black on a background of brown (Fig. 12-9A). *No* hues of red and blue.

Lentigo Maligna Melanoma The clinical change that indicates the transition of LM to LMM is the appearance of variegated red, white, and blue and of papules, plaques, or nodules (see Fig. 12-9B). Thus LMM is the same as LM *plus* (1) gray areas (indicate focal regression), and blue areas [indicating dermal pigment (melanocytes or melanin)], and (2) papules or nodules, which may be blue, black, or pink (Fig. 12-9B). Rarely, LMM may be nonpigmented. It is then skin-colored and patchy red and clinically not diagnosable (see Fig. 12-15A).

Distribution Single isolated lesion on the sun-exposed areas: forehead, nose, cheeks, neck, forearms, and dorsa of hands; rarely on lower legs. ✎

Other Skin Changes in Areas of Tumor Sun-induced changes: solar keratosis, freckling, telangiectasia, thinning of the skin, i.e., dermatoheliosis.

General Medical Examination Check for regional lymphadenopathy.

LABORATORY EXAMINATION

Dermatopathology LM shows increased numbers of atypical melanocytes distributed in a single layer along the basal layer and above the basement membrane of an epidermis that shows elongation of rete ridges. Atypical melanocytes are usually singly dispersed but may also aggregate to small nests and extend into the hair follicles, reaching the middermis, even in the preinvasive stage of LM. In LMM, they invade the dermis (vertical growth phase) and expand into the deeper tissues (Image 12-1).

TABLE 12-5	Cutaneous Melanoma: Stage Grouping and Prognosis						
Stage	**Clinical Staging**			**Pathologic Staging**			**Survival,%**
	T	N	M	T	N	M	
0	Tis	N0	M0	Tis	N0	M0	
IA	T1a	N0	M0	T1a	N0	M0	95
IB	T1b	N0	M0	T1b	N0	M0	90
	T2a	N0	M0	T2a	N0	M0	
IIA	T2b	N0	M0	T2b	N0	M0	78
	T3a	N0	M0	T3a	N0	M0	
IIB	T3b	N0	M0	T3b	N0	M0	65
	T4a	N0	M0	T4a	N0	M0	
IIC	T4b	N0	M0	T4b	N0	M0	45
III	Any T	N1	M0				
IIIA				T1–4a	N1a	M0	60
				T1–4a	N2a	M0	
IIIB				T1–4b	N1a	M0	
				T1–4b	N2a	M0	
				T1–4a	N1b	M0	52
				T1–4a	N2b	M0	
				T1–4a/b	N2c	M0	
IIIC				T1–4b	N1b	M0	
				T1–4b	N2b	M0	26
				Any T	N3	M0	
IV	Any T	Any N	Any M1	Any T	Any N	Any M1	7.5–11

Source: Adapted from CM Balch et al: J Clin Oncol 19:3622–34, 2001.

DIFFERENTIAL DIAGNOSIS

Variegate Tan-Brown Macule/Papule/Nodule
Seborrheic keratoses may be dark but are exclusively papules or plaques and have a characteristic stippled surface, often with a verrucous component, i.e., a "warty" but greasy surface that, when scratched, exhibits fine scales. *Solar lentigo*, although macular, does not exhibit the intensity or variegation of brown, dark brown, and black hues seen in LM. Dermoscopy is essential.

PROGNOSIS

Summarized in Tables 12-5 and 12-6.

MANAGEMENT

See also page 332.
1. Very early LM lesions: Imiquimod.
2. Excise with 1-cm beyond the clinically visible lesion where possible and provided the

TABLE 12-6 8-Year Survival Rates for Patients with Clinical Stage I Melanoma (In the Vertical Growth Phase) Based on Tumor Thickness

Thickness, mm	8-Year Survival Rate, %
<0.76	93.2
0.76–1.69	85.6
1.70–3.60	59.8
>3.60	33.3

Source: Adapted from WH Clark Jr et al: J Natl Cancer Inst 81:1893, 1989.

flat component does not involve a major organ. Use of Wood lamp and dermoscopy help in defining borders.

3. Sentinel node to be done in lesions >1.0 mm in terms of thickness.

SUPERFICIAL SPREADING MELANOMA   ICD-9:232 ∘ ICD-10:D02   ● ■

- Superficial spreading melanoma (SSM) is the most common melanoma (70%) type in persons with white skin.

- It arises most frequently on the upper back and occurs as a moderately slow-growing lesion over a period up to 2 years.

- SSM has a distinctive morphology: an elevated, flat lesion (plaque). The pigment variegation of

SSM is similar to, but more striking than, the variety of color present in most LMM. The color display is a mixture of brown, dark brown, black, blue, and red, with slate-gray or gray regions in areas of tumor regression.

- For most important clinical characteristics, see Table 12-4.

EPIDEMIOLOGY

Age of Onset   30 to 50 (median, 37) years of age.
Sex   Slightly higher incidence in females.
Race   In world surveys, white-skinned persons overwhelmingly predominate. Only 2% brown- or black-skinned. Furthermore, brown and black persons have melanomas usually occurring on the extremities; half of brown and black persons have primary melanomas arising on the sole of the foot (see below).
Incidence   SSM constitutes 70% of all melanomas arising in white persons.
Predisposing and Risk Factors (see Table 12-3)
In order of importance these are *presence of precursor lesions* (DN, CNMN; pages 300 and 304); *family history* of melanoma in parents, children, or siblings; *light skin color* (skin phototypes

I and II); and sunburns, especially during preadolescence. Especially increased incidence in young urban professionals, with a frequent pattern of intermittent, intense sun exposure ("weekenders") or winter holidays near the equator.

PATHOGENESIS

In the early stages of growth there is an intraepidermal, or radial, growth phase during which tumorigenic pigment cells are confined to the epidermis and thus cannot metastasize. At this stage SSM is an MIS (Fig. 12-8 and Image 12-2). This "grace period" of the radial growth phase, with potential for cure, is followed by the invasive vertical growth phase, in which malignant cells consist of a tumorigenic nodule that vertically invades the dermis with potential for metastasis (Image 12-2).

The pathophysiology of SSM is not yet understood. Certainly, in some considerable number of SSMs, sunlight exposure is a factor, and SSM is related to occasional bursts of recreational sun exposure during a susceptible period (<14 years). About 10% of the SSMs occur in high-risk families. The rest of the cases may occur sporadically among persons without a specific genetic risk.

CLINICAL MANIFESTATION

The usual history of SSM is a change in a previously existing pigmented lesion (mostly a DN). It should be noted, however, that 70% of melanomas arise in "normal" skin, but since initial growth is slow and melanomas often occur in persons with many nevi, an early SSM may be mistaken for a preexisting nevus by the patient. Often, a patient may offer a history of having had a mole at that particular site since childhood ("as long as I can remember"), but when a photograph of that particular age period and site is retrieved from a family album, no such "mole" can be detected.

The patient or a close relative may note a gradual darkening in one area of a "mole" (see Figs. 12-3, 12-8) or a change in shape; and as the dark areas increase there will develop variegation of color with mixes of brown, dark brown, and black. Also, the borders of a previously regularly shaped lesion may become irregular with pseudopods and a notch.

With the switch from the radial to a vertical growth phase (Image 12-2), and thus invasion into the dermis, there is the clinical appearance of a papule and later nodule on top of the slightly elevated plaque of an SSM. Since many SSMs initially have the potential for a tumor-infiltrating lymphocyte (TIL)-mediated regression, albeit only partial, other areas of the SSM plaque may sink to the level of surrounding normal skin and the color mixes of brown to black are expanded by the addition of red, white, and the tell-tale blue and blue-gray.

Skin Lesions (Figs. 12-10 and 12-11)
SSM is the lesion to which the ABCDE rule (page 310) best applies. Initially a very flat plaque 5–12 mm or smaller (Fig. 12-8); older lesions, 10–25 mm (Fig. 12-10). Asymmetric (one half unlike the other) (Figs. 12-10A, B, and C) or oval with irregular borders (Fig. 12-10D) and often with one or more indentations (notches) (Figs. 12-10 and 12-11). Sharply defined. Dark brown, black, with admixture of pink, gray, and blue-gray hues—with marked variegation and a haphazard pattern. White areas indicate regressed portions (Figs. 12-10C

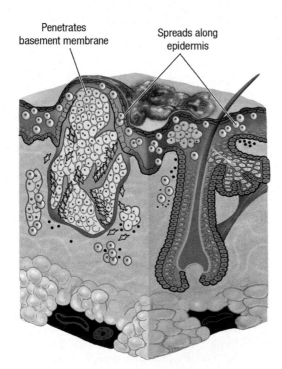

Penetrates basement membrane

Spreads along epidermis

IMAGE 12-2   Superficial spreading melanoma   The border is irregular and elevated throughout its entirety; biopsy of this plaque surrounding the large nodule shows a pagetoid distribution of large melanocytes throughout the epidermis in multiple layers, occurring singly or in nests, and uniformly atypical. On the left is a large nodule, and scattered throughout the surrounding portion of the plaque are smaller papular and nodular areas. The nodules may also show epithelioid, spindle cells or small malignant melanocytes as in lentigo maligna melanoma and nodular melanoma.

and *D*). An SSM is thus a flat plaque with all shades of brown to black plus the American flag or the tricolore (red, blue, white) (Fig. 12-10*D*). *No benign pigmented lesion has these characteristics.* As the vertical growth phase progresses, nodules appear; eventually erosions and even superficial ulceration develop (Figs. 12-11*C* and *D*).

Distribution Isolated, single lesions; multiple primaries are rare. Back (males and females); legs (females, between knees and ankles); anterior trunk and legs in males; relatively fewer lesions on covered areas, e.g., buttocks, lower abdomen, bra area. ⬛

Dermoscopy Increases diagnostic accuracy by over 50%.

General Examination Always search for enlarged regional nodes.

LABORATORY EXAMINATION

Dermatopathology Malignant melanocytes expand in a pagetoid pattern, i.e., in multiple layers within the epidermis (if confined to the epidermis, the lesion is an MIS) and superficial papillary body of the dermis—the radial growth phase. They occur singly and in nests (see Image 12-2) and are S-100 and HMB-45 positive. In the vertical growth phase, presenting clinically as small nodules, they expand further into the reticular dermis and beyond (Image 12-2). For microstaging see Table 12-7 and p. 331.

FIGURE 12-10 Superficial spreading melanoma, radial growth phase *A.* A flat-topped, elevated, asymmetric and irregular plaque with variegated color (brown, black) on the trunk with sharply demarcated margins. The surface is also irregular with a cobblestone pattern. *B.* An asymmetric, flat plaque with irregular and sharply defined margins and a cobblestone-like surface. The melanin pigmentation ranges from light brown to dark brown, black, and there are lighter areas interspersed. *C.* A highly irregular lesion with dark-brown to bluish-black papules forming a ring around a white macular area with a central brownish to bluish papule. This white area marks spontaneous regression. *D.* A relatively symmetric but large (8 cm) plaque with sharply defined and notched border and a considerable variegation of color: black, blue, red, and white.

TABLE 12-7 Melanoma TNM Classification		
T Classification	**Thickness, mm**	**Ulceration Status**
T1	≤1.0	a: Without ulceration and level II/III[a]
		b: With ulceration or level IV/V/T2[a]
T2	1.01–2.0	a: Without ulceration
		b: With ulceration
T3	2.01–4.0	a: Without ulceration
		b: With ulceration
T4	>4.0	a: Without ulceration
		b: With ulceration
N Classification	**No. of Metastatic Nodes**	**Nodal Metastatic Mass**
N1	1	a: Micrometastasis
		b: Macrometastasis
N2	2–3	a: Micrometastasis
		b: Macrometastasis
		c: In-transit met(s)/satellite(s) without metastatic nodes
N3	4 or more metastatic nodes, or matted nodes, or in-transit met(s)/satellite(s) with metastatic node(s)	
M Classification	**Site**	**Serum Lactate Dehydrogenase**
M1a	Distant skin, subcutaneous, or nodal metastases	Normal
M1b	Lung metastases	Normal
M1c	All other visceral metastases	Normal
	Any distant metastasis	Elevated

[a]Clark level I, Intraepidermal; level II, invades papillary dermis; level III, fills papillary dermis; level IV, invades reticular dermis; level V, invades subcutaneous fat.
Source: Adapted from CM Balch et al: J Clin Oncol 19:3635, 2001.

COURSE AND PROGNOSIS

Left untreated, SSM develops deep invasion (vertical growth) over months to years. Prognosis is summarized in Tables 12-5 and 12-6.

DIAGNOSIS

Clinically according to the ABCDE rule, verified by dermoscopy. In case of doubt, *biopsy*;

total excisional biopsy with narrow margins is optimal biopsy procedure. Incisional or punch biopsy acceptable when total excisional biopsy cannot be performed or when lesion is large, requiring extensive surgery to remove the entire lesion.

MANAGEMENT

Surgical Treatment   See page 332.

FIGURE 12-11 Superficial spreading melanoma, vertical growth phase **A.** An only minimally irregular plaque with variegate color (brown, black). In the center there is a small black, dome-shaped nodule. This is the switch to the vertical growth phase. **B.** An irregular very flat plaque with notched borders and highly variegated color (tan, brown, black, and red). Slightly off center there is a large partially crusted nodule (vertical growth phase). **C.** A highly irregular and asymmetric plaque with a cobblestone-like surface and variegated color (black, brown). On the right there is an excentric eroded black to blue nodule representing the vertical growth phase. **D.** A highly irregular, asymmetric bluish to black plaque with brown, red, and white (regression). Off center is an eroded black nodule (vertical growth).

NODULAR MELANOMA   ICD-9:232 ∘ ICD-10:D02   ■ ●

- Nodular melanoma (NM) is second in frequency after SSM.

- Occurring largely in middle life in persons with white skin and, as in SSM, on the less commonly exposed areas.

- The tumor from the beginning is in the vertical growth phase (Image 12-3).

- NM is uniformly elevated and presents as a thick plaque or an exophytic, polypoid or dome-shaped lesion.

- The color pattern is usually not variegated, and the lesion is uniformly blue or blue-black or, less commonly, can be very lightly pigmented or nonpigmented (amelanotic melanoma).

- NM is the one type of primary melanoma that arises quite rapidly (12 months to 2 years) from normal skin or from a melanocytic nevus as a nodular (vertical) growth without an adjacent epidermal component, as is always present in LMM and SSM (see Images 12-1 and 12-2).

For the most important clinical characteristics, see Table 12-4.

Primarily deep
invasion

IMAGE 12-3   Nodular melanoma   This arises at the dermal-epidermal junction and extends vertically in the dermis. The epidermis lateral to the areas of this invasion does not demonstrate atypical melanocytes. As in lentigo maligna melanoma and superficial spreading melanoma, the tumor may show large epithelioid cells, spindle cells, small malignant melanocytes, or mixtures of all three.

EPIDEMIOLOGY

Age of Onset   Middle life.

Sex   Equal incidence in males and females.

Race   NM occurs in all races, but in the Japanese it occurs eight times more frequently (27%) than SSM (3%).

Incidence   NM constitutes 15% (up to 30%) of the melanomas in the United States.

Predisposing and Risk Factors   See page 309 and Table 12-3.

PATHOGENESIS

Both SSM and NM occur in approximately the same sites (upper back in males, lower legs in females), and presumably the same pathogenetic factors are operating in NM as were described in SSM. For the growth pattern of NM, see Image 12-3. The reason for the high frequency of NM in the Japanese is not known.

CLINICAL MANIFESTATION

This type of melanoma may arise in a preexisting nevus, but more commonly arises de novo from normal skin. In contrast to SSM, NM evolves over a few months and is often noted by the patient as a new "mole" that was not present before.

Skin Lesions   Uniformly elevated "blueberry-like" nodule (Figs. 12-12*A* and *B*) or ulcerated or "thick" plaque; may become polypoid. Uniformly dark blue, black, or "thundercloud" gray (Fig. 12-12*A, B*); lesions may appear pink with a trace of brown or a black rim (amelanotic NM, see Fig. 12-15*C*). Surface smooth or scaly, eroded (Fig. 12-12*C*) or ulcerated (Fig. 12-12*D*). Early lesions are 1–3 cm in size but may grow much larger if undetected. Oval or round, usually with smooth, not irregular, borders, as in all other types of melanoma. Sharply defined, may be pedunculated (Fig. 12-12*D*).

Distribution   Same as SSM. In the Japanese, NM occurs on the extremities (arms and legs).

General Medical Examination   Always search for nodes.

LABORATORY EXAMINATIONS

Dermatopathology   Malignant melanocytes, which appear as epithelioid, spindle, or small atypical cells, show little lateral (radial) growth within and below the epidermis and invade vertically into the dermis and underlying subcutaneous fat (see Image 12-3). They are S-100 and usually HMB-45 positive. For microstaging, see page 331.

Serology   Serum levels of S-100 beta and melanoma-inhibiting activity (MIA), S-cysteinyldopa, and lactate dehydrogenase (LDH) levels are markers for *advanced* melanoma patients. LDH is to date the only statistically significant marker for *progressive* disease.

DIAGNOSIS

Clinical and with the help of dermoscopy. However, dermoscopy may fail in uniformly black lesions. In case of doubt, *biopsy*. Total excisional biopsy with narrow margins is optimal biopsy procedure, where possible. If biopsy is positive for melanoma, reexcision of site will be necessary (see Management, p. 332). Incisional or punch biopsy acceptable when total excisional biopsy cannot be performed or when lesion is large, requiring extensive surgery to remove the entire lesion.

DIFFERENTIAL DIAGNOSIS

Blue/Black Papule/Nodule   NM can be confused with *hemangioma* (long history) and *pyogenic granuloma* (short history—weeks) (see Fig. 12-12*C*) and is sometimes almost indistinguishable from *pigmented basal cell carcinoma*, although it is usually softer. However, any "blueberry-like" nodule of recent origin (6 months to 1 year) should be excised or, if large, an incisional biopsy is mandatory for histologic diagnosis.

PROGNOSIS

Summarized in Tables 12-5 and 12-6.

MANAGEMENT

Surgical Treatment   See page 332.

FIGURE 12-12   Nodular melanoma   A. A 9-mm dome-shaped smooth nodule with a flatter brownish rim arising on the back of a 38-year-old male. **B.** A 1-cm black papule on the posterior thigh of a 60-year-old female. The lesion had been present for less than 1 year. **C.** An eroded, bleeding, brown nodule having a mushroom-like configuration giving it a stuck-on appearance. Such lesions can be mistaken for a vascular lesion such as a pyo-genic granuloma. **D.** Large (5 cm) irregular, black, bleeding nodule sitting on the skin like a mushroom. The lesion had grown for over a half year and the 56-year-old male patient had not seen a physician out of fear "it might be melanoma."

DESMOPLASTIC MELANOMA (DM) □ ●

- The term *desmoplasia* refers to connective tissue proliferation and, when applied to malignant melanoma, describes (1) a dermal fibroblastic component of melanoma with only minimal melanocytic proliferation at the dermal-epidermal junction; (2) nerve-centered superficial malignant melanoma with or without an atypical intraepidermal melanocytic component; or (3) other lesions in which the tumor appears to arise in lentigo maligna or, rarely, in acral lentiginous melanoma or superficial spreading melanoma.

- Also, DM growth patterns have been noted in recurrent malignant melanoma.

- DM may be a variant of LMM in that most lesions occur on the head and neck in patients with dermatoheliosis.

- DM is more likely to recur locally and metastasize than LMM, however. DM is rare and occurs more frequently in women and persons >55 years old.

- At diagnosis DM lesions have been present from months to years. DM is asymptomatic, usually not pigmented and is therefore overlooked by the patient. Early lesions may appear as variegated lentiginous macules or plaques, at times with small blue-gray specks of color (Fig. 12-13*A*). Later lesions may appear as dermal nodules, and although they commonly lack any melanin pigmentation, they may have gray to blue papular elevations (Fig. 12-13*B*). Borders, when discernible, are irregular as in LM.

- The diagnosis requires an experienced dermatopathologist; S-100 immunoperoxidase-positive spindle cells need to be identified in the matrix collagen. HMB-45 staining may be negative. A typical junctional melanocytic proliferation, either individual or focal nests, occurs, resembling LM. S-100-positive spindle-shaped cells are embedded in matrix collagen that widely separates the spindle cell nuclei. Small aggregates of lymphocytes are commonly seen at the periphery of DM. Neurotropism is characteristic, i.e., fibroblast-like tumor cells around or within endoneurium of small nerves. Often, DM is seen with a background of severe solar damage to the dermis.

- There are mixed views about the prognosis of DM. In one series, approximately 50% of patients experienced a local recurrence after primary excision of DM, usually within 3 years of excision; some patients experienced multiple recurrences. Lymph node metastasis occurs less often than local recurrence. In one series, 20% developed metastases, and DM was regarded as a more aggressive tumor than LMM.

- For management see page 332.

A   *B*

FIGURE 12-13   **Desmoplastic melanoma**   *A.* Amelanotic desmoplastic melanoma. A flat, skin-colored nodule with a speck of brown in the center that appeared on the forehead of this 48-year-old female. *B.* A flat nodule with bluish-red and brown portion in an elderly male; lesions often are surrounded by a macular portion resembling lentigo maligna.

ACRAL LENTIGINOUS MELANOMA   ICD-9:232 ○ ICD-10:D02   ▣ ●

- Acral lentiginous melanoma (ALM) is a special presentation of cutaneous melanoma arising on the sole, palm, and fingernail or toenail bed.
- ALM occurs most often in Asians, sub-Saharan Africans, and African Americans, comprising 50–70% of the melanomas of the skin found in these populations.

- It occurs most often in older males (≥60 years) and often grows slowly over a period of years.
- The delay in development of the tumor is the reason these tumors are often discovered only when nodules appear or, in the case of nail involvement, the nail is shed; therefore, the prognosis is poor.

EPIDEMIOLOGY

Age of Onset   Median age is 65.
Incidence   7 to 9% of all melanomas; in whites, 2 to 8%.
Sex   Male:female ratio, 3:1.
Race   ALM is the principal melanoma in the Japanese (50–70%) and in American and sub-Saharan African blacks.

PATHOGENESIS

The pigmented macules that are frequently seen on the soles of African blacks could be comparable with DN. ALM has a similar growth pattern as LMM.

CLINICAL MANIFESTATION

ALM is slow growing (about 2.5 years from appearance to diagnosis). The tumors occur on the volar surface (palm or sole) and in their radial growth phase may appear as a gradually enlarging "stain." ALM as subungual (thumb or great toe) melanoma appears first in the nail bed and involves, over a period of 1 to 2 years, the nail matrix, eponychium, and nail plate. In the vertical growth phase nodules appear; often there are areas of ulceration, and nail deformity and shedding of the nail may occur.

Skin Lesions   Acral and Palm/Sole   Macular or slightly raised lesion in the radial growth phase (Fig. 12-14), with focal papules and nodules developing during the vertical growth phase. Marked variegation of color including brown, black, blue, depigmented pale areas (Fig. 12-14). Irregular borders as in LMM; usually well defined but not infrequently ill defined. This type of ALM occurs on soles, palms, dorsal and palmar/plantar aspects of fingers and toes (Figs. 12-14C and D).
Subungual   Subungual macule beginning at the nail matrix and extending to involve the

nail bed and nail plate. Papules, nodules, and destruction of the nail plate may occur in the vertical growth phase (Figs. 12-14B, 33-14). Dark brown or black pigmentation that may involve the entire nail and surrounding skin looking like LM (Figs. 12-14A and B). As the lesion switches to the vertical growth phase, a papule or nodule appears and the nail is shed (Figs. 12-14A and B). Often the nodules or papules are unpigmented. Amelanotic ALM is often overlooked for months and, since there are no pigmentary changes, may first present as nail dystrophy. ▨

DIFFERENTIAL DIAGNOSIS

ALM (plantar type) is not infrequently regarded as a "plantar wart" and treated as such. Dermoscopy is of decisive help. Also, often misdiagnosed as tinea nigra.
Subungual Discoloration   ALM (subungual) is usually considered to be traumatic bleeding under the nail, and subungual hematomas may persist for over 1 year; however, usually the whole pigmented area moves gradually forward. Distinction of ALM from subungual hemorrhage can easily be made by dermoscopy. With the destruction of the nail plate, the lesions are most often regarded as "fungal infection." When nonpigmented tumor nodules appear, they are misdiagnosed as pyogenic granuloma.

LABORATORY EXAMINATION

Dermatopathology   The histologic diagnosis of the radial growth phase of the volar type of ALM may be difficult and may require large incisional biopsies to provide for multiple sections. There is usually an intense lymphocytic inflammation at the dermal-epidermal junction. Characteristic large melanocytes along the basal cell layer may extend as large nests into the dermis, along eccrine ducts. Invasive malignant

FIGURE 12-14   Acral lentiginous melanoma   A. An ALM arising on the thumb. Lentiginous component on the dorsal skin of the thumb: macular, sharply and ill-defined brown and grey-bluish spots. Subungual and distal ulcerated nodular component. **B.** The tumor has replaced the entire nail bed and surrounding skin: macular and of variegated color resembling a lentigo maligna. The nail has been shed. This is ALM that has led to destruction of the nail matrix and was first diagnosed as nail dystrophy. **C.** ALM on the heel. There is a highly variegated macular component–brown to gray and black; the nodular component is hyperkeratotic, reddish, and ulcerated. **D.** Lentigo maligna melanoma on the sole. This is an advanced lesion with a macular component and a reddish, ulcerated nodule. The lesion measured 10 mm in depth, and there were enlarged inguinal lymph nodes.

melanocytes are often spindle shaped, so that ALM frequently has a desmoplastic appearance histologically.

PROGNOSIS

The volar type of ALM can be deceptive in its clinical appearance, and "flat" lesions may be quite deeply invasive. Five-year survival rates are <50%. The subungual type of ALM has a better 5-year survival rate (80%) than does the volar type, but the data are probably not accurate. Poor prognosis for the volar type of ALM may be related to inordinate delay in the diagnosis.

MANAGEMENT

In considering surgical excision, it is important that the extent of the lesion be ascertained by viewing the lesion with dermoscopy. Subungual ALM and volar-type ALM: amputation [toe(s), finger(s)]; volar and plantar ALM: wide excision with split skin grafting. Sentinel lymph node procedure necessary in most cases (see "Management of Melanoma," page 332).

AMELANOTIC MELANOMA   ICD-9:232 • ICD-10:D02   □ ●

- All types of melanoma can be amelanotic.
- Since they don't have the characteristic pigment marker they are a diagnostic challenge (Fig. 12-15).
- However, often there are pigmented clones in the tumor, which reveal its nature as a melanoma (Figs. 12-15B and C).

- In most cases only biopsy will reveal the correct diagnosis (Figs. 12-15A and D).

FIGURE 12-15   Amelanotic melanoma   A. Amelanotic LMM. The red nodule was soft and diagnosed as pyogenic granuloma and was excised. Histopathology revealed melanoma and subsequent punch biopsies performed in the erythematous skin of the cheek revealed lentigo maligna (LM). The outlines of the LM lesion as determined by further punch biopsies are marked with green circles. Note that over the mandible lesion is also nodular (vertical) growth. **B.** Amelanotic superficial spreading melanoma. The true nature of this red nodule is revealed by the blue crescent at its base and the variegated brown-red plaque with which it is contiguous. **C.** Amelanotic nodular melanoma. This cherry-red nodule has a brown, macular extension at 12 and 4 o'clock and a second, much smaller red nodule at 9 o'clock, giving away the correct diagnosis. **D.** Amelanotic ASM on the heel. This cherry-red lesion was clinically diagnosed as eccrine poroma. Biopsy revealed deeply invading ALM.

MALIGNANT MELANOMA OF THE MUCOSA   ICD-9:232 ∘ ICD-10:D02   □ ●

- Malignant melanomas arising in the mucosal epithelial lining of the respiratory tract and gastrointestinal and genitourinary tracts are very rare, with an annual incidence of 0.15% per 100,000 individuals.
- Major sites of the mucosal melanomas are the vulva and vagina (45%) and the nasal and oral cavity (43%).

- Mucosal melanomas are so rare that there are no large data bases compared to those for cutaneous melanoma.
- Therefore, pathologic microstaging has not been possible, and the fine-tuning of the prognosis that has been useful in cutaneous melanoma (Breslow thickness) has so far not been possible in mucosal melanoma.

Melanomas of the Oral Cavity

There is a delay in diagnosis of melanoma of the oral and nasal surfaces. Although melanosis of the mucosa is common in blacks and East Indians, it involves the buccal and gingival mucosa bilaterally (see "Disorders of the Mouth," Section 34); when there is a single area of melanosis (see Fig. 34–13), a biopsy should be performed to rule out melanoma; this is also true of pigmented nevi in the oral cavity, which should be excised (see Section 34).

Melanomas in the Genitalia

These melanomas mostly arise on the glans or prepuce (see Fig. 35-23) and the labia minora; there are fewer on the clitoris and the labia majora (see Fig. 35-24). Most tumors extend to the vagina at the mucocutaneous border. They look and evolve like LM and LMM (see Figs. 35-23, 35-24). Vulva melanomas are often flat like LMM with large areas of melanoma in situ, and this is important to ascertain in planning excision of all the lesion to prevent recurrence. Dermoscopy should be used to outline the periphery of the lesion, as is done in LMM (see "Disorders of the Genitalia, Perineum, and Anus," Section 35).

Anorectal Melanoma

Often presents with a localized, often polypoid or nodular primary tumor, but it may also present similarly to LMM.

METASTATIC MELANOMA

- Metastatic melanoma occurs in 15–26% of stage I and stage II melanoma (see below).

- The spread of disease from the primary site usually occurs in a stepwise sequence: primary melanoma ⟶ regional metastasis (Fig. 12-17*B*) ⟶ distant metastasis.

- Distant metastasis can occur, skipping the regional lymph nodes and indicating hematogenous spread.

- Distant metastases occur anywhere but usually in the following organs: lungs (18–36%), liver (14–29%), brain (12–20%), bone (11–17%), and intestines (1–7%).

- Most frequently, however, melanoma first spreads to distant lymph nodes, skin (Fig. 12-17*B*), and subcutaneous tissues (42 to 57%) (Fig. 12-17*D*).

- Local recurrence occurs if excision has not been adequate (Fig. 12-16) or it can involve the skin of an entire region both with and without adequate surgical treatment (Fig. 12-17*A, C*)

- Widespread metastasis can also lead to single metastatic melanoma cell lodgement in all organs with melanosis of the skin (Fig. 12-18), mucous membranes, liver, kidney, heart muscle and other tissues.

- *Metastatic melanoma without a primary tumor is rare, 1–6%. It is the result of metastasis from a melanoma that underwent total spontaneous regression.*

- *Melanoma may have a late recurrence (≥10 years). The usual time is 14 years, but there have been "very late" recurrences (>15 years) in one series at the Massachusetts General Hospital, with 0.072% (20 of 2766 Cases).*

- *Patients with a solitary metastasis confined to the subcutaneous, nonregional lymph nodes or lung are most likely to benefit from surgical intervention.*

ᗡ

A   *B*

FIGURE 12-16   Metastatic melanoma: recurring in excision scar   *A*. A pigmented lesion on the shin of a 35-year-old male, present for <2 years. Dermatopathology was initially interpreted as a spindle cell (Spitz) nevus. The primary lesion site was therefore not reexcised. ***B*.** Two papules are seen around the excision site scar, one of which has a blue-brown color. The histology from the excised lesion was reviewed and revised as a superficial spreading melanoma, and the histopathology of the two papules seen here was metastatic melanoma.

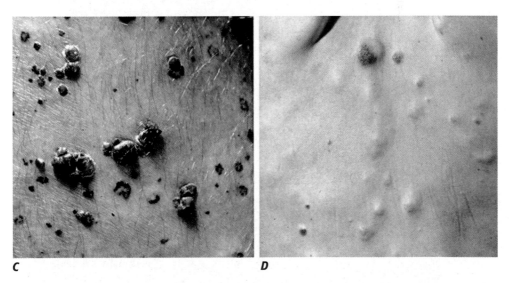

FIGURE 12-17 **Metastatic melanoma** **A.** Local recurrence and in-transit cutaneous metastases after excision of primary melanoma on the scalp and split skin grafting. Note: metastases are both in the surrounding skin and the graft. **B.** Advanced metastases in the axillary lymph nodes and in-transit metastases of the mammary skin. The primary tumor had been a pitch-black nodular melanoma and had been just lateral to the breast (the scar can still be seen). Note that both the in-transit and axillary nodules extending into the skin are amelanotic. **C.** Multiple melanoma metastases to the skin after hematogenous spread. **D.** Subcutaneous melanoma metastases by hematogenous spread. Since they are not bluish they are amelanotic. Primary and metastatic melanoma may differ with regard to pigmentation potential.

A

B

FIGURE 12-18 Universal melanosis due to metastatic melanoma ***A.*** Single-cell metastases are found throughout the skin and mucous membranes of the white patient and circulating metastatic melanoma cells were found in the blood. The urine was black (melanogenuria), and upon autopsy the internal organs were also black. ***B.*** The patient's hand is shown beside the hand of a nurse to demonstrate the difference in color.

STAGING OF MELANOMA

- Staging of melanoma depends on its TNM Classification (primary *tumor*, regional *nodes*, *metastases*, Table 12-7).
- *Clinical staging* of melanoma differentiates between local, regional, and distant disease and is based on microstaging of the melanoma and clinical and imaging evaluation for metastases.

- *Pathologic staging* consists of microstaging of the primary tumor and pathologic evaluation of regional lymph nodes (Tables 12-5 and 12-6). Staging of melanoma is strongly correlated with survival.

Microstaging

Microstaging is done according to Breslow method. The thickness of the primary melanoma is measured from the granular layer of the epidermis to the deepest part of the tumor. The thickness of melanoma (level of invasion) is the most important single prognostic variable and thus decisive for therapeutic decisions (Tables 12-6, 12-7).

Clark microstaging* according to tissue level of invasion is no longer considered a significant prognostic variable.

Sentinel Lymph Node Biopsy

Sentinel lymph node biopsy can predict the presence of clinically nondetectable metastatic melanoma within regional lymph nodes with the identification of malignant cells in H&E sections; staining for S-100 protein, HMB-45, and tyrosinase.

When the nodes are not palpated, it is not certain if there are micrometastases; these can be detected by the *sentinel node technique*. The hypothesis is that the *first* node draining a lymphatic basin, called the *sentinel node*, can predict the presence or absence of metastasis in other nodes in that basin. Either lymphatic mapping (LM) or sentinel lymphadenectomy (SL) is performed on the same day with a single injection of filtered ^{99m}Tc subcutaneously into the site of the primary melanoma for probe-directed LM and SL. Alternatively, one day after lymphoscintigraphy, sentinel node biopsy is performed, guided by a gamma probe and blue dye also injected into the primary site; the sentinel node is subjected to histopathology and immunohistochemistry. LM is very useful in locating the drainage areas, especially in primary

tumors on the trunk, which can drain on either side and to both the axillary and inguinal lymph nodes.

Lymph node dissection is performed only if micrometastasis is found in the sentinel node. The sentinel node technique is also essential in making a decision about the use of adjuvant therapy.

WORKUP OF MELANOMA

I   Primary melanoma: Stage I or II (no nodes palpated)
  A. Chest roentgenogram, sonography of lymph nodes
  B. Liver function tests, LDH
  C. Lymphatic mapping and sentinel lymphadenectomy in stage I thickness >1.0 mm

II Primary melanoma with local-regional disease
  A. Stage III, satellites and local recurrence
    1. Complete blood count
    2. Liver function tests, LDH
    3. Chest roentgenogram
    4. Ultrasound and CT scans: abdomen, pelvis (with disease below the waist), neck (with disease in the head and neck); positron emission tomography (PET) scan
  B. Stage IV
    1. Same as for stage III
    2. CT scan of the chest
    3. MRI of the brain
    4. Bone scan
    5. GI series (on the basis of symptoms)

---

*Clark level I, intraepidermal; level II, invades papillary dermis; level III, fills papillary dermis; level IV, invades reticular dermis; level V, invades subcutaneous fat.

PROGNOSIS OF MELANOMA

Prognosis of melanoma can be either excellent or grave, depending on whether the tumor is diagnosed early or late, when regional or distant metastases have occurred (Table 12-5). This emphasizes the importance of early diagnosis, of questioning patients for melanoma risks (Tables 12-2 and 12-3), of screening individuals belonging to risk groups, and of total-body examination of any patient seeing a physician for medical examination. Prognosis relating to stage grouping for cutaneous melanoma is shown in Table 12-5.

MANAGEMENT OF MELANOMA

The only curative treatment of melanoma is early surgical excision.

GUIDELINES FOR BIOPSY AND SURGICAL TREATMENT OF PATIENTS WITH MELANOMA

I. Biopsy
   A. Total excisional biopsy with narrow margins—optimal biopsy procedure, where possible.
   B. Incisional or punch biopsy acceptable when total excisional biopsy cannot be performed or when lesion is large, requiring extensive surgery to remove the entire lesion.
   C. When sampling the lesion: If raised, remove the most raised area; if flat, remove the darkest area.

II. Melanoma in situ
   A. Excise with 0.5-cm margin.

III. Lentigo maligna melanoma
   A. Excise with a 1-cm margin beyond the clinically visible lesion or biopsy scar—unless the flat component involves a major organ (e.g., the eyelid), in which case lesser margins are acceptable.
   B. Excise down to the fascia or to the underlying muscle where fascia is absent. Skin flaps or skin grafts may be used for closure.
   C. No node dissection is recommended unless nodes are clinically palpable and suspicious for tumor.
   D. See recommendation for sentinel node studies for thickness >1 mm (page 331).

IV. Superficial spreading melanoma, nodular melanoma, and acral lentiginous melanoma
   A. Thickness <1 mm
      1. Excise with a 1-cm margin from the lesion edge.
      2. Excise down to the fascia or to the underlying muscle where fascia is absent. Direct closure without graft is often possible.
      3. Node dissection is not recommended unless nodes are clinically palpable and suspicious for tumor.
   B. Thickness 1–4 mm
      1. Excise 2 cm from the edge of the lesion, except on the face, where narrower margins may be necessary.
      2. Excise down to the fascia or to the underlying muscle where fascia is absent. Graft may be required.
      3. The sentinel node procedure for tumors with thickness >1 mm is recommended.
      4. Lymphadenectomy is selectively performed and only for those nodal basins with occult tumor cells (i.e., positive sentinel lymph node). If the sentinel node is negative, then the patient is spared a lymph node dissection.
      5. Therapeutic nodal dissection is recommended if nodes are clinically palpable and suspicious for tumor.
      6. If regional node is positive and completely resected with no evidence of distant disease, adjuvant therapy with interferon-α-2b (IFN-α-2b) is considered.

ADJUVANT THERAPY

This is treatment of a patient after removal of all detectable tumor but the patient is considered at high risk for recurrence (i.e., stages IIb and III). As mentioned above, IFN-α-2b (both high and low dose) is subject to intensive investigation; however, despite early promising results to date no clear benefit on overall survival has been convincingly demonstrated.

Management of Distant Metastases (Stage IV)

Currently this can be considered palliative at best. Surgical removal of accessible metastases can provide excellent palliation. Chemotherapy encompasses a large list of drugs (dacarbazine/temozolomide, cisplatin, vindesine/vinblastine, fotemustine, taxol/taxotere) employed as single agents or in combination. Dacarbazine is still the most effective monotherapeutic agent, but all in all chemotherapeutic treatment of stage IV melanoma is disappointing, showing only a ≤20% response rate and no effect on overall survival. There are a large number of melanoma vaccination trials presently being performed, and the field is rapidly expanding to include gene-therapeutic approaches such as anti-Bcl-2 oligonucleotide therapy. Increase of overall survival has, however, not been shown to date. Radiotherapy has only palliative effects also, but stereotactive radiosurgery with the gamma-knife has shown considerable palliation.

FOLLOW-UP FOR PRIMARY MELANOMA

See Table 12-8.

TABLE 12-8 Follow-up for Primary Melanoma

Stage I (<1 mm)	Stages I (>1 mm) and II, Lymph Nodes Negative	Stage III, Lymph Nodes Positive
Every 3–6 months[a] for 3 years	Every 3–6 months[a] for 3 years	Every 3–6 months for 3 years; then 3–12 months for 2 years
Review of systems	Review of systems	Review of systems
Physical examination	Physical examination	Physical examination
	Liver function (LDH)	CBC, liver function (LDH)
	Chest x-ray and CT scans every 6 months	Chest x-ray and CT scans every 6 months
Annual examination for life	Annual examination for life	Annual examination for life

[a]Familial melanoma dysplastic nevus syndrome: every 3 months for 3 years, and then every 6 months for 5 years, and then annually for life.

PIGMENTARY DISORDERS

- Normal skin color is composed of a mixture of four biochromes, namely, (1) *reduced hemoglobin* (blue), (2) *oxyhemoglobin* (red), (3) *carotenoids* (yellow; exogenous from diet), and (4) *melanin* (brown).

- The principal determinant of the skin color is melanin pigment, and variations in the amount and distribution of melanin in the skin are the basis of the three principal human skin colors: black, brown, and white.

- These three basic skin colors are genetically determined and are called *constitutive melanin pigmentation*; the normal basic skin color pigmentation can be increased deliberately by exposure to ultraviolet radiation (UVR) or pituitary hormones, and this is called *inducible melanin pigmentation*.

- The combination of the constitutive and inducible melanin pigmentation determines what is called the *skin phototype* (SPT) (see Table 10–2). Ethnicity is not necessarily a part of the definition, e.g., African "black" ethnic persons can be SPT III and an East Indian Caucasian can be SPT IV or even V. *The skin phototype is a marker for skin cancer risk and should be recorded at the first patient visit.*

- Increase of melanin in the epidermis results in a state known as *hypermelanosis*. This reflects one of two types of changes:

- An increase in the number of melanocytes in the epidermis producing increased levels of melanin, which is called *melanocytotic hypermelanosis* (an example is *lentigo*).

- *No* increase of melanocytes but an increase in the production of melanin only, which is called *melanotic hypermelanosis* (an example is *melasma*).

- Hypermelanosis of both types can result from three factors: genetic; hormonal (as in Addison disease), when it is caused by an increase in circulating pituitary melanotropic hormones; and UVR (as in tanning).

- Hypomelanosis is a decrease of melanin in the epidermis. This reflects mainly two types of changes:
  - No decrease of melanocytes but a decrease of the production of melanin only that is called *melanopenic hypomelanosis* (an example is albinism).
  - A decrease in the number or absence of melanocytes in the epidermis producing no or decreased levels of melanin. This is called *melanocytopenic hypomelanosis* (an example is vitiligo).

- Hypomelanosis also results from genetic (as in albinism), from autoimmune (as in vitiligo), or other inflammatory processes (as in postinflammatory leukoderma in psoriasis).

VITILIGO   ICD-9:709.01 ○ ICD-10:L80

- Worldwide occurrence; 1% of population affected.
- A major psychological problem for brown or black persons, resulting in severe difficulties in social adjustment.
- A chronic disorder with multifactional predisposition and triggering factors.

- Clinically characterized by totally white macules, which enlarge and can affect the entire skin.
- Microscopically: complete absence of melanocytes.
- Associated with systemic autoimmune and/or endocrine disease.

EPIDEMIOLOGY

Sex   Equal in both sexes. The predominance in women suggested by the literature likely reflects the greater concern of women about cosmetic appearance.

Age of Onset   May begin at any age, but in 50% of cases it begins between the ages of 10 and 30 years. A few cases have been reported to be present at birth; onset in old age also occurs but is unusual.

Incidence   Common, worldwide. Affects up to 1% of the population.

Race   All races. The apparently increased prevalence reported in some countries and among darker-skinned persons results from a dramatic contrast between white vitiligo macules and dark skin and from marked social stigma in countries such as India, where even today the opportunities for advancement or marriage among affected individuals are limited.

Inheritance   Vitiligo has a genetic background; >30% of affected individuals have reported vitiligo in a parent, sibling, or child. Vitiligo in identical twins has been reported. Transmission is most likely polygenic with variable expression. The risk of vitiligo for children of affected individuals is unknown but may be <10%. Individuals from families with an increased prevalence of thyroid disease, diabetes mellitus, and vitiligo appear to be at increased risk for development of vitiligo.

PATHOGENESIS

Three principal theories have been presented about the mechanism of destruction of melanocytes in vitiligo:

1. The *autoimmune theory* holds that selected melanocytes are destroyed by certain lymphocytes that have somehow been activated.

2. The *neurogenic hypothesis* is based on an interaction of the melanocytes and nerve cells.

3. The *self-destruct hypothesis* suggests that melanocytes are destroyed by toxic substances formed as part of normal melanin biosynthesis.

While the immediate mechanism for the evolving white macules involves progressive destruction of selected melanocytes by cytotoxic T cells, other genetically determined cytobiologic changes and cytokines must be involved. Vitiligo may follow cytokine dermatitis after imiquimod. Because of differences in the extent and course of segmental and generalized vitiligo, the pathogenesis of these two types is probably different.

CLINICAL MANIFESTATION

Many patients attribute the onset of their vitiligo to physical trauma (where vitiligo appears at the site of trauma—Koebner phenomenon), illness, or emotional stress. Onset after the death of a relative or after severe physical injury is often mentioned. A sunburn reaction may precipitate vitiligo.

Skin Lesions   Macules, 5 mm to 5 cm *or more* in diameter (Figs. 13-1 and 13-2). "Chalk" or pale white, sharply marginated. The disease progresses by gradual enlargement of the old macules or by development of new ones. Margins are *convex* (as if the pathologic process of depigmentation were flowing into normally pigmented skin). Trichrome vitiligo (three colors: white, light brown, dark brown) represents different stages in the evolution of vitiligo. Newly developed macules may be "off-white" in color; this also represents a transitional phase. Pigmentation around a hair follicle in a white macule represents residual pigmentation or return of pigmentation (Fig. 13-3). Confetti-sized hypomelanotic macules may also be observed. *Inflammatory vitiligo* has an elevated erythematous margin and may be pruritic.

Distribution Two general patterns. The *focal* type is characterized by one or several macules in a single site; this may be an early evolutionary stage of one of the other types in some cases. *Generalized* vitiligo is more common and is characterized by widespread distribution of depigmented macules, often in a remarkable symmetry (Fig. 13-2). Typical macules occur around the eyes (Fig. 13-1) and mouth and on digits, elbows, and knees, as well as on the low back and in genital areas (Image 13-1). The *"lip-tip" pattern* involves the skin around the mouth as well as on distal fingers and toes; lips, nipples, genitalia (Fig. 35-6, tip of the penis), and anus may be involved. Confluence of vitiligo results in large white areas, and extensive generalized vitiligo may leave only a few normally pigmented areas of skin—*vitiligo universalis* (Fig. 13-4).

Segmental Vitiligo This is a special subset that usually develops in one unilateral region; usually does not extend beyond that initial onesided region (though not always); and, once present, is very stable. May be associated with vitiligo elsewhere.

Associated Cutaneous Findings White hair and prematurely gray hair. Circumscribed areas of white hair, analogous to vitiligo macules, are called *poliosis*. Alopecia areata and halo nevi. In older patients, photoaging as well as solar keratoses may occur in vitiligo macules in those with history of long exposures to sunlight. Squamous cell carcinoma, limited to the white macules, has rarely been reported.

General Examination Not uncommonly associated with thyroid disease (up to 30% of all vitiligo cases: Hashimoto thyroiditis, Graves disease); also diabetes mellitus—probably <5%; pernicious anemia (uncommon, but increased risk); Addison disease (uncommon); and multiple endocrinopathy syndrome (rare). Ophthalmologic examination may reveal evidence of healed chorioretinitis or iritis (probably <10% of all cases). Vision is unaffected. Hearing is normal. The *Vogt-Koyanagi-Harada syndrome* is vitiligo + poliosis + uveitis + dysacusis + alopecia areata.

LABORATORY EXAMINATIONS

Wood Lamp Examination This examination is required to evaluate macules, particularly in lighter skin types, and to identify macules in sun-protected areas in all but the darkest skin types.

Dermatopathology In certain difficult cases, a skin biopsy may be required. Established vitiligo macules show normal skin except for an absence of melanocytes. Use special stains to identify melanocytes. There may be a mild lymphocytic response. These changes are not diagnostic for vitiligo, however, only consistent with it.

Electron Microscopy Absence of melanocytes and of melanosomes in keratinocytes; also changes in keratinocytes: spongiosis, exocytosis, basilar vacuopathy, and apoptosis. Lymphocytes have been seen in the epidermis.

Laboratory Studies Thyroxine (T_4), thyroid-stimulating hormone (radioimmunoassay), fasting blood glucose, complete blood count with indices (pernicious anemia), ACTH stimulation test for Addison disease, if suspected.

DIAGNOSIS

Normally, diagnosis of vitiligo can be made readily on clinical examination of a patient with progressive, acquired, chalk-white, bilateral (usually symmetric), sharply defined macules in typical sites.

DIFFERENTIAL DIAGNOSIS OF VITILIGO

- *Pityriasis alba* (slight scaling, fuzzy margins, off-white color).

- *Pityriasis versicolor alba* (fine scales with greenish-yellow fluorescence under Wood lamp, positive KOH.

- *Chemical leukoderma* (history of exposure to certain phenolic germicides, confetti macules). This is a difficult differential diagnosis, as melanocytes are absent as in vitiligo.

- *Leprosy* (endemic areas, off-white color, usually ill-defined *anesthetic* macules).

- *Nevus depigmentosus* (stable, congenital, off-white macules, unilateral).

- *Hypomelanosis of Ito* [bilateral, Blaschko lines, marble cake pattern; 60–75% have systemic involvement–central nervous system (CNS), eyes, musculoskeletal system).

- *Nevus anemicus* (does not enhance with Wood lamp; does not show erythema after rubbing).

- *Tuberous sclerosis* (stable, congenital off-white macules polygonal, ash-leaf shape, - occasional segmental macules, and confetti macules).

FIGURE 13-1   Vitiligo: face   Extensive depigmentation of the central face. Involved vitiliginous skin has convex borders, extending into the normal pigmented skin. Note the chalkwhite color and sharp margination. *Note also, that the dermal nevomelanocytic nevus on the upper lip has retained its pigmentation.*

FIGURE 13-2   Vitiligo: knees   Depigmented, sharply demarcated macules on the knees. Apart from the loss of pigment, vitiliginous skin appears normal. There is striking symmetry. Note tiny follicular pigmented spots within the vitiligo areas that represent repigmentation.

- *Piebaldism* (congenital, white forelock, stable, dorsal pigmented stripe on back, distinctive pattern with large hyperpigmented macules in the center of the hypomelanotic areas).

- *Leukoderma associated with melanoma* (may not be true vitiligo inasmuch as melanocytes, although reduced, are usually present).

- *Postinflammatory leukoderma* [off-white macules (usually a history of psoriasis or eczema in the same macular area, see Fig. 13-14), lupus erythematosus not so sharply, defined].

- *Mycosis fungoides* (may be confusing as only depigmentation may be present and biopsy is necessary).

- *Vogt-Koyanagi-Harada syndrome* (vision problems, photophobia, bilateral dysacusis).

- *Waardenburg syndrome* (commonest cause of congenital deafness, white macules and white forelock, iris heterochromia).

COURSE AND PROGNOSIS

Vitiligo is a chronic disease. The course is highly variable, but rapid onset followed by a period of stability or slow progression is most characteristic. Up to 30% of patients may report some spontaneous repigmentation in a few areas—particularly areas that are exposed to the sun. Rapidly progressive, or "galloping," vitiligo may quickly lead to extensive depigmentation with a total loss of pigment in skin and hair, but not eyes.

The treatment of vitiligo-associated disease (i.e., thyroid disease) has no impact on the course of vitiligo. Surprisingly, there is less than expected number of solar keratoses, SCCIS, invasive SCC or BCE in vitiligo spots.

MANAGEMENT

The approaches to the management of vitiligo are as follows:

Sunscreens
The dual objectives of sunscreens are protection of involved skin from acute sunburn reaction and limitation of tanning of normally pigmented skin. Sunscreens with a sun protection factor >30 are reasonable choices to prevent sunburn for most patients and to limit the tanning reaction in fairer-skinned individuals. While all SPTs have a need for sun protection, sunscreens alone are often perfectly adequate management for those vitiligo patients with SPTs I, II, and sometimes III.

Cosmetic Coverup
The objective of coverup with dyes or makeup is to hide the white macules so that the vitiligo

FIGURE 13-3   Vitiligo repigmentation   A follicular pattern of repigmentation due to PUVA therapy occurring in a large vitiliginous macule on the lower abdomen. Melanocytes may persist in the hair follicle epithelium and serve to repopulate involved skin, spontaneously or with photochemotherapy.

FIGURE 13-4 Universal vitiligo Vitiliginous macules have coalesced to involve all skin sites with complete depigmentation of skin and hair in a female. The patient is wearing a black wig and has darkened the brows with eyebrow pencil and eyelid margins with eye liner.

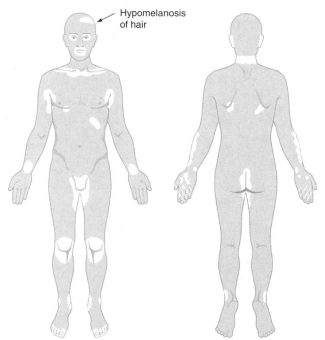

Hypomelanosis of hair

IMAGE 13-1 Vitiligo: predilection sites.

is not apparent. Over-the-counter preparations come in many color shades, are easy to apply, and do not rub off but gradually wash or wear off. So-called self-tanning agents, which contain dihydroxyacetone, are available in a number of formulations.

Repigmentation

The objective of repigmentation (Figs. 13-3 and 13-5) is the permanent return of normal melanin pigmentation. This may be achieved for local macules with topical glucocorticoids or topical psoralens and UVA (long-wave ultraviolet light) and for widespread macules with oral psoralens and UVA (PUVA).

- *Topical glucocorticoids* Initial treatment with intermittent (4 weeks on, 2 weeks off) topical class I glucocorticoid ointments is practical, simple, and safe for single or a few macules. If there is no response in 2 months, it is unlikely to be effective. Monitor for signs of early steroid atrophy.
- *Topical calcineurin inhibitors* Tacrolimus and pimecrolimus are effective in repigmenting vitiligo but only in sun-exposed areas. They are reported to be most effective when combined with UVB or excimer laser therapy (see below).
- *Topical photochemotherapy* Employs topical 8-methoxypsoralen (8-MOP) and UVA. This procedure should be undertaken for small macules only by experienced physicians and well-informed patients. As with oral psoralens, it may require ≥15 treatments to initiate response and ≥100 to finish.
- *Systemic photochemotherapy* For more widespread vitiligo, oral PUVA is more practical. Oral PUVA may be done using sunlight (in summer or in areas with year-round sunlight) and 5-methoxypsoralen (5-MOP) (available in Europe) or with artificial UVA and either 5-MOP or 8-MOP (Fig. 13-5). A response to PUVA is signaled by the appearance of tiny, usually follicular macules of pigmentation (Fig. 13-3). When this occurs, it is a good prognostic sign for successful repigmentation. Oral PUVA photochemotherapy with either 8-MOP or 5-MOP is up to 85% effective in >70% of patients with vitiligo of the head, neck, upper arms and legs, and trunk. However, at least 1 year of treatment is required to achieve this result. Distal hands and feet and the "lip-tip" variant of vitiligo are poorly responsive and, when present alone, are not usually worth treating. Genital areas should

be shielded and not treated. For risks of PUVA therapy see Section 3, "PUVA Therapy for Psoriasis."
- *Narrow-band UVB, 311 nm* This is just as effective as PUVA and does not require psoralens. It is the treatment of choice in children <6 years of age.
- Excimer laser (308 nm) This is effective but, as for PUVA, repigmentation is also slow. Produces best results in the face.

Minigrafting

Minigrafting (autologous Thiersch grafts, suction blister grafts, autologous minipunch grafts, transplantation of cultured autologous melanocytes) may be a useful technique for refractory and stable segmental vitiligo macules. PUVA may be required after the procedure to unify the color between the graft sites. The demonstrated occurrence of Koebnerization in donor sites in generalized vitiligo restricts this procedure to those who have limited cutaneous areas at risk for vitiligo. "Pebbling" of the grafted site may occur.

Depigmentation

The objective of depigmentation is "one" skin color in patients with extensive vitiligo or in those who have failed PUVA, who cannot use PUVA, or who reject the PUVA option.

Bleaching   Bleaching of *normally pigmented skin* with monobenzylether of hydroquinone 20% (MEH) cream is a permanent, irreversible process. Since application of MEH may be associated with satellite depigmentation, this treatment cannot be used selectively to bleach certain areas of normal pigmentation, since there is a real likelihood that new and distant white macules will develop over the months of use. The success rate is >90%. The end-stage color of depigmentation with MEH is chalk-white, as in vitiligo macules. The patient who may want bleaching with MEH is typically a skin phototype IV to VI with extensive repigmentation therapy–resistant vitiligo of the face and hands with residual areas of normal (dark) skin color who are happy with a uniform, albeit white skin color on the exposed regions. An occasional patient may wish to take 30–60 mg β-carotene per day to impart an off-white color to the vitiliginous skin.

All those who have bleached are at risk for sunburn from acute solar irradiation.

No long-term untoward effects have been reported from the use of MEH 20% cream, but note that the *depigmentation achieved is permanent.*

FIGURE 13-5 Vitiligo: therapy-induced repigmentation This 20-year-old Indian female is being treated with photochemotherapy (PUVA). There is slight erythema in the vitiliginous macules in the early phases (left) of therapy that will be followed by follicular pigmentation as in Fig. 13-3; after 1 year of treatment, vitiligo has completely repigmented but there is now hyperpigmentation of the knees (right). This, however, will fade with time and the color of the repigmented areas will blend with that of the surrounding skin.

ALBINISM   ICD-9 : 270.2 ○ ICD-10 : E70.3

- Albinism describes a group of genetic alterations of the melanin pigment system that affect skin, hair follicles, and eyes.

- It principally involves the synthesis of melanin in these sites, but a normal number of melanocytes are present.

- Albinism can affect the eyes: ocular albinism (OA); or the eyes and skin: oculocutaneous

albinism (OCA); or the skin and other organ systems; the CNS may also be affected in some forms.

- The classification of albinism is shown in Table 13-1.

- OCA is by far the most common form of albinism and is the only form discussed here.

OCULOCUTANEOUS ALBINISM (OCA)

EPIDEMIOLOGY

Classification See Table 13-1.

Prevalence Estimated 1:20,000. OCA1 and OCA2 account for 40–50%.

Inheritance Most autosomal recessive.

PATHOGENESIS

The defect in melanin synthesis has been shown to result from absence of the activity of the enzyme tyrosinase. Tyrosinase is a copper-containing enzyme that catalyzes the oxidation of tyrosine to dopa and the subsequent conversion of dopa to dopa-quinone. The mutations in the tyrosinase gene responsible for deficient tyrosinase activity in several types of albinism are shown in Table 13-1.

CLINICAL MANIFESTATION

Duration Present at birth. Patients with albinism avoid the sun because of repeated sunburns and bright light because of problems with vision; otherwise, they live an essentially normal life.

General Appearance "Poring" (eyes half closed, squinting) when in sunlight (Fig. 13-6).

Skin Varied, depending on the type: "Snow" white, creamy white, light tan (Fig. 13-6 and Table 13-1).

Hair White (tyrosinase-negative) (Fig. 13-6); yellow, cream, or light brown (tyrosinase-positive); red; platinum.

Eyes The eye changes are the essential physical finding that define the syndrome of OCA.

Nystagmus, a feature always present, results from hypoplasia of the fovea with reduction of visual acuity and alteration in the formation of the optic nerves; this misrouting of the optic paths is also associated with an alternating strabismus and diminished stereoacuity. The diagnostic features in the eye that identify albinism are therefore nystagmus and iris translucency (Fig. 13-7), reduction of visual acuity, decreased retinal pigment, foveal hypoplasia, and strabismus.

TABLE 13-1 Classification of Albinism

Type	Subtypes	Gene Locus	Includes	Clinical Findings
OCA1	OCA1A	*TYR*	Tyrosinase-negative OCA	White hair and skin, eyes (pink at birth → blue)
	OCA1B	*TYR*	Minimal pigment OCA	White to near-normal skin and hair pigmentation
			Platinum OCA	
			Yellow OCA	Yellow (pheomelanin) hair, light red or brown hair
			Temperature-sensitive OCA	May have near-normal pigment but not in axilla
			Autosomal recessive OCA (some)	
OCA2		*P*	Tyrosinase-positive OCA	Yellow hair, skin "creamy" white (Africa)
			Brown OCA	Light brown/tan skin (Africa)
OCA3		*TYRP1*	Autosomal recessive OCA (some)	
			Rufous OCA	Red and red-brown skin and brown eyes (Africa)
OCA4		*MATP*		
HPS		*HPS*	Hermansky-Pudlak syndrome	Skin/hair as in OCA1A or OCA1B or OCA2, bleeding diathesis (Puerto Rico)
CHS		*LYST*	Chédiak-Higashi syndrome	Silver hair/hypopigmentation/serious medical problems
OA1		*OA1*	X-linked OA	Normal pigmentation of skin and hair

NOTE: OCA, oculocutaneous albinism; TYR, tyrosinase; P, pink protein; TYRP1, tyrosinase-related protein 1; OA, ocular albinism; MATP, membrane-associated transporter protein; LYST, lysosome trafficking.

SOURCE: Modified from P Bahadoran et al, in IM Freedberg et al, (eds). *Fitzpatrick's Dermatology in General Medicine*, 6th ed. New York, McGraw-Hill, 2003.

FIGURE 13-6 Oculocutaneous albinism White skin, white eyelashes, eyebrows, and scalp hair. The irises appear translucent. Heme pigment gives the face a pinkish hue. There is squinting due to photophobia and nystagmus.

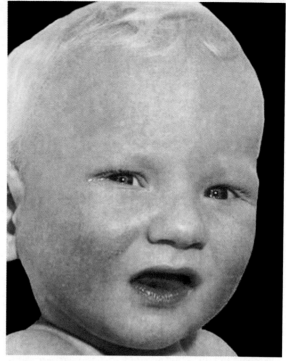

FIGURE 13-7 Iris translucency with albinism Iris translucency is a sine qua non in all types of oculocutaneous albinism, even in those patients in whom the iris is brown. The iris is rarely pink except in infants, and the diagnosis of albinism depends on the detection of iris translucency. This is best done in a dark room with a flashlight pointed at the sclera.

LABORATORY EXAMINATIONS

Dermatopathology *Light Microscopy* Melanocytes are present in the skin and hair bulb in all types of albinism. The dopa reaction is markedly reduced or absent in the melanocytes of the skin and hair, depending on the type of albinism (tyrosinase-negative or tyrosinase-positive).

Electron Microscopy Melanosomes are present in melanocytes in all types of albinism, but depending on the type of albinism, there is a reduction of the melanization of melanosomes, with many melanosomes being completely unmelanized in tyrosinase-negative albinism.

Molecular Testing Now available, and this makes it possible to classify the specific gene alteration in various types of albinism. However, it is not necessary for diagnosis or management of the problem.

DIAGNOSIS

White persons with very fair skin (SPT I), blond hair, and blue eyes may mimic albinos, but they do not have eye changes (iris translucency, nystagmus). Some persons with albinism who have constitutive black or brown skin color may have a dilution of their skin color from black to a light brown and have the capacity to tan; also, some types may have brown irides but still have iris translucency. Therefore, iris translucency and the presence of other eye findings in the fundus are the pathognomonic signs of albinism. The hair and skin color may vary from normal to absent melanin, and the various types are listed in Table 13-1. The special types of albinism are diagnosed on the basis of clinical presentation of the hair and skin pigmentation as well as hematologic studies (Hermansky-Pudlak and Chédiak-Higashi syndrome).

SIGNIFICANCE

Albinism is an important disease to recognize early in life in order to begin prophylactic measures to prevent dermatoheliosis and skin cancer, i.e., protective clothing, sunblocks, and sun avoidance in peak periods during the day.

COURSE AND PROGNOSIS

Albinos with tyrosinase-positive OCA form melanin pigment in the hair, skin, and eyes during early life, the hair becoming cream, yellow, or light brown, and the eye color changing from light gray to blue, hazel, or even brown.

Albinos living in central Africa who are unprotected from the sun develop squamous cell carcinomas early in life, and this significantly shortens their life span; few survive to the age of 40 years because of metastasizing squamous cell carcinoma. Dermatoheliosis and basal cell

carcinomas are frequent in albinos living in temperate climates. Melanomas are, curiously, very rare in albinos living in Africa; when they occur, they are usually amelanotic. Melanocytic nevi occur in albinism and may also be amelanotic but may be pigmented, depending on the type of albinism.

MANAGEMENT

Every albino should be under the care of an ophthalmologist for vision problems and a dermatologist to detect solar keratoses, skin cancers, and dermatoheliosis. Daily application of topical, potent, broad-spectrum SPF >30 sunblocks, including lip sunblocks. Avoidance of sun exposure in the high solar intensity season. Use of topical tretinoin for dermatoheliosis and for its possible prophylactic effect against sun-induced epithelial skin cancers. Treatment of solar keratoses to prevent the development of squamous cell carcinomas. Systemic β-carotene (30–60 mg thrice daily) imparts a more normal color to the skin and may have some protective effect on the development of skin cancers, although this has been proved only in mice. It is helpful for albinos to belong to a national volunteer group of albinos; in the United States it is called the *National Organization for Albinism and Hypomelanosis* (NOAH). (Noah, the builder of the ark in the Old Testament, was alleged to be an albino.) This group assists albinos in various ways, especially in dealing with vision problems: obtaining driver's license, etc.

MELASMA   ICD-9 : 709.69 ∘ ICD-10 : L81.1   ■ ○

- Melasma (Greek: "a black spot") is an acquired light- or dark-brown hyperpigmentation that occurs in the exposed areas, most often on the face, and results from exposure to sunlight.
- It may be associated with pregnancy, with ingestion of contraceptive hormones, or possibly with

certain medications such as diphenylhydantoin, or it may be idiopathic.
- *Synonyms*: Chloasma (Greek: "a green spot"), mask of pregnancy.

EPIDEMIOLOGY

Age of Onset   Young adults.
Sex   Females > males; about 10% of patients with melasma are men.

Race   Melasma is more apparent or more frequent in persons with brown or black constitutive skin color (persons from Asia, the Middle East, India, South America).
Incidence and Precipitating Factors   Very common, especially among persons with constitutive

brown skin color who are taking contraceptive regimens and who live in sunny areas. Pregnancy causes melasma. Melasma has recently been appearing in menopausal women as a result of regimens for prevention of osteoporosis using a combination of estrogens *and* progesterone; melasma does not appear in those women who are given estrogen replacement treatment but without progesterone. Also in patients on diphenylhydantoin. *Sun exposure required.*

PATHOGENESIS

Unknown.

CLINICAL MANIFESTATION

Duration of Lesions The pigmentation usually evolves quite rapidly over weeks, particularly after exposure to sunlight.
Skin Lesions Macular hyperpigmentation of the face, the hue and intensity depending largely on the skin phototype of the patient (Fig. 13-8). Light or dark brown or even black. Color is usually uniform but may be splotchy. Most often symmetric. Lesions have serrated, irregular, and geographic borders. Two-thirds

on central part of the face: cheeks (Fig. 13-8), forehead, nose, upper lip, and chin; a smaller percentage on the malar or mandibular areas of the face and occasionally the dorsa of the forearms.
Wood Lamp Examination A marked accentuation of the hyperpigmented macules. *This contrast is not accentuated in patients with a normal brown or black skin.*

DIFFERENTIAL DIAGNOSIS

Postinflammatory hypermelanotic macules.

SIGNIFICANCE

While this is a strictly cosmetic problem, it is very disturbing to both males and females, especially persons with brown skin color and good tanning capacity.

COURSE AND PROGNOSIS

Melasma may disappear spontaneously over a period of months after delivery or after cessation of contraceptive hormones. Melasma may or may not return with each subsequent pregnancy.

FIGURE 13-8   Melasma   Well-demarcated, hyperpigmented macules are seen on the cheek, nose, and upper lip.

MANAGEMENT

Topical   Commercially available preparations in the United States include: hydroquinone 3% solution and 4% cream; azelaic acid 20% cream; and a combination of flucinolone 0.01%, hydroquinone 4%, and tretinoin 0.05%. Hydroquinone 4% cream can be compounded with 0.05% tretinoin cream or glycolic acid by the pharmacist.

Under no circumstances should monobenzylether of hydroquinone or the other ethers of hydroquinone (monomethyl- or monoethyl-) be used in the treatment of melasma because these drugs can lead to a permanent loss of melanocytes with the development of a disfiguring spotty leukoderma.

Prevention   It is essential that the patient use, every morning, an *opaque* sunblock containing titanium dioxide and/or zinc oxide; the action spectrum of pigment darkening extends into the visible range, and even the potent transparent sunscreens (with high SPF) are completely ineffective in blocking visible radiation.

PIGMENTARY CHANGES FOLLOWING INFLAMMATION OF THE SKIN

HYPERPIGMENTATION   ICD-9:709.0 ○ ICD-10:L81.9

- *Postinflammatory epidermal melanin hyperpigmentation* is a major problem for patients with skin phototypes IV, V, and VI (Figs. 13-9 and 13-10). This disfiguring pigmentation can develop with acne (Fig. 13-9), psoriasis, lichen planus (Fig. 13-10), atopic dermatitis, or contact dermatitis or after any type of trauma to the skin. It may persist for weeks to months but does respond to topical hydroquinone, which accelerates its disappearance. Lesions are characteristically limited to the site of the preceding inflammation and have indistinct, feathered borders.

- Some drug eruptions may be associated with dermal melanin hyperpigmentation (Fig. 13-11), which may also be associated with lichen planus and cutaneous lupus erythematosus. This dermal hyperpigmentation may be persistent, and there is no treatment.

- *Riehl melanosis* (melanodermatitis toxica) is a reticular, confluent black to brown-violet pigmentation of the face and neck (Fig. 13-12). It may be a result of contact sensitivity or photocontact sensitivity related to chemicals, particularly fragrance in cosmetics.

  For *hypermelanosis due to phototoxic reactions* induced by psoralens (Berloque dermatitis), see Section 10, and for *non-melanin-based hyperpigmentation* due to drugs, see Section 22.

FIGURE 13-10   Postinflammatory hyperpigmentation   (Across facing page) This may follow a drug eruption, psoriasis, or lichen planus, especially in skin phototypes V and VI, as was the case in this middle-age East Indian male. Postinflammatory hyperpigmentation is a major problem in young females with skin phototypes V and VI.

A   **B**

FIGURE 13-9   **Hypermelanosis with acne**   **A.** This condition is a major complaint of this 18-year-old skin phototype III girl. The acne is not the problem now; it is the disfiguring hypermelanosis. This hyperpigmentation can be markedly reduced with topical hydroquinone (3%) cream or solution, best combined with tretinoin, applied daily. During the depigmentation, the patient must use an opaque sunblock daily to prevent the pigment darkening that occurs with daily sun exposure. **B.** In this 30-year-old Pakistani woman hypermelanosis due to acne, combined with melasma and hypopigmented acne scars, was considered a cosmetic disaster, not only by the patient but also her husband. She was successfully treated with 3% hydroquinone incorporated into a 0.05% tretinoin cream.

FIGURE 13-10

FIGURE 13-11   Postinflammatory dermal hyperpigmentation   This is shown on the hand of a skin phototype IV African woman following a fixed drug eruption.

A   *B*

FIGURE 13-12   Melanodermatitis toxica   *A.* A reticular confluent pigmentation on the face and neck of a 42-year-old female chemist who worked for a cosmetic industry and had applied, over years, most of the scented products she was involved in producing to her own skin. Since she lived in a sunny climate this increases the suspicion of a chronic photocontact sensitivity. ***B.*** In this Indian woman the mottled hyperpigmentation has coalesced to dark brown mottled hyperpigmentation of the cheeks. For professional reasons this patient had also excessively used cosmetics.

HYPOPIGMENTATION ICD-9:709.0 ∘ ICD-10:L81.9 ■ ○

- Postinflammatory hypomelanosis is always related to loss of melanin. It is a special feature of pityriasis versicolor (Fig. 13-13, see also Section 25), in which the hypopigmentation may also remain for weeks after the active infection has disappeared.

- Hypomelanosis is not uncommonly seen in atopic dermatitis, psoriasis (Fig. 13-14), guttate parapsoriasis, and pityriasis lichenoides chronica.

- It may also be present in cutaneous lupus erythematosus (Fig. 13-15), alopecia mucinosa, mycosis fungoides, lichen striatus, seborrheic dermatitis, and leprosy.

- Hypomelanosis may follow dermabrasion and chemical peels; in these conditions there is a "transfer block," in which melanosomes are present in melanocytes but are not transferred to keratinocytes, resulting in hypomelanosis. The lesions are usually not chalk white, as in vitiligo, but "off" white and have indiscrete margins.

- A common type of hypopigmentation is associated with *pityriasis alba* (Fig. 13-16). This is a macular hypopigmentation mostly on the face of children, off-white with a powdery scale. Relatively indistinct margins under Wood light and scaling distinguish this eczematous dermatitis from vitiligo. It is self-limited.

- Hypomelanosis not uncommonly follows intralesional glucocorticoid injections; but when the injections are stopped, a normal pigmentation develops in the areas.

- Depending on the associated disorder, postinflammatory hypomelanosis may respond to oral PUVA photochemotherapy.

A   *B*

FIGURE 13-13 Pityriasis versicolor *A.* Hypopigmented, sharply marginated, scaling macules on the back of an individual with skin phototype III. Gentle abrasion of the surface will accentuate the scaling. This type of hypomelanosis can remain long after the eruption has been treated and the primary process is resolved. *B.* Pityriasis versicolor in African skin. Lesions are perifollicular on the chest and coalesce to large confluent patches on the neck where the fine scaling can best be seen.

FIGURE 13-14   Postinflammatory hypomelanosis (psoriasis)   The hypomelanotic lesions correspond exactly to the antecedent eruption. There is some residual psoriasis within the lesions.

FIGURE 13-15 Postinflammatory hypopigmentation *Hypopigmentation* in a 33-year-old Vietnamese female. The patient had had chronic cutaneous lupus erythematosus. Residual inflammation of lupus is still seen on the upper lip.

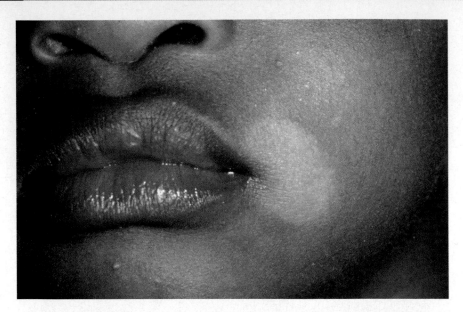

FIGURE 13-16 **Pityriasis alba** A common disfiguring hypomelanosis, which, as the name indicates, is a white area (alba) with very mild scaling (pityriasis). It is observed in a large number of children in the summer in temperate climates. It is mostly a cosmetic problem in persons with brown or black skin and commonly occurs on the face, as in this child. Among 200 patients with pityriasis alba, 90% ranged from 6–12 years of age. In young adults, PA quite often occurs on the arms and trunk.

PART II

DERMATOLOGY AND INTERNAL MEDICINE

THE SKIN IN IMMUNE, AUTOIMMUNE, AND RHEUMATIC DISORDERS

SYSTEMIC AMYLOIDOSIS   ICD-9 : 277.3 ∘ ICD-10 : E85.3

- Amyloidosis is an extracellular deposition in various tissues of amyloid fibril proteins and of a protein called *amyloid P component* (AP); the identical component of AP is present in the serum and is called *SAP*. These amyloid deposits can affect normal body function.

- *Systemic AL amyloidosis*, also known as *primary amyloidosis*, occurs in patients with B cell or plasma cell dyscrasias and multiple myeloma in whom fragments of monoclonal immunoglobulin light chains form amyloid fibrils.

- Clinical features of AL include a combination of macroglossia and cardiac, renal, hepatic, and gastrointestinal (GI) involvement, as well as carpal tunnel syndrome and *skin lesions*. These occur in 30% of patients, and since they occur early in the disease, they are an important clue to the diagnosis.

- *Systemic AA amyloidosis* (reactive) occurs in patients after chronic inflammatory disease, in whom the fibril protein is derived from the circulating acute-phase lipoprotein known as *serum amyloid A*.

- There are few or no characteristic skin lesions in AA amyloidosis, which usually affects the liver, spleen, kidneys, and adrenals.

- In addition, skin manifestations may also be associated with a number of (rare) heredofamilial syndromes.

- *Localized cutaneous amyloidosis* is not uncommon, presents with typical cutaneous manifestations, and has no systemic involvement.

SYSTEMIC AL AMYLOIDOSIS   ICD-9 : 277.3 ∘ ICD-10 : E85

- Rare
- Occurs in many but not all patients with multiple myeloma and B cell and plasma cell dyscrasias.

- Restrictive cardiomyopathy, renal function impairment, GI involvement with malabsorption, neuropathy.
- Prognosis poor

CLINICAL MANIFESTATION

Skin Lesions   Smooth, waxy papules (Fig. 14-1), but also nodules on the face, especially around the eyes (Fig. 14-2) and elsewhere. Purpura following trauma, "pinch" purpura in waxy papules (Fig. 14-2) sometimes also involving large surface areas without nodular involvement. Predilection sites are around the eyes, central face, extremities, body folds, axillae, umbilicus, anogenital area. *Nail changes*: Similar to lichen planus (see Section 33). *Macroglossia* : diffusely enlarged and firm, "woody" (Fig. 14-3).

Systemic Manifestations   Include fatigue, weakness, anorexia, weight loss, malaise, dyspnea; symptoms related to hepatic, renal, and GI involvement; paresthesia related to carpal tunnel syndrome, neuropathy.

General Examination   Kidney—nephrosis; nervous system—peripheral neuropathy, carpal tunnel syndrome; cardiovascular—partial heart block, congestive heart failure; hepatic—hepatomegaly;

GI—diarrhea, sometimes hemorrhagic, malabsorption; lymphadenopathy.

LABORATORY EXAMINATIONS

May reveal thrombocytosis >500,000/μL. Proteinuria and increased serum creatinine; hypercalcemia. Increased IgG. Monoclonal protein in two-thirds of patients with primary or myeloma-associated amyloidosis. Bone marrow: myeloma.

Dermatopathology Shows accumulation of faintly eosinophilic masses of amyloid in the papillary body near the epidermis, in the papillary and reticular dermis, in sweat glands, around and within blood vessel walls. Use thioflavin or congo red and examine the sections for an apple-green birefringence with a polarization microscope. Immunohistochemistry to assess the proportion of kappa and lambda light chains.

DIAGNOSIS

Made by the combination of purpuric skin lesions (Fig. 14-2), waxy papules (Fig. 14-1), macroglossia (Fig. 14-3), carpal tunnel syndrome, and cardiac symptoms. A tissue diagnosis can be made from the skin biopsy. Scintigraphy after injection of ^{123}I-labeled SAP will reveal the extent of the involvement and can serve as a guide for treatment, which is that of the underlying disease.

FIGURE 14-1 Systemic AL amyloidosis Waxy papules on the trunk of a 58-year-old male patient with myeloma.

FIGURE 14-2 Systemic AL amyloidosis: "pinch purpura" The topmost papule is yellowish and nonhemorrhagic; the lower portion is hemorrhagic. So-called pinch purpura of the upper eyelid can appear in amyloid nodules after pinching or rubbing the eyelid.

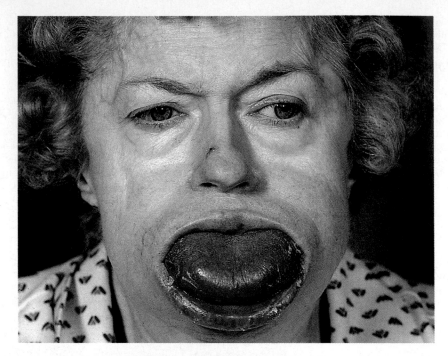

FIGURE 14-3   Systemic AA amyloidosis: macroglossia   Massive infiltration of the tongue with amyloid has caused immense enlargement; the tongue cannot be retracted completely into the mouth because of its size. (Courtesy of Evan Calkins, MD.)

SYSTEMIC AA AMYLOIDOSIS   ICD-9:277.3 ∘ ICD-10:E85

- A reactive type of amyloidosis.
- Occurs in any disorder associated with a sustained acute-phase response.
- 60% have inflammatory arthritis. The rest other chronic inflammatory infective or neoplastic disorders.
- Amyloid fibrils are derived from cleavage fragments of the circulating acute-phase reactant serum amyloid A protein.
- Presents with proteinuria followed by progressive renal dysfunction; nephrotic syndrome.
- There are no characteristic skin lesions in AA amyloidosis.

LOCALIZED CUTANEOUS AMYLOIDOSIS

- Three varieties of localized amyloidosis that are unrelated to the systemic amyloidoses.
- *Nodular amyloidosis*: single or multiple, smooth, nodular lesions with or without purpura on limbs, face, or trunk (Fig. 14-4*A*).
- *Lichenoid amyloidosis*: discrete, very pruritic, brownish-red papules on the legs (Fig. 14-4*B*).
- *Macular amyloidosis*: pruritic, gray-brown, reticulated macular lesions occurring principally on the upper back (Fig. 14-5); the lesions often have a distinctive "ripple" pattern.
- In lichenoid and macular amyloidosis the amyloid fibrils in skin are keratin-derived. Although these three localized forms of amyloidosis are confined to the skin and unrelated to systemic disease, the skin lesions of nodular amyloidosis are identical to those that occur in AL, in which amyloid fibrils derive from immunoglobulin light chain fragments.

A   **B**

FIGURE 14-4 **Localized cutaneous amyloidosis** ***A.*** Nodular. Two plaquelike nodules, waxy, yellowish-orange with hemorrhage. ***B.*** Lichenoid amyloidosis. Grouped confluent scaly papules of livid, violaceous color. This is a purely cutaneous disease.

FIGURE 14-5 **Macular amyloidosis** Gray-brown, reticulated pigmentation on the back of a 52-year-old Arabian male.

URICARIA AND ANGIOEDEMA   ICD-9 : 708.0 ∘ ICD-10 : L50   ■ ◑→●

- Urticaria is composed of wheals (transient edematous papules and plaques, usually pruritic and due to edema of the papillary body) (Figs. 14-6 and 14-7). The wheals are superficial, well defined.
- Angioedema is a larger edematous area that involves the dermis *and* subcutaneous tissue (Fig. 14-8) and is deep and ill defined. Urticaria and angioedema are thus the same edematous process but involving different levels of the cutaneous vascular plexus: papillary and deep.
  ICD-9 : 277.6 ∘ ICD-10 : D84.1
- Urticaria and/or angioedema may be acute recurrent or chronic recurrent.

- Other forms of urticaria/angioedema are recognized: IgE- and IgE receptor–dependent, physical, contact, mast cell degranulation–related, and idiopathic.
- In addition, angioedema/urticaria can be mediated by bradykinin, the complement system, and other effector mechanisms.
- Urticarial vasculitis is a special form of cutaneous necrotizing venulitis (see page 407).
- There are some syndromes with angioedema in which urticarial wheals are rarely present (e.g., hereditary angioedema).

EPIDEMIOLOGY AND ETIOLOGY

Incidence 15–23% of the population may have had this condition during their lifetime. Chronic urticaria is likely to be present at some time in about 25% of patients with urticaria.

Etiology Urticaria/angioedema is not a disease but a cutaneous reaction pattern. For classification and etiology, see Table 14-1.

CLINICAL TYPES

Acute Urticaria Acute onset and recurring over <30 days. Usually large wheals often associated with angioedema (Figs. 14-7 and 14-8); often IgE-dependent with atopic diathesis; related to foods, parasites, and penicillin. Also, complement-mediated in serum sickness–like reactions (whole blood, immunoglobulins, penicillin). Often accompanied by angioedema. Common. (See also "Drug-Induced Acute Urticaria," Section 22.)

Chronic Urticaria Recurring over <30 days. Small and large wheals (Fig. 14-9). Rarely IgE-dependent but often due to anti-FcεR autoantibodies; etiology unknown in 80% and therefore considered idiopathic. Intolerance to salicylates, benzoates. Common. Chronic urticaria affects adults predominantly and is approximately twice as common in women as in men. Up to 40% of patients with chronic urticaria of >6 months' duration still have urticaria 10 years later.

Symptoms *Pruritus* In angioedema of palms and soles pain. Angioedema of tongue, pharynx interferes with speech, food intake, and breathing. Angioedema of larynx may lead to asphyxia.

CLINICAL MANIFESTATION

Skin Lesions Sharply defined *wheals* (Fig. 14-6), small (<1 cm) to large (>8 cm), erythematous or white with an erythematous rim, round, oval, acriform, annular, serpiginous (Figs. 14-7 and 14-9), due to confluence and resolution in one area and progression in another (Fig. 14-7). Lesions are pruritic and transient.

Angioedema—skin-colored, transient enlargement of portion of face (eyelids, lips, tongue) (Figs. 14-8 and 22-7*A*, *B*), extremity, or other sites due to subcutaneous edema.

Distribution Usually regional or generalized. Localized in solar, pressure, vibration, cold urticaria/angioedema and confined to the site of the trigger mechanism (see below).

SPECIAL FEATURES/AS RELATED TO PATHOGENESIS

Immunologic Urticaria *IgE Mediated* Lesions in acute IgE-mediated urticaria result from antigen-induced release of biologically active molecules from mast cells or basophilic leukocytes sensitized with specific IgE antibodies (type I anaphylactic hypersensitivity). Released mediators increase venular permeability and modulate the release of biologically active molecules from other cell types. Often with atopic background. Antigens: food (milk, eggs, wheat, shellfish, nuts), therapeutic agents, drugs (penicillin) (see also "Drug-Induced Urticaria," Section 22), helminths. Most often acute (Figs. 14-8 and 22-6).

FIGURE 14-6   Urticaria   Wheals with white-to-light-pink color in the face in a close-up view. These are the classic lesions of urticaria. It is characteristic that they are transient and highly pruritic.

TABLE 14-1   Etiology and Classification of Urticaria/Angioedema

Immunologic	Urticaria due to mast cell–releasing agents, pseudoallergens, ACE inhibitors
IgE-mediated urticaria	Idiopathic urticaria
Complement-mediated urticaria	Nonimmune contact urticaria
Autoimmune urticaria	Urticaria associated with vascular/connective tissue autoimmune disease
Immune contact urticaria	Distinct angioedema (± urticaria) syndromes
Physical	Hereditary angioedema
Dermographism	Angioedema-urticaria-eosinophilia syndrome
Cold urticaria	
Solar urticaria	
Cholinergic urticaria	
Pressure angioedema	
Vibratory angioedema	

NOTE: ACE, angiotensin-converting enzyme.

FIGURE 14-7 **Acute urticaria** Small and large wheals with erythematous borders and a lighter color centrally. Well-defined. The lesion on the left upper arm is ill-defined at its lower border where it is regressing.

Complement Mediated By way of immune complexes activating complement and releasing anaphylatoxins that induce mast cell degranulation. Serum sickness, administration of whole blood, immunoglobulins. Acute.

Autoimmune Common, chronic. Autoantibodies against FcεRI and/or IgE. Positive autologous serum skin test. Clinically, patients with these autoantibodies (up to 40% of patients with chronic urticaria) are indistinguishable from those without them (Fig. 14-9). These autoantibodies may explain why plasmapheresis, intravenous immunoglobulins, and cyclosporine induce remission of disease activity in these patients.

Immunologic Contact Urticaria Usually in children with atopic dermatitis sensitized to environmental allergens (grass, animals) or individuals sensitized to wearing latex rubber gloves; can be accompanied by anaphylaxis.

Physical Urticarias ***Dermographism*** Linear urticarial lesions occur after stroking or scratching the skin; they itch and fade in 30 min (Fig. 14-10). 4.2% of the normal population have it; symptomatic dermographism is a nuisance.

Cold Urticaria Usually in children or young adults; urticarial lesions confined to sites exposed to cold occurring within minutes after rewarming. "Ice cube" test (application of an ice cube for a few minutes to skin) establishes diagnosis.

Solar Urticaria Urticaria after solar exposure. Action spectrum from 290–500 nm; whealing lasts for <1 h, may be accompanied by syncope; histamine is one of the mediators (see Section 10 and Fig. 10-10).

Cholinergic Urticaria Exercise to the point of sweating provokes typical small, papular, highly pruritic urticarial lesions (Fig. 14-11). May be accompanied by wheezing.

Aquagenic Urticaria Very rare. Contact with water of any temperature induces eruption similar to cholinergic urticaria.

Pressure Angioedema Erythematous swelling induced by sustained pressure (buttock swelling when seated, hand swelling after hammering, foot swelling after walking). Delayed (30 min to 12 h). Painful, may persist for several days, and interferes with quality of life. No laboratory abnormalities; fever may occur. Urticaria may occur in addition to angioedema.

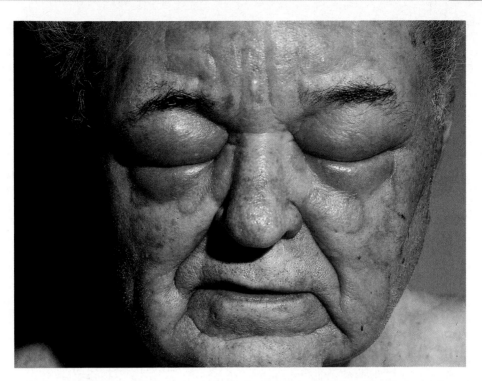

FIGURE 14-8 Acute urticaria and angioedema   Note that there are both superficial wheals and deep, diffuse edema. Occurred after the patient had eaten shellfish. He had similar episodes previously but never considered seafood as the cause.

FIGURE 14-9 Chronic urticaria   Chronic urticaria of 5-year duration in an otherwise healthy 35-year-old female. Eruptions occur on an almost daily basis and, as they are highly pruritic, greatly impair the patient's quality of life. Although suppressed by antihistamines, there is an immediate recurrence after treatment is stopped. Repeated laboratory and clinical examinations have not revealed an apparent cause.

Vibration Angioedema May be familial (autosomal dominant) or sporadic. Rare. It is believed to result from histamine release from mast cells caused by a "vibrating" stimulus—rubbing a towel across the back produces lesions, but direct pressure (without movements) does not.

Urticaria Due to Mast Cell–Releasing Agents and Pseudoallergens and Chronic Idiopathic Urticaria
Urticaria/angioedema and even anaphylaxis-like symptoms may occur with radiocontrast media and as a consequence of intolerance to salicylates, food preservatives and additives (e.g., benzoic acid and sodium benzoate), as well as several azo dyes, including tartrazine and sunset yellow (pseudoallergens) (Fig. 14-9); also to ACE inhibitors. May be acute and chronic. In chronic idiopathic urticaria, histamine derived from mast cells in the skin is considered the major mediator. Eicosanoids and neuropeptides may also play a part in producing the lesions.

Non-Immune Contact Urticaria Due to direct effects of exogenous urticants penetrating into skin or blood vessels. Localized to site of contact. Sorbic acid, benzoic acid in eye solutions and foods, cinnamic aldehydes in cosmetics, histamine, acetylcholine, serotonin in nettle stings.

Urticaria Associated with Vascular/Connective Tissue Autoimmune Disease Urticarial lesions may be associated with systemic lupus erythematosus (SLE) and Sjögren syndrome. However, in most instances they represent urticarial vasculitis (page 407). This is a form of cutaneous vasculitis associated with urticarial skin lesions that persist for >12 to 24 h. Slow changes in size and configuration, can be associated with purpura, and can show residual pigmentation due to hemosiderin after involution (see Fig. 14-41). Often associated with hypocomplementemia and renal disease.

Distinct Angioedema (± Urticaria) Syndromes
Hereditary Angioedema (HAE) A serious autosomal dominant disorder; may follow trauma (physical and emotional). Angioedema of the face (Fig. 14-12) and extremities, episodes of laryngeal edema, and acute abdominal pain caused by angioedema of the bowel wall presenting as surgical emergency. Urticaria rarely occurs. Laboratory abnormalities involve the complement system: decreased levels of C1-esterase inhibitor (85%) or dysfunctional inhibitor (15%), low C4 value in the presence of normal C1 and C3 levels. Angioedema results from bradykinin formation, since C1-esterase inhibitor is also the major inhibitor of the Hageman factor and kallikrein, the two enzymes

required for kinin formation. Episodes can be life threatening.

Angioedema-Urticaria-Eosinophilia Syndrome
Severe angioedema, only occasionally with pruritic urticaria, involving the face, neck, extremities, and trunk that lasts for 7–10 days. There is fever and marked increase in normal weight (increased by 10–18%) owing to fluid retention. No other organs are involved. Laboratory abnormalities include striking leukocytosis (20,000–70,000/µL) and eosinophilia (60–80% eosinophils), which are related to the severity of attack. There is no family history. This condition is rare, prognosis is good.

LABORATORY EXAMINATIONS

Dermatopathology Edema of the dermis or subcutaneous tissue, dilatation of venules but no evidence of vascular damage. Mast cell degranulation. The predominant perivascular inflammatory cell types are activated lymphocytes of the T helper phenotype.

Serology Search for hepatitis B-associated antigen, assessment of the complement system, assessment of specific IgE antibodies by radioallergosorbent test (RAST), anti-FcεRI autoantibodies. Serology for lupus and Sjögren syndrome. Autologous serum skin test for autoimmune urticaria.

Hematology The erythrocyte sedimentation rate (ESR) is often elevated in urticarial vasculitis, and there may be hypocomplementemia; transient eosinophilia in urticaria from reactions to foods, parasites, and drugs; high levels of eosinophilia in the angioedema-urticaria-eosinophilia syndrome.

Complement Studies Screening for functional C1 inhibitor in HAE.

Ultrasonography For early diagnosis of bowel involvement in HAE; if abdominal pain is present, this may indicate edema of the bowel.

Parasitology Stool specimen for presence of parasites.

DIAGNOSIS

A detailed history (previous diseases, drugs, foods, parasites, physical exertion, solar exposure) is of utmost importance. History should differentiate between *type of lesions*—urticaria, angioedema, or urticaria + angioedema; *duration of lesions* (<1 h or ≥1 h), *pruritus; pain* on walking (in foot involvement), *flushing, burning,* and *wheezing* (in cholinergic urticaria). *Fever* in serum sickness and in the

FIGURE 14-10   Urticaria: dermographism   Urticaria as it appeared 5 min after the patient was scratched on the back. The patient had experienced generalized pruritus for several months with no spontaneously occurring urticaria.

FIGURE 14-11   Cholinergic urticaria   Small urticarial papules on neck occurring within 30 min of vigorous exercise. Papular urticarial lesions are best seen under side lighting.

angioedema-urticaria-eosinophilia syndrome; in angioedema, *hoarseness, stridor, dyspnea. Arthralgia* (serum sickness, urticarial vasculitis), *abdominal colicky pain* in HAE. A careful history of medications including penicillin, aspirin, nonsteroidal anti-inflammatory drugs, and ACE inhibitors should be obtained. Autoimmune urticaria is tested by the autologous serum skin test and determination of anti-FcεRI antibody.

Dermographism is evoked by stroking the skin; pressure urticaria is tested by application of pressure (weight) perpendicular to the skin;

vibration angioedema by a vibratory stimulus, like rubbing the back with a towel. If *physical urticaria* is suspected, appropriate challenge testing should be performed. *Cholinergic urticaria* can best be diagnosed by exercise to sweating and intracutaneous injection of acetylcholine or mecholyl, which will produce micropapular whealing. *Solar urticaria* is verified by testing with UVB, UVA, and visible light. *Cold urticaria* is verified by a wheal response to the application to the skin of an ice cube or a test tube containing ice water. If urticarial wheals do not disappear in ≤24 h, urticarial vasculitis should be suspected

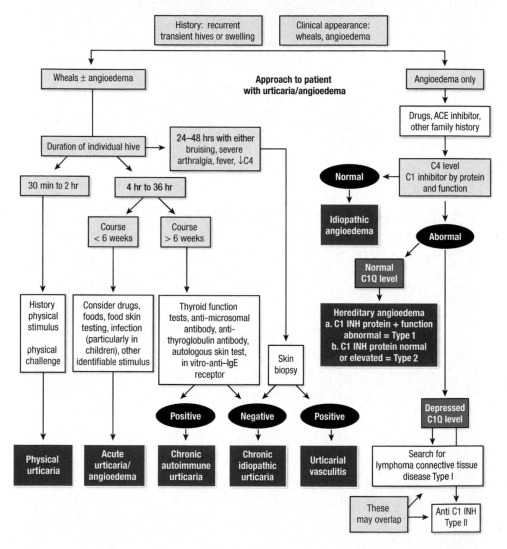

IMAGE 14-1   Approach to the patient with urticaria/angioedema. ACE angiotensin-converting enzyme; IgE, immunoglobulin E; INH, inhibitor; ↓, decreased. SOURCE: From AP Kaplan, in K Wolff et al (eds): *Fitzpatrick's Dermatology in General Medicine,* 7th ed. New York, McGraw-Hill, 2008, p 339.

A

B

FIGURE 14-12   Hereditary angioedema   A. Severe edema of the face during an episode leading to grotesque disfigurement. **B.** Angioedema will subside within hours. These are the normal features of the patient. The patient had a positive family history and had multiple similar episodes including colicky abdominal pain.

and a biopsy done. The person with *angioedema-urticaria-eosinophilia syndrome* has high fever, high leukocytosis (mostly eosinophils), a striking increase in body weight due to retention of water, and a cyclic pattern that may occur and recur over a period of years. *Hereditary angioedema* has a positive family history and is characterized by angioedema of the face and extremities as the result of trauma, abdominal pain, and decreased levels of C4 and C1-esterase inhibitor.

A practical approach to the diagnosis of urticaria/angioedema is shown in Image 14-1.

COURSE AND PROGNOSIS

Half the patients with urticaria alone are free of lesions in 1 year, but 20% have lesions for >20 years. Prognosis is good in most syndromes except HAE, which may be fatal if untreated.

MANAGEMENT

Prevention   Try to prevent attacks by elimination of etiologic chemicals or drugs: aspirin and food additives, especially in chronic recurrent urticaria—rarely successful; prevent trigger in physical urticarias.

Antihistamines H_1 blockers, e.g., hydroxyzine, terfenadine; or loratadine, cetirizine, fexofenadine. 180 mg/d of fexofenadine or 10–20 mg/d of loratadine usually controls most cases of chronic urticaria, but cessation of therapy usually results in a recurrence; if they fail, H_1 and H_2 blockers (cimetidine) and/or mast cell–stabilizing agents (ketotifen). Doxepin, a tricyclic antidepressant with marked H_1 antihistaminic activity, is valuable when severe urticaria is associated with anxiety and depression.

Prednisone   In *acute* urticaria with angioedema; also for angioedema-urticaria-eosinophilia syndrome.

Danazol or Stanozolol   Long-term therapy for hereditary angioedema; watch out for hirsutism, irregular menses; whole fresh plasma or C1-esterase inhibitor in the acute attack. A very effective bradikin-B_2-receptor antagonist for subcutaneous application is now available in Europe (Icatibant).

Other   In *chronic idiopathic* or *autoimmune* urticaria, if no response to antihistamines: switch to cyclosporine and taper gradually, if glucocorticoids are contraindicated or if side effects occur.

BEHÇET DISEASE   ICD-9 : 179.4 ○ ICD-10 : M35.2   ◧ ◑ → ●

- Rare; worldwide occurrence, but strongly variable ethnic prevalence.
- It is a perplexing multisystem vasculitic disease with multiorgan involvement.
- Main symptoms are recurrent oral aphthous ulcers, genital ulcers, erythema nodosum, superficial thrombophlebitis, skin pustules, iridocyclitis, and posterior uveitis.

- Additional symptoms may be arthritis, epididimitis, ileocecal ulcerations, vascular and central nervous system (CNS) lesions.
- Chronic relapsing progressive course with potentially poor prognosis.

EPIDEMIOLOGY

Age of Onset   Third and fourth decades.
Prevalence   Highest in Turkey (80–420 patients in 100,000), Japan, Southeast Asia, the Middle East, southern Europe. Rare in northern Europe, United States (0.12–0.33 in 100,000).
Sex   Males > females, but dependent on ethnic background.

PATHOGENESIS

Etiology unknown. In the eastern Mediterranean and East Asia, HLA-B5 and HLA-B51 association; in the United States and Europe, no consistent HLA association. The lesions are the result of leukocytoclastic (acute) and lymphocytic (late) vasculitis.

CLINICAL MANIFESTATION

Painful ulcers erupt in a cyclic fashion in the oral cavity and/or genital mucous membranes. Orodynophagia and oral ulcers may persist/recur weeks to months before other symptoms appear.
Skin and Mucous Membranes   *Aphthous Ulcers* Punched-out ulcers (3 to >10 mm) with rolled or overhanging borders and necrotic base (Fig. 14-13); red rim; occur in crops (2–10) on oral mucous membrane (100%) (Fig. 14-13; see also Fig. 34-xx), vulva, penis, and scrotum (Figs. 14-14, 14-15, 35-15); very painful.
Erythema Nodosum-Like Lesions   Painful inflammatory nodules on the arms and legs (40%) (see Section 7 and Fig. 7-23).
Other   Inflammatory pustules, superficial thrombophlebitis (see Fig. 16-6A), *inflammatory plaques* resembling those in Sweet syndrome

(acute febrile neutrophilic dermatosis) (see Fig. 7-30), *pyoderma gangrenosum-like lesions* (see Fig. 7-26), *palpable purpuric lesions* of necrotizing vasculitis (see Fig. 14-34).
Systemic Findings   *Eyes* Leading cause of morbidity. Posterior uveitis, anterior uveitis, retinal vasculitis, vitreitis, hypopyon, secondary cataracts, glaucoma, neovascular lesions.
Musculoskeletal   Nonerosive, asymmetric oligoarthritis.
Neurologic   Onset delayed, occurring in one quarter of patients. Meningoencephalitis, benign intracranial hypertension, cranial nerve palsies, brainstem lesions, pyramidal/extrapyramidal lesions, psychosis.
Vascular   Aneurysms, arterial occlusions, venous thrombosis, varices; hemoptysis. Coronary vasculitis: myocarditis, coronary arteritis, endocarditis, valvular disease.
GI Tract   Aphthous ulcers throughout.

LABORATORY EXAMINATIONS

Dermatopathology   Leukocytoclastic vasculitis with fibrinoid necrosis of blood vessel walls in acute early lesions; lymphocytic vasculitis in late lesions.
Pathergy Test   Positive pathergy test read by physician at 24 or 48 h, after skin puncture with a sterile needle. Leads to inflammatory pustule.
HLA Typing   Significant association with HLA-B5 and HLA-B51, in Japanese, Koreans, and Turks, and in the Middle East.

DIAGNOSIS AND DIFFERENTIAL DIAGNOSIS

Diagnosis is made according to the Revised International Criteria for Behçet disease (Image 14-2).

A   *B*

FIGURE 14-13   Behçet disease   Oral aphthous ulcers. **A.** These are highly painful, punched-out ulcers with a necrotic base on the buccal mucosa and lower and upper fornix in this 28-year-old Turkish male. **B.** A punched-out ulcer on the tongue of another patient.

FIGURE 14-14   Behçet disease: genital ulcers   Multiple large aphthous-type ulcers on the labial and perineal skin. In addition, this 25-year-old patient of Turkish extraction had aphthous ulcers in the mouth and previously experienced an episode of uveitis.

Differential Diagnosis   *Oral and genital ulcers*: Viral infection [herpes simplex virus (HSV), varicella-zoster virus (VZV)], hand-foot-and-mouth disease, herpangina, chancre, histoplasmosis, squamous cell carcinoma.

COURSE AND PROGNOSIS

Highly variable course, with recurrences and remissions; the mouth lesions are always present; remissions may last for weeks, months, or years. In the eastern Mediterranean and East Asia, severe course, one of the leading causes of blindness. With CNS involvement, there is a higher mortality rate.

MANAGEMENT

Aphthous Ulcers   Potent topical glucocorticoids. Intralesional triamcinolone, 3–10 mg/mL, injected into ulcer base. Thalidomide, 50–100 mg PO in the evening. Colchicine, 0.6 mg PO 2 to 3 times a day. Dapsone, 50–100 mg/d PO.

Systemic Involvement   Prednisone with or without azathioprine, cyclophosphamide, azathioprine alone, chlorambucil, cyclosporine.

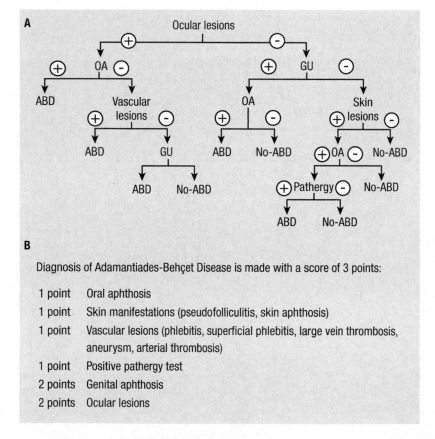

IMAGE 14-2   Revised International Criteria for Behçet Disease (International Team for the Revision of ICBD; coordinator: F. Davatchi) according to (**A**) the classification tree format, and (**B**) the traditional format ABD, Adamantiades-Behçet disease; GU, genital ulcer; OA, oral aphthous ulcer. SOURCE: CC Zouboulis: Adamantiades Behçet disease, in K Wolff et al (eds): *Fitzpatrick's Dermatology in General Medicine,* 7th ed. New York, McGraw-Hill, 2008, pp 1620–1622.

FIGURE 14-15 **Behçet disease** A large, punched-out ulcer on the scrotum of a 40-year-old Korean. The patient also had aphthous ulcers in the mouth and pustules on the thighs and buttocks.

DERMATOMYOSITIS   ICD-9 : 710.3 ∘ ICD-10 : M33.0   □ ●

- Dermatomyositis (DM) is a systemic disease belonging to the idiopathic inflammatory myopathies, a heterogeneous group of genetically determined autoimmune diseases targeting the skin and/or skeletal muscles.
- DM is characterized by violaceous (heliotrope) inflammatory changes +/− edema of the eyelids and periorbital area; erythema of the face, neck, and upper trunk; and flat-topped violaceous papules over the knuckles.

- It is associated with polymyositis, interstitial pneumonitis, and myocardial involvement.
- DM without myopathy (amyopathic DM) and polymyositis without skin involvement.
- Juvenile DM runs a different course and is associated with vasculitis and calcinosis.
- Adult-onset DM may be associated with internal malignancy.
- Prognosis is guarded.

EPIDEMIOLOGY AND ETIOLOGY

Rare. Incidence >6 cases per million, but this is based on hospitalized patients and does not include individuals without muscle involvement. Juvenile and adult (>40 years) onset.
Etiology   Unknown. In persons >55 years of age, may be associated with malignancy.
Clinical Spectrum   Ranges from DM with only cutaneous inflammation (amyopathic DM) to polymyositis with only muscle inflammation. Cutaneous involvement occurs in 30–40% of adults and 95% of children with dermatomyositis/polymyositis. For classification, see Table 14-2.

CLINICAL MANIFESTATION

± Photosensitivity. Manifestations in skin disease may precede myositis or vice versa; often, both are detected at the same time. Muscle weakness, difficulty in rising from supine position, climbing stairs, raising arms over head, turning in bed. Dysphagia; burning and pruritus of the scalp.
Skin Lesions   Periorbital heliotrope (reddish purple) flush, usually associated with some degree of edema (Fig. 14-16). May extend to involve scalp (+ nonscarring alopecia), entire face (Fig. 14-17A), upper chest, and arms.

In addition, papular dermatitis with varying degrees of violaceous erythema in the same sites. Flat-topped, violaceous papules (Gottron papule/sign) with various degrees of atrophy on the nape of the neck and shoulders and over the knuckles and interphalangeal joints (Fig. 14-17B). *Note*: In lupus, lesions usually occur in the interarticular region of the fingers (see Fig. 14-21A). Periungual erythema with

tel-angiectasia, thrombosis of capillary loops, infarctions. Lesions over elbows and knuckles may evolve into erosions and ulcers that heal with stellate scarring (particularly in juvenile DM with vasculitis). Long-lasting lesions may evolve into poikiloderma (mottled discoloration with red, white, and brown) (Fig. 14-18). Calcification in subcutaneous/fascial tissues common later in course of juvenile DM, particularly about elbows, trochanteric, and iliac region (calcinosis cutis); may evolve into calcinosis universalis. 🖉
Muscle   ± Muscle tenderness, ±muscle atrophy. Progressive muscle weakness affecting proximal/limb girdle muscles. Difficulty or inability to rise from sitting or supine position without using arms. Difficulty in raising arms above head and difficulty in climbing stairs. Intercostal muscles: difficulty in breathing.

Occasional involvement of facial/bulbar, pharyngeal, and esophageal muscles. Deep tendon reflexes within normal limits.
Other Organs   Interstitial pneumonitis, cardiomyopathy, arthritis, particularly in juvenile DM (20–65%).
Disease Association   Patients >50 years of age with DM have a higher than expected risk for malignancy, particularly ovarian cancer in females. Also carcinoma of the ovary, breast, bronchopulmonary, and GI tract. Most cancers detected within 2 years of diagnosis.

LABORATORY EXAMINATIONS

Chemistry   During acute active phase: elevation of creatine phosphokinase (65%), which is most specific for muscle disease; also, of aldolase (40%), lactate dehydrogenase, glutamic oxaloacetic transaminase.

FIGURE 14-16   Dermatomyositis   Heliotrope (reddish purple) erythema of upper eyelids and edema of the lower lids. This 55-year-old female had experienced severe muscle weakness of the shoulder girdle and presented with a lump in the breast that proved to be carcinoma.

TABLE 14-2   Comprehensive Classification of Idiopathic Inflammatory Dermatomyopathies

Dermatomyositis (DM)

- Adult onset
  - Classic DM: alone; with malignancy; as part of an overlap connective tissue disorder
  - Clinically amyopathic DM: amyopathic DM: hypomyopathic DM
- Juvenile onset
  - Classic DM
  - Clinically amyopathic DM: amyopathic DM; hypomyopathic DM

Polymyositis (PM)

- PM alone
- PM as part of an overlap connective tissue disorder
- PM associated with internal malignancy[a]

Inclusion Body Myositis
Other Clinical-Pathologic Subgroups of Myositis

- Focal myositis
- Proliferative myositis
- Orbital myositis
- Eosinophilic myositis
- Granulomatous myositis

[a] Although population-based European studies have now clearly confirmed that adult-onset classic DM is associated with a significant risk for internal malignancy, if such a relationship exists for PM, it is much weaker.

Autoantibodies   Autoantibodies to 155 kDa and/or Se in 80% to 140 kDa in 58% and to Jo-1 in 20% (both have a high specificity for DM) and to (low specificity) antinuclear antibodies (ANA, nuclear and speckled pattern) in 40%.

Urine   Elevated 24-h creatine excretion (>200 mg/24 h). Note: can also be elevated in glucocorticoid myopathy.

Electromyography   Increased irritability on insertion of electrodes, spontaneous fibrillations, pseudomyotonic discharges, positive sharp waves: excludes neuromyopathy. With evidence of denervation, suspect coexisting tumor.

MRI   MRI of muscles reveals focal lesions.

ECG   Evidence of myocarditis; atrial, ventricular irritability; atrioventricular block.

X-Ray   *Chest*: ± interstitial fibrosis. *Esophagus*: reduced peristalsis.

Pathology   *Skin*   Flattening of epidermis, hydropic degeneration of basal cell layer, edema of upper dermis, scattered inflammatory infiltrate, PAS-positive fibrinoid deposits at dermal-epidermal junction and around upper dermal capillaries, accumulation of acid mucopolysaccharides in dermis (all these are compatible with DM but are not diagnostic).

Muscle   Biopsy shoulder/pelvic girdle; one that is weak or tender, i.e., deltoid, supraspinatus, gluteus, quadriceps after marking by EMG or

A

B

FIGURE 14-17   Dermatomyositis   A. Violaceous erythema and edema on the face, particularly in the periorbital and malar regions. The patient could barely lift his arms and could not climb stairs. He had pulmonary carcinoma. **B.** Violaceous erythema and Gottron papules on the dorsa of the hands and fingers, especially over the metacarpopha-langeal and interphalangeal joints; the light-protected areas of the forearms of this 28-year-old male with severe muscle weakness were not involved. Periungual erythema and telangiectasis. This patient later developed severe calcinosis cutis.

FIGURE 14-18 Dermatomyositis, juvenile onset, poikiloderma There is mottled, reticular brownish pigmentation and telangiectasia plus small white scars. Note striae on trochanteric areas due to systemic glucocorticoid therapy.

MRI. Histology—segmental necrosis within muscle fibers with loss of cross-striations; waxy/coagulative type of eosinophilic staining; with or without regenerating fibers; inflammatory cells, histiocytes, macrophages, lymphocytes, plasma cells. Vasculitis is seen in juvenile DM. MRI-guided needle biopsy of muscle may replace conventional muscle biopsy in the future.

DIAGNOSIS AND DIFFERENTIAL DIAGNOSIS

Skin signs plus proximal muscle weakness with two of three laboratory criteria, i.e., elevated serum "muscle enzyme" levels, characteristic electromyographic changes, diagnostic muscle biopsy. Differential diagnosis is to seborrheic dermatitis, lupus erythematosus, mixed connective tissue disease, steroid myopathy, trichinosis, toxoplasmosis.

COURSE AND PROGNOSIS

Prognosis guarded but with treatment, it is relatively good except in patients with malignancy and those with pulmonary involvement.

With aggressive immunosuppressive treatment the 8-year survival rate is 70–80%. A better prognosis is seen in individuals who receive early systemic treatment. The early and aggressive use of glucocorticoids has reduced the mortality rates in children to <10%. The most common causes of death are malignancy, infection, cardiac and pulmonary disease. Successful treatment of an associated neoplasm is often followed by improvement/resolution of DM.

MANAGEMENT

Prednisone 0.5–1 mg/kg body weight per day, increasing to 1.5 mg/kg if lower dose ineffective. Taper when "muscle enzyme" levels approach normal. Best if combined with azathioprine, 2–3 mg/kg per day. *Note*: Steroid myopathy may occur after 4–6 weeks of therapy.
Alternatives Methotrexate, cyclophosphamide, cyclosporine, anti-tumor necrosis factor (TNF) α agents. High-dose IV immunoglobulin bolus therapy (2 g/kg body weight given over 2 days) at monthly intervals spares glucocorticoid doses to achieve or maintain remissions.

LIVEDO RETICULARIS   ICD-9 : 446.20 ∘ ICD-10 : L 95.0   □→■ ○→●

- Livedo reticularis (LR) is a mottled bluish (livid) discoloration of the skin that occurs in a netlike pattern. It is not a diagnosis in itself but a reaction pattern.
- Classification distinguishes between
  - *Idiopathic livedo reticularis* (ILR): a purple/livid discoloration of the skin in a netlike pattern disappearing after warming. A physiologic phenomenon. (*Synonym*: cutis marmorata.)

- *Secondary (symptomatic) livedo reticularis* (SLR): a purple discoloration occurring in a starburst or lightning-like pattern, netlike but with open (not annular) meshes; mostly, but not always, confined to the lower extremities and buttocks. A reaction pattern often indicative of serious systemic disease (Table 14-3). (*Synonym*: livedo racemosa.)

ETIOLOGY

ILR   A physiologic phenomenon.
SLR   That of associated disorder; following amantadine treatment for Parkinson disease.

PATHOGENESIS

ILR pattern due to vasospasm or obstruction of perpendicular arterioles, perforating dermis from below. Cyanotic periphery of each web of net caused by deoxygenated blood in surrounding horizontally arranged venous plexuses. When factors such as cold cause increased viscosity or flow rates in superficial venous plexus, further deoxygenation occurs and cyanotic reticular pattern becomes more pronounced. Elevation of limb decreases intensity of color due to increased venous drainage. SLR results from arteriolar disease causing obstruction to inflow and blood hyperviscosity or from obstruction to outflow of blood in venules.

CLINICAL MANIFESTATION

Appearance or worsening with cold exposure. ± Numbness, tingling associated. Worse during winter months.
Skin Lesions   *ILR*   A purple/livid discoloration of skin in netlike pattern (mesh diameter 3 cm) involving large areas of lower or upper extremities and trunk and disappearing after warming.
SLR   Blotchy, arborizing, lightning-like, starburst, or mottled pattern of cyanosis (Fig. 14-19). Netlike webs are open (semicircular), and within webs, skin is normal to pallid and

feels cool. Symmetric, arms/legs, buttocks; less commonly, body. On exposure to cold, livedo becomes more pronounced but never fades completely on warming. It never ulcerates. *Note*: When associated with *livedoid vasculitis* (see p. 475), ulceration about ankles and forefeet may occur.
General Examination   Symptoms of underlying disease in SLR (Table 14-3).

LABORATORY EXAMINATIONS

Laboratory   Varies with associated disorders.
Dermatopathology   Vascular pathology of underlying disease.

DIAGNOSIS AND DIFFERENTIAL DIAGNOSIS

Clinical diagnosis confirmed by laboratory data supporting diagnosis of associated disorder.
Differential Diagnosis   Cutis marmorata, ILR versus SLR, livedoid vasculitis (see page 475), erythema ab igne.

COURSE AND PROGNOSIS

Course/prognosis of SLR depends on that of associated disorder.

MANAGEMENT

- Keep from chilling. Pentoxifylline (400 mg PO three times a day), low-dose aspirin, and heparin may be helpful.
- Treat associated disorder.

FIGURE 14-19 Symptomatic livedo reticularis A netlike, arborizing pattern on the posterior thighs and buttocks defined by violaceous, erythematous streaks resembling lightning. The skin within the erythematous areas is normally pale. This occurred in a patient with labile hypertension and multiple cerebrovascular attacks and was thus pathognomonic for Sneddon syndrome.

TABLE 14-3 Disorders Associated with Symptomatic Livedo Reticularis

Vascular Obstruction	Viscosity Changes	Drugs
Atheroemboli	Thrombocythemia	Amantadine
Arteriosclerosis	Polyglobulinemia	Quinine
Polyarteritis nodosa	Cryoglobulinemia	Quinidine
Cutaneous polyarteritis nodosa	Cold agglutinemia	
Rheumatoid vasculitis	Disseminated intravascular	
Livedoid vasculitis	coagulation	
Sneddon syndrome	Lupus erythematosus	
	Anticardiolipin syndrome	
	Leukemia/lymphoma	

SNEDDON SYNDROME

- A potentially life-threatening disease of unknown etiology occurring more often in females than males and manifesting mainly in skin as SLR and in the CNS.

- Associated with transient ischemic attacks and cerebrovascular insult.

EPIDEMIOLOGY

Rare but underdiagnosed.

CLINICAL MANIFESTATION

Skin lesions precede neurologic symptoms, often by years.

Skin Lesions These represent classic SLR on lower extremities, buttocks, sometimes arms (Fig. 14-19). ± Angiomatosis (mottled-purple discoloration of the face and other parts of the body).

Note: Sneddon syndrome is not identical with antiphospholipid syndrome, although dermatologic manifestations (SLR) may be indistinguishable. May be associated with livedoid vasculitis—in this case, ulceration may occur around ankles or acrally (see page 475).

Neurologic Symptoms Include headaches, labile hypertension, transient ischemic attacks, transient amnesia, transient aphasia, palsy, and cerebrovascular insult.

LABORATORY EXAMINATION

Dermatopathology Endothelitis → proliferation of subendothelial myofibroblasts → vascular occlusion and fibrosis. Cytotoxic anti-endothelial cell antibodies in a small percentage of patients. There may be antiphospholipid antibodies.

MANAGEMENT

Longtime low-dose heparin, aspirin.

LUPUS ERYTHEMATOSUS (LE) ICD-9 : 695.4 ○ ICD-10 : L93

- LE is the designation of a spectrum of disease patterns that are linked by distinct clinical findings and distinct patterns of cellular and humoral autoimmunity.

- LE occurs more commonly in women (male to female ratio 1 : 9).

- LE ranges from life-threatening manifestations of acute systemic LE (SLE) to the limited and exclusive skin involvement in chronic cutaneous LE (CCLE) (Image 14-3). More than 85% of patients

  with LE have skin lesions, which can be classified into LE-specific and -nonspecific.

- An abbreviated version of Gilliam classification of LE-specific skin lesions is given in Table 14-4.

- Acute cutaneous LE (ACLE) is practically always associated with SLE, subacute cutaneous LE (SCLE) in about 50%, and chronic cutaneous LE (CCLE) most often has only skin disease. However, CCLE lesions can occur in SLE.

- ACLE and SCLE are highly photosensitive.

TABLE 14-4   Abbreviated Gilliam Classification of Skin Lesions of LE

I. LE-specific skin disease [cutaneous LE* (CLE)]

   A. Acute cutaneous LE [ACLE]

      1. Localized ACLE (malar rash; butterfly rash)

      2. Generalized ACLE (maculopapular lupus rash, malar rash, photosensitive lupus dermatitis)

   B. Subacute cutaneous LE [SCLE]

      1. Annular SCLE

      2. Papulosquamous SCLE (disseminated DLE, subacute disseminated LE, maculopapular photosensitive LE)

   C. Chronic cutaneous LE [CCLE]

      1. Classic discoid LE [DLE]: (a) localized DLE; (b) generalized DLE

      2. Hypertrophic/verrucous DLE

      3. Lupus profundus

      4. Mucosal DLE: (a) oral DLE; (b) conjunctival DLE

      5. Lupus tumidus (urticarial plaque of LE)

      6. Chilblains LE (chilblains lupus)

      7. Lichenoid DLE (LE/lichen planus overlap)

II. LE-nonspecific skin disease

   These range from necrotizing and urticarial vasculitis to livedo reticularis, Raynaud phenomenon, dermal mucinosis, and bullous lesions in LE.

*Alternative or synonymous terms are listed in parentheses; abbreviations are indicated in brackets.

SOURCE: Reprinted and modified from RD Sontheimer with permission from Stockton Journals, Macmillan Press, Ltd.

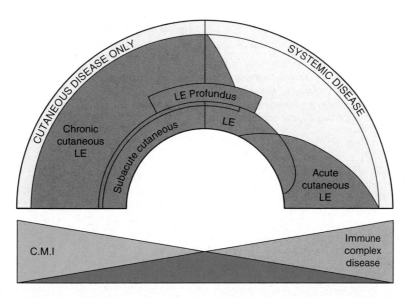

IMAGE 14-3   The spectrum of lupus erythematosus, as envisaged by the late Dr. James N. Gilliam. The left comprises conditions that define cutaneous disease only and it can be seen that chronic cutaneous lupus extends into the systemic disease section. This is also true for lupus profundus (lupus panniculitis) and subacute cutaneous lupus, whereas acute cutaneous lupus is characteristic for systemic disease only. The bottom shows that immune complex disease dominates systemic disease and cell-mediated immunity (CMI) is predominant in the cutaneous disease manifestations.

- This serious multisystem autoimmune disease is based on polyclonal B cell immunity, which involves connective tissue and blood vessels.
- More common in persons with black African heritage; male to female ratio 1:9.
- The clinical manifestations include fever (90%); skin lesions (85%); arthritis; CNS, renal, cardiac, and pulmonary disease.

- Skin lesions are those of ACLE and SCLE; not uncommonly of CCLE.
- SLE may uncommonly develop in patients with CCLE; on the other hand, lesions of CCLE are common in SLE (Image 14-3).

EPIDEMIOLOGY

Prevalence Ranges from 40 cases/100,000 Northern Europeans to more than 200/100,000 among blacks.
Age of Onset 30 (females), 40 (males).
Sex Male:female ratio 1:9.
Race More common in blacks.
Precipitating Factors Family history (<5%); sunlight (UVR) is the most effective precipitating factor. An SLE syndrome can be induced by drugs (hydralazine, certain anticonvulsants, and procainamide), but rash is a relatively uncommon feature of drug-induced SLE.

CLINICAL MANIFESTATION

Lesions present for weeks (acute), months (chronic). Sunlight may cause an exacerbation of SLE (36%). Pruritus, burning of skin lesions. Fatigue (100%), fever (100%), weight loss, and malaise. Arthralgia or arthritis, abdominal pain, CNS symptoms.
Skin Lesions Comprise ACLE lesions (Table 14-4) in the acute phases of the disease and SCLE and CCLE lesions. Whereas ACLE lesions occur only in acute or subacute SLE, SCLE and CCLE lesions are present in subacute and chronic SLE but may also occur in acute SLE. ACLE lesions are typically precipitated by sunlight.
ACLE *Butterfly Rash* Erythematous, confluent, macular butterfly eruption on the face (Fig. 14-20), sharply defined with fine scaling; erosions (acute flares) and crusts.
Generalized Erythematous, discrete, papular or urticarial lesions on the face, on the dorsa of hands (Fig. 14-21A), arms, and V of the neck.
Others *Bullae*, often hemorrhagic (acute flares). *Papules* and *scaly plaques* as in SCLE (Fig. 14-22) and *discoid plaques* as in CCLE (Fig. 14-23), predominantly on the face and

on the arms and scalp. Erythematous, sometimes violaceous, slightly scaling, densely set and *confluent papules* on the dorsa of the finger, usually with sparing of the articular regions (Fig. 14-21A). Note difference to dermatomyositis (Fig. 14-17B). *Palmar erythema*, mostly on fingertips (Fig. 14-21B), *nailfold telangiectasias*, microthrombi, erythema, edema of the periungual skin, (see Fig. 33-26). "Palpable" purpura (vasculitis), lower extremities (see Fig. 14-34). *Urticarial lesions* with purpura (urticarial vasculitis) (see Fig. 14-41).
Hair Diffuse alopecia or discoid lesions associated with patchy alopecia.
Mucous Membranes Ulcers arising in purpuric necrotic lesions on palate (80%), buccal mucosa, or gums (see Fig. 34-12).
Sites of Predilection Localized or generalized, preferentially in light-exposed sites. Face (80%); scalp (Fig. 32-17) (discoid lesions); presternal, shoulders; dorsa of the forearms, hands, fingers, fingertips (Fig. 33-31) (Image 14-4). ⌭
Extracutaneous Multisystem Involvement Arthralgia or arthritis (80%), renal disease (50%), pericarditis (20%), pneumonitis (20%), gastrointestinal (due to arteritis and sterile peritonitis), hepatomegaly (30%), myopathy (30%), splenomegaly (20%), lymphadenopathy (50%), peripheral neuropathy (14%), CNS disease (10%), seizures or organic brain disease (14%).

LABORATORY EXAMINATIONS

Pathology *Skin* Atrophy of epidermis, liquefaction degeneration of the dermal-epidermal junction, edema of the dermis, dermal lymphocytic infiltrate, and fibrinoid degeneration of the connective tissue and walls of the blood vessels.

FIGURE 14-20 **Acute systemic lupus erythematosus** Bright red, sharply defined erythema with slight edema and minimal scaling in a "butterfly pattern" on the face. This is the typical "malar rash." Note also that the patient is female and young.

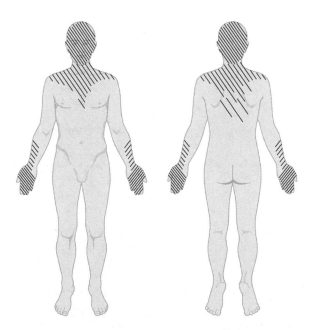

IMAGE 14-4 Predilection sites of cutaneous lupus erythematosus.

Immunofluorescence of Skin The lupus band test (LBT, direct immunofluorescence demonstrating IgG, IgM, C3) shows granular or globular deposits of immune reactants in a bandlike pattern along the dermal-epidermal junction. Positive in lesional skin in 90% and in the clinically normal skin (sun-exposed, 70–80%; non-sun-exposed, 50%).

Serology ANA positive (>95%); peripheral pattern of nuclear fluorescence. Anti-double-strand DNA antibodies, anti-Sm antibodies, and rRNP antibodies specific for SLE; low levels of complement (especially with renal involvement). Anticardiolipin autoantibodies (lupus anticoagulant) in a specific subset (anticardiolipin syndrome); SS-A(Ro) autoantibodies have a low specificity for SLE but are specific in the subset of SCLE (see below) (Table 14-5).

Hematology Anemia [normocytic, normochromic, or rarely, hemolytic Coombs-positive, leukopenia (>4000/µL)], lymphopenia, thrombocytopenia, elevated ESR.

Urinalysis Persistent proteinuria, casts.

DIAGNOSIS

Made on the basis of clinical findings, histopathology, lupus band test, and serology within the framework of the revised American Rheumatism Association (ARA) criteria for classification of SLE (Table 14-6).

PROGNOSIS

Five-year survival is 93%.

MANAGEMENT

General Measures Rest, avoidance of sun exposure.

Indications for Prednisone (60 mg/d in divided doses): (1) CNS involvement, (2) renal involvement, (3) severely ill patients without CNS involvement, (4) hemolytic crisis, (5) thrombocytopenia.

Concomitant Immunosuppressive Drugs Azathioprine, mycophenolate mofetil, methotrexate, cyclophosphamide, depending on organ involvement and activity of disease. In renal disease, cyclophosphamide IV bolus therapy.

Antimalarials Hydroxychloroquine is useful for treatment of the skin lesions in subacute and chronic SLE but does not reduce the need for prednisone. Observe precautions in the use of hydroxychloroquine. Alternative: chloroquine, quinacrine.

Investigational Ant-TNF agents; efalizumab, rituximab, leflunomide, anti-interferon α agents.

CUTANEOUS LUPUS ERYTHEMATOSUS

ACUTE CUTANEOUS LE

For skin lesions and systemic manifestations see "Systemic Lupus Erythematosus," above.

TABLE 14-5   Pathogenic Autoantibodies in Systemic Lupus Erythematosus

Antigen Specificity	Prevalence, %	Main Clinical Effects
Anti-double-strand DNA	70–80	Kidney disease, skin disease
Nucleosomes	60–90	Kidney disease, skin disease
Ro	30–40	Skin disease, kidney disease, fetal heart problems
La	15–20	Fetal heart problems
Sm	10–30	Kidney disease
NMDA receptor	33–50	Brain disease
Phospholipids	20–30	Thrombosis, pregnancy loss
α-Actinin	20	Kidney disease
C1q	40–50	Kidney disease

NOTE: NMDA, *N*-methyl-D-aspartate.
SOURCE: Abbreviated from A Rahman, DA Isenberg: N Engl J Med 358:929, 2008.

A

B

FIGURE 14-21   Acute SLE   *A.* Red-to-violaceous, well-demarcated papules and plaques on the dorsa of the fingers and hands, characteristically sparing the skin overlying the joints. This is an important differential diagnostic sign when considering dermatomyositis, which characteristically involves the skin over the joints (compare with Fig. 14-17*B*). ***B.*** Palmar erythema mainly on the fingertips. This is pathognomonic.

TABLE 14-6   1982 Revised ARA Criteria for Classification of Systemic Lupus Erythematosus[*]

Criterion	Definition
1. Malar rash	Fixed erythema, flat or raised, over the malar eminences, tending to spare the nasolabial folds.
2. Discoid rash	Erythematous raised patches with adherent keratotic scaling and follicular plugging; atrophic scarring may occur in older lesions.
3. Photosensitivity	Skin rashes as a result of unusual reaction to sunlight, by patient history or physician observation.
4. Oral ulcers	Oral or nasopharyngeal ulceration, usually painless, observed by a physician.
5. Arthritis	Nonerosive arthritis involving two or more peripheral joints, characterized by tenderness, swelling, or effusion.
6. Serositis	a. Pleuritis—convincing history of pleuritic pain or rub heard by a physician or evidence of pleural effusion *or*
	b. Pericarditis—documented by ECG or rub or evidence of pericardial effusion.
7. Renal disorder	a. Persistent proteinuria—0.5g/d or 3+ if quantitation not performed *or*
	b. Cellular casts—may be red cell, hemoglobin, granular, tubular, or mixed.
8. Neurologic disorder	a. Seizures—in the absence of offending drugs or known metabolic derangements, e.g., uremia, ketoacidosis, or electrolyte imbalance *or*
	b. Psychosis—in the absence of offending drugs or known metabolic derangements, e.g., uremia, ketoacidosis, or electrolyte imbalance.
9. Hematologic disorder	a. Hemolytic anemia—with reticulocytosis *or*
	b. Leukopenia—<4000/μL total on two or more occasions *or*
	c. Lymphopenia—<1500/μL on two or more occasions *or*
	d. Thrombocytopenia—<100,000/μL in the absence of offending drugs.
10. Immunologic disorder	a. Anti-DNA—antibody to native DNA in abnormal titer *or*
	b. Anti-Sm—presence of antibody to Sm nuclear antigen *or*
	c. Positive finding of antiphospholipid antibodies based on (1) an abnormal serum level of IgG or IgM anticardiolipin antibodies, (2) a positive test result for lupus anticoagulant using a standard method, or (3) a false-positive serologic test for syphilis known to be positive for at least 6 months and confirmed by negative *Treponema pallidum* immobilization or fluorescent treponemal antibody absorption test.
11. Antinuclear antibody	An abnormal titer of antinuclear antibody by immunofluorescence of an equivalent assay at any point in time and in the absence of drugs known to be associated with "drug-induced lupus" syndrome.

[*]The proposed classification is based on 11 criteria. For the purpose of identifying patients in clinical studies, a person shall be said to have SLE if any 4 or more of the 11 criteria are present, serially or simultaneously, during any interval of observation.
SOURCE: Reprinted from EM Tan et al: Arthritis Rheum 25:1271, 1982. Used by permission of the American College of Rheumatology.

SUBACUTE CUTANEOUS LUPUS ERYTHEMATOSUS (SCLE)

- Skin lesions of SCLE are annular or psoriasiform (Fig. 14-22).
- Patients with SCLE may have some of the criteria of SLE as defined by the ARA, including photosensitivity, arthralgias, serositis, renal disease, and serologic abnormalities. 50% of patients with SCLE have SLE.

- Practically all have anti-Ro (SS-A) and most have anti-La (SS-B) antibodies. The serious organ involvement of SLE is uncommon.
- The clinical skin lesions are the distinctive feature of SCLE.

EPIDEMIOLOGY

Age of Onset Young and middle age.
Race Uncommon in blacks or Hispanics.
Sex Females > males.
Incidence About 10% of the LE population.
Precipitating Factors Sunlight exposure.

CLINICAL MANIFESTATION

Rather sudden onset with annular or psoriasiform plaques erupting on the upper trunk, arms, dorsa of the hands, usually after exposure to sunlight; mild fatigue, malaise; some arthralgia, fever of unknown origin.

Skin Lesions *Two types*: (1) *Psoriasiform papulosquamous*, sharply defined, with slight delicate scaling (Fig. 14-22), evolving into bright red confluent plaques that are oval, arciform, or polycyclic, just as in psoriasis; and (2) *annular*, bright red annular lesions with central regression and little scaling. In both there may be telangiectasia, but there is no follicular plugging and less induration than in CCLE. Lesions resolve with slight atrophy (no scarring) and hypopigmentation.
Distribution Scattered, disseminated in light-exposed areas: shoulders, extensor surface of the arms, dorsal surface of the hands, upper back, V-neck area of the upper chest.

FIGURE 14-22 **Subacute cutaneous lupus erythematosus** Widely scattered, erythematous-to-violaceous, scaling, well-demarcated plaques on the trunk, neck, and arms, mimicking the clinical appearance of psoriasis vulgaris.

Other Lesions Periungual telangiectasia, diffuse nonscarring alopecia.

LABORATORY EXAMINATIONS

Dermatopathology and Immunopathology As in ACLE, LBT positive in 60%.
UV Testing Most patients have a lower than normal UVB minimum erythema dose (MED). Typical SCLE lesions may develop in UVB test sites.
Serology ANA present in 60–80%. Antibodies to Ro(SS-A) positive in > 80%, to La(SS-B) in 30–50%; high levels of circulating immune complexes.
Other Laboratory Tests Patients with SCLE, particularly those with manifest systemic involvement, may have a number of laboratory abnormalities, including anemia, leukopenia, lymphopenia, hematuria, proteinuria, and depressed complement levels.

DIAGNOSIS AND DIFFERENTIAL DIAGNOSIS

Clinical findings confirmed by histology and immunopathology. The extensive involvement is far more than is ever seen in CCLE, and the distinctive eruption is a marker for SCLE.

Differential Diagnosis Red plaques of dermatomyositis, secondary syphilis, psoriasis, seborrheic dermatitis, tinea corporis, polymorphic light eruption.

COURSE AND PROGNOSIS

A better prognosis than for SLE in general. Some patients with renal (and CNS) involvement have a guarded prognosis. The skin lesions can disappear completely, but occasionally, a vitiligo-like depigmentation remains for some months. Women with Ro(SS-A)-positive SCLE may give birth to babies with neonatal lupus and congenital heart block.

MANAGEMENT

Topical Anti-inflammatory glucocorticoids and topical pimecrolimus and tacrolimus are only partially helpful.
Systemic Systemic treatment usually required. *Thalidomide* (100–300 mg/d) is very effective for skin lesions but not for systemic involvement. *Hydroxychloroquine*, 400 mg/d; if this does not control the skin lesions, quinacrine hydrochloride, 100 mg/d, can be added. The bizarre yellow skin color caused by quinacrine can be somewhat modified by β-carotene, 60 mg tid.

CHRONIC CUTANEOUS LUPUS ERYTHEMATOSUS (CCLE) ICD-9:695.4 ∘ ICD-10:L93.0 ■ ◑

- This chronic, indolent skin disease is characterized by sharply marginated, scaly, infiltrated, and later atrophic red ("discoid") plaques, usually occurring on habitually exposed areas (Figs. 14-23, 14-24).
- This disorder, in most cases, is purely cutaneous without systemic involvement (Image 14-3).
- However, CCLE lesions may occur in SLE.
- CCLE may manifest as chronic discoid LE (CDLE; see below) or LE panniculitis (Table 14-4).

CLASSIC CHRONIC DISCOID LE (CDLE) ■ ◑

EPIDEMIOLOGY

Age of Onset 20–45 years.
Sex Females > males.
Race Possibly more severe in blacks.

CLINICAL MANIFESTATION

Can be precipitated by sunlight but to a lesser extent than ACLE or SCLE. Lesions last for months to years. Usually no symptoms,

FIGURE 14-23 **Chronic cutaneous lupus erythematosus** Well-demarcated, erythematous, hyperkeratotic plaques with atrophy, follicular plugging, and adherent scale on both cheeks. This is the classic presentation of chronic discoid LE.

FIGURE 14-24 **Chronic cutaneous lupus erythematosus: scarring** There are multiple scarred plaques that have a depressed center and an active, still erythematous and scaly margin in the face of this 60-year-old female farmer. Scarring has led to considerable disfigurement.

sometimes slightly pruritic or smarting. No general symptoms.

Skin Lesions Bright red papules evolving into plaques, sharply marginated, with adherent scaling (Fig. 14-23). Scales are difficult to remove and show spines on the undersurface (magnifying lens) resembling carpet tacks. Plaques are round or oval, annular or polycyclic, with irregular borders and expand in the periphery and regress in the center, resulting in depression of lesions, atrophy, and eventually scarring (Fig. 14-24). Follicular plugging and dilated follicles may persist in atrophic lesions but eventually disappear so that smooth, whitish scars result that are partially surrounded by a still active inflammatory and raised border (Fig. 14-24). "Burned out" lesions may be pink or white (hypomelanosis) macules and scars (Fig. 14-26), but scarred lesions may also show hyperpigmentation, especially in persons with brown or black skin (Fig. 14-25).

Distribution and Sites of Predilection CDLE may be localized or generalized, occurring predominantly on the face and scalp; dorsa of forearms, hands, fingers, toes, and less frequently, the trunk (Image 14-4) (Fig. 33-32).

Scalp Scarring alopecia with residual inflammation and follicular plugging (Fig. 14-26; see Section 32, Figs. 32-15, 32-16).

Mucous Membranes <5% of patients have lip involvement (hyperkeratosis, hypermelanotic scarring, erythema) and atrophic erythematous or whitish areas with or without ulceration on the buccal mucosa, tongue, and palate. *Nail apparatus* Nail dystrophy if nail matrix is involved.

LABORATORY EXAMINATIONS

Dermatopathology Hyperkeratosis, atrophy of the epidermis, follicular plugging, liquefaction degeneration of the basal cell layer. Edema, dilatation of small blood vessels, and perifollicular and periappendageal lymphocytic inflammatory infiltrate. Strong PAS reaction of the subepidermal, thickened basement zone.

Immunofluorescence LBT positive in 90% of active lesions at least 6 weeks old and not recently treated with topical glucocorticoids. LBT negative in burned-out (scarred) lesions and in the normal skin, both sun-exposed and nonexposed.

Serology Low incidence of ANA with titers >1:16.

Hematology Occasionally leukopenia (<4500/L).

DIAGNOSIS AND DIFFERENTIAL DIAGNOSIS

Clinical findings confirmed by histopathology and immunopathology. The discoid lesions of CDLE may closely mimic *actinic keratosis. Plaque psoriasis* and scaling discoid LE without atrophy and scarring may be difficult to distinguish, especially on the dorsa of the hands; histopathology permits distinction. *Polymorphous light eruption* LE (PMLE) may pose a problem. PMLE does not develop atrophy or follicular plugging, and does not occur in unexposed areas—mouth, hairy scalp. *Lichen planus* can be confusing, but the biopsy is distinctive. However, there is a lichen planus–LE, syndrome overlap of features. *Lupus vulgaris* and *tinea facialis.*

COURSE AND PROGNOSIS

Only 1–5% may develop SLE; with localized lesions, complete remission occurs in 50%; with generalized lesions, remissions are less frequent (<10%). *Note again*: CCLE lesions may be the presenting cutaneous sign of SLE.

MANAGEMENT

Prevention Topical sunscreens (SPF>30) routinely.

Local Glucocorticoids and Calcineurin Inhibitors Usually not very effective; topical fluorinated glucocorticoids with caution because of atrophy. Intralesional triamcinolone acetonide, 3–5 mg/mL, for small lesions.

Antimalarials Hydroxychloroqine, ≤6.5 mg/kg body weight per day. If hydroxychloroquine is ineffective, add quinacrine, 100 mg three times a day. Monitor for ocular side effects.

Retinoids Hyperkeratotic CDLE lesions respond well to systemic acitretin (0.5 mg/kg body weight).

Thalidomide 100–300 mg/d is effective. Observe contraindications.

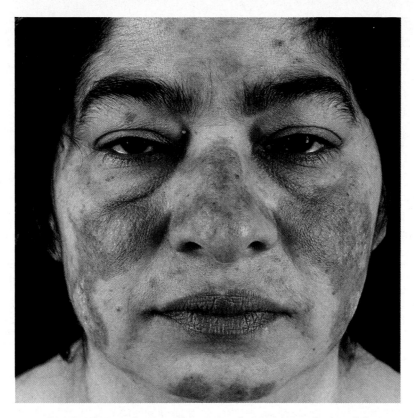

FIGURE 14-25   Chronic cutaneous lupus erythematosus: hyperpigmentation   As inflammatory lesions resolve there may be hyperpigmentation of the atrophic and partially scarred lesional skin, particularly in SPT III and IV patients. Although the skin lesions were CCLE, the patient had SLE.

FIGURE 14-26   Chronic cutaneous lupus erythematosus   Involvement of the scalp has led to complete hair loss with residual erythema, atrophy, and white scarring in this black male. Sharp demarcation of the lesions in the periphery indicates that these lesions originally were CDLE plaques.

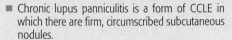

CHRONIC LUPUS PANNICULITIS

- Chronic lupus panniculitis is a form of CCLE in which there are firm, circumscribed subcutaneous nodules.
- Lead to subcutaneous atrophy and scarring resulting in sunken areas.

- Subcutaneous nodules occur both with and without DLE lesions of overlying skin.
- Usually a form of cutaneous lupus, but 35% of patients have mild SLE (see Image 14-3).
- *Synonym*: Lupus erythematosus profundus.

CLINICAL MANIFESTATION

May precede or follow the onset of discoid lesions by several years. Nodules are asymptomatic, tender, or sometimes painful.
Skin Lesions Deep-seated nodules or plate-like infiltrations with or without grossly visible epidermal changes or change of color; indolent and firm, sometimes tender or painful, and are better felt than seen. The overlying skin may be normal, erythematous, or brownish or exhibit typical lesions of CDLE. Lesions evolve into deep depressions (Fig. 14-27) but may also ulcerate; in this case there is scarring.
Distribution Scalp, face, upper arms (Fig. 14-27), trunk (especially the breasts), thighs, and buttocks.
Systems Review Mild SLE may be present (35%).

LABORATORY EXAMINATIONS

Dermatopathology Subcutaneous layer. Necrobiosis with fibrinoid deposits, dense lymphocytic infiltrates, and vasculitis; later, hyalinization of the fat lobules; fibrosis; there may be considerable mucinous deposits.
Other In patients with SLE there are typical hematologic and serologic abnormalities.

DIFFERENTIAL DIAGNOSIS

Morphea, erythema nodosum, sarcoid, miscellaneous types of panniculitis.

MANAGEMENT

- Antimalarials
- Thalidomide as for other forms of cutnaeous LE. Beware of contraindications.
  - Systemic glucocorticoids (short course)

FIGURE 14-27 Lupus panniculitis Chronic panniculitis with atrophy of the subcutaneous tissue, resulting in large sunken areas of overlying skin, representing resolving lesions. Where erythema is still visible, palpation reveals firm subcutaneous nodules and plaques. Also, some lesions reveal scarring in the center.

SCLERODERMA   ICD-9 : 710.1 ○ ICD-10 : M34   ◼ ◑ → ●

- Scleroderma is a not so rare multisystem disorder characterized by inflammatory, vascular, and sclerotic changes of the skin and various internal organs, especially the lungs, heart, and GI tract.
- Limited systemic scleroderma (lSSc) (60%) and diffuse systemic scleroderma (dSSc) are recognized.

- Clinical features always present are skin sclerosis and Raynaud phenomenon.
- Considerable morbidity; high mortality for dSSc
- *Synonyms*: Progressive systemic sclerosis, systemic sclerosis, systemic scleroderma.

EPIDEMIOLOGY

Prevalence   20 per million of U.S. population.
Age of Onset   30–50 years.
Sex   Female:male ratio, 4:1.

CLASSIFICATION

Systemic scleroderma can be divided into two subsets: *limited systemic scleroderma* (lSSc) and *diffuse systemic scleroderma* (dSSc). lSSc patients comprise 60%; patients are usually female; older than those with dSSc; and have a long history of Raynaud phenomenon with skin involvement limited to hands, feet, face, and forearms (acrosclerosis) and a high incidence of anticentromeric antibodies. lSSc includes the CREST syndrome, and systemic involvement may not appear for years; patients usually die of other causes. dSSc patients have a relatively rapid onset and diffuse involvement, not only of hands and feet but also of the trunk and face, synovitis, tendosynovitis, and early onset of internal involvement. Anticentromere antibodies are uncommon, but Scl-70 (antitopoisomerase I) antibodies are present in 33%.

ETIOLOGY AND PATHOGENESIS

Unknown. Primary event might be endothelial cell injury in blood vessels, the cause of which is unknown. Early in course, target organ edema occurs, followed by fibrosis; cutaneous capillaries are reduced in number; remainder dilate and proliferate, becoming visible telangiectasia. Fibrosis due to overproduction of collagen by fibroblasts.

CLINICAL MANIFESTATION

Raynaud phenomenon (see p. 394) with digital pain, coldness. Pain/stiffness of fingers, knees.

Migratory polyarthritis. Heartburn, dysphagia, especially with solid foods. Constipation, diarrhea, abdominal bloating, malabsorption, weight loss. Exertional dyspnea, dry cough.

Skin   *Hands/Feet*   *Early*: Raynaud phenomenon with triphasic color changes, i.e., pallor, cyanosis, rubor (Fig. 14-28*B*, see also Fig. 14-32). Precedes sclerosis by months and years. Nonpitting edema of hands/feet. Painful ulcerations at fingertips ("rat bite necrosis") (Fig. 14-29*A*), knuckles; heal with pitted scars. *Late*: sclerodactyly with tapering of fingers (madonna fingers) (Fig. 14-28*A*) with waxy, shiny, hardened skin, which is tightly bound down and does not permit folding or wrinkling; leathery crepitation over joints, flexion contractures; periungual telangiectasia, nails grow clawlike over shortened distal phalanges (Fig. 14-28*B*). Bony resorption and ulceration results in loss of distal phalanges.

As sclerosis proceeds proximally, there are loss of sweat glands with anhidrosis and thinning and complete loss of hair on distal extremities.

Face   *Early*: periorbital edema. *Late*: edema and fibrosis result in loss of normal facial lines, masklike (patients look younger than they are) (Fig. 14-30), thinning of lips, microstomia, radial perioral furrowing (Fig. 14-29*B*), beak-like sharp nose. Telangiectasia (Fig. 14-31) and diffuse hyperpigmentation.

Trunk   In dSSc the chest and proximal upper and lower extremities are involved early. Tense, stiff, and waxy appearing skin that cannot be folded. Impairment of respiratory movement of chest wall and of joint mobility.

Other Changes   *Cutaneous Calcification* Occurs on fingertips or over bony prominences or any sclerodermatous site; may ulcerate and exude white paste.

Color Changes   Hyperpigmentation that may be generalized and on the extremities may be accompanied by perifollicular hypopigmentation.

Mucous Membranes   Sclerosis of sublingual ligament; uncommonly, painful induration of gums, tongue.

Distribution of Lesions   *Early*: in lSSc early involvement is seen on fingers, hands, and face, and in many patients scleroderma remains confined to these regions. *Late*: the distal upper and lower extremities may be involved and occasionally the trunk. In dSSc sclerosis of the extremities and the trunk may start soon or soon after or concomitant with acral involvement.

Clinical Variant   CREST syndrome, i.e., *c*alcinosis cutis + *R*aynaud phenomenon + *e*sophageal dysfunction + *s*clerodactyly + *t*elangiectasia. Macular, matlike telangiectasia, especially the face (Fig. 14-31), upper trunk, and hands; also in the entire GI tract. Calcinosis over bony prominences, fingertips, elbows, and trochanteric regions.

GENERAL EXAMINATION

Esophagus   Dysphagia, diminished peristalsis, reflux esophagitis.

Gastrointestinal System   Small intestine involvement may produce constipation, diarrhea, bloating, and malabsorption.

Lung   Pulmonary fibrosis and alveolitis. Reduction of pulmonary function due to restricted movement of chest wall.

Heart   Cardiac conduction defects, heart failure, pericarditis.

Kidney   Renal involvement occurs in 45%. Slowly progressive uremia, malignant hypertension.

Musculoskeletal System   Carpal tunnel syndrome. Muscle weakness.

LABORATORY EXAMINATIONS

Dermatopathology   *Early*: mild cellular infiltrate around dermal blood vessels, eccrine coils, and at the dermal subcutaneous interphase. *Late*: broadening and homogenization of collagen bundles, obliteration and decrease of interbundle spaces, thickening of dermis with replacement of upper or total subcutaneous fat by hyalinized collagen. Paucity of blood vessels, thickening/hyalinization of vessel walls.

Autoantibodies   Patients with dSSc have circulating autoantibodies by ANA testing. Autoantibodies react with centromere proteins or DNA topoisomerase I; fewer patients have antinucleolar antibodies. Anticentromeric autoantibodies occur in 21% of dSSc and 71% of CREST patients, DNA topoisomerase I (Scl-70) antibodies in 33% of dSSc and 18% of CREST patients.

A   *B*

FIGURE 14-28   Scleroderma (lSSc): acrosclerosis   A. Hands and fingers are edematous (nonpitting); skin is without skin folds and bound down. Distal fingers are tapered (madonna fingers) **B.** Fingers show both bluish erythema and vasoconstriction (blue and white): Raynaud phenomenon. Fingers are edematous, the skin is bound down. Distal phalanges (index and third finger) are shortened, which is associated with bony resorption.

FIGURE 14-29 Scleroderma (lSSc): acrosclerosis *A.* Typical "rat bite" necroses and ulcerations of fingertips. ***B.*** Thinning of lips–microstomia (which would show better when patient attempts to open her mouth), radial perioral furrowing. Beaklike sharp nose.

DIAGNOSIS AND DIFFERENTIAL DIAGNOSIS

Clinical findings confirmed by dermatopathology.
Differential Diagnosis *Diffuse sclerosis:* mixed connective tissue disease, eosinophilic fasciitis, scleromyxedema, morphea, porphyria cutanea tarda, chronic graft-versus-host disease (GVHD), lichen sclerosus et atrophicus, polyvinyl chloride exposure, adverse drug reaction (pentazocine, bleomycin). Gadolinium and nephrogenic systemic fibrosis (see Section 17).

COURSE AND PROGNOSIS

Course characterized by slow, relentless progression of skin and/or visceral sclerosis; the 10-year survival rate is >50%. Renal disease is the leading cause of death, followed by cardiac and pulmonary involvement. Spontaneous remissions do occur. lSSc, which includes the CREST syndrome, progresses more slowly and has a more favorable prognosis; some cases do not develop visceral involvement.

FIGURE 14-30 Scleroderma (dSSc)   Masklike facies with stretched, shiny skin and loss of normal facial lines giving a younger appearance than actual age; the hair is dyed. Thinning of the lips and perioral sclerosis result in a small mouth. Sclerosis (whitish, glistening areas) and multiple telangiectases (not visible at this magnification) are also present.

MANAGEMENT

Systemic glucocorticoids may be of benefit for limited periods early in the disease. All other systemic treatments (EDTA, aminocaproic acid, D-penicillamine, *para*-aminobenzoate, colchicine) have not been shown to be of lasting benefit. Immunosuppressive drugs (cyclosporine, methotrexate, cyclophosphamide, mycophenolate mofetil) have shown improvement of skin score but only limited benefit for systemic involvement. Photopheresis: improvement in one third of patients. Immunoablation/stem cell transplantation and oral tolerization to type I collagen: ongoing studies.

FIGURE 14-31   Scleroderma: CREST syndrome   Numerous macular or matlike telangiectases on the forehead. Complete features include calcinosis cutis, Raynaud phenomenon, esophageal dysmotility, sclerosis, and telangiectasia.

SCLERODERMA-LIKE CONDITIONS □ ◑

- A dSSc-like condition occurs in persons exposed to polyvinyl chloride.
- Bleomycin also produces pulmonary fibrosis and Raynaud phenomenon but not skin sclerosis.
- Cutaneous changes indistinguishable from dSSc-like sclerosis of skin, accompanied by myalgia, pneumonitis, myocarditis, neuropathy, and encephalopathy, are related to the ingestion of certain lots of ʟ-tryptophan (*eosinophilia-myalgia syndrome*);
- The *toxic oil syndrome* that occurred in an epidemic in Spain in 1981 affecting 25,000 people

was due to the consumption of denatured rape seed oil. After an acute phase, with rash, fever, pneumonitis, and myalgia, the syndrome progresses to a condition with neuromuscular abnormalities and scleroderma-like skin lesions.

- Scleromyxedema and sclerema of Buschke are very rare, separate entities with guarded prognosis.
- lSSc-like sclerosis also occurs in porphyria cutanea tarda (see Section 10) and GVHD (see Section 21).

RAYNAUD PHENOMENON   ICD-9:443.0 ○ ICD-10:173.0   ■ ◑

- Raynaud phenomenon (RP) is digital ischemia that occurs on exposure to cold and/or as a result of emotional stress.
- Primary RP is a condition where no etiology is found; secondary RP is the designation for RP and underlying disease.
- The various causes of secondary RP are listed in Table 14-7. *Rheumatic disorders* [systemic scleroderma (85%), SLE (35%), dermatomyositis (30%), Sjögren syndrome, rheumatoid arthritis, polyarteritis nodosa], *diseases with abnormal blood proteins* (cryoproteins, cold agglutinins, macroglobulins), drugs (β-adrenergic blockers, nicotine), and *arterial diseases* (arteriosclerosis obliterans, thromboangiitis obliterans) are the most common.

EPIDEMIOLOGY

Age of Onset   Young adults or at menopause.
Sex   Female > male.
Incidence   As high as 20% in young women.
Occupation   May occur in persons using vibratory tools (chain saw users), meat cutters, typists, and pianists.
Precipitating Factors   Cold, mental stress, smoking, certain occupations (see above).

PATHOGENESIS

The vasomotor tone is regulated by the sympathetic nervous system. The centers for vasomotor tone are located in the brain, the spinal cord, and the peripheral nerves. Vasodilatation occurs only on withdrawal of the sympathetic activity. It is conjectured that there may be a "local fault" in which blood vessels are abnormally sensitive to cold.

CLINICAL MANIFESTATION

Numbness and/or pain worse in winter in temperate climates, in the cold (meat cutters); previous treatment (drugs), occupation (using vibratory tools) have to be explored. Careful review is important to detect diseases in which RP is associated: arthralgia, fatigue, dysphagia, muscle weakness, etc.

Types of Skin Changes *The Episodic Attack*   There is blanching or cyanosis of the fingers or toes, extending from the tip to various levels of the digits. The finger distal to the line of ischemia is white or blue and cold (Fig. 14-32); the proximal skin is pink and warm. When the digits are rewarmed, the blanching may be replaced by cyanosis because of slow blood flow; at the end of the attack, the normal color or a red color reflects the reactive hyperemic phase. To recapitulate, the sequence of color changes is white → blue → red (see Fig. 14-28B). Rarely, the tip of the nose, earlobes, or the tongue may be involved. Blanching may occur in one or two digits or in all the digits; often the thumb is spared. The feet are involved in only 40%.

Repeated or Persistent Vascular Vasospasm   Patients with RP often have a persistent vasospasm rather than episodic attacks. Skin changes include trophic changes with development of taut, atrophic skin, pterygium, clubbing and shortening of the terminal phalanges, sclerodactyly-like in lSSc (see Fig. 14-28). Acrogangrene is rare in RD (< 1%), but in RP associated with scleroderma, painful ulcers. Sequestration of the terminal phalanges or the development of gangrene (Fig. 14-33) may lead to autoamputation of the fingertips.

LABORATORY EXAMINATION

Serology   ANA should be determined.

DIAGNOSIS

Diagnosis is based on the vascular changes that are characteristic; ANA and other tests to rule out scleroderma and other conditions (Table 14-7). When no other disease is discovered, the diagnosis is primary RP.

PROGNOSIS

RP may disappear spontaneously; it progresses in about a third of patients.

FIGURE 14-32   Raynaud phenomenon   The left hand exhibits a distal cyanosis compared to the right hand; it is seen especially well in the nailbeds. Unilateral episodes such as this one may occur after contact with a cold object.

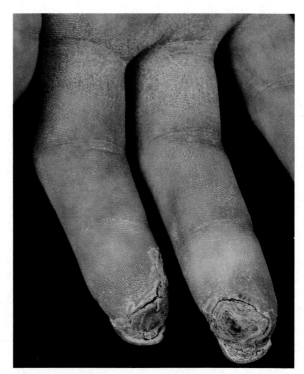

FIGURE 14-33   Raynaud phenomenon: acrogangrene   Persistent vasospasm of medium-sized arterioles can sometimes lead to gangrene of the terminal digits as illustrated in this patient with scleroderma.

MANAGEMENT

Prevention   Education regarding the use of loose-fitting clothing and avoiding cold and pressure on the fingers. Giving up smoking is mandatory.

Therapy   Drug therapy should be used in patients who have severe and progressive RP. Calcium channel blockers, anti-adrenergic drugs; intravenous prostacyclin (PGI_2); statins may benefit RP and digital ulcerations.

TABLE 14-7   Causes or Disorders Associated with Secondary Raynaud Phenomenon

- Connective tissue disease
  - Scleroderma
  - Systemic lupus erythematosus
  - Dermatomyositis and polymyositis
  - Undifferentiated connective tissue disease
  - Systemic vasculitis
  - Sjögren syndrome
  - Eosinophilic fasciitis
- Obstructive arterial disease
  - Atherosclerosis
  - Thromboangiitis obliterans (Buerger disease)
  - Thromboembolism
  - Thoracic outlet syndrome
- Drugs and toxins
  - β-Adrenergic blockers
  - Ergotamines
  - Oral contraceptives
  - Methysergide
  - Bleomycin and vinblastine
  - Clonidine
  - Bromocriptine
  - Cyclosporine
  - Amphetamines
  - Fluoxetine
  - Interferon-α

- Neurologic disorders
  - Carpal tunnel syndrome
  - Reflex sympathetic dystrophy
  - Hemiplegia
  - Poliomyelitis
  - Multiple sclerosis
  - Syringomyelia
- Occupation/environmental exposure
  - Vibration injury (lumberjacks, pneumatic hammer operators)
  - Posttraumatic injury (hypothenar hammer syndrome, crutch pressure)
  - Vinyl chloride disease
  - Cold injury
- Hyperviscosity disorders
  - Cryoproteins
  - Cold agglutinins
  - Macroglobulins
  - Polycythemia
  - Thrombocytosis
- Miscellaneous
  - Hypothyroidism
  - Infections (bacterial endocarditis, Lyme disease, viral hepatitis)
  - Neoplasms
  - Primary pulmonary hypertension
  - Arteriovenous fistula
  - Intra-arterial injections

SOURCE: JH Kippel: Raynaud phenomenon, in, K Wolff et al (eds): *Fitzpatrick's Dermatology in General Medicine* 7th ed. New York, McGraw-Hill, p 1646, 2008.

VASCULITIS   ICD-9:446.20 ∘ ICD-10:M31.0

HYPERSENSITIVITY VASCULITIS   ■ ◑ → ●

- Hypersensitivity vasculitis (HV) encompasses a heterogeneous group of vasculitides associated with hypersensitivity to antigens from infectious agents, drugs, or other exogenous or endogenous sources (Table 14-8).

- It is characterized pathologically by involvement of postcapillary venules and inflammation and fibrinoid necrosis (necrotizing vasculitis).

- Clinically, skin involvement is characteristic, manifested by "palpable purpura."

- Systemic vascular involvement occurs, chiefly in the kidney, muscles, joints, GI tract, and peripheral nerves.

- Schönlein-Henoch purpura is a type of HV associated with IgA deposits in skin.

- *Synonyms*: Allergic cutaneous vasculitis, necrotizing vasculitis.

EPIDEMIOLOGY AND ETIOLOGY

Age of Onset All ages.
Sex Equal incidence in males and females.
Etiology See Table 14-8; idiopathic 50%.

PATHOGENESIS

A postulated mechanism for necrotizing vasculitis is the deposition in postcapillary venules of circulating immune complexes. Initial alterations in venular permeability, due to the release of vasoactive amines from platelets, basophils, and/or mast cells, facilitate the deposition of immune complexes and these may activate the complement system or may interact directly with Fc receptors on endothelial cell membranes. When the complement system is activated, the generation of anaphylatoxins C3a and C5a can degranulate mast cells. Also, C5a can attract neutrophils that release lysosomal enzymes during phagocytosis of complexes and subsequently damage vascular tissue.

CLINICAL MANIFESTATION

A new drug taken during the few weeks before the onset of HV is a likely etiologic agent, as may be an infection, a known vascular/connective tissue disease, or paraproteinemia (Table 14-8). Onset and course: acute (days, as in drug-induced or idiopathic), subacute (weeks, especially urticarial types), chronic (recurrent over years). Symptoms are pruritus, burning pain; there may be no symptoms or there may be fever, malaise; symptoms of peripheral neuritis, abdominal pain (bowel ischemia), arthralgia, myalgia, kidney involvement (microhematuria), CNS involvement.

Skin Lesions The hallmark is *palpable purpura*. This term describes palpable petechiae that present as bright red, well-demarcated macules and papules with a central, dotlike hemorrhage (Fig. 14-34) (petechiae due to coagulation defects or thrombocytopenia are strictly macular and, therefore, not palpable). Lesions are scattered, discrete or confluent, and are primarily localized to the lower legs and the ankles (Fig. 14-34*A* and *B*) but may spread to the buttocks and arms. Stasis aggravates or precipitates lesions. Purpuric lesions do not blanch (with a glass slide). Red initially, they turn purple and even black in the center (Fig. 14-34*B*). In the case of massive inflammation, purpuric papules convert to hemorrhagic blisters, become necrotic (Fig. 14-34*B*), and even ulcerate.

LABORATORY EXAMINATIONS

Hematology Rule out thrombocytopenic purpura.
ESR Elevated.
Serology Serum complement is reduced or normal in some patients, depending on associated disorders.
Urinalysis RBC casts, albuminuria.
Others Depending on underlying disease.
Dermatopathology *Necrotizing vasculitis.* Deposition of eosinophilic material (fibrinoid) in

the walls of postcapillary venules in the upper dermis, and perivenular and intramural inflammatory infiltrate consisting predominantly of neutrophils. Extravasated RBC and fragmented neutrophils ("nuclear dust"). Frank necrosis of vessel walls. Intramural C3 and immunoglobulin deposition is seen with immunofluorescent techniques.

DIAGNOSIS AND DIFFERENTIAL DIAGNOSIS

Based on clinical appearance and histopathology. **Differential Diagnosis** Thrombocytopenic purpura, rash such as exanthematous drug eruption in setting of thrombocytopenia, disseminated intravascular coagulation (DIC) with purpura fulminans, septic vasculitis (rickettsial spotted fevers), septic emboli (infective endocarditis), bacteremia [disseminated gonococcal infection, meningococcemia (acute/chronic)],

pigmented purpura, other noninfectious vasculitides.

COURSE AND PROGNOSIS

Depends on underlying disease. In the idiopathic variant, multiple episodes can occur over the course of years. Usually self-limited, but irreversible damage to kidneys can occur.

MANAGEMENT

Antibiotics Antibiotics for patients in whom vasculitis follows bacterial infection.
Prednisone For patients with moderate to severe disease.
Cytotoxic Immunosuppressives Cyclophosphamide, azathioprine usually in combination with prednisone. Cyclosporine, intravenous high-dose immunoglobulin.

TABLE 14-8   Classification of Hypersensitivity Vasculitis

Associated with infections	Associated with neoplasms
Hepatitis B virus	Lymphoproliferative disease
Hepatitis C virus	Carcinoma of kidney
Group A hemolytic streptococcus (Schönlein-Henoch purpura)	Associated with autoimmune connective tissue disease
Staphylococcus aureus	SLE
Mycobacterium leprae (type 2 reaction, erythema nodosum leprosum)	Rheumatoid arthritis
Others	Sjögren syndrome
Associated with drugs	Associated with dysproteinemias
Sulfonamides	Cryoglobulinemia
Penicillin	Paraproteinemia
Serum	Hypergammaglobulinemia
Others	Congenital deficiencies of complement
	Idiopathic

A   *B*

FIGURE 14-34   **Hypersensitivity vasculitis**   *A.* Cutaneous vasculitis presents clinically as "palpable purpura" on the lower extremities. Although appearing to the eye as macules, the lesions can be palpated, and this contrasts with petechiae, for instance, in thrombocytopenic purpura. The lesions shown here have central punctum that is a darker red and do not blanch with a glass slide, indicating hemorrhage. *B.* This is a more advanced stage. Lesions have progressed to hemorrhagic bullae and some have become necrotic. The lesions may progress to ulceration.

SCHÖNLEIN-HENOCH PURPURA   ICD-9:287.0 ○ ICD-10:69.0   □ ●

- This is a specific subtype of hypersensitivity vasculitis that occurs mainly in children but also affects adults.

- There is a history of upper respiratory tract infection (75%), by group A streptococci.

- The disorder consists of palpable purpura (Fig. 14-35) accompanied by bowel angina (diffuse abdominal pain that is worse after meals), bowel ischemia, usually including bloody diarrhea, kidney involvement (hematuria and red cell casts), and arthritis.

- Histopathologically, there is necrotizing vasculitis and the immunoreactants deposited in skin are IgA.

- Long-term morbidity may result from progressive renal disease (5%).

FIGURE 14-35   Hypersensitivity vasculitis: Schönlein-Henoch purpura There is classic palpable purpura on the lower legs of a 19-year-old male. The patient had colicky abdominal pain, arthritis, and microhematuria and skin biopsy revealed IgA immunoreactivity around postcapillary venules.

POLYARTERITIS NODOSA   ICD-9:446.0 ∘ ICD-10:M30.0   □ ●

- Polyarteritis nodosa (PAN) is a multisystem, necrotizing vasculitis of small- and medium-sized muscular arteries with involvement of the renal and visceral arteries.
- Microscopic polyangitis (MPA) may be diffeent from PAN but this is not proven and therefore included in this discussion.

- Constitutional symptoms: fever, asthma, myalgia.
- Skin manifestations are palpable purpura, nodules and ulcers.
- *Synonyms*: Periarteritis nodosa, panarteritis nodosa.

EPIDEMIOLOGY AND ETIOLOGY

Age of Onset   Mean age 45 years.
Sex   Male:female ratio 2.5:1.
Etiology   Unknown.
Clinical Variants   *Cutaneous PAN* is a rare variant with symptomatic vasculitis limited to skin and at times peripheral nerves.

PATHOGENESIS

Necrotizing inflammation of small- and medium-sized muscular arteries; may spread circumferentially to involve adjacent veins. Lesions segmental, tend to involve bifurcations. About 30% of cases associated with hepatitis B and C antigenemia, i.e., immune complex formation.

A   *B*

FIGURE 14-36   Polyarteritis nodosa   A. Two dermal and subcutaneous nodules occurring on the pretibial aspects of the lower leg. **B.** A starburst pattern can be seen in the supra- and retromalleolar region of the right leg in another patient. These lesions represent cutaneous infarction with ulceration.

CLINICAL MANIFESTATION

Chronic Disease Syndrome With internal organ involvement and associated symptoms (see below).
Cutaneous PAN Pain in nodules, ulcers; aching during flares and physical activity. Myalgia. Neuralgia, numbness, mild paresthesia.
Skin Lesions Occur in 15% of cases. Subcutaneous inflammatory, bright red to bluish nodules (0.5–2 cm) that follow the course of involved arteries. Violaceous, become confluent to form painful subcutaneous plaques (Fig. 14-36*A*), and accompanied by livedo reticularis; "starburst" livedo is pathognomonic and marks a cluster of nodular lesions. Ulcers follow ischemia of nodules (Fig. 14-36*B*). Usually bilaterally on lower legs, thighs. Other areas: arms, trunk, head, neck, buttocks. Livedo reticularis may extend to trunk. Duration—days to months. Resolves with residual violaceous or postinflammatory hyperpigmentation. Skin lesions in systemic and cutaneous PAN are identical.

GENERAL EXAMINATION

Cardiovascular Hypertension; congestive heart failure, pericarditits, conduction system defects, myocardial infarction.
Neurologic Cerebrovascular accident. Peripheral nerves: mixed motor/sensory involvement with mononeuritis multiplex pattern.
Muscles Diffuse myalgias (excluding shoulder and hip girdle), lower extremities.
GI System Nausea, vomiting, abdominal pain, hemorrhage, infarction.
Eyes Hypertensive changes, ocular vasculitis, retinal artery aneurysm, optic disc edema/atrophy.
Kidney Renal failure, edema.
Testes Pain and tenderness.

LABORATORY EXAMINATIONS

Dermatopathology *Best yield: biopsy of nodular skin lesion* (deep wedge biopsy). Polymorphonuclear neutrophils infiltrate all layers of muscular vessel wall and perivascular areas; later, mononuclear cells. Fibrinoid necrosis of vessel wall with compromise of lumen, thrombosis, infarction of tissues supplied by involved vessel, with or without hemorrhage. Skin pathology is identical in systemic and cutaneous PAN.

CBC Commonly neutrophilic leukocytosis; rarely, eosinophilia; anemia of chronic disease. ± Elevated ESR.

Serology Antineutrophil cytoplasmic autoantibodies (p-ANCA) in some cases. In 60% of MPA patients, hepatitis B surface antigenemia; in 30% of cases, hepatitis C.

Chemistry Elevated creatinine, BUN.

Arteriography Aneurysms in small- and medium-sized muscular arteries of kidney/hepatic/visceral vasculature.

DIFFERENTIAL DIAGNOSIS

Other vasculitides and panniculitides.

COURSE AND PROGNOSIS

Untreated, very high morbidity and mortality rates characterized by fulminant deterioration or by relentless progression associated with intermittent acute exacerbations. Death from renal failure, bowel infarction and perforation, cardiovascular complications, intractable hypertension. *Cutaneous PAN*: chronic relapsing benign course.

MANAGEMENT

Systemic PAN *Combined therapy*: prednisone, 1 mg/kg body weight per day, and cyclophosphamide, 2 mg/kg per day.

Cutaneous PAN Nonsteroidal anti-inflammatory agents, prednisone. In severe cases, as for systemic PAN.

WEGENER GRANULOMATOSIS ICD-9:446.4 ∘ ICD-10:M31.3   □ ●

- Wegener granulomatosis (WG) is a systemic vasculitis, defined by a clinical triad of manifestations comprising involvement of the upper airways, lungs, and kidneys
- Skin manifestations are those of hypersensitivity vasculitis, nodulo-ulcerative lesions and oral/nasal ulcerations.

- A pathologic triad consisting of necrotizing granulomas in the upper respiratory tract and lungs, vasculitis involving both arteries and veins, and glomerulitis.

EPIDEMIOLOGY AND ETIOLOGY

Age of Onset Mean age 40 years, but occurs at any age.

Sex Male:female ratio 1.3:1.

Race Rare in blacks.

Etiology Unknown.

Clinical Variants One variant is limited to kidneys, i.e., glomerulitis occurs in 15% of cases; another is limited to respiratory tract.

PATHOGENESIS

Immunopathogenesis unclear. Possibly an aberrant hypersensitivity response to an exogenous or endogenous antigen that enters through or resides in upper airways. Clinical symptomatology caused by necrotizing vasculitis of small arteries and veins. Pulmonary involvement: multiple, bilateral, nodular infiltrates. Similar infiltrates in paranasal sinuses, nasopharynx.

CLINICAL MANIFESTATION

Chronic disease syndrome. Fever. Paranasal sinus pain, purulent or bloody nasal discharge. Cough, hemoptysis, dyspnea, chest discomfort.

PHYSICAL EXAMINATION

Skin Lesions Overall in 50% of patients but in only 13% of patients at initial presentation. *Ulcers with jagged, undermined borders* most typical; resemble pyoderma gangrenosum (Fig. 14-37). *Papules, vesicles, palpable purpura* as in hypersensitivity (necrotizing) vasculitis (Fig. 14-38), subcutaneous nodules, plaques, noduloulcerative lesions as in PAN. Most common on lower extremities. Also, face, trunk, upper limbs.

Mucous Membranes Oral ulcerations (Fig. 14-39). Often first symptom. ± Nasal mucosal ulceration, crusting, blood clots; nasal septal perforation; saddle-nose deformity. Eustachian

FIGURE 14-37 **Wegener granulomatosis** A pyoderma gangrenosum-like irregular ulceration on the cheek with jagged and undermined borders is often the first manifestation of Wegener gramulomatosis.

FIGURE 14-38 **Wegener granulomatosis** Palpable purpura with hemorrhagic and necrotic lesions on the legs as in hypersensitivity vasculitis.

tube occlusion with serous otitis media; ± pain. External auditory canal: pain, erythema, swelling. Marked gingival hyperplasia.
Eyes 65%. Mild conjunctivitis, episcleritis, scleritis, granulomatous sclerouveitis, ciliary vessel vasculitis, retroorbital mass lesion with proptosis.
Nervous System Cranial neuritis, mononeuritis multiplex, cerebral vasculitis.
Renal Disease 85%. Signs of renal failure in advanced WG.

DIFFERENTIAL DIAGNOSIS

Cutaneous Necrosis + Respiratory Tract Disease Other vasculitides, Goodpasture syndrome, tumors of the upper airway/lung, infectious/noninfectious granulomatous diseases (especially blastomycosis), midline granuloma, angiocentric lymphoma, allergic granulomatosis.

LABORATORY EXAMINATIONS

Hematology Mild anemia. Leukocytosis. ± Thrombocytosis.
ESR Markedly elevated.
Chemistry Impaired renal function.
Urinalysis Proteinuria, hematuria, RBC casts.
Serology Antineutrophil cytoplasmic autoantibodies (ANCA) are seromarkers for WG. Two ANCA patterns occur in ethanol-fixed neutrophils: cytoplasmic pattern (c-ANCA) and perinuclear pattern (p-ANCA). A 29-kDa protease (PR-3) is the major antigen for c-ANCA; myeloperoxidase, for p-ANCA. c-ANCA has been associated predominantly with WG and is considered specific for this condition; p-ANCA with microscopic polyarteritis, PAN, other vasculitides, idiopathic necrotizing and crescentic glomerulonephritis. Titers correlate with dis-

ease activity. Hypergammaglobulinemia, particularly IgA class.
Pathology All involved tissues including skin: necrotizing vasculitis of small arteries/veins with intra- or extravascular granuloma formation. Kidneys: focal/segmental glomerulonephritis.
Imaging *Paranasal sinuses*: opacification, with or without sclerosis. *Chest*: pulmonary infiltrates, nodules; consolidation, cavitation; upper lobes.

COURSE AND PROGNOSIS

Untreated, usually fatal because of rapidly progressive renal failure. With combination cyclophosphamide plus prednisone therapy, long-term remission is achieved in 90% of cases.

MANAGEMENT

Treatment of Choice Cyclophosphamide plus prednisone.
Cyclophosphamide 2 mg/kg body weight per day. Dose should be adjusted to keep leukocyte count > 5000/μL (neutrophil count 1500/μL) to avoid infections associated with neutropenia. Therapy should be continued for 1 year after complete remission, then tapered and discontinued. *Alternative drug*: azathioprine in similar doses if cyclophosphamide is not tolerated.
Prednisone 1 mg/kg body weight per day for 1 month, and then changed to alternate-day doses which are tapered and then discontinued after 6 months of therapy.
Rituximab In refractory patients.
Trimethoprim-Sulfamethoxazole As adjunctive therapy and/or prevention of upper airway bacterial infections that promote disease flare.

FIGURE 14-39 Wegener granulomatosis A large ulcer on the palate covered by a dense, adherent, necrotic mass; note accompanying edema of the upper lip. Similar lesions occur in the sinuses and tracheobronchial tree.

GIANT CELL ARTERITIS ICD-9:446.5 ○ ICD-10:μ31.5 □ ●

- Giant cell arteritis is a systemic granulomatous vasculitis of medium- and large-sized arteries, most notably the temporal artery and other branches of the carotid artery in elderly patients.

- Characterized by headaches, fatigue, fever, anemia, and high ESR.

- Cutaneous manifestations are necrosis and ulceration on the scalp.

- *Synonyms*: Temporal arteritis, cranial arteritis.

EPIDEMIOLOGY AND ETIOLOGY

Age of Onset Middle-age to elderly, usually > 55 years.
Sex Females > males.
Etiology Unknown. Probably via cell-mediated immunity.

CLINICAL MANIFESTATION

Fatigue. Fever. Chronic disease syndrome. Headache usually bilateral. Scalp pain. Claudication of jaw/tongue while talking/chewing. Eye involvement: transient impairment of vision, ischemic optic neuritis, retrobulbar neuritis, persistent blindness. Systemic vasculitis: claudication of extremities, stroke, myocardial infarction, aortic aneurysms/dissections, visceral organ infarction. *Polymyalgia rheumatica syndrome*: stiffness, aching, pain in the muscles of the neck, shoulders, lower back, hips, thighs.

PATHOGENESIS

Systemic vasculitis of multiple medium- and large-sized arteries. Symptoms secondary to ischemia.

Skin Lesions Superficial temporal arteries are swollen, prominent, tortuous, ± nodular thickenings. Tender. Initially, involved artery pulsates; later, occluded with loss of pulsation. ± Erythema of overlying skin. Gangrene, i.e., skin infarction of the area supplied by affected artery in the temporal/parietal scalp with sharp, irregular borders (Fig. 14-40A); ulceration with exposure of bone (Fig. 14-40B). Scars at sites of old ulcerations. Postinflammatory hyperpigmentation over involved artery.

General Examination Findings in other organ systems related to tissue ischemia/infarction. 🖉

LABORATORY EXAMINATIONS

CBC Normochromic/slightly hypochromic anemia.

ESR Markedly elevated.

Temporal Artery Biopsy Biopsy tender nodule of involved artery with or without overlying affected skin after Doppler flow examination. Lesions focal. Panarteritis with inflammatory mononuclear cell infiltrates within the vessel wall with frequent giant cell granuloma formation. Intimal proliferation with vascular occlusion, fragmentation of internal elastic lamina, extensive necrosis of intima and media.

COURSE AND PROGNOSIS

Untreated, can result in blindness secondary to ischemic optic neuritis. Excellent response to glucocorticoid therapy. Remission after several years.

MANAGEMENT

Prednisone First-line therapy. Initially, 40–60 mg/d; taper when symptoms abate; continue 7.5–10 mg/d for 1–2 years.

Methotrexate Low-dose (15–20 mg) methotrexate, once a week, has a considerable glucocorticoid-sparing effect.

A   *B*

FIGURE 14-40 **Giant cell arteritis** **A.** This elderly male had excruciating headaches and progressive impairment of vision. Necrosis developed bilaterally on the scalp. **B.** In this patient the necrotic tissue has been shed, revealing the bare bone of the skull.

URTICARIAL VASCULITIS □ ◑

- Urticarial vasculitis is a multisystem disease characterized by cutaneous lesions resembling urticaria, except that wheals persist for >24 h.

- Fever, arthralgia, elevated ESR, and histologic findings of a leukocytoclastic vasculitis are also present.

- The syndrome is often accompanied by various degrees of extracutaneous involvement.

- May be cutaneous manifestations of SLE.

Synonym: Urticaria perstans.

EPIDEMIOLOGY AND ETIOLOGY

Age of Onset Majority 30–50 years.
Sex Female:male ratio 3:1.
Etiology In patients with serum sickness; in collagen vascular diseases, in particular, LE; with certain infections (e.g., hepatitis B); and idiopathic.
Incidence <5% of patients with urticaria.

PATHOGENESIS

Thought to be an immune complex disease, similar to hypersensitivity vasculitis (see page 397).

CLINICAL MANIFESTATION

Lesions may be associated with itching, burning, stinging sensation, pain, tenderness. Fever (10–15%). Arthralgias with or without arthritis in one or more joints (ankles, knees, elbows, wrists, small joints of fingers). Nausea, abdominal pain. Cough, dyspnea, chest pain, hemoptysis. Pseudotumor cerebri. Cold sensitivity. Renal involvement: diffuse glomerulonephritis.
Skin Lesions Urticaria-like (i.e., edematous plaques and wheals), occasionally indurated, erythematous, circumscribed (Fig. 14-41); occasionally with angioedema. Eruption occurs in transient crops, usually lasting >24 h and up to 3–4 days. They change shape slowly, often reveal purpura on blanching (glass slide), and resolve with a yellowish-green color and hyperpigmentation.
General Examiation Extracutaneous manifestations: joints (70%), GI tract (20–30%), CNS (>10%), ocular system (>10%), kidneys (10–20%), lymphadenopathy (5%).

FIGURE 14-41 **Urticarial vasculitis** Erythematous plaques and wheals on the buttocks that, in part, do not blanch on diascopy (compression of the lesional skin with glass), which indicates hemorrhage. This contrasts with urticaria. Also, in contrast to lesions of urticaria, which usually resolve within 24 h, those of urticarial vasculitis persist for up to 3 days before resolving with residual hyperpigmentation (hemosiderin deposition). Lesions of urticaria change shape in a short time, while those of urticarial vasculitis change slowly.

LABORATORY EXAMINATIONS

Dermatopathology Inflammation of dermal venules primarily with neutrophils *without* necrotizing vasculitis. Later, frank leukocytoclastic vasculitis.
Urinalysis 10% of patients—microhematuria, proteinuria.
ESR Elevated.
Serologic Findings Hypocomplementemia (70%); circulating immune complexes.

DIAGNOSIS AND DIFFERENTIAL DIAGNOSIS

Clinical suspicion confirmed by skin biopsy. Urticaria, serum sickness, other vasculitides, SLE, urticaria in acute hepatitis B infection.
Disease Associations SLE and other collagen vascular autoimmune disease.

COURSE AND PROGNOSIS

Most often this syndrome has a chronic (months to years) but benign course. Episodes recur over periods ranging from months to years. Renal disease occurs only in hypocomplementemic patients.

MANAGEMENT

Rule out vascular/connective tissue disease.
First Line H_1 and H_2 blockers [doxepin (10 mg twice daily to 25 mg three times daily) *plus* cimetidine (300 mg three times daily)/ranitidine (150 mg twice daily)] *plus* a nonsteroidal anti-inflammatory agent [indomethacin (75–200 mg/d)/ibuprofen (1600–2400 mg/d)/naprosyn (500–1000 mg/d)].
Second Line Colchicine, 0.6 mg two or three times daily *or* dapsone, 50–150 mg/d.
Third Line Prednisone.
Fourth Line Cytotoxic immunosuppressive agents (azathioprine, cyclophosphamide).

NODULAR VASCULITIS ICD-9: O17.1 ∘ ICD-10: A18.4

- Nodular vasculitis is a form of lobular panniculitis associated with subcutaneous blood vessel vasculitis with subsequent ischemic changes that produce lipocyte injury, necrosis, inflammation, and granulation.

- Synonyms are *erythema induratum* and *Bazin disease*, but these terms are now reserved for those cases of nodular vasculitis that are associated with *Mycobacterium tuberculosis*.

EPIDEMIOLOGY AND ETIOLOGY

Age of Onset Middle-aged to older persons.
Sex Usually females.
Etiology Immune complex–mediated vascular injury due to bacterial antigens has been implicated. Immunoglobulins, complement, and bacterial antigens have been found by immunofluorescence and in some cases mycobacterial DNA sequences by polymerase chain reaction (PCR). Bacterial cultures are invariably negative.

CLINICAL MANIFESTATION

Chronic, recurrent, often bilateral, subcutaneous nodules and plaques with ulceration of the legs. Usually asymptomatic but may be tender. Often in middle-aged females with stubby column-like legs who work in the cold.

Skin Lesions Initially erythematous, tender, or asymptomatic subcutaneous nodules or plaques (Fig. 14-42) on the calves, rarely on shins and thighs. Lesions become bluish red in color, are firm, and fluctuate before ulcerating. Ulcers drain serous/oily fluid, are ragged, punched-out, and have violaceous or brown margins (Fig. 14-42). They persist for prolonged periods before healing with atrophic scars.
Associated Findings Follicular perniosis, livedo, varicose veins, and a cool, edematous skin.
General Examination Patients are usually healthy.

LABORATORY EXAMINATIONS

Dermatopathology Tuberculoid granulomas, foreign-body giant cell reaction, and necrosis

FIGURE 14-42   Nodular vasculitis   Multiple, deep-seated, brown to bluish nodules, particularly on the posterior aspects of both lower legs. The lesions, which are relatively asymptomatic, may undergo necrosis forming slowly healing ulcers. Varicose veins are also seen on the right calf.

of fat lobules. Medium-sized vessel vasculitis, predominantly venular but sometimes arterial, in the septal areas. Fibrinoid necrosis or a granulomatous chronic inflammatory infiltrate invades between the fat cells, replacing adipose tissue and leading to fibrosis.

Skin Testing   Patients with an association with *M. tuberculosis* infection are highly sensitive to tuberculin and purified protein derivative (PPD); therefore, skin testing to *M. tuberculosis* antigens should be performed. In such patients, *M. tuberculosis* DNA sequences can be found by PCR.

DIAGNOSIS AND DIFFERENTIAL DIAGNOSIS

By clinical findings and biopsy.

Differential Diagnosis   *Red nodules on legs*: Erythema nodosum, other forms of panniculitis, cutaneous panarteritis nodosa. *Note*: Erythema nodosum is hot, very tender, and never ulcerates.

COURSE AND PROGNOSIS

Chronic recurrent, scarring.

MANAGEMENT

Antituberculous therapy in those cases where *M. tuberculosis* etiology is proved. In other cases, bed rest, compression stockings, tetracyclines, and potassium iodide have proved effective. Systemic glucocorticoids are sometimes necessary for remission. In some cases dapsone is effective.

KAWASAKI DISEASE ICD-9:446.1 ∘ ICD-10:M30.3 □ (→■ *) ●

- Kawasaki disease (KD) is an acute febrile illness of infants and children.
- Characterized by cutaneous and mucosal erythema and edema with subsequent desquamation, cervical lymphadenitis.
- Bilateral bulbar non-exudative conjunctival injection, inflammation of oropharynx.
- Complications: coronary abnormalities, including aneurysms (30%), myocarditis, arthritis, urethritis, and aseptic meningitis.

- Immediate treatment with intravenous immunoglobulin and aspirin reduces coronary aneurysms.

Synonym: Mucocutaneous lymph node syndrome.

* This indicates that KD is common when there are epidemics.

EPIDEMIOLOGY AND ETIOLOGY

Age of Onset Peak incidence at 1 year, mean 2.6 years, uncommon after 8 years. Most cases of KD in adults probably represent toxic shock syndrome.
Sex Male predominance, 1.5:1.
Race In United States: Japanese > blacks > whites.
Etiology Unknown.
Season Winter and spring.
Geography First reported in Japan, 1961; United States, 1971. Epidemics.

PATHOGENESIS

Generalized vasculitis. Endarteritis of vasa vasorum involves adventitia/intima of proximal coronary arteries with ectasia, aneurysm formation, vessel obstruction, and distal embolization with subsequent myocardial infarction. Other vessels: brachiocephalic, celiac, renal, iliofemoral arteries. Increased activated helper T cells and monocytes, elevated serum interleukin (IL) 1, TNF-α, IL-6, adrenomedullin and vascular endothelial growth factor, anti-endothelial antibodies, and increased cytokine-inducible activation antigens on the vascular endothelium occur in KD. T cell response is driven by a superantigen.

CLINICAL MANIFESTATION/PHASES

Phase I: Acute Febrile Period Abrupt onset of fever, lasting approximately 12 days, followed (usually within 1–3 days) by most of the other principal features. Constitutional symptoms of diarrhea, arthritis, photophobia.

Phase II: Subacute Phase Lasts approximately until day 30 of illness; fever, thrombocytosis, desquamation, arthritis, arthralgia, carditis; highest risk for sudden death.
Phase III: Convalescent Period Begins within 8–10 weeks after onset of illness when all signs of illness have disappeared and ends when ESR returns to normal; very low mortality rate during this period.
Skin Lesions
Phase I Lesions appear 1–3 days after onset of fever. Duration 12 days average. Nearly all mucocutaneous abnormalities occur during this phase.
Exanthem Erythema usually first noted on palms/soles, spreading to involve trunk and extremities within 2 days. First lesions: erythematous macules; lesions enlarge and become more numerous (Fig. 14-43). Type: urticaria-like lesions most common; morbilliform pattern second most common; scarlatiniform and erythema multiforme–like in <5% of cases. Confluent macules to plaque-type erythema on perineum, which persist after other findings have resolved. Edema of hands/feet: deeply erythematous to violaceous; brawny swelling with fusiform fingers (Fig. 14-44). Palpation: lesions may be tender.
Mucous Membranes Bulbar conjunctivae: bilateral vascular dilatation (conjunctival injection); noted 2 days after onset of fever; duration, 1–3 weeks (throughout the febrile course). Lips: red, dry, fissured (Fig. 14-44), hemorrhagic crusts; duration, 1–3 weeks. Oropharynx: diffuse erythema. Tongue: "strawberry" tongue (erythema and protuberance of papillae of tongue).
Phase II Desquamation highly characteristic; follows resolution of exanthem (Fig. 14-45).

FIGURE 14-43 Kawasaki disease Blotchy erythema on the trunk of a child; bulbar conjunctivitis, lymphade-nopathy, and "strawberry" tongue were also present.

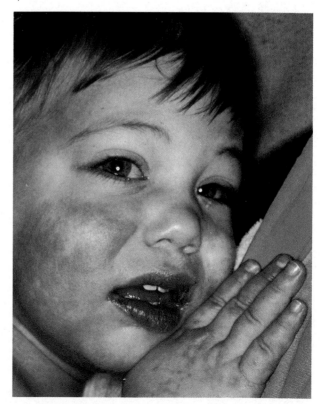

FIGURE 14-44 Kawasaki disease
Cherry-red lips with hemorrhagic fis-sures, in a little boy with prolonged high fever. This child also had a gener-alized morbilliform eruption, injected conjunctivae, and "strawberry" tongue (not shown). Note erythema and edema of fingertips.

Begins on tips of fingers and toes at junction of nails and skin; desquamating sheets of palmar/plantar epidermis are progressively shed.

Phase III Beau lines (transverse furrows on nail surface) may be seen (see Section 33). Possible telogen effluvium.

General Findings Meningeal irritation. Pneumonia. Lymphadenopathy, usually cervical nodes: ≥1.5 cm, slightly tender, firm. Arthritis/arthralgias, knees, hips, elbows. Pericardial tamponade, dysrhythmias, rubs, congestive heart failure, left ventricular dysfunction.

LABORATORY EXAMINATIONS

Chemistry Abnormal liver function tests.
Hematology Leukocytosis (>18,000/μL). Thrombocytosis after the tenth day of illness. Elevated ESR in phase II. ESR returns to normal in phase III.
Urinalysis Pyuria.
Dermatopathology Arteritis involving small and medium-sized vessels with swelling of endothelial cells in postcapillary venules, dilatation of small blood vessels, lymphocytic/monocytic perivascular infiltrate in arteries/arterioles of dermis.
Electrocardiography Prolongation of PR and QT intervals; ST-segment and T-wave changes.
Echocardiography and Angiography Coronary aneurysms in 20% of cases.

DIAGNOSIS AND DIFFERENTIAL DIAGNOSIS

Diagnostic criteria: fever spiking to >39.4°C, lasting ≥5 days without other cause, associated with four of five criteria: (1) bilateral conjunctival injection; (2) at least one of following mucous membrane changes: injected/fissured lips, injected pharynx, "strawberry" tongue; (3) at least one of the following extremity changes: erythema of palms/soles, edema of hands/feet,

generalized/periungual desquamation; (4) diffuse scarlatiniform or deeply erythematous maculopapular rash, iris lesions; and (5) cervical lymphadenopathy (at least one lymph node ≥1.5 cm in diameter).

Differential Diagnosis Adverse cutaneous drug eruption, juvenile rheumatoid arthritis, infectious mononucleosis, viral exanthems, leptospirosis, Rocky Mountain spotted fever, toxic shock syndrome, staphylococcal scalded-skin syndrome, erythema multiforme, serum sickness, SLE, reactive arthritis syndrome.

COURSE AND PROGNOSIS

Clinical course triphasic. Uneventful recovery occurs in majority. Cardiovascular system complications in 20%. Coronary artery aneurysms occur within 2–8 weeks, associated with myocarditis, myocardial ischemia/infarction, pericarditis, peripheral vascular occlusion, small-bowel obstruction, stroke. Case fatality rate, 0.5–2.8% of cases, and is associated with coronary artery aneurysms.

MANAGEMENT

Diagnosis should be made early and attention directed at prevention of the cardiovascular complications.
Hospitalization Recommended during the phase I illness, monitoring for cardiac and vascular complications.
Systemic Therapy *Intravenous Immunoglobulin* 2 g/kg as a single infusion over 10 h together with aspirin.
Aspirin 100 mg/kg per day until fever resolves or until day 14 of illness, followed by 5 to 10 mg/kg per day until ESR and platelet count have returned to normal.
Glucocorticoids Contraindicated Associated with a higher rate of coronary aneurysms.

FIGURE 14-45   Kawasaki disease   Shedding of the epidermis on the palm of this child 10 days after the acute illness.

REACTIVE ARTHRITIS (REITER SYNDROME)

- Reactive arthritis (RA) is defined by an episode of peripheral arthritis of >1 month's duration occurring in association with urethritis and/or cervicitis.
- Initiation by infection, usually in the genitourinary and gastrointestinal tract.
- *Salmonella, Campylobacter, Shigella, Yersinia,* and *Chlamydia* trigger RA, but other infections can also be initiators.

- Frequently accompanied by keratoderma blennorrhagicum, circinate balanitis, conjunctivitis, and stomatitis.
- The classic triad is arthritis, urethritis, and conjunctivitis.

ICD-9 : 711.0 ○ ICD-10 : M02.3

EPIDEMIOLOGY AND ETIOLOGY

Age of Onset   22 years (median) in the type following sexually transmitted infection (STI).
Sex   90% of patients are males (postvenereal type).
Race   Most common in Caucasians from northern Europe; rare in Asians and African blacks.
Genetic Diathesis   HLA-B27 occurs in up to 75% of Caucasians with RA but in only 8% of healthy Caucasians. Patients who are HLA-B27-negative have a milder course, with significantly less sacroiliitis, uveitis, and carditis.
Associated Disorders   Incidence of RA may be increased in HIV-infected individuals.
Etiology   Unknown.

PATHOGENESIS

RA appears linked to two factors: (1) *genetic factors*, i.e., HLA-B27 and (2) *enteric pathogens* such as *Salmonella enteritidis, S. typhimurium, S. heidelberg; Yersinia enterocolitica, Y. pseudotuberculosis; Campylobacter fetus; Shigella flexneri;* or genitourinary pathogens (such as *Chlamydia* or *Ureaplasma urealyticum*). Two patterns are observed: the *epidemic form*, which follows STI, the most common type in the United States and the United Kingdom; and the *postdysenteric form* following GI infection, the most common type in continental Europe and North Africa.

CLINICAL MANIFESTATION

Onset 1–4 weeks after infection: enterocolitis; nongonococcal urethritis. Urethritis and/or conjunctivitis usually first to appear, followed by arthritis.

Symptoms consist of malaise, fever, dysuria, urethral discharge. Eyes: red, slightly sensitive.

Arthritis: tendon/fascia inflammation results in pain over ischial tuberosities, iliac crest, long bones, ribs; heel pain at site of attachment of plantar aponeurosis (plantar fasciitis) and/or Achilles tendon; back pain; joint pains.

Skin Lesions   Resemble those of psoriasis, especially on palms/soles, glans penis.
Keratoderma blennorrhagicum: brownish-red papules or macules, sometimes topped by vesicles that enlarge; centers of lesions become pustular and/or hyperkeratotic, crusted (Fig. 14-46), i.e., resembling mollusk shells, mainly on palms and soles. Scaling erythematous, psoriasiform plaques on scalp, elbows, and buttocks. Erosive patches resembling pustular psoriasis may occur, especially on shaft of penis, scrotum. *Circinate balanitis* (Fig. 14-47): shallow erosions with serpiginous, micropustular borders if uncircumcised; crusted and/or hyperkeratotic plaques if circumcised, i.e., psoriasiform.
Nails   Small subungual pustules; → onycholysis and subungual hyperkeratosis.
Mucous Membranes   *Urethra*   Sterile serous or mucopurulent discharge.
Mouth   Erosive lesions on tongue or hard palate, resembling migratory glossitis.
Eyes   Conjunctivitis, mild, evanescent, bilateral; anterior uveitis.
Systemic Findings   Arthritis: oligoarticular, asymmetric; most commonly knees, ankles, small joints of feet; diffuse swelling of fingers and toes, enthesitis. (See Section 3, psoriatic arthritis).

LABORATORY EXAMINATIONS

Hematology   Nonspecific findings: anemia, leukocytosis, thrombocytosis, elevated ESR.
Culture   Urethral culture negative for gonococcus, may be positive for *Chlamydia* or

FIGURE 14-46   Reactive arthritis: keratoderma blennorrhagicum   Red-to-brown papules, vesicles, and pustules with central erosion and characteristic crusting and peripheral scaling on the dorsolateral and plantar foot.

FIGURE 14-47   Reactive arthritis: balanitis circinata   Moist, well-demarcated erosions with a slightly raised micropustular circinate border on the glans penis.

Ureaplasma. Stool culture: may be positive for *Shigella, Yersinia,* and others.

Serology   ANA, rheumatoid factor negative. HIV serology.

Dermatopathology   Spongiosis, vesiculation; later, psoriasiform epidermal hyperplasia, spongiform pustules, parakeratosis. Perivascular neutrophilic infiltrate in superficial dermis; edema.

DIAGNOSIS AND DIFFERENTIAL DIAGNOSIS

Clinical findings: arthritis and skin lesions ruling out other spondylo- and reactive arthropathies: psoriasis vulgaris with psoriatic arthritis, disseminated gonococcal infection, SLE, ankylosing spondylitis, rheumatoid arthritis, gout, Behçet disease.

COURSE AND PROGNOSIS

Only 30% develop complete triad of arthritis, urethritis, conjunctivitis; 40% have only one manifestation, i.e., incomplete RA. Majority have self-limited course, with resolution in 3–12 months. RA may relapse over many years in 30%. Chronic deforming arthritis in 10 to 20%.

MANAGEMENT

Prior Infection   Role of antibiotic therapy unproven in altering course of postvenereal RA.

Cutaneous Manifestations   Similar to management of psoriasis (see Section 3). Balanitis: low-potency glucocorticoids. Palmar/plantar: potent glucocorticoid preparations, which are more effective under plastic occlusion. Extensive or refractory disease: systemic retinoids (acitretin, 0.5–1 mg/kg body weight), photo therapy, and PUVA. Anti-TNF agents.

Prevention of Articular Inflammation/Joint Deformity   Rest, nonsteroidal anti-inflammatory agents. Occasionally, phenylbutazone is indicated, methotrexate, acitretin. In HIV/AIDS, antiretroviral therapy may ameliorate RA.

SARCOIDOSIS   ICD-9 : 135 ∘ ICD-10 : D86

- A systemic granulomatous disease of unknown cause.
- Primarily affecting the lungs (bilateral lymphadenopathy, pulmonary infiltration).
- Skin: papules, translucent yellow-red with apple jelly appearance on diascopy; nodules and bluish-red plaques.
- Often localizes in scars.
- Histologically, noncaseating, "naked" granulomas.
- Erythema nodosum is the most common nonspecific lesion in the skin in early sarcoidosis; it suggests a good prognosis.

EPIDEMIOLOGY

Age of Onset   Under 40 years (range 12–70 years).
Sex   Equal incidence in males and females.
Race   All races. In the United States and South Africa, much more frequent in blacks. The disease occurs worldwide; frequent in Scandinavia.
Other Factors   Etiology unknown. The disease can occur in families.

CLINICAL MANIFESTATION

Onset of lesions: days (presenting as acute erythema nodosum) or months (presenting as asymptomatic sarcoidal papules or plaques on skin or pulmonary infiltrate discovered on routine chest radiography). Constitutional symptoms such as fever, fatigue, weight loss, arrhythmia.
Skin Lesions   Earliest lesions are skin-colored papules, occuring periorifically on the face. Brownish or purple infiltrated plaques that may be annular, polycyclic, serpiginous, and occur mainly on extremities, buttocks, and trunk (Fig. 14-48). Central clearing with slight atrophy may occur. Multiple scattered maculopapular or papular lesions, 0.5–1 cm, yellowish brown, or purple occur mainly on the face (Fig. 14-49) and extremities. Occasionally, nodules, firm, purple or brown, may arise on the face, trunk, or extremities, particularly hands (Fig. 14-51). *Lupus pernio*: diffuse, violaceous, soft doughy infiltrations on the nose, cheeks, or earlobes (Fig. 14-50). Swelling of individual digits (Fig. 14-51). Sarcoidosis tends to infiltrate old scars, which then exhibit translucent purple-red or yellowish papules or nodules. *Note*: On blanching with glass slide, all cutaneous lesions of sarcoidosis reveal "apple jelly"

semitranslucent yellowish brown color. On the scalp sarcoidosis may cause scarring alopecia (see Section 32).
Systems Review   Enlarged parotids, pulmonary infiltrates, cardiac dyspnea, neuropathy, uveitis, kidney stones. *Loefgren syndrome*: erythema nodosum, fever, arthralgias, acute bilateral hilar adenopathy. *Heerford (-Waldenström) syndrome*: fever, parotitis, uveitis, facial palsy.

LABORATORY EXAMINATIONS

Dermatopathology   Large islands of epithelioid cells with a few giant cells and lymphocytes (so-called naked tubercles). Asteroid bodies in large histiocytes; occasionally fibrinoid necrosis.
Skin Tests   Intracutaneous tests for recall antigens usually but not always negative.
Imaging   Systemic involvement is verified radiologically by gallium scan and transbronchial, liver, or lymph node biopsy. In 90% of patients: hilar lymphadenopathy, pulmonary infiltrate. Cystic lesions in phalangeal bones (osteitis cystica).
Blood Chemistry   Increased level of serum angiotensin-converting enzyme, hypergammaglobulinemia, hypercalcemia.

DIAGNOSIS

Lesional biopsy of skin or lymph nodes is the best criterion for diagnosis of sarcoidosis.

MANAGEMENT

Systemic Sarcoidosis   Systemic glucocorticoids for active ocular disease, active pulmonary disease, cardiac arrhythmia, CNS involvement, or hypercalcemia.

FIGURE 14-48 **Sarcoidosis: granulomatous lesions**   Multiple, circinate, confluent, firm, brownish-red, infil-trated plaques that show a tendency to resolve in the center. Thus, the annular and multicentric appearance. The lesions are diascopy positive, i.e., an "apple-jelly" tan-pink color remains in lesions after compression with glass.

FIGURE 14-49 **Sarcoidosis**   Brownish-to-purple papules coalescing to irregular plaques, occurring on nose of this woman who also had massive pulmonary involvement. Blanching with a glass slide reveals "apple-jelly" color in the lesions.

Cutaneous Sarcoidosis *Glucocorticoids*
Local: intralesional triamcinolone, 3 mg/mL, effective for small lesions. *Systemic*: glucocorticoids for widespread or disfiguring involvement.

Hydroxychloroquine 100 mg twice daily for widespread or disfiguring lesions refractory to intralesional triamcinolone. Only sometimes effective.

Methotrexate Low-dose for widespread skin and systemic involvement. Not always effective.

Anti-TNF-α Agents, including thalidomide, anecdotally effective.

FIGURE 14-50   Sarcoidosis This is the classic appearance of "lupus pernio" with violaceous, soft, doughy infiltrations on cheeks and nose, which is grossly enlarged.

FIGURE 14-51   Sarcoidosis Papular brownish to violaceous lesions on the dorsa of the hands of a 40-year-old woman who also had pulmonary involvement. Note swelling of the fourth digit of the left hand and of the fifth digit of the right hand.

ENDOCRINE, METABOLIC, NUTRITIONAL, AND GENETIC DISEASES

SKIN DISEASES IN PREGNANCY

- Normal skin changes associated with pregnancy are darkening of linea alba (linea nigra), melasma (see Section 13), striae distensae (Fig. 15-1).
- Pruritus occurring in pregnancy may be due to a flare of preexisting dermatosis or a pregnancy-specific dermatosis.

- Pregnancy-specific dermatoses associated with fetal risk are cholestasis in pregnancy, pustular psoriasis of pregnancy (impetigo herpetiformis), and pemphigoid gestationis.
- Pregnancy-specific dermatoses not associated with fetal risk are polymorphic eruption of pregnancy and prurigo gestationis.

CHOLESTASIS OF PREGNANCY (CP)   ICD-9 : 646.7 ○ ICD-10 : K83.1   ■ ◐

- Occurs in the third trimester.
- Leading symptoms: pruritus, either localized (palms) or generalized. Most severe during the night.
- Cutaneous lesions invariably absent, but excoriations in severe cases.

- Elevation of serum bile acids.
- Fetal risks include prematurity, intrapartal distress, and fetal death.
- Treatment: ursodeoxycholic acid, plasmapheresis.

PUSTULAR PSORIASIS IN PREGNANCY   ICD-9 : 696.7 ○ ICD-10 : L40.1   □ ●

- Previously called *impetigo herpetiformis*.
- Clinically and histopathologically indistinguishable from pustular psoriasis of von Zumbusch
- Burning, smarting, not itching.

- May have hypocalcemia and decreased vitamin D levels.
- See "Pustular Psoriasis," Section 3.

PEMPHIGOID GESTATIONIS   ICD-9 : 646.8 ○ ICD-10 : O26.4   □ ●

Pemphigoid gestationis (PG) is a pruritic polymorphic inflammatory dermatosis of pregnancy and the postpartum period. It is an autoimmune process with circulating complement-fixing IgG antibodies in the serum. The condition is described in Section 6.

FIGURE 15-1   **Striae distensae in a pregnant woman (36 weeks of gestation)**

POLYMORPHIC ERUPTION OF PREGNANCY (PEP) ICD-9:709.8

- PEP is a distinct pruritic eruption of pregnancy that usually begins in the third trimester, most often in primigravidae (76%).
- There is no increased risk of fetal morbidity or mortality.
- The disease is common, estimated to be 1 in 120 to 240 pregnancies.
- The etiology and pathogenesis are not understood.
- Average time of onset is 36 weeks of gestation, usually 1–2 weeks before delivery. However, *symptoms and signs can start in the postpartum period.*
- Pruritus develops on the abdomen, often in the striae distensae, and is severe enough to disrupt sleep. *Skin lesions* consist of erythematous papules, 1–3 mm, quickly coalescing into urticarial plaques (Fig. 15-2) with polycyclic shape and arrangement; blanched halos around the periphery of lesions. Tiny vesicles, 2 mm, may occur in the plaques, but bullae are absent. Target lesions are observed in 19%. Although pruritus is the chief symptom, excoriations are infrequent. 50% of the women affected have papules and plaques in the striae distensae; the abdomen, buttocks,

thighs (Fig. 15-2), upper inner arms, and lower back may also be affected.
- The face, breasts, palms, and soles are rarely involved. The periumbilical area is usually spared. There are no mucous membrane lesions.
- Differential diagnosis includes all pruritic abdominal rashes in pregnancy: pemphigoid gestationis, adverse cutaneous drug reaction, allergic contact dermatitis, metabolic pruritus, atopic dermatitis.
- *Laboratory findings* are noncontributory, as are histopathology and immunohistopathology.
- The majority of women do not have a recurrence in the postpartum period, with subsequent pregnancies, or with the use of oral contraceptives. If a recurrence occurs, it is usually much milder
- Management consists of high-potency topical steroids that often can be tapered off after 1 week of therapy. Oral prednisone in doses of 10–40 mg/d has been used for severe cases; often the symptoms are relieved in 24 h. Oral antihistamines are generally ineffective.

Synonyms: Polymorphic eruption of pregnancy, toxemic rash of pregnancy, late-onset prurigo of pregnancy.

PRURIGO OF PREGNANCY AND ATOPIC ERUPTION OF PREGNANCY ICD-9:698-2]].782.1

- Prurigo of pregnancy is now reclassified as part of the *atopic eruption of pregnancy* (AEP) spectrum.[1]
- Very common.
- AEP consist of flares of atopic dermatitis (also in patients who previously did not have AD); present

either with eczematous or prurigo lesions (see Section 2).
- The cardinal symptom is pruritus (the algorithm on page 423 represents an approach to the pregnant patient with pruritus).

[1]CM Ambros-Rudolph et al. J Am Acad Dermatol 54:395, 2006.

FIGURE 15-2 **Polymorphic eruption of pregnancy [previously called pruritic urticarial papules and plaques of pregnancy (PUPPP)]** Urticarial papules are present on both thighs where they coalesce to urticarial plaques. Similar papules and urticarial lesions are present within striae distensae on the abdomen of this pregnant woman at 35 weeks of gestation. Lesions were extremely pruritic, causing sleepless nights and great stress, yet there are no excoriations.

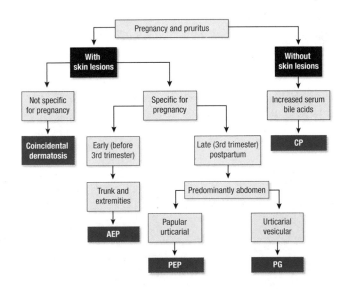

Algorithm of approach to patient with pruritus

SKIN MANIFESTATIONS OF OBESITY[2]

- Obesity is widely recognized as an epidemic in the Western world.
- Obesity is responsible for changes in skin barrier function, sebaceous glands and sebum production, sweat glands, lymphatics, collagen structure and function, wound healing, micro- and macro-circulation, and subcutaneous fat.
- Obesity is implicated in a wide spectrum of dermatologic diseases, including *acanthosis nigricans* (Section 5), acrochordons, keratosis pilaris (Section 4), *hyperandrogenism and hirsutism* (Section 32), *striae distensae, adipositas dolorosa* and fat redistribution, lymphedema (Section 16), *chronic venous insufficiency,* and *plantar hyperkeratosis* (Section 4).
- *Cellulitis, skin infections* (Section 24), *hidradenitis suppurativa* (Section 1), *psoriasis* (Section 3), *insulin resistance syndrome,* and *tophaceous gout* (p. 446).

DIABETES MELLITUS

SKIN DISEASES ASSOCIATED WITH DIABETES MELLITUS[3]

ACANTHOSIS NIGRICANS (p. 88) AND LIPODYSTROPHY[4]

Associated with insulin resistance in diabetes mellitus. Insulin-like epidermal growth factors may cause epidermal hyperplasia.

ADVERSE CUTANEOUS DRUG REACTIONS IN DIABETES (see Section 22)

Insulin: local reactions—lipodystrophy with decreased adipose tissue at sites of subcutaneous injection; Arthus-like reaction with urticarial lesion at site of injection.
Systemic insulin allergy: Urticaria, serum sickness–like reactions.
Oral hypoglycemic agents: Exanthematous eruptions, urticaria, erythema multiforme, photosensitivity.

CALCIPHYLAXIS (see Section 17, p. 482)

CUTANEOUS PERFORATING DISORDERS[4]

Rare conditions in which horny plugs perforate into the dermis or dermal debris is eliminated through the epidermis. Not always associated with diabetes (see Section 17).

DIABETIC BULLAE (Bullosis diabeticorum) (p. 425)

DIABETIC DERMOPATHY (p. 427)

ERUPTIVE XANTHOMAS (p. 438)

GRANULOMA ANNULARE (p. 134)

INFECTIONS (see Sections 24 and 25)

Poorly controlled diabetes associated with increased incidence of primary (furuncles, carbuncles) and secondary *Staphylococcus aureus* infections (paronychia, wound/ulcer infection), cellulitis (*S. aureus*, group A streptococcus), erythrasma, dermatophytoses (tinea pedis, onychomycosis), candidiasis (mucosal and cutaneous), mucormycosis with necrotizing nasopharyngeal infections.

NECROBIOSIS LIPOIDICA (p. 428)

PERIPHERAL NEUROPATHY (Diabetic foot) (p. 426)

PERIPHERAL VASCULAR DISEASE (see Section 16)

Small-vessel vasculopathy (microangiopathy): Involves arterioles, venules, and capillaries. Characterized by basement membrane thickening and endothelial cell proliferation. Presents clinically as acral erysipelas-like erythema, ± ulceration.

Large-vessel vasculopathy: Incidence greatly increased in diabetes. Ischemia is most often symptomatic on lower legs and feet with gangrene and ulceration. Predisposes to infections.

SCLEREDEMA DIABETICORUM[4]

Synonym: Scleredema adultorum of Buschke. Need not be associated with diabetes. Onset correlates with duration of diabetes and with presence of microangiopathy. Skin findings: poorly demarcated scleroderma-like induration of the skin and subcutaneous tissue of the upper back, neck, proximal extremities. Rapid onset and progression.

Scleroderma-Like Syndrome[4] Scleroderma-like thickening of skin and limited joint mobility ("prayer sign").

DIABETIC BULLAE   □ ◑

- Large, intact bullae arise spontaneously on the lower legs, feet, dorsa of the hands, and fingers on noninflamed bases (Fig. 15-3).
- When ruptured, oozing bright red erosions result but heal after several weeks.
- Localization on dorsa of hand and fingers suggests porphyria cutanea tarda, but abnormalities of porphyrin metabolism are not found.

- Neither trauma nor an immunologic mechanism has been implicated. Histologically, bullae show intra- or subepidermal clefting without acantholysis. ℮

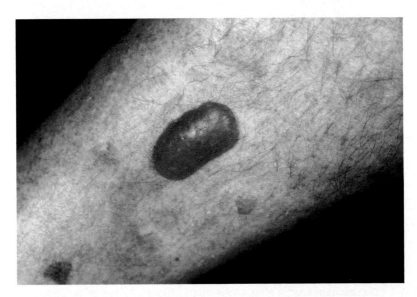

FIGURE 15-3   Diabetic bulla   A large, intact bulla is seen on the pretibial skin on the right lower leg. The patient had many of the vascular complications of diabetes mellitus, i.e., renal failure, retinopathy, and atherosclerosis obliterans resulting in amputation of the the left big toe.

"DIABETIC FOOT" AND DIABETIC NEUROPATHY   ICD-9:713.5 ∘ ICD-10:G63.2   ■ ◑

- Peripheral neuropathy is responsible for the "diabetic foot."

- Other factors are angiopathy, atherosclerosis, and infection and most often they are combined.

- Diabetic neuropathy is combined motor and sensory. Motor neuropathy leads to weakness and muscle wasting distally.

- Autonomic neuropathy accompanies sensory neuropathy and leads to anhidrosis, which may not be confined to the distal extremities.

- Sensory neuropathy predisposes to neurotropic ulcers over bony prominences of feet, usually on the great toe and sole as shown (Fig. 15-4).

- Ulcers are surrounded by a ring of callus and may extend to interlying joint and bone, leading to osteomyelitis. ⊘

FIGURE 15-4   Diabetic, neuropathic ulcer on the sole   A large ulcer overlying the second left metacarpophalangeal joint. The patient, a 60-year-old male with diabetes mellitus of 25 years' duration, has significant sensory neuropathy of the feet and lower legs as well as peripheral vascular disease, which resulted in the amputation of the fourth and fifth toes.

DIABETIC DERMOPATHY

- Circumscribed, atrophic, slightly depressed lesions on the anterior lower legs that are asymptomatic (Fig. 15-5).
- They arise in crops and gradually resolve, but new lesions appear and occasionally may ulcerate.

- The pathogenic significance of diabetic dermopathy remains to be established, but it is often accompanied by microangiopathy.

FIGURE 15-5 **Diabetic dermopathy** A crusted erosion at the site of traumatic injury and many old pink depressed areas and scars are seen on the anterior leg of a 56-year-old male with diabetes mellitus. The other leg had identical findings.

- Necrobiosis lipoidica (NL) is a cutaneous disorder often, but not always, associated with diabetes mellitus.
- The lesions are distinctive, sharply circumscribed, multicolored plaques occurring on the anterior and lateral surfaces of the lower legs.
- Lesions may ulcerate.

EPIDEMIOLOGY AND ETIOLOGY

Age of Onset   Young adults, early middle age, but not uncommon in juvenile diabetics.

Sex   Female: male ratio 3:1 in both diabetic and nondiabetic forms.

Incidence   From 0.3–3% of diabetic individuals. NL may occur in individuals without manifest diabetes. *Relationship to diabetes*: One-third of patients have clinical diabetes, one-third have abnormal glucose tolerance only, one-third have normal glucose tolerance.

Etiology   Unknown.

Precipitating Factors   A history of preceding trauma to the site can be a factor in the initial development of the lesions.

PATHOGENESIS

The arteriolar changes in the areas of necrobiosis of the collagen have been thought by some to be precipitated by aggregation of platelets. The granulomatous inflammatory reaction is believed to be due to alterations in the collagen. The severity of NL is not related to the severity of diabetes. Furthermore, control of the diabetes has no effect on the course of NL.

CLINICAL MANIFESTATION

Slowly evolving and enlarging over months, persisting for years. Cosmetic disfigurement; pain in lesions that develop ulcers.

Skin Lesions   Lesion starts as brownish-red or skin-colored papule that slowly evolves into a well-demarcated waxy plaque of variable size (Fig. 15-6A). The sharply defined and slightly elevated border retains a brownish-red color, whereas the center becomes depressed and acquires a yellow-orange hue. Through the shiny and atrophic epidermis, multiple telangiectasias of variable size are seen. Larger lesions formed by centrifugal enlargement or merging of smaller lesions acquire a serpiginous or polycyclic configuration. Ulceration may occur within the plaques (Fig. 15-6B), and healed ulcers result in depressed scars. Burned-out lesions appear as tan areas with telangiectasia.

Distribution   Usually 1 to 3 lesions; >80% occur on the shin; at times symmetric. Less commonly, on feet, arms, trunk, or face and scalp; rarely may be generalized. 🔖

LABORATORY EXAMINATIONS

Dermatopathology   Sclerosis, obliteration of the bundle pattern of collagen → necrobiosis, surrounded by concomitant granulomatous infiltration in lower dermis. Fat-containing foam cells are often present, imparting the yellow color to the clinical lesion. Dermal blood vessels show microangiopathy with endothelial thickening and focal deposits of PAS-positive material. Presence of immunoglobulins and complement (C3) in the walls of the small blood vessels.

Chemistry   Abnormal glucose tolerance test in two-thirds of patients.

DIAGNOSIS AND DIFFERENTIAL DIAGNOSIS

The lesions are so distinctive that biopsy confirmation is not necessary; however, biopsy may be required in early stages to rule out granuloma annulare (which frequently coexists with NL), sarcoidosis, or xanthoma.

COURSE AND PROGNOSIS

The lesions are indolent and can enlarge to involve large areas of the skin surface unless treated. The lesions are unsightly, and patients are often upset about the cosmetic appearance. Ulcerated areas within NL are painful.

A   *B*

FIGURE 15-6   Necrobiosis lipoidica diabeticorum   *A.* A large, symmetric plaque with active tan-pink, yellow, well-demarcated, raised, firm border and a yellow center in the pretibial region of a 28-year-old diabetic female. The central parts of the lesion are depressed with atrophic changes of epidermal thinning and telangiectasis against yellow background. ***B.*** Late lesion after healed ulceration. A very extensive plaque of necrobiosis lipoidica on the lower leg of a diabetic female. Apart from the features of necrobiosis lipoidica there is extensive scarring and atrophic depressed scars.

MANAGEMENT

Glucocorticoids *Topical* The application of potent glucocorticoids under occlusion is helpful in some cases; however, ulcerations may occur when NL is occluded.
Intralesional Intralesional triamcinolone, 5 mg/mL, into active lesions or lesion margins usually arrests extension of plaques of NL. This is the best treatment, with 3–5 mg/mL triamcinolone suspension.
Ulceration Most ulcerations within NL lesions heal with local wound care; if not, excision of entire lesion with grafting may be required.

CUSHING SYNDROME AND HYPERCORTICISM
ICD-9 : 255.0 ∘ ICD-10 : E24

- Cushing syndrome (CS) is characterized by truncal obesity, moon face, abdominal striae, hypertension, decreased carbohydrate tolerance, protein catabolism, psychiatric disturbances, and amenorrhea and hirsutism in females.

- It is associated with excess adrenocorticosteroids of endogenous or exogenous source.

- *Cushing disease* refers to CS associated with pituitary adrenocorticotropic hormone (ACTH)-producing adenoma.

- *CS medicamentosum* refers to CS caused by exogenous administration of glucocorticoids.

- Skin lesions: A plethoric obese person with a "classic" habitus that results from the redistribution of fat: moon facies (Fig. 15-7), "buffalo" hump, truncal obesity, and thin arms.

- Purple striae, mostly on the abdomen and trunk; atrophic skin with easy bruising and telangiectasia.

- Facial hypertrichosis with pigmented hairs and often increased lanugo hairs on the face and arms; androgenetic alopecia in females.

- Acne of recent onset (without comedones) or flaring of existing acne.

- General symptoms consist of fatigue and muscle weakness, hypertension, personality changes, amenorrhea in females, polyuria, and polydipsia.

- Workup includes determination of blood glucose, serum potassium, and free cortisol in 24-h urine. Abnormal dexamethasone suppression test with failure to suppress endogenous cortisol secretion when dexamethasone is administered. Elevated ACTH.

- CT scan of the abdomen and the pituitary. Assessment of osteoporosis.

- Management consists of elimination of exogenous glucocorticoids or the detection and correction of underlying endogenous cause. ℰ

FIGURE 15-7   Cushing syndrome   Plethoric moon facies with erythema and telangiectases of cheeks and forehead; the face and neck and supraclavicular areas (not depicted here) show increased deposition of fat.

GRAVES DISEASE AND HYPERTHYROIDISM
ICD-9 : 242.0 ∘ ICD-10 : E05.0

- Graves disease (GD) is a disorder with three major manifestations: hyperthyroidism with diffuse goiter, ophthalmopathy, and dermopathy.

- The manifestations often do not occur together, may not occur at all, and run courses that are independent of each other.

- *Dermopathy (pretibial myxedema)*: Early lesions: bilateral, asymmetric, firm, nonpitting nodules and plaques that are pink, skin-colored, or purple (Fig. 15-8C). Late lesions: confluence of early lesions, which symmetrically involve the pretibial regions and may, in extreme cases, result in grotesque involvement of entire lower legs and dorsa of feet; smooth surface with orange peel–like appearance, later becomes verrucous (Fig. 15-8C). *Note*: dermopathy may also occur *after* treatment of hyperthyroidism.

- *Fingers*: Fingers show acropachy, which represents diaphyseal proliferation of the periosteum and clubbing (Fig. 15-8B).

- *Ophthalmopathy*: GD ophthalmopathy has two components, spastic (stare, lid lag, lid retraction) and mechanical [proptosis (Fig. 15-8A), ophthalmoplegia, congestive oculopathy, chemosis, conjuctivitis, periorbital swelling, and potential complications of corneal ulceration, optic neuritis, optic atrophy]. Exophthalmic ophthalmoplegia: ocular muscle weakness with inward gaze, convergence, strabismus, diplopia.

- *Thyroid*: Diffuse toxic goiter, asymmetric, lobular. Asymmetric and lobular thyroid enlargement, often with the presence of a bruit.

- Management: *Thyrotoxicosis*: Antithyroid agents block thyroid hormone synthesis. Ablation of thyroid tissue, surgically or by radioactive iodine. *Ophthalmopathy*: Symptomatic treatment in mild cases. Severe cases: prednisone 100–120 mg/d initially, tapering to 5 mg/d. Orbital radiation. Orbital decompression. *Dermopathy*: Topical glucocorticoid preparations under plastic occlusion for several months are usually effective. Low-dose oral glucocorticoids (prednisone, 5 mg/d). Intralesional triamcinolone 3–5 mg/mL for smaller lesions.

HYPOTHYROIDISM AND MYXEDEMA
ICD-9 : 244.0-244.9 ∘ ICD-10 : E03.9

- Myxedema results from insufficient production of thyroid hormones and can be caused by multiple disturbances.

- Hypothyroidism may be *thyroprivic* (e.g., congenital, primary idiopathic, postablative); *goitrous* (e.g., heritable biosynthetic defects, maternally transmitted, iodine deficiency, drug-induced or chronic thyroiditis); *trophoprivic* (e.g., pituitary); or *hypothalamic* [e.g., infection (encephalitis), neoplasm].

- Early symptoms of *myxedema* are often overlooked: fatigue, lethargy, cold intolerance, constipation, stiffness and cramping of muscles, carpal tunnel syndrome, menorrhagia; slowing of intellectual and motor activity, decline in appetite, increase in weight, and deepening of voice.

- There is a dull, expressionless facies (Fig. 15-9), with puffiness of eyelids. Skin appears swollen, cool, waxy, dry, coarse, and pale with increased skin creases (Fig. 15-9).

- Palms and soles are yellow-orange due to carotenemia.

- The hair is dry, coarse, and brittle. Thinning of the scalp, beard (Fig. 15-9), and sexual areas. Eyebrows: alopecia of the lateral one-third.

- Nails brittle and slow growing.

- Large, smooth, red, and clumsy tongue.

- Workup includes thyroid function tests, thyroid-stimulating hormone (TSH), scintigraphic imaging, and serum cholesterol ($\uparrow$).

- Management is by replacement therapy.

FIGURE 15-8   Graves disease   _A._ Proptosis, lid retraction, and telangiectasia and hemorrhage in the bulbar conjunctiva. **_B._** Thyroid acropachy (osteoarthropathy) with clubbing. **_C._** The pink- and skin-colored papules, nodules and plaques in the pretibial region are called dermopathy (pretibial myxedema).

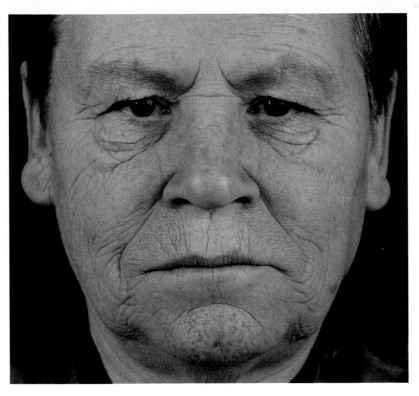

FIGURE 15-9   Myxedema   Dry, pale skin; thinning of the lateral eyebrows; puffiness of the face and eyelids; increased number of skin creases; dull, expressionless, beardless facies.

ADDISON DISEASE   ICD-9 : 255.41 ○ ICD-10 : E27.1   □ ◑

- Addison disease is a syndrome resulting from adrenocortical insufficiency.

- It is insidious and is characterized by progressive generalized brown hyperpigmentation, slowly progressive weakness, fatigue, anorexia, nausea, and, frequently, GI symptoms (vomiting and diarrhea).

- Suggestive laboratory changes include low serum sodium, high serum potassium, and elevation of the blood urea nitrogen. The diagnosis is confirmed by specific tests of adrenal insufficiency.

- Skin: the patient may appear completely normal except for a generalized brown hyperpigmentation: (1) in areas where pigmentation normally occurs either habitually or UV-induced: around the eyes, face, dorsa of hands (Fig. 15-10), nipples, in the linea nigra (abdomen), axillae, and anogenital areas in males and females (the intensity of the pigmentation is related to skin phototype); and (2) in new areas: gingival or buccal mucosa, creases of palms (Fig. 15-10B), bony prominences. Also in new scars following surgery.

- The differential diagnosis includes hemochromatosis; porphyria cutanea tarda; chronic renal failure; hepatic cirrhosis; benign endocrine tumors, such as chromophobe adenomas that produce ACTH and associated peptides [i.e., Nelson syndrome, metastatic cancers (especially lung), carcinoid]; vitamin B_{12} deficiency; chemotherapy (doxorubicin, busulfan, bleomycin, 5-fluorouracil); and systemic scleroderma.

- A screening test used for diagnosis is plasma cortisol 30–60 min after 250 μg cosyntropin intramuscularly or intravenously.

- This disease should be managed by an endocrinologist.

A   *B*

FIGURE 15-10   Addison disease   *A.* Hyperpigmentation representing an accentuation of normal pigmentation of the hand of a patient with Addison disease. ***B.*** Note accentuated pigmentation in the palmar creases.

METABOLIC AND NUTRITIONAL CONDITIONS

XANTHOMAS   ICD-9 : 272.2 ∘ ICD-10 : E78.5

- Cutaneous xanthomas are yellow-brown, pinkish, or orange macules, papules, plaques, nodules, or infiltrations in tendons.

- Histologically there are accumulations of xanthoma cells—macrophages containing droplets of lipids.

- Xanthomas may be symptoms of a general metabolic disease, a generalized histiocytosis, or a local fat phagocytosing storage process.

- The classification of metabolic xanthomas is based on this principle: (1) xanthomas due to hyperlipidemia and (2) normolipidemic xanthomas.

- The cause of xanthomas in the first group may be a primary hyperlipidemia, mostly genetically determined (Table 15-1), or secondary hyperlipidemia, associated with certain internal diseases such as biliary cirrhosis, diabetes mellitus, chronic renal failure, alcoholism, hyperthyroidism, and monoclonal gammopathy, or with intake of certain drugs such as beta-blockers and estrogens.

- Some of the xanthomas are associated with high plasma low-density lipoprotein (LDL)-cholesterol levels, and therefore with a serious risk of atheromatosis and myocardial infarction. For that reason laboratory investigation of plasma lipid levels is always necessary. In some cases an apoprotein deficiency is present.

- Table 15-2 shows correlations of clinical xanthoma type and lipoprotein disturbances.

TABLE 15-1 Classification of Genetic Hyperlipidemias

Frederickson Type	Classification	Lipid Profile
I	Familial lipoprotein lipase deficiency (hyperchylomicronemia, hypertriglyceridemia) (FLD)	TG++, C normal, CM++, HDL −/normal
IIa	Familial hypercholesterolemia (FH)	TG normal, C+, LDL+
IIb	Familial combined hyperlipidemia (FCHL)	TG+, C+, LDL+, VLDL+
III	Familial dysbetalipidemia (remnant particle disease) (FD)	TG+, C+, IDL+, CM remnants+
IV	Familial hypertriglyceridemia (FHTG)	TG+, C normal/+, LDL++, VLDL++
V	Familial combined hypertriglyceridemia (FHT)	TG+, C+, VLDL++, CM++

NOTE: TG, triglycerides; C, cholesterol; CM, chylomicrons; HDL, high-density lipoproteins; LDL, low-density lipoproteins; VLDL, very low-density lipoproteins; IDL, intermediate-density lipoproteins; +, raised; −, lowered.

TABLE 15-2 Clinical Presentations of Xanthomas

Type of Xanthoma	Genetic Disorders	Secondary Disorders
Eruptive	Familial lipoprotein lipase deficiency (type I)	Obesity
	Apo-C2 deficiency (type I)	Cholestasis
	Familial hypertriglyceridemia (type IV)	Diabetes
	Familial hypertriglyceridemia with chylomicronemia (type V)	Medications: Retinoids, estrogen therapy, protease inhibitors
Tuberous	Familial hypercholesterolemia (type II)	Monoclonal gammopathies
	Familial dysbetalipoproteinemia (type III)	
	Phytosterolemia	
Tendinous	Familial hypercholesterolemia (type II)	
	Familial defective apo-B	
	Familial dysbetalipoproteinemia (type III)	
	Phytosterolemia	
	Cerebrotendinous xanthomatosis	
Planar		
Palmar	Familial dysbetalipoproteinemia (type III)	
intertriginous	Familial homozygous hypercholesterolemia (type II)	Cholestasis
Diffuse		Monoclonal gammopathies, cholestasis
Xanthelasma	Familial hypercholesterolemia (type II)	Monoclonal gammopathies
	Familial dysbetalipoproteinemia (type III)	
Other		
Corneal arcus	Familial hypercholesterolemia (type II)	
Tonsillar	Tangier disease	

apo = apolipoprotein.

Source: LE White: Xanthomas and lipoprotein disorders, in K Wolff et. al. (eds): *Fitzpatrick's Dermatology in General Medicine*, 7th ed. New York, McGraw-Hill, 2008, P. 1272.

XANTHELASMA   ICD-9:374.51 ○ ICD-10:H02.6   ■ ○

- Most common of all xanthomas. In most cases an isolated finding unrelated to hyperlipidemia.
- Occurs in individuals >50 years; however, when in children or young adults, it is associated with familial hypercholesterolemia (FH) or familial dysbetalipoproteinemia (FD).
- Skin lesions are asymptomatic. Soft, polygonal yellow-orange papules and plaques localized to upper and lower eyelids (Fig. 15-11) and around inner canthus. Slow enlargement from tiny spots over months to years.

- Cholesterol should be estimated in plasma; if enhanced, screening for type of hyperlipidemia (FH or FD). If due to hyperlipidemia, complication with atherosclerotic cardiovascular disease may be expected.
- Laser, excision, electrodesiccation, or topical application of trichloroacetic acid. Recurrences are not uncommon.

Synonyms: Xanthelasma palpebrarum, periocular xanthoma. ⮩

XANTHOMA TENDINEUM   ICD-9:272.2   □ ◐

- These subcutaneous tumors are yellow or skin-colored and move with the extensor tendons (Fig. 15-12).
- They are a symptom of familial hypercholesterolemia (FH) that presents as type IIa hyperlipidemia.
- This condition is autosomal recessive with a different phenotype in the heterozygote and homozygote.
- In the homozygote, the xanthomata appear in early childhood and the cardiovascular complica-

tions in early adolescence; the elevation of the LDL content of the plasma is extreme. These patients rarely attain ages above 20 years.
- *Management*: A diet low in cholesterol and saturated fats, supplemented by cholestyramine or statins. In extreme cases, measures such as portacaval shunt or liver transplantation have to be considered.

Synonym: Tendinous xanthoma. ⮩

XANTHOMA TUBEROSUM   ICD-9:374.51 ○ ICD-10:E78.2   ◧ ◐

- This condition comprises yellowish nodules (Fig. 15-13) located especially on the elbows and knees by confluence of concomitant eruptive xanthomas.
- They are to be found in patients with FD, familial hypertriglyceridemia with chylomicronemia (type V) and FH (Table 15-2).

- In homozygous patients with FH, the tuberous xanthomas are flatter and skin colored. They are not accompanied by eruptive xanthomas.
- *Management*: Treatment of the underlying condition.

Synonym: Tuberous xanthoma. ⮩

FIGURE 15-13   Tuberous xanthoma   (Across facing page) Flat-topped, yellow, firm nodule with an erythematous margin.

FIGURE 15-11   Xanthelasma
Multiple creamy-orange, slightly elevated dermal papules on the eyelids of a normolipemic individual.

FIGURE 15-12   Tendinous xanthoma   Large subcutaneous tumor adherent to the Achilles tendon.

FIGURE 15-13

ERUPTIVE XANTHOMA ICD-9 : 272.2 ○ ICD-10 : E78.2

- These discrete inflammatory-type papules "erupt" suddenly and in showers, appearing typically on the buttocks, elbows, lower arms (Fig. 15-14) and knees.

- A sign of FHT, FD, the very rare familial lipoprotein lipase deficiency (FLD) (Table 15-2), and diabetes out of control.

- Papules are dome-shaped, discrete, initially red, then yellow center with red halo (Fig. 15-14).

- Lesions may be scattered, discrete, in a localized region [e.g., elbows, knees (Fig. 15-14), buttocks] or appear as "tight" clusters that become confluent to form nodular "tuberoeruptive" xanthomas.

- *Management*: React very favorably to a low-calorie and low-fat diet. ℮

A **B**

FIGURE 15-14 Papular eruptive xanthomas *A.* Multiple, discrete, red-to-yellow papules becoming confluent on the knees of an individual with uncontrolled diabetes mellitus; lesions were present on both elbows and buttocks. ***B.*** Higher magnification of xanthomas on the trunk of another patient.

XANTHOMA STRIATUM PALMARE

- This condition is characterized by yellow-orange, flat or elevated infiltrations of the volar creases of palms and fingers (Fig. 15-15).

- Pathognomonic for FD (type III) (Table 15-2). Next to xanthoma striatum palmare, FD also presents with tuberous xanthoma (Fig. 15-13) and xanthelasma palpebrarum (Fig. 15-11).

- Patients with FD are prone to atherosclerotic cardiovascular disease, especially ischemia of the legs and coronary vessels.

- *Management*: Patients with FD react very favorably to a diet low in fats and carbohydrates. If necessary, this may be supplemented with statins, fibrates, or nicotinic acid. ℮

FIGURE 15-15   Xanthoma striatum palmare   The palmar creases are yellow, often a subtle lesion noticeable only upon close examination.

NORMOLIPEMIC PLANE XANTHOMA   □ ●

- Xanthoma planum is a normolipemic xanthoma that consists of diffuse orange-yellow pigmentation and slight elevations of the skin (Fig. 15-16). There is a recognizable border.
- These lesions can be idiopathic or secondary to

leukemia, but the most common association is with multiple myeloma.
- The lesions may precede the onset of multiple myeloma by many years.

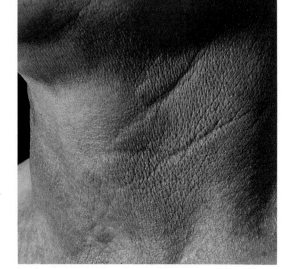

FIGURE 15-16   Plane xanthoma   Yellowish-red, slightly elevated plaques on the neck, noticeable mainly because of the accentuation of the skin texture in a normolipemic patient with lymphoma. Plane xanthomas occur most commonly on the upper trunk and neck and also occur in individuals with myeloma.

SCURVY   ICD-9 : 267 ∘ ICD-10 : E54   □ ●

- Scurvy is an acute or chronic disease of infancy and of middle and old age caused by dietary deficiency of ascorbic acid (vitamin C).
- Humans are unable to synthesize ascorbic acid and require it as an essential dietary vitamin. Total-body pool of vitamin C varies from 1.5–3 g. First symptoms of depletion occur when pool size is <0.5 g. Deficiency of vitamin C leads to impairment of peptidyl hydroxylation of procollagen, reduction in collagen formation with associated capillary fragility.
- Scurvy occurs in infants or children on a diet consisting of only processed milk with no added citrus fruit or vegetables as a result of parental neglect; or in edentulous adult persons who live alone, and do not eat salads and uncooked vegetables.
- *Precipitating factors*: Pregnancy, lactation, and thyrotoxicosis when there are increased requirements of ascorbic acid; most common in alcoholism.
- With no vitamin C intake, symptoms of scurvy occur after 1–3 months. Lassitude, weakness, arthralgia, and myalgia.
- *Skin lesions*: Petechiae, follicular hyperkeratosis with perifollicular hemorrhage, especially on the lower legs (Fig. 15-17*A*). Hair becomes fragmented and buried in these perifolliculár hyperkeratotic papules (corkscrew hairs); also, extensive ecchymoses (Fig. 15-17*B*), which can be generalized. Nails: splinter hemorrhages.

- Gingiva: swollen, purple, spongy, and bleeds easily; findings occur in more advanced scurvy. Loosening and loss of teeth.
- Hemorrhage occurring into periosteum of long bones and into joints causes painful swellings and, in children, epiphyseal separation. Sternum may sink inward: scorbutic rosary (elevation at rib margins).
- Retrobulbar, subarachnoid, intracerebral hemorrhage can cause death.
- *Differential diagnosis*: Includes thrombocytopenia, senile purpura, coagulopathy, anticoagulant drug therapy (warfarin, heparin), cryoglobulinemia, vasculitis and gingival hypertrophy due to poor dental hygiene, drug-induced gingival hyperplasia, leukemia, pregnancy.
- *Laboratory*: Normocytic, normochromic anemia. Folate deficiency, resulting in macrocytic anemia. Positive capillary fragility test. Platelet ascorbic acid level usually <25% of normal value; serum ascorbic acid level zero. X-ray findings are diagnostic.
- Unless treated, scurvy is fatal. On treatment, spontaneous bleeding ceases within 24 h, muscle and bone pain fade quickly, bleeding from gums stops in 2–3 days.
- *Management*: Ascorbic acid 100 mg 3–5 times daily until 4 g is given; then 100 mg/d is curative in days to weeks.

A *B*

FIGURE 15-17 **Scurvy** *A.* Perifollicular purpura on the leg. The follicles are often plugged by keratin (perifollicular hyperkeratosis). This eruption occurred in a 46-year-old alcoholic, homeless male, who also had bleeding gums and loose teeth. *B.* These extensive ecchymoses occurred in an edentulous 65-year-old male who lived alone and whose food intake consisted mainly of biscuits soaked in water.

ZINC DEFICIENCY AND ACRODERMATITIS ENTEROPATHICA ICD-9:269.9 ∘ ICD-10:E60 ☐ ●

- Acrodermatitis enteropathica (AE) is a genetic disorder of zinc absorption, presenting in infancy, characterized by a triad of acral dermatitis (face, hands, feet, anogenital area), alopecia, and diarrhea. (Fig. 15-18)

- Nearly identical clinical findings occur in older individuals with acquired zinc deficiency (AZD) due either to dietary deficiency or failure of intestinal absorption (Fig. 15-19).

- *AE* occurs in infants bottle-fed with bovine milk, days to few weeks. In breast-fed infants, soon after weaning. *AZD* in older individuals.

- Etiology: *AE*: autosomal recessive trait resulting in failure to absorb zinc. *AZD*: secondary to reduced dietary intake of zinc, malabsorption (regional enteritis, after intestinal bypass surgery for obesity), chronic alcoholism, increased urinary loss (nephrotic syndrome), hypoalbuminemic states, penicillamine therapy, high catabolic states (trauma, burns, surgery), hemolytic anemias; adolescents who eat dirt, prolonged parenteral nutrition without supplemental zinc.

- *Pathogenesis*: In AE, patients do not absorb enough zinc from the diet. The specific ligand involved in basic transport mechanisms for zinc that might be abnormal in AE is not known. The defect appears to be somewhere in the early stages of zinc nutriture, where zinc is presented to the intestinal brush border. This defect can be overcome by increased zinc supply in the diet. It is not known how zinc deficiency leads to skin and other lesions.

- *Skin Findings*: Patches and plaques of dry, scaly, sharply marginated and brightly red, eczematous dermatitis evolving into vesiculobullous, pustular, erosive, and crusted lesions (Figs. 15-18, and 15-19). Initially occur in the perioral and anogenital areas. Later, scalp, hands and feet, flexural regions, trunk. Fingertips glistening, erythematous, with fissures and secondary paronychia. Perlèche. Lesions become secondarily infected with *Candida albicans*, *S. aureus*. Impaired wound healing.
  - *Hair and nails:* Diffuse alopecia, graying of hair. Paronychia, nail ridging, loss of nails.
  - *Mucous membranes:* Red, glossy tongue; superficial aphthous-like erosions; secondary oral candidiasis.

- *General examination*: Photophobia; irritable, depressed mood. Children with AE whine and cry constantly. Failure of growth.

- *Laboratory*: Anemia, low serum/plasma zinc levels; reduced urinary zinc excretion.
  - *Dermatopathology:* Psoriasiform dermatitis with large, pale keratinocytes in the upper epidermis; prominent parakeratosis. There may be intraepidermal clefts with acantholysis and blisters. Sparse, superficial, perivascular lymphohistiocytic infiltrate and tortuous capillaries in the papillary dermis.

- *Course and prognosis*: After zinc replacement, severely infected and erosive skin lesions heal within 1–2 weeks (Fig. 15-18*B*), diarrhea ceases, and irritability and depression of mood improve within 24 h.

- *Management*: Dietary or IV supplementation with zinc salts in 2 to 3 times the required daily amount restores normal zinc status in days to weeks. ✐

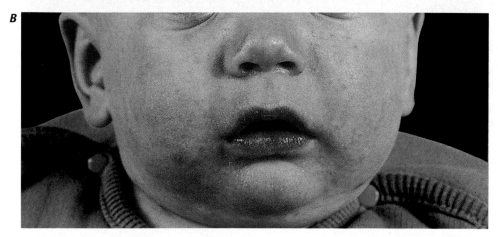

FIGURE 15-18   Acrodermatitis enteropathica   *A.* Sharply demarcated, symmetric, partially erosive, scaly, and crusted plaques on the face of an infant after weaning. Similar lesions were also found in the perigenital and perianal regions and on the fingertips. The child was highly irritable, whining, and crying and had diarrhea.
B. Within 24 h after zinc replacement, the irritability and diarrhea ceased and the infant's mood improved; and after 10 days (shown here) the perioral and perigenital lesions had healed.

FIGURE 15-19   Zinc deficiency   Well-demarcated, psoriasiform and eczematous–like plaques with scaling and erosions overlying the sacrum, intergluteal cleft, buttocks, and hip in a 60-year-old alcoholic female whose diet had consisted of pickles and cheap wine. She also had a similar eruption around the mouth, perlèche, atrophic glossitis, and had glistening, shiny, oozing fingertips.

PELLAGRA   ICD-9:265.2 ∘ ICD-10:E52   □ ◑

- Pellagra is related to niacin deficiency.

- Niacinamide is an important constituent of coenzyme I (NAD) and coenzyme II (NADP), which function in oxidation-reduction reactions as a hydrogen ion donor and acceptor, respectively.

- The essential amino acid tryptophan is converted in the body to niacin.

- Pellagra may arise from a diet deficient in niacin or tryptophan, or both. A predominantly maize-based diet is usually implicated, but only when the maize is steamed or cooked.

- Pellagra is characterized by the 3 Ds: *d*ermatitis, *d*iarrhea, and *d*ementia. Skin changes are determined by exposure to sunlight and pressure.

- The disorder begins with a symmetric itching and smarting erythema on the dorsa of the hands, neck, and face. Vesicles and bullae may erupt and break, so that crusting occurs and lesions become scaly (Fig. 15-20*A*). Later, skin becomes indurated, lichenified, rough, covered by dark scales and crusts; there are cracks and fissures and a sharp demarcation from normal skin (Fig. 15-20*B*).

- The distribution is striking: dorsa of hands and fingers ("gauntlet" of pellagra) (Fig. 15-20*B*), bandlike around the neck ("Casal necklace") (Fig. 15-20*A*), dorsa of feet up to malleoli with sparing of the heel, and butterfly region of the face.

- Diagnosis is verified by detection of decreased levels of urinary metabolites.

- *Management*: Oral administration of 100–300 mg niacinamide plus other vitamins of the B complex lead to complete resolution. ⊘

FIGURE 15-20   **Pellagra**   ***A.*** Scaly crusted bandlike plaque on the neck ("Casal necklace).

FIGURE 15-20   B. "Gauntlet" of pellagra; indurated, lichenified, pigmented, and scaly skin on the dorsa of the hands.

GOUT   ICD-9 : 274 ∘ ICD-10 : M10   ■ ◑

- A clinical syndrome occurring in a group of diseases characterized by the deposition of monosodium urate crystals in synovial fluid and joints.
- Acute gouty arthritis usually occurs in middle age and usually affects a single joint in the lower extremities, usually the first metatarsophalangial joint. Can also affect fingers (Fig. 15-21A).
- Intercritical gout describes the interval between attacks of gout. With time attacks tend to be polyarticular.

- In chronic tophaceous gout patients rarely have asymptomatic periods. Urate crystals are found in soft tissues, cartilage (Fig. 15-21B), and tendons.
- Gout may occur with and without hyperuricemia, renal disease, and nephrolithiasis.

FIGURE 15-21 ***A. Acute gouty arthritis*** affecting the distal interphalangeal joint of the fifth digit. ***B.*** Gouty tophi on helix.

GENETIC DISEASES

PSEUDOXANTHOMA ELASTICUM ICD-9:757.39 ○ ICD-10:Q82.8 ☐ ●

- Pseudoxanthoma elasticum (PXE) is a serious hereditary disorder of connective tissue that involves the elastic tissue in the skin, blood vessels, and eyes.

- *Incidence*: 1:40,000 to 1:100,000. *Inheritance*: Autosomal recessive (most common) and autosomal dominant.

- *Etiology and Pathogenesis*: Pathogenic mutation in the *ABCC6* gene, which encodes MRP6, a member of the ATPase-dependent transmembrane transporter family of proteins. MRP6 can serve as an efflux pump transporting small-molecular-weight glutathione conjugates, which may facilitate calcification of elastic fibers. This may result in fragmented elastic fibers in skin, eyes, arteries.

- The principal skin manifestations are a distinctive *peau d' orange* surface pattern resulting from closely grouped clusters of yellow (chamois-colored) papules in a reticular pattern on the neck, axillae, and other body folds (Fig. 15-22).

- The effects on the vascular system include GI hemorrhage, hypertension occurring in young persons and resulting from involvement of renal arteries, and claudication.

- Ocular manifestations ("angioid" streaks and retinal hemorrhages) can lead to blindness.

- *Dermatopathology*: Biopsy of a scar can detect characteristic changes of PXE *before typical skin changes are apparent*. Swelling and irregular clumping and basophilic staining of elastic fibers in reticular dermis; with von Kossa stain, elastic fibers appear curled and "chopped up" with calcium deposition.

- *Imaging*: X-ray: extensive calcification of the peripheral arteries of the lower extremities. Arteriography of symptomatic vessels.

- The course is inexorably progressive. Gastric artery hemorrhage occurs commonly, resulting in hematemesis. Peripheral vascular disease presents as premature cerebrovascular accidents, atherosclerosis obliterans, or bowel angina. Pregnancies are complicated by miscarriage, cardiovascular complications. Blindness. Life span is often shortened due to myocardial infarction or massive GI hemorrhage.

- *Management*: Genetic counseling. Evaluate family members for PXE. Obstetrician should be aware of PXE diagnosis and follow patient carefully. Regular reevaluation by primary care physician and ophthalmologist is mandatory.

- *Support organization*: PXE International, *www.pxe.org*

FIGURE 15-22 **Pseudoxanthoma elasticum** Multiple, confluent, chamois-colored or yellow papules (pseudoxanthomatous) created a large, circumferential, pebbled plaque on the neck of a 32-year-old woman. Changes in the connective tissue in this condition led to excessive folds on the lateral neck.

TUBEROUS SCLEROSIS (TS) ICD-9:759.5 ∘ ICD-10:Q85.1   ◧ ●

- Tuberous sclerosis is an autosomal dominant disease arising from a genetically programmed hyperplasia of ectodermal and mesodermal cells and manifested by a variety of lesions in the skin, CNS (hamartomas), heart, kidney, and other organs.

- The principal early manifestations are the triad of seizures, mental retardation, and congenital white spots.
- Facial angiofibromata are pathognomonic but do not appear until the third or fourth year.

EPIDEMIOLOGY

Incidence In mental institutions, 1:100 to 1:300; in general population, 1:20,000 to 1:100,000.
Age of Onset Infancy.
Sex Equal incidence.

Race All races.
Heredity Autosomal dominant. TS is caused by mutations in a tumor-suppressor gene, either *TSCS1* or *TSCS2*. *TSCS1* maps to chromosome 9q34. *TSCS2* maps to 16p13.3.

PATHOGENESIS

Genetic alterations of ectodermal and mesodermal cells with hyperplasia, with a disturbance in embryonic cellular differentiation.

CLINICAL MANIFESTATION

White macules are present at birth or appear in infancy (>80% occur by 1 year of age, 100% appear by 2 years); >20% of angiofibromata are present at 1 year of age, 50% occur by 3 years. Seizures (infantile spasms) occur in 86%; the earlier the onset of seizures, the worse the mental retardation. Mental retardation (49%).

Skin Lesions   96% incidence.

Hypomelanotic Macules   "Off-white"; one or many, usually more than three. Polygonal or "thumbprint," 0.5–2 cm; lance ovate or "ash-leaf" spots (Fig. 15-23*A*), 3–4 cm (up to 12 cm); tiny white "confetti" macules, 1–2 mm (Fig. 15-24). White macules occur on trunk (56%), lower extremities (32%), upper extremities (7%), head and neck (5%). White macules shine up with Wood light (Fig. 15-23*B*)

Angiofibromas   0.1–0.5 cm, dome-shaped and smooth, exhibiting red or skin color (Fig. 15-25). Occur in the center of the face. They are firm and disseminated but may coalesce; termed *adenoma sebaceum* but represent angiofibromas (present in 70%).

Plaques   Represent connective tissue nevi ("shagreen" patch), present in 40%; skin colored; occur on the back and buttocks (Fig. 15-26*B*).

Periungual Papules or Nodules   Ungual fibromas (Koenen tumors) present in 22%, arise late in childhood, and have the same pathology (angiofibroma) as the facial papules. (Fig. 15-26*A*).

ASSOCIATED SYSTEMS

CNS (tumors producing seizures), eye (gray or yellow retinal plaques, 50%), heart (benign rhabdomyomas), hamartomas of mixed cell type (kidney, liver, thyroid, testes, and GI system).

LABORATORY EXAMINATIONS

Dermatopathology   *White   Macules*   Decreased number of melanocytes, decreased melanosome size, decreased melanin in melanocytes and keratinocytes.

Angiofibromata   Proliferation of fibroblasts, increased collagen, angioneogenesis, capillary dilatation, absence of elastic tissue.

Brain Pathology   "Tubers" are gliomas.

Imaging   *Skull X-Ray*   Multiple calcific densities.
CT Scan   Ventricular deformity and tumor deposits along the striothalamic borders.
MRI   Subependymal nodules.
Electroencephalography   Abnormal.
Renal Ultrasound   Reveals renal hamartoma.

A   *B*

FIGURE 15-23   Tuberous sclerosis: ash-leaflet hypopigmented macules   *A.* Three well-demarcated, elongated (ash-leaflet shaped), hypomelanotic macules on the lower leg of a child with tan skin. ***B.*** Ash-leaflet hypomelanotic macules in pale skin are better visualized under Wood light where they light up.

FIGURE 15-24   Tuberous sclerosis: "confetti" macules   Multiple, discrete, small, confetti-like, hypopigmented macules of variable size on the leg. These lesions are pathognomonic.

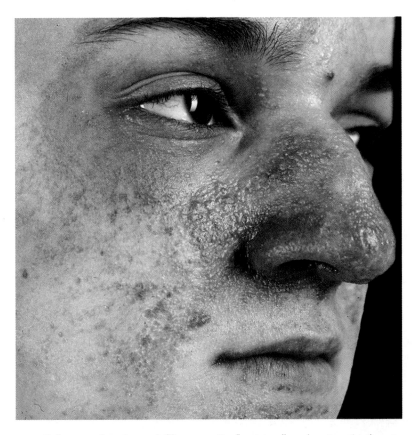

FIGURE 15-25   Tuberous sclerosis: angiofibromas   Confluent, small, angiomatous (erythematous, glistening) papules on the cheek and nose. These lesions were not present during the first few years of life; appeared only after the age of 4 years.

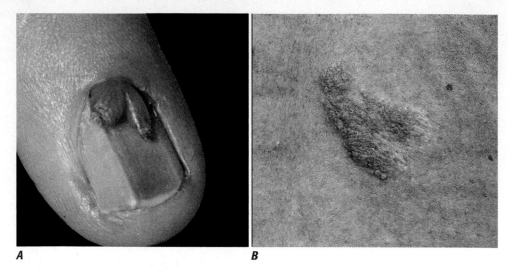

A   **B**

FIGURE 15-26 **Tuberous sclerosis** *A.* Periungual fibroma (Koenen tumor). *B.* Shagreen patch, slightly elevated, skin-colored. This represents a connective tissue nevus.

DIAGNOSIS

The diagnosis may be difficult or impossible in an infant or child if one or two white macules are the only cutaneous finding. More than five is highly suggestive. Even when typical white "ash-leaf" or "thumbprint" macules (Fig. 15-23) are present, it is necessary to confirm the diagnosis. Confetti spots (Fig. 15-24) are virtually pathognomonic. A pediatric neurologist can then evaluate the patient with a study of the family members and by obtaining various types of imaging as well as electroencephalography. Mental retardation and seizures may be absent.

DIFFERENTIAL DIAGNOSIS

White Spots Focal vitiligo, nevus anemicus, tinea versicolor, nevus depigmentosus, postinflammatory hypomelanosis.
Angiofibromas Tricholemmoma, syringoma, skin-colored papules on the face, dermal nevi.

Note: angiofibromata of the face (Fig. 15-25) have been mistaken for and treated as acne vulgaris or rosacea.
Periungual Fibromas Verruca vulgaris.

COURSE AND PROGNOSIS

A serious autosomal disorder that causes major problems in behavior, because of mental retardation, and in therapy, to control the serious seizure problem present in many patients.

In severe cases, 30% die before the fifth year of life, and 50–75% die before reaching adult age. Malignant gliomas are not uncommon. Genetic counseling is imperative.

MANAGEMENT

Prevention Counseling.
Treatment Laser surgery for angiofibromas.
Support organization: *http://www.support-group.com*

NEUROFIBROMATOSIS (NF) ICD-9:237.7 ○ ICD-10:Q85.0 ▮ ◖

- NF is an autosomal dominant trait manifested by changes in the skin, nervous system, bones, and endocrine glands. These changes include a variety of congenital abnormalities, tumors, and hamartomas.
- Two major forms of NF are recognized: (1) classic von Recklinghausen. NF, termed *NF1*; and (2) central, or acoustic NF, termed *NF2*.

- Both types have café-au-lait macules and neurofibromas, but only NF2 has *bilateral* acoustic neuromas (unilateral acoustic neuromas are a variable feature of NF1).
- An important diagnostic sign present only in NF1 is pigmented hamartomas of the iris (Lisch nodules).

Synonym: von Recklinghausen disease.

EPIDEMIOLOGY

Incidence *NF1*: 1:4000; *NF2*: 1:50,000.
Race All races.
Sex Males slightly more than females.
Heredity Autosomal dominant; the gene for NF1 is on chromosome 17 (q 1.2) and the gene codes for a protein named neurofibromin. The gene for NF2 is on chromosome 22 and codes for a protein called merlin.

PATHOGENESIS

Action of an abnormal gene on cellular elements derived from the neural crest: melanocytes, Schwann cells, endoneurial fibroblasts.

CLINICAL MANIFESTATION

Café-au-lait (CAL) macules are not usually present at birth but appear during the first 3 years; neurofibromata appear during late adolescence. Clinical manifestations in various organs are related to pathology: hypertensive headaches (pheochromocytomas), pathologic fractures (bone cysts), mental retardation, brain tumor (astrocytoma), short stature, precocious puberty (early menses, clitoral hypertrophy).
Skin Lesions *CAL Macules* Light or dark brown *uniform* melanin pigmentation with sharp margination. Lesions vary in size from multiple "freckle-like" tiny macules <2 mm (Fig. 15-27), to very large brown macules >20 cm (Fig. 15-28). The common size, however, is 2–5 cm. CAL macules also vary in number, from a few to hundreds. Tiny freckle-like lesions in the axillae are highly characteristic ("axillary freckling") (Fig. 15-27).
Papules/Nodules (Neurofibromas) Skin-colored, pink, or brown (Fig. 15-28); flat, dome-shaped or pedunculated (Fig. 15-29);

soft or firm, sometimes tender; "buttonhole sign"—invagination with the tip of the index finger is pathognomonic.
Plexiform Neuromas Drooping, soft, doughy (Fig. 15-30); may be massive, involving entire extremity, the head, or a portion of the trunk.
Distribution Randomly distributed (Figs. 15-28 and 15-29) but may be localized to one region (segmental NF1). The segmental type may be heritable or a localized hamartoma. ✍
Other Physical Findings *Eyes* Pigmented hamartomas of the iris (Lisch nodules) begin to appear at age 5 and are present in 20% of children with NF before age 6 but can be found in 95% of patients with NF1 in adolescence. They are not present in NF2. Lisch nodules are visible only with slit-lamp examination and appear as "glassy," transparent, dome-shaped, yellow-to-brown papules up to 2 mm. They do not correlate with the severity of the disease.
Musculoskeletal Cervicothoracic kyphoscoliosis, segmental hypertrophy.
Adrenal Pheochromocytoma Elevated blood pressure and episodic flushing.
Peripheral Nervous System Elephantiasis neuromatosa (gross disfigurement from neurofibromatosis of the nerve trunks).
Central Nervous System Optic glioma, acoustic neuroma (rare in NF1 and unilateral, but bilateral in NF2), astrocytoma, meningioma, neurofibroma.

LABORATORY EXAMINATIONS

Dermatopathology More than 10 *melanin macroglobules* per 5 high-power fields in "split" dopa preparations.
Wood Lamp Examination In white persons with pale skin, the CAL macules are more easily visualized with Wood lamp examination.

DIAGNOSIS AND DIFFERENTIAL DIAGNOSIS

Two of the following criteria:

1. Multiple CAL macules—more than six lesions with a diameter of 1.5 cm in adults and more than five lesions with a diameter of 0.5 cm or more in children younger than 5 years.
2. Multiple freckles in the axillary and inguinal regions.
3. Based on clinical and histologic grounds, two or more neurofibromas of any type, or one plexiform neurofibroma.
4. Sphenoid wing dysplasia or congenital bowing or thinning of long bone cortex, with or without pseudoarthrosis
5. Bilateral optic nerve gliomas
6. Two or more Lisch nodules on slit-lamp examination
7. First-degree relative (parent, sibling, or child) with NF1 by the preceding criteria

Differential Diagnosis   Brown CAL-type macules: Albright syndrome (polyostotic fibroma, dysplasia, and precocious puberty); a few CAL macules (three or less) may be present in 10–20% of normal population.

COURSE AND PROGNOSIS

It is important to establish the diagnosis in order to do genetic counseling and to follow patients for development of malignancy. Also, neurofibromatosis support groups help with social adjustment in severely affected persons.

There is variable involvement of the organs affected over time, from only a few pigmented macules to marked disfigurement with thousands of nodules, segmental hypertrophy, and plexiform neuromas. The mortality rate is higher than in the normal population, principally because of the development of neurofibrosarcoma during adult life. Other serious complications are relatively infrequent.

FIGURE 15-27   Neurofibromatosis (NF1)   Several larger (> 1 cm) café-au-lait macules on the upper chest and multiple small macules on the axillae (axillary "freckling") in a brown-skinned female. Myriads of early, small, pink-tan neurofibromas on the chest, breasts, and neck.

FIGURE 15-28   Neurofibromatosis (NF1)   Skin-colored and pink-tan, soft papules and nodules on the back are neurofibromas. The lesions first appeared during late childhood. Two large café-au-lait macules on the back. The large, soft, ill-defined, subcutaneous nodule on the right lower back and on the right posterior axillary line are plexiform neuromas.

MANAGEMENT

An orthopedic physician should manage the two major bone problems: kyphoscoliosis and tibial bowing. A plastic surgeon can do reconstructive surgery on the facial asymmetry. The language disorders and learning disabilities should be evaluated by a psychologist. Close follow-up annually should be mandatory to detect sarcomas that may arise within plexiform neuromas. Surgical removal of pheochromocytoma.

Support Group: *http://www.support-group. com*

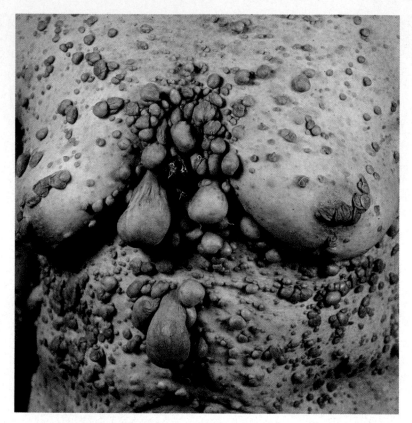

FIGURE 15-29   Neurofibromatosis (NF1)   An excessively large number of small and large, pedunculated neurofibromas on the chest of a 56-year-old woman who also had a severely distorted face due to multiple neurofibromas and plexiform neuromas.

FIGURE 15-30   Neurofibromatosis (NF1)   Plexiform neuroma on the sole of the foot of a child. This ill-defined subcutaneous mass is soft and asymptomatic. The patient has café-au-lait macules and multiple neurofibromas.

HEREDITARY HEMORRHAGIC TELANGIECTASIA   ICD-9 : 448.0 ∘ ICD-10 : I78.0   □ ◑

- Hereditary hemorrhagic telangiectasia is an autosomal dominant condition affecting blood vessels, especially in the mucous membranes of the mouth and the GI tract.

- The disease is frequently heralded by recurrent epistaxis that appears often in childhood.

- The diagnostic lesions are small, pulsating, macular and papular, usually punctate, telangiectases (Fig. 15-31) on the lips, tongue, face, palms/soles, fingers/toes, nail beds, tongue, conjunctivae, nasopharynx, and throughout the GI and genitourinary tracts. In the 18-year-old male, shown in Fig. 15-31*A*, there had been repeated epistaxis, but the telangiectasias had gone unnoticed until the patient was evaluated for anemia. Careful history then revealed that the patient's father had a minor form of the same condition.

- Pulmonary arteriovenous fistulas may occur.

- Chronic blood loss results in anemia.

- Electrocautery and pulse dye laser are used to destroy cutaneous and accessible mucosal lesions. Estrogens have been used to treat recalcitrant bleeding.

Synonym : Osler-Weber-Rendu syndrome.

A

B

FIGURE 15-31   Hereditary hemorrhagic telangiectasia   *A*. Multiple 1- to 2-mm, discrete, red macular and papular telangiectases on the lower lip and tongue. ***B*.** Multiple pinpoint telangiectases on the index finger of another patient. Using dermatoscopy or a glass slide the lesions can be shown to pulsate.

SKIN SIGNS OF VASCULAR INSUFFICIENCY

ATHEROSCLEROSIS, ARTERIAL INSUFFICIENCY, AND ATHEROEMBOLIZATION ■ ◑→●

- Atherosclerosis obliterans (ASO), especially of the lower extremities, is associated with spectrum of cutaneous findings of slowly progressive ischemic changes.

- Symptoms range from intermittent claudication with exertional muscle pain and fatigue to limb ischemia with rest pain and tissue damage and acute ischemia.

- Cutaneous findings range from dry skin, hair loss, onychodystrophy, gangrene, and ulceration.

- Atheroembolism is the phenomenon of dislodgment of atheromatous debris from a proximal affected artery or aneurysm with centrifugal microembolization and resultant acute ischemic and infarctive cutaneous lesions.

- More common with advanced age and invasive procedures.

- Manifestations are blue or discolored toes ("blue toe"), livedo reticularis, and gangrene.

ICD-9:440 ○ ICD-10:I70

EPIDEMIOLOGY

Age of Onset   Middle age to elderly.
Sex   Males > females.
Incidence   Atherosclerosis is the cause of 90% of arterial disease in developed countries, affecting 5% of men >50 years; 10% (20% of diabetics) of all men with atherosclerosis develop critical limb ischemia.
Risk Factors for Atherosclerosis   Cigarette smoking, hyperlipidemia, low high-density lipoprotein (HDL), high low-density lipoprotein (LDL), high cholesterol, hypertension, diabetes mellitus, hyperinsulinemia, abdominal obesity, family history of premature ischemic heart disease, personal history of cerebrovascular disease or occlusive peripheral vascular disease.
Diabetes Mellitus and Lower Leg Ischemia
Gangrene of lower extremities is estimated to be up to 150 times more frequent in diabetic than in nondiabetic individuals, most often occurring in those who smoke.

PATHOGENESIS

Atherosclerosis is the most common cause of arterial insufficiency and may be generalized or localized to the coronary arteries, aortic arch vessels to the head and neck, or those supplying the lower extremities, i.e., femoral, popliteal, anterior and posterior tibial arteries. Atheromatous narrowing of arteries supplying the upper extremities is much less common. Atheromatous deposits and thromboses occur commonly in the femoral artery in Hunter canal and in the popliteal artery just above the knee joint. The posterior tibial artery is most often occluded where it rounds the internal malleolus, the anterior tibial artery where it is superficial and becomes the dorsalis pedis artery. Atheromatous material in the abdominal or iliac arteries can also diminish blood flow to the lower extremities as well as break off and embolize downstream to the lower extremities (atheroembolization). Detection of atherosclerosis is often delayed until an ischemic event occurs, related to critical decrease in blood flow.

In addition to large-vessel arterial obstruction, individuals with diabetes mellitus often have microvasculopathy associated with endothelial cell proliferation and basement membrane thickening of arterioles, venules, and capillaries (see Section 15, pp 427).
Atheroembolism   Multiple small deposits of fibrin, platelet, and cholesterol debris embolize from proximal atherosclerotic lesions or aneurysmal sites. Occurs spontaneously or after intravascular surgery or procedures such as arteriography, fibrinolysis, or anticoagulation.

Emboli tend to lodge in small vessels of skin and muscle and usually do not occlude large vessels.

CLINICAL MANIFESTATION

Symptoms *Atherosclerosis of Lower Extremity Arteries* Pain on exercise, i.e., *intermittent claudication.* With progressive arterial insufficiency, pain and/or paresthesias at rest occur in leg and/or foot, especially at night. Individuals with arterial insufficiency of the lower extremities often have symptoms of ischemic heart disease (coronary artery disease or arteriosclerotic heart disease), diabetes mellitus.

Atheroembolism Acute pain and tenderness at site of embolization. "Blue toe," "purple toe" syndrome: peripheral ischemia, livedo reticularis of sudden onset may be accompanied by embolization to kidney, pancreas, muscle, etc.

Atherosclerosis/Arterial Insufficiency

Skin Lesions General findings associated with ischemia include pallor, cyanosis, livedoid vascular pattern (Fig. 16-1), loss of hair on affected limb. Earliest infarctive changes include well-demarcated maplike areas of epidermal necrosis. Later, dry black gangrene may occur over the infarcted skin (purple cyanosis → white pallor → black gangrene) (Fig. 16-2). Shedding of slough leads to well-demarcated ulcers in which underlying structures such as tendons can be seen.

General Examination *Pulses* Pulse of large vessels usually diminished or absent. In diabetics with mainly microangiopathy, gangrene may occur in the setting of adequate pulses. Temperature of foot: cool to cold.

Bürger Sign With significant reduction in arterial blood flow, limb elevation causes pallor (best noted on plantar foot); dependency causes delayed and exaggerated hyperemia. Auscultation over stenotic arteries reveals bruits.

Pain Ischemic ulcers are painful; in diabetics with neuropathy and ischemic ulcers, pain may be minimal or absent.

Distribution Ischemic ulcers may first appear between toes at sites of pressure and beginning on fissures on plantar heel. Dry gangrene of feet, starting at the toes or at pressure sites (Fig. 16-2). ✎

FIGURE 16-1 Atherosclerosis obliterans, early The great toe shows pallor and there is mottled, livedoid erythema on the tip of the toe. In this 68-year-old diabetic man, the iliac artery was occluded.

Atheroembolization

Skin Lesions   Violaceous livedo reticularis on legs, feet, but also as high up as buttocks. Ischemic changes with poor return of color after compression of skin. "Blue toe" (Fig. 16-3): indurated, painful plaques often following livedo reticularis on calves and thighs that may undergo necrosis (Fig. 16-4), become black and crusted, and ulcerate. Cyanosis and gangrene of digits. 🖉

General Examination   *Pulses*   Distal pulses may remain intact.

LABORATORY EXAMINATIONS

Hematology   Rule out anemia, polycythemia.
Lipid Studies   Hypercholesterolemia (>240 mg/ dL), often associated with rise in LDL. Hypertriglyceridemia (250 mg/dL), often associated with rise in very low-density lipoproteins (VLDLs) and remnants of their catabolism (mainly intermediate-density lipoprotein, IDL).
Dermatopathology of Atheroembolism   Deep skin and muscle biopsy specimen shows arterioles occluded by fibrosis with multinucleated giant cells surrounding biconvex, needle-shaped clefts corresponding to cholesterol crystal microemboli.
Doppler Studies   Show reduced or interrupted blood flow.
Digital Plethysmography   With exercise can unmask significant atherosclerotic involvement of lower extremity arteries.
X-Ray   Calcification can be demonstrated intramurally.
Arteriography   Atherosclerosis is best visualized by angiography. Ulceration of atheromatous plaques seen in abdominal aorta or more distally.

DIAGNOSIS AND DIFFERENTIAL DIAGNOSIS

Clinical suspicion confirmed by arteriography and deep skin biopsy (atheroembolism).
Differential Diagnosis   *Intermittent Claudication*   Pseudoxanthoma elasticum, Bürger disease (thromboangiitis obliterans), arthritis, gout.

A   *B*

FIGURE 16-2   **Atherosclerosis obliterans**   ***A.*** There is pallor of the forefoot and mottled erythema distally with incipient gangrene on the great toe and the second digit. This is a female diabetic with partial occlusion of the femoral artery. The patient was a smoker. ***B.*** More advanced gangrene of the second to the fifth toe, the great toe is ebony white and will also turn black.

Painful Foot Gout, interdigital neuroma, flat feet, calcanean bursitis, plantar fasciitis, rupture of plantar muscle.

Ischemic and Infarctive Lesions of Leg/Foot Vasculitis, Raynaud phenomenon (vasospasm), disseminated intravascular coagulation, cryoglobulinemia, hyperviscosity syndrome (macroglobulinemia), septic embolization (infective endocarditis), nonseptic embolization (ventricular mural thrombus with myocardial infarction, atrial thrombus with atrial fibrillation), aneurysms (dissecting, thrombosed), drug-induced necrosis (warfarin, heparin), ergot poisoning, intraarterial injection, livedo reticularis syndromes, external compression (popliteal entrapment).

COURSE AND PROGNOSIS

Arterial insufficiency is a slowly progressive disease, punctuated by episodes of complete occlusion or embolism. Approximately 5% per year of individuals with intermittent claudication progress to pain at rest or gangrene. A much higher percentage die from other complications of atherosclerosis such as ischemic heart disease.

Infection from interdigital tinea pedis, leg/foot ulcers, or small breaks and fissures in the skin. Chronic lymphedema, prior saphenous venous harvesting, and prior episodes of cellulitis increase the likelihood of cellulitis.

FIGURE 16-3 Atheroembolism after angiography A mottled ("blue toe"), violaceous, vascular pattern on the forefoot and great toe. The findings were noted after intravascular catheterization and angiography in an individual with ASO.

FIGURE 16-4 Atheroembolism with cutaneous infarction Violaceous discoloration and cutaneous infarctions with a linear arrangement on the medial thigh of a 73-year-old woman with atherosclerosis, heart failure, and diabetes.

Atherosclerosis of coronary and carotid arteries usually determines survival of patient, but involvement of lower extremity arteries causes significant morbidity. Balloon angioplasty, endarterectomy, and bypass procedure have improved prognosis of patients with atherosclerosis. Amputation rates have been lowered from 80% to <40% by aggressive vascular surgery. *Atheroembolism* may be a single episode if atheroembolization follows intraarterial procedure. May be recurrent if spontaneous and associated with significant tissue necrosis.

MANAGEMENT

Prevention   Goal of management is prevention of atherosclerosis.

Management of primary hyperlipidemia: Reduce intake of saturated fats and cholesterol as well as calories. *Exercise* is a useful adjunct to diet. Walking increases new collateral vessels in ischemic muscle. Reduce elevated blood pressure. *Discontinue cigarette smoking*. Correct anemia or polycythemia. *Drug therapy* is recommended for adults with LDL cholesterol >190 mg/dL or >160 mg/dL in the presence of two or more risk factors after an adequate trial of at least 3 months of diet therapy alone.

Medical Management   Encourage walking to create new collateral vessels. Position ischemic foot as low as possible without edema. Heparin and warfarin. IV prostacyclins. Analgesics.

Surgical Management   Endarterectomy or bypass for aortic iliac occlusions and for extensive femoral popliteal disease. Distal bypass surgery of crural arteries. Response to surgical revascularization or thrombolytic therapy often poor in atheroembolization. Debridement of necrotic tissue locally. Remove or bypass atherosclerotic vessel or aneurysm. Amputation of leg/foot: indicated when medical and surgical management has failed.

THROMBOANGIITIS OBLITERANS (TO)   ICD-9:443.1 ○ ICD-10:I73.1 ◻ ◑

- A rare inflammatory occlusive disease of medium-sized and small arteries and veins.
- Predominantly in males, 20–40 years of age.
- Very strong association with smoking.
- An angiitis clinically indistinguishable from TO occurs in persons consuming cannabis.
- Clinical manifestations are cold sensitivity; ischemia: claudication of leg, foot, arm, or hand.

- Peripheral cyanosis, ischemic ulcers, gangrene (Fig. 16-5), and superficial thrombophlebitis.
- Therapy: smoking cessation, analgesics, wound care; antiplatelet agents, prostacyclins, pentoxyphylin, angioplasty, sympathectomy, amputation.

Synonym: Bürger disease.

THROMBOPHLEBITIS AND DEEP VENOUS THROMBOSIS   ■ ◑→●

- Superficial phlebitis (SP) is an inflammatory thrombosis of a superficial *normal* vein, usually due to infection or trauma from needles and catheters.
- Inflammatory thrombosis of *varicose* vein usually in the context of the chronic venous insufficiency (CVI) syndrome.

ICD-9:671.2 ○ ICD-10:I 80

- Deep venous thrombosis (DVT) is due to thrombotic obstruction of a vein with or without an inflammatory response.
- Occurs due to slow blood flow, hypercoagulability, or changes in the venous walls.
- The most common causes are shown in Table 16-1

ICD-9:433.40 ○ ICD-10:I 80.2

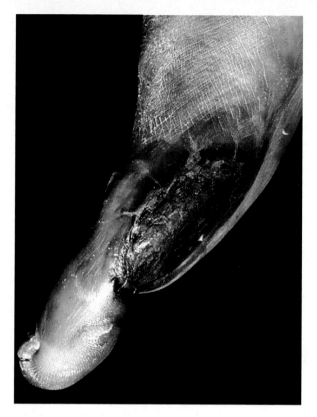

FIGURE 16-5   Thromboangiitis obliterans   Infarctive necrosis on the great toe of a 28-year-old man. The lesion is exquisitely painful. (The yellowish-brownish color is from iodine disinfection).

TABLE 16-1   Predisposing Factors in Deep Venous Thrombosis

Common Factors

Major surgery	Oral contraceptives
Fractures	Malignancies
Congestive heart failure	Venous varicosities
Acute myocardial infarction	Previous history of venous thrombosis
Stroke	Leiden factor V mutation
Pregnancy and postpartum	Severe pulmonary insufficiency
Spinal cord injuries	Prolonged immobilization
Shock	

Less Common Factors

Sickle cell anemia	Antithrombin III deficiency
Homocystinuria	Antiphospholipid antibodies
Protein C or S deficiency	Ulcerative colitis

Source: TD Coffman, RT Eberhardt, in IM Freedberg et al. (eds): *Fitzpatrick's Dermatology in General Medicine*, 6th ed. New York, McGraw-Hill, 2003.

ETIOLOGY AND PATHOGENESIS

The thrombus originates in an area of low venous flow. An occlusion of a vein by thrombus imposes a block to venous return, which leads to increased venous pressure and edema in the distal limb. An inflammatory response to the thrombus causes pain and tenderness. If the venous pressure is too high, arterial limb flow may rarely be compromised and ischemia of the distal limb may occur. The thrombus in the vein often has a free-floating tail, which may break off to produce a pulmonary embolus. Organization of the thrombus in the vein destroys the venous walls, and this leads to the postthrombotic syndrome.

CLINICAL MANIFESTATION

Patients complain of pain or aching in the involved limb or notice limb swelling. Some patients may have no symptoms. Pulmonary embolus may be the first indication of DVT.

Superficial thrombophlebitis is diagnosed by the characteristic induration of a superficial vein with redness, tenderness, and increased heat (Fig. 16-6A). DVT presents with a swollen, warm, tender limb (Fig. 16-6B) with prominent distended collateral veins. Pitting edema may occur but is not always present, and a tender cord may be felt where the vein is thrombosed. With iliofemoral thrombophlebitis the limb is swollen from the foot to the inguinal region and tenderness is not present in the limb, but collateral veins may form from the thigh to the abdominal wall. Two types are recognized: the limb may be very pale and painful (*phlegmasia alba dolens*) (Fig. 16-6B) or may be cyanotic and painful with cold digits if the arterial inflow is also compromised (*phlegmasia coerulea dolens*). In thrombosis of calf veins the calf and foot are swollen and warm, and there is deep tenderness of the calf, often without a palpable cord (Fig. 16-6B).

Migratory phlebitis describes an inflammatory induration of superficial veins that migrates within a defined region of the body; may be associated with thromboangiitis obliterans and malignancies. *Mondor disease* (sclerosing phlebitis) is an indurated, subcutaneous vein from the breast to the axillary region that during healing leads to a shortening of the venous cord, which puckers the skin.

LABORATORY EXAMINATIONS

Venous imaging by color-coded duplex ultrasound and Doppler examination reveals an absence of flow or of the normal respiratory venous flow variations in proximal venous occlusions. For thrombophlebitis of the calf veins, intravenous [^{125}I] fibrinogen or a venogram gives a definite diagnosis.

DIFFERENTIAL DIAGNOSIS

Lymphedema, cellulitis, erysipelas, superficial phlebitis, lymphangitis. An uncommon differential diagnosis is rupture of the plantar muscle, which produces pain, swelling, and ecchymotic areas in the dependent ankle area.

MANAGEMENT

The treatment of SP is compression, antiplatelet drugs, and nonsteroidal anti-inflammatory agents.

The treatment of DVT is anticoagulation. IV heparin at a loading dose of 5000 U and approximately 1000 U/h thereafter. The partial thromboplastin time (PTT) should be 1.5–2 times normal. Low-molecular-weight heparin is also effective. Warfarin can be started orally at the same time and should overlap heparin for 5 days until the necessary factors for blood clotting are depressed. Patients should be treated for at least 3 months with anticoagulation. Elastic stockings and compression are mandatory and should be worn for at least 3 months; zinc paste–impregnated bandages (Unna boot) and ambulation should be started as soon as symptoms subside.

A   *B*

FIGURE 16-6   Superficial phlebitis and deep venous thrombosis   *A*. A linear painful erythematous cord extending from the popliteal fossa to the mid-calf in a 35-year-old man who had moderate varicosities. Phlebitis occurred after a 15-h flight. ***B*.** The leg is swollen, pale, with a blotchy cyanotic discoloration, and is painful. The episode occurred after abdominal surgery (the circular marks are from a compression bandage).

CHRONIC VENOUS INSUFFICIENCY ICD-9:459.81 ∘ ICD-10:I87.2 ■ ◐

- Chronic venous insufficiency (CVI) results from failure of centripetal return of venous blood and increased capillary pressure.
- The resultant changes include edema, stasis dermatitis, hyperpigmentation, fibrosis of the skin

and subcutaneous tissue (lipodermatosclerosis) of the leg, and ulceration.
- Venous ulcers are the most common chronic wounds in humans.

EPIDEMIOLOGY AND ETIOLOGY

Varicose veins: peak incidence of onset 30–40 years. Varicose veins are three times more common in women than in men.
Etiology CVI is most commonly associated with varicose veins and the postphlebitic syndrome. Varicose veins are an inherited characteristic.

Aggravating Factors Pregnancy, increased blood volume, increased cardiac output, increased venocaval pressure, progesterone.

PATHOGENESIS

The damaged valves of the deep veins of the calf are incompetent at restricting backflow of blood. Damaged communicating veins connecting deep and superficial calf veins also cause CVI in that blood flows from deep veins to superficial venous plexus. Fibrin is deposited in the extravascular space and undergoes organization, resulting in sclerosis and obliteration of lymphatics and microvasculature. Perivascular fibrosis results in diminished nutrition of the epidermis, which breaks down with ulcer formation.

This cycle repeats itself: initial event → aggravation of venous stasis and varicose vein dilatation → lipodermatosclerosis → thrombosis → stasis dermatitis → ulceration.

CLINICAL MANIFESTATION

Prior episode(s) of superficial phlebitis and DVT. Risk factors are listed in Table 16-1.

CVI commonly associated with heaviness or aching of leg, which is aggravated by standing (dependency) and relieved by walking. Lipodermatosclerosis may limit movement of ankle and cause pain and limitation of movement, which in turn increases stasis. Leg edema aggravated by dependency (end of the day, standing), summer season. Shoes feel tight in the evening. Night cramps.

A simple staging system for CVI is shown in Table 16-2.

Skin Lesions
Varicose Veins Superficial leg veins are enlarged, tortuous, with incompetent valves; best evaluated with the patient standing (Fig. 16-7A). "Blow-out" at sites of incompetent communicating veins. Tourniquet test: A tourniquet is applied to the leg that has been elevated to empty the veins; when the patient stands up and the tourniquet is released, there is instant filling of a varicose vein due to absent or ill-functioning valves. Varicose veins may or may not be associated with starburst phlebectasia usually overlying the area of an incompetent communicating vein (Fig. 16-7B). These small venectasias per se have no pathogenic significance but are of cosmetic concern to the patient. Superficial venectasias (spider phlebectasia) without a starburst pattern occur also and far more commonly without CVI, usually on the thighs and lateral lower legs in women. ⬛

Edema Dependent; improved or resolved in the morning after a night in the horizontal position. Dorsa of feet, ankles, lower legs.

Eczematous (Stasis) Dermatitis Occurs in setting of CVI about the lower legs and ankles (Fig. 16-8). It is a classic eczematous dermatitis with inflammatory papules, scaly and crusted erosions; in addition, there is pigmentation, stippled with recent and old hemorrhages (Fig. 16-9); dermal sclerosis; and excoriations due to scratching. It must be distinguished from contact dermatitis secondary to topical agents, with which it is often combined. In addition, there may be concomitant irritant dermatitis due to secretion from stasis ulcer (see below) and bacterial colonization. If extensive, may be associated with generalized eczematous dermatitis, i.e., "id" reaction or autosensitization (see Section 2).

Atrophie Blanche Small ivory-white depressed plaques (Fig. 16-9) on the ankle and/or foot; stellate and irregular, coalescing; stippled

---

TABLE 16-2	Staging of CVI (CEAP Classification)

Clinical Picture (C)
- C_0 no clinical signs
- C_1 small varicose veins
- C_2 large varicose veins
- C_3 edema
- C_4 skin changes
- C_5 healed ulcer
- C_6 active ulcer

Anatomy (A)
- A_s superficial
- A_d deep
- A_p perforans (communicating vein)

Etiology (E)
- E_p primary
- E_s secondary
- E_c congenital

Pathophysiology (P)
- P_r reflux
- P_o obstruction
- $P_{r,o}$ reflux + obstruction

A   *B*

FIGURE 16-7   Varicose veins   A. There are meandering and convoluted irregular varicose veins on the thigh of a 70-year-old man who also had lipodermatosclerosis and stasis dermatitis on the lower legs. **B.** *Starburst venectasias on the calf.* This is an area overlying an insufficient communicating vein.

pigmentation; hemosiderin-pigmented border, usually within stasis dermatitis. Often following trauma. ⮌

Lipodermatosclerosis Inflammation, induration, pigmentation of lower third of leg creating "champagne bottle" or "piano leg" appearance with edema above and below the sclerotic region (Fig. 16–10). "Groove sign" created by varicose veins meandering through sclerotic tissue. A verrucous epidermal change can occur overlying the sclerosis; if combined with chronic lymphedema, it is referred to as *elephantiasis*

nostras verrucosa. In long-standing sclerosis, calcification can occur. ⮌

Ulceration Occurs in 30% of cases; very painful "hyperalgesic microulcer" in area of atrophie blanche; larger superficial or deep ulcers, sharply defined with deep margin, necrotic base surrounded by atrophie blanche, stasis dermatitis, and lipodermatosclerosis (Fig. 16-11). Venous ulcers usually occur medially and above ankles (Fig. 16-11). Venous ulcers and their differential diagnosis are discussed in more detail below (p. 470). ⮌

LABORATORY EXAMINATIONS

Doppler and Color-Coded Duplex Sonography These detect incompetent veins, venous occlusion due to thrombus.

Phlebography Contrast medium is injected into veins to detect incompetent veins and venous occlusion.

Imaging X-ray may show subcutaneous calcification (10% of chronic cases), i.e., postphlebitic subcutaneous calcinosis. Bony changes include periostitis underlying ulceration, osteoporosis as a result of disuse, fibrous ankylosis of ankle. Osteomyelitis.

Dermatopathology *Early*: small venules and lymphatic spaces appear dilated; edema of extracellular space with swelling and separation of collagen bundles. *Later*: capillaries dilated, congested with tuft formation and tortuousity of venules; deposition of fibrin. *Endothelial cell hypertrophy*: may be associated with venous thrombosis; angioendotheliomatous proliferation mimicking Kaposi sarcoma. In all stages, extravasation of red blood cells that break down forming hemosiderin, which is taken up by macrophages. Lymphatic vessels become encased in a fibrotic stroma, i.e., lipodermatosclerosis. Calcification of fat and fibrous tissue may occur.

DIAGNOSIS

Usually made on history, clinical findings, Doppler and color-coded Duplex sonography, phlebography.

MANAGEMENT

Prerequisite Compression dressings or stockings; Unna boot.

Atrophie Blanche Avoid trauma to area involved. Intralesional triamcinolone into painful lesions. Compression.

Stasis Dermatitis Topical gluscocorticoids (short term). Topical antibiotic treatments (e.g., mupirocin) when secondarily infected. Culture for methicillin-resistant *Staphylococcus aureus* (MRSA).

FIGURE 16-8 Stasis dermatitis in CVI *A* patch of eczematous dermatitis overlying venous varicosities on the medial ankle in a 59-year-old woman. The lesion is papular, scaly, and itching.

FIGURE 16-9 Chronic venous insufficiency. Atrophie blanche
An area of diffuse and mottled pigmentation due to hemosiderin and ivory-white patches of atrophie blanche. Such lesions are both itchy and painful.

A

B

FIGURE 16-10 Chronic venous insufficiency and lipodermatosclerosis The ankle is relatively thin and the upper calf edematous, creating a "champagne bottle" or "piano leg" appearance. **A.** Varicose veins are embedded in pigmented, sclerotic tissue. There are also areas of atrophie blanche. **B.** Varicose veins are less visible here but can be easily palpated in the sclerotic plaque encasing the entire calf ("groove" sign). There is also pigmentation and minor papular stasis dermatitis.

Varicose Veins *Injection Sclerotherapy* A sclerosing agent such as tetradecyl sulfate is injected into varicosities, followed by prolonged compression. Used mainly to treat minor branch varicosities not associated with saphenous incompetence and new branch vein varicosities developing after surgery. Recurrence is common within 5 years.

Vascular Surgery Incompetent perforating veins are identified, ligated, and cut, followed by stripping long and/or short saphenous veins out of the main trunk. Residual perforating veins are the main cause of recurrences after surgery. In patients with combined arterial and CVI, bypass or angioplasty may prove beneficial.

Endovascular Techniques These new technologies encompass endoscopic subfascial dissection of perforating veins (employed primarily in the elimination of insufficient perforating veins in CVI); and endoscopic endovenous diode laser or radiofrequency thermal heating, which leads to occlusion of varicose vein.

Venous Ulcers   See below.

A   *B*

FIGURE 16-11   Venous insufficiency   A. Two coalescing ulcers with a necrotic base in an area of atrophie blanche, lipodermatosclerosis, and stasis dermatitis. Scratch marks indicate itchiness of surrounding skin, while the ulcers are painful. **B.** A giant ulcer, well-defined with scalloped borders and a beefy red base in a leg with lipodermatosclerosis.

Venous Ulcers   The prevalence of venous ulcers is estimated to be approximately 1%. It rises with patient age, obesity, previous leg injury (fractures), DVT, and phlebitis. Patients complain of limb heaviness, swelling associated with standing and worsening in the evening, and pain. Venous ulcers are associated with at least one or all of the symptoms of CVI (Fig. 16-11 and Table 16-2) and may be single or multiple; they are commonly found on the medial lower aspect of the calf, especially over the malleolus (medial > lateral), in the area supplied by incompetent perforating veins (Fig. 16-11). They can be large, involving the circumference of the entire lower leg (Fig. 16-11B). They are sharply defined, irregularly shaped, relatively shallow with a sloping border, and usually painful. The base is usually covered by fibrin and necrotic material (Fig. 16-11A), and there is always secondary bacterial colonization. Stasis ulcers can also develop in the most dependent parts of a pendulous abdominal panniculus in a massively obese individual. Squamous cell carcinoma (SCC) can arise in a long-standing venous ulcer (Fig. 16-12) of the leg.

Arterial Ulcers   Arterial ulcers are associated with peripheral arterial disease (atherosclerosis obliterans, see p. 458). Associated with intermittent claudication and pain, even at rest, as disease progresses. Characteristically painful at night and often quite severe; may be worse when legs are elevated, improving on dependency. Occur on the lower leg, usually over sites of pressure and trauma: pretibial, supramalleolar (usually lateral), and at distant points, such as toes. Painful. Punched out, with sharply demarcated borders (Fig. 16-13). A tissue slough is often present at the base, under which tendons can be seen. Exudation minimal. Associated findings of ischemia: loss of hair on feet and lower legs, shiny atrophic skin. Stasis pigmentation and lipodermatosclerosis are absent. Pulses diminished or absent.

A special type of arterial ulcer is *Martorell ulcer*, which is associated with labile hypertension and lacks clinical signs of atherosclerosis obliterans. Ulcer(s) start with a black eschar surrounded by erythema and after sloughing of necrotic tissue are punched out with sharply demarcated borders, with surrounding erythema; very painful on the anterior lateral lower leg.

Combined Arterial and Venous Ulcers   These ulcers arise in patients who have both CVI and atherosclerosis obliterans and thus show a combination of signs and symptoms of both venous and arterial insufficiency and ulceration (Fig. 16–14). Symptoms include intermittent claudication, pain both at elevated and dependent position of the leg, both pallor and cyanosis of the foot, stasis dermatitis, and lipodermatosclerosis associated with both sloped and punched out ulcers reaching down to tendons (Fig. 16-14).

Neuropathic Ulcers   (See "Diabetic Foot," p 426) Soles, toes, heel. Most commonly associated with diabetes of many years' duration. Early symptoms of neuropathy include paresthesia, pain, anesthesia of leg and foot. Patients are often unaware of prior trauma that commonly precedes ulcerations of heel, plantar metatarsal area, or great toe. Neuropathic ulcers are discussed in Section 15 (see Fig. 15-4).

DIFFERENTIAL DIAGNOSIS

A differential diagnosis of the three main types of leg/foot ulcers is shown in Table 16-3. Other differential diagnostic considerations include ulcerated SCC (note that SCC can arise in a long-standing venous ulcer) (Fig. 16-12), basal cell carcinoma, injection drug use (skin popping), pressure ulcer (ski boot). Ulcerations also occur in vasculitis (particularly polyarteritis

TABLE 16-3　Differential Diagnosis of Three Major Types of Leg Ulcers

	Lesion	Site	Surrounding Skin	General Examination
Venous	Irregular	Malleolar and supramalleolar (medial)	Lipodermatosclerosis	Varicose veins
	Sloped borders		Stasis dermatitis	Pain, worse in dependent state
	Necrotic base		Atrophie blanche	
	Fibrin		Pigmentation	
			Lymphedema	
Arterial	Punched out	Pressure sites: distal (toes), pretibial, supramalleolar	Atrophic, shiny	Weak/absent pulses
	Necrotic base	(lateral)	Hair loss	Pallor on elevation of leg
			Pallor or reactive hyperemia	Pain worse on elevation of leg
Neuropathic	Punched out	Pressure sites	Callus before ulceration and surrounding ulcer	Peripheral neuropathy
		Plantar		Decreased sensation
				No pain

FIGURE 16-12　**Squamous cell carcinoma in chronic venous ulcer**　*A* venous ulcer had been present >10 years in an area of lipodermatosclerosis and stasis dermatitis. Eventually the base of the ulcer became elevated, hard, less painful. Deep biopsy (circular mark in the center) revealed necrosis and at the base invasive squamous cell carcinoma.

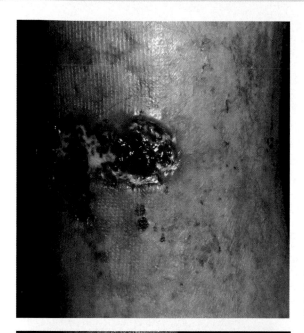

FIGURE 16-13 Chronic arterial insufficiency with a sharply defined, "punched out" ulcer with irregular outlines The extremity was pulseless, and there was massive ischemia on the toes.

FIGURE 16-14 Chronic arterial and venous insufficiency, "combined" arterial and venous ulcers Note pronounced lipodermatosclerosis and ulceration on the supramalleolar lower leg (venous component) and purple discoloration of forefoot and toes with punched-out ulcer revealing tendon over metatarsal site (arterial component).

nodosa), erythema induratum, calciphylaxis, and various infections [ecthyma, Buruli ulcer, *Mycobacterium marinum* infection, gumma, leprosy, invasive fungal infection, chronic herpes simplex virus (HSV) ulcer] and in sickle cell anemia, polycythemia vera, pyoderma gangrenosum, necrobiosis lipoidica with ulceration, factitia.

COURSE AND PROGNOSIS

Course and prognosis are dependent on underlying disease. With correction of underlying causes, ulcers heal with initial formation of pink granulation tissue at the base, which is reepithelialized by epithelium from either residual skin appendages or surrounding epidermis. Venous ulcers can heal with a pseudoepitheliomatous epidermal hyperplasia within the scar, which can mimic SSC.

MANAGEMENT

General Management   In general, factors such as anemia and malnutrition should be corrected to facilitate healing. Control hypertension, weight reduction in the obese, exercise; mobilize patient; correct edema caused by cardial, renal, or hepatic dysfunction. Of utmost importance is treatment of underlying disease. Arterial ulcers do not heal unless arterial blood flow is corrected by endarterectomy to remove localized atheromatous plaques or bypass of occluded areas (see "Management" of atherosclerosis obliterans, p. 462). Arterial ulcers at acral sites that do not heal despite arterial reconstruction or where arterial reconstruction cannot be performed may require amputation. Venous ulcers tend to be recurrent unless underlying risk factors are corrected, i.e., corrective surgery and/or elastic stockings worn on a daily basis (see "Management" of chronic venous insufficiency, p. 468). Beware of excess compression in patients with additional underlying arterial occlusion; leg elevation; intermittent pneumatic compression. In neuropathic ulcers, correct underlying diabetes. Rule out or treat underlying osteomyelitis. Distribute weight of pressure points with special shoes in neuropathic ulcers. *Note*: diabetic patients are particularly predisposed to ulcers and frequently have several etiologic factors in play, i.e., peripheral vascular disease, neuropathy, infection, and impaired healing.

Secondary infection should be treated with antibiotics both topically and systemically in all ulcers. Ulcers provide an easy portal of entry for systemic infection, which should be suspected if pain appears or increases in intensity. Infection can occur relatively superficially in ulcer base or more invasively with cellulitis and possible lymphangitis and bacteremia. Beware of MRSA.

Local Treatment of Ulcer and Surrounding Skin   Treat stasis dermatitis (or irritant, or allergic contact dermatitis) in CVI with wet dressings in the acute exudative phase and subsequently with moderate to potent glucocorticoid ointment. In all ulcers debride necrotic material mechanically (surgically) or by enzymatic debriding agents, including collagenase and papain; use antiseptics and antibiotics to counteract infection. Hydrocolloid dressings. Granulating but only slowly epithelializing ulcers are treated by surgical procedures either by pinch grafts, split-thickness skin grafts, epidermal grafts, cultured keratinocyte allografts, or composite grafts.

LIVEDOID VASCULITIS (LV)   ICD-10 : L95.0

- LV is a thrombotic vasculopathy of dermal vessels confined to the lower extremities and starting mostly in the ankle region.

- A triad of livedo reticularis, atrophie blanche, and very painful, small punched-out ulcers that have a very poor tendency for healing (Fig. 16-15).

- Atrophie blanche in livedoid vasculitis is clinically indistinguishable from that seen in CVI, except for varicose veins (compare Figs. 16-15 and 16-9). LV is a reaction pattern of the skin that often recurs in winter or summer ("livedo reticularis with winter and summer ulcerations").

- Histologically, there are fibrin thrombi in small and medium-sized dermal veins and arteries with wedge-shaped necrosis and hyalinization of the vessel walls (segmental hyalinizing vasculitis).

- LV may be idiopathic or may be associated with Sneddon syndrome (see Fig. 14-19, p. 375), antiphospholipid antibody syndrome, or conditions of hypercoagulability or hyperviscosity.

- Treatment: bed rest, analgesics, low-dose heparin, and platelet aggregation inhibitors. Pain can be relieved and healing accelerated by systemic glucocorticoids. Anabolic agents such as danazol and stanazolol have been anecdotally reported to be effective.

- Larger ulcers will have to be excised and grafted.

FIGURE 16-15   Livedoid vasculitis   This is characterized by the triad of livedo reticularis, atrophie blanche and small, painful, crusted ulcers. This is clinically indistinguishable from atrophie blanche seen in CVI except for the absence of varicose veins.

CHRONIC LYMPHATIC INSUFFICIENCY
ICD-9 : 459.81 ○ ICD-10 :I87.2

- Lymphedema in childhood and early adult life are genetic and are often caused by defects in vascular endothelial growth factor receptor (VEGFR3) and FoxC2, a transcription factor.

- Acquired lymphedema of adults may be related to chronic venous insufficiency; chronic, recurring soft tissue infections (erysipelas, cellulitis, see Section 24); node dissection and radiation after cancer; and in some geographic regions by filariasis.

- Depending on etiology acquired lymphedema most commonly occurs on the lower extremities but may also arise on the arm and hand.

- Clinical manifestations: swelling of extremities, pitting edema initially slowly evolving into nonpitting woody induration.

- Prolonged lymphedema may lead to grotesque enlargement of extremity; epidermal hyperplasia with verrucosis (Fig. 16-16).

- Secondary, soft tissue infection (erysipelas and cellulitis) is common, recurrent, and leads to worsening of the condition.

- Treatment is mainly compression (as in CVI) and manual lymphatic drainage; antibiotics in secondary infection.

- Lymphangiosarcoma (in postmastectomy-lymphedema) is a rare complication: Stewart-Treves syndrome

FIGURE 16-16   Chronic lymphatic insufficiency: lymphedema   Lower legs are thickened of woody consistency and three is massive hyperkeratosis. The 60-year-old patient had had innumerable episodes of erysipelas and cellulitis. There is also diabetes and atherosclerotic arterial insufficiency.

PRESSURE ULCERS ICD-9:707 ○ ICD-10:L89

- Pressure ulcers develop at body-support interfaces over bony prominences as a result of external compression of the skin, shear forces, and friction, which produce ischemic tissue necrosis.

- Occur in patients who are obtunded mentally or have diminished sensation (as in spinal cord

disease) in the affected region. Secondary infection results in localized cellulitis, which can extend locally into bone or muscle or into the bloodstream.

Synonyms: Pressure sore, bed sore, decubitus ulcer.

EPIDEMIOLOGY

Age of Onset Any age, but the greatest prevalence of pressure ulcers is in elderly, chronically bedridden patients.

Sex Equally prevalent in both sexes.

Prevalence Acute care hospital setting, 3–14%; long-term care settings, 15–25%; home-care settings, 7–12%; spinal cord units, 20–30%.

PATHOGENESIS

Risk factors: inadequate nursing care, diminished sensation/immobility (obtunded mental status, spinal cord disease), hypotension, fecal or urinary incontinence, presence of fracture, hypoalbuminemia, and poor nutritional status. The mean skin capillary pressure is approximately 25 mmHg. External compression with pressures >30 mmHg occludes the blood vessels so that the surrounding tissues become anoxic and eventually necrotic. Amount of damage is proportional to extent and duration of pressure. Secondary bacterial infection can enlarge the ulcer, extend to underlying structures (osteomyelitis), and invade the bloodstream, with bacteremia and septicemia. Infection also impairs or prevents healing.

CLINICAL MANIFESTATION

Ulcers often develop within the first 2 weeks of acute hospitalization and more rapidly if the patient experiences significant immobilization. Painful unless there is altered sensorium.

Skin Lesions *Clinical Categories of Pressure Ulcers* Early change: localized erythema that blanches on pressure.

Stage I: Nonblanching erythema of intact skin.

Stage II: Necrosis, superficial or partial-thickness involving the epidermis and/or dermis. Bullae → necrosis of dermis (black) → shallow ulcer.

Stage III: Deep necrosis, crateriform ulceration with full-thickness skin loss (Fig. 16-17); damage or necrosis can extend down to, but not through, fascia.

Stage IV: Full-thickness necrosis (→ ulceration) with involvement of supporting structures such as muscle and bone (Fig. 16-18). May enlarge to many centimeters. May or may not be tender. Borders of ulcers may be undetermined.

Well-established pressure ulcers are widest at the base and taper to a cone shape at the level of skin. Ulcers with devitalized tissue at the base (eschar) have a higher chance of secondary infection. Purulent exudate and erythema surrounding the ulcer suggest infection. Foul odor suggests anaerobic infection.

Distribution Occur over bony prominences: sacrum (60%) (Fig. 16-18) > ischial tuberosities, greater trochanter (Fig. 16-17), heel > elbow, knee, ankle, occiput.

General Examination Fever, chills, or increased pain of ulcer suggests possible cellulitis or osteomyelitis.

LABORATORY EXAMINATIONS

Hematologic Studies Elevated white blood cell count and erythrocyte sedimentation rate suggest infection (osteomyelitis or bacteremia).

Wound Culture Infection must be differentiated from colonization. Culture of the ulcer base detects only surface bacteria. Optimal culture technique: Deep portion of punch biopsy specimen obtained from the ulcer base is minced and cultured for aerobic and anaerobic bacteria. Most infections are polymicrobial and anaerobes may be present. Viral culture to rule out chronic herpes simplex virus ulcer.

Blood Culture Bacteremia often follows manipulation of ulcer (within 1–20 min of beginning the debridement); resolves within 30–60 min.

Pathology *Skin Biopsy* Epidermal necrosis with eccrine duct and gland necrosis. Deep ulcers show wedge-shaped infarcts of the subcutaneous tissue, obstruction of the capillaries with microthrombi, and endothelial cell swelling followed by endothelial cell necrosis and secondary inflammation.

Bone Biopsy Essential for diagnosing continuous osteomyelitis; specimen is examined histologically and microbiologically.

Imaging It is difficult to distinguish osteomyelitis from chronic pressure-related changes by radiogram or scan.

DIAGNOSIS AND DIFFERENTIAL DIAGNOSIS

Usually made clinically. Complications are assessed with data on cultures, biopsies, and imaging. Differential diagnosis includes infectious ulcer (actinomycotic infection, deep fungal infection, chronic herpetic ulcer), thermal burn, malignant ulcer (cutaneous lymphoma, basal cell carcinoma or SCC), pyoderma gangrenosum, rectocutaneous fistula.

COURSE AND PROGNOSIS

If pressure is relieved, some changes are reversible; intermittent periods of pressure relief increase resistance to compression. Osteomyelitis occurs in nonhealing pressure ulcers (32–81%). Septicemia is associated with a high mortality rate. Overall, patients with pressure ulcers have a fourfold risk of prolonged hospitalization and of dying when compared with patients without ulcers. With proper treatment, stages I and II ulcers heal in 1–4 weeks and stages III and IV ulcers heal in 6 to >12 weeks.

MANAGEMENT

Prophylaxis in At-Risk Patients Reposition patient every 2 h (more often if possible); massage areas prone to pressure ulcers while changing position of patient; inspect for areas of skin breakdown over pressure points.

- Use interface air mattress to reduce compression.
- Minimize friction and shear forces by using proper positioning, transferring, and turning techniques.
- Clean with mild cleansing agents, keeping skin free of urine and feces.
- Minimize skin exposure to excessive moisture from incontinence, perspiration, or wound drainage.
- Maintain head of the bed at a relatively low angle of elevation (<30°).
- Evaluate and correct nutritional status; consider supplements of vitamin C and zinc.
- Mobilize patients as soon as possible.

Stages I and II Ulcers Topical antibiotics (not neomycin) under moist sterile gauze may be sufficient for early erosions. Normal saline wet-to-dry dressings may be needed for debridement. Hydrogels or hydrocolloid dressings.

Stages III and IV Ulcers Surgical management: debridement of necrotic tissue, bony prominence removal, flaps and skin grafts.

Infectious Complications Prolonged course of antimicrobial agent depending on sensitivities, with surgical debridement of necrotic bone in osteomyelitis.

FIGURE 16-17 Pressure ulcer, stage III Well-demarcated crateriform ulcer with full thickness skin loss extending down to fascia over greater trochanteric region.

FIGURE 16-18 Pressure ulcer, stage IV Huge black necrosis over sacral area in a patient who had been bedridden after a stroke. The criss-cross marks in the necrotic area are from attempts to mechanically debride necrotic tissue. Surgical debridement of necrotic tissue under anesthesia revealed involvement of fascia and bone.

SKIN SIGNS OF RENAL INSUFFICIENCY

CLASSIFICATION OF SKIN CHANGES

- Acute renal failure
  - Edema
  - Uremic frost (deposition of urea crystals on skin surface in severe uremia)
- Chronic renal failure
  - Edema

- Uremic frost
- Calciphylaxis
- Bullous disease of hemodialysis (pseudoporphyria, see Section 22)
- Nephrogenic fibrosing dermopathy
- Acquired perforating dermatosis

CALCIPHYLAXIS ICD-9 : 275.49 □ ◑ → ●

- Calciphylaxis is characterized by progressive cutaneous necrosis associated with small- and medium-sized vessel calcification.
- It occurs in the setting of end-stage renal disease, diabetes mellitus, and hyperparathyroidism.
- Preinfarctive lesions show mottling or livedo reticularis pattern, dusky red.

- Turn into black, leathery eschar.
- Extremely painful.
- Extend to fascia and beyond.
- Lower extremities, abdomen, buttocks, penis.

EPIDEMIOLOGY

Age of Onset Middle to old age.
Sex Equal.

PATHOGENESIS

The pathogenesis is poorly understood. While vascular calcifications are common in patients with chronic renal failure and are asymptomatic, in calciphylaxis, there is sudden thrombosis in calcified vessels. In animal models, calciphylaxis is described as a condition of induced systemic hypersensitivity in which tissues respond to appropriate challenging agents with calcium deposition. Calciphylaxis is associated with chronic renal failure, secondary hyperparathyroidism, and an elevated calcium phosphate end product. Implicated "challenging agents" include glucocorticoids, albumin

infusions, intramuscular tobramycin, iron dextran complex, calcium heparinate, immunosuppressive agents, and vitamin D.

CLINICAL MANIFESTATION

Even early infarctive lesions are exquisitely tender and painful.
Disease Associations Occurs in end-stage renal disease. Onset often closely follows initiation of hemo- or peritoneal dialysis. Most patients are diabetic. Hyperparathyroidism.
Skin Lesions Initially preinfarctive ischemic plaques occur, appearing as mottling or having a livedo reticularis pattern, dusky red to violaceous (Fig. 17-1A). Bullae may form over ischemic tissue, which eventually becomes necrotic. Central infarcted sites have a tightly adherent black or yellowish, leathery slough (Fig. 17-1B). Lesions gradually enlarge over

A   **B**

FIGURE 17-1   Calciphylaxis A. *Early stage.*   An area of mottled erythema, starburst-like and reminiscent of livedo reticularis with two small ulcerations. Patient has chronic renal failure and is on hemodialysis. Even at this early stage lesions are extremely painful. **B.** Calciphylaxis, more advanced lesion. An area of jagged necrosis on the lower leg in a patient with diabetes and chronic renal failure who is on hemodialysis. The surrounding skin is indurated and represents a platelike subcutaneous mass that is appreciated only upon palpation.

weeks to months; when debrided, deep ulcers reaching down to the fascia result (Fig. 17-2). Ischemic skin frequently becomes secondarily infected; infection can remain localized or become invasive, causing cellulitis and bacteremia. In addition, large areas of induration can be defined on palpation as platelike subcutaneous masses that extend beyond infarcted or ulcerated areas (Fig. 17-2).
Distribution   Distal extremities, most commonly on the lateral and posterior calves; abdomen, buttocks; fingers; glans penis.

LABORATORY EXAMINATIONS

Chemistry   Azotemia. Calcium × phosphate ion product usually elevated.
Parathormone (PTH)   Levels usually, but not always, elevated.

Cultures   Rule out secondary infection. MRSA
Dermatopathology   Incisional, deep biopsy shows calcification of the media of small- and medium-sized blood vessels in the dermis and subcutaneous tissue. Intraluminal fibrin thrombi are present. Ischemia results in intralobular or septal fat necrosis, accompanied by a sparse lymphohistiocytic infiltrate.
Imaging   Radiographs of affected extremities show calcium deposition outlining small and large vessels. Microcalcification of calciphylaxis is difficult to visualize.

DIAGNOSIS AND DIFFERENTIAL DIAGNOSIS

Made on history of renal failure, clinical findings, elevated PTH level, elevated calcium × phosphate ion product, and histologic features.
Differential Diagnosis   Panniculitis, vasculitides, necrobiosis lipoidica with ulceration,

dystrophic calcinosis cutis, atheroembolization, atherosclerosis obliterans, disseminated intravascular coagulation (purpura fulminans), pyoderma gangrenosum, warfarin necrosis, heparin necrosis. *Vibrio vulnificus* cellulitis, other necrotizing cellulitides.

COURSE AND PROGNOSIS

Slowly progressive despite all therapeutic interventions. Pain is a constant feature. In advanced disease, gangrene of fingers, toes, and penis may result in autoamputation. Local infection and sepsis are common complications. Overall, the prognosis is poor, and the mortality rate is very high.

MANAGEMENT

Calciphylaxis is best managed by early diagnosis, treatment of renal failure, partial parathyroidectomy when indicated, aggressive debridement of necrotic tissue, and avoidance of precipitating factors.

FIGURE 17-2   Calciphylaxis, extensive   Lesions are ulcerated, the surrounding skin is indurated, best seen on left thigh where skin is hairless. Similar lesions are also found on the abdomen. Note edema of knees and lower legs.

NEPHROGENIC FIBROSING DERMOPATHY (NFD)

- NFD is a fibrosing disorder in patients with acute or chronic renal failure.

- Most patients receiving hemodialysis, peritoneal dialysis; in acute renal failure NFD occurs without dialysis.

- It is part of a wider spectrum of *nephrogenic systemic fibrosis* involving the heart, lungs, diaphragm, skeletal muscle, liver, genitourinary tract, and central nervous system.

- Etiology unknown but exposure to gadodiamid containing contrast media for MR angiography is a strong association. Gadodiamid is found only in lesions and not in normal tissue. Myofibroblasts and fibrogenic cytokines (e.g., transforming growth factor β) may be involved in the pathogenesis.

- NFD is characterized by acute onset, brawny indurations, plaquelike or nodular, bound down upon palpation (Fig. 17-3); up to 20 cm and more in diameter, with an uneven rippled surface.

- Mostly on lower extremities, less often on upper extremities and torso but not the face.

- Tingling, tender, often painful.

- Differential diagnosis: morphea, pretibial myxedema, lipodermatosclerosis, panniculitis.

- Course is chronic, unremitting; prognosis guarded.

- Therapy unknown. Imatinib may be beneficial

FIGURE 17-3   Nephrogenic fibrosing dermopathy   A brawny platelike induration bound down upon palpation, with an uneven surface on the legs. This patient had end-stage chronic renal failure and was on hemodialysis.

ACQUIRED PERFORATING DERMATOSIS (APD)* ☐ ○

- Occurs in chronic renal failure and diabetes mellitus; in up to 10% of patients undergoing hemodialysis.
- Chronic pruritic condition triggered by trauma.
- Umbilicated papules with central hyperkeratotic crust (Fig. 17-4).

- Transepidermal elimination of collagen.
- Relationship to other perforating disorders not clear. ✐

*See M Lebwohl, in K Wolff et al (eds): Fitzpatrick's *Dermatology in General Medicine*, 7th ed. New York, McGraw-Hill, 2008,). p 564.

FIGURE 17-4 **Acquired perforating dermatosis in a patient undergoing hemodialysis** There are purpuric umbilicated papules with a central hyperkeratotic crust.

SKIN SIGNS OF SYSTEMIC CANCERS

MUCOCUTANEOUS SIGNS OF SYSTEMIC CANCERS

- Mucocutaneous findings may suggest systemic cancers in several ways:
- Associations of heritable mucocutaneous disorders with systemic cancers.
- By action at a distance, i.e., paraneoplastic syndromes.

- Or spread of cancer to skin or mucosal sites by direct, lymphatic, or hematogenous extension (cutaneous metastasis).

ICD-9 : 199.0 ∘ ICD-10 : M8000/6

CLASSIFICATION OF SKIN SIGNS OF SYSTEMIC CANCER[1]

METASTATIC CANCERS

Persistent tumor. Lymphatic extension, hematogenous spread
Direct extension. Paget disease, extramammary Paget disease
Lymphomas with secondary skin involvement (Section 20)

HERITABLE DISORDERS

Cowden syndrome
Peutz-Jeghers syndrome
Neurofibromatosis (p. 453)
Tuberous sclerosis (p. 449)
Multiple endocrine neoplasia (MEN) (types 1 and 2b)

PARANEOPLASTIC SYNDROMES

Acanthosis nigricans, malignant, tripe palms
Acquired ichthyosis
Bazex syndrome
Carcinoid syndrome
Dermatomyositis (p. 14)
Ectopic ACTH syndrome
Erythema gyratum repens
Gardner syndrome
Glucagonoma syndrome
Hypertrichosis lanuginosa
Muir-Torre syndrome
Palmar keratoses
Paraneoplastic pemphigus
Pruritus (p. 7)
Pyoderma gangrenosum (p. 7)
Sweet syndrome (p. 14)
Vasculitis (p. 397)

[1]Conditions covered in this section are printed in **bold,** conditions dealt with in other sections are in *italics.* Numbers in parentheses indicate page numbers. Rare conditions not discussed in this book are described in CA deWitt et al, in K Wolff et al (eds): *Fitzpatrick's Dermatology in General Medicine* 7th ed. New York, McGraw-Hill, 2008, pp 1493–1507.

METASTATIC CANCER TO THE SKIN   ICD-9 : 199.0 ∘ ICD-10 : M8000/6

- Metastatic cancer to the skin is characterized by solitary or multiple dermal or subcutaneous nodules, occurring as metastatic cells from a distant noncontiguous primary malignant neoplasm.
- They are transported to and deposited in the skin or subcutaneous tissue by one of the following routes:

- Lymphatic routes.
- Hematogeneous spread.
- Contiguous spread across the peritoneal cavity or other tissues.
- For metastasis nonmelanoma *skin* cancers and melanoma, see Sections 11 and 12.

EPIDEMIOLOGY

Age of Onset   Any age, but usually older.
Sex   Frequency of primary tumors varies with sex.
Incidence   In principle almost any cancer can metastasize to skin. Skin metastases occur in up to 10% of all patients with cancer. The frequency of metastases according to type of tumor are shown in Table 18-1.

PATHOGENESIS

Includes detachment of cancer cells from primary tumor, invasion, intravasation into blood or lymphatic vessel, → circulation, stasis within vessel, attachment to endothelium, migration across vessel wall, invasion into tissue,

proliferation at metastatic site. The growth of metastases depends on proliferation of metastatic cells, cytokine and growth factor release from cancer and stromal cells, angiogenesis, and immune reactions. Three patterns of metastases are observed: mechanical tumor stasis (anatomic proximity and lymphatic draining), site-specific (selective attachment of tumor cells to specific organ), nonselective (independent of mechanical or organ-specific factors).

CLINICAL MANIFESTATION

Prior history of primary internal cancer or cancer chemotherapy or may be first sign of visceral cancer.

TABLE 18-1   Percent of Patients with Cutaneous Metastases

Type of Primary Malignancy	Patients with Cutaneous Metastases, %
Melanoma	44.8
Breast	30.0
Nasal sinuses	20.0
Larynx	16.3
Endocrine glands	12.5
Oral cavity	11.5
Esophagus	8.6
Kidney	4.6
Stomach	2.0

SOURCE: Adapted from DP Lookingbill et al: J Am Acad Dermatol 29:228, 1993.

Skin Lesions   Nodule (Figs. 18-1 and 18-2), raised plaque, thickened fibrotic area. First detected when <5 mm. Fibrotic area may resemble morphea; occurring on scalp, may produce alopecia. Initially, epidermis is intact, stretched over nodule; in time, surface may become ulcerated or hyperkeratotic (Fig. 18-4). May appear inflammatory, i.e., pink to red or hemorrhagic (Fig. 18-3). Note: Metastatic melanoma to dermis: blue to gray to black nodules (see Fig. 12-17). Firm to indurated. May be solitary, few, or multiple. May acquire considerable size and may be mistaken for a primary skin cancer (Fig. 18-4).

Distribution   Anywhere; specific sites discussed below.

Special Patterns of Cutaneous Involvement
Breast

Inflammatory metastatic carcinoma (carcinoma erysipelatoides): erythematous patch or plaque with an active spreading border (Fig. 18-5). Most often with breast cancer that may spread within lymphatics to skin of involved breast, resulting in inflammatory plaques resembling erysipelas (hence the designation *carcinoma erysipelatoides*). Breast most common primary (Fig. 18-5), but occurs with others as well [pancreas, parotid, tonsils, colon, stomach, rectum, melanoma, pelvic organs, ovary (Fig. 18-7), uterus, prostate, lung].

Telangiectatic metastatic carcinoma (*carcinoma telangiectaticum*): breast cancer appearing as pinpoint telangiectases with dilated capillaries within carcinoma erysipelatoides. Violaceous papules or papulovesicles resembling lymphangioma circumscriptum.

En cuirasse metastatic carcinoma: diffuse morphea-like induration of skin (Fig. 18-6). Usually local extension of breast cancer occurring in breast and presternal region. Sclerodermoid plaque may encase chest and resembles a metal breastplate of a cuirassier. Also occurs with primary of lung, GI tract, kidney.

Breast carcinoma of inframammary crease: cutaneous exophytic nodule resembling primary squamous cell carcinoma (SCC) or basal cell carcinoma of skin (Fig. 18-2B).

Paget disease: sharply demarcated plaque or patch of erythema and scaling occurring on nipple or areola associated with underlying breast cancer (see below).

FIGURE 18-1   Metastatic cancer to the skin: bronchogenic cancer   Dermal nodules on the scalp of a patient undergoing chemotherapy for metastatic lung cancer; the nodules were only apparent following loss of hair during chemotherapy. The nodule on the left is asymptomatic, erythematous, but noninflamed. The nodule on the right has a central depression marking a punch biopsy site.

A   **B**

FIGURE 18-2   Metastatic cancer to the skin   *A.* Adenocarcinoma of the colon. Two coalescent smooth firm nodules on the abdomen. ***B.*** *Breast cancer*: Large nodule on breast in a 40-year-old woman with breast cancer, present for 4 months.

FIGURE 18-3   Metastatic cancer to the skin, hypernephroma   Hypernephroma metastases often localize to the head and have an angiomatous appearance mimicking pyogenic granuloma, as in this lesion on the upper lip of a 66-year-old man. This was the first indication that the patient had cancer of the kidney.

FIGURE 18-4   Metastatic cancer to the skin   A. Bronchogenic carcinoma. Large ulcerated, crusted nodule on the scalp of a 69-year-old woman who had been a heavy smoker since the age of 19. The patient was otherwise asymptomatic and this tumor was originally diagnosed as primary squamous cell carcinoma of the skin. Biopsy revealed metastasis of moderately differentiated squamous cell carcinoma, and workup showed the primary cancer to be in the lung. **B.** Adenocarcinoma of the GI tract. This fungating mass was just the tip of the iceberg: a much larger mass was in the subcutis.

FIGURE 18-5 Metastatic cancer of the skin: inflammatory breast cancer (carcinoma erysipelatoides)
A large erythematous and only minimally indurated lesion covering the entire breast and presternal region; the lesion is red and sharply defined and thus looks like erysipelas. There was a 2 × 2 cm lump in the breast upon palpation.

Multiple smooth nodules on scalp: prostate adenocarcinoma, lung cancer, breast cancer (Fig. 18-1).

Alopecia neoplastica: On scalp, areas of hair loss resembling alopecia areata; well-demarcated, red-pink, smooth surface, flat.

Large Intestine Often presents on skin of abdomen or perineal regions; also, scalp or face. Most originate in rectum. May present with metastatic inflammatory carcinoma (like carcinoma erysipelatoides) of inguinal region, supraclavicular area, or face and neck. Less commonly, sessile or pedunculated nodules on buttocks, grouped vascular nodules of groin or scrotum, or facial tumor. Rarely, cutaneous fistula after appendectomy or resembling hidradenitis suppurativa.

Lung Carcinoma May produce a large number of metastatic nodules in a short period. Most commonly, reddish nodule(s) on scalp (Figs. 18-1 and 18-4*A*). Trunk: symmetric; along direction of intercostal vessels, may be zosteriform; in scar (thoracotomy site or needle aspiration tract).

Hypernephroma Can produce solitary lesion; also widespread. Usually appear vascular, ± pulsatile, ± pedunculated (Fig. 18-3); can resemble pyogenic granuloma. Most common on head (scalp) and neck; also trunk and extremities.

Carcinoma of Bladder, Ovary Can spread contiguously to abdominal and inguinal skin similarly to breast cancer, as described above, and look like erysipelas (Fig. 18-7).

Miscellaneous Patterns With dilation of lymphatics and superficial hemorrhage, may resemble lymphangioma. With lymph stasis and dermal edema, resembles pigskin or orange peel. May metastasize hematogenously to scalp, forming many subcutaneous nodules with "bag of marbles" feel to scalp.

Sister Mary Joseph nodule is metastatic carcinoma to umbilicus from intraabdominal carcinoma, most commonly stomach, colon, ovary, pancreas; however, primary may be in breast. Easier to detect by palpation than by visual detection. Can be firm to indurated nodule, ± fissuring, ± ulceration, ± vascular appearance, ± discharge. In 15% may be initial presentation of primary malignancy.

DIFFERENTIAL DIAGNOSIS

"Blueberry Muffin Baby" Neuroblastoma, congenital leukemia.

Multiple Smooth Nodules on Scalp Cylindromas (rare adnexal tumors of the scalp mimicking marbles tucked under the skin), trichilemmal (pilar) cysts.

Kaposi Sarcoma–Like Lesions Cancer of kidney.

Pyogenic Granuloma–Like Lesions Amelanotic melanoma, renal cancer.

Alopecia Areata–Like Lesions Breast cancer.

Lymphangioma-Like Lesions Cancer of breast, lung, cervix, ovary.

Morphea-Like Lesions Cancer of breast, stomach, lung, mixed tumors, lacrimal gland.

LABORATORY EXAMINATION

Dermatopathology At times, cell differentiation and architectural structure sufficient to predict primary site; however, many times cells anaplastic. Employ monoclonal antibodies to differentiate solid carcinoma metastases from lymphoma, neuroendocrine carcinoma, melanoma, anaplastic angiosarcoma, and sarcomas.

COURSE AND PROGNOSIS

In individuals with known cancer, cutaneous metastases are indicative of a poor prognosis. Average survival after detection of cutaneous metastasis only 3 months except for contiguous spread of breast cancer, which may last for years. In individuals with unknown cancer, skin metastases may help to detect primary tumor.

MANAGEMENT

With solitary or few lesions and if patient not terminal, excision may be indicated.

FIGURE 18-6 **Metastatic ovarian cancer** Manifesting as carcinoma erysipelatoides on the lower abdomen and inguinal region. Workup disclosed ovarian cancer with peritoneal carcinomatosis.

FIGURE 18-7 **Metastatic breast cancer: cancer en cuirasse** Both breasts are hard upon palpation—like an armor plate. There are multiple small and large, ulcerated nodules and there is a background of erysipelas-like erythema (carcinoma erysipelatoides).

PAGET DISEASE   ICD-9:174 ○ ICD-10:M542/3

MAMMARY PAGET DISEASE   ◼ ●

- Mammary Paget disease (MPD) is a malignant neoplasm that unilaterally involves the nipple or areola and simulates a chronic eczematous dermatitis.
- It represents contiguous spread of underlying intraductal carcinoma of the breast (1–4% of breast cancers).
- Usually occurring in females (>50 years), there are rare examples in males.
- Onset is insidious over several months or years. May be asymptomatic or there may be pruritus, pain, burning, discharge, bleeding, ulceration, nipple invagination.
- Skin lesion presents as red, scaling plaque, rather sharply marginated, oval with irregular borders. When scale is removed, the surface is moist and oozing (Fig. 18-8). Lesions range in size from 0.3–15 cm (Fig. 18-9). In early stages there is no induration of the plaque; later, induration and infiltration develop and nodules may be palpated in breast. At initial presentation an underlying breast mass is palpable in fewer than one-half of patients. May be bilateral. Lymph node metastases occur more often when MPD is associated with an underlying palpable mass.

- Differential diagnosis includes eczematous dermatitis, psoriasis, benign ductal papilloma, nipple-areola retention hyperkeratosis, impetigo, SCC in situ, familial pemphigus.

- *Eczematous dermatitis of the nipples* is usually bilateral; it is without any induration and responds rapidly to topical glucocorticoids. Nevertheless, be suspicious of Paget disease if "eczema" persists for >3 weeks. Diagnosis verified by biopsy showing neoplastic cells in epidermis following a pathognomonic pattern of spread. Define underlying intraductal carcinoma by mammography.

- Management consists of surgery, radiotherapy, and/or chemotherapy as in any other breast carcinomas. Lymph node dissection if regional nodes are palpable. Prognosis varies. When breast mass is not palpable, 92% of patients survive 5 years after excision; 82%, 10 years. When breast mass is palpable, 38% survive 5 years; 22%, 10 years. Prognosis worse when there is lymphadenopathy. ⊇

FIGURE 18-8 Mammary Paget disease A sharply demarcated red plaque mimicking eczema or psoriasis on the nipple. The plaque is slightly indurated and there is slight scaling; any red, eczema-like lesion on the nipple and areola that does not respond to topical glucocorticoids should be biopsied.

FIGURE 18-9 Mammary Paget disease A sharply defined psoriasiform plaque that has obliterated the areola and nipple. There was a lump in the breast and a small axillary mass.

EXTRAMAMMARY PAGET DISEASE □ ●

- Extramammary Paget disease (EPD) is a neoplasm of the anogenital and axillary skin, histologically identical and clinically similar to Paget disease of the breast.

- Often representing an intraepidermal extension of a primary adenocarcinoma of underlying apocrine glands or of the lower gastrointestinal, urinary, or female genital tracts.

- Often, however, it is unassociated with underlying cancer.

- The histogenesis of EPD not uniform. Occurs as an in situ upward extension of an in situ adeno-carcinoma in deeper glands (25%). Alternatively, EPD may have a multifocal primary origin in the epidermis and its appendages. Primary tumors in the anorectum can arise within the rectal mucosa or intramural glands.

- Insidious onset, slow spread, + itching. The lesion presents as erythematous plaque, + scaling, +erosion (Fig. 18-10), + crusting, + exudation; eczematous-appearing lesions but borders are sharply defined (Fig. 18-10, Fig. 35-25), geographic configuration. Lesions should always be biopsied.

- Histopathologically, Paget cells are dispersed between keratinocytes, occur in clusters, extend down into adnexal structures (hair follicles, eccrine ducts). Adnexal adenocarcinoma is often found when carefully searched for.

- In perineal/perianal EPD, underlying carcinoma should be searched for by *rectal examination, proctoscopy, sigmoidoscopy, barium enema*. In genital EPD, search for underlying carcinoma by *cystoscopy, intravenous pyelogram*; in vulvar EPD, by *pelvic examination*.

- Differential diagnosis includes all red plaques: eczematous dermatitis, lichen simplex chronicus, lichen sclerosus et atrophicus, lichen planus, intertriginous psoriasis, *Candida* intertrigo, SCC in situ (erythroplasia of Queyrat), human papilloma virus–induced SCC in situ, (amelanotic) superficial spreading melanoma.

- EPD is usually much larger than is apparent clinically. Surgical excision must be controlled histologically (Mohs micrographic surgery). If Paget cells are in dermis and regional lymph nodes are palpable, lymph node dissection may improve prognosis, which is related to underlying adenocarcinoma. EPD remains in situ in the epidermis and adnexal epithelium in >65% of cases. When no underlying neoplasm is present, there is nonetheless a high recurrence rate, even after apparently adequate excision; this is due to the multifocal origin in the epidermis and adnexal structures. ℰ

FIGURE 18-10 **Extramammary Paget disease** Moist, well-demarcated, eroded, oozing, erythematous plaque on the scrotum and inguinal fold in an older male. The lesion is commonly mistaken for *Candida* intertrigo and unsuccessfully treated as such.

COWDEN SYNDROME (MULTIPLE HAMARTOMA SYNDROME)

- Cowden syndrome (named after the propositus) is a rare, autosomal dominant heritable cancer syndrome with variable expressivity in a number of systems in the form of multiple hamartomatous neoplasms of ectodermal, mesodermal, and endodermal origin.
- Germ-line mutations in the tumor-suppressor gene *PTEN* are located on chromosome 10q22–23 in most cases.
- There is a special susceptibility for breast and thyroid cancers, and the skin lesions are important markers.
- Skin lesions may appear first in childhood but develop over time. They consist of *tricholemmomas*, skin-colored, pink (Fig. 18-11*B*), or brown papules having the appearance of flat warts on the central area of the face, perioral areas, lips near the angles of the mouth, and the ears; *translucent punctate keratoses* of the palms and soles; and *hyperkeratotic, flat-topped papules* on the dorsa of the hands and forearms. Mucous membrane lesions are characteristic: *papules* of the gingival, labial (Fig. 18-11*A*), and palatal surfaces that coalesce, giving a "cobblestone" appearance. *Papillomas* of the buccal mucosa and the tongue.

- In addition to breast cancer (20%), which is often bilateral, and thyroid cancer (8%), there are various internal hamartomas:
  - *Breast*: fibrocystic disease, fibroadenomas, adenocarcinoma, gynecomastia in males
  - *Thyroid*: goiter, adenomas, thyroglossal duct cysts, follicular adenocarcinoma
  - *GI tract*: hamartomatous polyps throughout tract but increased in large bowel, adenocarcinoma arising in polyp
  - *Female genital tract*: ovarian cysts, menstrual abnormalities
  - *Musculoskeletal*: craniomegaly, kyphoscoliosis, "adenoid" facies, high-arched palate
  - *CNS*: mental retardation, seizures, neuromas, ganglioneuromas, and meningiomas of the ear canal.
- It is important to establish the diagnosis of Cowden syndrome so that these patients can be followed carefully to detect breast and thyroid cancers.

ICD-9 : 759.6 ∘ ICD-10 : Q85.9

PEUTZ-JEGHERS SYNDROME   ICD-9 : 759.6 ∘ ICD-10 : Q85.8

- Peutz-Jeghers syndrome (PJS) is a familial (autosomal dominant, spontaneous mutation in 40%) polyposis characterized by many small, pigmented brown macules (lentigines) on the lips, oral mucous membranes (brown to bluish black), and on the bridge of the nose, palms, and soles.
- The gene has been mapped to 19p13.3.
- Macules on the lips may disappear over time, but not the pigmentation of the mouth; therefore the mouth pigmentation is the sine qua non for the diagnosis (Fig. 18-12).
- There are usually, but not always, multiple hamartomatous polyps in the small bowel, as well as in the large bowel and stomach, that cause abdominal symptoms such as pain, GI bleeding, anemia.

- Whereas pigmented macules are congenital or develop in infancy and early childhood, polyps come on in late childhood or before age 30.
- Adenocarcinoma may develop in polyps, and there is an increased incidence of breast, ovarian, and pancreatic cancer.
- There is a normal life expectancy unless carcinoma develops in the GI tract. Malignant neoplasms may be more frequent in Japanese patients with this syndrome, and prophylactic colectomy has been recommended for these patients.

A

B

FIGURE 18-11   Cowden syndrome A. Multiple reddish, confluent papules on the oral mucosa giving a cobblestone appearance. **B.** Multiple skin-colored warty papules on the face, which represent tricholemmonas.

FIGURE 18-12   Peutz-Jeghers syndrome Multiple, dark-brown lentigines on the vermilion border of the lip and the buccal mucosa. This patient had GI bleeding due to hamartomatous polyps in the small bowel.

GLUCAGONOMA SYNDROME ICD-9:211.7 ∘ ICD-10:M8152/0 ☐ ●

- Glucagonoma syndrome is a rare but well-described clinical entity caused by excessive production of glucagon in an α cell tumor of the pancreas.
- Characterized by superficial migratory necrolytic erythema (MNE) with erosions that crust and heal with hyperpigmentation.
- Inflammatory patches and red plaques (Figs. 18-13 and 18-14) of gyrate, circinate, arcuate, or annular shape that enlarge with central clearing, resulting in geographic areas that become confluent (Fig. 18-14). Borders show vesiculation to bulla formation, crusting, and scaling (Figs. 18-13 and 18-14).
- Lesions involve perioral and perigenital regions and flexures and intertriginal areas.
- Fingertips red, shining, erosive (Fig. 18-15).
- There is glossitis, angular cheilitis (Fig. 18-13), blepharitis.
- General examination reveals wasting, malnutrition.
- Most cases are associated with glucagonoma, but the pathogenesis of MNE is not known. There exists MNE without glucagonoma.
- *Differential diagnosis*: Includes all moist red plaque(s): acrodermatitis enteropathica, zinc deficiency, pustular psoriasis, mucocutaneous candidiasis, Hailey-Hailey disease (familial pemphigus).
- *Laboratory*: Fasting plasma glucagon level increased to >1000 ng/L (normal 50–250 ng/L) and makes the diagnosis. There is also hyperglycemia, reduced glucose tolerance. Associated findings include severe malabsorption, gross hypoaminoacidemia, low serum zinc. CT scan angiography will locate tumor within pancreas and metastases in the liver.
- Dermatopathology of early skin lesions shows bandlike upper epidermal necrosis with retention of pyknotic nuclei and pale keratinocyte cytoplasm.
- Prognosis depends on the aggressiveness of the glucagonoma. Hepatic metastases have occurred in 75% of patients at the time of diagnosis. If these are slow-growing, patients may have prolonged survival, even with metastatic disease.
- MNE responds poorly to all types of therapy. Some cases have responded partially to zinc replacement. MNE resolves after tumor excision. However, surgical excision of glucagonoma achieves cure in only 30% of cases because of persistent metastases (usually liver). Surgery also reduces tumor masses and associated symptoms. There is poor response to chemotherapy.

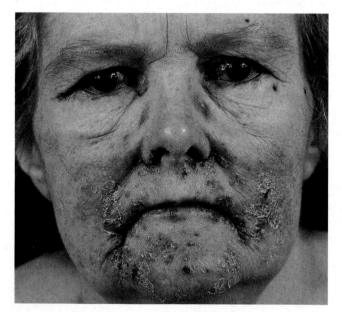

FIGURE 18-13 Glucagonoma syndrome: migratory necrolytic erythema Inflammatory dermatosis with angular cheilitis, inflammatory, scaly, erosive and crusted plaques and fissures around the nose, mouth, and medial aspects of the eyes. Marginal blepharitis.

FIGURE 18-14 **Glucagonoma syndrome: migratory necrolytic erythema** Polycyclic erosions in the anogenital gluteal and sacral regions. Sharply defined with necrotic flaccid epidermis still covering part of these erosions.

FIGURE 18-15 **Glucagonoma syndrome** Fingertips are red, glistening and partially erosive.

MALIGNANT ACANTHOSIS NIGRICANS　ICD-9 : 701.2 ○ ICD-10 : L83☐　●

- Like other forms of acanthosis nigricans (AN) (see Section 5), malignant AN starts as a diffuse, velvety thickening and hyperpigmentation chiefly on the neck, axillae and other body folds, as well as on the perioral and periorbital, umbilical, mamillary, and genital areas, giving the skin a dirty appearance (Fig. 18-16; see also Fig. 5-1).

- Hyperpigmentation and hyperkeratosis soon lead to a rugose, mamillated, and papillomatous surface (Fig. 18-16).

- Verrucous growths also involve the vermilion border of the lips (Fig. 18-17). On the oral mucous membranes there is a velvety texture with delicate furrows.

- The knuckles and the palms show maximal accentuation of the palmar ridges (tripe hands) (Fig. 18-18).

- Malignant AN differs from other forms of AN primarily because of (1) the more pronounced velvety hyperkeratosis and hyperpigmentation, (2) the pronounced mucosal involvement and involvement of the mucocutaneous junction, (3) tripe hands, and (4) weight loss and wasting due to the underlying malignancy.

- AN may precede by 5 years other symptoms of a malignancy, usually adenocarcinoma of the GI or GU tract, bronchocarcinoma, or, less commonly, lymphoma. Malignant AN is a truly paraneoplastic disease, and a search for underlying malignancies is imperative. Removal of malignancy is followed by regression of AN.

FIGURE 18-16　Acanthosis nigricans: malignant　Poorly defined, velvety, verrucous and papillomatous, dark chocolate-brown plaques on the medial thighs and scrotum. Similar changes were also present in the axillae and neck, and the vermilion border of the lips was covered with velvety, raspberry-like growths.

FIGURE 18-17　Acanthosis nigricans: malignant　Verrucous and mamillated growths on the vermilion border of the lips in a patient with carcinoma of the stomach. The gastric cancer was suspected because of these raspberry-like growths, acanthosis nigricans of the major skin folds, and weight loss. There is still a suture at the site of a biopsy.

PARANEOPLASTIC PEMPHIGUS (PNP)   ICD-9:694.4   □ ●

- Mucous membranes primarily and most severely involved.
- Lesions combine features of pemphigus vulgaris (page 106) and erythema multiforme (page 148), clinically, histologically, and immunopathologically.
- Most prominent clinical findings consist of severe oral (Fig. 18-19) and conjunctival erosions in a patient with an underlying neoplasm.
- These neoplasms are in order of frequency: non-Hodgkin lymphomas, chronic lymphatic leukemia, Castleman disease, thymoma, sarcoma, and Waldenström macroglobulinemia.
- Patients with PNP may also have clinical and serologic evidence of myasthenia gravis and autoimmune cytopenia.

- PNP sera contain autoantibodies to plakin antigens (in the intercellular plaque of desmosomes), envoplakin and periplakin, and to desmoplakin I and II. Less commonly patient sera may also recognize bullous pemphigoid antigen (230 kDa), plectin, and plakoglobin, and an unidentified 170-kDa antigen.
- Autoantibodies of PNP cause blistering in neonatal mice and are detected by indirect immunofluorescence on rodent urinary bladder epithelium.
- Treatment is directed toward elimination or suppression of malignancy but may also require systemic glucocorticoids.

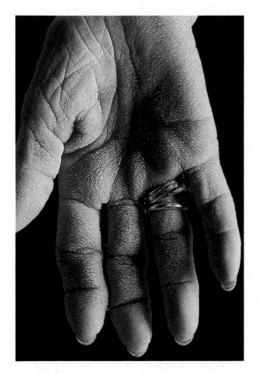

FIGURE 18-18   Acanthosis nigricans: tripe palm   The palmar ridges of the palm show maximal accentuation, thus resembling the mucosa of the stomach of a ruminant (tripe palm).

FIGURE 18-19   Paraneoplastic pemphigus   - Severe erosions covering practically the entire mucosa of the oral cavity with partial sparing of the dorsum of the tongue. Lesions are extremely painful, interfering with adequate food intake. This patient had non-Hodgkin lymphoma as underlying malignancy.

SKIN SIGNS OF HEMATOLOGIC DISEASE

THROMBOCYTOPENIC PURPURA

- Thrombocytopenic purpura (TP) is characterized by cutaneous hemorrhages occurring in association with a reduced platelet count.
- Hemorrhages are usually small (petechiae) but at times larger (ecchymoses).

- Occur at sites of minor trauma/pressure (platelet count < 40,000/µL) or spontaneously (platelet count < 10,000/µL).

ICD-9 : 287.31 ○ ICD-10 : D69.3

EPIDEMIOLOGY

Age of Onset Acute idiopathic thrombocytopenic purpura (ITP) mostly in children; drug-induced and autoimmune TP in adults.
Sex Both sexes; HIV-associated TP—homosexual men > heterosexual females.

ETIOLOGY AND PATHOGENESIS

Due to either decreased platelet production, splenic sequestration, or increased platelet destruction.
1. *Decreased platelet production.* Direct injury to bone marrow, drugs (cytosine arabinoside, daunorubicin, cyclophosphamide, busulfan, methotrexate, 6-mercaptopurine, vinca alkaloids, thiazide diuretics, ethanol, estrogens), replacement of bone marrow, aplastic anemia, vitamin deficiencies, Wiskott-Aldrich syndrome.
2. *Splenic sequestration.* Splenomegaly, hypothermia.
3. *Increased platelet destruction. Immunologic*: autoimmune TP, drug hypersensitivity (sulfonamides, quinine, quinidine, carbamazepine, digitoxin, methyldopa), after transfusion. *Nonimmunologic*: infection, prosthetic heart valves, disseminated intravascular coagulation, thrombotic thrombocytopenic purpura.

Platelet plugs by themselves effectively stop bleeding from capillaries and small blood vessels but are incapable of stopping hemorrhage from larger vessels. Platelet defects therefore produce problems with small-vessel hemostasis, small hemorrhages in the skin or in the CNS.

CLINICAL MANIFESTATION

Usually sudden appearance of asymptomatic hemorrhagic skin and/or mucosal lesions.

Skin Lesions *Petechiae*—small (pinpoint to pinhead), red, nonblanching macules that are not palpable and turn brown as they get older (Fig. 19-1); later acquiring a yellowish-green tinge. *Ecchymoses*—black and blue spots; larger area of hemorrhage. *Vibices*—linear hemorrhages (Fig. 19-1), due to trauma or pressure. Most common on legs and upper trunk, but may be anywhere.
Mucous Membranes *Petechiae*—most often on palate (Fig. 19-2), gingival bleeding.
General Examination Possible CNS hemorrhage, anemia.

LABORATORY EXAMINATIONS

Hematology Thrombocytopenia.
Bone Marrow Aspiration Defines state of platelet production.
Serology Rule out HIV disease.
Lesional Skin Biopsy May be contraindicated due to postoperative hemorrhage; however,

FIGURE 19-1 Thrombocytopenic purpura Multiple petechiae on the upper arm of an HIV-infected 25-year-old male were the presenting manifestation of his disease. The linear arrangement of petechiae at the site of minor trauma are called vibices.

FIGURE 19-2 Thrombocytopenic purpura Can first manifest on the oral mucosa or conjunctiva. Here multiple petechial hemorrhages are seen on the palate.

usually can be controlled by suturing biopsied site and applying pressure.

DIAGNOSIS

Clinical suspicion confirmed by platelet count.

DIFFERENTIAL DIAGNOSIS

Nonhemorrhagic Blanching Vascular Lesions Telangiectasia/erythema, spider nevi, Osler disease.
True Hemorrhagic Lesions Actinic or senile purpura, purpura of scurvy, progressive pigmentary purpura (Schamberg disease), purpura following severe Valsalva maneuver (coughing, vomiting/retching), traumatic purpura, factitial or iatrogenic purpura, Gardner-Diamond syndrome (autoerythrocyte sensitization

syndrome), palpable nonblanching purpura = *vasculitis*.

COURSE AND PROGNOSIS

Depends on and varies with the etiology.

MANAGEMENT

Identify underlying cause and correct, if possible. If platelet count is very low (< 10,000/μL), bed rest to reduce risk of hemorrhage.
Oral Glucocorticoids, High-Dose IV Immunoglobulins
Platelet Transfusions If the platelet count < 10,000/μL, platelet transfusion may be indicated.
Chronic ITP Splenectomy may be indicated.

DISSEMINATED INTRAVASCULAR COAGULATION

- Disseminated intravascular coagulation (DIC) is a widespread blood clotting disorder occurring within blood vessels.
- Associated with a wide range of clinical circumstances: bacterial sepsis, obstetric complications, disseminated malignancy, massive trauma.
- Manifested by purpura fulminans (cutaneous infarctions and/or acral gangrene) or bleeding from multiple sites.

- The spectrum of clinical symptoms associated with DIC ranges from relatively mild and subclinical to explosive and life-threatening.

Synonyms: Purpura fulminans, consumption coagulopathy, defibrination syndrome, coagulation-fibrinolytic syndrome.

ICD-9:256.8 ∘ ICD-10:D65

EPIDEMIOLOGY

Age of Onset All ages; occurs in children. Antecedent or concomitant infections due to bacteria (scarlet fever, group A streptococcal, staphylococcal, pneumococcal, vibrio, and meningococcal bacteremia; less commonly varicella.)

ETIOLOGY AND PATHOGENESIS

- *Events that initiate DIC* Tumor products, crushing trauma, extensive surgery, severe intracranial damage; retained contraception products, placental abruption, amniotic fluid embolism; certain snake bites; hemolytic

transfusion reaction; acute promyelocytic leukemia; burn injuries.
- *Extensive destruction of endothelial surfaces, exposure to foreign surfaces* Vasculitis in Rocky Mountain spotted fever, meningococcemia, or occasionally gram-negative septicemia; group A streptococcal infection, heat stroke, malignant hyperthermia; extensive pump oxygenation (repair of aortic aneurysm); eclampsia, preeclampsia; tufted angioma and Kaposiform hemangioendothelioma: Kasabach-Merritt syndrome; immune complexes; postvaricella purpura gangrenosa.
- *Events that complicate and propagate DIC* Shock, complement pathway activation.

Uncontrolled activation of coagulation results in thrombosis and consumption of platelets/

clotting factors II, V, VIII. Secondary fibrinolysis. If the activation occurs slowly, excess activated products are produced, predisposing to vascular infarctions/venous thrombosis. If the onset is acute, hemorrhage surrounding wound sites and IV lines/catheters or bleeding into deep tissues is usually seen.

CLINICAL MANIFESTATION

Hours to days; rapid evolution. Fever, chills associated with onset of hemorrhagic lesions.

Skin Lesions *Infarction (purpura fulminans)* (Figs. 19-3, 19-4, and 19-5): massive ecchymoses with sharp, irregular ("geographic") borders

FIGURE 19-3 Disseminated intravascular coagulation: purpura fulminans Extensive geographic area of cutaneous infarction with hemorrhage involving the hand. Similar lesions were on the face, the other hand, and the feet.

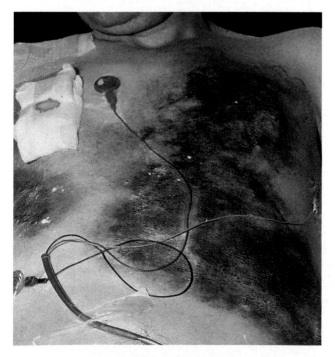

FIGURE 19-4 Disseminated intravascular coagulation: purpura fulminans Geographic cutaneous infarctions on the chest; lesions were also present on the hands, elbows, thighs, and feet. The patient was a diabetic with *Staphylococcus aureus* sepsis.

FIGURE 19-5   Extensive cutaneous infarction with hemorrhage involving the entire leg   This castas-trophic event followed sepsis after abdominal surgery.

with deep purple to blue color (Fig. 19-5) and erythematous halo, ± evolution to hemorrhagic bullae and blue to black gangrene (Fig. 19-4); multiple lesions are often symmetric; distal extremities, areas of pressure; lips, ears, nose, trunk; peripheral acrocyanosis followed by gangrene on hands, feet, tip of nose, with subsequent autoamputation if patient survives.

Hemorrhage from multiple cutaneous sites, i.e., surgical incisions, venipuncture or catheter sites. **Mucous Membranes**   Hemorrhage from gingiva. **General Examination**   High fever, tachycardia, ± shock. Multitude of findings depending on the associated medical/surgical problem.

LABORATORY EXAMINATIONS

Dermatopathology   Occlusion of arterioles with fibrin thrombi. Dense PMN infiltrate around infarct and massive hemorrhage. **Hematologic   Studies   *CBC*** Schistocytes (fragmented RBCs), arising from RBC entrap-ment and damage within fibrin thrombi, seen on blood smear; platelet count low. Leukocy-tosis. *Coagulation Studies*   Reduced plasma fi-brinogen; elevated fibrin degradation products;

prolonged prothrombin time, partial thrombo-plastin time, and thrombin time. **Blood Culture**   For bacterial sepsis.

DIAGNOSIS AND DIFFERENTIAL DIAGNOSIS

Clinical suspicion confirmed by coagulation studies. Differential diagnosis of *large cutaneous infarctions*: necrosis after initiation of warfarin therapy, heparin necrosis, calciphylaxis, athero-embolization.

COURSE AND PROGNOSIS

Mortality rate is high. Surviving patients re-quire skin grafts or amputation for gangrenous tissue. Common complications: severe bleeding, thrombosis, tissue ischemia/necrosis, hemolysis, organ failure.

MANAGEMENT

Correct reversible cause. Vigorous antibiotic therapy for infections. Control bleeding or thrombosis: heparin, pentoxifylline, protein C concentrate. Prevent recurrence in chronic DIC.

CRYOGLOBULINEMIA   ICD-9:273.2 ∘ ICD-10:D89.1   ◼ ◖

- Cryoglobulinemia (CG) is the presence of serum immunoglobulin (precipitates at low temperature and redissolves at 37°C) complexed with other immunoglobulins or proteins.
- Associated clinical findings include purpura in cold-exposed sites, Raynaud phenomenon, cold urticaria, acral hemorrhagic necrosis, bleeding disorders, vasculitis, arthralgia, neurologic manifestations, hepatosplenomegaly, and glomerulonephritis.

- Precipitation of cryoglobulins (when present in large amounts) causes vessel occlusion, also associated with hyperviscosity.
- Immune complex deposition followed by complement activation and inflammation.
- Platelet aggregation/consumption of clotting factors by cryoglobulins, causing coagulation disorder.
- Small-vessel thromboses and vasculitis produced by immune complexes.

ETIOLOGY AND PATHOGENESIS

Type I Cryoglobulins: Monoclonal immunoglobulins (IgM, IgG, IgA, light chains). *Associated with*: plasma cell dyscrasias such as multiple myeloma, Waldenström macroglobulinemia, lymphoproliferative disorders such as B cell lymphoma.

Type II Cryoglobulins: Mixed cryoglobulins: two immunoglobulin components, one of which is monoclonal (usually IgG, less often IgM) and one polyclonal; components interact and cryoprecipitate. *Associated with*: multiple myeloma, Waldenström macroglobulinemia, chronic lymphocytic leukemia; rheumatoid arthritis, systemic lupus erythematosus, Sjögren syndrome.

Type III Cryoglobulins: Polyclonal immunoglobulins that form cryoprecipitate with polyclonal IgG or a nonimmunoglobulin serum component occasionally mixed with complement and lipoproteins. Represents immune complex disease. *Associated with*: autoimmune diseases; connective tissue diseases; wide variety of infectious diseases, i.e., hepatitis B, hepatitis C, Epstein-Barr virus infection, cytomegalovirus infection, subacute bacterial endocarditis, leprosy, syphilis, streptococcal infections.

CLINICAL MANIFESTATION

There is cold sensitivity in <50% of cases. Chills, fever, dyspnea, diarrhea may occur following cold exposure. Purpura also may follow long periods of standing or sitting. Due to other organ system involvement, arthralgia, renal symptoms, neurologic symptoms, abdominal pain, arterial thrombosis.

- *Noninflammatory purpura* (usually type I), occurring at cold-exposed sites, e.g., helix (Fig. 19-6), tip of nose.
- *Acrocyanosis* and *Raynaud phenomenon*, with or without severe resultant gangrene of fingertips and toes or elsewhere on arms or legs (usually types I or II) (Fig. 19-7).
- *Palpable purpura* with bullae and necroses (usually types II and III) due to hypersensitivity

FIGURE 19-6   Cryoglobulinemia: monoclonal (type I) This noninflamed, purpuric lesion on the helix appeared on the first cold day in the fall.

A   **B**

FIGURE 19-7   Cryoglobulinemia: mixed (type II)   *A.* Extensive necrosis and hemorrhage on the skin of the forearm. There was also digital gangrene on hands and feet.   ***B.***   Extensive hemorrhagic necrosis on both legs. There was also acral gangrene on four toes.

FIGURE 19-8   Cryoglobulinemia: polyclonal (type III)   Palpable purpura with widespread hemorrhage blister formation and necrosis as in any other type of hypersensitivity vasculitis (compare with Fig. 14-34*B*).

vasculitis, occurring in crops on lower extremities with extension to thighs, abdomen; precipitated by standing up (Fig. 19-8), less commonly by cold.
- *Livedo reticularis* mostly on lower and upper extremities.
- *Urticaria* induced by cold, associated with purpura.
- *Systemic involvement:* Between 30 and 60% of individuals with essential mixed CG (type II) develop renal disease with hypertension, edema, or renal failure. Neurologic involvement manifests as peripheral sensorimotor polyneuropathy, presenting as paresthesias or foot drop. Arthritis. Hepatosplenomegaly.
- *Diagnosis* is confirmed by determination of cryoglobulins (blood drawn into warmed syringe, RBC removed via warmed centrifuge; plasma refrigerated in a Wintrobe tube at 4°C for 24–72 h, then centrifuged and cryocrit determined) and diagnosis of underlying disease.
- The *course* is characterized by cyclic eruptions induced by cold or fluctuations of the activity of the underlying disease.
- *Treatment* is that of the underlying disease.

LEUKEMIA CUTIS   ICD-9 : 205.3 ∘ ICD-10 : C92.3   ◼ ●

- Leukemia cutis (LC) is a localized or disseminated skin infiltration by leukemic cells. It is usually a sign of dissemination of systemic disease or relapse of existing leukemia.

- Incidence varies from <5 to 50%, depending on the type of leukemia, both acute and chronic, including the leukemic phase of non-Hodgkin lymphoma and hairy cell leukemia.

- Most commonly occurs with acute monocytic leukemia M5 and acute myelomonocytic leukemia M4.

- Pattern of presentation of skin lesions in LC is variable and may have features that overlap with other (inflammatory) eruptions. Most common lesions are small (2–5 mm) papules (Figs. 19-9 and 19-10), nodules (Figs. 19-11 and 19-12.), or plaques. LC lesions are usually somewhat more pink, violaceous, or darker than normal skin, always palpable, indurated, firm, or guttate psoriasiform or lymphomatoid papulosis-like lesions, but usually not tender.

- Localized or disseminated; usually on trunk (Fig. 19-9.), extremities (Fig. 19-11.), and face (Fig. 19-10.) but may occur at any site. May be hemorrhagic when associated with thrombocytopenia or may ulcerate (Fig. 19-12.). Erythroderma may (rarely) occur. Leukemic gingival infiltration (hypertrophy) occurs with acute monocytic leukemia. Similar lesional morphologies occur with different types of leukemia or a specific type of leukemia may present with a variety of morphologies.

- *Inflammatory disorders* occurring in patients with leukemia are modified by the participation of leukemic cells in the infiltrate, resulting in unusual presentations of such disorders, e.g., psoriasis with hemorrhage or erosions/ulcerations.

- Cutaneous inflammatory diseases that may be associated with leukemia are Sweet syndrome, bullous pyoderma gangrenosum, urticaria, and necrotizing vasculitis.

- Systemic symptoms are those associated with hematologic malignancy.

- The *diagnosis* is made by suspicion and verified by skin biopsy, immunophenotyping, and B or T cell receptor rearrangement studies. Hematologic studies with complete analysis of bone marrow aspirate and peripheral blood smear are then needed to make the diagnosis.

- The prognosis for LC is directly related to the prognosis for the systemic disease.

- *Therapy* is usually directed at the leukemia itself. However, systemic chemotherapy sufficient for bone marrow remission may not treat the cutaneous lesions effectively. Thus, a combination of systemic chemotherapy and local electron beam therapy or PUVA may be necessary for chemotherapy-resistant LC lesions.

FIGURE 19-9   Leukemia cutis   Hundreds of tan-pink papules and a nodule on the trunk of a female with acute myelogenous leukemia arose during a 1-week interval. Per se, these lesions are "nonspecific" and do not present a diagnosis; but when such an eruption is seen, one should perform a peripheral blood count and a biopsy.

FIGURE 19-10   Leukemia cutis   Multiple skin-colored and erythematous papules in a 38-year-old febrile woman that had erupted about 1 week before this picture was taken. The patient had acute myelogenous leukemia.

FIGURE 19-11 **Leukemia cutis** A large, dark brown nodule on the upper arm of a male with acute myelogenous leukemia; six similar nodules were also present on the trunk.

FIGURE 19-12 **Leukemia cutis: chloroma** Large, ulcerated, green-hued tumors (chloromas) in the inguinal and perineal regions of a female with acute myelogenous leukemia; similar lesions were also present in the axillae and on the tongue.

LANGERHANS CELL HISTIOCYTOSIS

- Langerhans cell histiocytosis (LCH) is an idiopathic group of disorders characterized histologically by proliferation and infiltration of tissue by Langerhans cell–type histiocytes that fuse into multinucleated giant cells and form granulomas with eosinophils.
- Etiology: a reactive versus neoplastic nature of LCH is debated.
- LCH is characterized clinically by cutaneous findings that range from soft tissue swelling to seborrheic dermatitis–like changes to papular, pustular lesions, erosions, and ulcerations.
- Systemic lesions affect bones (lytic erosions), and lungs, bone marrow, liver, spleen, and lymph nodes.
- The course is variable, ranging from localized self-healing forms to generalized and fatal cases.
- Therapy depends on extent of disease and systemic involvement.

ICD-9 : 202.5/277.89 ∘ ICD-10 : D76.0

CLASSIFICATION

The disorders of histiocytes are classified as Langerhans cell histiocytosis (LCH, formerly histiocytosis X), non-Langerhans cell histiocytosis,[1] and malignant histiocytosis (Table 19-1). LCH is best classified as shown in Table 19-2.

EPIDEMIOLOGY AND ETIOLOGY

Age of Onset   *Unifocal LCH*   Most commonly, childhood and early adulthood.
Multifocal LCH   Most commonly, childhood.
Letterer-Siwe Disease (LSD)   More commonly, infancy (LSD) and childhood. Also, adult form.

TABLE 19-1   Classification System for Histiocytosis Developed by the Histiocyte Society (1987 and 2004)

Class I: Langerhans cell histiocytosis

Class II: Histiocytosis of the mononuclear phagocyte system or non--Langerhans cell histiocytosis IIa: Histiocytosis involving dermal CD68+ and factor XIII+ dendrocytes (histiocytosis involving cells of dermal dendrocyte lineage) IIb: Histiocytosis involving cells other than Langerhans cells and cells of the dermal dendrocyte lineage

Class III: Malignant histiocytosis

TABLE 19-2   Classification of LCH

Unifocal LCH	Most commonly manifested by a single osteolytic bony or skin or soft tissue lesion.
Multifocal LCH	Bony lesions are multiple and interfere with function of neighboring structures. Multifocal LCH also involves skin (second most frequently involved organ), soft tissue, lymph nodes, lungs, and pituitary glands.
Clinical Syndromes:	
Eosinophilic Granuloma	Unifocal skin, mucous membranes or soft tissue lesions.
Hand-Schüller-Christian Disease (HSCD)	The chronic, progressive multifocal form of LCH.
Letterer-Siwe Disease (LSD)	The most aggressive multifocal LCH form, with skin and internal organ involvement.
Hashimoto-Pritzger Syndrome (HPS)	A benign, self-healing variant of LCH.

[1]For the non-Langerhans cell histiocytosis, the reader is referred to C Gelmeti, R Caputo in K Wolff et al (eds), *Fitzpatrick's Dermatology in General Medicine,* 7th ed. New York, McGraw-Hill, 2008, pp 1424–1434.

Hand-Schüller-Christian Disease (HSCD)
Also childhood, chronic progressive.
Hashimoto Pritzger Syndrome (HPS) Childhood, self-healing.
Sex Males > females.
Incidence Rare, 0.5 per 100,000 children (estimate).

ETIOLOGY AND PATHOGENESIS

The stimulus for the proliferation of Langerhans cells is unknown. A reactive versus neoplastic nature is debated.

CLINICAL MANIFESTATION

Unifocal LCH Systemic symptoms uncommon. Pain and/or swelling over underlying bony lesion. Disruption of teeth with mandibular disease, fracture, otitis media due to mastoid involvement.
Multifocal LCH Erosive skin lesions are exudative, pruritic, or painful and may have offensive odor. Otitis media caused by destruction of temporal and mastoid bones, proptosis due to orbital masses, loose teeth with infiltration of maxilla or mandible, pituitary dysfunction with involvement of sella turcica associated with growth retardation, diabetes insipidus. Lung involvement associated with chronic cough, pneumothorax.
LSD Child (or very rarely an adult) is systemically ill with a course that resembles a systemic infection or malignancy. Hepatomegaly, petechiae, and purpura, generalized skin eruption.

Skin Lesions
Unifocal LCH (Eosinophilic Granuloma)

- Swelling over bony lesion (e.g., humerus, rib, mastoid), tender.
- Cutaneous/subcutaneous nodule, yellowish, may be tender and break down, occurring anywhere.
- Sharply marginated ulcer, usually in genital and perigenital regions or oral mucous membrane (gingiva, hard palate). Necrotic base, draining, tender (Fig. 19-13).

Multifocal LCH As in unifocal LCH; in addition, regionally localized (head) or generalized (trunk) eruptions. Papulosquamous, seborrheic dermatitis–like (scaly, oily), eczematous dermatitis–like lesions (Fig. 19-14); sometimes vesicular or purpuric (Fig. 19-15A). Turn necrotic and may become heavily crusted. Removal of crusts leaves small, shallow punched-out ulcers (Fig. 19-15B.) that heal with scars. Intertriginous lesions coalesce, may be erosive and exudative, become secondarily infected, and ulcerate. Mandibular and maxillary bone involvement may result in loss of teeth (Fig. 19-13). Ulceration of vulva and/or anus (Fig. 19-16).
LSD Skin lesions as in multifocal LCH but more widespread, disseminated (Fig. 19-15.), and ulcerating in intertriginous regions (Fig. 19-16). 🕮

FIGURE 19-13 Langerhans cell histiocytosis: eosinophilic granuloma Solitary, ulcerated nodule with loss of teeth on the gingival ridge near the palate, associated with involvement of the maxillary bone. Lesion was asymptomatic and only when the molars were lost did the patient consult a physician.

FIGURE 19-14 **Langerhans cell histiocytosis** Erythema and small, yellow-pink papules with a greasy scale on the face and scalp in this infant. These were the only lesions at first presentation and were mistaken for infantile seborrheic dermatitis. After lesions proved refractory to topical treatment and additional purpuric and crusted lesions appeared on the trunk, a biopsy was performed and the correct diagnosis was established.

General Findings *Multifocal LCH* Bony lesions occur in calvarium, sphenoid bone, sella turcica, mandible, long bones of upper extremities, and vertebrae. Associated findings of pituitary involvement.
HSCD Lytic skull lesions, proptosis, diabetes mellitus, and skin lesions.
LSD Hepatosplenomegaly, lymphadenopathy, involvement of lungs and other organs and bone marrow; thrombocytopenia and widespread and ulcerating skin lesions (Figs. 19-15 and 19-16).

LABORATORY EXAMINATIONS

Histopathology Proliferation of Langerhans cells with abundant pale eosinophilic cytoplasm and indistinct cell borders; a folded, indented, kidney-shaped nucleus with finely dispersed chromatin; epidermotropism. Langerhans cells in LCH have to be recognized by morphologic, ultrastructural (Birbeck granules), histochemical, and immunohistochemical markers [S-100 protein, CD1a and CD207 (Langerin)].

DIAGNOSIS

Confirmation of diagnosis by biopsy (skin, bone, or soft tissue/internal organs). Since skin is the organ most frequently involved after bone, skin biopsies have great diagnostic significance.

COURSE AND PROGNOSIS

HPS Benign, selfhealing.
Unifocal LCH Benign course with excellent prognosis for spontaneous resolution but tissue destruction.
Multifocal LCH Spontaneous remissions possible. Prognosis poorer at extremes of age and with extrapulmonary involvement.
LSD Commonly fulminant and fatal. Current scoring systems for evaluation of prognosis are based on number of organs involved, presence or absence of organ dysfunction, and age. The worst prognosis is in the very young with multifocal LCH and organ dysfunction and in LSD.

FIGURE 19-15 **Langerhans cell histiocytosis: Letterer-Siwe disease** ***A.*** Erythematous papules and vesicles with purpura, crusting, becoming confluent on the abdomen of an infant. ***B.*** More advanced lesions in another infant that have led to ulcers and depressed scars.

MANAGEMENT

Unifocal LCH Curettage with or without bony chip packing. Low-dose (300–600 rad) radiotherapy. Extraosseous soft tissue lesions: surgical excision or low-dose radiotherapy.

Multifocal LCH Diabetes insipidus and growth retardation treated with vasopressin and human growth hormone. Low-dose radiotherapy to bony lesions. Systemic treatment with glucocorticoids and/or vinblastine,

given as single agents or in combination and etoposide. Nonresponders: polychemotherapy (vincristine and cytarabine and prednisone or vincristine and doxorubicine and prednisone). Bone marrow transplantation is an option.

Cutaneous lesions Glucocorticoids for discrete cutaneous lesions. Extensive or generalized: cutaneous lesions respond best to PUVA or topical nitrogen mustard but also to oral thalidomide.

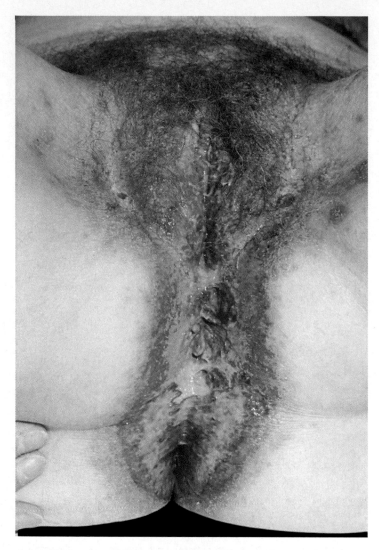

FIGURE 19-16 **Langerhans cell histiocytosis: Letterer-Siwe disease in an adult** Confluent erythematous plaques with necrosis and ulceration in the anogenital and perineal region in a 65-year-old female.

MASTOCYTOSIS SYNDROMES   ICD-9:757.33/202.6 ○ ICD-10:Q82.2 ■ ◑

- Mastocytosis is an abnormal accumulation of mast cells in the skin and at various systemic sites.
- An abbreviated World Health Organization (WHO) classification of mastocytosis is shown in Table 19-3.
- The skin is the most commonly involved organ system.
- Skin lesions are localized nodular or generalized maculopapular (Table 19-4).

- Because of the release of pharmacologically active substances, cutaneous symptoms are urticarial swelling or blistering with pruritus; systemic symptoms are blushing, vomiting, diarrhea, headache, syncope.
- Most patients with mastocytosis have only skin involvement, and most of these have no systemic symptoms. However, up to half of patients with systemic mastocytosis may not have any skin findings.

TABLE 19-3   Abbreviated WHO Classification of Mastocytosis

Cutaneous mastocytosis (CM)

Indolent systemic mastocytosis (ISM)

Systemic mastocytosis with an associated
clonal hematologic nonmast cell lineage disease (SM-AHNMD)

Aggressive systemic mastocytosis (ASM)

Mast cell leukemia (MCL)

Mast cell sarcoma (MCS)

Extracutaneous mastocytoma

Source: P Valent et. al.: WHO Classification of Tumors: Pathology and genetics of tumors of the hematopoietic and lymphoid tissues. ES Jaffe et.al. (eds). Lyon, IARC Press, 2001

TABLE 19-4   Classification of Cutaneous Mastocytosis (CM)

Localized	Nodular CM (mastocytoma, NCM)
Generalized	Maculopapular CM
	Papular plaque CM (PPCM)
	Urticaria pigmentosa (UP)
	Telangiectasia macularis eruptiva perstans (TMEP)
	Diffuse CM (DCM)

EPIDEMIOLOGY

Age of Onset   Between birth and 2 years of age (55%) (NCM, PPCM, UP), but mastocytosis can occur at any age; infancy-onset mastocytosis rarely associated with systemic mastocytosis.
Sex   Slight male: female predominance.
Prevalence   Unknown.

PATHOGENESIS

Human mast cell proliferation depends on Kit ligand and Kit is the receptor for stem cell factor. c-*kit* mutations have been identified in blood and tissues of patients with mastocytosis. Mast cells contain several pharmacologically active substances that are associated with the clinical findings in mastocytosis: histamine (urticaria, GI symptoms), prostaglandin D_2 (flush, cardiovascular symptoms, bronchoconstriction, GI symptoms), heparin (bleeding into tissue, osteoporosis), neutral protease/acid hydrolases (patchy hepatic fibrosis, bone lesions).

CLINICAL MANIFESTATION

Stroking lesion causes it to itch and to wheal (*Darier sign*). Various drugs are capable of causing mast cell degranulation and release of pharmacologically active substances that exacerbate skin lesions (whealing, itching) and cause flushing: alcohol, dextran, polymyxin B, morphine, codeine, scopolamine, D-tubocuratin, nonsteroidal anti-inflammatory drugs. Flushing episode can also be elicited by heat or cold and may be accompanied by headache, nausea, vomiting, diarrhea, dyspnea/wheezing, syncope. Systemic involvement may lead to symptoms of malabsorption; portal hypertension. Bone pain. Neuropsychiatric symptoms (malaise, irritability).

Skin Lesions (CM)   **Localized** *NCM* Macular to papular to nodular lesions (mastocytoma) (Fig. 19-17), often solitary; may be multiple, but few. Yellow to tan-pink, which become erythematous and raised (urticate) when stroked due to degranulation of mast cells (Darier sign); in some patients, lesions become bullous.
Generalized *PPCM* Tan, occasionally yellowish plaques, up to 2–5 cm, sharply defined with irregular outlines. Darier sign positive (Fig. 19-18). No scaling, occasionally with bulla formation after rubbing. Occurs mostly in infants and children.
UP Tan macules to slightly raised tan to brown papules (Fig. 19-19). Disseminated, few or >100 with widespread symmetric distribution. Darier sign (whealing) after rubbing; in infants may become bullous. Occurs in infancy and/or de novo in adults. Bright red diffuse flushing occurring spontaneously, after rubbing of skin, or after ingestion of alcohol or mast cell–degranulating agents.
TMEP Freckle-like, brownish to reddish macules (Fig. 19-20) with fine telangiectasia in long-standing lesions. Hundreds of lesions, trunk > extremities; lesions may be confluent. Urticate with gentle stroking. Dermatographism. Occur only in adults and very rare.
DCM Yellowish, thickened appearance of large areas of skin; "doughy." Smooth with scattered elevation, resembling leather,

"pseudoxanthomatous mastocytosis," skin folds exaggerated, especially in axilla/groin. Large bullae may occur after trauma or spontaneously. DCM may present as erythroderma (Fig. 19-21). Very rare, occurs at all ages. 🔲
Systemic Symptoms   Flushing, accompanied by wheezing, headache, asthma, nausea, vomiting, diarrhea, syncope. Bone pain/spontaneous fractures with osteolytic lesions. Neuropsychiatric symptoms, malaise, irritability. Malabsorption, weight loss.

LABORATORY EXAMINATIONS

Dermatopathology   Accumulation of normal-looking mast cells in dermis. Mast cell infiltrates may be sparse (spindle-shaped) or densely aggregated (cuboidal shape) and have a perivascular or nodular distribution. Pigmentation due to increased melanin in basal layer.
CBC   Systemic mastocytosis: anemia, leukocytosis, eosinophilia.
Blood   Tryptase levels↑, coagulation parameters.
Urine   Patients with extensive cutaneous involvement may have increased 24-h urinary histamine excretion.
Bone Scan and Imaging   Define bone involvement (lytic bone lesions, osteoporosis, or osteosclerosis), and endoscopy for small-bowel involvement.
Bone Marrow   Smear and/or biopsy for morphology and mast cell markers.

DIAGNOSIS

Clinical suspicion, positive Darier sign, confirmed by skin biopsy.

DIFFERENTIAL DIAGNOSIS

NCM   Juvenile xanthogranuloma, Spitz nevus.
Flushing   Carcinoid syndrome.
UP, PPCM, TMEP   Langerhans cell histiocytosis, secondary syphilis, papular sarcoid, generalized eruptive histiocytoma, non-Langerhans cell histiocytosis of childhood.
DCM   Cutaneous T cell lymphoma, pseudoxanthoma elasticum, forms of erythroderma.

COURSE AND PROGNOSIS

Most cases of solitary mastocytosis and generalized UP and PPCM in children resolve spontaneously. They rarely have systemic involvement.

FIGURE 19-17   Mastocytosis: solitary mastocytoma (NCM)   A solitary, tan plaque with poorly demarcated borders on the hand of an infant. When stroked very vigorously, the lesion became red, more elevated and a blister developed.

FIGURE 19-18   Mastocytosis: generalized (PPCM)   Multiple, flat-topped papules and small plaques of brownish to yellowish color on the buttocks of a child. Lesions are asymptomatic. Rubbing one of the lesions has resulted in urtication and an axon flare, a positive Darier sign, and itching.

Adults with onset of UP or TMEP with extensive cutaneous involvement have a higher risk for development of systemic mastocytosis (see Table 19-3). In young children, acute and extensive degranulation may be life-threatening (shock).

MANAGEMENT

Avoidance of drugs that may cause mast cell degranulation and histamine release (see above).

Antihistamines, both H_1 and H_2, either alone or with ketotifen. Disodium cromoglycate, 200 mg four times a day, may ameliorate pruritus, flushing, diarrhea, abdominal pain, and disorders of cognitive function but not skin lesions. PUVA treatment is effective for disseminated skin lesions, but recurrence is common. Vascular collapse is treated with epinephrine. NCM responds to potent glucocorticoid ointments under occlusion or to intralesional triamcinolone acetonide but may eventually recur.

A

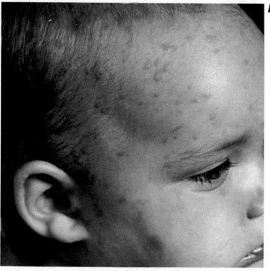

B

FIGURE 19-19   Mastocytosis: urticaria pigmentosa (UP)   *A.* Multiple, generalized tan to brown papules in a child. The patient had occasional syncopes, diarrhea, and wheezing; workup revealed systemic mastocytosis. ***B.*** Brown papules on the forehead of a 3-year-old boy who was otherwise asymptomatic.

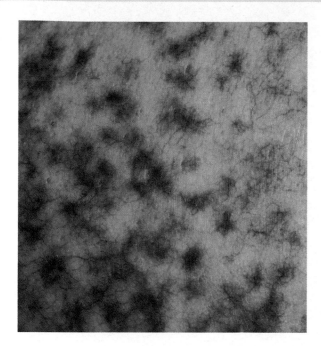

FIGURE 19-20 Mastocytosis: telangiectasia macularis eruptiva perstans Small, stellate erythematous macules and telangiectases on the back of a 45-year-old woman who had systemic (indolent) mastocytosis.

FIGURE 19-21 Mastocytosis: diffuse cutaneous mastocytosis The skin of this infant is uniformly erythematous (erythroderma) secondary to infiltrating mast cells with several spared, white areas of normal skin. In this child there were systemic symptoms associated with the flare of this erythroderma: syncope, wheezing, and diarrhea.

CUTANEOUS LYMPHOMAS AND SARCOMA

- Cutaneous lymphomas are clonal proliferations of neoplastic T or B cells, rarely natural killer cells or plasmacytoid dendritic cells. Cutaneous lymphomas are the second most common group of extranodal lymphomas. The annual incidence is estimated to be 1 per 100,000.
- The WHO-EORTC classification is shown in Table 20-1.

- For rare conditions not dealt with in this Atlas the reader is referred to C Assaf, W Sterry, in K Wolff et al (eds): *Fitzpatrick's Dermatology in General Medicine*, 7th ed. New York, McGraw-Hill, 2008, pp 1386–1402.

ADULT T CELL LEUKEMIA/LYMPHOMA ☐ ●

- Adult T cell leukemia/lymphoma (ATLL) is a neoplasm of CD4+/CD25+ T cells, caused by human T cell lymphotrophic virus I (HTLV-I).
- Manifested by skin infiltrates, hypercalcemia, visceral involvement, lytic bone lesions, and abnormal lymphocytes on peripheral smears.
- HTLV-I is a human retrovirus. Infection by the virus does not usually cause disease, which suggests that other environmental factors are involved. Immortalization of some infected CD4+ T cells, increased mitotic activity, genetic instability, and impairment of cellular immunity can all occur after infection with HTLV-I. These events may increase the probability of additional genetic changes, which, by chance, may lead to the development of leukemia 20-40 years after infection in some people (≤5%). Most of these effects have been attributed to the HTLV-I-encoded protein tax.
- ATLL occurs in southwestern Japan (Kyushu), Africa, the Caribbean Islands, southeastern United States. Transmission is by sexual intercourse, perinatally, or by exposure to blood or blood products (same as HIV).
- There are four main categories. In the relatively indolent *smoldering* and *chronic* forms, the median survival is ≥2 years. In the *acute* and *lymphomatous* forms, it ranges from only 4–6 months.
- Symptoms include fever, weight loss, abdominal pain, diarrhea, pleural effusion, ascites, cough,

sputum. Skin lesions occur in 50% of patients with ATLL. Single to multiple small, confluent erythematous, violaceous papules (Fig. 20-1), ±purpura; firm violaceous to brownish nodules (Fig. 20-2); papulosquamous lesions, large plaques, ±ulceration; trunk > face > extremities; generalized erythroderma; poikiloderma; diffuse alopecia. Lymphadenopathy (75%) sparing mediastinal lymph nodes. Hepatomegaly (50%) and splenomegaly (25%).

- Patients are seropositive (ELISA, Western blot) to HTLV-I; in IV drug users, up to 30% have dual retroviral infection with both HTLV-I and HIV. WBC ranges from normal to 500,000/µL. Peripheral blood smears show polylobulated lymphocytic nuclei ("flower cells"). *Dermatopathology* reveals lymphomatous infiltrates composed of many large abnormal lymphocytes, ±giant cells, ±Pautrier microabscesses. There is hypercalcemia—in 25% at time of diagnosis of ATLL and in >50% during clinical course; this is thought to be due to osteoclastic bone resorption.

- Management consists of various regimens of cytotoxic chemotherapy; the rates of complete response are <30% and responses lack durability, but good results have been obtained with the combination of oral zidovudine and subcutaneous interferon-α in acute and lymphoma-type ATLL patients. ✐

ICD-9 : 204.0/208.9 ∘ ICD-10 : C83/E88

TABLE 20-1 WHO-EORTC Classification of Primary Cutaneous Lymphomas

Cutaneous T-Cell and NK-Cell Lymphomas

- Mycosis fungoides
- Mycosis fungoides variants and sub-types
  - Folliculotropic mycosis fungoides
  - Pagetoid reticulosis
  - Granulomatous slack skin
- Sézary syndrome
- Adult T-cell leukemia/lymphoma
- Primary cutaneous CD30-positive lymphoproliferative disorders
  - Primary cutaneous anaplastic large-cell lymphoma
  - Lymphomatoid papulosis
- Subcutaneous panniculitis-like T-cell lymphoma
- Extra-nodal NK/T-cell lymphoma, nasal type
- Provisional entities of cutaneous T-cell lymphoma
  - Primary cutaneous aggressive epidermotropic CD8⁺ T-cell lymphoma
  - Cutaneous γ/δ T-cell lymphoma
  - Primary cutaneous CD4⁺ small or medium-sized pleomorphic T-cell lymphoma

Cutaneous B-Cell Lymphomas

- Primary cutaneous marginal zone B-cell lymphoma
- Primary cutaneous follicle center lymphoma
- Primary cutaneous diffuse lagre B-cell lymphoma, leg type
- Primary cutaneous diffuse large B-cell lymphoma, other
  - Intravascular large B-cell lymphoma (provisional)
- Precursor hematologic neoplasm
- CD4⁺/CD56⁺ hematodermic neoplasm (blastic NK-cell lymphoma)

NK, natural killer; WHO-EORTC, World Health Organization and European Organisation for Research and Treatment of Cancer.

FIGURE 20-1 **Adult T cell leukemia/lymphoma** A generalized eruption of small, confluent violaceous papules with a predilection for the trunk. The patient had fever, weight loss, abdominal pain, massive leukocytosis with "flower cells" in smear, lymphadenopathy, hepatosplenomegaly, and hypercalcemia.

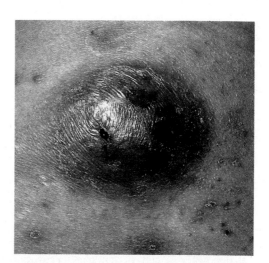

FIGURE 20-2 **Adult T cell leukemia/lymphoma** Firm, violaceous to brownish nodules as shown here are another cutaneous manifestation of ATLL. These nodules may ulcerate.

CUTANEOUS T CELL LYMPHOMA   ◧ ●

- Cutaneous T cell lymphoma (CTCL) is a term that applies to T cell lymphoma first manifested in the skin, but since the neoplastic process involves the entire lymphoreticular system, the lymph nodes and internal organs become involved in the course of the disease. CTCL is a malignancy of helper T cells (CD4+).
- In the classic form of CTCL, called *mycosis fungoides* (MF), the malignant cells are cutaneous

CD4+ cells, but the clinical entity of MF has now been expanded to the spectrum of CTCL including non-MF cutaneous T cell lymphomas.
- Whereas all MF is CTCL not all CTCLs are MF.
- Only the classic MF form is discussed here.

Synonym: Mycosis fungoides.

ICD-9 : 202.1/202.2 ∘ ICD-10 : C84.0/C84.1

MYCOSIS FUNGOIDES (MF)   ICD-9 : 202.1/202.0 ∘ ICD-10 : C84.0/C84.1   ◧ ●

- MF is the most common cutaneous lymphoma.
- Arising in mid to late adulthood with male predominance of 2:1.
- A clonal proliferation of skin-homing CTLA+ CD4+ T cells with an admixture of CD8+ T cells (antitumor response).
- Categorized as patch, plaque, or tumor stage.

- Related features are pruritus, alopecia, palmoplantar hyperkeratosis, and bacterial infections.
- Histologically, epidermotropism of T cells with hyperconvoluted nuclei. In the tumor stage dermal nodular infiltrates.
- Prognosis related to stage.
- Treatment: symptom-oriented and stage-adapted.

EPIDEMIOLOGY AND ETIOLOGY

Age of Onset   Median age at diagnosis 55–60 years.
Sex   Male:female ratio 2:1.
Incidence   Uncommon but not rare.
Etiology   Unknown. CTCL is a malignancy of skin-homing CTLA+ CD4+ T cells.

CLINICAL MANIFESTATIONS

For months to years, often preceded by various diagnoses such as psoriasis, nummular dermatitis, and "large plaque" parapsoriasis. Symptoms: pruritus, often intractable, but may be none.
Skin Findings   Skin lesions are classified into patches, plaques, and tumor stage. Patients may have simultaneously more than one type of lesions.

Patches   Randomly distributed, scaling or non-scaling patches in different shades of red (Fig. 20-3). Well or ill-defined; at first superficial, much like eczema or psoriasis (Figs. 20-3 and 20-4) or mimicking dermatophytosis ("mycosis"), and later becoming thicker.
Plaques   Round, oval, but often also arciform, annular, and of bizarre configuration (Figs. 20-3 and 20-5). Lesions are randomly distributed but in early stages often spare exposed areas.
Tumors: Later lesions consist of nodules (Figs. 20-5 and 20-6) and tumors, with or without ulceration (Fig. 20-7). Extensive infiltration can cause leonine facies (Fig. 20-8). Confluence may lead to erythroderma (see Section 8). There is palmoplantar keratoderma and there may be hair loss. Poikiloderma may be present from the onset or develop later (Fig. 20-9). ✐
General Examination   Lymphadenopathy, usually after thick plaques and nodules have appeared.

FIGURE 20-3   Mycosis fungoides   In early stages lesions consist of randomly distributed, well- and/or ill-defined patches and later plaques as shown here in a 37-year-old male. They may be scaly and appear in various shades of red. They mimic eczema, psoriasis, or dermatophytosis.

FIGURE 20-4   Mycosis fungoides: patches/plaque stage   More advanced stages show confluence of patches and plaques with irregular configuration. This patient had been treated unsuccessfully for psoriasis for 2 years. Morphologically, he could also have extensive, confluent dermatophytosis (see Section 25) but a negative KOH preparation ruled out this diagnosis. Only after a biopsy had been done was the correct diagnosis of MF made.

FIGURE 20-5   Mycosis fungoides   Plaque and early nodular stage with reddish-brownish scaly, and crusted plaques and flat nodules.

FIGURE 20-6   Mycosis fungoides: tumor stage   Scaly and crusted eczema-like plaques seen on the arm and chest have turned nodular on the shoulder. This patient had similar lesions elsewhere and was staged IIB (T_3 N_1 M_0).

FIGURE 20-7   Mycosis fungoides: tumors   Two large ulcerated tumors on the lower flank of a Vietnamese man. The tumors arose in a sea of ill-defined, scaly and crusted plaques. The patient had been treated for psoriasis for two years.

FIGURE 20-8   Mycosis fungoides: leonine facies   In this 50-year-old patient the disease had started with extremely pruritic, generalized eczema-like plaques on the trunk that had been treated as eczema over a course of 4 years. Massive nodular infiltration of the face occurred only recently leading to a leonine facies.

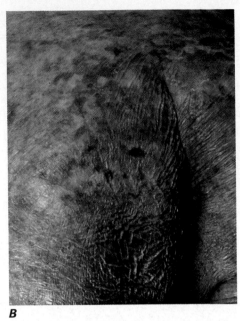

A   **B**

FIGURE 20-9   Mycosis fungoides: poikilodermatous lesions   *A.* Small reticulated, confluent papules mixed with superficial atrophy give the impression of poikiloderma. This patient had patches elsewhere on the body similar to those shown in Fig. 20-3. ***B.*** Poikiloderma in MF can also result from treatment. This patient had been treated with electron beam.

MYCOSIS FUNGOIDES VARIANTS

- *Folliculotropic MF*: With preferential involvement of head and neck, with or without mucinosis, degeneration of hair follicles (previously "mucinosis follicularis," "alopecia mucinosa") (Fig. 20-10).

- *Hypopigmented MF*: Hypopigmented patches in patients with dark skin.

- *Pagetoid reticulosis (Woringer-Kolopp disease)* This is a special variant of MF consisting of *localized* patches and plaques (Fig. 20-11), with a proliferation of neoplastic T cells, that expand intraepidermally following a pattern similar to Paget disease. Extracutaneous dissemination has not been observed, and there is an excellent prognosis.

- *Granulomatosus slack skin*: Rare subtype of MF with folds of lax skin in the major skin folds (Fig. 20-12).

- *Sézary syndrome*: A leukemic variant, see below p 534 and Section 8.

LABORATORY EXAMINATIONS

Dermatopathology In early stages repeated and multiple biopsies are often necessary to finally establish the diagnosis. Bandlike and patchy infiltrate in upper dermis of atypical lymphocytes (mycosis cells) extending to epidermis and skin appendages. The classic finding is the epidermotropism of this T cell infiltrate, which will form microabscesses in the epidermis (Pautrier microabscesses). In the plaque and tumor stage the infiltrate extends deep into the dermis and beyond. Mycosis cells are T cells with hyperchromatic, irregularly shaped (cerebriform) nuclei. Mitoses vary from rare to frequent.

FIGURE 20-10 **Folliculotropic MF** Multiple small follicular papules ("mucinosis follicularis").

FIGURE 20-11 **Pagetoid reticulosis** This singular plaque on the hip of a 62-year-old female looks like psoriasis. It was asymptomatic and had been present for 8 months. Histopathology revealed intraepidermal T cells in a pagetoid pattern.

Mycosis cells are activated monoclonal CTLA+ CD4+ T cells. However, lesions of MF often have a CD8+ T cell component, and these cells are considered to reflect an antitumor response; improved long-term prognosis has been correlated with the presence of such CD8+ tumor-infiltrating lymphocytes.

Hematology Eosinophilia, 6–12%, can increase to 50%. Buffy coat: abnormal circulating T cells (mycosis cell-type) and increased WBC (20,000/μL). Bone marrow examination is not helpful in early stages.

Chemistry Lactic dehydrogenase isoenzymes 1, 2, and 3 increased in erythrodermic stage.

Chest X-Ray Search for hilar lymphadenopathy.

Imaging In stage I and stage II disease, diagnostic imaging (CT, gallium scintigraphy, liver-spleen scan, and lymphangiography) does not provide more information than biopsies of lymph nodes.

CT Scan With more advanced disease, to search for retroperitoneal nodes in patients with extensive skin involvement, lymphadenopathy.

DIAGNOSIS AND DIFFERENTIAL DIAGNOSIS

In the early stages, the diagnosis of MF is a problem. Clinical lesions may be typical, but histologic confirmation may not be possible for years despite repeated biopsies. Tissue should be sent for immunophenotyping of infiltrating T cells by use of monoclonal antibodies and T cell receptor rearrangement studies. Lymphadenopathy and the detection of abnormal circulating T cells in the blood appear to correlate well with *internal* organ involvement.

Differential Diagnosis Mainly *scaling plaques* (see Figs. 20-3, 20-4, and 20-5). High index of suspicion is needed in patients with atypical or refractory "psoriasis," "eczema," and poikiloderma. MF often mimics psoriasis in being a scaly plaque and disappearing with exposure to sunlight.

Patient Evaluation in MF and Staging This has to focus on an evaluation of tumor burden, the degree of atypia of malignant cells, and the state of immunocompetence of the patient. Table 20-2 shows a flow sheet of patient evaluation, Table 20-3 shows the TNM classification and Table 20-4 the staging of mycosis fungoides.

TABLE 20-2   Patient Evaluation in MF

Skin
  Body surface area assessment
  Routine histology
  Immunophenotyping
  Polymerase chain reaction for T cell receptor rearrangement
Blood
  Complete blood count with smear examination
  Immunophenotyping
Lymph node
  Palpate all nodes
  Measure enlarged nodes by CT scan
  Biopsy enlarged nodes

TABLE 20-3   TNM Classification of Mycosis Fungoides (C532 TCL)

T: Skin	T_0	Clinically and/or histologically suspicious lesions
	T_1	Limited plaques, papules, or eczematous patches covering <10% of the skin surface
	T_2	Generalized plaques, papules, or erythematous patches covering >10% of the skin surface
	T_3	Tumors (1 or more)
	T_4	Generalized erythroderma
N: Lymph nodes	N_0	No clinically abnormal peripheral nodes, pathology negative for MF
	N_1	Clinically abnormal peripheral lymph nodes, pathology negative for MF
	N_2	No clinically abnormal peripheral lymph nodes, pathology positive for MF
	N_3	Clinically abnormal peripheral lymph nodes, pathology positive for MF
B: Blood	B_0	<5% atypical circulating lymphocytes
	B_1	>5% atypical circulating lymphocytes (Sézary)
M: Visceral organs	M_0	No visceral organ involvement
	M_1	Histologically proven visceral involvement

FIGURE 20-12   Granulomatous slack skin   Firm, platelike infiltrates on the neck and anterior chest and lax skin folds of the axillary and scapular region.

TABLE 20-4   Staging System for Mycosis Fungoides and Sézary Syndrome

Stage	T(Tumor)	N (Lymph Node)	M (Metastases)
IA	T1	N0	M0
IB	T2	N0	M0
IIA	T1 or T2	N1	M0
IIB	T3	N0 OR N1	M0
III	T4	N0 OR N1	M0
IVA	T1–T4	N2 OR N3	M0
IVB	T1–T4	N0–N3	M1

T1: patch/plaque ≤10% of body surface; T2: patch/plaque ≥ 10% of body surface; T3: skin tumor(s); T4 erythroderma; N0: normal nodes; N1: palpable nodes without histologic evidence of lymphoma; N2: no palpable nodes, but histologic evidence of lymphoma; N3: palpable nodes with histologic evidence of lymphoma; M0: no visceral involvement; M1: histologically confirmed visceral involvement.

COURSE AND PROGNOSIS

Unpredictable; MF (pre-MF) may be present for years. Course varies with the source of the patients studied. At the NIH there was a median survival time of 5 years from the time of the histologic diagnosis, while in Europe a less malignant course is seen (survival time, up to 10–15 years). This, however, may be due to patient selection. Prognosis is much worse when (1) tumors are present (mean survival, 2.5 years), (2) there is lymphadenopathy (mean survival, 3 years), (3) >10% of the skin surface is involved with pretumor-stage MF, and (4) there is a generalized erythroderma. Patients <50 years have twice the survival rate of patients >60 years.

MANAGEMENT

Therapy is symptom-oriented and extent of disease– and stage-adapted. In the pre-MF stage, in which the histologic diagnosis is only compatible, but not confirmed, PUVA photochemotherapy is the most effective treatment, but narrow-band UVB treatment is also effective. For histologically proven plaque-stage disease with no lymphadenopathy and no abnormal circulating T cells, PUVA photochemotherapy is also the method of choice, either alone or combined with oral isotretinoin or bexarotene or subcutaneous interferon-α. Also used at this stage are topical chemotherapy with nitrogen mustard in an ointment base (10 mg/dL), topical carmustine (BCNU) (for limited body surface area involvement), and total-body electron-beam therapy, singly or in combination. Isolated tumors that may develop should be treated with local x-ray or electron-beam therapy. For extensive plaque stage with multiple tumors or in patients with lymphadenopathy or abnormal circulating T cells, electron-beam plus chemotherapy is probably the best combination for now; randomized, controlled studies of various combinations are in progress. Also, extracorporeal PUVA photochemotherapy is being evaluated in patients with Sézary syndrome.

SÉZARY SYNDROME ICD-9:202.2 ∘ ICD-10:L84.1   □ ●

- Sézary syndrome is a rare special variant of MF characterized by universal erythroderma, peripheral lymphadenopathy, and cellular infiltrates of atypical lymphocytes (Sézary cells) in the skin and in the blood.

- The disease may arise de novo or, less commonly, result from extension of a preexisting circumscribed MF. It usually occurs in patients >60 years and more commonly in males than in females.

- Patients appear sick, shivering, and scared and there is generalized scaling erythroderma with considerable thickening of the skin. Because of the bright red color, the syndrome has been called the "red man syndrome" (see Section 8 and Fig. 8-3). There is diffuse hyperkeratosis of palms and soles, diffuse hair loss that can lead to baldness, and generalized lymphadenopathy.

- *Dermatopathology*: the same as MF. The lymph nodes may contain nonspecific inflammatory cells (dermatopathic lymphadenopathy) or there can be a complete replacement of the nodal pattern by Sézary cells. The cell infiltrates in the viscera are the same as are present in the skin. *Immunophenotyping*: CD4+ T cells; T cell receptor rearrangement: monoclonal process. There may be a moderate leukocytosis or a normal WBC. The buffy coat contains from 15–30% atypical lymphocytes (Sézary cells).

- Diagnosis rests on three features: erythroderma, generalized lymphadenopathy, and presence of increased numbers of atypical lymphocytes in the buffy coat.

- Note that any exfoliative dermatitis can mimic Sèzary syndrome (see Section 8).

- Without treatment, the course is progressive and patients die from opportunistic infections. Management is as in MF, plus appropriate supportive measures required for erythroderma (see Section 8).

LYMPHOMATOID PAPULOSIS ICD-10 : L41.2

- Lymphomatoid papulosis is an asymptomatic, chronic, self-healing, polymorphous eruption of unknown etiology.

- It is a low-grade, self-limited T cell lymphoma with a low but real risk of progression to more malignant forms of lymphoma.

- Incidence is 1.2–1.9 cases per million, occurring sporadically in both sexes from childhood to old age; average age 40 years.

- Characterized by recurrent crops of lesions that regress spontaneously, with histologic features of lymphocytic atypia.

- Pathogenesis Unknown; considered to be a low-grade lymphoma perhaps induced by chronic antigenic stimulation and controlled by host mechanisms. Begins as a chronic, reactive, polyclonal lymphoproliferative phenomenon that sporadically overwhelms host immune defenses and evolves into a clonal, antigen-independent, true lymphoid malignancy. It belongs in the spectrum of primary cutaneous CD30+ lymphoproliferative disorders.

- Close clinical resemblance to pityriasis lichenoides et varioliformis acuta (see Fig. 7-18). Erythematous to red-brown papules (Fig. 20-13) and nodules, 2–5 mm in diameter, which are initially smooth and hemorrhagic, later hyperkeratotic, with central, black necrosis, crusting (Fig. 20-13), and ulceration. Few to hundreds of lesions, asymptomatic or pruritic, arranged at random and often grouped, recurrent, primarily on trunk and extremities; rarely, oral and genital mucosa. Individual lesions evolve over a 2- to 8-week period and resolve spontaneously at any point in their evolution. Atrophic hyper- or hypopigmented scarring following ulcerated lesions.

- Other organ systems are uninvolved.

- *Dermatopathology:* Superficial or deep, perivascular or interstitial mixed cell infiltrate, wedge-shaped. Cytologically, atypical cells may comprise 50% of infiltrate. *Type A:* large CD30+, atypical histioid lymphocytes with abundant cytoplasm, convoluted nucleus with occasional binucleation, multipolar mitosis, and Reed-Sternberg cell appearance. Admixed with a dense inflammatory infiltrate. *Type B:* smaller CD30-, atypical lymphocytes with cerebriform nuclei, epidermotropism, and occasional mitosis. *Type C:* large CD30+ cells form sheets resembling cutaneous anaplastic large cell lymphoma (CALCL)

- *Differential diagnosis:* Based on typical histology and immunohistochemistry, lack of systemic involvement by history and physical examination.

- *Course:* May remit in 3 weeks or continue for decades. In 10–20% of patients, lymphomatoid papulosis is preceded by, associated with, or followed by another type of lymphoma: MF, Hodgkin disease, or CD30+ (CALCL). May persist despite systemic chemotherapy for concurrent lymphoma.

- No treatments have proved consistently effective, as is evidenced by the multiple reported therapies. Topical agents include glucocorticoids and carmustine (BCNU). Electron-beam irradiation. PUVA controls the disease but does not affect the long-term prognosis. Tetracyclines, sulfones, systemic glucocorticoids, and acyclovir have been anecdotally reported as effective. Also, retinoids, methotrexate, chlorambucil, cyclophosphamide, cyclosporine, and interferon-α2b, none with lasting effect.

CUTANEOUS ANAPLASTIC LARGE CELL LYMPHOMAS (CALCL)

- CALCL are cutaneous lymphomas consisting of large tumor cells that express CD30 antigen and have no evidence or history of lymphomatoid papulosis, mycosis fungoides, or other types of CTCL.

- They occur in adults and present as solitary, reddish to brownish nodules and tumors, which frequently tend to ulcerate (Fig. 20-14).

- The nodular infiltrates are nonepidermotropic, and neoplastic cells show an anaplastic morphology.

- At least 75% of the neoplastic cells are CD30+ and additionally express the CD4+ phenotype.

- CALCL have a favorable prognosis with a disease-related 5-year survival rate of 90%.

- Treatment is radiotherapy, but successful treatment with PUVA in combination with interferon-α has been reported.

ICD-9 : M9714/3

FIGURE 20-13   Lymphomatoid papulosis   Crops of reddish-brown papules appear in waves involving the entire body. Lesions are asymptomatic, become hyperkeratotic, crusted, and necrotic in the center. Since lesions arise asynchronously, all stages in this evolution are present simultaneously.

FIGURE 20-14   Anaplastic large cell lymphoma   A solitary violaceous, reddish nodule on the forearm of a 46-year-old male patient. Histopathology revealed nonepidermotropic anaplastic mononuclear cells, most of which were of the CD4+, CD30+ phenotype. The lesion was excised and there was no recurrence.

CUTANEOUS B CELL LYMPHOMA ICD-10 : C85.1 □ ●

- A clonal proliferation of B lymphocytes can be confined to the skin or more often is associated with systemic B cell lymphoma. Rare. Comprise 20% of all cutaneous lymphomas.

- Occurs in individuals >50 years.

- Crops of asymptomatic nodules and plaques, red to plum color (Fig. 20-15) with a smooth surface, firm, nontender, cutaneous or subcutaneous.

- Primary cutaneous follicle center cell lymphoma, primary cutaneous marginal zone lymphoma, and primary cutaneous large B cell lymphoma of the leg are special defined entities.

- *Dermatopathology*: Dense nodular or diffuse monomorphous infiltrates of lymphocytes usually separated from the epidermis by a zone of normal collagen ("grenz zone"). B cell–specific mono-clonal antibody studies facilitate differentiation of cutaneous B cell lymphoma from pseudolymphoma and cutaneous T cell lymphoma and permit more accurate classification of the cell type. Most cases react with CD19, 20, 22, and 79A. Gene-typing studies confirm diagnosis with immunoglobulin gene rearrangement.

- Patients should be investigated thoroughly for nodal and extracutaneous disease; if found, bone marrow, lymph node, and peripheral blood studies will show morphologic, cytochemical, and immunologic features similar to those of the cutaneous infiltrates.

- *Management*: Consists of x-ray therapy to localized lesions and chemotherapy for systemic disease. ℓ

FIGURE 20-15 **Cutaneous B cell lymphoma** Smooth, cutaneous and subcutaneous nodules on the lower leg. One is ulcerated. They were asymptomatic and firm and were the first signs of B cell lymphoma.

KAPOSI SARCOMA (KS) ICD-9 : 176 ○ ICD-10 : C46

- KS is a multifocal systemic tumor of endothelial cell origin.
- Invariably linked with human herpesvirus 8 infection.
- Four clinical variants: classic KS, endemic African KS, immunosuppressive therapy–related KS and HIV/AIDS-related KS.

- Stage- and variant-dependent localized and/or generalized disease: patches, plaques, nodules.
- Systemic involvement: mainly GI tract.
- Responds to radiation and chemotherapy.

ETIOPATHOGENESIS

DNA of human herpesvirus type 8 (HHV-8) has been identified in tissue samples of all variants of KS. There is seroepidemiologic evidence that this virus is involved in the pathogenesis.

CLASSIFICATION AND CLINICAL VARIANTS

Classic or European KS Occurs in elderly males of eastern European heritage (Mediterranean and Ashkenazi Jewish). Not so uncommon in eastern and southern Europe; rare in the United States. Peak incidence after sixth decade. Males > females. Predominantly arises on the legs but also occurs in lymph nodes and abdominal viscera; slowly progressive.
African-Endemic KS Between 9 and 12.8% of all malignancies in Zaire. Two distinct age groups: young adults, mean age 35; and young children, mean age 3 years. Males > females. No evidence of underlying immunodeficiency. Four clinical patterns (see below).
Iatrogenic Immunosuppression-Associated KS Rare. Most commonly in solid-organ transplant recipients as well as individuals treated chronically with immunosuppressive drugs. Arises on average 16.5 months after transplantation. Resolves on cessation of immunosuppression.
HIV/AIDS-Associated KS In HIV-infected individuals, the risk for KS is 20,000 times that of the general population, 300 times that of other immunosuppressed individuals. Early in the HIV/AIDS epidemic in the United States and Europe, 50% of homosexual men at the time of initial diagnosis of AIDS had KS; currently, the incidence is 18% in this risk group. Young adults. HIV/AIDS-associated KS occurs almost exclusively in homosexual males; rarely women may have HIV/AIDS-associated KS when they acquire HIV infection via heterosexual exposure from a bisexual male. Associated with HIV infection, rapid progression, extensive systemic involvement. At the time of initial presentation, one in six HIV-infected individuals with KS have CD4+ T cell counts of ≤500/μL.

PATHOGENESIS

KS cells likely are derived from the endothelium of the blood/lymphatic microvasculature. Initially not a true malignancy but rather a widespread reactive polyclonal proliferation in response to angiogenic molecules. Later becomes monoclonal. KS lesions produce factors that promote their own growth as well as the growth of other cells, but it is not known how HHV-8 induces/promotes proliferation of endothelial cells.

CLINICAL MANIFESTATION

Mucocutaneous lesions are usually asymptomatic but are associated with significant cosmetic stigma. At times lesions may ulcerate and bleed easily. Large lesions on palms or soles may impede function. Lesions on the lower extremities that are tumorous, ulcerated, or associated with significant edema often give rise to moderate to severe pain. Urethral or anal canal lesions can be associated with obstruction. GI involvement rarely causes symptoms. Pulmonary KS can cause bronchospasm, intractable coughing, shortness of breath, progressive respiratory failure.
Skin Lesions KS most often begins as an ecchymotic-like macule (Figs. 20-16 and 20-19). Macules evolve into patches, papules, plaques (Figs. 20-16, 20-17, and 20-18), nodules, and tumors that are violaceous, red, pink, or tan and become purple-brownish (Figs. 20-16 and 20-17) with a

FIGURE 20-16 **Classic Kaposi sarcoma**
Ecchymotic purple-brownish confluent macules
and a 1-cm nodule on the dorsum of the hand of
a 65-year-old male of Ashkenazi-Jewish extraction.
The lesion was originally mistaken for a bruise
as were similar lesions on the feet and on the
other hand. The appearance of brownish nodules
together with additional macules prompted a refer-
ral of this otherwise completely healthy patient to
a dermatologist who diagnosed Kaposi sarcoma,
which was verified by biopsy. There is also onychomycosis of all fingernails.

FIGURE 20-17 **Classic Kaposi sarcoma** Brownish confluent papules on the dorsum of the foot. Involvement of lymphatics has led to pronounced edema of the forefoot, which indicates that the disease process is
further advanced.

greenish hemosiderin halo as they age. Almost all KS lesions are palpable, feeling firm to hard even when they are in a patch stage. Often oval initially, and on the trunk often arranged parallel to skin tension lines (Fig. 20-20). Lesions may initially occur at sites of trauma, usually in the acral regions (Fig. 20-18). In time, individual lesions may enlarge and become confluent, forming tumor masses. Secondary changes to larger nodules and tumors include erosion, ulceration, crusting, and hyperkeratosis.

Lymphedema usually occurs on the lower extremities (Fig. 20-17) and results from confluent masses of lesions due to deeper involvement of lymphatics and lymph nodes. Distal edema may initially be unilateral but later becomes symmetric and involves not only the lower legs but also the genitalia and/or face.

Distribution   Widespread or localized. In classic KS, lesions almost always occur on the feet and legs or the hands and slowly spread centripetally (Figs. 20-16 and 20-17). Tip of nose (Fig. 20-19), periorbital areas, ears, and scalp as well as penis (Fig. 35-26) and legs may also be involved, but involvement of the trunk is rare. In HIV/AIDS-associated KS there is early involvement of the face (Fig. 20-19) and widespread distribution on the trunk (Fig. 20-20). 🖉

Mucous Membranes   Oral lesions are the first manifestation of KS in 22% of cases; in HIV/AIDS-associated KS often a marker for CD4+ T cell counts of <200/µL. Very common (50% of individuals) on hard palate, appearing first as a violaceous stain, which evolves into papules and nodules with a cobblestone appearance. Lesions also arise on soft palate, uvula, pharynx, gingiva, and tongue. Conjunctival lesions uncommon. 🖉

Special Features of African-Endemic KS   (Non-HIV-associated) Four clinical patterns are recognized:

Nodular type: Runs a rather benign course with a mean duration of 5–8 years and resembles classic KS.

Florid or vegetating type: Characterized by more aggressive biologic behavior; is also nodular but may extend deeply into the subcutis, muscle, and bone.

Infiltrative type: Shows an even more aggressive course with florid mucocutaneous and visceral involvement.

Lymphadenopathic type: Predominantly affects children and young adults. Frequently confined to lymph nodes and viscera, but occasionally also involves the skin and mucous membrane.

General Examination   *Viscera*   KS lesions of the viscera, though common, are often asymptomatic. This is particularly true for classic KS. At autopsy of HIV-infected individuals with mucocutaneous KS, 75% have visceral involvement (bowel, liver, spleen, lungs).

Lymph Nodes   Lymph nodes are involved in half of cases of HIV/AIDS-associated KS and in all cases of African lymphadenopathic type KS.

Urogenital Tract   Prostate, seminal vesicles, testes, bladder, penis, scrotum.

Lung   Pulmonary infiltrates, particularly in HIV-associated KS.

GI Tract   GI hemorrhage, rectal obstruction, protein-losing enteropathy can occur.

Other   Heart, brain, kidney, adrenal glands.

LABORATORY EXAMINATIONS

Skin Biopsy   Vascular channels lined by atypical endothelial cells among a network of reticulin fibers and extravasated erythrocytes with hemosiderin deposition. Three histologic stages:

Patch stage: Proliferation of small, irregular, and jagged endothelial-lined spaces surrounding normal dermal vessels and adnexal structures; variable, inflammatory lymphocytic infiltrate (±plasma cells).

Plaque stage: Spindle cells throughout dermal collagen bundles forming irregular, cleftlike, angulated vascular channels that contain variable numbers of RBCs. Hemosiderin deposits; eosinophilic hyaline globules. Peripheral perivascular inflammatory infiltrate.

Nodular stage: Spindle cells in sheets and fascicles with mild to moderate cytologic atypia, single cell necrosis, trapped RBCs within an extensive network of slitlike vascular spaces.

Imaging   For internal organ involvement.

DIAGNOSIS AND DIFFERENTIAL DIAGNOSIS

Confirmed on lesional skin biopsy.

Differential Diagnosis   Includes single pigmented lesions: dermatofibroma, pyogenic granuloma, hemangioma, bacillary (epithelioid) angiomatosis, melanocytic nevus, ecchymosis, granuloma annulare, insect bite reactions, stasis dermatitis.

COURSE AND PROGNOSIS

Classic KS   Average survival, 10-15 years; death usually from unrelated causes. Secondary malignancies arise in >35% of cases.

FIGURE 20-18 Classic Kaposi sarcoma of the feet Brownish to blue nodules and plaques, partially hyperkeratotic on the soles and lateral aspects of the feet. This is a typical localization of early classic KS.

FIGURE 20-19 HIV/AIDS-associated Kaposi sarcoma Multiple bruiselike purplish and brownish macules, papules and nodules are present not only on the face but also on the trunk and the extremities of this 29-year-old male homosexual with AIDS. Note also swelling of the nose. Early involvement of the face is typical for HIV/AIDS-associated KS.

African-Endemic KS   Mean survival in young adults, 5–8 years; young children, 2–3 years.

Iatrogenic Immunosuppression-Associated KS Course may be chronic or rapidly progressive; KS usually resolves after immunosuppressive drugs are discontinued.

HIV/AIDS-Associated KS   (See also Section 31) HIV-infected individuals with high CD4+ T cell counts can have stable or slowly progressive disease for many years. Rapid progression of KS can occur after decline of CD4+ T cell counts to low values, prolonged systemic glucocorticoid therapy, or illness such as *Pneumocystis carinii* pneumonia. KS of the bowel and/or lungs is the cause of death in 10–20% of patients. Patients with only a few lesions, present for several months, without history of opportunistic infections, and CD4+ T cell counts >200/μL tend to respond better to therapy and have a better overall prognosis. At time of initial diagnosis, 40% of KS patients have GI involvement; 80% at autopsy. Reduced survival rate in patients with GI involvement. Pulmonary KS has high short-term mortality rate, i.e., median survival <6 months.

MANAGEMENT

The goal of therapy for KS is to control symptoms of the disease, not cure. A number of local and systemic therapeutic modalities are effective in controlling symptoms. Classic KS responds well to radiotherapy of involved sites. African-endemic KS, when symptomatic, responds best to systemic chemotherapy. Immunosuppressive drug–associated KS regresses or resolves when drug dosages are reduced or discontinued. HIV/AIDS-associated KS usually responds to a variety of local therapies; for extensive mucocutaneous involvement or visceral involvement, chemotherapy is indicated.

Local therapy is usually directed at individual lesions that are cosmetically disturbing (e.g., on the face), bulky, bleeding, cause functional disturbance on the palms or soles, or cause lymphatic obstruction and lymphedema.

Limited Intervention

Radiotherapy   Indicated for tumorous lesions, confluent lesions with a large surface area, large lesions on distal extremity, large oropharyngeal lesions. Dosing: 8 Gy in a single fraction for small lesions, 800–3000 rad in single or divided dose.

Cryosurgery   Indicated for deeply pigmented, protruding nodules. Best results with two freeze-thaw cycles. Pain is moderate during freeze cycle. Treated lesions heal with crust formation. KS often persists in deeper portions of lesion. Violaceous lesion is replaced with a white scar. Secondary infection is uncommon.

Laser Surgery   Pulsed-dye laser effective for small superficial lesion.

Photodynamic Therapy   For small superficial lesions.

Electrosurgery   Effective for ulcerated, bleeding nodular lesion; must use a smoke evacuator in conjunction.

Excisional Surgery   Effective for selected small lesions. Not a realistic approach to the patient with many lesions.

Intralesional Cytotoxic Chemotherapy *Vinblastine*   0.1 mg (0.5 mL of a 0.2-mg/mL solution) injected per square centimeter of lesion; for refractory lesions, incremental doses of up to 0.2 mg/cm^2 can be given. Most effective for small, early, papular lesions. Larger nodular lesions respond more slowly. The maximal total vinblastine dose injected should not exceed 2 mg per clinic visit. Some lesions heal with blister formation, crusting, and scarring. Inadvertent injection near a cutaneous sensory nerve can result in a neuritic pain that can last up to a month.

Vincristine and Bleomycin   These have also been used for intralesional therapy.

Aggressive Intervention
Single-Agent Chemotherapy

- Adriamycin, 20 mg/m^2.
- Vinblastine, IV bolus 0.1 mg/kg weekly.
  - Lipid formulations of daunorubicin and doxorubicin.
  - Etoposide (VP16), given orally.
- Paclitaxel (Taxol), given IV every 3 weeks.

Combination Chemotherapy

- Vincristine (2 mg) + bleomycin (15 U/m^2) + adriamycin (20 mg/m^2) is given every other week in patients with relatively advanced KS.
- Interferon-α (15 million U/d) + zidovudine (600 mg/d).

Type-Specific Therapy

- *Classic KS*: Any of the above.
- *African KS*: Any of the above.
- *Immunosuppression-related KS*: Reduction of immunosuppression, replacement of calcineurin inhibitors by rapamycine.
- *HIV/AIDS-related KS*: Any of the above, preferably liposomal anthracyclines intravenously every 2 to 4 weeks plus HAART.

FIGURE 20-20 **HIV/AIDS-associated Kaposi sarcoma** Multiple purplish plaques and nodules on the trunk of a homosexual AIDS patient. The patient had CD4+ T cell counts <200/μL and marked mucous membrane involvement, *Pneumocystis carinii* pneumonia, and *Candida*.

SKIN DISEASES IN ORGAN AND BONE MARROW TRANSPLANTATION

- Organ transplant recipients are chronically immunosuppressed and their T cell function is impaired.
- Ensuing diseases are mostly infections and are similar to those occurring in other conditions associated with T cell impairment, such as AIDS.

- In addition, organ transplant recipients are at great risk for developing nonmelanoma skin cancer and other cancers.
- Bone marrow and stem cell graft recipients are candidates for graft-versus-host disease (GVHD).

MOST COMMON INFECTIONS ASSOCIATED WITH ORGAN TRANSPLANTATION*

- Bacterial pathogens: (see Section 24)

  Staphylococcus, Streptococcus, Salmonella, Listeria, Nocardia, Mycobacterium avium-intracellulare, M. tuberculosis, Legionella

- Viral pathogens (see Sections 27 and 31)

  Cytomegalovirus (CMV), herpes simplex virus (HSV), varicella zoster virus (VZV), molluscum contagiosum virus, human papilloma virus (HPV), Epstein-Barr virus (EBV)

- Fungal pathogens (see Sections 25 and 31)

  Candida, Cryptococcus, Histoplasma, Coccidioides, Blastomyces, Dermatophytes (onychomycosis), Aspergillus

  *Clinical manifestations are discussed in their respective sections.

SKIN CANCERS ASSOCIATED WITH ORGAN TRANSPLANTATION*

- Nonmelanoma skin cancer is the most common malignancy in adult solid organ transplant patients.

- The majority are squamous cell carcinomas (SCC) (Section 11).

- The risk of developing SCC increases exponentially with the length of immunosuppression.

- The cumulative incidence is 80% after 20 years of immunosuppression in renal transplantation. SCC in posttransplant patients are aggressive.

- HPV infection is implicated in the pathogenesis.

- Other epithelial proliferative lesions are actinic keratoses, keratoacanthomas, porokeratosis, appendage tumors, and Merkel cell carcinomas (Section 11).

- Children with organ transplants may also be at higher risk for the development of melanoma (Section 12).

- Lymphoproliferative disorders are common in graft recipients and related to Epstein-Barr virus (EBV)-mediated proliferation of B cells and most are lymphomas of B cell origin. Cutaneous T cell lymphomas account for 30% of cutaneous lymphomas in transplant patients (Section 20).

- Kaposi sarcoma occurs in immunosuppressed transplant recipients with an incidence of 0.5–5%. All cases are associated with Kaposi sarcoma–associated herpesvirus (KSHV) infection (Section 20).

*Clinical manifestations are discussed in their respective sections.

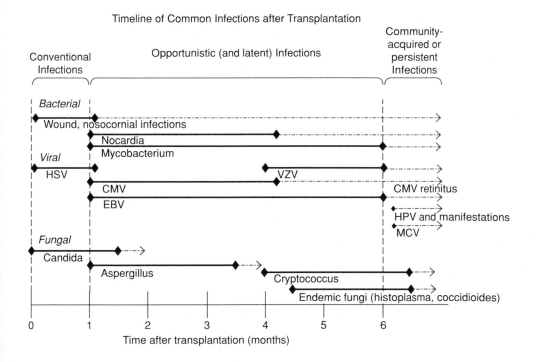

Timeline of Common Infections after Transplantation

GRAFT-VERSUS-HOST DISEASE   ICD:9:996.85 ○ ICD-10:T86.0   ◻ ●

- GVHD is the totality of organ dysfunction caused by the action of histoincompatible, immunocompetent donor cells against the tissues of an immunocompetent host.
- Graft-versus-host reaction (GVHR) is the expression of GVHD in a specific organ (e.g., cutaneous GVHR).
- Acute cutaneous GVHR is the earliest and most frequent GVHR. Liver and GI tract GVHR are also common.

- Acute cutaneous GVHR, usually occurring 10–30 days after bone marrow transplantation (BMT), is characterized by faint erythematous macules, often in perifollicular pattern progressing to confluent erythema, erythroderma, or toxic epidermal necrolysis (TEN).
- Chronic cutaneous GVHR occurs >60 days after allogeneic BMT and manifests as lichenoid and sclerodermoid changes.

EPIDEMIOLOGY

Incidence Allogeneic BMT: 20–80% of successful engraftments. Autologous BMT: mild cutaneous GVHR occurs in 8%. Low incidence after blood transfusion in immunosuppressed patients, maternal-fetal transfer in immunodeficiency disease.

ACUTE CUTANEOUS GVHR   ◻ ●

PATHOGENESIS

With successful engraftment, there is replacement of host marrow by immunocompetent donor cells capable of mounting an inflammatory reaction against the-"foreign" tissue antigens of the host. GVHR of specific host organs—skin, liver, or GI tract. Severity of GVHD related to histocompatibility match between donor and recipient and preparatory regimen used.

CLINICAL MANIFESTATION

During the first 2 months after BMT (usually between 10 and 30 days): mild pruritus, localized/generalized; pain on pressure, palms/soles.

Nausea/vomiting, abdominal pain; watery diarrhea. Jaundice; dark yellow urine.

Skin Lesions Initially, subtle, discrete macules and/or papules on upper trunk, hands/feet (Fig. 21-1), especially palms/soles. Painful. Mild edema with violaceous hue, periungual and on pinna. Erythema often in perifollicular array. If controlled/resolved, erythema diminishes with subsequent desquamation (Fig. 21-2) and postinflammatory hyperpigmentation. If it progresses, macules/papules become generalized, confluent (Fig. 21-3), and evolve into erythroderma. Subepidermal bullae, especially over pressure/trauma sites, palms/soles. Positive Nikolsky sign. If bullae widespread with rupture/erosion, TEN-like form of acute cutaneous GVHR (see Section 8) (Fig. 21-4). For staging, see Table 21-1.

TABLE 21-1   Clinical Staging of Acute Cutaneous GVHR

1. Erythematous maculopapular eruption involving <25% of body surface
2. Erythematous maculopapular eruption involving 25–50% of body surface
3. Erythroderma
4. Bulla formation

TABLE 21-2   Histologic Grading Scheme for Acute Cutaneous GVHR

Grade	Description
0	Normal skin or changes not referable to graft-versus-host disease
1	Basal vacuolization of the dermal-epidermal junction
2	Basal vacuolization, necrotic epidermal cells, lymphocytes in the dermis and/or epidermis
3	Sub-epidermal cleft formation plus grade 2 changes
4	Separation of epidermis from dermis plus grade 2 changes

Adapted from Lerner KG et al: Histopathology of graft-versus-host reaction (GVHR) in human recipients of marrow from HLA-matched sibling donors. *Transplantation* 18:367, 1974.

FIGURE 21-1 **Acute cutaneous GVHR** Discrete and confluent erythematous, blanching macules and rarely elevated papules with indistinct borders involving hands and trunk. Note relative sparing over the metacarpophalangeal and proximal interphalangeal joints.

FIGURE 21-2 **Acute cutaneous GVHR, remitting** The maculopapular lesions have acquired a brownish hue and there is slight scaling.

Mucosa   Lichen planus–like lesions in buccal mucosa; erosive stomatitis, oral and ocular sicca-like syndrome; esophagitis/esophageal strictures. Keratoconjunctivitis.

General Findings   Fever, jaundice, nausea, vomiting, right upper quadrant pain/tenderness, cramping, abdominal pain, diarrhea, serositis, pulmonary insufficiency, dark urine.

LABORATORY EXAMINATIONS

Chemistry   Elevated SGOT, bilirubin, alkaline phosphatase.

Dermatopathology   Focal vacuolization of basal cell layer, apoptosis of individual keratinocytes; mild perivenular mononuclear cell infiltrate. Apposition of lymphocytes to necrotic keratinocytes (satellitosis); vacuoles coalesce to form subepidermal clefts → subepidermal blister formation. Endothelial cell swelling. Immunocytochemistry: HLA-DR expression of keratinocytes precedes morphologic changes and thus represents important, early diagnostic sign (for grading see Table 21-2).

DIAGNOSIS AND DIFFERENTIAL DIAGNOSIS

Clinical findings confirmed by skin biopsy.

Differential Diagnosis   Exanthematous drug reaction, viral exanthem, TEN, erythroderma.

FIGURE 21-3   Acute cutaneous GVHR involving the face of a 10-year-old boy   The individual lesions are confluent, there is slight desquamation, and there are erosions on the lips. The mucous membranes were severely involved.

FIGURE 21-4 Acute GVHR, TEN-like Confluent epidermal necrosis with wrinkling and dislodgment of the necrotic epidermis, erosions, and hemorrhagic crusts. This severe reaction involved the entire skin and is indistinguishable from TEN. It occurred after allogeneic BMT and is clearly a very severe condition.

COURSE AND PROGNOSIS

Mild to moderate GVHR responds well to treatment. Prognosis of TEN-like GVHR is grave. Severe GVHD susceptible to infections—bacterial, fungal, viral (CMV, HSV, VZV). Acute GVHD is primary or associated cause of death in 15–70% of BMT recipients.

MANAGEMENT

Topical   Glucocorticoids.
Physical   PUVA, extracorporeal photopheresis.
Systemic   Methylprednisolone 2 mg/kg per day, tacrolimus 4–20 mg/d, cyclosporine 12–15 mg/kg per day PO; mycophenolate mofetil 2 g/d, etanercept 25 mg twice daily, infiximab 10 mg/kg per week.

CHRONIC CUTANEOUS GVHR   ▢ ■ ●

CLINICAL MANIFESTATION

>60 days after BMT. Evolving from acute GVHR or arising de novo. Acute GVHR not always followed by chronic GVHR. Clinical classification thus distinguishes between quiescent onset, progressive onset, and de novo chronic cutaneous GVHR. Chronic GVHR occurs in 25% of recipients of marrow from an HLA-identical sibling who survive >100 days.

Skin Lesions
Flat-topped (lichen planus–like) papules of violaceous color, initially on distal extremities but later generalized (Fig. 21-5) and/or confluent areas of dermal sclerosis (Fig. 21-6) with overlying scale resembling scleroderma mainly on trunk, buttocks, hips, and thighs. With more severe disease, severe generalized sclerodermoid changes also involving face (Fig. 21-6A) with necrosis and ulceration on acral and pressure sites. Hair loss; anhidrosis; nails: dystrophy, anonychia; vitiligo-like hypopigmentation.

Mucosa   Like erosive/ulcerative lichen planus.
General Findings   Chronic liver disease, general wasting.

LABORATORY EXAMINATIONS

Chemistry   Elevated ALT, AST, γ-glutamyltransferase.
Dermatopathology   Like *lichen planus*: hyperkeratosis, hypergranulosis, mild irregular acanthosis or atrophy, moderate basal vacuolization and epidermal apoptosis, mild perivascular mononuclear cell infiltrate, melanin incontinence; like *scleroderma*: dense dermal sclerosis. Loss of hair follicles, entrapment of sweat glands.

COURSE AND PROGNOSIS

Sclerodermoid GVHR with tight skin/joint contracture may result in impaired mobility, ulcerations. Permanent hair loss; xerostomia, xerophthalmia, corneal ulcers, blindness. Malabsorption. Mild chronic cutaneous GVHR may resolve spontaneously. Chronic GVHR may be associated with recurrent and occasionally fatal bacterial infections.

DIAGNOSIS AND DIFFERENTIAL DIAGNOSIS

Clinical, history, and histopathology. Differentiate from lichen planus, lichenoid drug reaction, scleroderma, all types of poikiloderma.

MANAGEMENT

Topical glucocorticoids, PUVA, and extracorporeal photopheresis are effective. *Systemic immunosuppression* with prednisone, cyclosporine, azathioprine, mycophenolate mofetil, methotrexate, tacrolimus, and thalidomide.

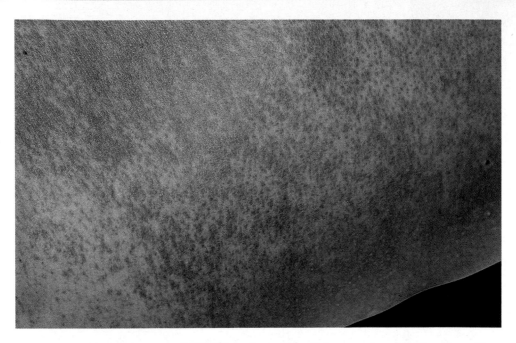

FIGURE 21-5   Chronic cutaneous GVHR, lichen planus–like   Violaceous to brownish, lichen planus–like perifollicular papules becoming confluent on the trunk, occurring 3 months after allogeneic BMT.

A   *B*

FIGURE 21-6   Chronic cutaneous GVHR, sclerodermoid   A. Ebony-white bound down skin and telangiectasias in the 10-year-old boy shown in Fig. 21-3. In this case acute GVHR evolved directly into chronic GVHR and involved the entire skin of the trunk and extremities. **B.** Close-up view of the back of the same patient with poikilodermatous changes (hypo- and hyperpigmentation) and telangiectasias in the sclerotic skin.

ADVERSE CUTANEOUS DRUG REACTIONS*

■ Adverse cutaneous drug reactions (ACDRs) are common in hospitalized (2–3%) as well as in ambulatory patients (>1%).

■ Most reactions are mild, accompanied by pruritus, and resolve promptly after the offending drug is discontinued.

■ Severe, life-threatening ACDRs do occur and are unpredictable.

■ *Drug eruptions can mimic virtually all the morphologic expressions in dermatology and must* *be the first consideration in the differential diagnosis of a suddenly appearing eruption.*

■ Drug eruptions are caused by immunologic or nonimmunologic mechanisms and are provoked by systemic or topical administration of a drug.

■ The majority are based on a hypersensitivity mechanism and are thus immunologic and may be of types I, II, III, or IV.

ICD-9 : 995.2 ∘ ICD : 10 : T88.7

CLASSIFICATION

Immunologically Mediated ACDR See Table 22-1. It should be noted, however, that classification of immunologically mediated ACDR according to the Gell and Coombs classification is an oversimplification because in most reactions both cellular and humoral immune reactions are involved. Nonimmunologic reactions are summarized in Table 22-2.

GUIDELINES FOR ASSESSMENT OF POSSIBLE ACDRs

• Exclude alternative causes, especially infections, in that many infections (especially viral) are difficult to distinguish clinically from the adverse effects of drugs used to treat infections.
• Examine interval between introduction of a drug and onset of the reaction.
• Note any improvement after drug withdrawal.
• Determine whether similar reactions have been associated with the same compound.
• Note any reaction on readministration of the drug.

FINDINGS INDICATING POSSIBLE LIFE-THREATENING ACDR

• Skin pain
• Confluent erythema
• Facial edema or central facial involvement
• Palmar/plantar painful erythema
• Concomitant erosive mucous membrane involvement
• Blisters of epidermal detachment
• Positive Nikolsky sign
• Mucous membrane erosions
• Urticaria
• Swelling of the tongue
• High fever (temperature > 40 °C)
• Enlarged lymph nodes
• Arthralgia
• Shortness of breath, wheezing, hypotension
• Palpable purpura
• Skin necrosis

*Skin reactions or changes regularly occurring after high dose or prolonged administration of certain drugs like glucocorticoids, retinoids, cyclosporine, and others are not discussed in this section but throughout the book whenever these drugs are discussed in greater detail.

TABLE 22-1   Immunologically Mediated Adverse Cutaneous Drug Reactions*

Type of Reaction	Pathogenesis	Examples of Causative Drug	Clinical Patterns
Type I	IgE-mediated; immediate-type immunologic reactions	Penicillin, other antibiotics	Urticaria/angioedema of skin/mucosa, edema of other organs, and anaphylactic shock
Type II	Drug + cytotoxic antibodies cause lysis of cells such as platelets or leukocytes	Penicillin, sulfonamides, quinidine, isoniazid	Petechiae due to thrombocytopenic purpura, drug-induced pemphigus
Type III	IgG or IgM antibodies formed to drug; immune complexes deposited in small vessels activate complement and recruitment of granulocytes	Immunoglobulins, antibiotics, rituximab, infliximab	Vasculitis, urticaria, serum sickness
Type IV	Cell-mediated immune reaction; sensitized lymphocytes react with drug, liberating cytokines, which trigger cutaneous inflammatory response Contact sensitivity†	Sulfamethoxazole, anticonvulsants, allopurinol	Morbilliform exanthematous reactions, fixed drug eruption, lichenoid eruptions, Stevens-Johnson syndrome, toxic epidermal necrolysis

*After the Gell and Coombs classification of immune reactions.
†See Section 2.

TABLE 22-2   Nonimmunologic Drug Eruptions

Idiosyncrasy	Reactions due to hereditary enzyme deficiencies
Individual idiosyncrasy to a topical or systemic drug	Mechanisms not yet known
Cumulation	Reactions are dose dependent, based on the total amount of drug ingested: pigmentation due to gold, amiodarone, or minocycline
Reactions due to combination of a drug with ultraviolet irradiation (photosensitivity)	Reactions have a toxic pathogenesis but can also be immunologic in nature (see Section 10)
Irritancy/toxicity of a topically applied drug	5-Fluorouracil, imiquimod
Atrophy by topically applied drug	Glucocorticoids

CLINICAL TYPES OF ADVERSE DRUG REACTIONS

ACDRs can be exanthematous and can manifest as urticaria/angioedema, anaphylaxis and anaphylactoid reactions, or serum sickness; they can mimic or cause dermatoses that can also have other causes; they can present as cutaneous necrosis, pigmentation, alopecia, hypertrichosis; and they can induce nail changes. An overview is presented in Table 22-3.

TABLE 22-3 Types of Clinical ACDRs

Type	Drugs	Comment
BASIC REACTIONS		
Exanthematous reactions	Any	Most common; initial reaction usually <14 days after drug intake; recurs after rechallenge (see page 563); drug hypersensitivity syndrome, initially indistinguishable (see page 568) (Figs. 22-1 and 22-2)
Fixed drug eruptions	See Table 22-5	See p. 566
Urticaria/angioedema	Aspirin, nonsteroidal anti-inflammatory drugs (NSAIDs), codeine, penicillin, opiates, amphetamine, polymyxine B, atropine, hydralazine, infliximab, pentamidine, quinine, radiocontrast media, angiotensin-converting enzyme (ACE) inhibitors (see Table 22-4)	Second most common; usually within 36 h after initial exposure; within minutes after rechallenge (see page 563) (Figs. 22-6 and 22-7)
Anaphylaxis and anaphylactoid reactions	Antibiotics, extracts of allergens, radiocontrast media, monoclonal antibodies (see Table 22-4)	Most serious type of ACDR, within minutes and hours; more common with oral than parenteral drug administration. Intermittent administration of drug may predispose to anaphylaxis
Serum sickness	IVIg, antibiotics, bovine serum albumin (used for oocyte retrieval in in vitro fertilization), cefaclor, cefprozil, bupropion, minocycline, rituximab, infliximab	5 to 21 days after initial exposure *Minor form*: fever, urticaria, arthralgia *Major (complete) form*: fever, urticaria, angioedema, arthralgia, arthritis, lymphadenopathy, eosinophilia, ± nephritis, ± endocarditis.
ACDR MIMICRY OF OTHER DERMATOSES		
Acneiform eruption	Glucocorticoids, anabolic steroids, contraceptives, halogens, isoniazid, lithium, azathioprine, danazol	See Section 1 and Fig. 22-5
Bullous eruptions	Naproxene, nalidixic acid, furosemide, oxaprozin, penicillamine, piroxicam, tetracyclines	Fixed drug eruption, (Fig. 22-8*B*) drug-induced vasculitis, Stevens-Johnson syndrome (SJS), toxic epidermal necrolysis (TEN), porphyria, pseudoporphyria, drug-induced pemphigus, drug-induced pemphigoid, drug-induced linear IgA disease, bullae over pressure areas in sedated patients (Fig. 22-19)
Dermatomyositis-like reactions	Penicillamine, NSAIDs, carbamazepine	See Section 14

Type	Drugs	Comment
Drug hypersensitivity syndrome	Antiepileptic drugs, sulfonamides, and others	Mimics exanthematous reactions; systemic involvement (see page 568) (Fig. 22-10)
Eczematous eruptions	Ethylenediamine, antihistamines, aminophylline/aminophylline suppositories; procaine/benzocaine; iodides, iodinated organic compounds, radiographic contrast media/iodine; streptomycin, kanamycin, paramomycin, gentamicin/neomycin sulfate; nitroglycerin tablets/nitroglycerin ointment; disulfiram/thiuram	Systemic administration of a drug to an individual who has been previously sensitized to the drug by topical application can provoke a widespread eczematous dermatitis (systemic contact-type dermatitis, see Section 2) or urticaria
Erythema multiforme, SJS, TEN	Anticonvulsants, sulfonamides, allopurinol, NSAIDs (piroxicam)	See Sections 7 and 8
Erythema nodosum	Sulfonamides, other antimicrobial agents, analgesics, oral contraceptives, granulocyte colony-stimulating factor (G-CSF)	See Section 7
Exfoliative dermatitis and erythroderma	Sulfonamides, antimalarials, phenytoin, penicillin	See Section 8
Lichenoid eruptions	Gold, beta blockers, ACE inhibitors, especially captopril; see also Table 7-1	See Sections 7 and 21. May be extensive, occurring weeks to months after initiation of drug therapy; may progress to exfoliative dermatitis Adnexal involvement may result in alopecia, anhidrosis Resolution after discontinuation slow, 1–4 months; up to 24 months after gold May be photodistributed or bullous Oral involvement occurs with some drugs
Lupus erythematosus (LE)	Procainamide, hydralazine, isoniazid, minocycline, acebutolol, Ca^{2+} channel blockers, ACE inhibitors, docetaxel	See Section 14. 5% of cases of systemic LE are drug-induced Cutaneous manifestations, including photosensitivity; however, urticaria, erythema multiforme-like lesions, Raynaud phenomenon are not common
Photosensitivity	See Tables 10-4 to 10-6	See Section 10 Phototoxic, photoallergic, or photocontact
Pityriasis rosea–like eruptions	Gold, captopril, imatimib, and others	For clinical appearance, see Section 7
Pseudolymphoma	Phenytoin, carbamazepine, allopurinol, antidepressants, phenothiazines, benzodiazepam, antihistamines, beta blockers, lipid-lowering agents, cyclosporine, D-penicillamine	Papular eruptions with a histology mimicking lymphoma

(*continued*)

TABLE 22-3 (*Continued*)

Type	Drugs	Comment
Pseudoporphyria	Tetracycline, furosemide, naproxene	See Section 10 and page 574, (Fig. 22-13)
Psoriasiform eruption	Antimalarials, beta-blockers, lithium salts, NSAIDs, interferon, penicillamine, methyldopa	See Section 3
Purpura	Penicillin, sulfonamides, quinine, isoniazid	See Section 19. Hemorrhage into morbilliform ACDR occurs not uncommonly on the legs Progressive pigmented purpura also reported associated with drugs (see Section 7)
Pustular eruptions	Ampicillin, amoxicillin, macrolides, tetracyclines, beta blockers, Ca^{2+} channel blockers EGFR inhibitors (Fig. 22-5)	Acute generalized exanthematous pustulosis (AGEP, page 561) Must be differentiated from pustular psoriasis; eosinophil in the infiltrate suggests AGEP
Scleroderma-like reactions	Penicillamine, bleomycin, bromocryptine, Na-valproate, 5-hydroxytryptophan, docetaxel, gemcitabine, acetanilide-containing rapeseed cooking oil	See Section 14
Sweet syndrome	All-*trans* retinoic acid, contraceptives, G-CSF, granulocyte-macrophage CSF (GM-CSF), minocycline, imatinib, trimethoprim-sulfamethoxazole	See Section 7
Vasculitis	Propylthiouracil, hydralazine, G-CSF, GM-CSF, allopurinol, cefaclor, minocycline, penicillamine, phenytoin, isotretinoin	See Section 14
ACDR-RELATED PIGMENTATION		
ACDR pigmentation	Amiodarone, minocycline, clofazimine, zidovudine, hydantoins, cytotoxic agents, heavy metals, hormones, chlorpromazine, bleomycin	See page 570 Associated with postinflammatory hyperpigmentation, increased melanin synthesis, increased lipofuscin synthesis, or cutaneous deposition of drug-related material (Fig. 22-11, 22-12)
ACDR-RELATED NECROSIS		
ACDR necrosis	Warfarin, heparin, interferon-α, cytotoxic agents	See page 575 (Figs. 22-14, 22-15, 22-16).
Others		
ACDR related to chemotherapy		See page 579
Alopecia		See Section 32
Hypertrichosis		See Section 32
Nail changes		See Section 33

LABORATORY EXAMINATIONS

Hematology   Eosinophil count > 1000/μL. Lymphocytosis with atypical lymphocytes.
Chemistry   Abnormal results of liver function tests.

DIAGNOSIS

Usually made on clinical findings. Lesional skin biopsy is helpful in defining the type of reaction pattern occurring but not in identifying the offending drug. Skin tests and radioallergosorbent tests are helpful in diagnosing IgE-mediated type I hypersensitivity reactions, more specifically to penicillins.

MANAGEMENT

In most cases, the implicated or suspected drug should be discontinued. In some, such as with morbilliform eruptions, the offending drug can be continued and the eruption may resolve. In cases of urticaria/angioedema or early Stevens-Johnson syndrome (SJS)/toxic epidermal necrolysis (TEN), the ACDR can be life-threatening, and the drug must be discontinued.

EXANTHEMATOUS DRUG REACTIONS   ICD-9:995.2 ∘ ICD-10:T88.7■

- An exanthematous drug reaction (eruption) is an adverse hypersensitivity reaction to an ingested or parenterally administered drug.
- Cutaneous eruption that mimics a measles-like viral exanthem.

- Systemic involvement is low.

Synonyms: Morbilliform drug reaction, maculopapular drug reaction.

EPIDEMIOLOGY

Age of Onset   Less common in the very young.
Incidence   Most common type of cutaneous drug reaction.

ETIOLOGY AND PATHOGENESIS

Drugs with a high probability of reaction (3 –5%): penicillin and related antibiotics, carbamazepine, allopurinol, gold salts (10–20%). *Medium probability*: sulfonamides (bacteriostatic, antidiabetic, diuretic), nonsteroidal anti-inflammatory drugs (NSAIDs), hydantoin derivatives, isoniazid, chloramphenicol, erythromycin, streptomycin. *Low probability* (<1%): barbiturates, benzodiazepines, phenothiazines, tetracyclines (Table 22-3).

Exact mechanism unknown. Probably delayed hypersensitivity. In Epstein-Barr virus (EBV) and cytomegalovirus (CMV) mononucleosis, exanthematous drug reactions occur very frequently but are probably not allergic.

CLINICAL MANIFESTATIONS

Mononucleosis   Up to 100% of patients with primary EBV or CMV infection (infectious mononucleosis syndrome) given ampicillin or amoxicillin develop an exanthematous drug eruption.
HIV/AIDS Infection   50–60% of HIV-infected patients who receive sulfa drugs (i.e., trimethoprim-sulfamethoxazole) develop an eruption. With immune restitution with highly-active antiretroviral therapy (HAART), previously tolerant individuals may develop ACDR as CD4+ cell count rises.
Drug History   Increased incidence of reactions in patients on allopurinol given ampicillin/amoxicillin.
Prior Drug Sensitization   Patients with prior history of exanthematous drug eruption

will most likely develop a similar reaction if rechallenged with same drug. About 10% of patients sensitive to penicillins who are given cephalosporins will exhibit cross-drug sensitivity and develop eruption. Patients sensitized to one sulfa-based drug may cross-react with another category of the drug in 20% of cases.

Onset   *Early Reaction*   In previously sensitized patient, eruption starts within 2 or 3 days after readministration of drug.

Late Reaction   Sensitization occurs during administration or after completing course of drug; peak incidence at ninth day after administration. However, ACDR may occur at any time between the first day and 3 weeks after the beginning of treatment. Reaction to penicillin can begin ≥2 weeks after drug is discontinued.

Skin Symptoms   Usually quite pruritic, disturbs sleep. Painful skin lesions suggest development of a more serious ACDR, such as TEN.

Systems Review   ± Fever, chills.

Skin Lesions   Macules and/or papules, a few millimeters to 1 cm in size (Figs. 22-1 and 22-2). Bright or "drug" red. Resolving lesions have hues of tan and purple. In time, lesions become confluent forming large macules, polycyclic/gyrate erythema, reticular eruptions, sheet-like erythema (Fig. 22-1), erythroderma; also erythema multiforme–like. Purpura may be seen in lesions of lower legs. In individuals with thrombocytopenia, exanthematous eruptions can mimic vasculitis because of intralesional hemorrhage. Scaling and/or desquamation may occur with healing.

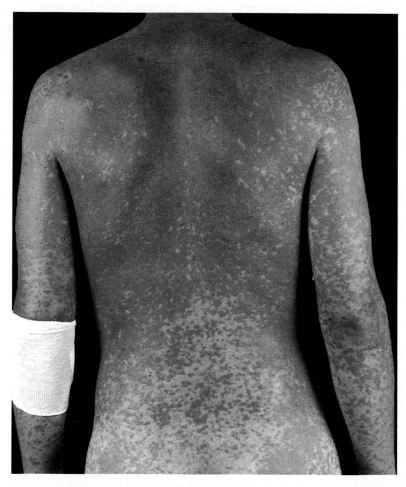

FIGURE 22-1   **Exanthematous drug eruption: ampicillin**   Symmetrically arranged, brightly erythematous macules and papules, discrete in some areas and confluent in others, on the trunk and the extremities.

Distribution Symmetric (Fig. 22-1). Almost always on trunk and extremities. Confluent lesions in intertriginous areas, i.e., axilla, groin, inframammary area. Palms and soles variably involved. In children, may be limited to face and extremities. May spare face, nipple, periareolar area, surgical scar. Reactions to ampicillin usually appear initially on the elbows, knees, and trunk, extending symmetrically to most areas of the body. 🖱

Mucous Membranes Enanthem on buccal mucosa.

Reactions to Specific Drugs (*Selected*) ***Ampicillin, Amoxicillin*** In up to 100% of patients with EBV or CMV mononucleosis syndrome.

NSAIDS Incidence: 1–3%. Site: trunk, pressure areas. Onset: 1–2 weeks after beginning therapy.

Barbiturates Site: face, trunk. Onset: few days after initiation of therapy. Cross-reactivity with other barbiturates: not universal.

Nitrofurantoin Associated findings: fever, peripheral eosinophilia, pulmonary edema, chest pain, dyspnea. Onset: 2 weeks after initiation of therapy; within hours if previously sensitized.

Hydantoin Derivatives Macular or confluent erythema. Begins on face, spreads to trunk and extremities. Onset: 2 weeks after initiation of therapy. Associated findings: fever, peripheral eosinophilia; facial edema; lymphadenopathy (can mimic lymphoma histologically).

Isoniazid Morbilliform; may evolve to exfoliative dermatitis. Associated findings: fever; hepatitis.

Benzodiazepines Rare. Onset: few days after initiation of therapy. Rechallenge: frequently rash does not occur.

Phenothiazines Begins on face, spreads to trunk (mainly back) and extremities. Onset: between second and third weeks after initiation of therapy. Associated findings: periorbital edema. Rechallenge: rash may not occur. Crossreactivity: common.

Carbamazepine Morphology: diffuse erythema; severe erythroderma may follow. Site: begins on face, spreads rapidly to all areas; may occur in

FIGURE 22-2 Exanthematous drug eruption: ampicillin in a patient with EBV mononucleosis
Confluent maculopapular lesions, generalized.

photodistribution. Onset: 2 weeks after initiation of therapy. Associated findings: facial edema.

Sulfonamides Incidence: common in up to 50–60% of HIV/AIDS-infected patients. Morphology: morbilliform, erythema multiforme-like.

Allopurinol Incidence: 5%. Morphology: morbilliform. Begins on face, spreads rapidly to all areas; may occur in photodistribution. Onset: 2–3 weeks after initiation of therapy. Associated findings: facial edema; systemic vasculitis, especially involving kidneys. Rash may fade in spite of continued administration.

Gold Salts Incidence: 10–20% of patients; dose-related. Morphology: diffuse erythema; exfoliative dermatitis, lichenoid, hemorrhagic, bullous, or pityriasis rosea–like eruptions may follow.

General Examination Drug fever. Findings associated with the indication for drug administration.

LABORATORY EXAMINATIONS

Hemogram Peripheral eosinophilia.
Dermatopathology Perivascular lymphocytes and eosinophils.

DIAGNOSIS AND DIFFERENTIAL DIAGNOSIS

Clinical diagnosis, at times confirmed by histologic findings, correlated with history of drug administration.

Differential Diagnosis Includes all exanthematous eruptions: Viral exanthem (often begins on face, progresses to trunk; may be accompanied by conjunctivitis, lymphadenopathy, fever), secondary syphilis, atypical pityriasis rosea, early widespread allergic contact dermatitis.

COURSE

After discontinuation of drug, rash usually fades; however, it may worsen for a few days.

The eruption may also begin after the drug has been discontinued. Occasionally fades even though drug is continued. Eruption usually recurs with rechallenge, although not always. In some cases of exanthematous ampicillin reactions, readministration of the drug does not cause the eruption. Duration of ampicillin eruption after discontinuation of drug: 3–5 days. If drug is continued, exfoliative dermatitis may develop. Of more concern, a morbilliform eruption may be the initial presentation of a more serious eruption, i.e., SJS, TEN, drug hypersensitivity syndrome, or serum sickness.

MANAGEMENT

The definitive step in management is to identify the offending drug and discontinue it.

Indications for Discontinuation of Drug Urticaria (concern for anaphylaxis), facial edema, pain, blisters, mucosal involvement, ulcers, palpable or extensive purpura, fever, lymphadenopathy.

Symptomatic Treatment Oral antihistamine to alleviate pruritus.

Glucocorticoids *Potent Topical Preparation* May help speed resolution of eruption.

Oral or IV Provides symptomatic relief. If offending drug cannot be substituted or omitted, systemic glucocorticoids can be administered to treat the ACDR; also, to induce more rapid remission.

Prevention Patients must be aware of their specific drug hypersensitivity and that other drugs of the same class can cross-react. Although an exanthematous drug eruption may not recur if the drug is given again, readministration is best avoided by using a different agent. Wearing a medical alert bracelet is advised.

PUSTULAR ERUPTIONS   ICD-9:995.2 ○ ICD-10:T88.7

■ *Acute generalized exanthematous pustulosis* (AGEP) is an acute febrile eruption that is often associated with leukocytosis (Fig. 22-3). After drug administration, it may take 1–3 weeks before skin lesions appear; however, in previously sensitized patients, the skin symptoms may occur within 2–3 days.

■ Onset is acute, most often following drug intake, but viral infections can also trigger the disease.

■ AGEP typically presents with nonfollicular sterile pustules occurring on a diffuse, edematous erythema (Fig. 22-3).

■ May be irregularly dispersed (Fig. 22-3) or grouped (Fig. 22-4), usually starting in the folds and/or the face.

■ Fever and elevated blood neutrophils are common.

■ Histopathology typically shows spongiform subcorneal and/or intraepidermal pustules; a marked edema of the papillary dermis; and eventually vasculitis, eosinophils, and/or focal necrosis of keratinocytes.

■ Pustules resolve spontaneously in <15 days and generalized desquamation occurs approximately 2 weeks later.

■ Differential diagnosis includes pustular psoriasis, the hypersensitivity syndrome reaction with pustulation, subcorneal pustular dermatosis (Sneddon-Wilkinson disease), pustular vasculitis, or TEN, especially in severe cases of AGEP.

■ The estimated incidence rate of AGEP is approximately 1–5 cases per million per year.

■ *Acneiform eruptions* (see Section 1) are associated with iodides, bromides, adrenocorticotropic hormone (ACTH), glucocorticoids, isoniazid, androgens, lithium, actinomycin D, phenytoin. The EGFR tyrosine kinase inhibitors erlotinib, gefitinib, cetuximab, panitumumab produce pustules that are not acneiform and erupt in the face (Fig. 22-5) but can erupt also in atypical areas, such as on the arms and legs, and are most often monomorphous. Comedones are usually absent.

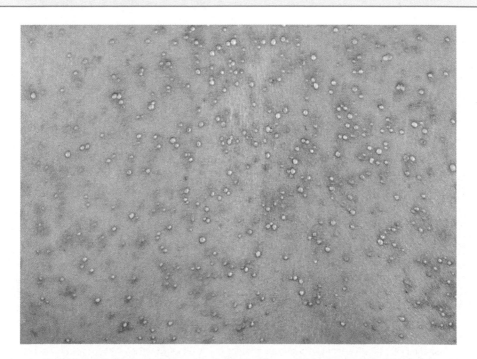

FIGURE 22-3   Pustular drug eruption: acute generalized exanthematous pustulosis (AGEP)   Multiple tiny nonfollicular pustules against the background of diffuse erythema that first appeared in the large folds and then covered the entire trunk and the face.

FIGURE 22-4   Pustular drug eruption: AGEP   Multiple sterile pustules surrounded by fiery-red erythema in a 58-year-old female who had fever and leukocytosis. In contrast to the disseminated pustules in Fig. 22-3, here the pustules show a tendency for grouping. Differential diagnosis of von Zumbusch pustular psoriasis (compare with Figs. 3-13 and 3-14).

A

B

FIGURE 22-5   Pustular drug eruption: erlotinib   This pustular eruption occurred in a patient who had received an anti-EGR monoclonal antibody for cancer of the colon. Although these eruptions usually are not associated with comedones, this patient did have comedones on the nose but not in the other "seborrheic" areas such as the forehead and the cheeks.

DRUG-INDUCED ACUTE URTICARIA, ANGIOEDEMA, EDEMA, AND ANAPHYLAXIS (See also Section 14)

- Drug-induced urticaria and angioedema occur due to a variety of mechanisms (see Table 22-1) and are characterized clinically by transient wheals and larger edematous areas that involve the dermis and subcutaneous tissue (angioedema).

- In some cases, cutaneous urticaria/angioedema is associated with systemic anaphylaxis, which is manifested by respiratory distress, vascular collapse, and/or shock.

- Drugs causing urticaria/angioedema and anaphylaxis are listed in Table 22-4.

CLASSIFICATION OF URTICARIAL/ ANGIOEDEMA ACDRs

- Immune-mediated
  - IgE-mediated: penicillin
  - Complement- and immune complex–mediated: penicillin, immunoglobulins, whole blood
- Nonallergic urticarial ACDR
  - Analgesics/NSAIDs inhibit/block cyclooxygenase in prostaglandin synthesis
  - Radio contrast media
  - ACE inhibitors: inhibition of kinin metabolism
  - Calcium channel blockers
  - Drugs releasing histamine

CLINICAL MANIFESTATION

Time from Initial Drug Exposure to Appearance of Urticaria *IgE-Mediated* Initial sensitization, usually 7–14 days; urticaria may occur while the drug is still being administered or after it is discontinued. In previously sensitized individuals, usually within minutes or hours.

TABLE 22-4 Drugs Causing Urticaria/Angioedema/Anaphylaxis

Drug Type	Specific Drugs
Antibiotics and chemotherapeutic agents	Penicillins: ampicillin, amoxicillin, dicloxacillin, mezlocillin, penicillin G, penicillin V, tricarcillin. Cephalosporins, including third-generation sulfonamides and derivatives
Cardiovascular drugs	Amiodarone, procainamide
Immunotherapeutics, vaccines	Antilymphocyte serum, levamisole, horse serum, monoclonal antibodies
Cytostatic agents	L-Asparaginase, bleomycin, cisplatin, daunorubicin, 5-fluorouracil, procarbazine, thiotepa
Angiotensin-converting enzyme inhibitors	Captopril, enalopril, lininopril
Calcium-channel blockers	Nifedipine, diltiazem, verapamil
Drugs releasing histamine	Centrally acting drugs: morphine, meperidine, atropine, codeine, papaverine, propanidid, alfaxalone
	Muscle relaxants: D-tubocurarine, succinylcholine
	Sympathomimetics: amphetamine, tyramine
	Hypotensive agents: hydralazine, tolazoline, trimethaphan camsylate
	Antimicrobial agents: pentamidine, propamidine, stilbamidine, quinine, vancomycin
	Radiographic contrast media and others

Immune Complex–Mediated Initial sensitization, usually 7–10 days, but as long as 28 days; in previously sensitized individuals, symptoms appear 12–36 h after drug is readministered.

Analgesics/Anti-Inflammatory Drugs Occurs after administration of drug by 20–30 min (up to 4 h).

Prior Drug Exposure *Radiographic Contrast Media* 25–35% probability of repeat reaction in individuals with history of prior reaction to contrast media.

Duration of Lesions Hours.

Skin Symptoms Pruritus, burning of palms/soles, auditory canal. With airway edema, difficulty breathing.

Constitutional Symptoms IgE-mediated: flushing, sudden fatigue, yawning, headache, weakness, dizziness; numbness of tongue, sneezing, bronchospasm, substernal pressure, palpitations; nausea, vomiting, crampy abdominal pain, diarrhea.

Systems Review Arthralgia.

Skin Lesions Urticaria and angioedema are described in Section 14. *Urticaria*: Large wheals (Fig. 22-6) that appear and resolve within a few hours, spontaneously or with therapy. *Angioedema*: Extensive tissue swelling with involvement of deep dermal and subcutaneous tissues. Often pronounced on face with skin-colored enlargement of portion of face (eyelids, lips) (Fig. 22-7*A*) or mucous membranes (tongue, Fig. 22-7*B*). 🖉

General Findings *IgE-Mediated Reactions* Hypotension. Bronchospasm, laryngeal edema.

LABORATORY EXAMINATIONS

Dermatopathology As in urticaria.

Complement Levels Decreased in serum sickness.

Ultrasonography For early diagnosis of bowel involvement; presence of abdominal pain may indicate edema of the bowel.

DIAGNOSIS

Clinical diagnosis. *Differential diagnosis* is of acute edematous red pruritic plaque(s): Allergic contact dermatitis (poison ivy, poison oak dermatitis), cellulitis, insect bite(s).

COURSE AND PROGNOSIS

Drug-induced urticaria/angioedema usually resolves within hours to days to weeks after the causative drug is withdrawn.

MANAGEMENT

The offending drug should be identified and withdrawn as soon as possible.

Prevention *Previously Sensitized Individuals* The patient should carry information listing drug sensitivities (wallet card, bracelet).

Radiographic Contrast Media Avoid use of contrast media known to have caused prior reaction. If not possible, pretreat patient with antihistamine and prednisone (1 mg/kg) 30–60 min before contrast media exposure.

Treatment of Acute Severe Urticaria/Anaphylaxis

Epinephrine 0.3–0.5 mL of a 1:1000 dilution subcutaneously, repeated in 15–20 min. Maintain airway. Intravenous access.

Antihistamines H_1 blockers or H_2 blockers or combination.

Systemic Glucocorticoids *Intravenous* Hydrocortisone or methylprednisolone for severe symptoms.

Oral Prednisone, 70 mg, tapering by 10 or 5 mg daily over 1–2 weeks, is usually adequate.

FIGURE 22-6   Drug-induced urticaria: penicillin   Large, urticarial wheals on the abdomen, thigh, and other areas such as the back and the face.

A

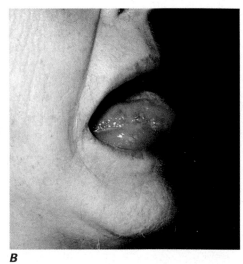

B

FIGURE 22-7   Drug-induced angioedema: penicillin   *A.* Angioedema has led to closure of right eye.   ***B.*** Sublingual angioedema in another patient interfered with breathing, talking, and eating and caused great concern.

FIXED DRUG ERUPTION   ICD-9:995.2 ○ ICD-10:T88.7

- A fixed drug eruption (FDE) is an adverse cutaneous reaction to an ingested drug, characterized by the formation of a solitary (but at times multiple) erythematous patch or plaque.
- If the patient is rechallenged with the offending drug, the FDE occurs repeatedly at the identical skin site (i.e., fixed) within hours of ingestion.

- Lesion can become bullous and erosive.
- Most commonly implicated agents are listed in Table 22-5.

PATHOGENESIS

Unknown.

CLINICAL MANIFESTATION

Drug History   Patients frequently give a history of identical lesion(s) occurring at the identical location. FDEs may be associated with the following: (1) a headache for which the patient takes a barbiturate containing analgesic, (2) constipation for which the patient takes a phenolphthalein-containing laxative, or (3) a cold for which the patient takes an over-the-counter medication containing a yellow dye. The offending "drug" in food dye–induced FDE may be difficult to identify, e.g., yellow dye in Galliano liqueur or phenolphthalein in maraschino cherries; quinine in tonic water.

Skin symptoms: Usually asymptomatic. May be pruritic, painful, or burning. Painful when eroded. *Time to onset of lesion(s)*: Occur from 30 min to 8 h after ingestion of drug in previously sensitized individual. *Duration of lesion(s)*: Lesions persist if drug is continued. Resolve days to few weeks after drug is discontinued.

Skin Lesions   The characteristic early lesion is a sharply demarcated macule (Fig. 22-8*A*), round or oval in shape, occurring within hours after ingestion of the offending drug. Initially erythema, then dusky red to violaceous (Figs. 22-8*A* and 22-9*A*). Most commonly, lesions are solitary (Fig. 22-9*A*) and can spread to become quite large (Fig. 22-9*A*), but they may be multiple (Fig. 22-9*B*) with random distribution; numerous lesions may simulate TEN. Lesions become edematous, thus forming a plaque, which may evolve to become a bulla (Fig. 22-8*B*) and then an erosion. Eroded lesions, especially on genitals or oral mucosa, are quite painful. After healing, dark brown with violet hue postinflammatory hyperpigmentation. Genital skin (Fig. 35-19) is frequently involved site, but any site may be involved; perioral, periorbital (Fig. 22-8*A*). Occur in conjunctivae, oropharynx.

TABLE 22-5   Most Commonly Implicated Agents in Fixed Drug Eruptions

Antimicrobial agents	Psychoactive agents
Tetracyclines (tetracycline, minocycline)	Barbiturates, including Fiorinal, Quaalude, Doriden
Sulfonamides, including	Oral contraceptives
"nonabsorbable" drugs;	Quinine (including quinine in tonic water), quinidine
cross-reactions with antidiabetic and diuretic	Phenolphthalein
sulfa drug may occur	Food coloring (yellow): in food or medications
Metronidazole	
Nystatin	
Anti-inflammatory agents	
Salicylates	
NSAIDs	
Phenylbutazone	
Phenacetin	

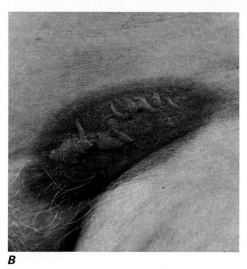

A   **B**

FIGURE 22-8   Fixed drug eruption   A. Tetracycline. Two well-defined periorbital plaques with edema. This was the second such episode following ingestion of a tetracycline. No other lesions were present. **B.** Tylenol. A large oval violaceous lesion with blistering in the center. Erosive mouth lesions were also present.

A   **B**

FIGURE 22-9   Fixed drug eruption   A. Phenolphthalein. A large area of dusky, violaceous erythema covering the entire groin and suprapubic region and extending to the upper thighs. It followed the ingestion of a phenolphthalein-containing laxative. **B.** Doxycycline. Multiple lesions. Similar violaceous plaques were also on the anterior and posterior trunk.

LABORATORY EXAMINATIONS

Dermatopathology   Similar to findings in erythema multiforme and/or TEN.

Patch Test   Suspected drug can be placed as a patch test at a previously involved site; an inflammatory response occurs in only 30% of cases.

DIAGNOSIS AND DIFFERENTIAL DIAGNOSIS

Made on clinical grounds. Readministration of the drug confirms diagnosis but should be avoided.

Solitary genital erosion to be differentiated from recurrent herpetic lesion; multiple erosions from SJS, TEN; oral erosion(s) from aphthous stomatitis, primary herpetic gingivostomatitis, erythema multiforme.

COURSE AND PROGNOSIS

FDE resolves within a few weeks of withdrawing the drug. Recurs within hours after ingestion of a single dose of the drug.

MANAGEMENT

Identify and withhold the offending drug. Noneroded lesions can be treated with a potent topical glucocorticoid ointment. Eroded cutaneous lesions can be treated with an antimicrobial ointment and a dressing until the site is reepithelialized. For widespread, generalized, and highly painful mucosal lesions, oral prednisone 1 mg/kg body weight tapered over a course of 2 weeks.

DRUG HYPERSENSITIVITY SYNDROME   ▪ ◑→●

- Drug hypersensitivity syndrome is an idiosyncratic adverse drug reaction that begins acutely in the first 2 months after initiation of drug and is characterized by fever, malaise, and facial edema or an exfoliative dermatitis.
- Skin lesions are a maculopapular exanthem.
- Lymphadenopathy, hematologic abnormalities (eosinophilia, atypical lymphocytes), and organ involvement (hepatitis, carditis, interstitial nephritis, or interstitial pneumonitis).

- The mortality rate is 10% if unrecognized and untreated.
- Lesional biopsy specimens show a lymphocytic infiltrate, at times mimicking a cutaneous lymphoma.

Synonym: Drug rash with eosinophilia and systemic symptoms (DRESS).

ICD-9 : 995.2 ∘ ICD.0 : I88.7

EPIDEMIOLOGY AND ETIOLOGY

Race   Reactions to antiepileptic drugs may be higher in black individuals.

Etiology   Most commonly: antiepileptic drugs (phenytoin, carbamazepine, phenobarbital; cross-sensitivity among the three drugs is common) and sulfonamides (antimicrobial agents, dapsone, sulfasalazine). Less commonly: allopurinol, gold salts, sorbinil, minocycline, zalcitabine, calcium-channel blockers, ranitidine, thalidomide, mexiletine.

PATHOGENESIS

Some patients have a genetically determined inability to detoxify the toxic arene oxide metabolic products of anticonvulsant agents. Slow *N*-acetylation of sulfonamide and increased susceptibility of leukocytes to toxic hydroxylamine metabolites are associated with higher risk of hypersensitivity syndrome.

CLINICAL MANIFESTATION

Onset   2–6 weeks after drug is initially used, and later than most other serious skin reactions.

Prodrome   Fever. rash.

Systems Review   Fever, malaise.

Skin Lesions   *Early*: morbilliform eruption (Fig. 22–10) on face, upper trunk, upper extremities; cannot be distinguished from exanthematous drug eruption. May progress to generalized exfoliative dermatitis/erythroderma, especially if drug is not discontinued. Eruption becomes infiltrated with edematous follicular accentuation. Facial edema (especially periorbitally) is characteristic. Dermal edema may result in blister formation. Sterile folliculocentric as well as nonfollicular pustules may occur. Eruption may become purpuric on legs. Scaling and/or desquamation may occur with healing.

Distribution Symmetric. Almost always on trunk and extremities. Lesions may become confluent and generalized.

Mucous Membranes Cheilitis, erosions, erythematous pharynx, enlarged tonsils.

General Examination Elevated temperature (drug fever).

Lymph Nodes Lymphadenopathy frequent ± tender; usually due to benign lymphoid hyperplasia.

Other Involvement of liver, heart, lungs, joints, muscles, thyroid, brain also occurs.

LABORATORY EXAMINATIONS

Hemogram and Chemistries Eosinophilia (30% of cases). Leukocytosis. Mononucleosis-like atypical lymphocytes. Signs of hepatitis and nephritis.

Histology *Skin* Lymphocytic infiltrate, dense and diffuse or superficial and perivascular. ± Eosinophils or dermal edema. In some cases, bandlike infiltrate of atypical lymphocytes with epidermotropism, simulating cutaneous T cell lymphoma.

Lymph Nodes Benign lymphoid hyperplasia. Uncommonly atypical lymphoid hyperplasia, pseudolymphoma.

Liver Eosinophilic infiltrate or granulomas.

Kidney Interstitial nephritis.

DIAGNOSIS

Proposed Diagnostic Criteria (1) Cutaneous drug eruption; (2) hematologic abnormalities (eosinophilia ≥ 1500/μL or atypical lymphocytes); (3) systemic involvement [adenopathies ≥ 2 cm in diameter or hepatitis (SGOT ≥ 2 N) or interstitial nephritis or interstitial pneumonitis or carditis]. Diagnosis is confirmed if three criteria are present.

DIFFERENTIAL DIAGNOSIS

Early That of morbilliform eruptions. Can mimic early measles or rubella.

Later Serum sickness, drug-induced vasculitis, Henoch-Schönlein purpura, cryoglobulin-associated vasculitis, vasculitis associated with infection, and collagen vascular diseases.

Rash Plus Lymphadenopathy Rubella, primary EBV or CMV mononucleosis syndrome.

FIGURE 22-10 Drug hypersensitivity syndrome: phenytoin Symmetric, bright red, exanthematous eruption, confluent in some sites; the patient had associated lymphadenopathy.

COURSE AND PROGNOSIS

Rash and hepatitis may persist for weeks after drug is discontinued. In patients treated with systemic glucocorticoids, rash and hepatitis may recur as glucocorticoids are tapered. Lymphadenopathy usually resolves when drug is withdrawn; however, rare progression to lymphoma has been reported. Rarely, patients die from systemic hypersensitivity such as with eosinophilic myocarditis. Clinical findings recur if drug is given again.

MANAGEMENT

Identify and discontinue the offending drug.
Symptomatic Treatment Oral antihistamine to alleviate pruritus.

Glucocorticoids *Topical* High-potency topical glucocorticoids applied twice a day are usually helpful in relieving cutaneous symptoms of pruritus but do not alter systemic hypersensitivity.
Systemic Prednisone (0.5 mg/kg per day) usually results in rapid improvement of symptoms and laboratory parameters.
Future Drug Therapy Cross-sensitivity between various aromatic antiepileptic drugs occurs, making it difficult to select alternative anticonvulsant therapy.
Prevention The individual must be aware of his or her specific drug hypersensitivity and that other drugs of the same class can cross-react. These drugs must never be readministered. Patient should wear a medical alert bracelet.

DRUG-INDUCED PIGMENTATION   ICD-9:995.2 ∘ ICD-10:T88.7

- Drug-induced alterations in pigmentation are relatively common.
- They result from the deposition of a variety of endogenous and exogenous pigments in the skin.

- Can be of significant cosmetic concern to the patient.

DRUGS CAUSING HYPERPIGMENTATION

The following drugs are capable of inducing hyperpigmentation of skin and/or mucosa:

- Antiarrhythmic: amiodarone
- Antimalarial: chloroquine, hydroxychloroquine, quinacrine, quinine
- Antimicrobial: minocycline, clofazimine, zidovudine
- Antiseizure: hydantoins
- Cytostatic: bleomycin, cyclophosphamide, doxorubicin, daunorubicin, busulfan, 5-fluorouracil, dactinomycin
- Heavy metals: silver, gold, mercury
- Hormones: ACTH estrogen/progesterone
- Psychiatric: chlorpromazine

CLINICAL MANIFESTATION

Skin Findings
Amiodarone > 75% of patients after 40-g cumulative dose after >4 months of therapy. More common in skin phototypes I and II. Low-grade or minimal photosensitivity; phototoxic erythema limited to the light-exposed areas in a small proportion (8%) of patients. Dusky-red erythema and, later, blue-gray dermal melanosis (ceruloderma) (Fig. 22-11) in exposed areas (face and hands). Lipofuscin-type pigment deposited in macrophages and endothelial cells.
Other Adverse Effects of Amiodarone Pulmonary fibrosis, pneumonitis, hepatotoxicity, thyroid dysfunction, neuropathy, and myopathy.

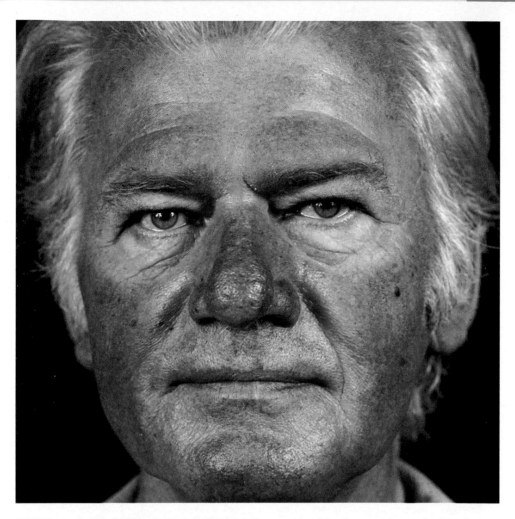

FIGURE 22-11   Drug-induced pigmentation: amiodarone   A striking slate-gray pigmentation in a photo-distribution of the face. The blue color (ceruloderma) is due to the deposition of melanin and lipofuscin contained in macrophages and endothelial cells in the dermis. The brown color is due to melanin. The pigmentation is reversible, but it may take up to a year or more to complete resolution. In this patient it took 16 months for the ceruloderma to disappear.

Course The low-grade photosensitivity disappears 12–24 months after drug is discontinued; the long period results from the gradual elimination of the photoactive drug from the lysosomal membranes. The pigmentation also disappears after 1–3 years if drug is discontinued and sun is avoided.

Minocycline Onset delayed, usually after total dose of >50 g, but may occur after a small dose. Not melanin but an iron-containing brown pigment, located in the dermal macrophages; stippled or diffuse. Blue-gray or slate-gray pigmentation (Fig. 22-12). Distributed on extensor legs, ankles, dorsa of feet, face, especially around eyes; sites of trauma or inflammation such as acne scars, contusions, abrasions; hard palate, teeth; nails.

Internal Sites Bones, cartilage, thyroid ("black thyroid").

Course Discoloration gradually disappears over a period of months after drug is discontinued.

Clofazimine Orange, reddish brown (range, pink to black) discoloration, ill-defined on light-exposed areas; conjunctivae; accompanied by red sweat, urine, feces. Subcutaneous fat is orange.

Zidovudine Brown macules on lips or oral mucosa; longitudinal brown bands in nails.

Antimalarials (Chloroquine, Hydroxychloroquine, Quinacrine) Occurs in 25% of individuals who take the drug for >4 months. Brownish, gray-brown, and/or blue-black discoloration due to melanin, hemosiderin. With quinacrine: yellow, yellow-green due to quinacrine-containing complexes. Over shins; face, nape of neck; hard palate (sharp line of demarcation at soft palate); under finger- and toenails (see Fig. 33-36); may also occur in cornea and retina; quinacrine: skin and sclerae (resembling icterus); yellow-green fluorescence of nail bed with Wood lamp. Discoloration disappears within a few months after drug is discontinued; quinacrine dyschromia can fade after 2–6 months even though drug is continued.

Phenytoin High dose over a long period of time (> 1 year). *Discoloration* is spotty, resembling melasma, in light-exposed areas and is due to melanin.

Bleomycin Mechanism unknown. Tan or brown to black and due to increase in epidermal melanin at sites of minor inflammation, i.e., parallel linear streaks at sites of dermatographism induced by excoriation ("flagellate" pigmentation), most commonly on the back, elbows, small joints, nails.

Cyclophosphamide Brown. Diffuse or discrete macules on elbows; palms with Addisonian-like pigmentation (see Fig. 15-10) and macules.

Busulfan Occurs in 5% of treated patients. Addisonian-like pigmentation. Face, axillae, chest, abdomen, oral mucous membranes.

ACTH Addisonian pigmentation of skin and oral mucosa. First 13 amino acids of ACTH are identical to α-melanocyte-stimulating hormone (MSH) (see Fig. 15-10*A*, *B*).

Estrogens/Progesterone Caused by endogenous and exogenous estrogen combined with progesterone, i.e., during pregnancy or with oral contraceptive therapy. Sunlight causes marked darkening of pigmentation. Tan/brown (melasma or chloasma) (see Fig. 13-8).

Chlorpromazine and Other Phenothiazines Occurs after long-term (> 6 months), high-dose (> 500 mg/d) therapy. Phototoxic reaction. Slate-gray, blue-gray, or brownish in areas exposed to light, i.e., chin and cheeks. After discontinuation of drug, discoloration usually fades slowly.

Silver (Argyria or Argyrosis) *Source*: Silver nitrate nose drops; silver sulfadiazine applied as an ointment. Silver sulfide (silver nitrate converted into silver sulfide by light, as in photographic film). Blue-gray discoloration. Primarily areas exposed to light, i.e., face, dorsa of hands, nails, conjunctiva; also diffuse.

Gold (Chrysiasis) *Source*: Organic colloidal gold preparations used in therapy of rheumatoid arthritis. 5–25% of all treated patients. Dose-dependent. In high-dose therapy, appears in a short time; with lower dose, occurs after months. Blue-gray to purple discoloration. In light-exposed areas; sclerae. Persists long after drug is discontinued.

Iron *Source*: IM iron injections; multiple blood transfusions. Brown or blue-gray discoloration. Generalized; also, local deposits at site of injection.

Carotene Ingestion of large quantities of β-carotene-containing vegetables; β-carotene tablets. Yellow-orange discoloration. Most apparent on palms and soles.

FIGURE 22-12   Drug-induced pigmentation: minocycline   Stippled, blue-gray macular pigmentation on the lower legs. The patient had taken minocycline for years for rosacea. The pigmentation was much more pronounced on the left leg, associated with varicose veins, chronic venous insufficiency, and chronic edema. A melon-sized inguinal hernia was also present with striking pigmentation of the enlarged scrotum.

PSEUDOPORPHYRIA

- Pseudoporphyria is a condition that clinically presents with cutaneous manifestations of porphyria cutanea tarda (PCT) (see Section 10) without the characteristic abnormal porphyrin excretion.
- It is a bullous drug-induced photosensitivity reaction.
- Develops on the dorsa of hands and feet with characteristic tense bullae that rupture and leave erosions (Fig. 22-13) and heal with scars and milia formation.

- Pseudo-PCT is associated with ingestion of drugs such as furosemide and nalidixic acid (Table 22-6).
- It is characterized by subepidermal blistering with little or no dermal inflammation and, in contrast to true PCT, little or no deposition of immunoreactants around upper dermal blood vessels and capillary walls.
- A bullous dermatosis that is morphologically and histologically indistinguishable from pseudoporphyria also occurs in patients with chronic renal failure receiving maintenance hemodialysis (see Section 17).

TABLE 22-6	Drugs Causing Pseudoporphyria
Naproxen	Diflunisal
Nabumetone	Celecoxib
Oxaprozin	Tetracyclines
Ketoprofen	Nalidixic acid
Mefenamic acid	Amiodarone
Tiaprofenic acid	Furosemide

FIGURE 22-13   Pseudoporphyria: nonsteroidal anti-inflammatory agents   In this 20-year-old male blisters appeared on the dorsa of both hands that led to erosions, crusting, and were clinically indistinguishable from porphyria cutanea tarda. However, there was no urinary fluorescence, and porphyrin studies were negative. The patient had taken an NSAID for arthritis and had impaired kidney function.

ACDR-RELATED NECROSIS   ICD-9 : 995.2 ∘ ICD-10 : T88.7   □ ◑ ➔ ●

- Drugs can cause cutaneous necrosis when given orally or at sites of injection.
- *Warfarin-induced cutaneous necrosis* is a rare reaction with onset between the third and fifth days of anticoagulation therapy with the warfarin derivatives and indandione compounds, manifested by sharply demarcated, purpuric cutaneous infarction.
- *Risk factors*: higher initial dosing, obesity, female sex; individuals with hereditary deficiency of protein C, protein S or antithrombin III deficiency. Idiosyncratic reaction. In individuals with hereditary deficiency of protein C, a natural anticoagulant protein, warfarin greatly depresses protein C levels before decreasing other vitamin K–dependent coagulation factors, inducing a transient hypercoagulable state and thrombus formation.
- Lesions vary with severity of reaction: petechiae to ecchymoses to tender hemorrhagic infarcts to extensive necrosis: well-demarcated, deep purple to black (Fig. 22-14). Deep tissue sloughing and ulceration if lesions are not debrided and grafted. Often single; may present as two lesions. *Distribution*: areas of abundant subcutaneous fat: breasts (Fig. 22-14), buttocks, abdomen, thighs, calves; acral areas are spared.
- *Coagulation studies*: Usually within normal limits.
- *Differential diagnosis*: Purpura fulminans (disseminated intravascular coagulation), hematoma/

ecchymosis in overly anticoagulated patient, necrotizing soft tissue infection, vasculitis, rare necrosis after vasopressin treatment, brown recluse spider bite. Depending on severity of reaction, lesions may subside, heal by granulation, or require surgical intervention. If area of necrosis is large in an elderly, debilitated patient, may be life-threatening. If warfarin is inadvertently readministered, reaction recurs.
- *Heparin* can cause cutaneous necrosis, usually at the site of subcutaneous injection (Fig. 22-15).
- *Interferon-*α can cause necrosis and ulceration at injection sites, often in the lower abdominal panniculus or thighs (Fig. 22-16).
- *Ergotism* can cause necrosis. Ergotamine-containing medications lead to acral gangrene, ergotamine-containing suppositories after prolonged use cause extremely painful anal and perianal black eschars that, after having been shed, leave deep painful ulcers (Fig. 22-17).
- *Embolia cutis medicamentosa*: Deep necrosis developing at the site of intramuscular injection of oily drugs inadvertently injected into an artery (Fig. 22-18).
- Necrosis also develops in obtunded or deeply sedated patients at pressure sites (Fig. 22-19).

FIGURE 22-14   ACDR-related cutaneous necrosis: warfarin   Bilateral areas of cutaneous infarction with purple-to-black coloration of the breast surrounded by an area of erythema occurred on the fifth day of warfarin therapy.

FIGURE 22-15   ACDR-related cutaneous necrosis: heparin   Two lesions of irregular dark-red erythema with central hemorrhagic necrosis on the abdomen occurring postoperatively in a female injected with heparin.

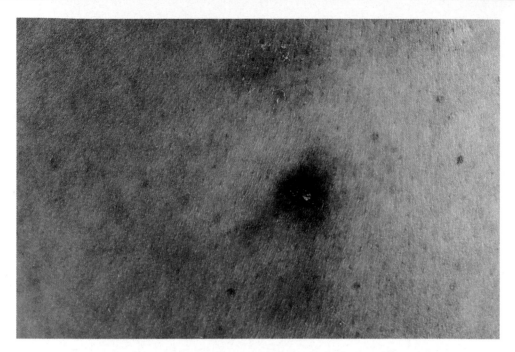

FIGURE 22-16 ACDR-related cutaneous necrosis: interferon-α An ulcer on the thigh at the site of interferon injection.

FIGURE 22-17 ACDR-related cutaneous necrosis: ergotamine This 60-year-old male had used ergot-containing suppositories for pain relief over many months. Painful black necrosis followed by ulceration developed on the anus and perianally and extended into the rectum.

FIGURE 22-18   ACDR-related necrosisa following intramuscular injection   Embolia acutis medica mentosa. The drug (an oily preparation of testosterone) had been inadvertently administered intraarterially.

FIGURE 22-19   ACDR-related necrosis with hemorrhagic blistering after an overdose of barbiturates
This patient had attempted suicide.

ACDR RELATED TO CHEMOTHERAPY   ICD-9:995.2 ○ ICD-10:T88.7■ ◑

- Chemotherapy may induce local and systemic skin toxicity with a wide range of cutaneous manifestations from benign to life threatening.

- The ACDR can be related to overdose, pharmacologic side effects, cumulative toxicity, delayed toxicity, or drug-drug interactions.

- Clinical manifestations range from alopecia (see Section 32) and nail changes (see Section 33, Figs. 33-23, 33-35) to mucositis and acral erythema, often with sensory abnormalities: palmoplantar dysesthesia (capecitabine, cytaribine, doxorubicin, fluorouracil).

- Chemotherapeutic agents are also responsible for inflammation and ulceration at sites of extravasation of intravenous medications, such as doxorubicin or taxol, which can be followed by skin necrosis with ulceration (Fig. 22-20A).

- Other reactions are radiation recall or enhancement (as with methotrexate), erosion or ulceration of psoriasis due to an overdose of methotrexate, inflammation and sloughing of actinic keratosis due to 5-fluorouracil or fludarabine, or erosions due to cisplatin plus 5-fluorouracil (Fig. 22-20B).

- Table 22-7 lists newer chemotherapeutics including "biologicals" and their ACDR.

A   *B*

FIGURE 22-20   ACDR-related cellulitis and erosions   A. *Cellulitis caused by taxol.* This extremely painful cellulitis appeared after a paravenous taxol infusion. **B.** *Erosions resulting from cisplatin and 5-fluorouracil (5FU).* This patient had received chemotherapy with cisplatin and 5FU. Painful erosive lesions appeared on the scrotum and there was also erosive mucositis.

TABLE 22-7 Newer Chemotherapeutic Agents and their ACDR

Class	Agents	ACDR[1]
Spindle inhibitor	Taxanes: docetaxel, paclitaxel	Hand-foot skin reaction[2]; combined with sensory abnormalities: erythrodysesthesia; radiation recall urticaria, exanthems, mucositis, alopecia, nail changes (see Section 33); scleroderma-like changes on lower extremities; subacute cutaneous lupus erythematosus
	Vinca alkaloids: vincristine, vinblastine, vinorelbine	Phlebitis, alopecia, acral erythema, extravasation reactions (including necrosis)
Antimetabolites	Fludarabine	Macular, papular exanthem, mucositis, acral erythema, paraneoplastic pemphigus
	Cladribine	Exanthem, TEN (?)
	Capecitabine	Hand-foot skin reaction[2] acral hyperpigmentation, palmoplantar keratoderma, pyogenic granuloma, inflammation of actinic keratoses
	Tegafur	Hand-foot skin reaction[2] acral hyperpigmentation; pityriasis lichenoides et varioliformis acuta
	Gemcitabine	Mucositis, alopecia, maculopapular exanthem, radiation recall, linear IgA, bullous dermatosis, pseudoscleroderma, lipodermatosclerosis, erysipelas-like plaques, pseudolymphoma, lymphomatoid papulosis (?)
	Pemetrexed	Exanthema, radiation recall, urticarial vasculitis
Genotoxic agents	Carboplatin	Alopecia, hypersensitivity reaction (erythema, facial swelling, dyspnea, tachycardia, wheezing), palmoplantar erythema, facial flushing
	Oxaliplatin	Hypersensitivity reaction (see above); irritant extravasation reaction; radiation recall
	Liposomal doxorubicin	Acral erythema, palmoplantar erythrodysesthesia neutrophilic eccrine hidradenitis, hyperpigmentation (blue-gray), mucositis, alopecia, exanthems, radiation recall, ultraviolet light recall
	Liposomal daunorubicin	Alopecia, mucositis, extravasation reactions
	Idarubicin	Radiation recall; alopecia, acral erythema, mucositis, nail changes, extravasation reactions
	Topotecan	Maculopapular exanthem, alopecia, neutrophilic hidradenitis
	Irinotecan	Mucositis, alopecia
Signal transduction inhibitors	EGFR antagonists: gefitinib, cetuximab, erlotinib, panitumumab	Papulopustular eruptions in seborrheic areas (Fig. 22-5*A+B*), erythematous plaques, telangiectasias; xerosis, paronychia; hair abnormalities (trichomegaly, curling, fragility, see Section 32)

Class	Agents	ACDR[1]
	Multikinase inhibitors:	Maculopapular exanthem, edema imatinib (face, forearms, ankles), exfoliative dermatitis, graft-versus-host reaction–like reaction, erythema nodosum, vasculitis, SJS, AGEP; hypopigmentation, hyperpigmentation, darkening of hair, nail hyperpigmentation, lichen planus-like eruption (skin and oral mucosa), follicular mucinosis, pityriasis rosea–like eruption, Sweet syndrome, exacerbation of psoriasis, palmoplantar hyperkeratosis, porphyria cutanea tarda, primary cutaneous EBV-related B cell lymphoma
	Dasatinib and nilotinib	Localized and generalized erythema, maculopapular exanthem, mucositis, pruritus, alopecia, xerosis "acne," urticaria, panniculitis
	Sorafenib and sunitinib	Rash/desquamation, hand-foot skin reaction[2] pain, alopecia, mucositis, xerosis, flushing edema, seborrheic dermatitis, yellow skin coloration (sunitinib), subungual splinter hemorrhages, pyoderma gangrenosum
Proteasome inhibitor	Bortezomib	Erythematous nodules and plaques, morbilliform exanthem, ulceration, vasculitis

SOURCE: Collated from: N Haidary et al: J Am Acad Dermatol 58:545, 2008.
[1]Only cutaneous adverse reactions are listed here.
[2]Hand-foot skin reaction: erythema, hyperkeratotic with halo of erythema, tender, localized to areas of pressure on finger tips, toes, heels.

DISORDERS OF PSYCHIATRIC ETIOLOGY

CLASSIFICATION OF DISORDERS OF PSYCHIATRIC ETIOLOGY

- Dysmorphic syndrome
- Delusions of parasitosis

- Compulsive habits
  - ○ Neurotic excoriations
  - ○ Trichotillomania
- Factitious syndromes
- Cutaneous signs of injecting drug use

BODY DYSMORPHIC SYNDROME (BDS)   ICD-9:300.7 ○ ICD-10:F45.2 □ ◑

- Patients with dysmorphic syndrome regard their image as distorted in the eyes of the public; this becomes almost an obsession.

- The patient with BDS does not consult a psychiatrist but a dermatologist or plastic surgeon. The typical patient with BDS is a single, female, young adult who is an anxious and unhappy person.

- Common dermatologic complaints are facial (wrinkles, acne, scars, hypertrichosis, dry lips), scalp (incipient baldness, increased hair growth), genital [normal sebaceous glands on the penis, red scrotum (males), red vulva, vaginal odor (females)], hyperhidrosis, and bromhidrosis.

- Management is a problem. One strategy is for the dermatologist to agree with the patient that there is a problem and thus establish rapport; in a few visits the complaint can be explored and further discussed.

- If the patient and physician do not agree that the complaint is a vastly exaggerated skin or hair change, then the patient should be referred to a psychiatrist; this latter plan is usually not accepted, in which case the problem may persist indefinitely.

DELUSIONS OF PARASITOSIS   ICD-9:300.29 ○ ICD-10:F22.0 □ ◑

- This rare disorder, which occurs in adults and is present for months or years, is associated with pain or paresthesia and is characterized by the presence of numerous skin lesions, mostly excoriations, which the patient truly believes are the result of a parasitic infestation (Fig. 23-1).

- The onset of the initial pruritus or paresthesia may be related to xerosis or, in fact, to a previously treated infestation.

- Patients pick with their fingernails or dig into their skin with needles or tweezers to remove the "parasites" (Fig. 23-1).

- It is important to rule out other causes of pruritus. This problem is serious; patients truly suffer and are opposed to seeking psychiatric help. Patients may sell their houses to move away from the offending parasite.

- The patient should see a psychiatrist for at least one visit and for recommendations of drug therapy: pimozide plus an antidepressant. Treatment is difficult and usually unsuccessful.

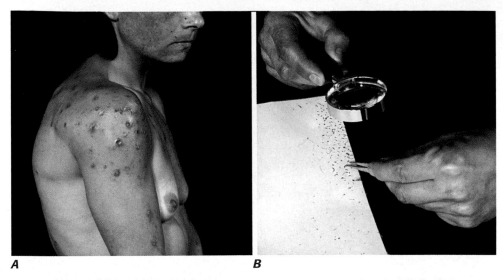

A   *B*

FIGURE 23-1   **Delusions of parasitosis**   ***A.*** Usually patients collect small pieces of debris from their skin by scratching with their nails or an instrument and submit them to the doctor for examination for parasites. In this case pointed tweezers were used and the result are ulcers, crusted lesions, and scars. ***B.*** Occasionally this can progress to an aggressive behavior such as depicted in this case where the patient posed to demonstrate how she collects the "parasites" from her skin on a piece of paper. In the majority of cases, patients are not dissuaded from their monosymptomatic delusion.

NEUROTIC EXCORIATIONS AND TRICHOTILLOMANIA

- *Neurotic excoriations* are not an uncommon problem, occurring in females more than in males and in the third to fifth decades.

- They may relate the onset to a specific event or to chronic stress; patients deny picking and scratching.

- The clinical lesions are an admixture of several types of lesions, principally excoriations, all produced by habitual picking of the skin with the fingernails; most common on the face (Fig. 23-2), back (Fig. 23-3), and extremities but also at other sites (see Figs. 33-5, 33-6). There may be depigmented atrophic or hyperpigmented macules → scars (Fig. 23-3).

- *The lesions are located only on sites that the hands can reach, thus often sparing the center of the back.*

- The diagnosis can be deceptive, and what prima facie appears to be neurotic excoriations could be a serious cause of pruritus.

- Psychiatric guidance may be necessary if the problem is not solved, as it can be very disfiguring on the face and disruptive to the patient and the family. The course is prolonged, unless life adjustments are made.

- Pimozide has been helpful but must be used with caution and with the advice and guidance of a psychopharmacologist. Also, antidepressant drugs may be used.

- Trichotillomania is a compulsive desire or habit to pluck hair. Can be on the scalp or any other hairy region (e.g., beard). Confluence of areas with very short sparse hairs, small bald areas, and normal area of scalp (Fig. 23-4). More pronounced on side of dominant hand. Can be combined with neurotic excoriations induced by vigorous plucking with tweezers. Microscopically, anagen hairs, bluntly broken hairs. Treatment as for neurotic excoriations.

ICD-9 : 698.4 ∘ ICD-10 : L 98.1

FIGURE 23-2   Neurotic excoriations   Several erythematous and crusted macules and erosions on the lower cheek and upper lip of a 19-year-old female with mild facial acne. No primary lesions are seen. The patient, who is moderately depressed, has mild acneiform lesions, which she compulsively picks with her fingernails.

FIGURE 23-3   Neurotic excoriations: back   Excoriations of the upper, mid-back and gluteal areas and linear areas of postinflammatory hyperpigmentation, crusting, and scarring in a 66-year-old diabetic female. Lesions have been present for at least 10 years but the ulcerated crusted lesion resolved with cloth tape occlusion. Once the protection was removed, the patient resumed excoriating the sites.

FIGURE 23-4 **Trichotillomania** This extensive alopecia has resulted from pulling and plucking hairs by the 17-year-old patient. She appeared balanced but mildly depressed and had considerable conflict with her parents. She admitted pulling hairs after considerable questioning.

FACTITIOUS SYNDROMES (MÜNCHAUSEN SYNDROME)

- The term *factitious* means "artificial," and in this condition there is a self-induced dermatologic lesion(s); either the patient claims no responsibility or admits deliberately mutilating the skin.

- It occurs in young adults, females > males. The history is vague ("hollow" history) of the evolution of the lesions.

- The lesions may be present for weeks to months to years (Fig. 23-5).

- Patient may be normal looking and act normally in every respect, although frequently there is a strange affect and bizarre personality.

- The skin lesions consist of cuts, ulcers, dense adherent necrotic membrane (Fig. 23-6). The shape of the lesions may be linear (Fig. 23-5), bizarre shapes, geometric patterns, single or multiple. The diagnosis can be difficult, but the nature of the lesions (bizarre shapes) may immediately suggest an artificial etiology.

- It is important to rule out every possible cause—chronic infections, granulomas, and vasculitis—perform a biopsy before assigning the diagnosis of *dermatosis artefacta,* both for the benefit of the patient and because the physician may be at risk for malpractice if he or she fails to diagnose a true pathologic process.

- There is often serious personality and/or psychosocial stress, or a psychiatric disease.

- The condition demands the utmost tact on the part of the physician, who can avert a serious outcome (i.e., suicide) by attempting to gain enough empathy with the patient to ascertain the cause. This varies with the nature of the psychiatric problem.

- The condition may persist for years in a patient who has selected his or her skin as the target organ of his or her conflicts. Consultation and management with a psychiatrist are mandatory in most patients.

ICD-9 : 301.51 ∘ ICD-10 : F 68.1

FIGURE 23-5 Factitious syndrome   These linear cuts were self-inflicted with a razor blade by a patient with a borderline syndrome. Similar, much deeper cuts were on the forearm.

FIGURE 23-6 **Factitious syndrome** These necroses were self-inflicted by the covert application of diluted sulfuric acid and tightly fitting bandages. The patient appeared well-adjusted and refused to see a psychiatrist.

CUTANEOUS SIGNS OF INJECTING DRUG USE ICD-9:999.3

- Injecting drug users often develop cutaneous stigmata as a result of their habit, whether injecting subcutaneously or intravascularly.

- Cutaneous lesions range from foreign body response to injected material, infections, and scars.

Cutaneous Injection Reactions *Cutaneous Injury* Multiple punctures at sites of cutaneous injection, often linear over veins (Fig. 23-7).
Foreign Body Granuloma Subcutaneous injection of adulterants (talc, sugar, starch, baking soda, flour, cotton fibers, glass, etc.) can elicit a foreign body response ± cellulitis ± granuloma ± ulceration. (Fig. 23-8)
Intravascular Injection Reactions *Venous Injury* Intravenous injection can result in thrombosis, thrombophlebitis, septic phlebitis. Chronic edema of the upper extremity is common.
Arterial Injury Chronic intraarterial injection can result in injection site pain, cyanosis, erythema, sensory and motor deficits, and vascular compromise (vascular insufficiency/gangrene).

Infections *Transmission of Infectious Agents* Injecting drug use can result in transmission of HIV, hepatitis B virus (HBV), and hepatitis C virus (HCV) with subsequent life-threatening systemic infections.
Injection Site Infections Local infections include cellulitis (Fig. 23-8), abscess formation, lymphangitis, septic phlebitis/thrombophlebitis. The most common organisms are those from the drug users, e.g., *S. aureus* and GAS. Less common microbes: enteric organisms, anaerobes, *Clostridium botulinum*, oral flora, fungi (*Candida albicans*), and polymicrobial infections.
Systemic Infections Intravenous injection of microbes can result in infection of vascular

endothelium, most commonly heart valve with infectious endocarditis.

Scars *Linear Scars* Multiple cutaneous punctures result in linear scarring along the course of veins, i.e., "needle tracks" (Fig. 23-7). These are found on the forearms, dorsum of the hands, wrists, antecubital/popliteal fossae, penis.

Atrophic Punched-Out Scars Result from subcutaneous injections (i.e., "skin popping") after an inflammatory (sterile or infected) response to injected material.

Tattoos Carbon on needles (after flame sterilization) can result in inadvertent tattooing and pigmented linear scars.

FIGURE 23-7 Injecting drug use: injection tracks over veins on the dorsum of the hand Linear tracks with punctures, fibrosis, and crusts were created by daily injections into the superficial veins.

FIGURE 23-8 Injecting drug use: cellulitis and foreign body response at injection site The patient injected into the subcutaneous tissue as well as veins of the forearm, resulting in foreign body response and *S. aureus* cellulitis with associated bacteremia and infectious endocarditis.

PART III

DISEASES DUE TO MICROBIAL AGENTS

BACTERIAL INFECTIONS INVOLVING THE SKIN

■ Coagulase-negative staphylococci (CoNS) normally colonize skin, more heavily in occluded than nonoccluded sites (axillae, anogenitalia)

■ Erythrasma, pitted keratolysis, trichomycosis, and infectious intertrigo are common superficial cutaneous infections

■ *Staphylococcus aureus* colonizes the nares and intertriginous skin intermittently, can penetrate the stratum corneum, and can cause infection, e.g., impetigo, folliculitis

■ Methicilllin-resistant *S. aureus* (MRSA) has become an important pathogen for community-acquired (CA-MRSA) and health care-acquired (HA-MRSA) infections
  ▪ Erythrasma: intertriginous sites of webspaces of feet, groins, axillae
  ▪ Pitted keratolysis: plantar feet and webspaces of feet
  ▪ Trichomycosis: axillae, pubis

■ *S. aureus* and group A streptococcus (GAS) cause cutaneous infections and systemic intoxications

■ Etiology: overgrowth of normal flora at sites of skin occlusion

---

• Normal skin is heavily colonized by bacterial flora (harmless commensals) such as coagulase negative staphylococci (CoNS). Colonization is more dense in intertriginous and occluded sites.

• Pathogens *Staphylococcus aureus* and, less commonly, group A β-hemolytic streptococcus (GAS) (*Streptococcus pyogenes*) colonize, and infect the skin. They cause a variety of syndromes, including skin and soft tissue infections (SSTIs), bacteremia, and systemic intoxications. An intact stratum corneum is the most important defense against invasion of pathogenic bacteria.

• Predispositon to infection:
  ◦ Chronic *S. aureus* carrier state (nares, axillae, perineum, vagina)
  ◦ Warm weather/climate, high humidity
  ◦ Skin disease, especially atopic dermatitis, familial pemphigus
  ◦ Social situation: poor hygiene, crowded living conditions, neglected minor trauma
  ◦ Chronic disease: obesity, diabetes mellitus, HIV/AIDS, especially MRSA infection, solid organ transplant recipient, iatrogenic immunosuppression
  ◦ Immunodeficiency: cancer chemotherapy, bactericidal defects (e.g., chronic granulomatous disease), chemotactic defects, hyper-IgE syndrome (Job syndrome)

• Coagulase negative staphylococci (CoNS), colonizing the skin shortly after birth, have been subdivided into 32 species, 15 of which are indigenous to humans. The most common CoNS are *S. epidermidis* (65–90% of individuals), *S. hominis. S. haemolyticus, S. warneri,* and *S. lugdunensis.* CoNS have lower pathogenicity in the skin and mucosa but increasingly cause infection of artificial devices such as percutaneous intravenous catheter (PIC) lines and heart valves.

• Group A streptococcus (GAS) usually colonizes the skin first and then the nasopharynx. Group B (*Streptococcus agalactiae*) and group G β-hemolytic streptococci (GBS, GGS) colonize the perineum of some individuals and may cause superficial and invasive infections.

• *S. aureus* does not normally reside on human skin (not one of the normal resident flora), but may be present transiently, inoculated from colonized sites such as the nares. Colonization and infection follow contact with shedding human lesions, fomites contaminated from these lesions, and human respiratory tract and skin. The nares of pets can also be colonized. *S. aureus* of mucous membranes of the anterior nasopharynx (nares) of 30% of otherwise healthy persons; other commonly colonized sites include axillae, vagina (5–15%; up to 30% during menses), damaged skin, perineum. Colonization is usually intermittent; 10–20% of individuals have persistent colonization; 10–20% are never colonized. Colonization rates higher among health care workers, dialysis patients, patients with type 1 diabetes, injection drug users, persons with HIV/AIDS disease, those with atopic dermatitis (90% in dermatitis, 70% of nonlesional skin).

- Methicillin-resistant *S. aureus* (MRSA) emerged in the 1960s as a cause of infections among patients in health care settings (operating rooms, intensive care units, cancer chemotherapy wards, newborn nurseries, chronic care facilities). Currently, MRSA infections are acquired in health care settings and in the community (healthy individuals, those with chronic disease, prisoners, intravenous-drug users, athletes, military trainees, men who have sex with men). Community-associated MRSA cause SSTIs, sepsis, and necrotizing pneumonia. Compared with health care–associated MRSA (HA-MRSA) isolates, community-associated MRSA (CA-MRSA) isolates tend to be resistant to fewer antibiotics, to produce different toxins, and to have different types of the gene complex known as staphylococcal cassette chromosome mec (SCCmec); this complex contains the mecA gene that confers methicillin resistance. In some metropolitan areas in the United States, MRSA causes the majority of SSTIs. Clindamycin, trimethoprim–sulfamethoxazole, rifampin, and doxycycline are recommended for outpatient empirical treatment of CA-MRSA SSTI. Combination rifampin plus trimethoprim–sulfamethoxazole eradicates CA-MRSA colonization and treats infection.

- Drugs for serious invasive MRSA infections: vancomycin, clindamycin, daptomycin, tigecycline, linezolid. Partial vancomycin resistance may result in failures among MRSA infections.

- MRSA is the most common identifiable cause of SSTI among patients presenting to emergency departments in many large U.S. cities. When antimicrobial therapy is indicated for the treatment of SSTIs, clinicians should consider obtaining cultures and modifying empirical therapy to provide MRSA coverage.

STAPHYLOCOCCUS AUREUS: INFECTIONS AND INTOXICATIONS

- Skin and soft tissue infections (SSTIs): impetigo/ecthyma; folliculitis; furuncle/carbuncle; cellulitis; mastitis; wound infections

- Musculoskeletal infections: septic arthritis, pyomyositis, psoas abscess

- Respiratory tract infections: ventilator-associated or nosocomial pneumonia, septic pulmonary emboli, postviral pneumonitis (e.g., influenza), empyema

- Bacteremia and its complications: sepsis/septic shock; metastatic infections (joints, bone, kidney, lung, paraspinal, brain); infective endocarditis (injection drug-use associated, native valve, prosthetic valve, nosocomial)

- Device-related infections: IV catheters, prosthetic joints

- Toxin-mediated illnesses: toxic shock syndrome, staphylococcal scalded-skin syndrome; food poisoning

STREPTOCOCCUS PYOGENES [GROUP A STREPTOCOCCUS (GAS)]: INFECTIONS AND INTOXICATIONS

- Skin and soft tissue infections: impetigo/ecthyma; erysipelas, cellulitis; necrotizing fasciitis (streptococcal gangrene); wound infection

- Bacteremia and its complications: sepsis/septic shock; metastatic infections; infective endocarditis

- Toxin-mediated illnesses: scarlet fever, streptococcal toxic shock syndrome

- Poststreptococcal diseases: rheumatic fever, glomerulonephritis

SUPERFICIAL BACTERIAL EPIDERMAL COLONIZATIONS AND INFECTIONS

- Three superficial bacterial "infections" occur in the stratum corneum and hair follicles:
  - Erythrasma: intertriginous sites of webspaces of feet, groins, axillae
  - Pitted keratolysis: plantar feet and webspaces of feet

- Trichomycosis: axillae, pubis
- Predisposition: high surface humidity
- Etiology: overgrowth of normal flora at sites of skin occlusion

ERYTHRASMA   ICD-9:039.0 ∘ ICD-10:L08.1   ■ ○

- From the Greek: "red spot"
- Etiology: *Corynebacterium minutissimum*
- Distribution: intertriginous areas of webspaces of feet, groins, axillae, submammary areas
- Clinical findings: well-demarcated red or tan patches, ± scale

- Distinguish from dermatophytosis and noninfectious intertrigo
- Diagnosis: Wood lamp examination shows coral-red fluorescence

EPIDEMIOLOGY

Age of Onset   Adults.

Etiology   *C. minutissimum,* gram-positive (diphtheroid), non–spore-forming, aerobic or facultatively anaerobic bacillus; part of normal skin flora, which causes superficial epidermal infection under certain conditions.

Predisposing Factors   Humid cutaneous microclimate: warm and/or humid climate or season; occlusive clothing/shoes; obesity, hyperhidrosis.

CLINICAL MANIFESTATION

Symptoms   Usually asymptomatic. Duration: weeks to months to years. Frequently misdiagnosed as tinea cruris or pedis.

Skin Lesions   Patches, sharply marginated (Fig. 24-1). Scaling at sites not continuously occluded. In webspaces of feet, may be macerated (Fig. 24-2), eroded, or fissured. Often symmetric or in multiple webspaces. Red or brownish red; postinflammatory hyperpigmentation in more heavily melanized individuals. If pruritic, secondary changes of excoriation, lichenification. Dermatophytosis, candidiasis, and pseudomonal webspace infection may also be present.

Sites of Predilection   Toe webspaces (Fig. 24-2) >> inguinal folds > axillae; also, intertriginous skin under panniculus, intergluteal, inframammary (submammary). ✐

DIFFERENTIAL DIAGNOSIS

Well-Demarcated Intertriginous Plaque   Dermatophytosis, intertriginous candidiasis, pityriasis versicolor, pitted keratolysis (webspace of feet), intertriginous psoriasis, acanthosis nigricans, familial pemphigus (inguinal, axillary).

LABORATORY EXAMINATIONS

Wood Lamp   Characteristic coral-red fluorescence (attributed to coproporphyrin III). May not be present if patient has bathed recently.

Direct Microscopy   Negative for fungal forms on KOH preparation of skin scraping. In the webspaces of the feet, concomitant interdigital tinea pedis may also be present. Gram or Giemsa stains may show fine bacterial filaments.

Bacterial Culture   Heavy growth of *Corynebacterium.* Rules out *Staphylococcus aureus,* group A or group B streptococcus, and *Candida* infection. In some cases, concomitant *Pseudomonas aeruginosa* webspace infection (feet) is also present.

DIAGNOSIS

Clinical findings, absence of fungi on direct microscopy, positive Wood lamp examination.

COURSE

Relapse occurs if predisposing causes are not corrected. Secondary prophylaxis usually indicated. Very rarely, *C. minutissimum* reported to cause invasive infection with bacteremia and its complications.

MANAGEMENT

Prevention/Prophylaxis   Wash with benzoyl peroxide. Medicated powders (do not use corn starch powder). Topical antiseptic alcohol gels: isopropyl, ethanol.

Topical Therapy   Preferable. Benzoyl peroxide (2.5%) gel daily, after showering, for 7 days. Topical erythromycin or clindamycin solution twice daily for 7 days. Sodium fusidate ointment, mupirocin ointment or cream. Topical antifungal agents; clotrimazole, miconazole, or econazole.

Systemic Antibiotic Therapy   A macrolide or a tetracycline for 7 days.

FIGURE 24-1   Erythrasma: groins   Sharply marginated, red patch in the axilla (infectious intertrigo). Wood lamp examination shows bright coral-red, differentiating erythrasma from intertriginous psoriasis. KOH preparation was negative for hyphae.

FIGURE 24-2   Erythrasma: webspace   This macerated interdigital webspace (infectious intertrigo) appeared bright coral-red when examined with Wood lamp; KOH preparation was negative for hyphae. The webspace is the most common site for erythrasma in temperate climates. In some cases, interdigital tinea pedis and/or pseudomonal intertrigo may coexist.

PITTED KERATOLYSIS (KERATOLYSIS SULCATA)   ▮ ○

- Etiology: *Kytococcus sedentarius*
- Distribution: plantar feet, webspaces of feet
- Predisposition: hyperhidrosis and occlusive footwear

- Clinical findings: defects in thickly keratinized skin with eroded pits of variable depth

EPIDEMIOLOGY

Etiology   *K. sedentarius.* Age of onset: young adults. Sex: males > females. Predisposing factors: hyperhidrosis of the feet; occlusive footwear. *K. sedentarius* produces two extracellular proteases that can digest keratin. Incidence reported to be 43% of paddy field workers in India.

CLINICAL MANIFESTATION

Skin Symptoms   Usually asymptomatic. Foot odor. Sliminess of feet. Uncommonly, itching, burning, tenderness. Often mistaken for tinea pedis.

Skin Lesions   Crater-like pits in stratum corneum, 1–8 mm in diameter (Figs. 24-3, 24-4).

FIGURE 24-3   Pitted keratolysis: plantar   The stratum corneum of the anterior plantar foot shows loss of keratinization with well-dermarcated scalloped margins, formed by the confluence of multiple, confluent "pits" (defects in the stratum corneum).

Pits can remain discrete or, more often, become confluent, forming large areas of eroded stratum corneum. Involved areas are white when stratum corneum is fully hydrated. Symmetric or asymmetric involvement of both feet.
Distribution Pressure-bearing areas, ventral aspect of toe, ball of foot, heel. Friction areas: interface of toes.

DIFFERENTIAL DIAGNOSIS

Erosion in Multiple Webspaces of Feet Interdigital tinea pedis, *Candida* intertrigo, erythrasma, *Pseudomonas* webspace infection.

LABORATORY EXAMINATIONS

Direct Microscopy KOH preparation negative for hyphae.
Wood Lamp Examination Negative for bright coral-red fluorescence (erythrasma).
Culture In some cases, rule out *S. aureus*, group A streptococcus (GAS), or *P. aeruginosa* infection.

DIAGNOSIS

Clinical diagnosis ruling out other causes.

COURSE AND PROGNOSIS

Persists and recurs until the underlying predisposing factors are corrected. Secondary prophylaxis usually indicated.

FIGURE 24-4   Pitted keratolysis: toe Deeply pitted epidermis of an intertriginous toe, associated with hyperhidrosis. Pits are defects in the stratum corneum, becomng confluent in the occluded webspace.

MANAGEMENT

See "Erythrasma," above. Intradermal botulinum toxin injection is effective for hyperhidrosis and has been reported to be effective for pitted keratolysis.

TRICHOMYCOSIS   ICD-9:039.0 ○ ICD-10:A48.8/L08.8

- Etiology: *Corynebacterium*; gram-positive diphtheroid. *Not* fungus.
- Distribution: axillae (trichomycosis axillaris), pubic hair (trichomycosis pubis)
- Predisposition: hyperhidrosis and occlusive footwear
- More common in males than females; adults

- Clinical findings: granular concretions (yellow, black, or red) on hair shaft. Hair appears thickened, beaded, firmly adherent.
- Insoluble adhesive may erode cuticular and cortical keratin.
- Management: shave off affected hair. Benzoyl peroxide wash. Alcohol gel. Topical erythromycin or clindamycin. ☒

NONSPECIFIC INTERTRIGO   ICD-9:695.89 ∘ ICD-10:L30.4

- Intertrigo (Latin *inter,* "between," *trigo,* "rubbing")
- Nonspecific inflammation of opposed skin (inframammary regions, axillae, groins, gluteal folds, redundant skin folds of obese individuals.
- Clinical findings: Erythema ± symptoms of pruritus, tenderness, or increased sensitivity, excluding infectious causes.
- Rule out infectious intertrigo: bacteria [GAS (Figs. 24-5, 24-6) and group B streptococcus (GBS) (Fig. 24-7)], *C. minutissimum* (erythrasma), *P. aeruginosa,* (Fig. 24-8), and fungi [dermatophytes, *Candida, Malassezia furfur* (pityriasis versicolor)]
- Rule out dermatoses: psoriasis vulgaris, seborrheic dermatitis, atopic dermatitis
- Predisposition: high surface humidity

- Management:
  - Symptomatic relief: moist dressings and/or Castellani paint
  - Powders with antibacterial/antifungal activity are helpful for preventing recurrence.
  - Zinc oxide ointment reduces friction at involved sites and protects skin from urine or feces (anogenital intertrigo)
  - Topical glucocorticoid preparations best avoided because of risk of cutaneous atrophy at these naturally occluded sites
  - Pimecrolimus cream and tacrolimus ointment may be effective, without risk of atrophy.
  - Weight reduction
  - Panniculectomy may be indicated after extreme weight reduction.

FIGURE 24-5   Intergluteal intertrigo: group A streptococcus (GAS)   A painful moist erythematous plaque in a male with intertriginous psoriasis, with foul odor. Infection resolved with penicillin VK.

FIGURE 24-6   Perineal intertrigo: group A streptococcus   Well-dermarcated erythema and erosion in the perineum of an 8-year-old boy associated with pruritus and tenderness (perianal streptococcal "cellulitis").

FIGURE 24-7   Inguinal intertrigo: group B streptococcus (GBS)   Painful foul-smelling intertrigo in the left inguinal area was present for several days in a morbidly obese diabetic female. Culture reported heavy growth of GBS, which commonly colonized the anogenital area. Symptoms resolved with penicillin VK.

FIGURE 24-8   Webspace intertrigo: _P. aeruginosa_   Erosion of a webspace of the foot with a bright red base and surrounding erythema. Tinea pedis (interdigital and moccasin-patterns) and hyperhidrosis were also present, which facilitated growth of _Pseudomonas_.

PYODERMA   ICD-9 : 684 ∘ ICD-10 : L01

IMPETIGO AND ECTHYMA   ICD-9 : 686.80 ∘ ICD-10 : B08.0

- Etiology: _S. aureus;_ also, GAS
- Infections of the epidermis (impetigo), which may extend into the dermis (ecthyma)
- Clinical findings:
  - Impetigo: crusted erosions
  - Ecthyma: crusted deep erosions or ulcers

- Portal of entry
  - Primary infections in minor superficial breaks in the skin
  - Secondary infections of preexisting dermatoses (impetiginization, or secondary infection)

EPIDEMIOLOGY AND ETIOLOGY

Age of Onset   Primary infections more common in children. Secondary infections, any age. Bullous impetigo: neonates, especially; children <5 years old.

Etiology

- _S. aureus_ most commonly
- GAS
- Bullous impetigo: epidermolytic toxin A-(etA) gene producing _S. aureus_, which also causes staphylococcal scalded skin syndrome.

Predisposing Factors Topical glucocorticoids have little effect on the microflora of the skin, except in those with atopic dermatitis; topical glucocorticoids applied to atopic dermatitis usually reduce the density of *S. aureus.* Ecthyma: lesion of neglect—develops in excoriations; insect bites; minor trauma in diabetics, elderly patients, soldiers, and alcoholics.

Portals of Entry of Infection

Primary Impetigo Minor breaks in the skin.

Secondary Impetigo (Impetiginization) Underlying dermatoses; traumatic breaks and wounds of the epidermis.

- *Inflammatory dermatoses*: Atopic dermatitis, stasis dermatitis, psoriasis vulgaris, chronic cutaneous lupus erythematosus, pyoderma gangrenosum.
- *Bullous disease*: Bullous pemphigoid, sunburn, porphyria cutanea tarda.
- *Insect bites*
- *Ulcers*: Pressure, venous insufficiency
- *Chronic lymphedema*
- *Cutaneous infections* (impetigo is superinfection): Herpes simplex, varicella, herpes zoster; dermatophytosis (tinea pedis, tinea capitis).
- *Trauma/wounds*: Surgical wounds; abrasion; laceration; puncture; bites (human, animal, insect); burns; ulcers; umbilical stump.

CLINICAL MANIFESTATION

Duration of Lesions Impetigo: days to weeks. Ecthyma: weeks to months.

Symptoms Impetigo: variable pruritus, especially associated with atopic dermatitis. Ecthyma: pain, tenderness.

Skin Lesions *Impetigo* Small erosions with crust (Figs. 24-9, 24-10). Golden-yellow crusts are often seen in impetigo but are not pathognomonic (Fig. 24-11). 1- to 3-cm lesions; central healing often apparent if lesions present for several weeks (Fig. 24-12). *Arrangement*: scattered, discrete lesions; without therapy, lesions may become confluent; satellite lesions occur by autoinoculation. Secondary impetiginization of various dermatosis is common (Figs. 24-13, 24-14). ▨

Bullous Impetigo Vesicles and bullae containing clear yellow or slightly turbid fluid ± surrounding erythema, arising on normal-appearing skin. With rupture, bullous lesions decompress. If roof of bulla is removed, shallow moist *erosion* forms (Fig. 24-15). *Distribution*: more common in intertriginous sites. ▨

Ecthyma Ulceration with a thick adherent crust (Fig. 24-16). Lesions may be tender, indurated. *Distribution*: more common on distal extremities. ▨

Miscellaneous Physical Findings

At times, lymphangitis and/or regional lymphadenopathy.

DIFFERENTIAL DIAGNOSIS

Erosion ± Crust/Scale-Crust Excoriation, allergic contact dermatitis, herpes simplex, epidermal dermatophytosis, scabies. *The majority of lesions with "honey-colored crusts" are not impetigo.*

FIGURE 24-9 Nostril colonization and impetigo: methicillin-sensitive *S. aureus* (MSSA): nasal colonization and impetigo of nares Colonization of the nares is usually asymptomatic. This patient had tenderness, erythema, and crusting of the skin adjacent to the nares, indicative of superficial infection extending from colonization of the nostril.

FIGURE 24-10   Impetigo: MSSA   Crusted erythematous erosion on the moustache area in an 8-year-old girl. Multiple scattered other lesions were also present.

FIGURE 24-11   Impetigo: MSSA   Crusted erythematous erosions becoming confluent on the nose, cheek, lips, and chin in a child with nasal carriage of *S. aureus* and mild facial eczema.

Intact Bulla(e)   Allergic contact dermatitis, insect bites, thermal burns, herpes simplex, herpes zoster, bullous pemphigoid, porphyria cutanea tarda (PCT) (dorsa of hands), pseudo-porphyria.

Ulcer ± Crust/Scale-Crust   Prurigo nodularis, chronic herpetic ulcers, excoriated insect bites, neurotic excoriations, cutaneous diphtheria, PCT, venous (stasis) and ischemic ulcers (legs).

LABORATORY EXAMINATIONS

Gram Stain   Gram-positive cocci, in chains or clusters, within neutrophils.

Culture   *S. aureus*, commonly; GAS. Failure of oral antibiotic suggests MRSA.

Dermatopathology   Impetigo: gram-positive cocci in blister fluid, acantholysis, erosion, or ulceration.

DIAGNOSIS

Clinical findings confirmed by Gram stain or culture.

FIGURE 24-12   Impetigo: methicillin-resistant *S. aureus* (MRSA)   A 22-year-old diabetic male being treated with isotretinoin for acne with erythema of lips and lower face with crusted erosions. Shaving has debrided crusts. Blood glucose was 500 mg/dL at the time of examination. Cheilitis is universal during isotretinoin treatment, and *S. aureus* secondary infection, common.

FIGURE 24-13   Secondary impetiginization of grafted burn site: MSSA   Extensive erythema and crusting are seen on hypertrophic scars and normal skin of a 10-year-old boy with prior severe thermal burns.

COURSE AND PROGNOSIS

Untreated, lesions of impetigo progress for several weeks. Untreated or neglected impetigo can progress to ecthyma. With adequate treatment, prompt resolution. Lesions can progress to invasive infection with lymphangitis, suppurative lymphadenitis, cellulitis or erysipelas, bacteremia, septicemia. Nonsuppurative complications of GAS infection include guttate psoriasis, scarlet fever, and glomerulonephritis. Ecthyma often heals with scar. Recurrent

FIGURE 24-14   Secondary impetiginization of factitial ulcers: MRSA   60-year-old female with endstage-renal disease (ESRD) and generalized pruritus has large self-induced excoriations and ulcers, which are secondarily infected.

FIGURE 24-15   Bullous impetigo: MSSA   Secondary infection of atopic dermatitis in the antecubital area. Bullae have ruptured, forming crusted erosion (same patient as in Fig. 24-10).

FIGURE 24-16   Ecthyma: MSSA   Thickly crusted erosion/ulcer on the nose had been present for 6 weeks, arising at the site of a small wound. The crust was adherent and the site bled with debridement.

S. aureus or GAS infections can occur because of failure to eradicate microbe or by recolonization from a family member, pet, or health care worker. Undiagnosed MRSA infection does not respond to usual antibiotics given for methicillin-sensitive *S. aureus* (MSSA). MRSA infection has higher morbidity and mortality.

MANAGEMENT

Prevention Daily bath. Benzoyl peroxide wash (bar). Check family members for signs of impetigo. Ethanol or isopropyl gel for hands and/or involved sites.

Topical Treatment Mupirocin and retapamulin ointment is highly effective in eliminating both *S. aureus*, including MRSA, from the nares and cutaneous lesions. Apply twice daily to involved skin and to nares for 7–10 days.

Systemic Antimicrobial Treatment See Tables 24-1, 24-2. For MRSA, sensitivities of the isolated organism and personal history of antibiotic allergies determine drug of choice and alternatives.

TABLE 24-1 Organisms, Antimicrobial Agents of Choice, and Alternatives

Infecting Organism	Antimicrobial Agent(s) of First Choice	Alternative Antimicrobial Agents
Staphylococcus aureus* or *epidermidis Non-penicillinase producing	Penicillin G or V	A cephalosporin; clindamycin; vancomycin; imipenem; a fluoroquinolone
Penicillinase- producing	A penicillinase-resistant penicillin. PO: dicloxacillin, cloxacillin. IV for severe infections; nafcillin, oxacillin	A cephalosporin; vancomycin; amoxicillin/clavulanic acid; ticarcillin/clavulanic acid; piperacillin/tazobactam; ampicillin/sulbactam; imipenem; clindamycin; a fluoroquinolone
Methicillin-resistant	Vancomycin ± gentamicin ± rifampin	Trimethoprim-sulfamethoxazole; a fluoroquinolone; minocycline; linezolid; quinupristin/dalfopristin
***Streptococcus pyogenes* (group A) and groups C and G**	Penicillin G or V	An erythromycin, clarithromycin, azithromycin; a cephalosporin; vancomycin; clindamycin
***Streptococcus*, group B**	Penicillin G or ampicillin	A cephalosporin, vancomycin, an erythromycin
***Streptococcus pneumoniae* (pneumococcus)**	Penicillin G or V	A cephalosporin erythromycin; azithromycin; clarithromycin; a fluoroquinolone; meropenem; imipenem; trimethoprim-sulfamethoxazole; clindamycin; a tetracycline
Penicillin-susceptible (MIC <0.1 μg/mL)	Penicillin G IV (12 million U/d for adults) *or* ceftriaxone *or* cefotaxime	Levofloxacin; vancomycin; clindamycin
Penicillin–intermediate resistance	Meningitis: vancomycin + ceftriaxone *or* cefotaxime ± rifampin	Meropenem; imipenem; clindamycin
Penicillin–high-level resistance (MIC ≥ 2 μg/mL)	Other infections: varicomycin ± ceftriaxone *or* cefotaxime; *or* levofloxacin	Quinupristin/dalfopristin; linezolid

Infecting Organism	Antimicrobial Agent(s) of First Choice	Alternative Antimicrobial Agents
Erysipelothrix rhusiopathiae	Penicillin G	Erythromycin, a cephalosporin, a fluoroquinolone
Haemophilus influenzae Meningitis, epiglottitis, arthritis, and other serious infections	Cefotaxime *or* ceftriaxone	Cefuroxime (not for meningitis); chloramphenicol; meropenem
Upper respiratory infections and bronchitis	Trimethoprim-sulfamethoxazole	Cefuroxime; amoxicillin/clavulanic acid; cefuroxime axetil; cefpodoxime; cefaclor; cefotaxime, ceftizoxime; ceftriaxone; cefixime; a tetracycline; clarithromycin; azithromycin; a fluoroquinolone; ampicillin or amoxicillin
Pasteurella multocida	Penicillin G	A tetracycline; a cephalosporin; amoxicillin/clavulanic acid; ampicillin/sulbactam
Pseudomonas aeruginosa	Ciprofloxacin; ticarcillin, mezlocillin *or* piperacillin + tobramycin, gentamicin *or* amikacin	Carbenicillin, ticarcillin, piperacillin *or* mezlocillin; ceftazidime; cefepime; imipenem *or* meropenem; aztreonam; tobramycin; gentamicin; amikacin
Vibrio vulnificus	A tetracycline	Cefotaxime
Neisseria gonorrhoeae (gonococcus)	Ceftriaxone *or* cefixime *or* ciprofloxacin *or* ofloxacin	Cefotaxime; spectinomycin; penicillin G; ceftizoxime; ceftriaxone
Neisseria meningitidis (meningococcus)	Penicillin G	Chloramphenicol; a sulfonamide; a fluoroquinolone
Mycobacterium tuberculosis	Isoniazid + rifampin + pyrazinamide + ethambutol *or* streptomycin	Levofloxacin, ofloxacin *or* ciprofloxacin; cycloserine; capreomycin *or* kanamycin *or* amikacin; ethionamide; clofazimine; aminosalicylic acid
Mycobacterium fortuitum/ chelonae complex	Amikacin + clarithromycin	Cefoxitin; rifampin; a sulfonamide; doxycycline; ethambutol
Mycobacterium marinum (balnei)	Minocycline	Trimethoprim-sulfamethoxazole; rifampin; clarithromycin; doxycycline
Mycobacterium leprae (leprosy)	Dapsone + rifampin + clofazimine	Minocycline; ofloxacin; sparfloxacin; clarithromycin
Actinomyces israelii (actinomycosis)	Penicillin G	A tetracycline; erythromycin; clindamycin
Nocardia	Trimethoprim-sulfamethoxazole	Sulfasoxazole; amikacin; a tetracycline; imipenem *or* meropenem; cycloserine

TABLE 24-2 Oral Antimicrobial Agents for Bacterial Infections

Antimicrobial Agent	Dosing (PO Unless Indicated), Usually For 7–14 Days
Natural penicillins	
Penicillin V	250–500 mg 3 or 4 times a day for 10 days
Penicillin G	600,000–1.2 million U IM daily for 7 days
Benzathine penicillin G	600,000 U IM in children ≤6 years, 1.2 million units if ≥7 years, if compliance is a problem
Penicillinase-resistant penicillins	
Cloxacillin	250–500 mg (adults) 4 times a day 10 days
Dicloxacillin	250–500 mg (adults) 4 times a day for 10 days
Nafcillin	1.0–2.0 g IV q4h
Oxacillin	1.0–2.0 g IV q4h
Aminopenicillins	
Amoxicillin	500 mg 3 times a day or 875 mg q12h
Amoxicillin plus clavulanic acid (β-lactamase inhibitor)	875/125 mg twice a day; 20 mg/kg per day 3 times a day for 10 days
Ampicillin	250–500 mg 4 times a day for 7–10 days
Cephalosporins	
Cephalexin	250–500 mg (adults) 4 times a day for 10 days; 40–50 mg/kg per day (children) for 10 days
Cephradine	250–500 mg (adults) 4 times a day for 10 days; 40–50 mg/kg per day (children) for 10 days
Cefaclor	250–500 mg q8h
Cefprozil	250–500 mg q12h
Cefuroxime axetil	125–500 mg q12h
Cefixime	200–400 mg q12–24h
Erythromycin group	
Erythromycin ethylsuccinate	250–500 mg (adults) 4 times a day for 10 days; 40 mg/kg per day (children) 4 times a day for 10 days
Clarithromycin	500 mg twice a day for 10 days
Azithromycin	500 mg on day 1, then 250 mg/d on days 2–5
Clindamycin	150–300 mg (adults) 4 times a day for 10 days; 15 mg/kg per day (children) 4 times a day for 10 days
Tetracylines	
Minocycline	100 mg twice a day for 10 days
Doxycycline	100 mg twice a day
Tetracycline	250–500 mg 4 times a day
Miscellaneous agents	
Trimethoprim-sulfamethoxazole	160 mg TMP + 800 mg SMX twice a day
Metronidazole	500 mg 4 times a day
Ciprofloxacin	500 mg twice a day for 7 days

ABSCESS, FURUNCLE, AND CARBUNCLE ICD-9:680.9/682.9 ∘ ICD-10:L02 ■ ◑

- *Abscess:* acute or chronic localized inflammation, associated with a collection of pus and tissue destruction.
- *Folliculitis* (staphylococcal): infection of hair follicle with ± pus in the ostium of follicle (see Section 32)
- *Furuncle:* acute, deep-seated, red, hot, tender nodule or abscess that evolves from a staphylococcal folliculitis.

- *Carbuncle:* deeper infection composed of interconnecting abscesses usually arising in several contiguous hair follicles.
- *Synonym:* Boil

EPIDEMIOLOGY AND ETIOLOGY

Age of Onset Children, adolescents, and young adults.

Sex More common in boys.

Etiology MSSA, MRSA. Much less commonly, other organisms. Sterile abscess can occur as a foreign-body response (splinter, ruptured inclusion cyst, injection sites). Cutaneous odontogenic sinus can appear anywhere on the lower face, even at sites distant from the origin (see Fig. 34-16).

Predisposing Factors

- Chronic *S. aureus* carrier state (nares, axillae, perineum, vagina)
- Diabetes mellitus
- Obesity
- Poor hygiene
- Bactericidal defects (e.g., chronic granulomatous disease)
- Chemotactic defects
- Hyper-IgE syndrome (Job syndrome)
- HIV/AIDS, especially MRSA infection

PATHOGENESIS

Folliculitis, furuncles, and carbuncles represent a continuum of severity of *S. aureus* infection. Portal of entry: hair follicle, break in the integrity of skin. MRSA infections often have high morbidity due to delay in administration of effective antibiotic. Control/eradication of carrier state treats/prevents folliculitis, furuncle, and carbuncle formation.

CLINICAL MANIFESTATION

Duration of Lesions Days to weeks to months.

Skin Symptoms Throbbing pain. Tenderness.

Constitutional Symptoms Carbuncles may be accompanied by low-grade fever and malaise.

Skin Lesions Lesions are red, hot, and painful/tender.

Abscess May arise in any organ or structure. Abscesses that present on the skin arise in the dermis, subcutaneous fat, muscle, or a variety of deeper structures. Initially, a tender red nodule forms. In time (days to weeks), pus collects within a central space (Fig. 24-17). A well-formed abscess is characterized by fluctuance of the central portion of the lesion and can occur at any cutaneous site. At sites of trauma. Upper back for abscesses in ruptured inclusion cysts. Single or multiple.

Folliculitis (Staphylococcal) See "Infectious Folliculitis," Section 32 and Figs. 32-27, 32-28, and 32-31.

Furuncle Initially, a firm tender nodule, up to 1–2 cm in diameter (Fig. 24-18). In many individuals, furuncles occur in setting of staphylococcal folliculitis in beard area or neck. Nodule becomes fluctuant, with abscess formation ± central pustule. Nodule with cavitation remains after drainage of abscess. A variable zone of cellulitis may surround the furuncle. Distribution: any hair-bearing region: beard area, posterior neck and occipital scalp, axillae, buttocks. Single or multiple (Figs. 24-19, 24-20*A, B*). ✏

Carbuncle Evolution is similar to that of furuncle. Composed of several to multiple, adjacent, coalescing furuncles (Fig. 24-21). Characterized by multiple loculated dermal and subcutaneous abscesses, superficial pustules, necrotic plugs, and sieve-like openings draining pus. ✏

DIFFERENTIAL DIAGNOSIS

Painful Dermal/Subcutaneous Nodule Ruptured epidermoid or pilar cyst, hidradenitis suppurativa (axillae, groin, vulva), necrotizing lymphangitis.

LABORATORY EXAMINATIONS

Gram Stain   Gram-positive cocci within polymorphonuclear (PMN) leukocytes.

Bacterial Culture   Culture of pus isolates *S. aureus*. Sensitivities to antimicrobial agents may determine management.

Antibiotic Sensitivities   Identifies MRSA and need for changing usual antibiotic therapy.

Dermatopathology   Pyogenic infection arising in hair follicle and extending into deep dermis and subcutaneous tissue (furuncle) and with loculated abscesses (carbuncle).

DIAGNOSIS

Clinical findings confirmed by findings on Gram stain and culture.

FIGURE 24-17   Abscess: MSSA   A very tender abscess with surrounding erythema on the heel. The patient was a diabetic with sensory neuropathy; a sewing needle in the heel had provided a portal of entry.

FIGURE 24-18   Follicultis and Furunculosis: MRSA   Multiple follicular papules, pustules, and large nodules on the medial thigh in a 41-year-old male with HIV/AIDS.

FIGURE 24-19   Furuncle in HIV/AIDS: MRSA   Large fluctuant abscess on the buttock of a male with HIV/AIDS. He was initially empirically treated without culture. The abscess was drained, and MSSA isolated. Sensitivities reported resistance to all orally administered antibiotic except for linezolid. The lesion resolved with linezolid, 600 mg bid for 10 days.

FIGURE 24-20   Multiple furuncles and cellulitis: MRSA   A 64-year-old male developed multiple furuncles on the dorsum of the left hand (**A**) and forearm (**B**). He was being treated with hemodialysis for end-stage renal disease (ESRD) associated with Alport syndrome. *S. aureus* colonization of the nares is common in persons being dialyzed.

COURSE AND PROGNOSIS

Most cases resolve with treatment (see below). At times, however, furunculosis is complicated by bacteremia and possible hematogenous seeding of heart valves, joints, spine, long bones, and viscera (especially kidneys). *S. aureus* can disseminate hematogenously via venous drainage to cavernous sinus with resultant cavernous venous thromboses and meningitis. Some individuals are subject to recurrent furunculosis, particularly diabetics.

MANAGEMENT

The treatment of an abscess, furuncle, or carbuncle is incision and drainage plus systemic antimicrobial therapy.

Prevention   Mupirocin ointment is effective for eliminating nasal carriage.

Surgery   Incision and drainage are often adequate for treatment of abscesses, furuncles, or carbuncles. Scissors or scalpel blade can be used to drain loculated pus in carbuncles; if this is not done, resolution of pain and infection can be delayed despite systemic antibiotic therapy. Dental abscesses are often associated with devitalized tooth pulp, which must be removed or the tooth extracted. All foreign matter must be removed: comedone, keratinaceous debris, foreign body.

Adjunctive Therapy   Application of heat to the lesion promotes localization/consolidation and aids early spontaneous drainage.

Systemic Antimicrobial Treatment   Systemic antibiotics speed resolution in healthy individuals and are mandatory in any individual at risk for bacteremia (e.g., immunosuppressed patients). See Table 24-2.

Recurrent Furunculosis   Usually related to persistent *S. aureus* in the nares, perineum, and body folds.

Topical Therapy   Shower with providone iodine soap or benzoyl peroxide (bar or wash). Apply mupirocin ointment daily to the inside of nares and other sites of *S. aureus* carriage. Retapamulin ointment applied on infected sites is also effective.

Systemic Therapy   Appropriate antibiotic treatment is continued until all lesions have resolved. Secondary prophylaxis may be given once a day for many months.

Carrier State   Rifampin: 600 mg PO for 7–10 days for eradication of carrier state.

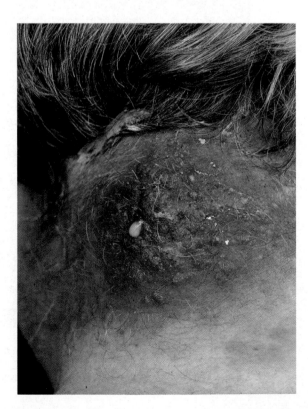

FIGURE 24-21   Carbuncle: MSSA
A very large, inflammatory plaque studded with pustules, draining pus, on the nape of the neck. Infection extends down to the fascia and has formed from a confluence of many furuncles.

SOFT TISSUE INFECTIONS (STIs)

- Characterized by an acute, diffuse, spreading, edematous, suppurative inflammation of the dermis and subcutaneous tissues
- Often associated with systemic symptoms of malaise, fever, and chills
- Nonnecrotizing STIs are treated with antibiotics, drainage of abscesses, and supportive measures
- Necrotizing STIs are often life-threatening and require, in addition, extensive surgical debridement.

CLASSIFICATION/DEFINITIONS

Erysipelas A distinct type of superficial cutaneous cellulitis with marked dermal lymphatic vessel involvement presenting as a painful, bright red, raised, edematous, indurated plaque with advancing raised borders, sharply marginated from the surrounding normal skin (Figs. 24-22 to 24-24). Usually caused by group A β-hemolytic streptococcus (GAS) (very uncommonly group C or G streptococcus) and rarely due to *S. aureus*.

Cellulitis Has many of the features of erysipelas but extends into the subcutaneous tissues. Cellulitis is differentiated from erysipelas by two physical findings: cellulitis lesions are primarily not raised, and demarcation from uninvolved skin is indistinct. The tissue feels hard on palpation and is extremely painful. In some cases, bulla formation (see Fig. 24-25) or necrosis. Infection may localize in the soft tissue, with dermal and subcutaneous abscess formation (see Fig. 24-26) or necrotizing fasciitis. *S. aureus* and GAS are by far the most common etiologic agents, but other bacteria are implicated.

Lymphangitis Inflammation of the lymphatic vessels, usually beginning on acral sites such as hands or feet; presents as erythematous streaking on the volar or dorsal aspect of the arm proximal to a finger or hand infection (Figs. 24-27 and 24-28).

Gangrenous Cellulitis Characterized by necrosis of the dermis, subcutaneous fat (hypodermis), fascia, or muscle. Classified as *necrotizing fasciitis, clostridial soft tissue infections,* and *progressive bacterial synergistic gangrene.*

Necrotizing Soft Tissue Infection (NSTI) Differs from other variants because of significant tissue necrosis, lack of response to antimicrobial treatment alone, and need for surgical debridement of devitalized tissues. Starts with erythema and painful induration of underlying soft tissues; rapid development of black eschar, which transforms into liquefied black and malodorous necrotic mass (see Fig. 24-31). Divided into three categories: *necrotizing cellulitis, necrotizing fasciitis, myonecrosis.* NSTI in the genital area is called *Fournier gangrene.*

Ecthyma Gangrenosum An NSTI, most commonly caused by *P. aeruginosa,* characterized by a cutaneous infarction progressing to large ulcerated gangrenous lesions (see Fig. 24-29).

ERYSIPELAS AND CELLULITIS   ICD-9:035 ○ ICD-10:A46.0

- Acute, spreading infections of dermal and subcutaneous tissues
- Characterized by a red, hot, tender area of skin
- Often originating at the site of bacterial entry
- Caused most frequently by GAS (erysipelas) or *S. aureus.*

EPIDEMIOLOGY AND ETIOLOGY

Age of Onset Any age. Children <3 years; older individuals.

Etiology Adults: *S. aureus,* GAS. Children: *H. influenzae* type b (Hib), GAS, *S. aureus* (Table 24-3).

Less Commonly Group B streptococci (GBS), pneumococci, *E. rhusiopathiae* (erysipeloid). In patients with diabetes or impaired immunity: *E. coli, Proteus mirabilis, Acinetobacter, Enterobacter, P. aeruginosa, Pasteurella multocida, Vibrio vulnificus; Mycobacterium fortuitum* complex, *C. neoformans.* In children: pneumococci, *N. meningitidis* group B (periorbital).

TABLE 24-3   Etiology of Soft Tissue Infections (STIs)

Type of Infection	Most Common Cause(s)	Uncommon Causes
Erysipelas	Group A streptococcus (GAS)	Group B, C, and G streptococci (GBS, GCS, GGS) *S. aureus*
Cellulitis	*S. aureus*, GAS	GBS, GCS, GGS
		Erysipelothrix rhusiopathiae
		Pneumococcus
		Haemophilus influenzae (children)
		Escherichia coli
		Campylobacter jejuni
		Moraxella
		Serratia, Proteus, other Enterobacteriaceae
		Cryptococcus neoformans
		Legionella pneumophila, L. micdadei
		Bacillus anthracis (anthrax)
		Aeromonas hydrophila
		Vibrio vulnificus, V. alginolyticus
Cellulitis in children	*S. aureus*, GAS	GBS (neonates)
Facial/periorbital cellulitis	*H. influenzae* (young children)	*Neisseria meningitidis*
Perianal cellulitis	GAS	*S. aureus*
Cellulitis secondary to bacteremia	*P. aeruginosa*	*V. vulnificus*
		Streptococcus pneumoniae, GAS, GBS
Crepitant cellulitis	*Clostridia* spp. *(C. perfringens, C. septicum)*	*Bacteroides* spp.
		Peptostreptococci
		E. coli, Klebsiella
Cellulitis associated with water exposure	*E. rhusiopathiae* (erysipeloid)	Seal finger (etiology unknown)
	V. vulnificus	
	Aeromonas hydrophila	
	Mycobacterium marinum (nodular lymphangitis)	
	M. fortuitum complex	
Gangrenous cellulitis (infectious gangrene)		
Necrotizing fasciitis (NF) Streptococcal gangrene	GAS	GBS, GCS, GGS
Nonstreptococcal NF	Mixed infection with one or more anaerobes (*Peptostreptococcus* or *Bacteroides*) plus at least one facultative species (non-group A streptococci; members of the Enterobacteriaceae such as *Enterobacter* or *Proteus*)	*Bacillus cereus* (agranulocytic patient)

Opportunistic Pathogens *Helicobacter cinaedi* (HIV/AIDS); *C. neoformans*; *Fusarium, Proteus, Pseudomonas* spp.

Dog and Cat Bites *P. multocida* and other *Pasteurella* spp.; *S. aureus, Capnocytophaga canimorsus* (DF–2)

Human Bites Most common in young males. Most bites occur on the hands: clenched-fist or occlusional injuries. Multiple organisms often isolated from wound site, including *Streptococcus anginosus, S. aureus, E. corrodens, Fusobacterium nucleatum,* and *Prevotella melaninogenica. Fusobacterium, Peptostreptococcus,* and *Candida* spp. more frequently from occlusional bites than from clenched-fist injuries.

Portals/Source of Infection Mucocutaneous, subjacent, bacteremic. (See Table 24-4.)

Mucocutaneous

- *Underlying dermatoses*: Bullous disease (pemphigus pemphigoid, sunburn); chronic lymphedema; dermatophytosis (epidermal dermatophytosis/ tinea pedis, tinea capitis, tinea barbae); viral infections (herpes simplex, varicella, herpes zoster); inflammatory dermatoses (atopic dermatitis, contact dermatitis, stasis dermatitis, pyoderma gangrenosum); superficial pyoderma (impetigo, folliculitis, furunculosis, carbuncle, ecthyma); ulcers (pressure, chronic venous insufficiency, ischemic, neuropathic); umbilical stump
- *Trauma*: Abrasion; bites (human, animal); insect bites; burns; laceration; puncture
- *Surgical wound*: Surgical incisions; PIC lines
- *Mucosal infection*: Oropharynx, nasal mucosa; middle ear
- *Injecting drug use (IDU)*: "Skin popping" sites
- Water exposure: *V. vulnificus, V. cholerae* non-01 and non-0139. *Aeromonas hydrophilia.*

Subjacent Osteomyelitis, cutaneous odontogenic sinus, abdominal infection.

Bacteremic Sepsis, infectious endocarditis. *S. pneumoniae, V. vulnificus,* and *C. neoformans.*

Risk Factors Drug and alcohol abuse, cancer and cancer chemotherapy, chronic lymphedema (postmastectomy, postcoronary artery grafting, previous episode of cellulitis/erysipelas), cirrhosis, diabetes mellitus, nephritic syndrome, iatrogenic immunosuppression, neutropenia, immunodeficiency syndromes, malnutrition, renal failure, systemic atherosclerosis.

PATHOGENESIS

After entry, infection spreads to tissue spaces and cleavage planes as hyaluronidases break down polysaccharide ground substances, fibrinolysins digest fibrin barriers, lecithinases destroy cell membranes. Local tissue devitalization, e.g., trauma, is usually required to allow for significant anaerobic bacterial infection. The number of infecting organisms is usually small, suggesting that cellulitis may be more of a reaction to cytokines and bacterial superantigens than to overwhelming tissue infection.

CLINICAL MANIFESTATION

Incubation Period Few days.

Prodrome Malaise, anorexia; fever, chills can develop rapidly, before cellulitis is apparent clinically. Higher fever (38.5° C) and chills usually associated with GAS.

Immune Status Immunocompromised patients susceptible to infection with pathogens of low pathogenicity.

History Local pain and tenderness. Necrotizing infections associated with more local pain and systemic symptoms.

Skin Lesions

Portals of Entry Red, hot, edematous and shiny plaque, and very tender area of skin of varying size (Figs. 24-22, 24-24); borders usually sharply defined, irregular, and slightly elevated; bluish purple color with *H. influenzae* (Fig. 24-23). Vesicles, bullae, erosions, abscesses, hemorrhage, and necrosis may form in plaque. Lymphangitis. *Lymph nodes*: Can be enlarged and tender, regionally.

Distribution *Adults* Lower leg (Fig. 24-24); most common site, following interdigital tinea (Fig. 24-25). Arm: in young male, consider IV drug use; in female, postmastectomy (Fig. 24-27). Trunk: operative wound site. Face: following rhinitis, conjunctivitis. 🔳

Children Cheek, periorbital area, head, neck most common: usually *H. influenzae*. Extremities: *S. aureus*, GAS. 🔳

Variants in Infecting Organism

S. aureus Often a portal of entry is apparent; usually a focal infection. Most common pathogen in injection drug user. Toxin syndromes [scalded-skin syndrome, toxic shock syndrome (TSS)] may occur. Endocarditis may follow bacteremia.

Group A Streptococcus Incidence of invasive GAS infections is increasing. The morbidity and mortality rates are significant: 37% of patients have necrotizing fasciitis and 25% meet the criteria for streptococcal TSS; mortality rate reported to be 21%.

Group B Streptococcus (*S. agalactiae*) Colonizes anogenital region. Causes anogenital cellulitis, which may extend into pelvic tissues. Following childbirth, known as *puerperal sepsis.* Cellulitis occurs in neonates; high morbidity and mortality.

S. pneumoniae (Pneumococcus) Occurs more commonly in individuals with systemic lupus erythematosus, complement deficiency, HIV/AIDS, glucocorticoid therapy, drug or alcohol abuse. Infected sites show bulla formation, brawny erythema, violaceous hue.

E. rhusiopathiae: Erysipeloid Painful, swollen plaque with sharply defined irregular raised border occurring at the site of inoculation, i.e., finger or hand (Fig. 24-28), spreading to wrist and forearm. Color: purplish red acutely; brownish with resolution. Enlarges peripherally with central fading. Usually no systemic symptoms. Uncommonly, associated with bacteremia and aortic valvulitis. Occurs in individuals who handle game, poultry, fish.

P. aeruginosa (See "Cutaneous *P. aeruginosa* infections") Ecthyma gangrenosum begins as

FIGURE 24-22   Erysipelas of face: group A streptococcus   Painful, well-defined, shiny, erythematous, edematous plaques involving the central face of an otherwise healthy male. On palpation the skin is hot and tender.

FIGURE 24-23   Cellulitis of cheek: H. influenzae   Erythema and edema of the cheek of a young child, associated with fever and malaise. *H. influenzae* was isolated on culture of the nasopharynx. (Courtesy of Sandy Tsao, MD.)

FIGURE 24-24 Erysipelas of leg: MSSA The lower leg is red, hot, tender, and edematous. Erythematous plaque is well defined (blue mark). The infection is recurrent with interdigital tinea pedis as the portal of entry.

FIGURE 24-25 Recurrent cellulitis of foot: MSSA Interdigital tinea pedis was the portal of entry for this recurrent cellulitis, in the setting of chronic edema. The foot is edematous, erythematous with bulla formation.

FIGURE 24-26 Cellulitis of the arm: MSSA Erosion on the elbow in a plaque of psoriasis was the portal of entry for infection. Well-demarcated erythema, edema, and abscess formation are seen.

erythematous macule (cutaneous ischemic lesion) that quickly evolves to a bluish or gunmetal gray plaque with an erythematous halo (infarction) (Fig. 24-29A, B). The epidermis overlying the ischemic area forms a bulla. Epidermis eventually sloughs, forming an ulcer. *Distribution:* most commonly in the axilla, groin, perineum. Usually occurs as solitary lesion but may occur as a few lesions. Lesions associated with *Pseudomonas* septicemia: rose spotlike lesions (erythematous macules and/or papules on trunk as in typhoid fever, occur with *Pseudomonas* infection of GI tract, i.e., diarrhea, headache, high fever); painful clustered vesicular to bullous lesions; multiple painful nodules representing small embolic lesions.

H. influenzae Occurs mainly in children <2 years. Cheek, periorbital area, head, neck most common sites (Fig. 24-23). Clinically, swelling, characteristic violaceous erythema hue. Use of Hib vaccine has dramatically reduced incidence.

***V. vulnificus, V. cholerae* non-01 and non-0139** Underlying disorders: cirrhosis, diabetes, immunosuppression, hemochromatosis, thalassemia. Follows ingestion of raw/undercooked seafood, gastroenteritis, bacteremia with seeding of skin; also exposure of skin to sea water. Characterized by bulla formation, necrotizing vasculitis (Fig. 24-30). Usually on the extremities; often bilateral.

A. hydrophila Water-associated trauma; preexisting wound. Immunocompromised host. Lower leg. Necrotizing STIs.

C. canimorsus Immunosuppression or asplenia; exposure to a dog.

P. multocida Follows cat bite.

***Clostridium* Spp.** Associated with trauma, contamination by soil or feces, malignant intestinal tumor. Infection may be characterized by gas (crepitation on palpation), marked systemic toxicity.

***M. chelonei–M. fortuitum* Complex** History of recent surgery, injection, penetrating wound. Low-grade cellulitis. Systemic findings lacking.

C. neoformans Patient always immunocompromised. Red, hot, tender, edematous plaque on extremity. Rarely multiple noncontiguous sites.

Mucormycosis   Usually occurring in individual with uncontrolled diabetes.

General Findings
Fever, signs of sepsis.

DIFFERENTIAL DIAGNOSIS

Erysipelas/Cellulitis   Deep vein thrombophlebitis, stasis dermatitis, early contact dermatitis, giant urticaria, insect bite (hypersensitivity response), fixed drug eruption, erythema nodosum, acute gout, erythema migrans (Lyme borreliosis), prevesicular herpes zoster, Wells syndrome (eosinophilic cellulitis), familial Mediterranean fever–associated cellulitis-like erythema, cutaneous anthrax, pyoderma gangrenosum, Sweet syndrome (acute febrile neutrophilic dermatosis), Kawasaki disease, carcinoma erysipeloides.

Necrotizing STIs   Vasculitis, embolism with infarction of skin, peripheral vascular disease, purpura fulminans, calciphylaxis, warfarin necrosis, traumatic injury, cryoglobulinemia, fixed drug eruption, pyoderma gangrenosum, brown recluse spider bite.

FIGURE 24-27   Recurrent cellulitis of arm with chronic lymphedema: MSSA   Right breast cancer had been treated with mastectomy and lymph node excision 10 years previously. Lymphedema of the right arm followed. Hand dermatitis was secondarily infected with MSSA. Cellulitis occurred repeatedly in the setting of chronic lymphedema.

LABORATORY EXAMINATIONS

Direct Microscopy *Smears* Gram stain of exudate, pus, bulla fluid, aspirate, or touch preparation may show bacteria. GAS: chains of gram-positive cocci. *S. aureus:* clusters of gram-positive cocci. Clostridia: gram-negative rods, few neutrophils.

"Touch" Preparation Lesional skin biopsy specimen touched to microscope slide. Potassium hydroxide applied; examined for yeast and mycelial forms of fungus; detects *Candida, Cryptococcus, Mucor.* Gram stain: detects bacteria.

Cultures *Cellulitis:* aspirate or biopsy of leading edge of inflammation, identifies pathogen in up to 20% of cases. Fungal and mycobacterial cultures indicated in atypical case. *Portal of entry* (ulcers, etc.), adjacent to cellulitis: similar result to culture of cellulitis. *Blood cultures:* yield very low, ≤2–4%, highest in GAS infections. Yields higher in the setting of chronic lymphedema and in patients with buccal or periorbital cellulitis.

Hematology White blood count (WBC) and erythrocyte sedimentation rate (ESR) may be elevated.

Dermatopathology Frozen sections of lesional biopsies may be helpful in ruling out noninfectious inflammatory dermatoses. Open surgical inspection with debridement defines the extent and severity of NF; tissue is obtained for histologic examination, Gram staining, and

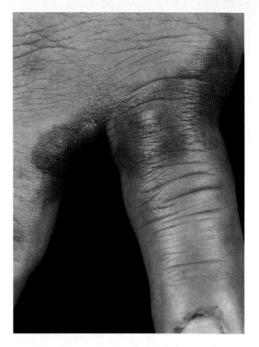

FIGURE 24-28 Erysipeloid of hand A well-demarcated, violaceous, cellulitic plaque (without epidermal changes of scale or vesiculation) on the dorsa of the hand and fingers, occurred following cleaning fish; the site was somewhat painful, tender, and warm.

A

B

FIGURE 24-29 Ecthyma gangrenosum of buttock: *P. aeruginosa* A 30-year-old male with advanced HIV/AIDS and neutropenia. ***A.*** An extremely painful, infarcted area with surrounding erythema present for 5 days. This primary cutaneous infection was associated with bacteremia. ***B.*** Two weeks later, the lesion had progressed to a large ulceration. The patient died 3 months later of *P. aeruginosa pneumonitis* associated with chronic neutropenia.

culture. In necrotizing STI: vasculitis without thrombosis, paucity of neutrophils at site of infection; bacilli found in media and adventitia, but usually not in intima, of vessel. Helpful with cryptococcal cellulitis.

Imaging MRI may be helpful in diagnosis of severe acute infectious cellulitis, identifying pyomyositis, necrotizing fasciitis, and infectious cellulitis with or without subcutaneous abscess formation. Soft tissue radiography, CT, MRI, and ultrasonographic imaging can detect localized abscess, gas in tissue, and subjacent osteomyelitis but do not define NF or myonecrosis.

DIAGNOSIS

Clinical diagnosis based on morphologic features of lesion and the clinical setting [travel history, animal exposure, history of bite, age, underlying disease(s)]. Confirmed by culture in only 29% of cases in immunocompetent patients. Suspicion of NF requires immediate deep biopsy and frozen-section histopathology.

COURSE AND PROGNOSIS

When occurring as a local infection in the absence of bacteremia, prognosis is much more favorable. Dissemination of infection (lymphatics, hematogenously) with metastatic sites of infection occurs if treatment is delayed. Abnormal or prosthetic heart valve may be colonized and infected. In the preantibiotic era, the mortality rate was very high. In immuncompromised patients, prognosis depends on prompt restoration of altered immunity, usually on correction of neutropenia. Without surgical debridement, NF is fatal. If neutropenia exists, prognosis depends on recovery of neutrophil count.

MANAGEMENT

See guidelines for the treatment of skin and soft tissue infections by the Infectious Diseases Society of America at *http://www.journals.uchicago.edu./IDSA/guidelines/*

Prophylaxis *Primary* Status postsaphenous vein harvest (especially with tinea pedis): Wash with benzoyl peroxide bar daily or apply topical antifungal cream or alcohol gel. *Pneumococcus*: Immunize those at risk. *Hib*: Chemoprophylaxis for household contacts <4 years of age if unimmunized. *Vibrio* spp.: Diabetics, alcoholics, cirrhotics should avoid eating undercooked seafood.

Secondary *Individuals with prior episodes of cellulitis* (especially in sites of chronic lymphedema): Support stockings or sleeve, antiseptics to skin (Purell), chronic secondary antimicrobial

FIGURE 24-30 Bilateral cellulitis of legs: *V. vulnificus* Bilateral hemorrhagic plaques and bullae on the legs, ankles, and feet of an older diabetic with cirrhosis. Unlike other types of cellulitis in which microorganisms enter the skin locally, that which is caused by *V. vulnificus* usually follows a primary enteritis with bacteremia and dissemination to the skin. Most cases initially diagnosed as bilateral cellulitis are inflammatory (eczema, stasis dermatitis, psoriasis) rather than infectious.

prophylaxis (penicillin G, dicloxacillin, or erythromycin, 500 mg/d). *Interdigital tinea pedis*: Treat and institute prophylaxis against recurrent tinea pedis.

Supportive   Rest, immobilization, elevation, moist heat, analgesia.

Dressings   Cool sterile saline dressings for removal of purulent exudate and necrotic tissue.

Surgical Intervention   Drain abscesses. Debride necrotic tissue. Early/aggressive surgical exploration/debridement is lifesaving in suspected necrotizing STIs. Deep structures are visualized, necrotic tissue removed, compartment decompressed, tissues obtained for Gram stain and aerobic and anaerobic cultures.

Antimicrobial Therapy   In that most cases of cellulitis are caused by *S. aureus* and streptococci, β-lactam antibiotics with activity against penicillinase-producing *S. aureus* are the usual drugs of choice.

Indications for Initial IV Therapy   Lesion spreading rapidly, systemic response is prominent (chills, fever of ≥37.8 °C), clinically significant coexisting conditions (immunocompromise, neutropenia, asplenia, preexisting edema, cirrhosis, cardiac failure, renal insufficiency).

Oral Therapy   In healthy persons with early infection in the absence of systemic symptoms and following initial IV therapy, oral antibiotics are given (Table 24-4).

In immunocompetent hosts: treat gram-positive cocci (*S. aureus*, GAS). In diabetics, greater range of potential pathogens, especially arising in diabetic ulcers: *S. aureus*, GAS, enterococci; gram-negative aerobes (*Proteus, Klebsiella, Enterobacter, Acinetobacter*). *P. aeruginosa*; anaerobes (*Bacterioides, Peptococcus*).

TABLE 24-4   Initial Treatment for Cellulitis at Specific Sites or Particular Exposures

Variable	Bacterial Spp. to Consider	Standard Antimicrobial Therapy	Alternative Antimicrobial Agent
Buccal cellulitis	*H. influenzae*	Ceftriaxone (1–2 g/d IV)	Meropenem *or* imipenem-cilastatin
Limb-threatening diabetic foot ulcer	Aerobic gram-negative bacilli	Ampicillin-sulbactam (3 g IV q6h)	Meropenem or imipenem-cilastatin clindamycin + a broad-spectrum fluoroquinolone (ciprofloxacin or levofloxacin); metronidazole + fluoroquinolone or ceftriaxone
Human bites	Oral anaerobes	Amoxicillin-clavulanate (500 mg PO q8h)	Penicillin + a cephalosporin
Dog and cat bites	*P. multocida* etc; see "Etiology"	Amoxicillin-clavulanate (500 mg PO q8h)	Moxifloxacin + clindamycin
Exposure to salt water at site of abrasion or laceration	*V. vulnificus*	Doxycycline (200 mg IV initially, followed by 100–200 mg/d IV in divided doses. Give along with antimicrobial agents for common pathogens)	Cefotaxime; ciprofloxacin
Exposure to fresh water at site of abrasion or laceration or after therapeutic use of leeches	*Aeromonas* spp.	Ciprofloxacin (400 mg IV q12h) *or* ceftazidime + gentamycin	Meropenem *or* imipenem-cilastatin
Working as butcher, fish or clam handler, veterinarian, housewife	*E. rhusiopathiae*	Amoxicillin (500 mg PO q8h for mild skin infections; penicillin G (12 million–20 million U IV daily) for bacteremic infections *or* endocarditis	Ciprofloxacin *or* cefotaxime *or* imipenem-cilastatin

NECROTIZING SOFT TISSUE INFECTIONS

- Characterized by rapid progression of infection with extensive necrosis of subcutaneous tissues and overlying skin.
- Clinical variants of NSTIs differ with the
  - Causative organism
  - Anatomic location of the infection
  - Predisposing conditions.
- Correct diagnosis is imperative in understanding pathogenesis and deciding on the appropriate antimicrobial and surgical therapies.
- *When skin necrosis is not obvious, diagnosis must be suspected if there are signs of severe sepsis* (accelerated heart or respiratory rates, oliguria, mental confusion) and/or some of the following local symptoms/signs:
  - Severe spontaneous pain
  - Indurated edema

- Bullae
- Cyanosis
- Skin pallor
- Absence of lymphangitis
- Skin hypesthesia
- Crepitation
- Muscle weakness
- Foul smell of exudates.
- May be associated with toxic shock syndrome.
- *Risk factors for necrotizing fasciitis* (NF): local lesion of skin or mucous membrane (acute or chronic disease, trauma, surgery), diabetes, arteriopathy, alcoholism, obesity, immunosuppression, use of nonsteroidal anti-inflammatory drugs (NSAIDs).

CLINICAL VARIANTS

NF Caused by group A streptococcus (GAS) (Rarely, Groups B, C, or G)

- Often begins deep at site of nonpenetrating minor trauma (bruise, muscle strain).
- May develop at the site of a break in the epidermis
  - Minor trauma, laceration, needle puncture, or surgical incision) on an extremity
  - Postoperative abdominal incisions.
- GAS may be seeded to this site during transient bacteremia
- Most cases occur in otherwise healthy persons, often in children and the elderly.
- Myonecrosis occurs concomitantly in 50% of NF cases.
- Streptococcal necrotizing myositis occurs as a primary myositis.
- Streptococcal toxic shock syndrome may occur with GAS NF.
- Group B streptococcus (GBS) may cause NF:
  - Infected episiotomy incisions
  - Adult diabetics

Clinical Findings

Initially, findings of acute cellulitis (local redness, edema, heat, and pain in the involved area), typically occur on an extremity. Characteristic findings appear within 36–72 h after onset: the involved area becomes dusky blue in color; vesicles or bullae appear containing initially yellowish, then red-black fluid. Infection spreads rapidly along fascial planes resulting in extensive necrotic sloughs (Fig. 24-31). Bullae rupture, and extensive, sharply demarcated cutaneous gangrene develops. At this point the area may be numb, and the black necrotic eschar with surrounding irregular border of erythema resembles a third-degree burn. The eschar sloughs off by the end of 1 week to 10 days. Peripheral areas of involvement develop about the initial site of infection.

Fever and other constitutional symptoms are prominent as the inflammatory process extends rapidly over the next few days. Streptococcal TSS occurs with GAS, GBS, GCS, GGS. Metastatic abscesses may occur as a consequence of bacteremia, resembling purpura fulminans but then evolving to dark-colored blebs containing streptococci. Secondary thrombophlebitis is common, but lymphangitis and lymphadenitis are not.

DIFFERENTIAL DIAGNOSIS

Pyoderma gangrenosum, purpura fulminans (disseminated intravascular coagulation), calciphylaxis, ischemic necrosis (atherosclerosis obliterans, thromboembolism), fixed drug eruption, warfarin necrosis, heparin necrosis, pressure ulcer, amebic (*Entamoeba histolytica*) skin gangrene after bowel surgery, brown recluse spider bite.

MANAGEMENT

Surgical Debridement   Requires early and complete surgical debridement of necrotic tissue in combination with high-dose antimicrobial agents.

Antimicrobial Therapy   See Table 24–2.

FIGURE 24-31   Necrotizing fasciitis of buttock   Erythematous, edematous plaque involving the entire buttock with rapidly progressive area of necrosis.

LYMPHANGITIS   ICD-9:457-2 ○ ICD-10:189-1

- An inflammatory process involving the subcutaneous lymphatic channels
- Etiology:
  - Acute: Most often due to GAS; also *S. aureus*; rarely, *P. multocida* or herpes simplex virus
  - Subacute: *Mycobacterium marinum*, other nontuberculous mycobacteria (NTM), *Sporotrix schenkii, Nocardia brasiliensis*
- Clinical findings:
  - Acute: portal of entry of infection on distal extremity associated with ascending linear streak; ± tender lymphadenopathy.
  - Subacute: Nodular or sporotrichoid lymphangitis; ± lesion at portal of entry with erythematous nodules with linear arrangement; ± lymphadenopathy.

CLINICAL MANIFESTATION

Portal of Entry   Break in skin, wound, infected blister, *S. aureus* paronychia, herpes simplex.

Local Symptoms   Pain and/or erythema proximal to break in the skin.

Systemic Symptoms   May occur either before any evidence of infection is present at the site of inoculation or after the initial lesion has subsided. May be more prominent than expected from degree of local pain and erythema.

Skin Findings   Red linear streaks and palpable lymphatic cords, which may be up to several centimeters in width, extend from the local lesion toward the regional lymph nodes (Figs. 24-32 and 24-33), which are usually enlarged and tender. Acute sporotrichoid lymphangitis can occur with *S. aureus* or GAS infection. Breakdown of overlying skin and ulceration occur in course of bacterial lymphangitis; rare in the antibiotic era.

DIFFERENTIAL DIAGNOSIS

Linear Lesions on Extremities   Phytoallergic contact dermatitis (poison ivy or oak), phyto-photodermatitis, superficial thrombophlebitis, cat-scratch disease.

Subacute   Sporotrichoid   Lymphangitis *S. schenckii, N. brasiliensis, M. marinum, Leishmania* spp. are the most common pathogens.

LABORATORY FINDINGS

Culture   Isolate *S. aureus* or GAS from portal of entry.

DIAGNOSIS

The combination of a peripheral lesion with proximal tender/painful red linear streaks leading toward regional lymph nodes is diagnostic of lymphangitis.

COURSE AND PROGNOSIS

Bacteremia with metastatic infection in various organs may occur.

MANAGEMENT

See Table 24-2.

FIGURE 24-32   Acute lymphangitis of forearm: *S. aureus*   A small area of cellulitis on the volar wrist with a tender linear streak extending proximally up the arm; the infection spreads from the portal of entry within the superficial lymphatic vessels.

FIGURE 24-33   Acute lymphangitis of forearm: HSV   Primary herpes simplex virus infection of the palm with lymphangitis of the forearm.

WOUND INFECTIONS

■ ◑ → ●

■ Loss of the integrity of the skin provides a portal of entry for infection.

■ All wounds are colonized by bacteria.

■ Wound infection (purulence, erythema, warmth, tenderness) must be diagnosed on clinical and cultural grounds and treated appropriately.

CLASSIFICATION OF WOUNDS

- Chronic ulcers
  ∘ Arterial insufficiency
  ∘ Venous insufficiency
  ∘ Neuropathic ulcers/diabetes mellitus
  ∘ Pressure ulcers (bedsores)

- Trauma
- Bites
  ∘ Animal
  ∘ Human
  ∘ Insect

- Surgical wounds
  ∘ Class I/clean
  ∘ Class II/clean-contaminated
  ∘ Class III/contaminated
  ∘ Class IV/dirty-infected
- Burn wounds
  ∘ Burn wound impetigo
  ∘ Open burn–related surgical wound infection
  ∘ Burn wound cellulitis
  ∘ Invasive infection in unexcised burn wounds

EPIDEMIOLOGY AND ETIOLOGY

Etiology Health care–associated MRSA (HA-MRSA) is currently the most common pathogen isolated in wounds cultured in hospital environment. MSSA, *Streptococcus*, and *Pseudomonas* spp. are also commonly isolated. Others: *E. coli*, *Enterococcus* spp., *Proteus* spp., coagulase-negative *Staphylococcus* (CoNS), fungi, vancomycin-resistant enterococci, other enterobacteriaceae, *Klebsiella* spp. Anaerobes may constitute more than one-third of antimicrobial isolates.

For *human, dog, and cat bites*, see page 611.

Predisposing Factors

- *General factors*: Age, obesity, malnutrition; endocrine/metabolic factors; hypoxia, anemia; malignant disease; immunosuppression.
- *Local factors*: Necrotic tissue, foreign bodies, tissue ischemia, hematoma formation, poor surgical technique.

- *Microbial contamination*: Type/virulence of organism; size of bacterial inoculum, antibiotic resistance.

Risk Factors Surgical wound infection is up to 10 times more likely among patients who harbor *S. aureus* in nares. The vast majority of postoperative wound infections are caused by a strain of *S. aureus* that was present in nares before surgery. Presurgical clearance of carriage with topical or systemic antibiotics decreases incidence of postoperative staphylococcal infection. Postoperative infection: prolonged operative time, diabetes, obesity, chronic lung disease, male sex, treatment with glucocorticoids, social deprivation.

Nosocomial Infections Hospital-acquired or health care–associated infections (most commonly surgical wound infections) are the most common complication affecting hospitalized patients. 5–10% of patients admitted to acute care hospitals acquire one or more infections (2 million patients annually in the United States), resulting in 90,000 deaths.

Definition of Surgical Wound Infection

Types of Surgical Wound Infections

- Surgical site infection
- Superficial incisional infection
- Deep incisional infections
- Organ space infections

Surgical site infections must fulfill the following criteria:

- Infection must occur within 30 days of surgery
- Infection must involve only the skin and subcutaneous tissue
- There must be at least one of the following:
  ∘ Purulent discharge from a superficial infection
  ∘ Organisms isolated from aseptically obtained wound culture

- Must be at least one of the following signs of infection:
  ∘ Pain or tenderness
  ∘ Localized swelling
  ∘ Redness or heat

PATHOGENESIS

Wounds are initially colonized by skin flora or introduced organisms. In some cases, these organisms proliferate, causing a host inflammatory response defined as infection. Skin and soft tissue infections (SSTIs) include superficial conditions, such as erysipelas, cellulitis, folliculitis, and furuncles, as well as deeper infections, such as abscesses, necrotizing fasciitis, myositis, and gas gangrene.

DIFFERENTIAL DIAGNOSIS

Allergic contact dermatitis (e.g., topical antibiotic such as neomycin), herpes zoster; herpes simplex, pyoderma gangrenosum, vasculitis, peripheral vascular disease (infarction), disseminated intravascular coagulation (DIC) (purpura fulminans), warfarin necrosis.

CLINICAL MANIFESTATION

Symptoms   Local infection: tenderness, purulent drainage. Invasive infection: malaise, anorexia, sweats; fever, chills.
Skin Findings   Purulent drainage, erythema, warmth, induration, tenderness.
Systemic Findings   Sepsis syndrome (fever, hypotension).
Types of Surgical Infections   Superficial infection of wound (Fig. 24-36), impetigo/ecthyma (Figs. 24-34, 24-37, 24-38), cellulitis (Figs. 24-35, 24-39), erysipelas, soft tissue abscess (see Fig. 24-17), NSTIs, tetanus.

FIGURE 24-34   Surgical excision wound infection: MSSA   Surgical site was the portal of entry for infection 7 days after the procedure, with subsequent cellulitis. Dehiscence of the wound has occurred. Necrotic tissue is seen in the resultant ulcer/wound.

FIGURE 24-35   Surgical excision/graft infection: MRSA   Cellulitis of the eyelids occurred following excision and grafting of lentigo maligna of the cheek.

LABORATORY EXAMINATIONS

Direct Microscopy Gram stain of exudate, pus, bulla fluid, aspirate, or touch preparation may show bacteria.

Culture and Sensitivities Indications: wounds with classic signs of infection [purulent drainage, signs of inflammation (erythema, increased warmth, induration, tenderness)]. Specimens: exudates and necrotic tissue.

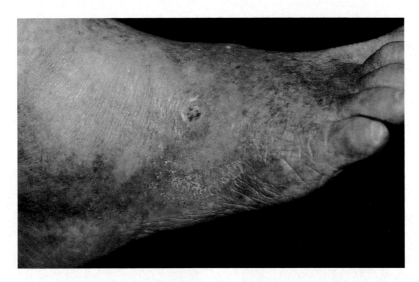

FIGURE 24-36 Surgical wound infection: MRSA Invasive squamous cell carcinoma was removed by disc excision with electrosurgery to the base. The patient had prior MRSA infections. The wound became painful 7 days following the procedure. MRSA was isolated and reported to be sensitive only to linezolid and vancomycin. The infection resolved with linezolid, 600 mg bid for 7 days. Nasal carriage was treated with mupirocin ointment. There is also tinea pedis

FIGURE 24-37 Laceration infection in renal transplant recipient: MRSA A laceration on the lower leg has become painful with surrounding erythema and edema. Two invasive squamous cell carcinomas are also seen on the calf. He has been immunosuppressed for 22 years.

DIAGNOSIS

Because all open wounds become colonized with microorganisms, diagnosing infection relies on the clinical characteristics of the wound. Wounds with classic signs of infection: Gram stain of exudates helpful initially. Cultures are definitive.

MANAGEMENT

Although all wounds require treatment, only infected lesions require antimicrobial therapy.

Prevention of Wound Infection *Exogenous* Sterilization of instruments, sutures, etc.; positive pressure ventilation; laminar air flow; exclusion of staff with infections.

Endogenous Skin preparation; antibiotic prophylaxis, good surgical technique.

Wound Care Adjunctive treatments include weight off-loading, topical agents, special dressings, control of edema, revascularization.

Surgical Debridement Treating infected wounds often requires surgical procedures (e.g., debridement), especially for deep or necrotic wounds. Modern burn wound therapy centered on early excision and closure of the wound.

Antimicrobial Therapy Virtually all infected wounds require antimicrobial therapy. See Table 24-2.

Topical Antimicrobial Therapy May be sufficient for superficial lesions.

FIGURE 24-38 Infection in chronic lymphedema: MSSA   Multiple painful ulcers with surrounding erythema on a very edematous lower leg and foot. The patient has idiopathic retroperitoneal fibrosis with progressive lymphedema and ulceration. He was treated with cephalexin as secondary prophylaxis.

FIGURE 24-39 Infection of factitial ulcers: MRSA   A 53-year-old male with obsessive-compulsive disorder scratched extremities in the evening. He was being treated by a psychiatrist who lacked insight into the origin of the ulcers. MRSA infections occurred repeatedly. Ulcers resolved with oral clindamycin, doxepin, and Unna boots applied weekly.

GRAM-POSITIVE COCCAL INFECTIONS ASSOCIATED WITH TOXIN PRODUCTION (INTOXICATIONS)

- *S. aureus*, group A streptococcus (GAS), *B. anthracis*, *C. diphtheriae*, and *C. tetani* produce toxins that have local mucocutaneous and systemic effects.
- Clinical syndrome caused by these toxins:
  - Bullous impetigo
  - Staphylococcal scalded-skin syndrome (SSSS)

- Staphylococcal toxic shock syndrome (TSS)
- Staphylococcal food poisoning (enterotoxin)
- Scarlet fever (SF)
- Streptococcal TSS
- Anthrax
- Diphtheria
- Tetanus

Staphylococcal Toxins

- Toxic shock syndrome toxin 1 (TSST-1)
  - Induces fever directly on the hypothalamus or indirectly via interleukin 1 (IL-1) and tumor necrosis factor (TNF) production
  - Promotes T lymphocyte "superantigenization" and overstimulation
  - Induces interferon production
  - Enhances delayed hypersensitivity
  - Suppresses neutrophil migration and immunoglobulin secretion
  - Enhances host susceptibility to endotoxins
- Exfoliatin type A and B (ET-A, ET-B).
  - ET-A is responsible for the pathogenic changes of the SSSS.
  - These toxins bind directly to desmoglein-1, a desmosomal cadherin
  - Results in interdesmosomal splitting and causes blistering and denudation by disruption of the epidermal granular cell layer.
- Staphylococcal enterotoxins B and C (SEB, SEC) have a biochemical structure almost identical to that of TSST-1.

Streptococcal Toxins

- Streptolysin S: leukocidin
- Streptolysin O: leukocidin
- NADase: leukotoxic
- Hyaluronidase: digests host connective tissue hyaluronic acid
- Streptokinases: participate in fibrin lysis.
- Streptodornases A–D: possess deoxyribonuclease activity. Streptodornases B and D: possess deoxyribonuclease and ribonuclease activity
- Protease activity similar to that in *S. aureus* has been shown in strains causing soft tissue necrosis or toxic shock syndrome.

- Streptococcal pyrogenic exotoxins (SPE) (formerly known as erythrogenic toxin) types A, B, C

Superantigens

- Group of bacterial and viral proteins
  - Act as globular intact proteins
  - Presented by class II major histocompatibility complex (MHC) molecules
  - Bind to conserved amino acid residues that are on the outer walls of peptide antigen-binding groove
  - Bind to variable region of T cell receptor β chain (Vβ)
  - Activate a large percentage of T cells expressing relevant T cell receptor Vβ chains
  - Superantigen-mediated T cell activation generates increased numbers of T cells expressing the skin homing receptor cutaneous lymphocyte antigen (CLA)
  - Superantigens lead to massive release of cytokines, a cytokine storm:
    - TNF-α
    - IL-1
    - IL-6
  - Cytokines cause capillary leak syndrome and clinical manifestations of superantigen-mediated diseases
- Bind directly to MHC class II molecules on the surface of antigen-presenting cells
- Can stimulate 10–20% of T cells (conventional antigen can stimulate 1/10,000 T cells)
- Massive T cell stimulation results in release of
  - IL-1 and -2
  - TNF
  - Interferon γ

- Staphylococcal superantigens include SEs, TSST-1, some ETs.

Syndromes associated with staphylococcal exfoliative toxin do not have significant systemic symptoms. However, syndromes due to superantigens are characterized by systemic manifestations. Superantigen-mediated toxin syndromes can be divided according to the relative amounts of systemic toxicity:

- Intermediate cutaneous and systemic: recalcitrant desquamating disorder (REDD), recurrent toxin-mediated erythema (recurrent perineal erythema)
- Predominantly systemic: scarlet fever, TSS

STAPHYLOCOCCAL SCALDED-SKIN SYNDROME (SSSS)   ICD-9:695.81

- Etiology: *S. aureus*.
- Age: occurs mainly in newborns and infants < 2 years. Also, older immunocompromised persons
- Pathogenesis: toxin-mediated epidermolytic disease
- Clinical syndromes: Erythema and widespread detachment of the superficial layers of the epidermis, resembling scalding

- Severity ranges from:
  - Localized form: bullous impetigo
  - Generalized form with extensive epidermolysis and desquamation: generalized scalded-skin syndrome
  - Abortive form (scarlatiniform variant) (staphylococcal scarlet fever)
- Management: systemic antibiotic to treat infection and stop toxin production

---

EPIDEMIOLOGY AND ETIOLOGY

Age of Onset   Most common in neonates during first 3 months of life. Infants and young children <5 years. Rarely in immunocompromised adults.

Etiology   *S. aureus* of phage group 2 (types 71 and 55). *S. aureus* produces exotoxins:

- Exfoliatin A and B (ET-A and ET-B)
  - Serine proteases that bind to cell adhesion molecule, resulting in loss of cell-cell adhesion
  - Epidermolysis takes place between stratum corneum and stratum granulosum
- Exfoliatin B (ET-B); produced by plasmid (pieces of self-replicating DNA that often code for secondary characteristics, such as antibiotic resistance and toxin production).
- Exotoxins are proteases that cleave desmoglein-1, which normally hold the granulosum and spinulosum layers together.

Risk Factors   Age <5 years. Adults: renal failure, systemic immunosuppression.

PATHOGENESIS

In newborns and infants, *S. aureus* colonizes nose, conjunctivae, or umbilical stump with or without causing clinically apparent infection, producing ETs that are transported hematogenously to the skin. In bullous impetigo, ET is produced in impetigo lesion. Specific antistaphylococcal antibody, metabolic differences, or the greater ability to localize, metabolize, and excrete in individuals >5 years probably accounts for decreased incidence of SSSS with older age. At times purulent conjunctivitis, otitis media, or occult nasopharyngeal infection occurs at site of toxin production. ET causes acantholysis and intraepidermal cleavage within the stratum granulosum. Local effects of the ET result in bullous impetigo, but with absorption of the toxin, a mild scarlatiniform rash accompanying the bullous lesions may appear. Conversely, local effects of the toxin may be absent, with systemic absorption resulting in a staphylococcal scarlet fever syndrome. More extensive epidermal damage is characterized by sloughing of superficial epidermis in SSSS. Healing occurs spontaneously in 5–7 days.

CLINICAL MANIFESTATION

Skin Symptoms   SSSS: early erythematous areas are very tender.

Skin Lesions

Localized Form   See "Bullous Impetigo" (p. 598). Intact flaccid purulent bullae, clustered. Rupture of the bullae results in moist red and/or crusted erosive lesions. Lesions are often clustered in an intertriginous area.

Generalized Form ET-induced changes: micro-macular scarlatiniform rash (staphylococcal scarlet fever syndrome) or diffuse, ill-defined erythema (Fig. 24-40) and a fine, stippled, sandpaper appearance occur initially. In 24 h, erythema deepens in color and involved skin becomes tender. Initially periorificially on face, neck, axillae, groins; becoming more widespread in 24–48 h. Initial erythema and later sloughing of superficial layers of epidermis are most pronounced periorificially on face and in flexural areas on neck, axillae, groins, antecubital area, back (pressure points). With epidermolysis, epidermis appears wrinkled and can be removed by gentle pressure (skin resembles wet tissue paper) (Nikolsky sign) (Fig. 24-40). In some infants, flaccid bullae occur. Unroofed epidermis forms erosions with red, moist base. (Fig. 24-41*A*). Desquamation occurs with healing (Fig. 24-41*B*).

Mucous Membranes Uninvolved in SSSS.

General Examination Possible low-grade fever. Irritable child, pain.

DIFFERENTIAL DIAGNOSIS

TSS, Kawasaki syndrome, drug-induced toxic epidermal necrolysis (TEN).

LABORATORY EXAMINATIONS

Direct Microscopy *Gram Stain*

- Bullous impetigo: pus in bullae, clumps of gram-positive cocci within PMN.
- SSSS: gram-positive cocci only at colonized site, not in areas of epidermolysis.

Bacterial Culture

- Bullous impetigo: *S. aureus* isolated from involved site.

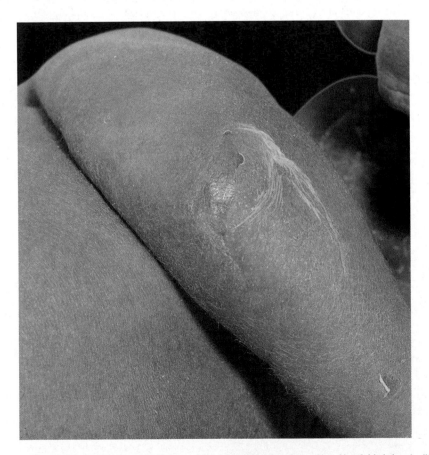

FIGURE 24-40 Staphylococcal scalded-skin syndrome: Nikolsky sign The skin of this infant is diffusely erythematous; gentle pressure to the skin of the arm has sheared off the epidermis, which folds like tissue paper.

- SSSS: *S. aureus* only at site of infection (i.e., site of toxin production)—umbilical stump, ala nasi, nasopharynx, conjunctivae, external ear canal, stool. *S. aureus* is not recovered from sites of sloughing skin or bullae.

Dermatopathology   Intraepidermal cleavage with splitting occurring beneath and within stratum granulosum.

DIAGNOSIS

Clinical findings confirmed by bacterial cultures. Tzanck smear reveals acantholytic keratinocytes.

COURSE AND PROGNOSIS

In late phases of SSSS, and in an accelerated manner, after adequate antibiotic treatment, the superficially denuded areas heal in 3–5 days associated with generalized desquamation in large sheets of skin (Fig. 24-42); there is no scarring. Death can occur in neonates with extensive disease.

MANAGEMENT

Prophylaxis   Prevent spread of toxigenic *S. aureus* in neonatal care units.

General Care   Hospitalization is recommended for neonates and young children, especially if skin sloughing is extensive and parental compliance questionable. Discharge home when significant improvement is apparent. If case is mild and home care reliable, children can be treated with oral antibiotic.

Topical Therapy   Baths or compresses for debridement of necrotic superficial epidermis. Topical antimicrobial agents for impetigo lesions: mupirocin, retapamulin, bacitracin, or silver sulfadiazine ointment.

Systemic Antimicrobial Therapy   See Table 24-2.

Adjunctive Therapy   Replace significant water and electrolyte loss intravenously in severe cases.

A

B

FIGURE 24-41   Staphylococcal scalded-skin syndrome: desquamation   In this infant, painful, tender, diffuse erythema was followed by generalized epidermal sloughing and erosions. *S. aureus* had colonized the nares with perioral impetigo, the site of exotoxin production. **A.** Extensive desquamation is seen on the face and anterior trunk. **B.** Desquamation on buttocks and legs.

TOXIC SHOCK SYNDROME   ICD-9 : 040.82 ∘ ICD-10 : A48.3

- Etiology: Toxin-producing *S. aureus* and GAS
- Clinical setting
  - Staphylococcal TSS
    - Menstrual (MTSS) (rare after 1984)
    - Nonmenstrual (NMTSS)
  - Streptococcal TSS
    - Skin or soft tissue infection with toxin production

- Clinical manifestations
  - Rapid onset of fever and hypotension
  - Skin findings
    - Early: generalized skin and mucosal erythema
    - Late: desquamation in early convalescence
  - Organ hypoperfusion and multisystem failure
- Management: systemic antibiotic to treat infection and stop toxin production. Supportive.

EPIDEMIOLOGY AND ETIOLOGY

Age of Onset   MTSS: 23 years (mean age); NMTSS: 27 years (mean age).
Sex   Prior to 1984, >99% of cases were in females; after 1984, equal sex distribution. 8–10% of women are vaginal carriers of *S. aureus*.
Race   In the United States, 97% of MTSS in whites; 87% of NMTSS in whites.
Etiology   Toxin-producing *S. aureus* producing TSST-1, GAS
Underlying Disorders   NMTSS can occur secondary to a wide variety of primary *S. aureus* and GAS infections as well as secondary infection of underlying dermatoses.

Site of TSST-1 Production

- Mentrual-associated: Use of vaginal tampon of high absorbency. Usually present on 3rd to 5th day of menses.
- Nonmenstrual
  - Wounds
    - Nonsurgical wounds (burns, skin ulcers, cutaneous and ocular injuries, insect bites, body piercing site)
    - Surgical wounds: *median* time of onset of postoperative NMTSS
  - Superinfection of varicella
  - Postpartum infections
  - Vaginal nonmenstrual origin (contraceptive sponge, contraceptive diaphragm)
  - Nasal packing
  - Superinfection after influenza or acute sinusitis

Streptococcal TSS superantigen production
Soft tissue infections: cellulitis, necrotizing fasciitis.

PATHOGENESIS

S. aureus multiplies foreign body, around, in minor wound infection, or mucosal surface, elaborating the TSST-1 and staphylococcal enterotoxin B. Toxins are absorbed and act as superantigens that allow the nonspecific binding of MHC II with T cell receptors, resulting in polyclonal T cell activation, causing secretion of massive amounts of cytokines. Cytokines result in the clinical syndrome of fever, hypotension, rash, organ hypoperfusion/multiorgan failure. The individual must be colonized or infected with toxigenic strain of *S. aureus* or GAS and must lack a protective level of antibody to the toxin made by that strain. >90% of adults have antibodies to TSS toxins.

CLINICAL MANIFESTATION

Incubation Period   Shorter in NMTSS. After surgical procedure, <4 days.
Symptoms   Recurrent symptoms in MTSS in untreated cases; tampon use. Sudden onset of fever, hypotension. Tingling sensation in hands and feet. Maculopapular eruption, pruritic. Generalized myalgias, muscle tenderness and weakness; headache, confusion, disorientation, seizures; profuse diarrhea; dyspnea.

Skin Lesions

- Generalized scarlatiniform erythroderma, most intense around infected area. Blanching erythema, "painless sunburn." Fades within 3 days of appearance.
- Edema, extensive generalized, nonpitting; most marked on face (Fig. 24-42), hands, feet.

- One week after onset of skin lesions, desquamation begins with scaling of skin of torso, face, and extremities, followed by desquamation of palms, soles, fingers/toes.

Cutaneous Sites of Infection/Colonization

- Soft tissue infection: Cellulitis, necrotizing fasciitis, puerperal sepsis
- Varicella in children with superinfection
- Rarely asymptomatic streptococcal pharyngitis

Mucous Membranes

- Forgotten or retained vaginal tampon.
- Eyes: Intense erythema and injection of bulbar conjunctivae (Fig. 24-42). Subconjunctival hemorrhages.
- Mouth: Erythema of mucous membranes of mouth, tongue, pharynx, tympanic membranes. Strawberry tongue. Ulcers: mouth, esophagus.
- Genital: vagina erythema, ulcers.

General Findings

- Fever.
- Organ hypoperfusion results in renal and myocardial dysfunction, fluid overload, and adult respiratory distress syndrome (ARDS).
- Late complications include peripheral gangrene, muscle weakness, lingering asthenia, neuropsychiatric dysfunction.

DIFFERENTIAL DIAGNOSIS

Toxin-Mediated Infections SSSS, scarlet fever, Kawasaki disease.
Erythema + Multisystem Disease SSSS, Kawasaki syndrome, Rocky Mountain spotted fever (RMSF), gram-negative sepsis, exanthematous viral syndromes; severe adverse drug reactions (Stevens-Johnson syndrome, TEN), acute systemic lupus erythematosus (SLE).

LABORATORY EXAMINATIONS

Direct Microscopy *Gram Stain* Vaginal, wound exudate: many leukocytes and gram-positive cocci in clusters.
Culture *S. aureus*: vaginal, wound exudate, foreign body. GAS: blood or primary site of infection.
Biopsy Confluent epidermal necrosis, vacuolar alteration of dermal-epidermal junction, subepidermal vesiculation, little or no inflammatory infiltrate in dermis.

DIAGNOSIS

Case Definition of TSS
An Illness with the Following Clinical Manifestations

- *Fever*: Temperature ≥38.9°C (102°F)
- *Rash*: Diffuse macular erythroderma
- *Desquamation*: 1–2 weeks after onset of illness, particularly on the palms and soles
- *Hypotension*: Systolic blood pressure (BP) ≤90 mmHg (adults) or less than fifth percentile for age (children <16 years of age); or orthostatic hypotension (orthostatic drop in diastolic BP by 15 mmHg, orthostatic dizziness, or orthostatic syncope)
- *Systemic involvement* (three or more of the following):
  ○ Gastrointesinal: vomiting or diarrhea at onset of illness
  ○ Muscular: severe myalgias or serum creatine phosphokinase level at least twice the upper limit of normal
  ○ Mucosal hyperemia: vaginal, oropharyngeal, conjunctiva
  ○ Renal: blood urea nitrogen or creatinine at least twice the upper limit of normal for laboratory or urinary sediment with pyuria (≥5 leukocytes per high-power field) in the absence of urinary tract infection
  ○ Hepatic: total bilirubin, alanine aminotransferase enzyme, or aspartate aminotransferase enzyme levels at least twice the upper limit of normal for laboratory
  ○ Hematologic: platelet count <100,000/μL
  ○ CNS: disorientation or alterations in consciousness without focal neurologic signs when fever and hypotension are absent

Laboratory Criteria: Negative Results on the Following Tests, if Obtained

- Blood, throat, or cerebrospinal fluid cultures (blood culture may be positive for *S. aureus*)
- Rise in titer to Rocky Mountain spotted fever, leptospirosis, or measles.

Case Classification
Probable A case in which four of the five clinical findings described above are present.
Confirmed A case in which all five of the clinical findings described above are present, including desquamation, unless the patient dies before desquamation occurs.

FIGURE 24-42 Toxic shock syndrome Erythema of the bulbar conjunctivae associated with facial erythema and edema in a female with menstrual TSS.

COURSE AND PROGNOSIS

Diagnosis of NMTSS is often delayed because of the wide variety of clinical settings and associated symptomatology. Complications: refractory hypotension, ARDS, cardiomyopathy, arrhythmias, encephalopathy, acute renal failure, metabolic acidosis, liver necrosis, DIC. Recurrence of untreated MTSS is possible. Antibiotic therapy and discontinuance of tampons significantly reduce risk. Recurrences after NMTSS are rare. Among cases reported to the Centers for Disease Control and Prevention (CDC) (1985–1994), case fatality rate was 2.5% for menstrual cases, and 6.4% for nonmenstrual cases.

Streptococcal TSS: associated with mortality rate of 25–50%.

MANAGEMENT

Local Infection Remove potentially foreign bodies. Drain and irrigate infected sites.
Systemic Antimicrobial Therapy (See Table 24-2.) IV antistaphylococcal antibiotic. Clindamycin, 900 mg IV q8h. Nafcillin or oxacillin, first-generation cephalosporin. Vancomycin for MRSA.
Adjunctive Therapy Aggressive monitoring and management of specific organ system failure (i.e., management of fluid, electrolyte, metabolic, and nutritional needs). Methylprednisolone for severe cases.

SCARLET FEVER ICD-9:034 ∘ ICD-10:A38   ☐ ◑

- Etiology: Group A streptococcus (GAS), exotoxin-producing strains
- Clinical syndromes
  - Infection: tonsils, skin, soft tissues, other
  - Toxin syndrome: scarlatiniform exanthem in the nonimmune individual
- Severe infection and toxin production causes streptococcal toxic shocklike syndrome (TSLS)
- Management: systemic antibiotic to treat infection and prevent nonsuppurative sequelae
- *Synonym*: Scarlatina

EPIDEMIOLOGY AND ETIOLOGY

Age of Onset Children.
Incidence Much less than in the past.
Etiology Usually group A β-hemolytic *S. pyogenes* (GAS). Uncommonly, ET-producing *S. aureus*.

PATHOGENESIS

Scarlet fever occurs in the nonimmune person. Production of streptococcal pyrogenic exotoxins [erythrogenic toxin (ET)] A, B, or C depends on the presence of a temperate bacteriophage. The development of SF rash may reflect hypersensitivity reaction requiring prior exposure to toxin. *S. aureus* can synthesize an ET, producing a scarlatiniform exanthem. In addition to ET, GAS also produces streptolysins O and S. Antibodies to antistreptolysin O can be used to assess recent GAS infection. SF seems to be less severe than a century ago due to decrease in virulence of GAS or the advent of antimicrobial therapy.

CLINICAL MANIFESTATION

Incubation Period   Rash appears 1–3 days after onset of infection.

Exposure   Household member(s) may be a streptococcal carrier.

Symptoms   Fever, sore throat, fatigue, headache, flushing, tachycardia, enlarged cervical lymph nodes.

Skin Lesions   *Site of GAS Infection*

- Pharyngitis; tonsillitis.
- Infected surgical or other wound.
- Impetiginized (secondarily infected) skin lesion.

Exanthem

- Face: flushed with perioral pallor.
- Finely punctate erythema is first noted on the upper part of the trunk (Fig. 24-43); may be accentuated in skin folds such as neck, axillae, groin, antecubital and popliteal fossae (Pastia lines).
- Palms/soles usually spared.
- Initial punctate lesions become confluently erythematous, i.e., scarlatiniform.
- Linear petechiae (Pastia sign) occur in body folds.
- Intensity of the exanthem varies from mild to moderate erythema confined to the trunk due to an extensive purpuric eruption.

Petechiae   Scattered petechiae occur (Rumpel-Leede test for capillary fragility positive).

Desquamation   Exanthem fades within 4–5 days and is followed by desquamation on the body and extremities and by sheet-like exfoliation on the palms/fingers and soles/toes. In subclinical or mild infections, exanthem and pharyngitis may pass unnoticed. In this case patient may seek medical advice only when exfoliation on the hand and soles is noted.

Mucous Membranes   *Site of GAS Infection*   Acute follicular or membranous tonsillitis.

May be asymptomatic or mild and go undetected.

Enanthem

- Pharynx beefy red.
- Forchheimer spots: Small red macules on hard/soft palate, uvula.
- Punctate erythema and petechiae may occur in the palate.
- Tongue
  - White tongue: Initially is white with scattered red, swollen papillae (white strawberry tongue) (Fig. 24-44).
  - Red strawberry tongue: By the fourth or fifth day, the hyperkeratotic membrane is sloughed, and the lingular mucosa appears bright red (Fig. 24-44).

General Examination   Patient may appear acutely ill with high fever, fatigue, sore throat, headache, nausea, vomiting, tachycardia. Anterior cervical lymphadenitis associated with pharyngitis/tonsillitis.

Streptococcal TSLS   Toxemia, organ failure, and a scarlatiniform rash associated with GAS cellulitis or necrotizing fasciitis.

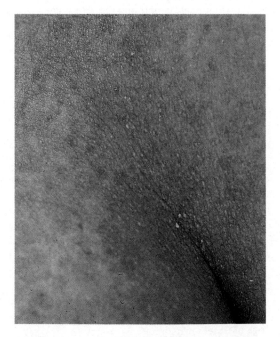

FIGURE 24-43   Scarlet fever: exanthem   Finely punctated erythema has become confluent (scarlatiniform); petechiae can occur and have a linear configuration within the exanthem in body folds (Pastia line).

DIFFERENTIAL DIAGNOSIS

Generalized Exanthem Staphylococcal SF (pharyngitis, tonsillitis, strawberry tongue, and palatal enanthem *not* seen), staphylococcal or streptococcal TSS, Kawasaki syndrome, viral exanthem, adverse cutaneous drug eruption.

LABORATORY EXAMINATIONS

Direct Microscopy *Gram Stain* Gram-positive cocci in chain (GAS) or clusters (*S. aureus*) identified in smear from infected wound or impetiginized skin lesion.
Rapid Direct Antigen Tests (DATs) Used to detect GAS antigens in throat swab specimens.
Culture Isolate GAS on culture of specimen from throat or wound. Blood cultures are rarely positive.
Hematology Leukocytosis with neutrophilia, elevated ESR.
Serology Elevated antistreptolysin O titer.

DIAGNOSIS

Clinical findings confirmed by detecting streptococcal antigen in a rapid test and/or culturing GAS from throat or wound.

Centor clinical criteria for the diagnosis of streptococcal pharyngitis:

- Temperature > 38°C
- Tender anterior cervical adenopathy
- Lack of a cough
- Pharyngotonsillar exudate.

COURSE AND PROGNOSIS

Suppurative Complications

- Peritonsillar cellulitis
- Peritonsillar abscess
- Retropharyngeal abscess
- Otitis media
- Acute sinusitis
- Suppurative cervical lymphadenitis
- Bacteremia/septicemia with streptococcal TSS
- Metastatic foci of infection

Nonsuppurative Sequelae of Streptococcal Infections

- Acute rheumatic fever (onset 1–4 weeks after onset of pharyngitis). Incidence of acute rheumatic fever is about 3%; has markedly decreased during the past five decades

FIGURE 24-44 Scarlet fever: white and red strawberry tongue Bright red tongue with prominent papillae on the fifth day after onset of group A streptococcal pharyngitis in a child. The white patches at the back of the tongue represent residua of the initial white strawberry tongue.

- Acute glomerulonephritis (more common after impetigo with nephritogenic strain of GAS (types 4, 12, 2, 49, and 60)
- Guttate psoriasis (see Section 3)
- Erythema nodosum may follow if the infection goes untreated (see Section 7)

MANAGEMENT

Symptomatic Therapy Aspirin or acetaminophen for fever and/or pain.
Systemic Antimicrobial Therapy *Penicillin is the drug of choice* because of its efficacy in prevention of rheumatic fever. Goal is to eradicate GAS throat carriage.
Follow-Up Reculture of throat recommended for individuals with history of rheumatic fever or if a family member has history of rheumatic fever.

GRAM-POSITIVE BACILLARY INFECTIONS ASSOCIATED WITH TOXIN PRODUCTION (INTOXICATIONS)

- *Anthrax toxins*: Three proteins secreted by virulent strains of *Bacillus anthracis*. Three proteins act together in a synergistic way in which they are endocytosed and translocated into the cytoplasm of a macrophage, where it disrupts cellular signaling and induces cell death, allowing the bacteria to evade the immune system.
  - Protective antigen (PA)
  - Edema factor (EF)
  - Lethal factor (LF)
- *Diphtheria toxin*: A single polypeptide chain of 535 amino acids consisting of two subunits linked by disulfide bridges. Binding to the cell surface of the less stable of these two subunits allows the more stable part of the protein to penetrate the host cell. Extraordinarily potent. The lethal dose for humans is about 0.1 µg of toxin per kg of bodyweight. A massive release of toxin into the body will likely cause lethal necrosis of the heart and liver.
- *Tetanus toxin*: Tetanospasmin. Molecular weight of 150 kDa. It is made up of two parts: a 100-kDa heavy or B-chain and a 50-kDa light or A-chain.

CUTANEOUS ANTHRAX (CA)   ICD-9:022 ○ ICD-10:A22

- Etiology: *Bacillus anthracis*
- Zoonosis
- Pathogenesis: toxin-mediated
- Portal of entry:
  - Skin: cutaneous abrasions
  - Inhalations (woolsorters' disease)
  - Ingestion
- Cutaneous anthrax accounts for 95% of anthrax cases in United States
- Clinical findings of cutaneous anthrax:
  - Black eschar surrounded by edema and purple vesicles
- Management: systemic antibiotic to treat infection and stop toxin production
- *Synonym*: Malignant pustule

http://www.bt.cdc.gov/agent/anthrax/

EPIDEMIOLOGY AND ETIOLOGY

Etiology

- B. anthracis, a nonmotile, gram-positive, aerobic rod 1.2–10 µm in length and 0.5–2.5 µm in width.
- Spores can remain dormant in soil for decades.
- Anthrax spores have been developed as a biologic weapon. (See Appendix B)

Occupation   Farmers, herders; slaughterhouse and textile workers.

Transmission   Zoonosis of mammals, especially herbivores. Human infections result from contact with contaminated wild and domestic animals (herbivores, i.e., cattle, sheep, goats, camels, antelopes) or animal products (hides, hair, wool, bone, meal). Human-to-human transmission does not occur. Bioterrorism (2001) in the United States resulted in cases of both cutaneous and inhalation anthrax.

Geography   "Anthrax zones": soil rich in organic matter and dramatic changes in climate (abundant rainfall followed by prolonged drought). Most common in agricultural regions where it occurs in animals: South/Central America, Southern/Eastern Europe, Asia, Africa, the Caribbean, Middle East.

Recent outbreaks in Zimbabwe (1979–1980), Paraguay (1987). Accidental release of weapons-grade anthrax spores in Sverdlovsk (1979) resulted in 66 deaths.

PATHOGENESIS

Introduced endospores are phagocytosed by macrophages, carried to regional lymph nodes, and germinate inside the macrophages and become vegetative bacteria. The vegetative bacilli are released from macrophages, multiply in the lymphatic system, and enter the bloodstream, causing massive septicemia, associated with production of edema and lethal exotoxins. Low-level germination occurs at the primary site, resulting in local edema and necrosis. Gastrointestinal anthrax follows ingestion of endospore-contaminated meat from diseased animals.

CLINICAL MANIFESTATION

- Cutaneous anthrax: Occupational exposure to animals or animal products. Incubation period: 1–10 days (in bioterrorism attack); usually no prodrome.
- Inhalation anthrax: early symptoms resemble those of common cold; shortness of breath and shock follow.
- GI anthrax follows consumption of contaminated meat; associated with nausea/vomiting, fever, abdominal pain, diarrhea.

Skin Lesions *Portal of Entry*

- Cut or abrasion.
- Nondescript, painless, pruritic papule (resembling insect bite) appears 3–5 days after introduction of endospores.
- In 1–2 days, evolves to vesicle(s) ± hemorrhage + necrosis.
- Vesicles rupture to form depressed ulcers, often with local edema (Fig. 24-45A), ultimately forming dry eschars (1–3 cm).
- Satellite lesions can form in a sporotrichoid pattern proximally on edematous extremity (Fig. 24-45B).
- Edema more extensive on head/neck.

Also see: http://www.bt.cdc.gov/agent/anthrax/anthrax-images/cutaneous.asp

Distribution Exposed sites of head, neck, extremities.

Mucous Membranes Oropharyngeal anthrax can occur following ingestion of contaminated meat, presenting with cervical edema and local lymphadenopathy, with dysphagia and respiratory difficulties.

General Findings Possible fever and/or other systemic signs. Pain is not a feature of cutaneous anthrax. Fever in cutaneous anthrax usually indicates superinfection of the cutaneous lesion with streptococci or staphylococci. Lymph nodes in adjacent area may enlarge.

Variants Inhalation anthrax, gastrointestinal anthrax.

DIFFERENTIAL DIAGNOSIS

Cutaneous anthrax should be considered in any patient with a *painless* ulcer with vesicles, edema, without regional lymphadenopathy, and a history of exposure to animals or animal products.

Painless, Blackened, Necrotic Eschar ± Regional Lymphadenopathy Brown recluse spider bite, ecthyma, ulceroglandular tularemia, vaccinia, necrotic herpes simplex infection, orf, glanders.

LABORATORY EXAMINATIONS

Cultures Gram stain and culture recommended; prior antibiotic treatment rapidly renders the site culture negative. Gentle sampling with a moist, sterile cotton tip applicator is preferred; the rate of positive cultures is about 65%. Expressing eschar fluid is not recommended because it can cause dissemination of the pathogen. Blood cultures with systemic anthrax are always positive.

Biopsy Biopsy edge of lesion; examine by silver staining and immunohistochemical testing. May facilitate systemic dissemination.

Dermatopathology Nonsuppurative necrosis and massive edema with lymphocytic infiltrates. Gram stain of tissue shows bacilli in dermis and subcutaneous tissue.

DIAGNOSIS

Isolation of *B. anthracis* from blood, skin lesions, or respiratory secretions or by measuring specific antibodies in blood of persons with suspected symptoms.

COURSE AND PROGNOSIS

- About 20% of untreated cases of cutaneous anthrax result in death.
- 80% of cases are self-limiting and usually resolve without scarring.
- Pain in cutaneous anthrax usually indicates streptococcal or staphylococcal superinfection.
- 10% of cases of cutaneous anthrax progress to systemic anthrax.
- Malignant edema is a rare complication, usually involving the head and neck and manifested by severe edema, induration, multiple bullae, and shock.
- Inhalation anthrax is nearly always fatal.

MANAGEMENT

Cutaneous anthrax can be self-limited, but antibiotic therapy is recommended. *Drug of choice*: Ciprofloxacin, 400 mg IV q12h, or doxycycline, 100 mg IV q12h, is optimal. *Alternatives*: None. Surgery for excision of eschar is contraindicated. **Anthrax Vaccine**   Indicated for persons at risk for exposure to anthrax spores: laboratory personnel working with *B. anthracis*, persons who work with imported animal hides/fur if exposure to anthrax is possible, veterinarians who travel to endemic areas, military personnel deployed to area with high risk of exposure. Protection against inhalation anthrax has not been tested. Animals are immunized in endemic regions.

Postexposure Prophylaxis   Doxycycline, 100 mg twice daily, or ciprofloxacin, 500 mg twice daily, for 8 weeks. Amoxicillin (three times/ day) for children and lactating women.

A

B

FIGURE 24-45   Cutaneous anthrax   A 40-year-old farmer with anthrax. *A.* A black eschar at the site of inoculation with a central hemorrhagic ulceration on the thumb associated with massive edema of the hand. *B.* A nodular lymphangitis extending proximally from the primary lesion on the thumb.

CUTANEOUS DIPHTHERIA ICD-9:032 ∘ ICD-10:A30

- Etiology: *Corynebacterium diphtheriae*
- Incidence in industrialized countries: extremely rare.
- Epidemic in former Soviet Union in 1990: >190,000 affected.
- Pathogenesis: localized infection caused by toxigenic and nontoxigenic strains, which produce exotoxin.
- Acute infection of the respiratory tract but may involve any mucous membrane or skin wound.
- Unlike in the pharynx, cutaneous diphtheria is nonspecific and the diagnosis is made by culture from the wound
- Essentials of diagnosis:
  - Tenacious gray membrane at portal of entry in pharynx.
  - Sore throat, nasal discharge, hoarseness, malaise, fever.
  - Myocarditis causes arrythmias, heart block, and heart failure.
- Neuropathy usually involves cranial nerves first: diplopia, slurred speech, and difficulty in swallowing.
- Culture confirms the diagnosis.
- Diphtheria toxin causes:
  - Myocarditis
  - Polyneuritis
  - Other toxic systemic effects
  - Respiratory diphtheria is usually caused by toxicogenic (*tox+*) strains.
  - Cutaneous diphtheria is frequently caused by nontoxicogenic (*tox–*) organisms.
- Vaccination: immunity to vaccine wanes over time. Decennial boosters are recommended.
- Diphtheria antitoxin is available in the United States through the CDC. Should be given in all cases where diphtheria is suspected.
- Either penicillin, 250 mg, or erythromycin, azithromycin or clarithromycin
- Treat contacts to a case

TETANUS ICD-9:037 ∘ ICD-10:A33

- Etiology: *Clostridium tetani*
- Neurologic disorder, characterized by increased muscle tone and spasms caused by tetanospasmin, a powerful protein toxin elaborated by *C. tetani.*
- *C. tetani* spores survive in soil for years.
- Vegetative cells produce tetanospasmin, which mediates binding to nerve cell receptors and entry into these cells and blocks neurotransmitter release.
- Skin is portal of entry, but there are no skin lesions specific for tetanus
- Incubation period is 5 days to 15 weeks; average 8–12 days.
- Site of infection: an acute injury (puncture wound, laceration, abrasion; the injury is usually trivial); secondary infection of breaks in skin [injecting drug use ("skin popping")]; skin ulcers, gangrene, frostbite, burns, surgical wounds, childbirth, abor-
tion; superinfection (abscesses, middle-ear infection).
- Tetanus affects nonimmunized persons, partially immunized persons, or fully immunized individuals who fail to maintain adequate immunity with booster doses of vaccine.
- At risk: elderly, newborns, migrant workers, injecting drug users. Activities: farming, gardening, and other outdoor activities.
- Globally, tetanus is common in areas where soil is cultivated, in rural areas, in warm climates, during summer months, and among males.
- Spores germinate in wounds with low oxidation-reduction potential (devitalized tissue, foreign bodies, or active infection).
- Without immunization, tetanus occurs predominantly in neonates and other young children (490,000 neonates died of tetanus worldwide in 1994).

INFECTIVE ENDOCARDITIS, SEPSIS, AND SEPTIC SHOCK

- Infective endocarditis (IE), sepsis, and septic shock are very serious systemic infections with high associated morbidity and mortality rates.
- Clinical findings are often acute in onset and relatively nonspecific in nature.

- Cutaneous findings extremely helpful in making the correct diagnosis.
- Early recognition of clinical findings, diagnosis, and initiation of therapy increase the likelihood of a positive outcome.

INFECTIVE ENDOCARDITIS (IE)   ICD-9:421 ∘ ICD-10:I33

- Infection of the endocardium or endarterium
- A vegetation forms at the site of IE, a mass of fibrin, platelets, microcolonies of microorganisms, and few inflammatory cells.
- *Infective endocarditis* occurs most commonly on:
  - Heart valves: native prosthetic
  - Low-pressure side of a ventricular septum at a defect site

- Mural endocardium
- Cardiac devices.
- *Infective endarteritis* occurs in
  - Arteriovenous shunts
  - Arterioarterial shunts
  - Coarctation of the aorta

EPIDEMIOLOGY AND ETIOLOGY

Incidence Subacute bacterial endocarditis (SBE) is now much less common because of the decreased incidence of rheumatic heart disease; the incidence is increasing in the elderly and in injecting drug users (IDUs), and with prosthetic valve use.

Temporal Evolution of Disease

- *Acute endocarditis* rapidly damages cardiac structures, hematogenously seeds extracardiac sites, and may progress to death in a few weeks.
- SBE causes structural damage slowly, rarely causes metastatic infection, and is gradually progressive unless complicated by a major embolic event or ruptured mycotic aneurysm.

Etiology Varies with native valve IE, prosthetic valve IE, and endocarditis in IDUs. IE is more often due to gram-positive than gram-negative bacteria, possibly because of differences in adherence to damaged valves or because of differences in their susceptibility to serum-induced killing.

- *Community-acquired native valve IE*: Mouth, skin, and upper respiratory tracts are the respective primary portals for the viridans streptococci, staphylococci, and HACEK organisms (*Haemophilus, Actinobacillus,*

Cardiobacterium, Eikenella, Kingella). GI tract: *Streptococcus bovis*. GU tract: enterococci.
- *Nosocomial native valve IE*: Associated with bacteremia arising from intravascular catheters; less commonly, nosocomial wound and genitourinary (GU) infection. IE complicates 6–25% of episodes of catheter-associated *S. aureus* bacteremia.
- *Prosthetic valve IE*: 1–5% of cases of IE. Onset within 2 months of valve surgery associated with intraoperative contamination or postoperative bacteremia: coagulase staphylococcus (CoNS), *S. aureus*, facultative gram-negative bacilli, diphtheroids, fungi. Onset 2–12 months after surgery: nosocomial (CoNS); 85% are MRSA; decreases to 25% resistance >12 months after valve surgery. Onset >12 months after surgery: similar to community-acquired native valve IE, i.e., streptococci, HACEK.
- *IE in IDUs*: Incidence increase. 60–80% of patients have no known preexisting valve lesions. Pathogen usually originates in skin: *S. aureus, P. aeruginosa,* and fungi. Tricuspid valve (>50% of cases): *S. aureus*, usually MSRA. Left-sided valve (aortic 25%; mitral 20%): *P. aeruginosa, Candida* spp. Polymicrobial. Others: *Bartonella, Salmonella, Listeria.*

Transmission During transient bacteremia: dental procedures, IDU various infections, induced abortions, intrauterine contraceptive devices, temporary transvenous pacemakers, percutaneous intravenous catheter lines, endoscopic procedures.

Groups at Risk   IDUs (median age, 30–40 years) (estimated risk for IE in United States, 2–5% per year), elderly people with valve sclerosis, patients with intravascular prostheses, those exposed to nosocomial disease, and those undergoing hemodialysis.

Nosocomial Endocarditis   Complicates 6–25% of episodes of catheter-associated *S. aureus* bacteremia. Associated with catheters and medicosurgical procedures. Mortality >50%. In 1999, 37% of cases caused by CoNS.

Hemodialysis   Two to three times more common in hemodialysis than peritoneal dialysis patients. >50% of cases due to *S. aureus.*

PATHOGENESIS

Bacterial adherence to damaged valves, which occurs during transient bacteremia, is the primary event. Bacteria grow within the cardiac lesion(s), with local extension and cardiac damage. Subsequently, septic embolization occurs to skin, kidney, spleen, brain, etc. Microulcerations and local inflammation (resembling arteriosclerosis) occur in degenerative valve lesions (occur in up to 25% of patients >40 years). IDUs, injecting impure materials; prior IE can damage right-sided valves. *S. aureus* is most likely to invade cardiac tissue, resulting in abscess formation. Circulating immune complexes may result in glomerulonephritis, arthritis, or various mucocutaneous manifestations of vasculitis. This leads to:

- Constitutional symptoms associated with cytokine production
- Damage to intracardiac structures
- Embolization of vegetative fragments leading to infection/infarction of remote tissues
- Hematogenous infection of sites during bacteremia
- Tissue injury due to deposited bacterial antigens

CLINICAL MANIFESTATION

Symptoms

- Fever (80–90%)
- Chills/sweats (40–75%)
- Anorexia/weight loss/malaise (25–50%)
- Myalgias/arthralgias (15–30%)
- Back pain (7–15%).

General Findings   Consider IE in any patient with fever and heart murmur or injecting drug use.

- Heart murmur (80–85%)
- New/worsened regurgitant murmur (80–85%)
- Arterial emboli (10–40%)
- Splenomegaly (15–50%)
- Neurologic manifestations (20–40%)
- Clubbing of fingers
- IDUs: 50% of cases are limited to tricuspid valve; pulmonary findings include cough, pleuritic chest pain, pulmonary infiltrates.

Skin Lesions   Peripheral manifestations occur in 2–5% (Fig. 24-46).
Embolic Lesions   *Osler Nodes* (Table 24-5) Palpable, tender, and almost always in the pulp of the fingers distally and occasionally on the toes. Red, hemorrhagic and infarcted. Occasionally white center. In acute IE (*S. aureus*), may be more inflammatory than in SBE. In SBE (e.g., viridans strep), lesions usually more vasculitic than septic. 🔲
Janeway Lesions   Red, macular, papular, infarctive, nontender, and almost always on the palms or soles; usually part of the vasculitis of SBE (Fig. 24-46).
Septic Embolism   Painful, hemorrhagic macules, papules, or nodules (Fig. 24-47), usually acral location.
Subungual Splinter Hemorrhages   Septic embolic phenomenon. Linear in the *middle* of the nailbed in acute IE (see Fig. 33-30). (Distal hemorrhages are traumatic.) Common in acute *S. aureus* IE.
Petechial Lesions   Small, nonblanching, reddish-brown macules. Occur on extremities,

TABLE 24-5   Cutaneous Manifestations and Characteristics of Infective Endocarditis

Cutaneous Manifestations	Palpation	Morphologic Findings
Osler node	Tender	Erythematous papules and nodules with white centers; may become necrotic
Janeway lesions	Nontender	Hemorrhagic papules
Splinter hemorrhages	Nontender	Subungual hemorrhagic streaks

FIGURE 24-46 **Infective endocarditis, acute: Janeway lesions** Hemorrhagic, infarcted papules on the volar fingers in a patient with *S. aureus* endocarditis.

upper chest, mucous membranes [conjunctivae (Fig. 24-48), palate]. Occur in crops. Fade after a few days (20–40%).
Roth Spots Retinitis septica—a white spot in the retina close to the optic disk, often surrounded by hemorrhages; also seen in pernicious anemia, leukemia.
Gangrene of Extremities Secondary to embolization.
Pustular/Purulent Petechiae With *S. aureus.*
Hematogenously Seeded Focal Infection Skin, spleen, kidneys, skeletal system, meninges.
Embolization with Infarction Extremities, spleen, kidneys, bowel, brain.
Neurologic Complications Embolic strokes, meningitis, intracranial hemorrhage, seizures, encephalopathy.
For further clinical images see. 🖥

DIFFERENTIAL DIAGNOSIS

Fever with Skin Lesions Meningococcemia, DIC, acute rheumatic fever, marantic endocarditis, SLE with cardiac involvement, systemic vasculitis, dysproteinemia, atrial myxoma, organizing left atrial thrombus, atheromatous embolism.

LABORATORY EXAMINATION

Imaging Echo-Doppler study demonstrates vegetations, acute severe mitral or aortic regurgitation. Evidence of septic pulmonary emboli suggests tricuspid valve IE. Systemic embolization can occur from aortic or mitral valve.

DIAGNOSIS

Modified Duke criteria for diagnosis of IE are based on both microbiologic data and echocardiographic imaging.[1] Demonstration on histologic and microbiological examination of pathogens in vegetations.
Definite Diagnosis of IE Either two major criteria *or* one major criterion and three minor criteria *or* five minor criteria.

[1]See P Moreillon, Y-A Que: Lancet 363:139, 2004.

FIGURE 24-47 **Septic vasculitis associated with bacteremia** Dermal nodule with hemorrhage and necrosis on the dorsum of a finger. This type of lesion occurs with bacteremia (e.g., *S. aureus*, gonococcus) and fungemia (e.g., *Candida tropicalis*).

FIGURE 24-48   Infective endocarditis, acute: subconjunctival hemorrhage Submucosal hemorrhage of the lower eyelid in an elderly diabetic with enterococcal endocarditis; splinter hemorrhages in the midportion of the nailbed and Janeway lesions were also present on the volar fingers. Infection followed urosepsis.

Major Criteria

- Positive blood culture
  - Typical microorganism for IE from two separate blood cultures
    - Viridans streptococci, *S. bovis,* HACEK group, *S. aureus, or*
    - Community-acquired enterococci in the absence of a primary focus, *or*
  - Persistently positive blood culture, defined as recovery of a microorganism consistent with IE from:
    - Blood cultures drawn ≥12 h apart; *or*
    - All of three or a majority of four or more separate bood cultures, with first and last drawn at least 1 h apart

- Evidence of endocardial involvement
  - Positive echocardiogram [Transesophageal echocardiography (TEE) recommended for assessing possible prosthetic valve endocarditis or complicated endocarditis]
    - Occilating intracardiac mass or valve or supporting structures or in the path of regurgitant jets or in implanted material, in the absence of an alternative anatomic explanation, *or*
    - Abscess, *or*
    - New partial dehiscence of prosthetic valve, *or*
  - New valvular regurgitation (increase or change in preexisting murmur not sufficient)

Minor Criteria

- Predisposition: predisposing heart condition or injection drug use
- Fever ≥ 38.0°C (≥100.4°F)
- Valvular phenomena: major arterial emboli, septic pulmonary infarcts, mycotic aneurysms, intracranial hemorrhage, conjunctival hemorrhage, Janeway lesions
- Immunologic phenomena: glomerulonephritis, Osler nodes, Roth spots, rheumatoid factor
- Microbiologic evidence: positive blood culture but not meeting major criterion or serologic evidence of active infection with organism consistent with IE.

COURSE AND PROGNOSIS

Acute course in IE is common with β-hemolytic streptococci, *S. aureus,* pneumococcal infection; also, *Staphylococcus lugdunensis* and enterococci in some cases. Subacute typically occurs in IE caused by viridans streptococci, enterococci, CoNS, HACEK. Course varies with the underlying cardiac disease and baseline health of the patient, as well as with the complications that occur. Complications: congestive heart failure, stroke, other systemic embolizations, septic pulmonary embolization. Aortic valve involvement has higher risk of death or need for surgery. In HIV/AIDS-infected IDUs, mortality rises inversely to the CD4 count.

MANAGEMENT

Prophylaxis Identify patients at risk, procedures that might provoke bacteremia, and the most effective prophylactic regimen. Balance between risk of adverse effects of prophylaxis and of developing disease.

Treatment Depends on multidisciplinary approach, involving specialists in infectious disease, cardiologists, and cardiac surgeons.[1]

Cure of IE requires eradication of all microbes from vegetation(s). Microbicidal drug regimens must produce high enough concentrations for long enough duration to sterilize vegetation(s).

Antimicrobial Therapy Appropriate IV antibiotic therapy, depending on the sensitivity of the infecting organism.

Surgery Most common indication, congestive heart failure. Valve replacement.

SEPSIS AND SEPTIC SHOCK   ICD-9:995.91 ∘ ICD:A40

- Sepsis and septic shock constitute the inflammatory response to microbial invasion, manifesting with an extremely wide range of clinical findings: fever or hypothermia, tachypnea, tachycardia.
- Spectrum of clinical findings: bacteremia, septicemia, systemic inflammatory response syndrome (SIRS), sepsis, severe sepsis (similar to "sepsis syndrome"), septic shock, refractory septic shock, multiple-organ dysfunction syndrome (MODS)

- SIRS: infectious or noninfectious etiology
  - Fever or hypothermia
  - Leukocytosis or leukopenia
  - Tachypnea
  - Tachycardia
- Early sepsis is reversible; septic shock has high morbidity.

Synonym: Blood poisoning

EPIDEMIOLOGY AND ETIOLOGY

Age of Onset For *N. meningitidis* (NM), highest incidence in children aged 6 months to 3 years (peak, 6–12 months); lowest in persons >20 years.

Incidence In the United States; 750,000 cases annually, with 210,000 deaths. Two-thirds of cases occur in patients hospitalized for other illnesses. Increasing incidence in the United States attributable to aging population, with increasing longevity of patients with chronic diseases.

Etiology See Table 24-6.

Risk Groups Those with influenza A virus infection; absence of spleen or functional asplenia; alcoholism; complement deficiency, especially impaired alternative pathway activation.

TABLE 24-6   Microorganisms Involved in Episodes of Severe Sepsis at Eight Academic Medical Centers

Microorganisms	Episodes with Bloodstream Infection, % (*n* = 436)	Episodes with Documented Infection but No Bloodstream Infection, % (*n* = 430)	Total Episodes, % (*n* = 866)
Gram-negative bacteria[a]	35	44	40
Gram-positive bacteria[b]	40	24	31
Fungi	7	5	6
Polymicrobial	11	21	16
Classic pathogens[c]	<5	<5	<5

[a]Enterobacteriaceae, pseudomonads, *Haemophilus* spp., other gram-negative bacteria.

[b]*Staphylococcus aureus*, coagulase-negative staphylococci, enterococci, *Streptococcus pneumoniae*, other streptococci, other gram-positive bacteria.

[c]Such as *Neisseria meningitidis, S. pneumoniae. H. influenzae*, and *Streptococcus pyogenes*.

Source: Adapted from KE Sands et al: Epidemiology of sepsis syndrome in 8 academic medical centers. JAMA 278:234, 1997

Risk Factors Increasing age and preexisting comorbidity. Widespread use of antimicrobial agents, immunosuppressive drugs, indwelling catheter and mechanical devices, mechanical ventilation. HIV/AIDS. Malnutrition.

- *Gram-negative bacillary bacteremia*: Diabetes mellitus, lymphoproliferative disease, cirrhosis, burns, invasive procedures or devices, treatment with drugs that cause neutropenia.
- *Gram-positive bacteremia*: Vascular catheterization, presence of indwelling mechanical devices, burns, IDU.
- *Fungemia*: Immunosuppressed patients with neutropenia, often after broad-spectrum antimicrobial therapy.

Risk Factors for Severe Sepsis in Patients with Bacteremia Age (>50 years) and primary pulmonary, abdominal, or neuromeningeal site of infection.

PATHOGENESIS

Septic response triggered when microorganisms spread from skin or GI tract into contiguous tissues. Localized infection may then lead to bacteremia or fungemia. Microbes can also be introduced into bloodstream directly from such routes as venous access lines. In some cases, however, no primary site of infection is apparent. Septic response occurs when invading microbes have circumvented host's innate and acquired immune defenses. Lipopolysaccharide (LPS) (endotoxin) is the most potent gram-negative bacterial signal molecule. Septic response involves complex interaction among microbial signal molecules, leukocytes, humoral mediators, and vascular endothelium. Many of the characteristics of sepsis (fever, tachycardia, tachypnea, leukocytosis, myalgias, somnolence) are produced by release of TNF. Intravenous fibrin deposition, thrombosis, and DIC are important features of septic response. C5a and other products of complement activation may promote neutrophil reactions such as chemotaxis, aggregation, degranulation, and oxygen-radical production. The underlying mechanism of tissue damage is widespread vascular endothelial injury, with fluid extravasation and microthrombosis that decrease oxygen and substrate utilization by affected tissues. Nitric oxide is a mediator of septic shock.

CLINICAL MANIFESTATION

The majority of patients experience septic response superimposed on underlying illness and primary infection. Fever may be absent in neonates, the elderly, those with uremia, and alcoholics.

Skin Lesions

- Cutaneous infections as source of sepsis
  - Pyodermas
  - Soft tissue infections
  - Wounds

- Specific skin lesions
  - *Exanthem*: See meningococcemia and Rocky Mountain spotted fever.
  - *Petechiae*: Cutaneous/oropharyngeal location suggests meningococcal infection; less commonly *H. influenzae*. In patient with tick bite living in endemic area, Rocky Mountain spotted fever (RMSF).
  - *Ecthyma gangrenosum*: See Fig. 24-29A, B. *P. aeruginosa* most commonly; also *Aeromonas hydrophila*.
  - *Hemorrhagic bullous lesions*: *Vibrio vulnificus* in patient (diabetes mellitus, liver disease) with history of eating raw oysters (Fig. 24-30); *Capnocytophaga canimorsus* or *C. cynodegmi* following dog bite (Fig. 24-49).

- Generalized erythema due to toxins, e.g., TSS
- Findings with hypotension
  - Extremities cool, acrocyanosis
  - Ischemic necrosis of peripheral tissue, most often digits (Fig. 24-49).

- Findings with DIC and purpura fulminans (see Section 19).

General Examination
Fever May be absent in neonates, elderly patients, persons with uremia, alcoholism.
GI Manifestations Nausea, vomiting, diarrhea, ileus; stress ulcer. Liver; cholestatic jaundice; hepatocellular/canalicular dysfunction. Prolonged hypotension: acute hepatic injury; ischemic bowel necrosis.
Less Common Manifestations Arthritis (5–10%), pneumonia, sinusitis, otitis media,

conjunctivitis, endophthalmitis, endocarditis, pericarditis, urethritis, endometritis.

DIFFERENTIAL DIAGNOSIS

Sepsis and Shock   Acute bacteremia and endocarditis, acute "hypersensitivity" vasculitis, enteroviral infections, RMSF, TSS.

LABORATORY EXAMINATIONS

Direct Microscopy   Examine skin/mucosal surfaces. Gram stain of material from primary site of infection or from infected cutaneous lesions. In overwhelming infection (pneumococcal sepsis in splenectomized patient or fulminant meningococcemia), microorganisms can be seen in buffy coat. In meningococcemia, scrapings from nodular lesions show gram-negative diplococci.
Hematology   Leukocytosis with left shift, thrombocytopenia; later, leukopenia. Neutrophils contain toxic granules, Döhle bodies, cytoplasmic vacuoles.
Clotting Studies   Prolonged thrombin time, decreased fibrinogen, presence of D-dimers.
Chemistry   Hyperbilirubinemia, increased creatinine.
Cultures   *Blood*   Obtain at least two blood samples (from different venipuncture sites) for culture. Gram-negative bacteremia is low grade; multiple blood cultures or prolonged incubation of cultures may be necessary. *S. aureus* grows rapidly and is most easily detectable. Negative blood cultures may reflect prior antibiotic administration, slow-growing or fastidious organisms, or absence of microbial invasion of bloodstream. Acute meningococcemia, NM in nearly 100%; meningitis, one-third positive.
Skin/Soft Tissue   Obtain cultures from sites of possible cutaneous infection.
Cerebrospinal Fluid (CSF) Culture   Acute meningococcemia, usually positive.
Culture of Lesional Skin Biopsy Specimen   Up to 85%.

DIAGNOSIS

Definitive etiologic diagnosis requires isolation of microorganism from blood or local site of infection.

COURSE AND PROGNOSIS

Ventilation-perfusion mismatching produces ARDS. Severe decrease in systemic vascular resistance results in generalized maldistribution of blood flow, functional hypovolemia, diffuse capillary leakage of intravascular components. Cardiac output may intially be elevated; subsequent cardiac dysfunction common. Renal failure occurs due to hypotension and capillary injury. Platelet counts low in patients with DIC; low counts reflect diffuse endothelial injury. Approximately 25–35% of patients with severe sepsis and 40–45% of those with septic shock die within 30 days; others die within the ensuing 5 months.

MANAGEMENT

Requires urgent measures to treat local infection, provide hemodynamic and respiratory support, and eliminate offending organism. Outcome depends on underlying disease.
Prevention   Reduce number of invasive procedures, limit use of indwelling vascular and bladder catheters, reduce incidence and duration of profound neutropenia (<500 neutrophils/mL), aggressively treat localized nosocomial infections.
Surgery   Removal or drainage of focal source of infection is essential.
Antimicrobial Therapy   In the absence of an obvious source of infection, antimicrobial regimen differs in the following types of patients: immunocompetent adult, neutropenic patient, splenectomized patient, injecting drug user, HIV/AIDS patient. Any febrile patient with a petechial rash should be considered to have *N. meningitidis* infection; blood culture should be obtained; treatment begun without awaiting confirmation.
Antibiotic Therapy of Sepsis Due to Other Microbes   Depends on the sensitivity of the infecting organism (see Table 24-2).
Hemodynamic, Respiratory, Metabolic Support   Primary goal is to restore adequate oxygen and substrate delivery to tissues. Adequate fluids should be infused to treat intravascular volume depletion. Adrenal insufficiency should be considered in patients with refractory hypotension, fulminant meningococcemia, prior glucocorticoid use, disseminated tuberculosis, HIV/AIDS disease. Ventilator therapy is indicated for progressive hypoxia, hypercapnia, neurologic deterioration, respiratory muscle failure.

FIGURE 24-49 Septic shock: ischemic necrosis of acral sites *Capnocytophaga canimorsus* sepsis (dog bite) with prolonged hypotension and hypoperfusion resulted in infarction of fingers and nose.

NEISSERIA

- Genus of gram-negative bacteria; diplococci that resemble coffee beans.
- *N. meningitidis* (meningococcus)
  - Colonizes oropharyngeal mucosa
  - Clinical syndromes
    - Local infection: meningitis, pericarditis, arthritis
    - Meningococcemia (meningococcal septicemia)

- *N. gonorrhoeae* (gonococcus)
  - Colonizes anogenital or oropharyngeal mucosa
  - Cinical syndrome
    - Local infection: gonorrhea
    - Pelvis inflammatory disease
    - Gonococcemia (gonococcal septicemia)
- Eight nonpathogenic species of *Neisseria*

NEISSERIA MENINGITIDIS INFECTION   ICD-9:036.9 ∘ ICD-10:A39

- Etiology: *Neisseria meningitidis*, the meningococcus
- Colonizes mucosa
- Epidemiology: sporadic cases, institutional outbreak, epidemic
- Dominant proinflammatory molecule in the meningococcal cell wall is the endotoxin or lipooligosaccharides; concentrations of endotoxin detected in the blood of patients with fulminant meningococcemia are 10- to 1000-fold higher than those found in the blood of patients with bacteremia due to other gram-negative bacteria.
- Clinical syndromes dependent on rate of replication of microbe within blood stream:
  - Intermittent bacteremia: chronic meningococcemia
  - Slow replication seeds various organs: meninges; pericardium and large joints

- More rapid replication causes rapid inflammatory response: meningococcemia with shock and death
- Clinical findings of a variable spectrum of:
  - Meningitis, pericarditis, arthritis
  - Meningococcemia and shock; characteristic hemorrhagic skin lesions
  - Meningitis and meningococcemia
- Meningococcemia and meningitis are associated with high morbidity and mortality.
- Fulminant meningococcemia is the most rapidly lethal form of septic shock. Differs from most other forms of septic shock by the prominence of hemorrhagic skin lesions (petechiae, purpura) and the consistent development of DIC.
- Prevention: vaccination partially effective

ETIOLOGY

Meningococcus is a gram-negative, encapsulated coccus. Only a minority of nasopharyngeal isolates cause invasive disease. 13 serogroups, which are classified according to antigenicity of capsular polysaccharides. Five serogroups (A, B, C, Y, and W-135) are responsible for >90% of cases of meningococcal disease worldwide. Polymerase chain reaction (PCR) also used for identification of strains associated with outbreaks of disease. *Worldwide*: serogroups A, B, C account for most cases; *America, Europe*: most outbreaks caused by serogroups B, C; *Asia/Africa*: A, C. *The United States, Sweden, Israel*: also have group Y.

Confined to humans; natural habitat is nasopharynx. Nasopharyngeal carrier rate: in nonepidemic periods, 10%; in closed populations, up to 60–80%. Carriage persists for a few months. Invasive infection usually occurs within first few days of carriage, before development of protective antibodies.

EPIDEMIOLOGY

Age of Onset   Highest incidence is in children ages 6 months to 3 years (peak, 6–12 months) (protective antibodies have not yet developed). Increasing in adolescents and young adults; 28% of cases are in 12- to 29-year olds.

Transmission Person-to-person through inhalation of droplets of aerosolized infected nasopharyngeal secretions; direct or indirect oral contact.

Season Highest incidence in midwinter, early spring; lowest in midsummer.

Demography Worldwide; 300,000–500,000 cases annually. Major outbreaks reported in Africa, China, South America. African savannah from Ethiopia to east of Senegal: "meningitis belt." Largest epidemic occurred in 1996–1997 in sub-Saharan Africa: >300,000 cases with 30,000 deaths caused by serogroup A. In the United States 2500–3000 cases annually.

Risk Factors for Colonization and Meningococcal Disease Residence in household of person who has meningococcal disease or is a carrier; household or institutional crowding; exposure to tobacco smoke; recent viral upper respiratory infection (URI).

Black race, low socioeconomic status, military recruits, college freshmen living in dormitories. Persons with deficiency of antibody-dependent complement-mediated immune lysis, functional/anatomic asplenia, properdin deficiency, deficiency of terminal complement components, HIV/AIDS are most susceptible.

Incidence Occurs worldwide as (1) isolated (sporadic) case; (2) institution- or community-based outbreaks, (3) large epidemics.

PATHOGENESIS

Meningococci colonizing mucosa of the upper respiratory tract are internalized by nonciliated mucosal cells and can traverse to submucosa and to blood vessels. The clinical syndrome depends on the rate of multiplication within the bloodstream:

- Slow replication: seeds local sites such as meninges, joint, or pericardium. Host inflammatory reaction limited to seed site.
- More rapid replication: fulminant meningococcemia occurs with hemorrhagic skin lesions (petechiae, purpura), DIC, and shock. Host inflammatory response in blood signs of sepsis and shock.

Fulminant meningococcemia is the most rapidly lethal form of septic shock experienced by humans. It differs from most other forms of septic shock by the prominence of hemorrhagic skin lesions (petechiae, purpura) and the consistent development of DIC (see Section 19). Extremely high blood levels of both proinflammatory mediators (TNF, IL-1, interferon, IL-8) and anti-inflammatory mediators (IL-1 receptor antagonist, soluble IL-1 receptors, soluble TNF receptors, and IL-10).

CLINICAL MANIFESTATIONS

Meningococcemia Fever, chills, nausea, vomiting, myalgias; prostration. Stupor, hemorrhagic lesions, hypotension within a few hours of onset of symptoms (fulminant disease).

Meningitis Headache; stiffness of neck; altered mental status; agitated, maniacal behavior. Some patients (10–30%) with meningococcal disease have both meningococcemia and meningitis.

Skin Lesions of Fulminant Meningococcemia

- Early exanthem
  ○ Occurs soon after onset of disease in 75% of cases; pink, 2- to 10-mm macules/papules
    ▪ Sparsely distributed on trunk/lower extremities as well as face, arms (Fig. 24-50).
    ▪ Mucous membranes (palate, conjunctivae)
  ○ Petechiae may coalesce into hemorrhagic bullae or may undergo necrosis and ulcerate.

- Later lesions
  ○ Petechiae appear in center of macules.
  ○ Lesions become purpuric/hemorrhagic within hours.
  ○ In severe cases, petechiae may become confluent and develop into hemorrhagic bullae with extensive ulcerations.
  ○ *Fulminant*: purpura, ecchymoses, and confluent, often bizarre-shaped, grayish to black necrosis (purpura fulminans) associated with DIC in fulminant disease (Fig. 24-51) (see also Section 19).
  ○ With severe coagulopathy, ischemia of extremities and/or digits occurs, often with a sharp line of demarcation between normal and ischemic tissue.

General Examination

High fever, tachypnea, tachycardia, mild hypotension. Patient appears acutely ill with marked prostration.

- *Meningitis*: 50–88% of patients with meningococcemia develop meningitis. Sudden onset of fever, signs of meningeal irritation. Signs of increased intracranial pressure (bulging fontanelle in infant).
- *Meningococcemia*: Rapid progression/overwhelming character. Occurs in 10–20% of

cases of meningococcal disease; characterized by development of shock, DIC, hypotension, peripheral vasoconstriction with cold cyanotic extremities, and multiorgan failure. Peripheral gangrene may occur, requiring amputation in those who survive.

- *Complications*: Intercurrent infections, CNS damage. Patients who recover may have necrosis of skin, distal extremities, tips of ears/nose.
- *Less common manifestations*: Arthritis (5–10%), pneumonia, sinusitis, otitis media, conjuctivitis, endophthalmitis, endocarditis, pericarditis, urethritis, endometritis.
- *Chronic meningococcemia*: Rare. Episodic fever, rash (macules, papules, petechial), arthralgias. Duration: weeks to months. Splenomegaly. If untreated, meningitis, fulminant meningococcemia, or endocarditis may occur.

DIFFERENTIAL DIAGNOSIS

Acute Meningococcemia and Meningitis Gonococcemia, infectious endocarditis, acute hypersensitivity, vasculitis, enteroviral infections, RMSF, endemic typhus.

LABORATORY EXAMINATIONS

Direct Microscopy Pus from nodular lesions shows gram-negative diplococci. In fulminant meningococcemia, meningococci can be seen in buffy coat. In 85% of cases of meningitis, meningococci can be seen in CSF.

Clotting Studies Prolonged thrombin time, decreased fibrinogen, presence of D-dimers.

Cultures *Blood* Acute meningococcemia, meningococci in nearly 100%; meningitis, one-third positive.

CSF Acute meningococcemia, usually positive.

DIAGNOSIS

Definitive etiologic diagnosis requires isolation of meningococci from blood or local site of infection.

COURSE AND PROGNOSIS

Case fatality rate for fulminant meningococcemia is 20–40%; for meningococcal meningitis, 3–10%. In Africa, mortality is 10%, but many patients die before reaching hospital. In 1996, an epidemic in the meningitis belt reported 160,000 cases with 16,000 deaths.

MANAGEMENT

Immunization <20% of meningococci isolates from associated disease belong to serogroups for which vaccines are available: A, C, W-135, Y.

Prophylaxis of Contacts of Primary Cases Rifampin, minocycline, or ciprofloxacin.

FIGURE 24-50   Acute meningococcemia: early exanthem Discrete, pink-to-purple macules and papules as well as purpura on the face of this young child. These lesions represent early disseminated intravascular coagulation with its cutaneous manifestation, purpura fulminans.

FIGURE 24-51 Acute meningococcemia: purpura fulminans Maplike, gray-to-black areas of cutaneous infarction of the leg in a child with NM meningitis and disseminated intravascular coagulation with purpura fulminans.

Antimicrobial Therapy Any febrile patient with a petechial rash should be considered to have meningococcal infection; blood culture should be obtained and treatment begun without awaiting confirmation.
Acute Meningococcemia Third-generation cephalosporin: cefotaxime (2 g IV q8h) or ceftriaxone (1 g IV q12h). *Alternative*: Penicillin G (4 million U IV q4h). *Chloramphenicol* in penicillin-allergic individuals.
Hemodynamic, Respiratory, Metabolic Support Primary goal is to restore adequate oxygen and substrate delivery to tissues. Adequate fluids should be infused to treat intravascular volume depletion.

NEISSERIA GONORRHOEAE INFECTIONS ☐ → ■ ◐

- Etiology: *N. gonorrhoeae,* the gonococcus
- Colonize mucosa: oropharynx, anogenital
- Epidemiology: sexually transmitted infection (STI). Shares clinical spectrum of *C. trachomatis*; symptoms are usually more severe with gonococcal infections.
- Symptoms
  - Males: urethritis often symptomatic
  - Females: cervicitis often asymptomatic; pain with deeper infection
  - Newborns: conjunctivitis

- Clinical findings:
  - Local infections: urethritis, cervicitis, proctitis, pharyngitis, conjunctivitis
  - Invasive tissue infections: pelvic inflammatory disease (PID)
  - Bloodstream invasion: gonococcemia with seeding of multiple sites, i.e., joints and skin resulting in disseminated gonococcal infection (DGI)
- Complications
  - Tubal scarring, infertility, ectopic pregnancy
  - Secondary infections of preexisting dermatoses (impetiginization, or secondary infection)

EPIDEMIOLOGY AND ETIOLOGY

Etiology

- *N. gonorrhoeae*, the gonococcus.
- Humans are the only natural reservoir of the organism.
- Strains that cause DGI tend to cause minimal genital inflammation.
- In the United States, these strains have occurred infrequently during the past decade.

Age of Onset Young, sexually active. In newborns, conjunctivitis.

Sex

- Young females; males who have sex with males.
- Symptomatic infection more common in males.
- Pharyngeal and anorectal in homosexual males.

Race In the United States; highest incidence in blacks, lowest in those of Asian/Pacific Island descent.

Transmission

- *Sexually,* from partner who either is asymptomatic or has minimal symptoms.
- *Neonate* exposed to infected secretions in birth canal.
- About 1% of patients with untreated mucosal gonococcal infection develop DGI (see below). Gonorrhea may enhance HIV/AIDS transmission.

Co-infection   Up to 40% of persons co-infected with *C. trachomatis.* Gonorrhea enhances transmission as well as acquisition of HIV/AIDS.

Demography   Worldwide. In Africa, median prevalence of gonorrhea in pregnant women is 10%. Incidence of DGI varies with local incidence of DGI strains of gonococcus (see below).

Incidence   Highest in developing countries. Prevalence of DGI in pregnant women: 10% in Africa; 5% in Latin America; 4% in Asia.

PATHOGENESIS

- Gonococcus has affinity for columnar epithelium; stratified and squamous epithelia are more resistant to attack.

- Epithelium is penetrated between epithelial cells, causing a submucosal inflammation with polymorphonuclear (PMN) leukocyte reaction with resultant purulent discharge.
- Strains of gonococcus that cause DGI tend to cause little genital inflammation and thereby escape detection. Most signs and symptoms of DGI are manifestations of immune complex formation and deposition.
- Multiple episodes of DGI may be associated with abnormality of terminal complement component factors (see below).

LABORATORY STUDIES

See below: *N. gonorrhoeae.*

MANAGEMENT

See Table 30-4 and pages 653-654. For Centers for Disease Control and Prevention (CDC) STD treatment guidelines—2002, see http://www.cdc.gov/mmwr/preview/mmwrhtml/rr5106 a1.htm

---

NEISSERIA GONORRHOEAE: LOCAL INFECTIONS (GONORRHEA)   ICD-9:098 ∘ ICD-10:A54   ■ ◑

- ■ *N. gonorrhoeae* infects mucocutaneous surfaces of the lower genitourinary tract, anus, and rectum and the oropharynx.
- ■ The most common presentation in males is a purulent urethral discharge.
- ■ In females, cervical infection is most common and is often asymptomatic

- ■ If untreated, infection can spread to deeper structures with abscess formation and disseminated gonococcal infection (DGI) (see Section 24)

Synonyms: Clap, blennorrhagia, blennorrhea.

CLINICAL MANIFESTATIONS

Incubation Period

- *Males:* 90% of males develop urethritis within 5 days of exposure.
- *Females:* Usually >14 days when symptomatic; however, up to 75% of women are asymptomatic.

Skin Symptoms

- *Urethra:* discharge, dysuria.
- *Vagina:* discharge; deep pelvic or lumbar pain.

- *Anus/rectum:* Copious purulent anal discharge; burning or stinging pain on defecation; tenesmus; blood in/on stool.
- *Oropharynx:* Mild sore throat.

Mucocutaneous Findings
External Genitalia
Males

- Urethral discharge ranging from scanty and clear to purulent and copious (Figs. 24-52, 24-53).

- *Edema*: meatus, prepuce, or penis.
- Balanoposthitis with subpreputial discharge in uncircumcised men; balanitis in circumcised men.
- Folliculitis or cellulitis of thigh or abdomen.
- *Deeper structures*: Prostatitis, epididymitis, vesiculitis, cystitis.

Females

- Periurethral edema, urethritis.
- Purulent discharge from cervix but no vaginitis.
- In prepubescent females, vulvovaginitis. Bartholin abscess.
- *Deeper structures*: Pelvic inflammatory disease (PID) with signs of peritonitis, endocervicitis, endosalpingitis, endometritis.

Anorectum

- With receptive anal intercourse, proctitis with pain and purulent discharge.
- In female, can spread from cervicitis.

Pharynx

- Occurs secondary to oral-genital sexual exposure.
- In females and homosexual males, pharyngitis with erythema.
- Always coexists with genital infection.

Eyes

- Conjunctivitis, swollen eyelid, severe hyperemia, chemosis, profuse purulent discharge; rarely, corneal ulcer and perforation.
- In newborn, organism is transmitted as newborn passes through birth canal.
- Usually occurs in the absence of genital infection, copious purulent conjunctival discharge.
- Can be complicated by corneal ulceration and perforation.

General Examination
Disseminated Gonococcal Infection See below.

DIFFERENTIAL DIAGNOSIS

Urethritis Genital herpes with urethritis, *C. trachomatis* urethritis, *Ureaplasma urealyticum* urethritis, *Trichomonas vaginalis* urethritis, Reiter's syndrome.
Cervicitis *C. trachomatis* or HSV cervicitis.

FIGURE 24-52 *Neisseria gonorrhoeae:* Gram stain Multiple, gram-negative diplococci within polymorphonuclear leukocytes as well as in the extracellular areas of a smear from a urethral discharge.

FIGURE 24-53 Gonorrhea Purulent, creamy urethral discharge from the distal urethra of a male.

LABORATORY EXAMINATIONS

Gram Stain Gram-negative diplococci intracellularly in polymorphonuclear leukocytes in exudate (Fig. 24-52).
Culture Isolation on gonococcal-selective media, i.e., chocolatized blood agar, Martin-Lewis medium, Thayer-Martin medium. Antimicrobial susceptibility testing important due to resistant strains.
Specimen Collection Sites *Heterosexual men*: Urethra, oropharynx. *Homosexual men*: Urethra, rectum, oropharynx. *Women*: Cervix, rectum, oropharynx. *DGI*: Blood.
Serologic Tests None available for gonorrhea. All patients should have a Serologic test for syphilis and should be offered HIV/AIDS testing.

DIAGNOSIS

Clinical suspicion, confirmed by laboratory findings, i.e., presumptively by identifying gram-negative diplococci intracellularly in PMNs in smears, confirmed by culture.

COURSE AND PROGNOSIS

- Most infections among men produce symptoms that cause the person to seek curative treatment soon enough to prevent serious sequelae—but not soon enough to prevent transmission to others.
  - If not treated, complications due to ascending infection occur: Prostatitis—pain on defecation
  - Epididymitis—swelling of epididymis and pain in walking.
  - Cystitis.
- Many infections among women do not produce recognizable symptoms until complications such as PID occur.
  - PID, whether symptomatic or asymptomatic, can cause tubal scarring, leading to infertility or ectopic pregnancy.
- Because gonococcal infections among women are often asymptomatic, a primary measure for controlling gonorrhea in the United States has been screening of high-risk women.
- DGI more common in
  - Women with asymptomatic cervical, endometrial, or tubal infection
  - Homosexual men with asymptomatic rectal or pharyngeal gonorrhea.

MANAGEMENT

See CDC updated recommended regimens:
http://www.cdc.gov/std/treatment
See Table 30-4.
See pages 653-654 for management of disseminated gonococcal infections.

DISSEMINATED GONOCOCCAL INFECTION   ICD-9 : 098.89   ☐ ◑ → ●

- DGI is a systemic infection that follows the hematogenous dissemination of gonococcus from infected mucosal sites to skin, tenosynovium, and joints.
- Characterized by fever, petechial or pustular acral lesions, asymmetric arthralgias, tenosynovitis, or septic arthritis.

- Occasionally complicated by perihepatitis and, rarely, endocarditis or meningitis.

Synonyms: Gonococcemia, gonococcal arthritis–dermatitis syndrome

---

CLINICAL MANIFESTATION

Incubation Period 7–30 days of mucosal infection (range, from a few days to 1 year). Varies with host factors such as menstruation, invasiveness of infecting organism.
Prodrome Fever, anorexia, malaise, shaking chills, polyarthralgias (knees, elbows, distal joints).

Other Factors Recurring symptoms around menses, migratory polyarthralgias.

Mucocutaneous Findings

- 1- to 5-mm erythematous macules evolving to hemorrhagic pustules (Fig. 24-54) within 24–48 h in 75% of cases.
- Centers at times hemorrhagic/necrotic, 5–40 in number.

- Rarely, large hemorrhagic bullae.
- *Distribution*: Acral (Fig. 24-54), arms more often than legs, near small joints of hands or feet. Difficult to detect in black patients; look in webspaces. Face spared.
- *Mucous membranes*: Usually asymptomatic colonization of oropharynx, urethra, anorectum, endometrium.

Fever 38°C to 39°C usual. Severity varies:

- DGI with skin lesions alone
- Classic DGI with skin lesions and tenosynovitis
- DGI with septic arthritis
- DGI with metastatic infection at other sites.

Tenosynovitis

- Common
- Single or few sites, acrally
- Extensor/flexor tendons and sheaths of hands/feet
- Erythema, tenderness, swelling along tendon sheath aggravated by moving tendon

Septic Arthritis

- Red, hot, tender with effusion; asymmetric
- Most commonly involved: knee, wrist, ankle, elbow, metacarpophalangeal/interphalangeal joints of hand, shoulder, hip
- Usually only one to two joints involved

Other

- Hepatitis, perihepatitis (Fitz-Hugh–Curtis syndrome), myopericarditis, endocarditis, meningitis, perihepatitis
- Rarely, pneumonitis, ARDS, osteomyelitis

DIFFERENTIAL DIAGNOSIS

Scant, Acral, Hemorrhagic Pustules Bacteremia: meningococcemia, other bacteremias, endocarditis.
Tenosynovitis/Arthritis Infectious arthritis, infectious tenosynovitis, reactive syndrome, psoriatic arthritis, SLE.

LABORATORY EXAMINATIONS

Dermatopathology Immunofluorescence of skin lesion biopsy shows gonococci in 60%.
Gram Stain From the male urethra or cervix, may show gonococci.
Culture Mucosal sites yield 80–90% positive cultures. Skin biopsy: ≤5% chance of positive culture; joint fluid, blood also low yield.

DIAGNOSIS

Made on clinical criteria, confirmed by culture of gonococcus from mucosal sites.

COURSE AND PROGNOSIS

Untreated, skin/joint lesions often gradually resolve; endocarditis usually fatal.

MANAGEMENT

Recommended regimen
   Ceftriaxone, 1 g IM or IV every 24 h
Alternative regimens
   Cefotaxime, 1 g IV every 8 h, *or*
   Ceftizoxime, 1 g IV every 8 h, *or*
   Ciprofloxacin, 400 mg IV every 12 h, *or*
   Ofloxacin, 400 mg IV every 12 h, *or*
   Levofloxacin, 250 mg IV daily, *or*
   Spectinomycin, 2 g IM every 12 h

FIGURE 24-54 Disseminated gonococcal infection Hemorrhagic, painful pustules on erythematous bases on the palm and the finger of the other hand. These lesions occur at acral sites and are few in number.

All of the preceding regimens should be continued for 24–48 h after improvement begins, at which time therapy may be switched to one of the following regimens to complete at least 1 week of antimicrobial therapy:

Cefixime, 400 mg orally twice daily, *or*
Ciprofloxacin, 500 mg orally twice daily, *or*
Ofloxacin, 400 mg orally twice daily, *or*
Levofloxacin, 500 mg orally once daily

GRAM-NEGATIVE INFECTIONS

BARTONELLA INFECTIONS ○ ◑

- Etiology: *Bartonella* spp.; tiny gram-negative bacilli that can adhere to and invade mammalian cells such as endothelial cells and erythrocytes (Table 24-7).
- Transmission by: cat scratch or bite, body louse, sandfly bite
- Manifestations vary with the immune status of the host
  - *B. henselae*
    - Immunocompetent host: cat-scratch disease (CSD)
    - HIV/AIDS: bacillary angiomatosis (BA)
- *B. bacilliformis*
  - Nonimmune, nonresidents of endemic area: Oroya fever with severe febrile illness, profound anemia
  - Immune person after convalescence: verruga peruana with red-purple cutaneous lesions (Peruvian warts; resemble angiomatous lesions of BA
- *Trench fever* is caused by *B. quintana*, presenting as a febrile systemic illness with prolonged bacteremia; no cutaneous manifestations.

PATHOGENESIS

Bartonella (Table 24-7) species cause vascular proliferation (angiogenesis), histologically resembling Kaposi sarcoma: *B. bacilliformis* causes verruga peruana, *B. henselae* and *B. quintana* cause bacillary angiomatosis. *B. henselae* is associated with hepatosplenic disease (peliosis hepatitis) and infection of lymph nodes. *B. quintana* is associated with bony and subcutaneous lesions.

MANAGEMENT

See Table 24-8.

TABLE 24-7   Major Diseases Caused by *Bartonella* Species

Disease	Organism	Risk factor
Cat-scratch disease	*B. henselae*	Cat scratch or bite
Bacillary angiomatosis	*B. quintana, B. henselae*	Cat scratch or bite
Bacillary peliosis	*B. henselae*	Cat scratch or bite
Trench fever	*B. quintana*	Homelessness, body louse infestation, alcoholism
Endocarditis	*B. quintana, B. henselae, B. elizabethae*	As for cat-scratch disease and trench fever
Bartonellosis	*B. bacilliformis*	Sandfly bite

SOURCE: From DH Spach, E Darby, in AS Fauci et al (eds): *Harrison's Principles of Internal Medicine*, 17th ed. New York, McGraw-Hill, 2008.

TABLE 24-8   Treatment of Adults with Disease Caused by *Bartonella* Species[a]

Disease	Treatment
Cat-scratch disease	
Lymphadenopathy	Consider azithromycin (500 mg PO on day 1, then 250 mg PO qd for 4 days)
Retinitis	Doxycycline (100 mg PO bid for 4–6 weeks) *plus*
	Rifampin (300 mg PO bid for 4–6 weeks)
Bacillary angiomatosis	Erythromycin (500 mg PO qid for 3 months) *or*
	Doxycycline (100 mg PO bid for 3 months)
Bacillary peliosis	Erythromycin (500 mg PO qid for 4 months) *or*
	Doxycycline (100 mg PO bid for 4 months)
Bartonella endocarditis	
Suspected	Gentamicin (3 mg/kg qd IV for 14 days) *plus* ceftriaxone (2g IV qd for 6 weeks) *with or without*
	Doxycycline (100 mg PO bid for 6 weeks)
Confirmed	Gentamicin (3 mg/kg qd IV for 14 days) *plus*
	Doxycycline (100 mg PO bid for 6 weeks)
Trench fever	Doxycycline (200 mg PO qd for 4 weeks) *plus*
	Gentamicin (3 mg/kg qd IV for 14 days)
Bartonellosis	
Oroya fever	Chloramphenicol (500 mg PO or IV *qid* for 14 days) *plus* a β-lactam agent *or*
	Ciprofloxacin (500 mg bid for 10 days)
Verruga peruana	Rifampin (10 mg/kg qd PO for 14 days) *or*
	Streptomycin (15–20 mg/kg qd IM for 10 days)

SOURCE: From JM Rolain et al: Recommendations for treatment of human infections caused by *Bartonella* species. *Antimicrob Agents Chemother* 48:1921, 2004; with permission.

CAT-SCRATCH DISEASE (CSD)   ICD-9:078.30 ∘ ICD-10:A28.1

- Etiology: *B. henselae*
- Transmission: scratch from or contact with a cat
- Clinical findings:
  - Inoculation site: skin or conjunctival lesion after cat scratches or contact with a cat
  - Lymph nodes: acute to subacute tender regional lymphadenopathy

- Conjunctival inoculation: unilateral conjunctival lesion with preauricular lymphadenopathy (Parinaud oculoglandular syndrome)
- Systemic involvement uncommon: nervous system, visceral organs, bone

Synonym: Cat-scratch fever

EPIDEMIOLOGY AND ETIOLOGY

Etiology   *B. henselae*.
Reservoir   Domestic cat.
Vector   Cat flea (*Ctenocephalides felis*).
Host   Immunocompetent.
Transmission   Associated with exposure to young cats with fleas. Blood cultures of kittens are frequently positive for *B. henselae*. Fleas transmit infection between cats.
Season   Late fall, winter, or early spring in cooler climates; July and August in warmer climates. Worldwide.
Age of Onset   Majority (60%) of cases occur in children. 40% in adults.

Sex   Males > females.

Incidence   20,000 cases annually in the United States, of whom 2000 are hospitalized.

PATHOGENESIS

B. henselae causes granulomatous inflammation in healthy individuals (CSD) and angiogenesis in immunocompromised persons.

CLINICAL MANIFESTATION

Incubation Period

- Primary lesion at bite/scratch site: 3–5 days after inoculation; occurs in about half of cases.
- Regional lymphadenopathy: 1–2 weeks after inoculation.

Prodrome   Mild fever and malaise occur in fewer than half the patients. Chills, general aching, and nausea are infrequently present.

Mucocutaneous Lesions
Inoculation Site

- Innocuous-looking, small (0.5 to 1-cm) papule, vesicle, or pustule 3–5 days after inoculation; may ulcerate; skin color pink to red; firm, at times tender (Fig. 24-55).
- Residual linear cat scratch.
- Persists for 1–3 weeks.
- *Distribution*: Exposed skin of face, hands.
- *Mucous membranes*: If portal of entry is the conjunctiva, 3- to 5-mm whitish-yellow granulation on palpebral conjunctiva associated with tender preauricular and/or cervical lymphadenopathy (Parinaud oculoglandular syndrome).

Uncommonly: urticaria, transient maculopapular eruption, vesiculopapular lesions, erythema nodosum.

General Examination   Most patients do not have fever. Systemic symptoms common: malaise, anorexia, weight loss.

Regional Lymphadenopathy

- (Fig. 24-56) Evident within 2–3 weeks after inoculation in 90% of cases; primary lesion, if present, may have resolved by the time lymphadenopathy occurs.
- Nodes are usually solitary, moderately tender, freely movable. Involved lymph nodes: epitrochlear, axillary, pectoral, cervical.
- Nodes may suppurate. Usually resolved within 3 months.
- Generalized lymphadenopathy or involvement of the lymph nodes of more than one region is unusual.

Other   Encephalitis (seizures, coma in children), meningitis, transverse myelitis, pneumonitis, thrombocytopenia, osteomyelitis, granulomatous hepatitis, abscesses in liver or spleen, disseminated infection.

DIFFERENTIAL DIAGNOSIS

Distal Cutaneous Lesion with Regional Lymphadenopathy   Suppurative bacterial lymphadenitis, nontuberculous mycobacteria (NTM), sporotrichosis, tularemia, tumors, sarcoidosis, lymphogranuloma venereum, coccidioidomycosis.

Other Cat-Associated Infections   *Pasteurella multocida*, bite infection; *Capnocytophaga* (DF-2) spp., bite infection, sporotrichosis; *Microsporum canis*, dermatophytosis; *Toxocara cata*, larva migrans; *Dirofilaria repens*, subcutaneous nodules.

LABORATORY EXAMINATIONS

Hematology   WBC usually normal; ESR commonly elevated.

Dermatopathology   Granulomatous inflammation with stellate necrosis; no angiogenesis. Demonstration of small, pleomorphic bacilli in Warthin-Starry–stained sections of primary skin lesion, conjunctiva, or lymph nodes.

Culture   *B. henselae* rarely isolated from lymph node aspirates.

Serology   Antibodies to *B. henselae* usually positive ≥1:64.

PCR   Done on tissue from lymph node; preferred over culture.

DIAGNOSIS

Suggested by regional lymphadenopathy developing over 2–3 weeks in an individual with cat

FIGURE 24-55   Bartonellosis: cat-scratch disease with primary lesion   Erythematous nodule of the cheek of a 9-year-old girl at the site of cat-scratch. Diagnosis was made on the histologic findings of the excised specimen.

contact and a primary lesion at the site of contact; confirmed by identification of *B. henselae* from tissue or serodiagnosis.

COURSE AND PROGNOSIS

- Self-limiting, usually within 1–2 months.
- Uncommonly, prolonged morbidity with persistent high fever, suppurative lymphadenitis, severe systemic symptoms.
- May be confused with lymphoma. Uncommonly, cat-scratch encephalopathy occurs.
- Antibiotic therapy has not been very effective in altering the course of the infection.

MANAGEMENT

In the immunocompetent host, CSD resolves spontaneously.
Antimicrobial Therapy   Antibiotic therapy may hasten resolution of lymphadenopathy. See Table 24-2.
Surgical Therapy   Draining of lymph nodes may be required.

FIGURE 24-56   Bartonellosis: cat-scratch disease with axillary adenopathy   Acute, very tender, axillary lymphadenopathy in a child; cat scratches were present on the dorsum of the ipsilateral hand. (Courtesy of Howard Heller, MD.)

BARTONELLA INFECTIONS IN HIV/AIDS

- Infection by *B. henselae* and *B. quintana* in immunocompromised HIV/AIDS-infected individuals can cause
  - Bacillary angiomatosis (BA) with cutaneous angiomatous lesions
- Systemic infections with peliosis hepatitis, osteomyelitis, fever of unknown origin, bacteremia, endocarditis.
- Visceral infection can be fatal if not diagnosed and treated appropriately.

BACILLARY ANGIOMATOSIS   ICD-9:088.0 ○ ICD-10:A44.8   ☐ ◑

- Etiology: *B. henselae, B. quintana*
  - Both cause cutaneous angiomas
  - *B. quintana* causes subcutaneous nodules and lytic bone lesion
- HIV/AIDS-infected persons with CD4 T cell counts ≤ 100 /uL
- Incidence: uncommon. Incidence decreased with prophylaxis of opportunistic infection and antiretroviral therapy (ART)
- Risk factors
  - *B. henselae*: contact with cats and/or cat fleas (*C. felis*)
  - *B. quintana*: low income, homelessness, body louse (*P. humanis corporis*) infestation
- Clinical findings:
  - Skin: red angiomatous papules, nodules, tumors; usually multiple. Subcutaneous nodules.
  - Systemic involvement: liver, spleen, bone

CLINICAL MANIFESTATION

Cutaneous BA   Lesions may be painful.
Disseminated BA   Skin lesions usually absent. Presents with nausea, vomiting, diarrhea, fever, chills. Bony lesions may cause focal bone pain.
Skin Lesions   Papules or nodules resembling angiomas (red, bright red, violaceous, or skin-colored) (Fig. 24-57); up to 2–3 cm in diameter; usually situated in dermis with thinning or erosion of overlying epidermis surrounded by a collarette of scale. Larger lesions may ulcerate. Pyogenic granuloma–like lesions (Fig. 24-57). Subcutaneous nodules, 1–2 cm in diameter, resembling cysts. Uncommonly, abscess formation. Papules/nodules range from solitary lesions to >100 and, rarely, >1000. Firm, nonblanching. Lesions may be nontender or painful, a finding not seen in nodular lesions of Kaposi sarcoma.
Distribution   Any site, but palms and soles are usually spared. Occasionally, lesions occur at the site of a cat scratch. A solitary lesion may present as dactylitis.
Mucous Membranes   Angioma-like lesions of lips and oral mucosa. Laryngeal involvement with obstruction.

Systemic Findings   Infection may spread hematogenously or via lymphatics to become systemic, commonly involving the liver and spleen (hepatosplenomegaly, liver abscesses, necrotizing splenitis, hepatic/splenic necrotizing granulomata). Lesions may also occur in the heart (cardiac lesions, endocarditis), bone marrow, lymph nodes, muscles, soft tissues, and CNS (brain abscess, aseptic meningitis, encephalopathy).

DIFFERENTIAL DIAGNOSIS

Multiple Cutaneous Angiomatous Papules/Nodules in HIV/AIDS disease   Kaposi sarcoma, pyogenic granuloma, cherry angioma, sclerosing hemangioma.

LABORATORY EXAMINATIONS

Dermatopathology   Lobular vascular proliferations composed of plump "epithelioid" endothelia. Neutrophils scattered throughout the lesion, especially around eosinophilic granular aggregates, which are masses of bacteria (visualized by Warthin-Starry staining or electron microscopy).

Liver Biopsy Associated with higher morbidity and mortality rates in that the lesions are vascular tumors. Dilated capillaries or multiple blood-filled cavernous spaces; myxoid stroma containing an admixture of inflammatory cells and granular clumps (*Bartonella*).

Culture *Bartonella* can be isolated from lesional skin biopsy specimens, blood, or other infected tissues on endothelial-cell monolayer.

PCR Detects *Bartonella* DNA in tissue.

Chemistry Bacillary peliosis hepatitis associated with elevated aminotransferase, alkaline phosphatase.

Serology Anti-*Bartonella* antibodies detected by indirect fluorescent-antibody testing (detected by the CDC). Also, enzyme immunoassay for detection of IgG antibodies to *B. henselae*.

Imaging Lesions can be visualized by conventional radiographs and nuclear imaging. Lesions regress with appropriate therapy. CT scan shows hepatomegaly, ± splenomegaly.

DIAGNOSIS

Clinical findings confirmed by demonstration of *Bartonella* bacilli on silver stain of lesional biopsy specimen or culture or antibody studies.

COURSE AND PROGNOSIS

Rarely seen in HIV/AIDS individuals successfully treated with ART. In untreated HIV/AIDS disease, course variable. In some individuals, lesions regress spontaneously. Untreated systemic infection causes significant morbidity and mortality. With effective antimicrobial therapy, lesions resolve within 1–2 weeks. As with other infections occurring in HIV/AIDS, relapse

FIGURE 24-57 Bartonellosis: bacillary angiomatosis 3- to 5-mm cherry hemangioma-like papules and a larger pyogenic granuloma-like nodule on the shin of a male with advanced HIV disease. Subcutaneous nodular lesions were also present.

may occur and require lifelong secondary prophylaxis. Azithromycin given for *Mycobacterium avium* complex (MAC) prophylaxis seems to prevent BA as well.

MANAGEMENT

Prevention HIV/AIDS individuals should avoid contact with cats, especially kittens, to minimize the risk for acquiring BA, as well as toxoplasmosis.

Antimicrobial See page 657.

TULAREMIA ICD-9:021 ∘ ICD-10:A21   □ ○ → ●

- Etiology: *Francisella tularensis*, types A and B
- Transmission by:
  - Handling flesh of infected animals
  - Bite of insect vectors
  - Inoculation of conjunctiva
  - Ingestion of infected food
  - Inhalation

- Clinical syndromes
  - Ulceroglandular
  - Oculoglandular
  - Typhoidal
  - Pulmonary
- *Synonyms*: Rabbit fever, deerfly fever, Ohara fever, Francis disease

Historical Fact   Named after Tulare County, CA

EPIDEMIOLOGY AND ETIOLOGY

Age of Onset/Sex   Young males.
Etiology

- *F. tularensis*, a pleomorphic gram-negative intracellular coccobacillus.
- Two subspecies:
  - Type A common in North America, highly virulent in animals and humans;
  - Type B causes all human cases in Asia and Europe.

- One of the most infectious bacteria known.

Occupation   Rabbit hunters, butchers, cooks, agricultural workers, trappers, campers, sheep herders and shearers, mink ranchers, muskrat farmers, laboratory technicians.
Insect Vector   Ticks (*Ixodes, Dermacentor*), deer flies, body lice, other arthropods.
Animal Reservoir   Rabbits, hares, muskrats, prairie dogs, foxes, squirrels, skunks, voles, beavers.
Transmission   As few as 10 organism can cause infection.

- Arthropod bites: deer flies, ticks, or other insects carrying the disease.
- Handling infected animal tissue or fluids. Small abrasion or puncture wound. Conjunctival inoculation.
- Eating or drinking food or water contaminated by the bacteria
- Breathing in the bacteria. Inhaling particles from an infected rabbit ground up in a lawnmower (Martha's Vineyard). Transporting hay.
- Laboratory exposure.
- Biological weapon: Strains suitable for inhalation have been developed. See Appendix B.

Season   Most U.S. cases occur June–September when arthropod transmission is most common.
Geography   Throughout northern hemisphere: North America, parts of Europe, Asia. United States: south-central and western states.
Biological Weapon   Could be used; aerosol release would have the greatest adverse medical and public health consequences. Pleuropneumonitis; ocular tularemia; ulceroglandular or glandular disease. (See Appendix B.)
http://www.bt.cdc.gov/agent/tularemia/tularemia-biological-weapon-abstract.asp

Incidence   Rare. <200 cases reported in United States per year; underdiagnosed, underreported.
Clinical Syndromes

- Ulceroglandular (75% of cases)
- Glandular
- Pulmonary
- Oropharyngeal
- Oculoglandular
- Typhoidal
- Biological weapon

PATHOGENESIS

- Facultative intracellular organism; multiplies in macrophages.
- Major targets: lymph nodes, lungs and pleura, spleen, liver, kidney.
- After inoculation into skin, mucous membrane, lung (inhalation), or GI tract *F. tularensis* reproduces and spreads through lymphatic channels to lymph nodes and bloodstream.
- Suppurative lesions become granulomatous with central necrosis and ± caseation.

CLINICAL MANIFESTATION

Incubation Period   2–10 days.
Symptoms   Prodrome: headache, malaise, myalgia, high fever. About 48 h after inoculation, pruritic papule develops at the site of trauma or insect bite followed by enlargement of regional lymph nodes.
Mucocutaneous Lesions

- At inoculation site: erythematous tender papule evolving to a vesicopustule, enlarging to crusted ulcer with raised, sharply demarcated margins (96 h) (Fig. 24-58).
- Depressed center that is often covered by a black eschar (chancriform).
- Primary lesion on finger/hand at site of trauma/insect bite; groin/axilla after tick bite.
- After bacteremia, exanthem (trunk and extremities) with macules, papules, petechiae; erythema multiforme (Fig. 24-59); erythema nodosum.
- *Mucous membranes*: In oculoglandular tularemia, *F. tularensis* is inoculated into conjunctiva, causing a purulent conjunctivitis with pain, edema, congestion. Small yellow nodules occur on conjunctivae and ulcerate.

http://www.logicalimages.com/resourcesBTAgentsTularemia.htm

FIGURE 24-58 Tularemia: primary lesion and regional adenopathy A crusted ulcer at the site of inoculation is seen on the dorsum of the left ring finger with associated axillary lymph node enlargement (chancriform syndrome). The infection occurred after the patient killed and skinned a rabbit.

General Findings

- Fever to 41°C.
- Regional lymph nodes
  - As the ulcer develops, nodes enlarge and become tender (chancriform syndrome) (Fig. 24-58).
  - If untreated, become suppurating buboes.
  - Lung consolidation, splenomegaly, generalized lymphadenopathy, hepatomegaly may occur.
- Variants
  - "Typhoidal" form occurs with ingestion of *F. tularensis*, resulting in ulcerative or exudative pharyngotonsillitis with cervical lymphadenopathy.
  - Tularemic pneumonia occurs after bacteremia or inhalation of *F. tularensis*.

DIFFERENTIAL DIAGNOSIS

Cutaneous Inoculation Site Furuncle, paronychia, spotted fever, anthrax, *Pasteurella multocida* infection, sporotrichosis, *M. marinum* infection.
Tender Regional Adenopathy Herpes simplex virus lymphadenitis, plague, cat-scratch disease,

FIGURE 24-59 Tularemia: erythema multiforme An exanthem on the chest with features of erythema multiforme syndrome, a hypersensitivity to *Francisella tularensis*.

melioidosis or glanders, lymphogranuloma venereum.

LABORATORY EXAMINATIONS

Cultures Routine culture media do not support the growth of *F. tularensis* from clinical specimens.
Serology Diagnosis usually confirmed by demonstrating a fourfold rise in acute and convalescent *F. tularensis* antibody titers.

DIAGNOSIS

Clinical diagnosis in a patient with chancriform syndrome with appropriate animal exposure or insect exposure and systemic manifestations. Disease in pneumonic presentation has "flu-like" symptomatology and is fatal if unrecognized.

COURSE AND PROGNOSIS

Untreated, mortality rate for ulceroglandular form is 5%; 1% if therapy initiated promptly; for typhoidal and pulmonary forms, 30%.

MANAGEMENT

Prevention Avoid contact with wild rabbits. In tick-infested areas, wear tight wristbands and pants tucked into boots to prevent tick attachment. Inspect for ticks at day's end. Live vaccine available for high-risk groups. Wear rubber gloves when handling or processing wild rabbits.
Drug of Choice Gentamycin or streptomycin.
Alternatives Doxycycline, chloramphenicol, ciprofloxacin.
http://www.bt.cdc.gov/agent/tularemia/
http://www.cidrap.umn.edu/idsa/bt/tularemia/
biofacts/tularemiafactsheet.html

PSEUDOMONAS SPECIES

- Heterogeneous group of gram-negative bacteria (pseudomonads)
  - *Pseudomonas*
  - *Burkholderia*
  - *Stenotrophomonas*
- Pathogenicity: usually opportunistic, nosocomial
- *Pseudomonas aeruginosa* is the major pathogen for skin infections.

CUTANEOUS *PSEUDOMONAS AERUGINOSA* INFECTIONS

- Nonfastidious, motile; produce pyocyanin and pyoverdin, pigments that cause yellow to dark green to bluish color.
- Environmental sources: moist ecological niches of soils, plants, vegetables, tap water.
- Risk factors: hospitalization, cancer, cytotoxic chemotherapy, neutropenia, broad-spectrum antibiotic therapy, chronic wounds, HIV/AIDS, immunocompromise, glucocorticoids, catheters (IV, urethral), debilitation; mucosal ulceration; cystic fibrosis.
- Cutaneous infections in healthy persons
  - Pseudomonal folliculitis: occurs in healthy individuals exposed to contaminated hot-tubs (hot-tub folliculitis)
  - Gram-negative webspace intertrigo: occurs with hyperhidrosis, often with concomitant tinea pedis
- Green nail: grows as a biofilm on the undersurface of onycholytic nail plate such as with psoriasis or onychomycosis; colonization not infection.
- Local invasion can follow colonization of any mucocutaneous site with local wound infection, soft tissue infection, and subsequent hematogenous dissemination.
- Cutaneous infection in compromised patients:
  - Wound infection, e.g., burns, pressure ulcers, surgical sites
  - Ecthyma gangrenosum (EG) is the necrotizing soft tissue infection that occurs after local tissue invasion or bacteremic seeding, associated with blood vessel invasion, septic vasculitis, vascular occlusion, and infarction of tissue.

EPIDEMIOLOGY

Ecology

- Widespread in nature, inhabiting water, soil, plants, and animals, preferring moist environments.
- Carriage rate is low in healthy individuals.
- Colonizes skin, external ear, upper respiratory tract, and/or large bowel in those who are naturally or iatrogenically compromised, have received antimicrobial therapy, and/or been exposed to a hospital environment.

Transmission

- Most infections are hospital acquired.
- Pseudomonal carriage increases with length of hospital stay and antibiotic administration.
- Transmitted to patients via hands of hospital personnel or via fomites.
- Entry sites for bacteremia at breaks in mucocutaneous barriers: sites of trauma, foreign bodies (IV or urinary catheter), aspiration/aerosolization into respiratory tract, skin ulcers, thermal burns.

Risk Factors for Invasive Infection *P. aeruginosa* is primarily a nosocomial pathogen—the fourth most commonly isolated—accounting for 10% of all hospital-acquired infections.

PATHOGENESIS

- Most infections are both invasive and toxigenic. Infection occurs in three stages:
  - Bacterial attachment and colonization
  - Local invasion and damage of tissue
  - Disseminated systemic disease
- Infection may stop at any stage
- *P. aeruginosa* rarely causes disease in the healthy host. Infections occur when:
  - Normal cutaneous or mucosal barriers have been breached or bypassed (e.g., burn injury, penetrating trauma, surgery, endotracheal intubation, urinary bladder catheterization, IV drug abuse)
  - Immunologic defense mechanisms have been compromised (e.g., by chemotherapy-induced neutropenia, hypogammaglobulinemia, extremes of age, diabetes mellitus, cystic fibrosis, cancer, HIV/AIDS disease)
  - Protective function of normal bacterial flora has been disrupted by broad-spectrum antimicrobial therapy

  - When a patient has been exposed to reservoirs associated with hospital environment.
- Blood vessel and bloodstream invasion, dissemination, SIRS (sepsis syndrome), multiorgan dysfunction, and, ultimately, death may follow localized infection.
- The organism and/or its products may cause tissue injury at primary and secondary sites of infection; release of systemically acting toxins or inflammatory mediators of infected host may contribute directly or indirectly to SIRS.

CLINICAL MANIFESTATION

Cutaneous Infections
Nail Colonization *P. aeruginosa* grows within a biofilm on the undersurface of onycholytic nails, e.g., psoriasis, onychomycosis; the under surface of the nail plate has a surface green discoloration that can easily be abraded (see Section 33, Fig. 33-3). The onycholytic nail plate can be trimmed to eliminate the abnormal space.

Folliculitis *P. aeruginosa* can infect multiple hair follicles in healthy individuals after aqueous exposure in contaminated hot tubs ("hot-tub folliculitis," see Fig. 32-30) or physiotherapy pools, presenting as multiple follicular pustules on the trunk (see Section 32). The infection is self-limited.

Toe Webspace Infection Intertrigo of toe webspaces. Webspace(s) macerated, moist often with green color (see Fig. 25-3); usually in setting of hyperhidrosis, ± macerated interdigital tinea pedis, ± erythrasma, ± keratoderma.

Primary and Secondary Pyoderma *P. aeruginosa* can cause primary infection of hair follicles or small breaks in skin, or secondary infections of sites of trauma, burn injury, inflammatory dermatoses, ulcers. With deeper invasion, necrotizing infection (due to blood vessel invasion and occlusion) occurs, i.e., EG. These pyodermas have a typical blue-green exudate and characteristic fruity odor. In thermal burn injury, black, dark brown, or violaceous discoloration of burn eschar may occur.

External Otitis "Swimmer's ear." Moist environment of external auditory canal provides medium for superficial infection, presenting as pruritus, pain, discharge; usually self-limited. Malignant external otitis occurs in elderly diabetics most commonly; may progress to deeper invasive infection.

Invasive Infections

Ecthyma Gangrenosum Begins as an erythematous macule (cutaneous ischemic lesion that quickly evolves to an infarction) (see Fig. 24-29*A, B*). The epidermis overlying the ischemic area may slough with formation of erosion/ulcer. EG usually occurs as a solitary lesion but may occur as a few lesions. EG can occur as a complication of primary or secondary pyoderma or of bacteremia. Initially erythematous, progressing to hemorrhagic bluish (so-called gunmetal gray). Fully evolved EG: blackish central necrosis with erythematous halo. Lesions usually tender, but may be painless. Most common sites: axillae, groin, perianal; may occur anywhere, including lip and tongue.

Disseminated Nodule Hematogenous dissemination of *P. aeruginosa* can seed the dermis, resulting in multiple tender subcutaneous nodules.

DIFFERENTIAL DIAGNOSIS

Necrotic Skin Lesion(s) Vasculitis, cryoglobulinemia, fixed drug eruption, pyoderma gangrenosum.

LABORATORY EXAMINATIONS

Cultures In most cases, *P. aeruginosa* can be cultured from both blood and ecthymatous skin lesions. However, EG can remain a localized cutaneous infection, not accompanied by systemic infection; in this case, only culture of exudate or biopsy specimen from the lesion is positive for *P. aeruginosa*.

Dermatopathology Vasculitis without thrombosis; paucity of neutrophils at site of infection; bacilli found in media and adventitia, but usually not in intima, of vessel.

DIAGNOSIS

Clinical suspicion confirmed by blood and skin exudate/biopsy specimen culture.

COURSE AND PROGNOSIS

- The heterogeneity of infections accounts for substantial differences in short-term and long-term prognosis.
- Prognosis depends on prompt restoration of altered immunity, usually on correction of neutropenia.
- When occurring as a local infection in the absence of bacteremia, prognosis is much more favorable.
- *Bacteremia*: may be associated with SIRS; fever, tachypnea, tachycardia, prostration, hypotension.
- *Endocarditis*: left-sided infections present with embolic phenomena: large emboli, ecthyma gangrenosum, Osler nodes, Janeway lesions (see Figs. 24-46 and 24-48).
- *Gastrointestinal infection*: "rose" spotlike lesions: erythematous macules and/or papules on trunk as in typhoid fever; occur with *Pseudomonas* infection of GI tract, i.e., diarrhea, headache, high fever (Shanghai fever).

MANAGEMENT OF INVASIVE INFECTIONS

Correct Predisposing Factors White cell transfusion or granulocyte colony-stimulating factor for granulocytopenia.

Antimicrobial Therapy Antibiotic and dosage are adjusted according to sensitivities and results of cultures.

Surgery After control of infection, areas of infarction should be debrided.

MYCOBACTERIAL INFECTIONS

- Mycobacteria are rod-shaped or coccobacilli; acid-fast bacilli (AFB); acid-fastness associated with composition of their cell walls
- >120 species identified; relatively few associated with human disease
- Mycobacterial infections
  - Tuberculosis
  - Leprosy (Hansen disease)

- Infections due to nontuberculous mycobacteria (NTM). Buruli ulcer disease (*M. ulcerans*) is the third most common mycobacterial disease globally.
- Tuberculosis due to BCG immunization

CLASSIFICATION OF MYCOBACTERIA AND MYCOBACTERIAL INFECTIONS

- *M. tuberculosis* complex: pathogenic in otherwise healthy individuals; however, tuberculosis is much more florid in immunocompromised hosts.
  - *M. tuberculosis*
  - *M. bovis*
  - *M. africanum*
- *M. leprae* causes disease in humans exclusively. Otherwise-healthy individuals become infected with this mycobacterium; clinical manifestations vary tremendously according to the host's immune response to the organism.

- Nontuberculous mycobacteria (NTM) exist in the environment; identification in human tissue, unlike *M. tuberculosis* or *M. leprae,* is not a sine qua non of etiology of a disorder.
  - Slow-growing NMT facultative human pathogens: *M. marinum*; *M. scrofulaceum*; *M. avium-intracellulare* complex; *M. haemophilum*; *M. ulcerans*
  - Fast-growing NMT facultative human pathogens: *M. fortuitum*; *M. chelonae*; *M. abscessus*

EPIDEMIOLOGY

With the advent of HIV/AIDS disease, tuberculosis and NTM infections have been brought to the forefront of clinical medicine. Concurrent HIV/AIDS and *M. tuberculosis* infections can result in severe infections; disseminated infections with NTM are extremely common in advanced HIV/AIDS disease.

LEPROSY   ICD-9:030 ∘ ICD-10:A30   □ → ■ ◑

- Etiology: *M. leprae*
- Chronic granulomatous disease principally acquired during childhood/young adulthood.
- Sites of infection: skin, peripheral nervous system, upper respiratory tract, eyes, testes
- Clinical manifestations, natural history, and prognosis of leprosy are related to the host response

- Various types of leprosy (tuberculoid, lepromatous, etc.) represent the spectra of the host's immunologic response (cell-mediated immunity).

Synonym: Hansen disease.

CLINICOPATHOLOGIC CLASSIFICATION OF LEPROSY

(Based on clinical, immunologic, and bacteriologic findings)

- *Tuberculoid (TL)*: Localized skin involvement and/or peripheral nerve involvement; few organisms.
- *Lepromatous (LL)*: Generalized involvement including skin, upper respiratory mucous membrane, reticuloendothelial system, adrenal glands, testes; many bacilli.
- *Borderline (or "dimorphic") (BL)*: Has features of both TL and LL. Usually many bacilli present, varied skin lesions: macules, plaques; progresses to TL or regresses to LL.

- *Indeterminate forms.*
- *Transitional forms*: See "Pathogenesis," below.

ETIOLOGY AND EPIDEMIOLOGY

Etiology   *M. leprae.* Obligate intracellular acid-fast bacillus; reproduces maximally at 27°C–30°C. Organism cannot be cultured in vitro. Infects skin and cutaneous nerves (Schwann cell basal lamina). In untreated patients, only 1% of organisms are viable. Grows best in cooler tissues (skin, peripheral nerves, anterior chamber of eye, upper respiratory tract, testes), sparing warmer areas of the skin (axilla, groin, scalp, and mid-line of back).

Age of Onset Incidence rate peaks at 10–20 years; prevalence peaks at 30–50 years.

Sex Males > females.

Race Inverse relationship between skin color and severity of disease; in black African, susceptibility is high, but there is predominance of milder forms of the disease, i.e., TL vis-à-vis LL.

Hosts Humans are main reservoirs of *M. leprae*. Wild armadillos (Louisiana) as well as mangabey monkeys and chimpanzees are naturally infected with *M. leprae*; armadillos can develop lepromatous lesions.

Transmission Uncertain; possible transmission includes nasal droplet infection, contact with infected soil, insect vectors. Sneeze from untreated LL patient may contain 10^{10} organisms. 20% of asymptomatic individuals in endemic areas may have *M. leprae* in the nose, identified by PCR. Portals of entry of *M. leprae* are poorly understood but include inoculation via skin (bites, scratches, small wounds, tattoos) or inhalation into nasal passages or lungs.

Demography Disease of developing world:

- 600,000 new cases annually
- 1.5–8 million total cases worldwide
- >80% of cases occur in India, China, Myanmar, Indochina, Indonesia, Brazil, Nigeria.
- In the United States: 4000 cases, 100–200 new cases annually; most cases are in immigrants from Mexico, Southeast Asia, Philippines, Caribbean; diagnosed in California, Texas, New York, and Hawaii
- Risk factors: poverty, rural residence, HAV/AIDS disease
- Most individuals have natural immunity and do not develop disease.

PATHOGENESIS

Clinical spectrum of leprosy depends exclusively on variable limitations in host's capability to develop effective cell-mediated immunity (CMI) to *M. leprae*. Organism is capable of invading and multiplying in peripheral nerves and infecting and surviving in endothelial and phagocytic cells in many organs. Subclinical infection with leprosy is common among residents in endemic areas. Presumably the subclinical infection is handled readily by the host's CMI response. Clinical expression of leprosy is development of a granuloma; patient may develop a "reactional state," which may occur in some form in >50% of certain groups of patients.

Granulomatous Spectrum of Leprosy

- High-resistance tuberculoid response (TT)
- Low- or absent-resistance lepromatous pole (LL)
- Morphic or borderline region (BB)
- Two intermediary regions
  - Borderline lepromatous (BL)
  - Borderline tuberculoid (BT)

In order of decreasing resistance, the spectrum is TT, BT, BB, BL, LL.

Immunologic Responses Immune responses to *M. leprae* can produce several types of reactions associated with a sudden change in the clinical status.

Lepra Type 1 Reactions (Downgrading and Reversal Reactions) Individuals with BT and BL develop inflammation within existing skin lesions. Can be associated with low-grade fever, new multiple small "satellite" maculopapular skin lesions, and/or neuritis. Downgrading reactions occur before therapy. Reversal reactions occur in response to therapy.

Lepra Type 2 Reactions (Erythema Nodosum Leprosum, ENL) Seen in half of LL patients, usually occurring after initiation of antilepromatous therapy, generally within the first 2 years of treatment. Massive inflammation with erythema nodosum–like lesions.

Lucio Reaction Individuals with diffuse LL develop shallow, large polygonal sloughing ulcerations on the legs. The reaction appears to be either a variant of ENL or secondary to arteriolar occlusion.

CLINICAL MANIFESTATION

Incubation Period 2–40 years (most commonly 5–7 years).

Onset Insidious and painless; first affects peripheral nervous system with persistent or recurrent painful paresthesias and numbness without any visible clinical signs. At this stage there may be transient macular skin eruptions; blister, but lack of awareness of trauma.

Systems Review Neural involvement leads to muscle weakness, muscle atrophy, severe neuritic pain, and contractures of the hands and feet.

Lepra Type 1 Reactions Acute or insidious tenderness and pain along affected nerve(s), associated with loss of function.

Tuberculoid Leprosy (TT, BT) *Skin* Most common form in India, Africa. Few well-defined hypopigmented hypesthetic macules (Fig. 24-60)

FIGURE 24-60 Leprosy: tuberculoid type Well-defined, hypopigmented, slightly scaling, anesthetic macules and plaques on the posterior trunk.

with raised edges and varying in size from a few millimeters to very large lesions covering the entire trunk. Erythematous or purple border and hypopigmented center. Sharply defined, raised; often annular; enlarge peripherally. Central area becomes atrophic/depressed. Advanced lesions are anesthetic, devoid of skin appendages (sweat glands, hair follicles). Any site including the face. *TT:* Lesions may resolve spontaneously; not associated with lepra reactions. *BT:* Does not heal spontaneously; type 1 lepra reactions may occur. *Nerve Involvement* May be a thickened nerve on the edge of the lesion; large peripheral nerve

enlargement frequent (ulnar). Skin involvement is absent in *neural leprosy.* Test pinprick, temperature, vibration.
Borderline BB Leprosy *Skin* Lesions are intermediate between tuberculoid and lepromatous and are composed of macules, papules, and plaques (Figs. 24-61 and 24-62). Anesthesia and decreased sweating are prominent in the lesions. 🖉
Lepromatous Leprosy (LL, BL) *Skin* Skin-colored or slightly erythematous papules/nodules. Lesions enlarge; new lesions occur and coalesce. Later: symmetrically distributed

nodules, raised plaques, diffuse dermal infiltrate, which on face results in loss of hair (lateral eyebrows and eyelashes) and leonine facies (lion's face). *Diffuse lepromatosis*, occurring in western Mexico, Caribbean, presents as diffuse dermal infiltration and thickened dermis. 🔲

Distribution of Lesions Bilaterally symmetric involving earlobes, face, arms, and buttocks, or less frequently the trunk and lower extremities. Tongue: nodules, plaques, or fissures.

Nerve Involvement More extensive than in TT.

Reactional States Immunologically mediated inflammatory states, occurring spontaneously or after initiation of therapy.

Lepra Type 1 Reactions Downgrading and reversal reactions. Occur in borderline disease. Skin lesions become acutely inflamed, associated with edema and pain; may ulcerate. Edema most severe on face, hands, and feet.

Lepra Type 2 Reactions (ENL) Occur in 50% of LL. 90% of cases occur after initiation of therapy. Present as painful red skin nodules arising superficially and deeply, in contrast to true erythema nodosum; lesions form abscesses or ulcerate. Lesions occur most commonly on face and extensor limbs.

Lucio Reaction Occurs only in patients from Mexico/Caribbean with diffuse LL. Presents as irregularly shaped erythematous plaques; lesions may resolve spontaneously or undergo necrosis with ulceration.

General Findings *Extremities* Sensory neuropathy, plantar ulcers, secondary infection; ulnar and peroneal palsies (Fig. 24-63), Charcot joints. Squamous cell carcinoma can arise in chronic foot ulcers (Fig. 11-13)

A

FIGURE 24-61 Leprosy: borderline-type A 31-year-old Vietnamese female. ***A.*** Geographic shaped plaque on the buttock with raised red indurated margins and central clearing. There is extension of the infection indicated by the erythematous papules beyond the margins. ***B.*** Similar geographic plaque on the legs with raised red margins and central clearing.

B

Nose Chronic nasal congestion, epistaxis; destruction of cartilage with saddle-nose deformity (Fig. 24-63).

Eyes Cranial nerve palsies, lagophthalmus, corneal insensitivity. In LL, anterior chamber can be invaded with uveitis, glaucoma, cataract formation. Corneal damage can occur secondary to trichiasis and sensory neuropathy, secondary infection, and muscle paralysis.

Testes May be involved in LL with resultant hypogonadism.

Amyloidosis Secondary with hepatic/renal abnormalities.

Complications Invasive squamous cell carcinoma (SCC) can arise in chronic neurotrophic ulcers on the lower extremities (see Fig. 11-13). The tumors are usually low-grade malignancies but can metastasize to regional lymph nodes and cause death.

DIFFERENTIAL DIAGNOSIS

Hypopigmented Lesions with Granulomas Sarcoidosis, leishmaniasis, lupus vulgaris, NTM infection, lymphoma, syphilis, yaws, granuloma annulare, necrobiosis lipoidica.

LABORATORY EXAMINATIONS

Slit-Skin Smears A small skin incision is made; the site is then scraped to obtain tissue fluid from which a smear is made and examined after Ziehl-Neelsen staining. Specimens are usually obtained from both earlobes and two other active lesions. Negative BIs are seen in paucibacillary cases, treated cases, and cases examined by an inexperienced technician.

Nasal Smears or Scrapings No longer recommended.

Culture *M. leprae* has not been cultured in vitro; however, it does grow when inoculated into the mouse foot pad. Routine bacterial cultures to rule out secondary infection.

PCR *M. leprae* DNA detected by this technique makes the diagnosis of early paucibacillary leprosy and identifies *M. leprae* after therapy.

Dermatopathology TL shows epithelioid cell granulomas forming around dermal nerves; AFB are sparse or absent. LL shows an extensive cellular infiltrate separated from the epidermis by a narrow zone of normal collagen. Skin appendages are destroyed. Macrophages are filled with *M. leprae*, having abundant foamy or vacuolated cytoplasm (lepra cells or Virchow cells).

A

B

FIGURE 24-62 Leprosy: borderline-type A 26-year-old Vietnamese male. **A.** Well-demarcated, infiltrated, erythematous plaques on the face. **B.** Identical red plaques on the lower back.

DIAGNOSIS

Made if one or more of the cardinal findings are detected: patient from endemic area, skin lesions characteristic of leprosy with diminished or loss of sensation, enlarged peripheral nerves, finding of *M. leprae* in skin or, less commonly, other sites.

COURSE AND PROGNOSIS

After the first few years of drug therapy, the most difficult problem is management of the changes secondary to neurologic deficits—contractures and trophic changes in the hands and feet. Uncommonly, secondary amyloidosis with renal failure can complicate long-standing leprosy. Lepra type 1 reactions last 2–4 months in individuals with BT and up to 9 months in those with BL. Lepra type 2 reactions (ENL) occur in 50% of individuals with LL and 25% of those with BL within the first 2 years of treatment. ENL may be complicated by uveitis, dactylitis, arthritis, neuritis, lymphadenitis, myositis, orchitis. Lucio reaction or phenomenon occurs secondary to vasculitis with subsequent infarction.

MANAGEMENT

General principles of management:

- Eradicate infection with antilepromatous therapy (Table 24-9).
- Prevent and treat reactions.
- Reduce the risk of nerve damage.
- Educate patient to deal with neuropathy and anesthesia.
- Treat complications of nerve damage.
- Rehabilitate patient into society.

Management involves a broad multidisciplinary approach including orthopedic surgery, podiatry, ophthalmology, and physical therapy.

FIGURE 24-63 Leprosy: lepromatous type A 60-year-old Vietnamese female with treated advanced disease. Ulnar palsy, loss of digits on right hand, and saddle-nose deformity associated with loss of nasal cartilage are seen.

TABLE 24-9 Antimicrobial Regimens Recommended for Treatment of Leprosy in Adults

Form of Leprosy	More Intensive Regimen	WHO-Recommended Regimen (1982)
Tuberculoid (paucibacillary)	Dapsone (100 mg/d) for 5 years	Dapsone (100 mg/d unsupervised) *plus* rifampin (600 mg/month supervised) for 6 months
Lepromatous (multibacillary)	Rifampin (600 mg/month) for 3 years *plus* dapsone (100 mg/d) indefinitely	Dapsone (100 mg/d) *plus* (300 mg) clofazimine (50 mg/d, unsupervised); and rifampin (600 mg) *plus* clofazimine monthly (supervised) for 1 year

Therapy of Reactions *Lepra Type 1 Reactions* Prednisone, 40–60 mg/d; the dosage is gradually reduced over a 2- to 3-month period. Indications for prednisone: neuritis, lesions that threaten to ulcerate, lesions appearing at cosmetically important sites (face).
Lepra Type 2 Reactions (ENL) Prednisone, 40–60 mg/d, tapered fairly rapidly; thalidomide for recurrent ENL, 100–300 mg/d.
Lucio Reaction Neither prednisone nor thalidomide is very effective. Since there is no other

alternative, prednisone, 40–60 mg/d, tapered fairly rapidly.
Systemic Antimicrobial Agents Secondary infection of ulcerations should be identified and treated with appropriate antibiotics to prevent deeper infections such as osteomyelitis.
Orthopedic Care Splints should be supplied to prevent contractures of denervated regions. Careful attention to foot care to prevent neuropathic ulceration.

CUTANEOUS TUBERCULOSIS (CTB) ICD-9:017.0 ∘ ICD-10:A18.4

- Etiology: *Mycobacterium tuberculosis* complex; *M. tuberculosis* (MTb); *M. bovis, M. caprae, M. africanum, M. microti, M. pinnipedii, M. canetti;* occasionally bacillus Calmette-Guérin (BCG)
- Transmission: airborne spread of droplet nuclei from those with infectious pulmonary Tb
- Demography
  - Up to 10% of those infected with MTb will develop active Tb in their lifetime
  - Incidence of Tb highest in late adolescence and early adulthood
  - One-third of global population infected
  - In United States, estimated that 15 million are infected
  - 8–9 million new infections annually
  - 2–3 million TB-related deaths annually worldwide
  - Children: 1.5 million new cases; 500,000 deaths
  - Globally, main cause of death in HIV/AIDS
- Predisposing factors (exogenous factor) for acquiring MTb infection: poverty, crowding, HIV/AIDS pandemic, social disruption
- Factors for developing tuberculous disease (endogenous):
  - Innate immunologic and nonimmunologic defenses
  - Level of function of cell-mediated immunity (CMI)

- Sites of infection
  - Most commonly infected lungs
  - Cutaneous infection
    - Cutaneous inoculation (rare)
    - Direct extension (e.g., from joint)
    - Lymphatic spread
    - Hematogenous spread
- Risk factors for active Tb among MTb-infected persons
- Recent infection (<1 year)
  - Fibrotic lesions
  - Comorbidity: HIV/AIDS, immunosuppressive therapy, posttransplantation (solid organ, i.e., kidney, liver, heart, lung), silicosis, end-stage renal disease/hemodialysis, diabetes, injecting drug use, gastrectomy, jejunoileal bypass
  - Malnutrition
- Diagnosis: clinical findings, histopathology, relevant mycobacteria in tissue or culture, host reaction to MTb antigen
- Course/prognosis
  - Properly treated, caused by drug-susceptible strains curable in virtually all cases
  - Untreated, may be fatal within 5 years
  - Multidrug resistant (MDR) Tb is an emerging infection
- Treatment: standard multidrug regimens

Synonyms: Phthisis, consumption

CLASSIFICATION OF CUTANEOUS TUBERCULOSIS

- Exogenous inoculation: Skin inoculation
  - Primary inoculation tuberculosis (PIT), i.e., tuberculous chancre: occurs at inoculated site in nonimmune host.

- Tuberculosis verrucosa cutis (TVC): occurs at inoculated site in individual with prior tuberculosis infection.
- Endogenous spread: Lymphatics, hematogenous, bodily fluids (sputum, feces, urine)
  - Lupus vulgaris (LV)
  - Scrofuloderma (SD)

° Metastatic tuberculosis abscess (MTA)
° Acute miliary tuberculosis (AMT)
° Orificial tuberculosis (OT)

• Tuberculosis due to BCG immunization

EPIDEMIOLOGY AND ETIOLOGY

Type of clinical lesion depends on route of cutaneous inoculation and immunologic status of the host. Cutaneous inoculation results in a tuberculous chancre in the nonimmune host but TVC in the immune host. Modes of endogenous spread to skin include the following: direct extension from underlying tuberculous infection, i.e., lymphadenitis or tuberculosis of bones and joints, results in SD; lymphatic spread to skin, results in LV; hematogenous dissemination, results in AMT, LV, or MTA; autoinoculation from body fluids (sputum, urine, feces).

Age of Onset   AMT more common in infants and adults with advanced immunodeficiency. PIT more common in infants. SD more common in adolescents, elderly. LV affects all ages.

Sex   LV more common in females. TVC more common in males.

Occupation   TVC: historically in physicians, medical students, and pathologists as verruca necrogenica, anatomist's wart, postmortem wart; in butchers and farmers from *M. bovis*.

Incidence   CTb has declined steadily worldwide, paralleling decline of pulmonary tuberculosis. Always rare in the United States compared with Europe. Incidence of various types of CTb varies geographically; LV, SD most common types in Europe; LV, verrucous lesions more common in tropics; TVC a common type in developing countries. Currently, the incidence of CTb has been increasing, associated with HIV/AIDS disease.

Tuberculosis in HIV/AIDS Disease   Tuberculosis is the most common opportunistic infection occurring in HAV/AIDS-infected individuals who reside in developing nations; CTb has been reported in these individuals. Problem of multidrug resistance (MDR) is also common in these persons.

PATHOGENESIS

Clinical lesions occurring in skin depend on whether host has had prior infection with *M. tuberculosis*, and therefore delayed hypersensitivity to the organism, and inoculation route and mode of spread.

CLINICAL MANIFESTATION

Primary Inoculation Tuberculosis (Tuberculous Chancre)   Initially, papule occurs at the inoculation site 2–4 weeks after the wound. Lesion enlarges to a painless ulcer, i.e., a tuberculous chancre (up to 5 cm) (Fig. 24-64), with shallow granular base and multiple tiny abscesses or may be covered by thick crust. Undermined margins; older ulcers become indurated with thick crusts. Deeper inoculation results in subcutaneous abscess. Most common on exposed skin at sites of minor injuries. Oral lesions occur after ingestion of bovine bacilli in nonpasteurized milk; in the past, lesions in male babies have occurred on the penis after ritual circumcision. Intraoral inoculation results in ulcers on gingiva or palate. Regional lymphadenopathy occurs within 3–8 weeks.

Tuberculosis Verrucosa Cutis   Initial papule with violaceous halo. Evolves to hyperkeratotic, warty, firm plaque (Fig. 24-65). Clefts and fissures occur from which pus and keratinous material can be expressed. Border often irregular. Lesions are usually single, but multiple lesions occur. Most commonly on dorsolateral hands and fingers. In children, lower extremities, knees. No lymphadenopathy.

Lupus Vulgaris   Initial papule ill defined and soft and evolves into well-defined, irregular plaque (Fig. 24-66). Reddish-brown: diascopy (i.e., use of glass slide pressed against skin) reveals an "apple jelly" (i.e., yellowish-brown) color. Consistency is characteristically soft; if lesion is probed, instrument breaks through overlying epidermis. Surface is initially smooth or slightly scaly but may become hyperkeratotic. Hypertrophic forms result in soft tumorous nodules. Ulcerative forms present as punched-out, often serpiginous ulcers surrounded by soft, brownish infiltrate. Usually solitary, but several sites may occur. Most lesions on the head and neck, most often on nose and ears or scalp. Lesions on trunk and extremities rare. Disseminated lesions after severe viral infection (measles) (*lupus postexanthematicus*). Involvement of underlying cartilage but not bone results in its destruction (ears, nose). Scarring is prominent, and, characteristically, new brownish infiltrates occur within atrophic scars.

Scrofuloderma   Firm subcutaneous nodule that initially is freely movable; lesion then becomes doughy and evolves into irregular, deep-seated node or plaque that liquefies and perforates (Fig. 24-67). Ulcers and irregular sinuses, usually of linear or serpiginous shape,

FIGURE 24-64 Primary inoculation tuberculosis A large, ulcerated nodule at the site of *Mycobacterium*. Tuberculosis inoculation on the right thigh associated with inguinal lymphadenopathy. The erythematous papules on the left forearm occurred at the site of tuberculin testing.

discharge pus or caseous material (Fig. 24-68). Edges are undermined, inverted, and dissecting subcutaneous pockets alternating with soft, fluctuating infiltrates and bridging scars. Most often occurs in the parotidal, submandibular, and supraclavicular regions; lateral neck; SD most often results from contiguous spread from affected lymph nodes or tuberculous bones (phalanges, sternum, ribs) or joints.

Metastatic Tuberculosis Abscess Also called *tuberculous gumma*. Subcutaneous abscess, nontender, "cold," fluctuant. Coalescing with overlying skin, breaking down and forming fistulas and ulcers. Single or multiple lesions, often at sites of previous trauma.

Acute Miliary Tuberculosis Exanthem. Disseminated lesions are minute macules and papules or purpuric lesions. Sometimes vesicular and crusted. Removal of crust reveals umbilication. Disseminated on all parts of body, particularly trunk.

Orificial Tuberculosis Small yellowish nodule on mucosa breaks down to form painful

FIGURE 24-65 Tuberculosis verrucosa cutis Crusted and hyperkeratotic plaque arising at the site of inoculation in an individual previously infected with *M. tuberculosis*. There is no associated lymphadenopathy.

FIGURE 24-66   Lupus vulgaris   Reddish-brown plaque, which on diascopy exhibits the diagnostic yellow-brown apple-jelly color. Note nodular infiltration of the earlobe, scaling of the helix, and atrophic scarring in the center of the plaque.

circular or irregular ulcer (Fig. 24-69) with undermined borders and pseudomembranous material, yellowish tubercles, and eroded vessels at base. Surrounding mucosa swollen, edematous, and inflamed. Since OT results from autoinoculation of mycobacteria from progressive tuberculosis of internal organs, it is usually found on the oral, pharyngeal (pulmonary tuberculosis), vulvar (genitourinary tuberculosis), and anal (intestinal tuberculosis) mucous membranes. Lesions may be single or multiple, and in the mouth most often occur on the tongue, soft and hard palate, or lips. OT may occur in a tooth socket after tooth extraction. 🖊

DIFFERENTIAL DIAGNOSIS

Primary Inoculation Tuberculosis   Chancriform syndrome: primary syphilis with chancre, cat-scratch disease, sporotrichosis, tularemia, *M. marinum* infection.
Tuberculosis Verrucosa Cutis   Verruca vulgaris, *M. marinum* infection, blastomycosis, chromomycosis, ecthyma, hypertrophic lichen planus, squamous cell carcinoma (SCC).
Lupus Vulgaris   Sarcoidosis, lymphocytoma, lymphoma, chronic cutaneous lupus erythematosus, tertiary syphilis, leprosy, blastomycosis, lupoid leishmaniasis.
Scrofuloderma   Invasive fungal infections, sporotrichosis, nocardiosis, actinomycosis, tertiary syphilis, acne conglobata, hidradenitis suppurativa.
Metastatic Tuberculosis Abscess   Panniculitis, invasive fungal infections, hidradenitis, tertiary syphilis.
Orificial Tuberculosis   Aphthous ulcers, histoplasmosis, syphilis, SCC.

FIGURE 24-67   Scrofuloderma: clavicle area
Large abscess near the clavicular head, which on pressure extrudes pus and caseous material. A tuberculous lymphadenitis undergoes necrosis with abscess formation, subsequently draining to the skin surface.

FIGURE 24-68   Scrofuloderma: lateral chest wall.   Two ulcers on the chest wall and axilla are associated with underlying sinus tracts.

FIGURE 24-69   Orificial tuberculosis: lips   A large, very painful ulcer on the lips of this patient with advanced cavitary pulmonary tuberculosis.

LABORATORY EXAMINATIONS

Dermatopathology   PIT: initially nonspecific inflammation; after 3–6 weeks, epithelioid cells, Langhans giant cells, lymphocytes, caseation necrosis. AMT: nonspecific inflammation and vasculitis. All other forms of CTb show more or less typical tuberculous histopathology; TVC is characterized by massive pseudoepitheliomatous hyperplasia of epidermis and abscesses. Mycobacteria are found in PIT, SD, AMT, MTA, and OT but only with difficulty or not at all in LV and TVC.

Culture   Yields mycobacteria also from lesions of LV and TVC.

PCR   Can be used to identify *M. tuberculosis* DNA in tissue specimens.

Skin Testing   PIT: Patient converts from intradermal skin test negative to positive (Fig. 24-70) during the first weeks of the infection. AMT: usually negative. SD, MTA, and OT: may be negative or positive depending on state of immunity. LV and TVC: positive.

DIAGNOSIS

Clinical, histologic findings, confirmed by isolation of *M. tuberculosis* on culture or by PCR.

COURSE AND PROGNOSIS

The course of CTb is quite variable, depending on the type of cutaneous infection, amount of inoculum, extent of extracutaneous infection, age of the patient, immune status, and therapy. PIT: without treatment, usually resolves within 12 months, with some residual scarring. Rarely, LV develops at site of PIT. Tuberculosis due to BCG immunization: depends on general state of immunity. It may assume appearance and course of PIT, LV, or SD; in immunocompromised may lead to MTA or AMT.

MANAGEMENT

Only PIT and TVC limited to the skin. All other patterns of CTb are associated with systemic infection that has disseminated secondarily to skin. As such, therapy should be aimed at achieving a cure, avoiding relapse, and preventing emergence of drug-resistant mutants.

Antituberculous Therapy   Prolonged antituberculous therapy with at least two drugs is indicated for all cases of CTb except for TVC that can be excised.

- Standard antituberculous therapy:
  - Isoniazid (5 mg/kg daily) *plus*
  - Rifampin (600 mg/kg daily)

- Supplemented in initial phases with:
  - Ethambutol (25 mg/kg daily) *and/or*
  - Streptomycin (10–15 mg/kg daily) *and/or*
  - Pyrazinamide (15–30 mg/kg daily)

Isoniazid and rifampin for at least 9 months; can be shortened to 6 months if four drugs are given during the first 2 months.

Multidrug Resistant (MDR) Tb   Incidence is increasing.

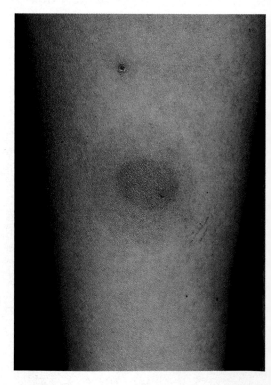

FIGURE 24-70   Purified protein derivative or Mantoux test: positive test   A 31-year-old Taiwanese female with psoriasis, with a negative skin test one year previously, was retested prior to beginning entanercept. She had become infected while visiting her father, who had pulmonary tuberculosis, in Taiwan. A red plaque with surrounding erythema is seen at the test site.

NONTUBERCULOUS MYCOBACTERIAL INFECTIONS ICD-9 : 031.1 ○ ICD-10 : A31.1

- Nontuberculous mycobacteria (NTM) defined as mycobacteria other than *M. tuberculosis* complex and *M. leprae*
- The original classification of NTM depended on speed of growth, morphology, and pigmentation of colonies on solid media as well as biochemical reactions (Table 24-10). Currently, however, molecular probes are used for rapid identification of the most important species in a positive culture; hybridization of the probe to specific sequences of the mycobacteria.
- Occur naturally in the environment
- Capable of causing primary infections in otherwise healthy individuals and more serious infection in immunocompromised, e.g., *M. marinum, M. ulcerans,* and *M. fortuitum* complex

- Immunocompetent individuals: primary cutaneous infections at sites of inoculation. Nodules, lymphocutaneous or sporotrichoid lesions. Furunculosis.
- Immunocompromised host: disseminated mucosal and cutaneous lesions
- Diagnosis: detection of mycobacteria histochemically or by culture on specific media
- New molecular techniques based on DNA amplification accelerate diagnosis, identify common sources of infection, reveal new types of NTM
- Treatment: clarithromycin, rifampicin, fluoroquinolones, minocycline

Synonyms: Atypical mycobacteria, mycobacteria other than tuberculosis (MOTT)

TABLE 24-10   Species of Nontuberculous Mycobacterium (NTM) Causing Cutaneous Infection

Species	Growth on Solid Media	Environmental Reservoir	Cutaneous Infection
M. marinum	Slow	Fish tanks, salt water	Most common
			Verrucous nodule/plaque
			Chancriform lesion
			Sporotrichoid infections
			Solitary plaque on face
M. ulcerans	Slow	Natural water	Ulcerous osteomyelitis
M. abscessus	Rapid	Natural and potable water; soil	Inflammatory plaque at injection site
M. fortuitum	Rapid	Natural and potable water; soil	Mycobacterial furunculosis
M. chelonae	Rapid	Natural and potable water; soil	Nodules, ulcerated nodules
M. haemophilum	Slow Fastidious	Unknown	Cutaneous nodules, ulcerated nodules, sporotrichoid pattern, myositis, lymphadenitis, disseminated infection in immunocompromised patients

MYCOBACTERIUM MARINUM INFECTION

- Etiology: *M. marinum*
- Exposure in aqueous environment, i.e., fish tank, pool, water
- Infection follows traumatic inoculation
- Clinical findings:
  - Nodule(s): verrucous, eroded.
  - Lymphocutaneous extension with sporotrichoid pattern.
  - Tenosynovitis

- Diagnosis: Isolate *M. marinum* on culture
- Treatment: Clarithromycin or minocycline. Combination antituberculous therapy

Synonyms: Fish tank granuloma, swimming pool granuloma

EPIDEMIOLOGY

Age of Onset   Second to fourth decades.
Sex   Males > females.
Etiology   *M. marinum.*
Exposure   Tropical fish tanks; lesions usually on dominant hand. Chlorination has reduced transmission in swimming pools.

CLINICAL MANIFESTATION

Incubation Period   Variable: usually 1 week to 2 months after inoculation.
Duration of Lesions   Weeks to months.

Symptoms   Commonly asymptomatic. Possible local tenderness; limitation of movement if lesion over a joint; with deeper extension, pain.
Skin Lesions   Inoculation site: papule(s) enlarging to inflammatory, red to red-brown nodule or plaque 1–4 cm in size on dominant hand. Surface of lesions may be hyperkeratotic/verrucous (Fig. 24-71). May become ulcerated: superficial crust, granulation tissue base, ± serosanguineous or purulent discharge. In some cases, small satellite papules, draining sinuses, fistulas may develop. Usually solitary, over bony prominence. More extensive soft tissue infection may occur, with osteomyelitis,

FIGURE 24-71   *M. marinum*: inoculation site infection on the foot   A 31-year-old male with painful indurated plaque on the lateral dorsal foot. The lesion arose at the site of a small blister one year ago while in Afghanistan. Three previous biopsies and tissue cultures had been unsuccessful at making a diagnosis. After intralesional injection of triamcinolone 1.5 mg/mL, acid–fast bacilli were identified in the biopsy specimen and *M. marinum* isolated on culture. He was successfully treated with four antimycobacterial agents. Old World leishmaniasis was on the differential diagnosis of this lesion.

in the immunocompromised host. Atrophic scarring follows spontaneous regression or successful therapy. 🖉

Sporotrichoid or Lymphocutaneous Pattern Deep-seated nodules in a linear configuration on hand and forearm exhibit lymphocutaneous spread (Fig. 24-72). Boggy inflammatory reaction may mimic bursitis, synovitis, or arthritis about the elbow, wrist, or interphalangeal joints. Tenosynovitis.

Disseminated Infection Rare. May occur in immunocompromised host.

Lymph Nodes Regional lymphadenopathy uncommon.

DIFFERENTIAL DIAGNOSIS

Solitary Verrucous/Ulcerated Lesion on Extremity Verruca vulgaris, sporotrichosis, blastomycosis, erysipeloid, tularemia, tuberculosis verrucosa cutis, nocardiosis, leishmaniasis, syphilis, yaws, iododerma, bromoderma, foreign-body response to sea urchin or barnacle, benign or malignant skin tumors.

Sporotrichoid Lesion Staphylococcal or group A streptococcal lymphangitis, sporotrichosis, tularemia, leishmaniasis, nocardiosis, actinomycosis.

LABORATORY EXAMINATIONS

Skin Tests Intradermal tuberculin test (PPD-S) often positive.

Skin Biopsy Suggestive but not pathognomonic. Older lesions: More typical tuberculoid architecture is developed with epithelioid cells and Langhans giant cells. Acid-fast stain demonstrates *M. marinum* only in approximately 50% of cases.

Direct Microscopy

Smears of Exudate or Pus Acid-fast bacilli can be demonstrated in some cases.

Culture *M. marinum* grows at 32°C (but not at 37°C) in 2–4 weeks. Early lesions yield numerous colonies. Lesions 3 months or older generally yield few colonies.

DIAGNOSIS

History of trauma in an aqueous environment, clinical findings, confirmed by isolation of *M. marinum* on culture.

COURSE AND PROGNOSIS

Most usually benign and self-limited but can remain active for a prolonged period. Single papulonodular lesions resolve spontaneously within 3 months to 3 years, whereas sporotrichoid form can persist for years. In the immunocompromised host, most extensive deep infection can occur.

FIGURE 24-72 *M. marinum*: **lymphocutaneous infection beginning on finger** A 48-year-old female with painful swelling of the right middle finger for 4 months. She recalled cleaning a fish tank several weeks before the distal digital became red and tender. The finger and hand became progressively more inflamed and red nodules appeared on the forearm. Slight enlargement of axillary nodes was detected.

MANAGEMENT

Prophylaxis Wear waterproof gloves when working in fish tank.

Antibiotics Drug of first choice: clarithromycin and either rifampin or ethambutol for 1–2 months after lesion(s) have resolved (3–4 months). Minocycline alone may be effective. Susceptibility testing is not routinely recommended and should be reserved for cases of treatment failure.

Surgical Debridement May be required for deep tissue involvement, especially in immunocompromised host.

MYCOBACTERIUM ULCERANS INFECTION ICD-9:031.1 ∘ ICD-10:A31.1 □→□ ◑

- Etiology: *M. ulcerans*
- Transmission: insect bite, i.e., mosquitoes; traumatic inoculation
- Geography: occurs in >30 countries. Tropical regions of west Africa; Australia, Papua New Guinea; Central Mexico. Climate: humid, hot.
- Pathogenesis: *M. ulcerans* produces mycolactone, which has a toxic effect on tissue and inhibits immune response
- Age: 10–14 years; 75–79 years.
- Sex: more common in males in older individuals
- Incidence: third most common mycobacterial infection after tuberculosis and leprosy

- Clinical findings:
  - Lesions: papules evolving to large ulcers. May be multiple. Osteomyelitis.
  - Distribution: extremities; lower more often than upper
- Diagnosis: identification of microbe on culture or by PCR
- Course: ulcers in older age may be reactivation of latent infection. Spontaneous healing may occur.

Synonyms: Buruli ulcer, Buruli ulcer disease (BUD) (Africa); Bairnsdale or Daintree ulcer (Australia)

EPIDEMIOLOGY

Age of Onset Children, young adults.

Etiology *M. ulcerans.* An environmental habitat for the organism has not been established. Progenitor of *M. ulcerans* thought to be *M. marinum.*

Sex Females > males.

Transmission Inoculation probably via minor trauma occurring in wet, marshy, or swampy sites. Bites of aquatic insects; *M. ulcerans* replicates in insect salivary glands; in endemic areas, 5–10% of aquatic insects have microbe in salivary gland.

Demography Tropics, most infections in Africa and Australia.

PATHOGENESIS

A secreted polyketide toxin, mycolactone, suppresses immune response to microbe.

CLINICAL MANIFESTATION

Incubation Period Approximately 3 months.

Symptoms The early nodule at site of trauma and subsequent ulceration are usually painless.

Skin Lesions A painless subcutaneous swelling occurs at the site of inoculation. Papule(s), nodule(s), plaques often overlooked. Lesion enlarges and ulcerates. The ulcer extends into the subcutaneous fat, and its margin is deeply undermined (Fig. 24-73). Ulcerations may enlarge to involve an entire extremity. Legs more commonly involved (sites of trauma). Any site may be involved. Soft tissue and bony involvement can occur. As ulcerations healed, scarring and disabling deformities may occur.

Systemic Findings Fever, constitutional findings are usually absent. Regional lymph nodes usually not enlarged. Underlying destructive osteomyelitis.

DIFFERENTIAL DIAGNOSIS

Subcutaneous Induration Panniculitis, phycomycosis, nodular vasculitis, pyomyositis.

Large Cutaneous Ulceration Blastomycosis, sporotrichosis, nocardiosis, actinomycosis, mycetoma, chromomycosis, pyoderma gangrenosum, basal cell carcinoma, squamous cell carcinoma, necrotizing soft tissue infections.

FIGURE 24-73 *M. ulcerans:* **Buruli ulcer** A 15-year-old Ugandan male with a huge ulcer with a clean base and undermined margins extends into the subcutaneous tissue. (Courtesy of M. Dittrich, MD.)

LABORATORY EXAMINATIONS

Bacterial Culture Rule out secondary bacterial infection.
Mycobacterial Culture *M. ulcerans* grows optimally at 32°–33°C.
PCR Reported to be effective.
Dermatopathology Necrosis originates in the interlobular septa of the subcutaneous fat. Poor inflammatory response despite clusters of extracellular bacilli. Ulceration is surrounded by granulation tissue with giant cells but no caseation necrosis or tubercles. Acid-fast bacilli are always demonstrable.

DIAGNOSIS

Clinical findings confirmed by isolation of *M. ulcerans* from lesional skin biopsy specimen.

COURSE AND PROGNOSIS

Because of delay in diagnosis and treatment, lesions are often extensive at presentation. Ulcerations tend to persist for months to years.

Spontaneous healing occurs eventually in many patients. Ulceration and healing can be complicated by scarring, contracture of the limb, and lymphedema. Malnutrition and anemia delay healing.

MANAGEMENT

Prevention Cover exposed extremities with clothing; bed netting. Avoid mosquito bites. Insect repellants. Immediately wash minor skin wounds.
Symptomatic In that *M. ulcerans* prefers cooler temperatures, application of heat to the involved site has been reported to be effective. Improve nutritional status.
Antimycobacterial Drug Therapy WHO recommends rifampicin and streptomycin (requires IM injection) combined with surgery. Combination of rifampicin and ciprofloxacin may be effective. Streptomycin. 8 weeks of antibiotic treatment may reverse local immunosuppression.
Surgery Excision of the infected tissue with a small rim of normal tissue, usually followed by grafting. Reconstructive surgery.

MYCOBACTERIUM FORTUITUM COMPLEX (MFC) INFECTIONS   ICD-9:031.1 ∘ ICD-10:A31.1

- Etiology: *M. fortuitum, M. chelonae, M. abscessus*
- Natural reservoirs: water, soil, nosocomial environments
- Cutaneous infection account for 60% of MFC infections

- Clinical findings:
  - Immunocompetent individuals: localized infection in traumatic or surgical wounds, injections sites
  - Immunosuppressed individuals: disseminated cutaneous infection
- Treatment: Antibiotic(s) ± surgery

EPIDEMIOLOGY

Age of Onset   Children, young adults.
Sex   Females > males.
Etiology   MFC organisms include *M. fortuitum, M. chelonae, M. abscessus.*
Natural Reservoirs   The organisms are widely distributed in soil, dust, and water. Can be isolated from tap water, municipal water supplies, moist areas in hospitals, contaminated biologicals, aquariums, domestic animals, marine life.
Transmission   Inoculation via traumatic puncture wounds or surgical procedures/injections. Silicone injections. Whirlpool footbaths in nail salons (*M. fortuitum*).

CLINICAL MANIFESTATION

Incubation Period   Usually within 1 month (range 1 week to 2 years).
History   Surgical wound infections follow augmentation mammaplasty, median sternotomy, and percutaneous catheterizations.
Symptoms   Infection presents as a painful traumatic or surgical wound infection.
Skin Lesions   Postinjection abscesses. Traumatic wound infections (Fig. 24-74) present as dark red, infiltrated nodule, ± abscess formation, ± drainage of serous exudate. Linear lesions, commonly at incision sites. Traumatic infection occurs more commonly on the extremities. Surgical infections occur in scars of median sternotomy and augmentation mammaplasty. Foot baths associated with furunculosis. In immunocompromised individuals, infection can disseminate hematogenously to skin (multiple recurring abscesses on the extremities) and joints.
General Findings   Other primary MFC infections include pneumonitis, osteomyelitis, lymphadenitis, postsurgical endocarditis.

DIFFERENTIAL DIAGNOSIS

Traumatic and Postoperative Wound Infection   *S. aureus* and group A streptococcus infections, various other bacteria, foreign-body reaction, allergic contact dermatitis to topically applied agent, *Candida albicans* infection, *Aspergillus* spp. infection.

LABORATORY EXAMINATIONS

Bacterial Culture   Rule out secondary bacterial infection.
Mycobacterial Culture   MFC organisms usually can be isolated on primary culture in 2–30 days.
PCR   May be diagnostic if available
Dermatopathology   Polymorphonuclear microabscesses and granuloma formation with foreign-body–type giant cells (dimorphic inflammatory response) are seen. Necrosis is often present without caseation. AFB can be seen within microabscesses.

DIAGNOSIS

Clinical findings confirmed by isolation of MFC from lesional skin biopsy specimen or identifiy by PCR.

COURSE AND PROGNOSIS

The infection becomes chronic unless treated with antimycobacterial therapy, ± surgical debridement.

MANAGEMENT

Antimycobacterial Chemotherapy   Depends on species and sensitivities. Effective agents include clarithromycin, amikacin, cefoxitin, imipenem, doxycycline, fluoroquinolone.
Surgery   Debridement with delayed closure is effective for localized infections.

FIGURE 24-74 *M. fortuitum* **infection** A 45-year-old female with erythematous tender nodules on the lower legs. The lesions occurred several weeks after a pedicure in a foot care salon. Shaving of legs may have facilitated the infection. *M. fortuitum* was isolated on culture of skin biopsy specimen.

LYME BORRELIOSIS (LB)   ICD-9:088.81 ∘ ICD-10:A69.2   ■ ◑

- A complex, multisystem disease
- Etiologic agent: *Borrelia* spirochetes
- Transmitted to humans by the bite of an infected ixodid tick
- Three stages of LB:
  - Stage 1 is localized
- Stage 2 (untreated stage 1) is disseminated
- Stage 3 is persistent infection, developing months or years later
- The clinical findings associated with each stage are listed in Table 24-11.
- *Synonym*: Lyme disease

EPIDEMIOLOGY AND ETIOLOGY

Etiologic Agent   *B. burgdorferi* sensu lato (*B. burgdorferi* in the general sense); 13 closely related species have been identified. LB is caused by three pathogenic genospecies. Clinical variations of disease occurring in North America, Europe, and Asia may be related to differences in the various causative strains. *B. burgdorferi* has been identified in 19 states in the United States.

Vector   Infected nymphal tick of genus *Ixodes racinus* complex. Three stages of tick development: larval, nymphal, adult; each stage requires blood meal. Preferred host for larval and nymphal *I. scapularis* is white-footed mouse (and certain other rodents). The tiny nymphal tick transmits *B. burgdorferi* to humans in early summer. Preferred host of adult *I. scapularis* (Fig. 24-75) is white-tailed deer, which is not involved in life cycle of spirochete but is critical to the survival of the tick. In United States, *I. scapularis* also transmits babesiosis and human anaplasmosis. In Europe and Asia, *I. ricinus* and *I. persulcatus* also transmit tick-borne encephalitis.

Transmission   Ticks cling to vegetation; are most numerous in brushy, wooded, or grassy habitats; not found on open sandy beaches. *B. burgdorferi* is transmitted to humans after biting and feeding of nymphs or, less commonly, adult ticks. Transmission to humans occurs in association with hiking, camping, or hunting trips and with residence in wooded or rural areas.

Season   In the midwestern and eastern United States, late May through early fall (80% of early LB begins in June and July). In the Pacific Northwest, January through May.

Risk for Exposure   Strongly associated with prevalence of tick vectors and proportion of those ticks that carry *B. burgdorferi*. In the northeastern United States with endemic disease, the infection rate of the nymphal *I. scapularis* tick with *B. burgdorferi* is commonly 20–35%. Risk associated with hiking, camping, or hunting trips and with residence in wooded or rural area.

Incidence   LB is the most common vector-borne infection in the United States, with >20,000 cases reported annually.

PATHOGENESIS

After inoculation into the skin as nymphal tick feeds, spirochetes replicate and migrate outward, producing the erythema migrans (EM) lesion, and invade vessels, spreading hematogenously to other organs. The spirochete has a particular trophism for tissues of the skin, nervous system, and joints. The organism persists in affected tissues during all stages of the illness. The immune response to the spirochete develops gradually. Specific IgM antibodies peak between the third and sixth weeks after disease onset. The specific IgG response develops gradually over months. Proinflammatory cytokines TNF-α, and IL-1 are produced in affected tissues.

CLINICAL MANIFESTATION

Incubation Period   EM: 3–32 days after tick bite. Cardiac manifestations: 35 days (3 weeks to >5 months after tick bite). Neurologic manifestions: average 38 days (2 weeks to months) after tick bite. Rheumatologic manifestations: 67 days (4 days to 2 years) after bite.

Prodrome   With disseminated infection (stage 2), malaise, fatigue, lethargy, headache, fever, chills, stiff neck, arthralgia, myalgia, backache, anorexia, sore throat, nausea, dysesthesia, vomiting, abdominal pain, photophobia.

History   Because of small size of nymphal tick, most patients are unaware of tick bite. Ixodid tick bites are asymptomatic. Removal of the pinhead-sized tick within 18 h of attachment

TABLE 24-11 Staging of LYME Borreliosis	
Stage	**Clinical Findings**
Early infection: stage 1 (localized infection)	Erythema migrans (EM)
	Lymphocytoma
Early infection: stage 2 (disseminated)	Systemic symptoms (fever, chills, myalgia, infection, headaches, weakness, photophobia)
	Secondary EM
	Carditis
	Meningitis, cranial neuritis, radiculoneuropathy
	Arthralgia/myalgia
Late infection: stage 3 (persistent infection)	Arthritis
	Encephalomyelitis
	Acrodermatitis chronica atrophicans (ACA)

may preclude transmission. EM may be associated with burning sensation, itching, or pain. Only 75% of patients with LB exhibit EM. Joint complaints more common in North America. Neurologic involvement more common in Europe. With persistent disease, chronic fatigue.

Skin Findings See Table 24-11.

Stage 1 Localized Infection *Erythema Migrans* Initial erythematous macule or papule enlarges within days to form an expanding annular lesion with a distinct red border and partially clearing middle, i.e., a migrating erythema, at the bite site (Fig. 24-76). Maximum median diameter is 15 cm (range 3–68 cm). The expanding lesion may have several rings of varying shades of red (targetoid or bull's eye). At times, concentric rings form. When occurring on the scalp, only a linear streak may be evident on the face or neck. Multiple EM lesions are seen with multiple bite sites. Most common sites: thigh, groin, axilla. Center may become indurated, vesicular, or necrotic. Less common: central hemorrhagic vesiculation or necrosis, lymphangitic streaks. Hypersensitivity to various tick antigens, other pathogens, and outer borrelial surface proteins occur in some individuals. As EM evolves, postinflammatory erythema or hyperpigmentation, transient alopecia, and desquamation may occur. 25% of patients do not exhitit EM lesion. 🔲

Borrelial Lymphocytoma Mainly seen in Europe. Usually arises at the site of tick bite. Some patients have a history of EM; others may show concomitant EM located around or near the lymphocytoma. Usually presents

FIGURE 24-75 *Ixodes scapularis* **(deer tick) feeding** A nymph with its mouth parts attached to skin with surrounding erythema; this inflammation is a response to the bite itself and is not necessarily indicative of infection. Transmission of *Borrelia burgdorferi* usually occurs only after prolonged attachment and feeding (>18 h).

FIGURE 24-76   Lyme borreliosis: erythema migrans (EM) on upper thigh   A 75-year-old male noted an asymptomatic red plaque on his thigh the day of the examination. He felt well, and was unaware of tick bite. **A.** Red plaque with fading margins (erythema migrans). The day after beginning doxycycline, 100 mg bid, he experienced flulike symptoms (Jarisch-Herxheimer reaction). **B.** Four days after beginning treatment, the EM lesion is much larger; symptoms had resolved.

as a solitary bluish-red nodule (Fig. 24-77) or plaque. Sites of predilection: earlobe (children), nipple/areola (adults), areola, scrotum; 3–5 cm in diameter. Usually asymptomatic.

Other Cutaneous Findings Malar rash, diffuse urticaria, subcutaneous nodules (panniculitis).

Stage 2 Disseminated Infection *Secondary Lesions* Present in 17–50% of patients with early disseminated LB in North America; more common in Europe. Lesions range in number from 2 to >100 and thus may present as rash. Secondary lesions resemble EM but are smaller, migrate less, and lack central induration and may be scaly (Fig. 24-78). Lesions occur at any site except the palms and soles; can become confluent. When face, hands, feet are involved, mild swelling can occur.

Stage 3 Persistent Infection: Acrodermatitis Chronica Atrophicans (ACA) Associated with *B. afzelii* infection in Europe and Asia. More common in elderly women.

Early Inflammatory Phase (Months to Years) Initially, diffuse or localized violaceous erythema, usually on one extremity, accompanied by mild to prominent edema, most commonly involving the extensor surfaces and periarticular areas. Asymptomatic dull red infiltrated plaques arise on the extremities, more commonly on lower legs than forearms, which slowly extend centrifugally over several months to years, leaving central areas of atrophy.

Endstage Skin becomes atrophic, veins and subcutaneous tissue become prominent, easily lifted and pushed into fine accordion-like folds,

i.e., "cigarette paper" or "tissue paper" skin (Fig. 24-79). Lesions may be single or multiple. 🔎

Sclerotic or Fibrotic Plaques and Bands Localized fibromas and plaques are seen as subcutaneous nodules around the knees and elbows; may involve the joint capsule with subsequent limitation of movement of joints in hands, feet, or shoulders. Fibrotic/sclerotic band along ulna is pathognomonic ("ulnar band").

General Findings See Table 24-11. 🔎

Stage 1 None.

Stage 2 (Disseminated Infection) Fever: in adults, low-grade; in children, may be high and persistent. Regional lymphadenopathy, generalized lymphadenopathy.

Neurologic Involvement Occurs in 10–20% of untreated LB cases, 1–6 weeks (or longer) after the tick bite. Manifested as meningitis (excruciating headache, neck pain), subtle encephalitic signs (sleep disturbances, difficulty concentrating, poor memory, irritability, emotional lability, dementia), cranial neuritis (including bilateral facial palsy), motor or sensory radiculoneuropathy, mononeuritis multiplex, or myelitis. In the United States, most common presentation is fluctuating symptoms of meningitis accompanied by facial palsy and peripheral radiculoneuropathy. In Europe and Asia, the first sign is characteristically radicular pain followed by CSF pleocytosis (Bannwarth syndrome); meningeal and encephalitic signs are often absent. Early neurologic manifestations usually resolve within months; chronic neurologic disease may occur later.

FIGURE 24-77 Lyme borreliosis: lymphocytoma cutis Solitary, red-purple nodule on the characteristic site of the ear.

Cardiac Involvement Occurs in 8% of un-treated cases, usually within 4 weeks. Mani-fested by fluctuating degrees of atrioventricular block, myopericarditis, and left ventricular dys-function. Usually transient and not associated with long-term sequelae.

Musculoskeletal Involvement Common. Mi-gratory pain in joints, tendons, bursae, muscles, or bones. Pain lasts hours or days, affecting one or two locations at a time.

Stage 3 (Persistent Infection) Fever: in adults, low-grade; in children, may be high and presist-ent. Regional lymphadenopathy, generalized lymphadenopathy.

Chronic Neuroborreliosis May become ap-parent months or years after onset of latent infection. Less common than arthritis. Most common presentation is subtle encephalopathy (altered memory, mood, or sleep), often ac-companied by axonal polyneuropathy (distal paresthesias, spinal radicular pain). Prolonged course resembles that of tertiary syphilis.

Arthritis More common in United States, occurring in 60% of untreated cases. Charac-terized by intermittent attacks of oligoarticular arthritis in large joints (especially knees), last-ing weeks to months. In a small percentage of cases, involvement of large joints (usually one or both knees) becomes chronic and may lead to destruction of cartilage and bone.

DIFFERENTIAL DIAGNOSIS

EM Insect bite (annular erythema caused by ticks, mosquitoes, Hymenoptera), epidermal dermatophytoses, allergic contact dermatitis, herald patch of pityriasis rosea, granuloma annulare, early inflammatory morphea, cellu-litis, urticaria, erythema multiforme, erythema annulare centrifugum, involuting psoriasis le-sion, lichen simplex chronicus, fixed drug eruption.

LB-like illness with exposure in midwest and southern United States transmitted by Lone Star tick (*Amblyomma americanum*); referred to as *Southern tick-associated rash illness* (STARI).

Secondary Lesions Secondary syphilis, pityria-sis rosea, erythema multiforme, urticaria.

Lymphocytoma Insect bite reaction, pseud-olymphoma, cutaneous lymphoma.

ACA Arterial insufficiency of the lower leg, ve-nous insufficiency with stasis dermatitis, venous thrombosis/thrombophlebitis.

Fibrotic Nodules Rheumatic nodules, gouty tophi, erythema nodosum.

LABORATORY EXAMINATIONS

Skin Biopsy *EM* Deep and superficial perivascular and interstitial infiltrate contain-ing lymphocytes and plasma cells with some degree of vascular damage (mild vasculitis or hypervascular occlusion). Spirochetes can be demonstrated in up to 40% of EM biopsy specimens.

ACA Early, perivascular inflammatory infil-trate with plasma cells and dermal edema. Subsequently, infiltrate broadens to a dense middermal bandlike infiltrate. Ultimately, epi-dermal and dermal atrophy, dilated dermal blood vessels, plasma cell infiltrate, elastin and collagen defects.

Serology CDC recommends a two-step ap-proach in which samples are first tested by enzyme-linked immunosorbent assay (ELISA) and equivocal or positive results are then tested by Western blotting. During the first month of infection, both IgM and IgG responses to the spirochete should be determined, preferably in both acute- and convalescent-phase serum samples. Approximately 20–30% of patients have a positive response detectable in acute-phase samples; about 70–80% have positive re-sponse during convalescence (2–4 weeks later). After that time, the great majority of patients continue to have a positive IgG antibody re-sponse, and a single test (that for IgG) is usually sufficient. According to current criteria adopted by the CDC, an IgM Western blot is considered positive if two of the following three bands are present: 23, 39, and 41 kDa.

Positive serology indicates past infection. It does not distinguish between an abortive infec-tion, a successfully treated past infection, or an active infection.

Culture *B. burgdorferi* can be isolated from lesional skin biopsy specimen on modified Barbour-Stoenner-Kelly medium. Permits de-finitive diagnosis.

PCR Detects *B. burgdorferi* DNA in lesional skin biopsy specimen, blood, or joint fluid. Not routinely available.

DIAGNOSIS

CDC surveillance criteria:

- *Early LB*: Made on characteristic clinical find-ings in a person living in or having visited an endemic area; does not require laboratory confirmation.

- *Late LB*: Confirmed by specific serologic tests.
- *ACA*: Made on clinical findings confirmed by lesional biopsy.

COURSE AND PROGNOSIS

Untreated EM and secondary lesions fade in median time of 28 days, but the range is from 1 day to 14 months. Both EM and secondary lesions can fade and recur during this time. However, after adequate treatment, early lesions resolve within two weeks, and late manifestations are prevented. Late manifestations identified early usually clear after adequate antibiotic therapy; however, delay in diagnosis may result in permanent joint or neurologic disabilities.

FIGURE 24-78 Lyme borreliosis: secondary erythema migrans on trunk A 78-year-old male was sent in by his wife when she noted a trunk rash. The patient was blind, was not aware of tick bite, and felt well. On examination, confluent large red warm plaques (4 days' duration) are seen on the back and buttocks; lesions were also present on the anterior trunk and groin. *Borrelia* disseminates hematogenously from the primary EM (inoculation) site, resulting in secondary EM lesions in some persons. These lesions are analogous to lesions of secondary syphilis. Lyme serology was positive. Lesions resolved several days after beginning doxycycline.

ACA shows little response to adequate antibiotic therapy once atrophy has supervened. Adequately treated patients have declining titers of anti-*B. burgdorferi* antibody within 6–12 months.

EM (short duration of infection) treated with antimicrobial agents does not confer protective immunity. If LB goes untreated for months, immunity may develop that protects against reinfection for years.

MANAGEMENT

Prophylaxis

- Avoid known habitats of *I. scapularis* and *I. pacificus* (United States). Other preventive measures include wearing long pants and long-sleeved shirts, tucking pants into socks.
- Apply tick repellents containing *N, N*-diethyl-*m*-toluamide ("DEET") to clothing and/or exposed skin.
- Check regularly for ticks and promptly remove any attached ticks.
- Acaricides containing permethrin kill ticks on contact and can provide further protection when applied to clothing.
- After a recognized tick bite, the risk of infection with *B. burgdorferi* is low, and antibiotic prophylaxis is not routinely indicated. Therapy with amoxicillin or doxycycline for 10 days may be given to prevent Lyme disease in the following circumstances: Tick engorged (feeding for > 24 h), *Ixodes* nymph from a hyperendemic area, pregnancy, immunocompromised status, follow-up difficult, patient anxious.
- Temperature of > 38°C may represent human anaplasmosis or babesiosis transmitted with tick bite.

Immunization The vaccine for LB is no longer manufactured.
Antimicrobial Treatment See Fig. 24-80.
Centers for Disease Control and Prevention: Lyme Disease Home Page
http://www.cdc.gov/ncidod/dvbid/lyme/index.htm

Lyme Disease Network
http://www.lymenet.org/

FIGURE 24-79 Lyme borreliosis: acrodermatitis chronica atrophicans: endstage Advanced atrophy of the epidermis and dermis with associated violaceous erythema of legs and feet; the visibility of the superficial veins is striking.

TREATMENT OF LYMEBORRELIOSIS

Skin	Joint	Heart	Nervous system
Erythema migrans Acrodermatitis	Arthritis	AV block	Facial palsy alone — Meningitis Radiculoneuritis Encephalopathy Polyneuropathy

1°, 2°   3°

Oral therapy

First choice
 Age ≥ 9 years, not pregnant:
 doxycycline, 100 mg bid
 Age < 9 years: amoxicillin,
 50 mg/kg per day
Second choice for adults:
 amoxicillin, 500 mg tid
Third choice for all ages:
 cefuroxime axetil, 500 mg bid
Fourth choice for all ages:
 erythromycin, 250 mg qid

Intravenous therapy

First choice:
 ceftriaxone, 2 g qd
Second choice:
 cefotaxime, 2 g q8h
Third choice:
 Na penicillin G, 5 million
 U q6h

Guidelines for duration of therapy

Localized skin infection: 14 days
Early disseminated infection:
 21 days
Acrodermatitis: 30 days
Arthritis: 30–60 days*

Neurologic involvement:
 14–28 days
Cardiac involvement:
 28 days complete course
 with oral therapy when
 patient is no longer in
 high-degree AV block

FIGURE 24-80   Algorithm for the treatment of the various acute or chronic manifestations of Lyme borreliosis   Relapse may occur with any of these regimens, and a second course of treatment may be necessary. AV, atrioventricular. [AC Steere: Chap. 157 in *Harrison's Principles of Internal Medicine,* 16ed, D Kasper et al (eds). New York, McGraw-Hill, 2005.

FUNGAL INFECTIONS OF THE SKIN AND HAIR

- Superficial fungal infections are caused by numerous fungi that are capable of superficially invading the following:
  - Skin
    - Epidermis
    - Hair/hair follicles
    - Nail apparatus
  - Mucosal sites
    - Oropharynx
    - Anogenitalia
  - These fungi are commensural organisms that frequently colonize normal epithelium.
    - Dermatophytes
    - *Candida* species
    - *Malassezia* species
  - Infections can extend more deeply in the immunocompromised host.
- Deeper, chronic cutaneous fungal infections can occur after cutaneous inoculation.

- Mycetoma
- Chromomycosis
- Sporotrichosis
- Systemic fungal infections with cutaneous dissemination; these infections occur most often in the immunocompromised host.
  - Primary lung infection; can disseminate hematogenously to multiple organ systems, including the skin.
    - Cryptococcosis
    - Histoplasmosis
    - North American blastomycosis
    - Coccidioidomycosis
    - Penicillinosis
  - Primary gastrointestinal (GI) infection; neutropenic host
    - Disseminated candidiasis commonly arises in the GI tract.

SUPERFICIAL FUNGAL INFECTIONS   ICD-9 : 111 ∘ ICD-10 : B36

- Superficial fungal infections are the most common of all mucocutaneous infections, often caused by overgrowth of transient or resident flora associated with a change in the microenvironment of the skin.
- Fungi causing these infections:
  - Dermatophytes: infect keratinized epithelium, hair follicles, and nail apparatus

- *Candida* spp.: Require a warm humid environment.
- *Malassezia* spp.: Require a humid microenvironment and lipids for growth.
- *Trichosporon* spp
- *Hortaea* (*Exophiala* or *Phaeoannellomyces*) *werneckii*: Tinea nigra

DERMATOPHYTOSES ICD-9:110 ∘ ICD-10:B35.0-B36

- Dermatophytes are a unique group of fungi capable of infecting nonviable keratinized cutaneous structures including stratum corneum, nails, and hair.
- *Dermatophytosis* denotes an infection caused by dermatophytes.
- Clinical infection by structure involved:
  - *Epidermomycosis* (epidermal dermatophytosis)
  - *Trichomycosis* (dermatophytosis of hair and hair follicles)
  - *Onychomycosis* (dermatophytosis of the nail apparatus)

- The pathogenesis of epidermomycosis vs trichomycosis leading to different clinical manifestations is schematically depicted in Image 25-1.
- The term *tinea* is best used for dermatophytoses and is modified according to the anatomic site of infection, e.g., tinea pedis.
- "Tinea" versicolor is called *pityriasis versicolor* outside of the United States; it is not a dermatophytosis but rather an infection caused by the yeast *Malassezia*.

EPIDEMIOLOGY AND ETIOLOGY

Age of Onset

- Children have scalp infections (*Trichophyton, Microsporum*).
- Young and older adults have intertriginous infections.
- The incidence of onychomycosis is correlated directly with age; in the United States, up to 50% of individuals age 75 years have onychomycosis.

Race

- Adult blacks may have a lower incidence of dermatophytosis.
- Tinea capitis is more common in black children.

Etiology

- Three genera of dermatophytes:
  - *Trichophyton*
  - *Microsporum*
  - *Epidermophyton.*
- More than 40 species are currently recognized; approximately 10 spp. are common causes of human infection.
- *T. rubrum* is the most common cause of epidermal dermatophytosis and onychomycosis in industrialized nations.
  - Currently, 70% of the U.S. population experience at least one episode of *T. rubrum* infection (usually tinea pedis).
  - *T. rubrum* is indigenous to Southeast Asia, the Australian outback, and western Africa.

A

B

IMAGE 25-1 The pathogenesis of epidermomycosis (A) and trichomycosis (B) are different because they involve different structures leading to different clinical manifestations. In epidermomycosis, dermatophytes (red dots and lines) within the stratum corneum not only disrupt the horny layer and thus lead to scaling, but also elicit an inflammatory response (black dots symbolize inflammatory cells), which may then manifest as erythema, papulation, and even vesiculation. On the other hand, in trichomycosis the hair shaft is involved (red dots) resulting in the destruction and breaking off of the hair. If the dermatophyte infection extends farther down into the hair follicle, it will elicit a deeper inflammatory response (black dots) and this will manifest as deeper inflammatory nodules, follicular pustulation, and abscess formation. (See also Fig. 25-19.)

Visitors/colonizers from Europe and North America became infected in these areas, developing tinea pedis and onychomycosis; these conditions did not occur in natives, who were barefoot or wore open moccasins. These visitors/colonizers and soldiers (World Wars I and II, and the Vietnam conflict) brought *T. rubrum* to North America and Europe.

- Soldiers wearing occlusive boots in tropical climates developed "jungle rot"—extensive tinea pedis with secondary bacterial infection.
- Presently, *T. rubrum* infection can be acquired by contact with contaminated floors (homes, health clubs, athletic locker rooms, or hotel rooms).

- The etiology of tinea capitis in children varies geographically.
  - North America and Europe: *T. tonsurans* is the most common cause, having replaced *M. audouinii*.
  - Europe, Asia, and Africa: *T. violaceum*.
- In U.S. adults, *T. rubrum* is the most common cause of dermatophytic folliculitis.

Demography Some species have a worldwide distribution; others are restricted to particular continents or regions. However, *T. concentricum*, the cause of tinea imbricata, is endemic to the South Pacific and parts of South America. *T. rubrum* was endemic to Southeast Asia, western Africa, and Australia but now occurs most commonly in North America and Europe.

Transmission

- Dermatophyte infections can be acquired from three sources:
  - Most commonly from another person [usually by fomites, less so by direct skin-to-skin contact (tinea gladiatorum)]
  - From animals such as puppies or kittens
  - Least commonly from soil.
- Based on their ecology, dermatophytes are also classified as follows:
  - *Anthropophilic*: Person-to-person transmission by fomites and by direct contact. *Trichophyton* spp.: *T. rubrum, T. mentagrophytes* (var. *interdigitale*), *T. schoenleinii, T. tonsurans, T. violaceum. Microsporum audouinii. Epidermophyton floccosum.*
  - *Zoophilic*: Animal-to-human by direct contact or by fomites. *Trichophyton* spp.: *T. equinum, T. mentagrophytes* (var. *mentagrophytes*), *T. verrucosum. M. canis.*

- *Geophilic*: Environmental. *Microsporum* spp.: *M. gypseum, M. nanum.*

Predisposing Factors

- Atopic diathesis: Cell-mediated immune deficiency for *T. rubrum.*
- Topical immunosuppression: with prolonged application of topical glucocorticoids, there can be marked modification in the usual banal character of dermatophytosis (tinea incognito); this is especially true of the face, groin, and hands.
- Systemic immunocompromise:
  - Patients have a higher incidence and more intractable dermatophytoses.
  - Abscesses and granulomas may occur (Majocchi granuloma).

CLASSIFICATION

In vivo, dermatophytes grow only on or within keratinized structures and, as such, involve the following:

- *Dermatophytoses of keratinized epidermis (epidermal dermatophytosis, epidermomycosis)*: Tinea facialis, tinea corporis, tinea cruris, tinea manus, tinea pedis.
- *Dermatophytoses of nail apparatus (onychomychosis)*: Tinea unguium (toenails, fingernails). Onychomycosis (more inclusive term, including nail infections caused by dermatophytes, yeasts, and molds).
- *Dermatophytoses of hair and hair follicle (trichomycosis)*: Dermatophytic folliculitis, Majocchi (trichophytic) granuloma, tinea capitis, tinea barbae.

PATHOGENESIS

Dermatophytes synthesize keratinases that digest keratin and sustain existence of fungi in keratinized structures. Cell-mediated immunity and antimicrobial activity of polymorphonuclear leukocytes restrict dermatophyte pathogenicity.

- *Host factors that facilitate dermatophyte infections*: atopy, topical and systemic glucocorticoids, ichthyosis, collagen vascular disease
- *Local factors favoring dermatophyte infection*: sweating, occlusion, occupational exposure, geographic location, high humidity (tropical or semitropical climates)

The clinical presentation of dermatophytoses depends on several factors: site of infection, immunologic response of the host, species of fungus. Dermatophytes (e.g., *T. rubrum*) that initiate little inflammatory response are better able to establish chronic infection. Organisms such as *M. canis* cause an acute infection associated with a brisk inflammatory response and spontaneous resolution. In some individuals, infection can involve the dermis, as in kerion and Majocchi granuloma.

LABORATORY EXAMINATIONS

Direct Microscopy (Fig. 25-1)
Sampling

- *Skin*: Collect scale with a no. 15 scalpel blade, edge of a glass microscope slide, brush (tooth or cervical brush). Scales are placed on center of microscope slide, swept into a small pile, and covered with a coverslip. Recent application of cream/ointment or powder often makes identification of fungal element difficult/impossible.
- *Nails*: Keratinaceous debris is collected with a no. 15 scalpel blade or small curette. Distal lateral subungual onychomycosis (DLSO): debride from the undersurface of nail of most proximally involved site; avoid nail plate. Superficial white onychomycosis (SWO): superficial nail plate. Proximal subungual onychomycosis (PSO): undersurface of proximal nail plate; obtain sample by using a small punch biopsy tool, boring through involved nail plate to undersurface; obtain keratin from undersurface.

- *Hair*: Remove hairs by epilation of broken hairs with a needle holder or forceps. Place on microscope slide and cover with glass coverslip. Skin scales from involved hairy site can be obtained with a brush (tooth or cervical).

Preparation of Sample *Potassium hydroxide 5 to 20% solution* is applied at the edge of coverslip. Capillary action draws solution under coverslip. The preparation is gently heated with a match or lighter until bubbles begin to expand, clarifying the preparation. Excess KOH solution is blotted out with bibulous or lens paper. Condenser should be "racked down." Epidermal dermatophytosis: positive unless patient is using antifungal therapy. DLSO: 90% of cases positive. Variations of KOH with fungal stains: Swartz-Lampkins stain, chlorazol black E stain.
Microscopy Dermatophytes are recognized as septated, tubelike structures (hyphae or mycelia) (Fig. 25-1).
Wood Lamp Hairs infected with *Microsporum* spp. fluoresce. Greenish. Darken room and illuminate affected site with Wood lamp. Coral red fluorescence of intertriginous site confirms diagnosis of erythrasma.
Fungal Cultures Specimens collected from scaling skin lesions, hair, nails. Scale and hair from the scalp are best harvested with tooth or cervical brush; the involved scalp is brushed vigorously; keratinaceous debris and hairs then placed into fungal culture plate. Culture on Sabouraud's glucose medium. Repeat cultures recommended monthly.
Dermatopathology DLSO: periodic acid–Schiff (PAS) or methenamine silver stains are more sensitive than KOH preparation or fungal culture in identification of fungal elements in DLSO.

FIGURE 25-1 Potassium hydroxide (KOH) preparation Multiple, septated, tube-like structures (hyphae or mycelia) and spore formation in scales from an individual with epidermal dermatophytosis. In contrast, KOH preparation in candidiasis shows elongated yeast forms (pseudohyphae) without true septations. (Compare with Fig. 25-22.)

MANAGEMENT

Prevention	Apply powder containing imidazoles or tolnaftate to areas prone to fungal infection after bathing.
Topical antifungal preparations	*These preparations may be effective for treatment of dermatophytoses of skin but not for those of hair or nails.*
	Preparation is applied bid to involved area optimally for 4 weeks including at least 1 week after lesions have cleared.
	Apply at least 3 cm beyond advancing margin of lesion.
	These topical agents are comparable. Differentiated by cost, base, vehicle, and antifungal activity.
Imidazoles	Clotrimazole (Lotrimin, Mycelex)
	Miconazole (Micatin)
	Ketoconazole (Nizoral)
	Econazole (Spectazole)
	Oxiconizole (Oxistat)
	Sulconizole (Exelderm)
	Sertaconazole (Ertaczo)
Allylamines	Naftifine (Naftin)
	Terbinafine (Lamisil)
Naphthionates	Tolnaftate (Tinactin)
Substituted pyridone	Ciclopirox olamine (Loprox)
Systemic antifungal agents	*For infections of keratinized skin*: use if lesions are extensive or if infection has failed to respond to topical preparations.
	Usually required for treatment of tinea capitis and tinea unguium. Also may be required for inflammatory tineas and hyperkeratotic moccasin-type tinea pedis.
Terbinafine	250-mg tablet. Allylamine. Most effective oral antidermophyte antifungal; low efficacy against other fungi.
Azole/imidazoles	Itraconazole and ketoconazole
Itraconazole	100-mg capsules; oral solution (10 mg/mL): Intravenous. Triazole. Needs acid gastric pH for dissolution of capsule. Raises levels of digoxin and cyclosporine. Approved for onychomycosis in the United States.
Fluconazole	100-, 150-, 200-mg tablets; oral suspension (10 or 40 mg/mL); 400 mg IV.
Ketoconazole	200-mg tablets. Needs acid gastric pH for dissolution of tablet. Take with food or cola beverage; antacids and H2 blockers reduce absorption. The most hepatotoxic of azole drugs; hepatotoxicity occurs in an estimated one of every 10,000–15,000 exposed persons. Not approved for treatment of dermatophyte infections in the United States.
Griseofulvin	*Micronized*: 250- or 500-mg tablets; 125 mg/teaspoon suspension. *Ultramicronized*: 165- or 330-mg tablets. Active only against dermatophytes; less effective than triazoles. Adverse effects include headache, nausea/vomiting, photosensitivity; lowers effect of crystalline warfarin sodium. *T. rubrum* and *T. tonsurans* infection may respond poorly. Should be taken with fatty meal to maximize absorption. In children, CBC and LFTs recommended if risk factors for hepatitis exist or treatment lasts longer than 3 months.

Note: CBC, complete blood count; LFTs, liver function tests.

DERMATOPHYTOSES OF EPIDERMIS

- Epidermal dermatophytoses are the most common dermatophytic infection.
- May be followed/accompanied by dermatophytic infection of hair/hair follicles and/or the nail apparatus.

Synonyms: Ringworm, epidermomycosis.

TINEA PEDIS ICD-9 : 110.4 ∘ ICD-10 : B35.3 ■ ▢

- Dermatophytic infection of the feet
- Clinical findings: erythema, scaling, maceration, and/or bulla formation
- In most cases of epidermal dermatophytosis, the infection occurs initially on the feet (*T. rubrum*), and, in time, spreads to sites such as the
  - Inguinal area (tinea cruris)
  - Trunk, arms, legs (tinea corporis)
  - Hands (tinea manuum)

- Tinea pedis often provides breaks in the integrity of the epidermis through which bacteria such as *Staphylococcus aureus* or group A streptococcus (GAS) can invade, causing skin or soft-tissue infection (cellulitis or lymphangitis).

Synonyms: Athlete's foot. Jungle rot

EPIDEMIOLOGY

Age of Onset Late childhood or young adult life. Most common, 20–50 years.
Sex Males > females.
Predisposing Factors Hot, humid weather; occlusive footwear; excessive sweating.
Transmission Walking barefoot on contaminated floors. Arthrospores can survive in human scales for 12 months.

CLINICAL MANIFESTATION

Duration Months to years or lifetime. Often, prior history of tinea pedis, tinea unguium of toenails. May flare if in hot climate.
Skin Symptoms Usually asymptomatic. Pruritus. Pain with bacterial superinfection.

Skin Lesions
Interdigital Type
- Two patterns:
  ∘ Dry scaling (Fig. 25-2)
  ∘ Maceration, peeling, fissuring of toe webs (Fig. 25-3). Hyperhidrosis common.
- Most common site: between fourth and fifth toes.

- Infection may spread to adjacent areas of feet.

Moccasin Type
- Well-demarcated erythema with minute papules on margin, fine white scaling, and hyperkeratosis (Fig. 25-4) (confined to heels, soles, lateral borders of feet).
- *Distribution*: Sole, involving area covered by a ballet slipper.
- One or both feet may be involved with any pattern; bilateral involvement more common.

Inflammatory/Bullous Type
- Vesicles or bullae filled with clear fluid (Fig. 25-5).
- Pus usually indicates superinfection with *S. aureus* infection or GAS.
- After rupturing, erosions with ragged ringlike border.
- May be associated with "id" reaction (autosensitization or dermatophytid).
- *Distribution*: Sole, instep, webspaces.

Ulcerative Type
- Extension of interdigital tinea pedis onto dorsal and plantar foot.

FIGURE 25-2   Tinea pedis: interdigital dry type   The interdigital space between the toes shows erythema and scaling; the toenail is thickened, indicative of associated distal subungual onychomycosis.

FIGURE 25-3   Tinea pedis: interdigital macerated type   A 48-year-old male with athlete's foot and hyperhidrosis for years. The skin of the webspace between the 4th and 5th toes is hyperkeratotic and macerated (hydration of the stratum corneum). The KOH+ preparation shows septated hyphae, confirming the diagnosis of dermatophytosis. Wood lamp demonstrated coral-red fluorescence confirming concomitant erythrasma. *Pseudomonas aeruginosa* was isolated on bacterial culture.

FIGURE 25-4 Tinea pedis: moccasin type A 65-year-old female with scaling feet for years. Sharply marginated erythema of the foot with a mild keratoderma associated with distal/lateral subungual onychomycosis, typical of *T. rubrum* infection.

FIGURE 25-5 Tinea pedis: bullous type A 72-year-old female with pruritic scaling feet for months, treating with clobetasol cream. Erythema, scaling, and blister formation on the dorsum of the foot. The initial diagnosis was eczema that was treated with clobetasol ointment, which facilitated the growth of dermatophyte, so-called tinea incognito. Bullous tinea pedis is usually caused by *T. mentagrophytes*.

- Often complicated by bacterial superinfection: *S. aureus* [Methicillin-sensitive *S. aureus* (MSSA) or Methicillin-resistant *S. aureus* (MRSA)], GAS, group B streptococcus (GBS), *Pseudomonas aeruginosa*; erythrasma; *Candida albicans*.

DIFFERENTIAL DIAGNOSIS

Interdigital Type Erythrasma, impetigo, pitted keratolysis, *Candida* intertrigo, *P. aeruginosa* webspace infection.

Moccasin Type Psoriasis vulgaris, eczematous dermatitis (dyshidrotic, atopic, allergic contact), pitted keratolysis, various keratodermas.

CLASSIFICATION

Type	Clinical Features	Etiology
Interdigital (acute and chronic)	Most common type; frequently overlooked two patterns: dry and moist with maceration	*T. rubrum* most common cause of chronic tinea pedis; *T. mentagrophytes* causes more inflammatory lesions
Dry	Scaling of webspace, may be erosive	*T. rubrum*
Moist (macerated)	Hyperkeratosis of webspace with maceration of stratum corneum	*T. mentagrophytes*
Moccasin (chronic hyperkeratotic or dry)	Keratoderma	Most often caused by *T. rubrum*, especially in atopic individuals; also *Epidermophyton floccosum*
Inflammatory or bullous (vesicular)	Blisters in nonoccluded skin	Least common type; usually caused by *T. mentagrophytes* var. *mentagrophytes* (granular). Resembles an allergic contact dermatitis
Ulcerative	An extension of interdigital type into dermis due to maceration and secondary (bacterial) infection	*T. rubrum, E. floccosum, T. mentagrophytes, C. albicans*
Dermatophytid	Presents as a vesicular eruption of the fingers and/or palmar aspects of the hands secondary to inflammatory tinea pedis. A combined clinical presentation also occurs. *Candida* and bacteria *(S. aureus,* GAS, *P. aeruginosa)* may cause superinfection.	*T. mentagrophytes, T. rubrum*

Inflammatory/Bullous Type   Bullous impetigo, allergic contact dermatitis, dyshidrotic eczema, bullous disease.

LABORATORY EXAMINATIONS

Direct Microscopy   (Fig. 25-1). In bullous type, examine scraping from the inner aspect of bulla roof for detection of hyphae.
Wood Lamp   Negative fluorescence usually rules out erythrasma in interdigital infection. Erythrasma and interdigital tinea pedis may coexist.

Culture

• *Fungal:* Dermatophytes can be isolated in 11% of normal-appearing interspaces and 31% of macerated toe webs. *Candida* spp. may be copathogens in webspaces.

• *Bacterial:* In individuals with macerated interdigital space, *S. aureus, P. aeruginosa,* and diphtheroids are commonly isolated. *S. aureus* and GAS can cause superinfection.

DIAGNOSIS

Demonstration of hyphae on direct microscopy, isolation of dermatophyte on culture.

COURSE AND PROGNOSIS

• Tends to be chronic, with exacerbations in hot weather.
• May provide portal of entry for lymphangitis or cellulitis, especially in patients whose leg veins have been used for coronary artery bypass surgery and have chronic low-grade edema of leg.
• Without secondary prophylaxis, recurrence is the rule.

MANAGEMENT

Prevention	Use of shower shoes while bathing at home or in public facility. Washing feet with benzoyl peroxide bar directly after shower. Diabetics and those who have undergone coronary artery bypass with harvesting of leg veins are especially subject to secondary bacterial infection (impetiginization, lymphangitis, cellulitis).
Special considerations by type of infection	
Macerated interdigital	Acute: Burow's wet dressings; Castellani paint. Chronic: aluminum chloride hexahydrate 20% bid to reduce sweating.
Moccasin	Most difficult to eradicate. Many patients have a minor defect in cell-mediated immune response: stratum corneum thick, making it difficult for topical antifungal agents to penetrate, often associated with tinea unguium, a source of reinfection of skin. Keratolytic agent (salicylic acid, lactic acid, hydroxy acid) with plastic occlusion useful in reducing hyperkeratosis. Nail reservoir must be eradicated to cure moccasin-type infection.
Inflammatory/bullous	Acutely, use cool compresses. If severe, systemic glucocorticoids are indicated.
Antifungal agents	
Topical	See "Management", page 696. Apply to all affected sites twice daily. Treat for 2–4 weeks.
Systemic	Indicated for extensive infection, for failures of topical treatment, or for those with tinea unguium and moccasin-type tinea.
Terbinafine	250 mg daily for 14 days
Itraconazole	200 mg twice daily for 7 days *or* 200 mg daily for 14 days
Fluconazole	150–200 mg daily for 4–6 weeks
Secondary prophylaxis	Important in preventing recurrence of interdigital and moccasin types of tinea pedis. Daily washing of feet while bathing with benzoyl peroxide bar is effective and inexpensive. Antifungal powders, alcohol gels.

TINEA MANUUM   ICD-9:110.2 ∘ ICD-10:B35.2

- Chronic dermatophytosis of the hand(s).
- Often unilateral, most commonly on the dominant hand.
- Usually associated with tinea pedis.

CLINICAL MANIFESTATION

Duration Months to years.
Skin Symptoms Frequently symptomatic. Pruritus. Pain if fissured. *Dyshidrotic type:* Episodic symptoms of pruritus.

Skin Lesions

- Well-demarcated scaling patches, hyperkeratosis, and scaling confined to palmar creases, fissures on palmar hand (Fig. 25-6). Borders well demarcated; central clearing.
- May extend onto dorsum of hand with follicular papules, nodules, pustules with dermatophytic folliculitis.
- *Dyshidrotic Type*: Papules, vesicles, bullae (uncommon on the margin of lesion) on palms and lateral fingers, similar to lesions of bullous tinea pedis.
- *Secondary Changes*: Lichen simplex chronicus, prurigo nodules, impetiginization.
- *Distribution*: Diffuse hyperkeratosis of the palms with pronounced involvement of palmar creases or patchy scaling on the dorsa and sides of fingers; 50% of patients have unilateral involvement (Fig. 25-7). Usually associated with tinea pedis (Fig. 25-6), tinea cruris. If chronic, often associated with tinea unguium of fingernails.

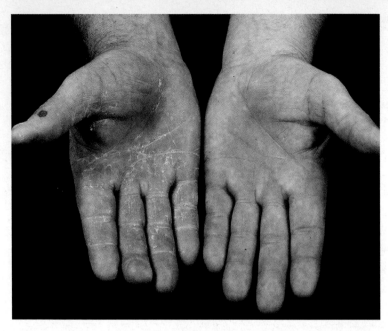

FIGURE 25-6 **Tinea manuum** Erythema and scaling of the right hand, which was associated with bilateral tinea pedum; the "one-hand, two-feet" distribution is typical of epidermal dermatophytosis of the hands and feet. In time, distal/lateral subungual onychomycosis occurs on the fingernails.

FIGURE 25-7 **Tinea manuum, tinea pedis, and onychomycosis** A 54-year-old male with hepatitis C infection presented with a rash on examination. A large erythematous scaling plaque with sharp margination on the dorsum of the left hand associated with tinea pedis and distal subungual onychomycosis. Tinea facialis involving the face and right ear were also present.

DIFFERENTIAL DIAGNOSIS

Erythema/Scaling Hands Atopic dermatitis, lichen simplex chronicus, allergic contact dermatitis, irritant contact dermatitis, psoriasis vulgaris.

COURSE

- Chronic, does not resolve spontaneously.
- After treatment, recurs unless onychomycosis of fingernails, feet, and toenails is eradicated.
- Fissures and erosions provide portal of entry for bacterial infections.

MANAGEMENT

Prevention Must eradicate tinea unguium of fingernails as well as toenails; also tinea pedis and tinea cruris, otherwise, tinea manuum will recur.

Antifungal Agents *Topical* See "Management," page 696. Failure common.

Systemic

- Because of thickness of palmar stratum corneum, and especially if associated with tinea unguium of fingernails, tinea manuum is impossible to cure with topical agents.
- Oral agents eradicate dermatophytoses of hands, feet, and nails:
  - *Terbinafine:* 250 mg daily for 14 days
  - *Itraconazole:* 200 mg daily for 7 days
  - *Fluconazole:* 150 to 200 mg daily for 2 to 4 weeks
- *Note:* Eradication of fingernail onychomycosis requires longer use.

TINEA CRURIS ICD-9 : 110.3 ∘ ICD-10 : B35.6

- Subacute or chronic dermatophytosis of the groin, pubic regions, and thighs.
- "Always" associated with tinea pedis, the source of the infection.

- *Synonym:* "Jock itch."

EPIDEMIOLOGY AND ETIOLOGY

Age of Onset Adult.
Sex Males > females.
Etiology *T. rubrum, T. mentagrophytes.*
Predisposing Factors Warm, humid environment: tight clothing worn by men; obesity. Chronic topical glucocorticoid application.

CLINICAL MANIFESTATION

Duration Months to years. Often, history of long-standing tinea pedis and prior history of tinea cruris.
Skin Symptoms Often none. In some persons, pruritus causes patient to seek treatment.

Skin Lesions

- Usually associated with tinea pedis, tinea unguium of toenails.
- Large, scaling, well-demarcated dull red/tan/brown plaques (Fig. 25-8).
- Central clearing.
- Papules, pustules may be present at margins: dermatophytic folliculitis.
- Treated lesions: lack scale; postinflammatory hyperpigmentation in darker-skinned persons.
- In atopics, chronic scratching may produce secondary changes of lichen simplex chronicus.

Distribution Groins and thighs; may extend to buttocks. Scrotum and penis are rarely involved.

DIFFERENTIAL DIAGNOSIS

Erythema/Scaling in Groins Erythrasma, intertrigo, *Candida* intertrigo, intertriginous psoriasis, pityriasis versicolor, Langerhans cell histiocytosis.

FIGURE 25-8   Tinea cruris: tinea incognito   A 60-year-old renal transplant recipient has been treating thigh rash with topical corticosteroid for several months. Blotchy erythema with areas of atrophy and scale on the right medial upper thigh bordering the inguinal area. Tinea pedis and onychomycosis were also present. KOH preparation showed septated hyphae. Topical steroid facilitates dermatophyte growth, suppressing the immune response, creating an undiagnosed infection, tinea incognito.

MANAGEMENT

Prevention   After eradication of tinea cruris, tinea pedis, and tinea unguium, reinfection can be minimized by wearing shower shoes when using a public or home (if family members are infected) bathing facility; using antifungal powders; benzoyl peroxide wash; alcohol gels.

Antifungal Agents   *Topical*   See "Management," page 696.

Systemic   If recurrent, if dermatophytic folliculitis is present, or if it has failed to respond to adequate topical therapy. See "Management," page 696.

TINEA CORPORIS   ICD-9:110.5 ∘ ICD-10:B35.4

- Dermatophyte infections of the trunk, legs, arms, and/or neck, excluding the feet, hands, and groin.

EPIDEMIOLOGY AND ETIOLOGY

Age of Onset   All ages.
Occupation   Animal (large and small) workers.
Etiology

- *T. rubrum* most commonly
- *M. canis:* inflammatory
- *T. tonsurans* in parents of black children with tinea capitis

Transmission

- Autoinoculation from other parts of the body, i.e., from tinea pedis and tinea capitis.
- Direct or indirect with another person, e.g., in wrestlers, tinea gladiatorum.
- Contact with animals or contaminated soil.

Geography   More common in tropical and subtropical regions.

Predisposing Factors Most commonly, infection is spread from dermatophytic infection of the feet (*T. rubrum, T. mentagrophytes*). Infection can also be acquired from an active lesion of an animal (*T. verrucosum, M. canis*) or, rarely, from soil (*M. gypseum*).

CLINICAL MANIFESTATION

Incubation Period Days to months.
Duration Weeks to months to years.
Symptoms Often asymptomatic. Mild pruritus.

Skin Lesions

- Small to large (Fig. 25-9), scaling, sharply marginated plaques with or without pustules or vesicles, usually at margins.
- Peripheral enlargement and central clearing (Fig. 25-10) produce annular configuration with concentric rings or arcuate lesions (Fig. 25-11); fusion of lesions produces gyrate patterns.
- Single and occasionally scattered multiple lesions.
- Psoriasiform plaques.
- Verrucous lesions.

- Lesions of zoophilic infection (contracted from animals) are more inflammatory, with marked vesicles (Fig. 25-12), pustules, crusting at margins.
- Papules, nodules, pustules: dermatophytic folliculitis, i.e., Majocchi granuloma.

DIFFERENTIAL DIAGNOSIS

Well-Demarcated Scaling Plaque(s) Allergic contact dermatitis, atopic dermatitis, annular erythemas, psoriasis, seborrheic dermatitis, pityriasis rosea, pityriasis alba, pityriasis versicolor, erythema migrans, subacute lupus erythematosus, mycosis fungoides (CTCL).

LABORATORY EXAMINATIONS

See "Direct Microscopy," page 695, and culture.

MANAGEMENT

Antifungal Agents See "Management," page 696, for topical and systemic treatment.

FIGURE 25-9 Tinea corporis: tinea incognito An 80-year-old male with a rash on buttocks for one year. Erythematous patches on the buttocks, some with sharp margination, others with clearing, and excoriations. He had been treating the pruritus with topical corticosteroid. Tinea cruris, tinea pedis, and onychomycosis were also present.

FIGURE 25-10   Tinea corporis: tinea incognito   A 101-year-old male with bullous pemphigoid was treated with topical clobetasol by caregivers. Blotchy erythematous scaling patches are seen on the back.

FIGURE 25-11   Tinea corporis   A 10-year-old female with pruritic rash on back for 5 weeks. Well-demarcated scaling plaques are seen on the upper back. Mild scalp scaling was present. *T. tonsurans* was detected on fungal culture.

FIGURE 25-12   Tinea corporis: inflammatory   A 13-year-old female with inflammatory lesion on the arm for one week. A younger sibling had tinea capitis. Acutely inflamed edematous exudative annular plaque on the upper arm.

TINEA FACIALIS

- Dermatophytosis of the glabrous facial skin
- Well-circumscribed erythematous patch

- More commonly misdiagnosed than any other dermatophytosis.
Synonym: Tinea faciei

EPIDEMIOLOGY AND ETIOLOGY

Age of Onset More common in children.
Etiology *T. tonsurans* associated with tinea capitis in black children and their parents. *T. mentagrophytes, T. rubrum* most commonly; also *M. audouinii, M. canis.*
Predisposing Factors Animal exposure, chronic topical application of glucocorticoids.

CLINICAL MANIFESTATION

Skin Symptoms Most commonly asymptomatic. At times, pruritus and photosensitivity.

Skin Lesions

- Well-circumscribed macule to plaque of variable size; elevated border and central regression (Fig. 25-13).
- Scaling is often minimal (Fig. 25-14) but can be pronounced.
- Pink to red.
- In black patients, hyperpigmentation.
- Any area of face but usually not symmetric.

DIFFERENTIAL DIAGNOSIS

Scaling Facial Patches Seborrheic dermatitis, contact dermatitis, erythema migrans, lupus erythematosus, polymorphous light eruption, phototoxic drug eruption, lymphocytic infiltrate.

LABORATORY EXAMINATIONS

See page 695 and culture.

MANAGEMENT

Antifungal Agents See "Management," page 696, for topical and systemic therapy.

FIGURE 25-13 Tinea facialis A 32-year-old female with pruritic lesions on the face for one week; she had acquired a new kitten 2 weeks previously. Multiple small red scaling patches are seen on the lower face. KOH preparation detected septated hyphae; *M. canis* on dermatophyte culture.

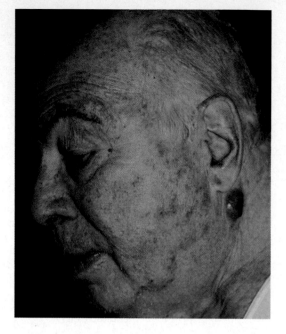

FIGURE 25-14 Tinea facialis An 83-year-old immunosuppressed male with a history of prednisone treatment for polymyalgia rheumatica and chronic lymphatic leukemia. Note a facial rash and a new nodule. Well-demarcated erythema and scaling in the beard area. SCC in situ is present on the left eyebrow. The tumor on the left neck is B-cell lymphoma; this lesion regressed when prednisone was tapered.

TINEA INCOGNITO

- Epidermal dermatophytosis, often associated with dermatophytic folliculitis.
- Occurs after the topical application of a glucocorticoid preparation to a site colonized or infected with dermatophyte.
- Occurs when an inflammatory dermatophytosis is mistaken for psoriasis or an eczematous dermatitis (Figs. 25-8 to 25-10).
- Lesions are usually aymptomatic but may be very pruritic or even painful.

- Involved sites often have exaggerated features of epidermal dermatophytoses, being a deep red or violaceous with follicular papules or pustules.
- Epidermal atrophy caused by chronic glucocorticoid application may be present.
- Systemic antifungal therapy may be indicated due to deep involvement of the hair apparatus.

DERMATOPHYTOSES OF HAIR (TRICHOMYCOSIS)

- Dermatophytes are capable of invading hair follicles and hair shafts, causing dermatophytic trichomycosis
  - Tinea capitis
  - Tinea barbae

- Dermatophytic folliculitis
- Majocchi granuloma
- Two types of hair involvement are seen (Image 25-2).

Ectothrix Endothrix

IMAGE 25-2 Dermatophytic folliculitis. Ectothrix type: mycelia and arthroconidia are seen on the surface of the hair follicle (extrapilary). Endothrix type: hyphae and arthroconidia occur within the hair shaft (intrapilary).

TINEA CAPITIS ICD-9:110.5 ∘ ICD-10:B35.0

- Dermatophytic trichomycosis of the scalp
- Predominantly a disease of preadolescent children
- Clinical presentations vary widely:
  - Noninflammatory scaling
  - Scaling and broken-off hairs

- Severe, painful inflammation with painful, boggy nodules that drain pus (kerion) and result in scarring alopecia

Synonyms: Ringworm of the scalp, tinea tonsurans

EPIDEMIOLOGY AND ETIOLOGY

Age of Onset Toddlers and school-age children. Most common at 6–10 years of age; less common after age 16. In adults it occurs most commonly in a rural setting.

Race Much more common in blacks than in whites.

Etiology/Demography

- Varies from country to country and from region to region.
- Species change in time due to immigration.
- Infections can become epidemic in schools and institutions, especially with overcrowding.
- United States: Random fungal cultures in urban study detected a 4% infection rate and a 12.7% colonization rate among black children

Epidemiology
United States and Western Europe

- 90% of cases of tinea capitis caused by *T. tonsurans*.
- Less commonly, *M. canis*.
- Formerly, most cases were caused by *M. audouinii*. Less commonly, *M. gypseum*, *T. mentagrophytes, T. rubrum.*

Eastern and Southern Europe, North Africa
T. violaceum

Transmission Person-to-person, animal-to-person, via fomites. Spores are present on asymptomatic carriers, animals, or inanimate objects.

Risk Factors For favus (see below): debilitation, malnutrition, chronic disease

CLASSIFICATION

Ectothrix infection	Invasion occurs outside hair shaft. Hyphae fragment into arthroconidia, leading to cuticle destruction. Caused by *Microsporum* spp. (*M. audouinii* and *M. canis*) (Image 25-2).
Endothrix infection	Infection occurs within hair shaft without cuticle destruction (Image 25-2). Arthroconidia found within hair shaft. Caused by *Trichophyton* spp. (*T. tonsurans* in North America; *T. violaceum* in Europe, Asia, parts of Africa).
"Black dot" tinea capitis	Variant of endothrix resembling seborrheic dermatitis.
Kerion	Variant of endothrix with boggy inflammatory plaques.
Favus	Variant of endothrix with arthroconidia and airspaces within hair shaft. Very uncommon in western Europe and North America. In some parts of the world (Middle East, South Africa), however, it is still endemic.

PATHOGENESIS

- Scalp hair traps fungi from the environment or fomites.
- Asymptomatic colonization is common.
- Trauma assists inoculation.
- Dermatophytes initially invade stratum corneum of scalp, which may be followed by hair shaft infection. Spread to other hair follicles then occurs.
  - Noninflammatory lesions:
    - Invasion of hair shaft by the dermatophytes.
    - Principally *M. audouinii* (child-to-child, via barber, hats, theater seats), *M. canis* (young pets-to-child and then child-to-child), or *T. tonsurans*.
  - Inflammatory lesions:
    - *T. tonsurans, M. canis, T. verrucosum,* and others.
    - Spores enter through breaks in hair shaft or scalp to cause clinical infection.
- Eventually, infection regresses with or without an inflammatory response.
- Clinical appearance varies with type of hair invasion, level of host resistance, degree of inflammatory host response:
  - Few dull gray, broken-off hairs with little scaling to severe painful inflammatory mass covering entire scalp.
  - Partial hair loss with inflammation in all cases.
  - Kerion is associated with a high degree of hypersensitivity to fungal hapten.
- Two types of hair invasion:
  - *Microsporum* types:
    - Small-spored ectothrix; hair shaft is invaded in mid-follicle. Intrapilary hyphae grow inward toward hair bulb. Secondary extrapilary hyphae burst, growing over surface of hair shaft.
    - Large-spored ectothrix have similar arrangement.
  - *Trichophyton* types:
    - Large-spored ectothrix (in chains); arthrospores spherical, arranged in straight chains, confined to external surface of hair shaft. Spores are all larger than those of small-spored *Microsporum* ectothrix.
    - Endothrix type; intrapilary hyphae fragment into arthroconidia within hair shaft, making it fragile, with subsequent breakage close to scalp surface.

CLINICAL MANIFESTATION

Duration of Lesions   Weeks to months.
Skin Symptoms

- Inflammatory tinea capitis:
  - Pain, tenderness
  - ± Alopecia

- Noninflammatory infection:
  - Scaling
  - Scalp pruritus
  - Diffuse or circumscribed alopecia
  - Occipital or posterior auricular adenopathy

Skin Lesions and Hair Changes
Small-Spored Ectothrix Tinea Capitis

- "Gray patch" tinea capitis (Fig. 25-15). Partial alopecia, often circular in shape, showing numerous broken-off hairs, dull gray from their coating of arthrospores. Fine scaling with fairly sharp margin. Hair shaft becomes brittle, breaking off at or slightly above scalp. Small patches coalesce, forming larger patches.

FIGURE 25-15 Tinea capitis: "gray patch" type A large, round, hyperkeratotic plaque of alopecia due to breaking off of hair shafts close to the surface, giving the appearance of a mowed wheat field on the scalp of a child. Remaining hair shafts and scales exhibit a green fluorescence when examined with Wood lamp. *M. canis* was isolated on culture.

Inflammatory response minimal, but massive scaling.
- Several or many patches, randomly arranged, may be present.
- *M. audouinii, M. ferrugineum, M. canis* infections show green fluorescence with Wood's lamp.

Endothrix Tinea Capitis

- *"Black dot" tinea capitis:* Broken-off hairs near surface give appearance of "dots" (Fig. 25-16) (swollen hair shafts) in dark-haired patients. Dots occur as affected hair breaks at surface of scalp. Tends to be diffuse and poorly circumscribed.
- Low-grade folliculitis may be present.
- Resembles seborrheic dermatitis, chronic cutaneous lupus erythematosus.
- Usually caused by *T. tonsurans, T. violaceum.*
- Onychomycosis also occurs in 2–3% of cases.
- *Kerion*:
  ◦ Inflammatory mass in which remaining hairs are loose.
  ◦ Characterized by boggy, purulent, inflamed nodules and plaques (Fig. 25-17).

◦ Usually extremely painful; drains pus from multiple openings, like honeycomb.
◦ Hairs do not break off but fall out and can be pulled without pain. Follicles may discharge pus; sinus formation; mycetoma–like grains.
◦ Thick crusting with matting of adjacent hairs.
◦ A single plaque is usual, but multiple lesions may occur with involvement of entire scalp.
◦ Frequently, associated lymphadenopathy is present.
◦ Usually caused by zoophilic (*T. verrucosum, T. mentagrophytes* var. *mentagrophytes*) or geophilic species.
◦ Heals with scarring alopecia.

- *Agminate folliculitis*:
  ◦ Less severe inflammation than kerion with sharply defined, dull red plaques studded with follicular pustules.
  ◦ Caused by zoophilic species.

- *Favus*:
  ◦ Early cases show perifollicular erythema and matting of hair.

◦ Later, thick yellow adherent crusts (scutula) composed of skin debris and hyphae that are pierced by remaining hair shafts (Fig. 25-18).
◦ Fetid odor.
◦ Shows little tendency to clear spontaneously.
◦ Often results in cutaneous atrophy, scar formation, and scarring alopecia.
◦ Caused by *T. schoenleinii.*

DIFFERENTIAL DIAGNOSIS

"Gray Patch" Tinea Capitis   Seborrheic dermatitis, psoriasis, atopic dermatitis, lichen simplex chronicus, alopecia areata.
"Black Dot" Tinea Capitis   Seborrheic dermatitis, psoriasis, seborrhiasis, atopic dermatitis, lichen simplex chronicus, chronic cutaneous lupus erythematosus, alopecia areata.
Kerion   Cellulitis, furuncle, carbuncle.
Favus   Impetigo, ecthyma, crusted scabies.

LABORATORY EXAMINATIONS

Wood Lamp

• Should be performed in any patient with scaling scalp lesions or hair loss of undetermined origin.
• *T. tonsurans,* the most common cause of tinea capitis in the United States, does not fluoresce.
• *M. canis* and *M. audouinii,* which previously were the most common causes of tinea capitis, could be diagnosed by Wood lamp examination, by bright green hair shafts with ectothrix infection.

Direct Microscopy

• Specimens should include hair roots and skin scales.
• Pluck hairs and use toothbrush to gather specimens.
• Skin scales contain hyphae and arthrospores.
• Hair
  ◦ *Ectothrix:* arthrospores can be seen surrounding the hair shaft in cuticle.
  ◦ *Endothrix:* spores within hair shaft.
  ◦ *Favus:* loose chains of arthrospores and airspaces in hair shaft.

FIGURE 25-16   Tinea capitis: "black dot" variant   A subtle, asymptomatic patch of alopecia due to breaking off of hairs on the frontal scalp in a 4-year-old black child. The lesion was detected because her infant sister presented with tinea corporis. *Trichophyton tonsurans* was isolated on culture.

FIGURE 25-17   Kerion   An extremely painful, boggy, purulent inflammatory nodule on the scalp of this 4-year-old child. The lesion drains pus from multiple openings and there is retroauricular, tender lymphadenopathy. Infection was due to *T. verrucosum* contracted from an infected rabbit.

FIGURE 25-18   Tinea capitis: favus   Extensive hair loss with atrophy, scarring, and so-called scutula, i.e., yellowish adherent crusts present on the scalp; remaining hairs pierce the scutula. *Trichophyton schoenleinii* was isolated on culture.

Fungal Culture   With brush-culture technique, a dry toothbrush or brush used for cervical Pap testing is rubbed over area of scale or alopecia; bristles are then inoculated into fungal medium. A wet cotton swab can also be rubbed in affected area, which is then implanted into medium. The cotton-tipped swab from a bacterial culturette, moistened with water, can also be used to collect the specimen and sent to a commercial laboratory. Growth of dermatophytes usually seen in 10 to 14 days.

Endothrix   *T. tonsurans, T. violaceum, T. sou-danense,* and *T. schoenleinii*
Ectothrix   *Microsporum* spp., *T. mentagro-phytes, T. verrucosum*

Favus   *T. schoenleinii,* most commonly; also *T. violaceum, M. gypseum*
Bacterial Culture   Rule out bacterial superinfection, usually *S. aureus* or GAS.

MANAGEMENT

Prevention	Important to examine home and school contacts of affected children for asymptomatic carriers and mild cases of tinea capitis. Ketoconazole or selenium sulfide shampoo may be helpful in eradicating the asymptomatic carrier state.
Topical antifungal agents	Topical agents are ineffective in management of tinea capitis. Duration of treatment should be extended until symptoms have resolved and fungal cultures negative.
Oral antifungal agents	Griseofulvin is considered the drug of choice in the United States. Short-term terbinafine, itraconazole, and fluconazole have been shown to be comparable in efficacy and safety to griseofulvin.
Griseofulvin	**Pediatric Dose**
	• Microsized: 15 mg/kg per day; maximum 500 mg/d
	• Ultramicrosized: 10 mg/kg per day
	Treatment duration: at least 6 weeks to several months; better absorption with fatty meal.
	Adult Dose
	• "Gray patch" tinea capitis: 250 mg twice daily for 1 or 2 months
	• "Black dot" tinea capitis: longer treatment and higher doses continued until KOH and cultures are negative
	For kerion:
	250 mg twice daily for 4–8 weeks, hot compresses; antibiotics for accompanying staphylococcal infection
Terbinafine	250 mg/d. Reduce dosing according to weight in pediatric patients.
Itraconazole	100-mg capsules or oral solution (10 mg/mL). Treatment duration: 4–8 weeks.
	Pediatric Dose 5 mg/kg per day
	Adult Dose 200 mg/d
Fluconazole	100-, 150-, 200-mg tablets; oral solution (10 mg/mL, 40 mg/mL). 6–8 mg/kg per day. Treatment duration: 3–4 weeks (in some cases 2).
	Pediatric Dose 6 mg/kg per day
	Daily for 2 weeks; repeat at 4 weeks if indicated
	Adult Dose 200 mg/d
Ketoconazole	200-mg tablets. Treatment duration: 4–6 weeks.
	Pediatric Dose 5 mg/kg per day
	Adult Dose 200–400 mg/d
Adjunctive therapy	
Prednisone	1 mg/kg per day for 14 days for children with severe, painful kerion.
Systemic antibiotics	If culture shows superinfection with *S. aureus* or GAS, oral antibiotic according to sensitivities of organism. Drain pus from kerion lesions.
Surgery	Drain pus from kerion lesions.

COURSE

- Chronic untreated kerion and favus, especially if infected with *S. aureus*, result in scarring alopecia.
- Regrowth of hair is the rule if treated with systemic antifungal agents.

- Favus may persist until adulthood. Radiotherapy was used to treat tinea capitis in the 1930s and 1940s; the incidence of non-melanoma skin cancer is increased fourfold in these individuals.

TINEA BARBAE   ICD-9 : 110.0 ∘ ICD-10 : B35.0   ☐ ◑

- Dermatophytic trichomycosis involving the beard and moustache areas.
- Resembles tinea capitis, with invasion of the hair shaft.

Synonym: Ringworm of the beard.

EPIDEMIOLOGY AND ETIOLOGY

Age of Onset   Adult.
Sex   Males only.
Etiology

- *T. verrucosum, T. mentagrophytes* var. *mentagrophytes*, most commonly.
- May be acquired through animal exposure.
- *T. rubrum* an uncommon cause.

Predisposing Factors   More common in farmers.

CLINICAL MANIFESTATION

Skin Symptoms   Pruritus, tenderness, pain.

Skin Lesions

- Pustular folliculitis (Fig. 25-19), i.e., hair follicles surrounded by red inflammatory papules or pustules, often with exudation and crusting.
- Involved hairs are loose and easily removed.
- With less follicular involvement, there are scaling, circular, reddish patches (tinea facialis) in which hair is broken off at the surface.
- Papules may coalesce to inflammatory plaques topped by pustules.
- Kerion: boggy purulent nodules and plaques as with tinea capitis (Fig. 25-20).
- Beard and moustache areas, rarely, eyelashes, eyebrows.

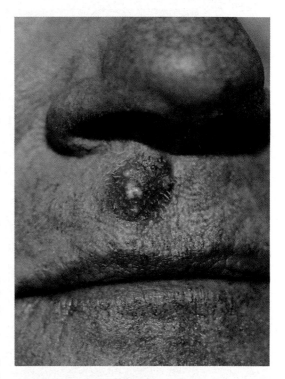

FIGURE 25-19   Tinea barbae   A 63-year-old male with pustules in beard area for several months. A large pustule in an inflammatory nodule is seen on the moustache area. Extensive subtle tinea facialis was also present. Tinea pedis, onychomycosis, and tinea cruris were present as well. KOH preparation was positive; *T. rubrum* was detected on dermatophyte culture. Bacterial culture was negative for pathogens. Facial lesions resolved with oral terbinafine.

Systemic Findings Regional lymphadenopathy, especially if of long duration and if superinfected.

DIFFERENTIAL DIAGNOSIS

Beard Folliculitis *S. aureus* folliculitis, furuncle, carbuncle, acne vulgaris, rosacea, pseudofolliculitis.

LABORATORY EXAMINATIONS

See "Laboratory Examinations," page 712.

MANAGEMENT

Topical Agents Ineffective.
Systemic Agents See "Management," page 714.

DERMATOPHYTIC FOLLICULITIS

See "Infectious Folliculitis" in Section 32.

FIGURE 25-20   Tinea barbae and tinea facialis   Confluent, painful papules, nodules, and pustules on the upper lip. Epidermal dermatophytosis (tinea facialis) with sharply marginated erythema and scaling is present on the cheeks, eyelids, eyebrows, and forehead. *Trichophyton mentagrophytes* was isolated on culture. In this case, the organism caused two distinct clinical patterns (epidermal involvement, tinea facialis versus follicular inflammation, tinea barbae), depending on whether glabrous skin or hairy skin was infected. (See also Image 25-1.)

MAJOCCHI GRANULOMA ■ ☐

- Deep dermatophytic folliculitis, with foreign-body granuloma occurring in response to dermatophytes in the dermis.
- Etiology: Most commonly *T. rubrum, T. tonsurans*
- Risk factors
  - Topical glucocorticoid application
  - Systemic immunocompromise
    - Atopic dermatitis
    - Chemotherapy for leukemia, lymphoma
    - Autoimmune disease
    - Solid-organ transplant recipient
- Pathogenesis: foreign-body response to keratin
- Clinical findings:

- Types
  - Follicular type with local immunosuppression (topical glucocorticoid use)
  - Subcutaneous nodular type with systemic immunocompromise (Fig. 25-21). Solitary or multiple
- Folliculocentric papules and pustules arise within an area of epidermal dermatophytosis such as tinea incognito (Fig. 25-8).
- Distribution: Any hair-bearing area; scalp, face, forearms, dorsum of hands/feet, shaved legs.

Synonym: Dermatophytic or trichophytic granuloma

FIGURE 25-21   Dermatophytic folliculitis: Majocchi granuloma   A 55-year-old diabetic male renal transplant recipient with painful nodules on left lower thigh. Eroded papules with crusting above the knee. Tinea pedis and onychomycosis were also present. *T. rubrum* was isolated on dermatophyte culture. He was treated with voriconazole.

CANDIDIASIS   ICD-9 : 112 ◦ ICD-10 : B37.0

- Etiology
  - Most most commonly caused by the yeast *Candida albicans*
  - Less often by other *Candida* spp.
- Clinical types and risk factors
  - Superficial infections of mucosal surface
    - Common in otherwise healthy individuals in the oropharynx and genitalia.
    - Occur in the setting of significant immunocompromise in the esophagus and tracheobronchial tree.
- Cutaneous candidiasis occurs on moist occluded skin.
- Disseminated candidemia
  - Occurs in immunocompromised individuals
  - Usually after invasion of the GI tract

Synonyms: Candidosis, moniliasis

EPIDEMIOLOGY AND ETIOLOGY

Etiology

- *C. albicans*
  - An oval yeast varying in size (2–6 μm by 3–9 μm).
  - Polymorphism is displayed as: yeast forms, budding yeast, pseudohyphae, true hyphae.
- Besides *C. albicans*, >100 species of the genus have been identified, most of which are neither commensal nor pathogenic for humans.
- Other pathogenic species, usually in the setting of immunocompromise, include: *C. tropicalis, C. parapsilosis, C. guilliermondii, C. krusei, C. pseudotropicalis, C. lusitaneae, C. glabrata.*

Ecology

- *C. albicans* and other species frequently colonize the GI tract. Colonization may occur during birthing from the birth canal, during infancy, or later.
- Oropharyngeal colonization is present in approximately 20% of healthy individuals, the rate being higher in hospitalized patients.
- Fecal colonization is higher than oral, with a rate of 40–67%; the rate increases after treatment with antibacterial agents.
- Serologic and skin test studies indicate that a significant proportion of those not colonized have been exposed to *Candida* in the past.
- Antibiotic therapy increases the incidence of carriage, the number of organisms present, and the chances for tissue invasion.
- Approximately 13% of women are colonized vaginally with *C. albicans*; antibiotic therapy, pregnancy, oral contraception, and intrauterine devices increase the incidence of carriage.

- *C. albicans* may transiently colonize the skin but is not one of the permanent flora and is seldom recovered from skin of normal individuals.
- Candidiasis *is* usually an endogenous infection.
- With balanitis, *Candida* may be transmitted from sexual partner.

Age of Onset   The young and old are more likely to be colonized.

Host Factors

- Immunocompromise
- Diabetes mellitus
- Obesity
- Hyperhidrosis, heat, maceration
- Polyendocrinopathies
- Systemic and topical glucocorticoids
- Chronic debilitation.

Immunologic Factors

- Reduced cell-mediated immunity is the most significant factor.
- Decreased specific anti-*Candida* IgA salivary antibody may be a factor.
- Defects in neutrophil or macrophage functions are factors in invasive disseminated candidiasis.

LABORATORY EXAMINATIONS

Direct Microscopy   KOH preparation visualizes pseudohyphae and yeast forms (Fig. 25-22).
Culture   *Fungal*   Identifies species of *Candida*; however, the presence in culture of *C. albicans* does not make the diagnosis of candidiasis; *Candida* is a normal inhabitant of the GI tract. Identifying *Candida* in the absence of symptoms

should not lead to treatment, because 10–20% of normal women harbor *Candida* spp. and other yeasts in the vagina. Sensitivities to antifungal agents can be performed on isolate in cases of recurrent infection.
Bacterial Rule out bacterial superinfection.

CLASSIFICATION

See Table 25-1.

MANAGEMENT

Oral Antifungal Agents Indicated for infections resistant to topical modalities of therapy.
Fluconazole Tablets: 50, 100, 150, 200 mg. Oral suspension: 50 mg/5 mL. Parenteral: for injection or IV infusion.
Itraconazole Capsules: 100 mg. Oral solution: 10 mg/mL
Ketoconazole Tablets: 200 mg

TABLE 25-1 Classification of Candidiasis

Type	Site	Clinical presentation
Occluded site (where occlusion and maceration create warm, moist microecology)	Body folds	Axillae, submammary, groin, intergluteal, abdominal panniculus Webspace: hands (erosio interdigitale blastomycetica), feet Angular cheilitis; often associated with oropharyhgeal candidiasis
	Genital	Balanitis, balanoposthitis Vulvitis, vulvovaginitis
	Occluded skin	Under occlusive dressing, under cast, back in hospitalized patient
	Folliculitis	Back; in hospitalized patient
	Area occluded under diaper	Diaper dermatitis
Nail apparatus	Paronychium	Chronic paronychia
	Nail plate	Onychia
	Hyponychium	Secondary infection with onycholysis
Chronic mucocutaneous	Extensive, multiple or 20 nail	Individuals with congenital immunologic (T cell defects) or endocrinologic disorders (hypoparathyroidism, hypoadrenalism, hypothyroidism, diabetes mellitus) develop persistent or recurrent mucosal, cutaneous, and/or paronychial/nail infections.
Genitalia	Vulva, vagina; preputial sac	Erythema, erosions, white plaques of candidal colonies
Mucosal	Oropharynx	Thrush; atrophic candidiasis; hyperplastic candidiasis
	Esophagus	Inflamed, eroded plaques
	Trachea, bronchi	Inflamed, eroded plaques
Candidemia	Skin, viscera	Skin: erythematous papules, ± hemorrhage

FIGURE 25-22 *Candida albicans:* **KOH preparation** Budding yeast forms and sausage-like pseudohyphal forms.

CUTANEOUS CANDIDIASIS   ■ ◑

- Cutaneous candidiasis occurs in moist, occluded cutaneous sites.
- Many patients have predisposing factors.

CLINICAL MANIFESTATION

Intertrigo Erythema. Pruritus, tenderness, pain.
Occluded Skin Under occlusive dressing, under cast, on back in hospitalized patient.
Diaper Dermatitis Irritability, discomfort with urination, defecation, changing diapers.

Skin Lesions
Intertrigo

- Initial pustules on erythematous base become eroded and confluent.
- Subsequently, fairly sharply demarcated, polycyclic, erythematous, eroded patches with small pustular lesions at the periphery (satellite pustulosis).
- Distribution: Inframammary (submammary) (Fig. 25-23), axillae, groins (Fig. 25-24), perineal, intergluteal cleft.

Interdigital

- Erosio interdigitalis candidomycetica.
- Most common in obese elderly.
- Initial pustule becomes eroded, with formation of superficial erosion or fissure, surrounded by thickened white skin (Fig. 25-25).
- May be associated with *Candida* paronychia.

- *Distribution*:
  - ◦ Hands: usually between third and fourth fingers (Fig. 25-25)
  - ◦ Feet: maceration in webspace

Diaper Dermatitis

- Erythema, edema with papular and pustular lesions; erosions, oozing, collarette-like scaling at the margins of lesions
- Perigenital and perianal skin, inner aspects of thighs and buttocks (Fig. 25-26).

Follicular Candidiasis

- Small, discrete pustules in ostia of hair follicles.
- Usually in occluded skin.

DIFFERENTIAL DIAGNOSIS

Intertrigo/Occluded Skin Nonspecific intertrigo, streptococcal intertrigo, intertriginous psoriasis, erythrasma, dermatophytosis, pityriasis versicolor.
Diaper Dermatitis Atopic dermatitis, psoriasis, irritant dermatitis, seborrheic dermatitis.
Folliculitis Bacterial (*S. aureus, P. aeruginosa*) folliculitis, *Pityrosporum* folliculitis, acne.

FIGURE 25-23   Cutaneous candidiasis: intertrigo   Small peripheral "satellite" papules and pustules that have become confluent centrally, creating a large eroded area in the submammary region.

FIGURE 25-24   Cutaneous candidiasis: intertrigo   Erythematous papules with a few pustules, becoming confluent on the medial thigh. The lesions occurred during a holiday trip to the Caribbean.

LABORATORY EXAMINATIONS

See "Laboratory Examination," page 718.

DIAGNOSIS

Clinical findings confirmed by direct microscopy or culture.

MANAGEMENT

See Table 25-2.

■ **TABLE 25-2** Management of Cutaneous Candidiasis	
Prevention	Keep intertriginous areas dry (often difficult). Washing with benzoyl peroxide bar may reduce *Candida* colonization. Powder with imidazole applied daily.
Topical treatment	
Castellani paint	Brings almost immediate relief of symptoms, i.e., candidal paronychia.
Glucocorticoid preparation	Judicious short-term use speeds resolution of symptoms.
Topical antifungal agents	Antifungal preparation: Nystatin, azole, or imidazole cream twice daily or more often with diaper dermatitis. Tolnaftate not effective for candidiasis. Terbinafine may be effective.
Nystatin cream	Effective for *Candida* only; not effective for dermatophytosis.
Imidazole creams	Effective for candidiasis, dermatophytosis, and pityriasis versicolor.
Oral antifungal agents	Eliminate bowel colonization. Azoles treat cutaneous infection.
Nystatin (suspension, tablet, pastille)	Not absorbed from the bowel. Eradicates bowel colonization. May be effective in recurrent candidiasis of diaper area, genitals, or intertrigo.
Systemic antifungal agents	See "Management," page 727.

FIGURE 25-25   Cutaneous candidiasis: interdigital intertrigo   An 80-year-old male with plexiform neurofibroma of the left-hand noted painful erosion in the webspace of the hand. Erosion with erythema is seen in the webspace between two fingers; the neurofibroma has created an intertriginous space.

FIGURE 25-26   Candidiasis: diaper dermatitis   Confluent erosions, marginal scaling, and "satellite pustules" in the area covered by a diaper in an infant. Atopic dermatitis or psoriasis also occurs in this distribution and may be concomitant.

- Occurs with minor variations of host factors such as
  - Antibiotic therapy
  - Glucocorticoid therapy (topical or systemic)
  - Age (very young, very old)
  - Significant immunocompromise.
- Esophageal and/or tracheobronchial candidiasis may be associated with OPC

- Always occurs in the setting of advanced immunocompromise.
- *Candida* can invade through eroded mucosa, with resultant candidemia.

Synonym: Thrush

EPIDEMIOLOGY AND ETIOLOGY

Etiology

- *C. albicans*, one of the resident flora of the mouth, overgrows in association with various local or systemic factors.
- In some cases, an exogenous infection.
- After chronic antifungal therapy, especially with advanced immunocompromise, fluconazole-resistant strains of *Candida* spp. can evolve and cause infection resistant to oral/intravenous azole therapy.

Incidence Although a number of risk factors exist (see below) and almost obligatory involvement occurs in immunocompromised patients, the vast majority of mucosal candidiasis occurs in otherwise healthy individuals.
HIV Disease In the absence of effective antiretroviral therapy (ART):
- OPC occurs in 50% of HIV-infected patients
- 80–95% of those with AIDS
- 60% relapse within 3 months after treatment.
- Esophageal candidiasis occurs in 10–15% of persons with AIDS.

Bone Marrow Transplant Recipients 30–40% develop superficial mucosal candidiasis.
CDC Surveillance Case Definition for AIDS Candidiasis of the esophagus, trachea, bronchi, or lungs is an AIDS-defining condition if the patient has no other cause of immunodeficiency and is without knowledge of HIV antibody status.

CLASSIFICATION OF MUCOSAL CANDIDIASIS

Superficial mucosal candidiasis: may be associated with mild to moderate impairment of cell-mediated immunity
Oropharyngeal candidiasis: pseudomembranous candidiasis (thrush);

erythematous (atrophic) candidiasis; candidal leukoplakia (hyperplastic candidiasis); angular cheilitis
Deep mucosal candidiasis: occurs in states of advanced immunocompromise (AIDS-defining):
esophageal candidiasis; tracheobronchial candidiasis, both of which are AIDS-defining conditions; bladder

CLINICAL MANIFESTATION

Symptoms
Oropharynx

- Often symptomatic.
- Burning or pain on eating spices/acidic foods, diminished taste sensation.
- Cosmetic concern about white curds on tongue.
- Odynophagia.
- In HIV/AIDS, may be the initial presentation; OPC is a clinical marker for disease progression, first noted when CD4+ cell count is 390/μL.

Esophagus

- Often asymptomatic.
- Occurs when CD4+ cell count is low (<200/μL) and is an AIDS-defining condition.
- Odynophagia, resulting in difficulty eating and malnutrition.

Mucosal Lesions
Type *Pseudomembranous Candidiasis (Thrush)* (Figs. 25-27 and 25-28)

- White-to-creamy plaques on any mucosal surface; vary in size from 1–2 mm to extensive and widespread.
- Removal with a dry gauze pad leaves an erythematous mucosal surface.

- Distribution: Dorsum of tongue, buccal mucosa, hard/soft palate, pharynx extending down into esophagus and tracheobronchial tree.

Erythematous (Atrophic) Candidiasis

- Smooth, red, atrophic patches (Fig. 25-29).
- Areas of thrush may also be present.

- Distribution: Hard/soft palate, buccal mucosa, dorsal surface of tongue.

Candidal Leukoplakia

- White plaques that cannot be wiped off but regress with prolonged anticandidal therapy.
- Distribution: buccal mucosa, tongue, hard palate.

FIGURE 25-27   Oral candidiasis: thrush White curdlike material on the mucosal surface of the lower lip of a child; the material can be abraded with gauze (pseudomembranous), revealing underlying erythema.

FIGURE 25-28   Oral candidiasis: thrush Extensive cottage cheeselike plaques, colonies of *Candida* that can be removed by rubbing with gauze (pseudomembranous), on the palate and uvula of an individual with advanced HIV/AIDS. Patches of erythema between the white plaques represent erythematous (atrophic) candidiasis. Involvement may extend into the esophagus and become associated with dysphagia.

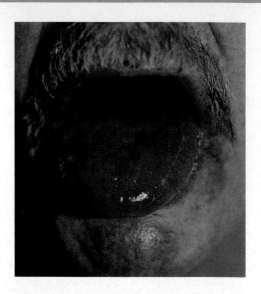

FIGURE 25-29   Oral candidiasis: atrophic glossitis with angular cheilitis   A 67-year-old alcoholic male with sore tongue. The surface of the tongue is atrophic and shiny; an intertrigo is present at the angles of the lips.

Angular Cheilitis

- Intertrigo at the corner (angles) of lips (Fig. 25-29).
- Erythema; slight erosion
- White colonies of *Candida* in some cases
- Usually associated with oropharyngeal colonization with *Candida*

General Findings
Invasive Disseminated Candidiasis

- In individuals with severe prolonged neutropenia
- Portal of entry of *Candida*
  ○ GI tract
    ▪ Invades submucosa and blood vessels
  ○ Intravascular catheter
- Candidemia: hematogenous dissemination to skin and viscera

DIFFERENTIAL DIAGNOSIS

Pseudomembranous Candidiasis (Thrush)   Oral hairy leukoplakia, condyloma acuminatum, geographic tongue, hairy tongue, lichen planus, bite irritation.
Atrophic (Erythematous) Candidiasis   Lichen planus

LABORATORY EXAMINATIONS

See "Candidiasis," page 718.
Endoscopy   Documents esophageal and/or tracheobronchial candidiasis.

DIAGNOSIS

Clinical suspicion confirmed by KOH preparation of scraping from mucosal surface.

COURSE AND PROGNOSIS

- Most cases respond to correction of the precipitating cause (e.g., use of inhaled glucocorticoids).
- Topical agents effective in most cases.
- Clinical resistance to antifungal agents may be related to patient noncompliance, severe immunocompromise, drug-drug interaction (rifampin-fluconazole).
- Bone marrow transplant recipients
  ○ 30–40% develop superficial mucosal candidiasis;
  ○ 10–25% develop deep invasive candidiasis, of whom some develop chronic visceral candidiasis, and 25% die from the infection.

- HIV/AIDS
  ○ Oropharyngeal and esophageal candidiasis have been reported with primary HIV infection.
  ○ In later HIV/AIDS without effective ART
    ▪ OPC is nearly universal.
    ▪ Esophageal infection occurs in 10–20% of patients.
    ▪ Relapse after topical or systemic treatment is expected.
    ▪ Virtually all HIV/AIDS-infected individuals with CD4+ cell counts of 100/μL are colonized with *Candida*.

MANAGEMENT

Topical Therapy   These preparations are effective in the immunocompetent individual but relatively ineffective with decreasing cell-mediated immunity.

Nystatin   (Note: Nystatin is not absorbed from the GI tract)

- Oral tablets: 100,000 units four times a day dissolved slowly in the mouth, are the most effective preparation.
- Oral suspension: 1–2 teaspoons, held in mouth for 5 min and then swallowed, may be effective.

Clotrimazole

- Oral tablets (troche), 10 mg, one tablet 5 times daily may be effective.

HIV Disease   Responds to topical and/or systemic therapy; however, recurrence is the rule. May become refractory to intermittent therapy, requiring daily chemoprophylaxis with either topical or systemic treatment. Increase dose with resistant disease.

Systemic Therapy

Fluconazole

- Oral
  - 200 mg PO once followed by 100 mg/d for 2–3 weeks, then discontinue.
  - Increase the dose to 400–800 mg in resistant infection.
- IV: Also available

Itraconazole

- Capsules or oral solution
- 100 mg PO daily or twice daily for 2 weeks
- Increase dose with resistant disease

Ketoconazole

- 200 mg PO daily or twice daily for 1–2 weeks

Fluconazole-Resistant Candidiasis

- Defined as clinical persistence of infection after treatment with fluconazole, 100 mg/d PO for 7 days.
- Occurs most commonly in HIV-infected individuals with CD4+ cell counts <50/μL who have had prolonged fluconazole exposure.
- Chronic low-dose fluconazole treatment (50 mg/d) facilitates emergence of resistant strains; 50% of resistant strains sensitive to itraconazole.
- Amphotericin B for severe resistant disease. Liposomal preparations are effective and less toxic.
- Recurrence is the rule; maintenance therapy is often required.

GENITAL CANDIDIASIS   ICD-9 : 112.1/112.2 ∘ ICD-10 : B37.3/B37.4   ■ ◐

- Occurs on the nonkeratinized genital mucosa
  - Vulva, vagina
  - Preputial sac of the penis
- Usually represents overgrowth of endogenous colonizing *Candida* rather than from exogenous source (sexual partner)

Synonym: Yeast infection

EPIDEMIOLOGY AND ETIOLOGY

Etiology   >20% of normal women have vaginal colonization with *Candida*. *C. albicans* accounts for 80–90% of genital isolates.

Incidence

- Most vaginal candidiasis (VC) occurs in the normal population.
- 75% of women experience at least one episode of VC during their lifetime.
- 40–45% experience two or more episodes.
- Often associated with vulvar candidiasis, i.e., vulvovaginal candidiasis (VVC).
- A small percentage of women (probably <5%) experience recurrent VVC (RVVC).

Risk Factors   Diabetes, HIV/AIDS

- Females
  - Often none
  - Pregnancy
  - Usually sexually active, but also in sexually inactive, young, elderly
- Males
  - Uncircumcised

Transmission

- In neonatal OPC, *C. albicans* is acquired from the genital tract of mother.
- To males from colonized sexual partners.

CLINICAL MANIFESTATION

Symptoms
Vulvitis/ Vulvovaginitis

- Onset often abrupt, usually the week before menstruation.
- Symptoms may recur before each menstruation.
- Pruritus, vaginal discharge, vaginal soreness, vulvar burning, dyspareunia, external dysuria.

Balanoposthitis, Balanitis Burning, itching, redness

Mucosal Lesions
Vulvitis

- Erosions, pustules, erythema (Fig. 25-30), swelling, removable curdlike material

Vulvitis/Vulvovaginitis

- Vaginitis with white discharge.
- Vaginal erythema and edema; white plaques that can be wiped off on vaginal and/or cervical mucosa.
- May be associated with candidal intertrigo of inguinal folds and perineum. Subcorneal pustules at periphery with fringed, irregular margins.
- In chronic cases, vaginal mucosa glazed and atrophic.

Balanoposthitis, Balanitis

- Glans and preputial sac: papules, pustules, erosions (Fig. 25-31).
- Maculopapular lesions with diffuse erythema.
- Edema, ulcerations, and fissuring of prepuce, usually in diabetic men; white plaques under foreskin.

DIFFERENTIAL DIAGNOSIS

VC/VVC Trichomoniasis (caused by *T. vaginalis*), bacterial vaginosis (caused by replacement of normal vaginal flora by an overgrowth of anaerobic microorganisms and *Gardnerella vaginalis*), lichen planus, lichen sclerosus et atrophicus.
Balanoposthitis Psoriasis, eczema, lichen planus

LABORATORY EXAMINATIONS

See "Candidiasis," page 718.

DIAGNOSIS

Clinical suspicion confirmed by KOH preparation of scraping from mucosal surface.

COURSE AND PROGNOSIS

Recurrent VVC

- Defined as three or more episodes of symptomatic VVC annually.
- Affects a small proportion of women (<5%).
- The natural history and pathogenesis of recurrent VVC are poorly understood.
- The majority of women with RVVC have no apparent predisposing conditions.

MANAGEMENT

VC/VVC Topical Therapy

- Azoles/imidazoles
  - More effective than nystatin
  - Result in relief of symptoms and negative cultures among 80–90% of patients after therapy is completed.

Recommended Regimens Single-dose regimens probably should be reserved for cases of uncomplicated mild to moderate VVC. Multiday regimens (3- to 7-day) are the preferred treatment for severe or complicated VVC.

- Butoconazole: 2% cream 5 g intravaginally for 3 days *or*
- Clotrimazole: 1% cream 5 g intravaginally for 7–14 days *or* 100-mg vaginal tablet for 7 days *or* 100-mg vaginal tablet, two tablets for 3 days *or* 500-mg vaginal tablet, one tablet in a single application *or*

FIGURE 25-30   Candidiasis: vulvitis Psoriasiform, erythematous lesions becoming confluent on the vulva with erosions and satellite pustules on the thighs.

FIGURE 25-31   Candidiasis: balanoposthitis A 52-year-old uncircumcised male with penile pain for 7 days; topical application of hydrocortisone cream worsened symptoms. Erythema and a curdlike matter is seen on the glans penis and foreskin.

- Miconazole: 2% cream 5 g intravaginally for 7 days *or* 200-mg vaginal suppository, one suppository for 3 days *or* 100-mg vaginal suppository, one suppository for 7 days *or*
- Tioconazole: 6.5% ointment 5 g intravaginally in a single application *or*
- Terconazole: 0.4% cream 5 g intravaginally for 7 days *or* 0.8% cream 5 g intravaginally for 3 days *or* 80-mg suppository, one suppository for 3 days
- Fluconazole: 150 mg PO as a single dose

Recurrent VVC   Weekly dosing with the following may be effective:

- Clotrimazole: 500-mg vaginal tablet, one tablet in a single application *or*

- Fluconazole: 150 mg PO as a single dose
- Itraconazole: 100 mg PO bid

Balanitis, Balanoposthitis

- Azole cream twice daily.
- Treat sexual partner if recurrent.

Systemic Treatment   See page 727.

CANDIDIASIS OF THE NAIL APPARATUS

See "Disorders of the Nail Apparatus," Section 33.

CHRONIC MUCOCUTANEOUS CANDIDIASIS (CMC)   ICD-9 : 112.3 ∘ ICD-10 : B37.7   □ ●

- Characterized by persistent/recurrent *Candida* infections of the oropharynx, skin, and nail apparatus (Figs. 25-32 and 25-33).
- Usually associated with
  - Underlying immunocompromise
  - Onset in infancy or early childhood.
- Oropharyngeal candidiasis:
  - Refractory to conventional therapy
  - Relapsing after successful therapy
  - Chronic infection results in hypertrophic (leukoplakic) candidiasis.
- Cutaneous candidiasis manifests as:
  - Intertrigo
  - Widespread infection (Figs. 25-32, 25-33) of the trunk and/or extremities

- Lesions become hypertrophic in chronic untreated cases.
- Infection of the nail apparatus is universal with
  - Chronic paronychia
  - Nail plate infection and dystrophy
  - Eventually total nail dystrophy.
- Many patients also have dermatophytosis and cutaneous warts.
- Six types of CMC have been defined:
  - Chronic oral candidiasis
  - Chronic candidiasis with endocrinopathy
  - Chronic candidiasis without endocrinopathy
  - Chronic localized mucocutaneous candidiasis
  - Chronic diffuse candidiasis
  - Chronic candidiasis with thymoma.

CANDIDEMIA AND DISSEMINATED CANDIDIASIS

See "Systemic Fungal Infections with Dissemination to Skin," below.

FIGURE 25-32 Mucocutaneous candidiasis Persistent candidiasis in an immunocompromised infant manifesting as erosions covered by scales and crusts, oropharyngeal candidiasis, and widespread infection of the trunk.

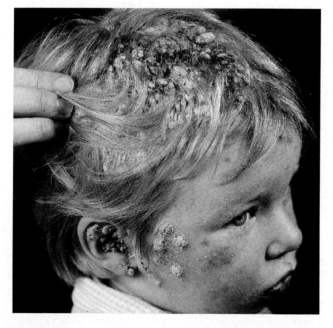

FIGURE 25-33 Mucocutaneous candidiasis This 3-year-old child with hypothyroidism had oral thrush, intertriginous candidiasis, warty hyperkeratoses, and crusts on the scalp and face; and also, candidal onychomycosis. The warty growths shown in the photo consisted of dried pus, serum, and pure cultures of *Candida*.

MALASSEZIA INFECTIONS

- Clinical syndromes
  - Pityriasis or tinea versicolor
- *Malassezia* folliculitis
- Seborrheic dermatitis (implicated in pathogenesis)

PITYRIASIS VERSICOLOR (PV)   ICD-9 : 111.0 ∘ ICD-10 : B36.0

- Chronic asymptomatic scaling epidermomycosis
- Associated with the superficial overgrowth of the hyphal form of *Malassezia furfur*
- Clinical findings:
  - Well-demarcated scaling patches
- Variable pigmentation: hypo- and hyperpigmented; pink
- Most commonly on the trunk.

Synonym: Tinea versicolor

EPIDEMIOLOGY AND ETIOLOGY

Etiology

- *M. furfur* (previously known as *Pityrosporum ovale, P. orbiculare*)
- Lipophilic yeast that normally resides in the keratin of skin and hair follicles of individuals at puberty and beyond.
- An opportunistic organism, causing pityriasis versicolor and *Malassezia* folliculitis; it is implicated in the pathogenesis of seborrheic dermatitis.
- *Malassezia* infections are not contagious.
- Overgrowth of resident cutaneous flora occurs under certain favorable conditions.

Age of Onset   Young adults. Less common when sebum production is reduced or absent; tapers off during fifth and sixth decades.

Predisposing Factors

- Warm season or climates; tropical climate
- Hyperhidrosis; aerobic exercise
- Oily skin
- Glucocorticoid treatment
- Immunodeficiency
- Application of lipids such as cocoa butter predisposes young children to PV

Season

- Temperate zones
  - More common in summertime
  - 2% of population
  - May regress during cooler months
  - In physically active individuals, may persist year round.
- Subtropical and tropical zones
  - Year round
  - 20% of population

PATHOGENESIS

- *Malassezia* changes from the blastospore form to the mycelial form under the influence of predisposing factors (see above).
- Dicarboxylic acids formed by enzymatic oxidation of fatty acids in skin surface lipids inhibit tyrosinase in epidermal melanocytes and thereby lead to hypomelanosis.
- The enzyme is present in *M. furfur*.

CLINICAL MANIFESTATION

Duration of Lesions   Months to years.
Skin Symptoms

- Usually none.
- Occasionally, mild pruritus.
- Individuals with PV usually present because of cosmetic concerns about the dyspigmentation.

Skin Lesions

- Macules, sharply marginated (Figs. 25-34 through 25-36), round or oval in shape, varying in size.
- Fine scaling is best appreciated by gently abrading lesions with a no. 15 scalpel blade or the edge of a microscope slide.
- Treated or burned-out lesions lack scale.
- Some patients have findings of *Malassezia* folliculitis and seborrheic dermatitis.
- Color:
  - In untanned skin, lesions are light brown (Fig. 25-35).
  - On tanned skin, hypopigmented (Fig. 25-36).
  - In brown- or black-skinned persons, dark brown macules (Fig. 25-34). Brown of varying intensities and hues; off-white macules.

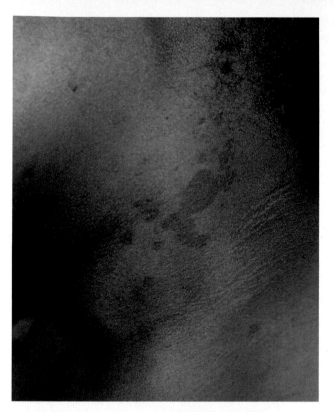

FIGURE 25-34   Pityriasis versicolor: hyperpigmented   A 23-year-old obese black female with discoloration of the neck for 1 year. Sharply marginated brown scaling macules on the left side of the neck. The velvety texture and hyperpigmentation of the skin of the neck is acanthosis nigricans associated with obesity.

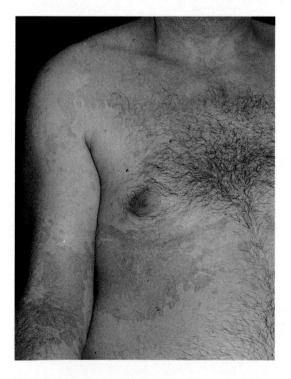

FIGURE 25-35   Pityriasis versicolor: hyperpigmented   A 36-year-old male with pigmented patches on trunk and arms for several years. Multiple pink, well-demarcated scaling macules becoming confluent on the upper and lateral trunk, neck and arm.

∘ Some PV lesions are pink (Fig. 25-35).
∘ In time, individual lesions may enlarge, merge, forming extensive geographic areas.
∘ Distribution:
  ▪ Upper trunk, upper arms, neck, abdomen, axillae, groins, thighs, genitalia.
  ▪ Facial, neck, and/or scalp lesions occur in patients applying creams/ointments or topical glucocorticoid preparations.

DIFFERENTIAL DIAGNOSIS

Hypopigmented PV   Vitiligo, pityriasis alba, postinflammatory hypopigmentation, tuberculoid leprosy.
Scaling Lesions   Tinea corporis, seborrheic dermatitis, pityriasis rosea, guttate psoriasis, nummular eczema.

LABORATORY EXAMINATIONS

Direct Microscopic Examination of Scales Prepared with KOH

• Filamentous hyphae and globose yeast forms, termed *spaghetti and meatballs*, are seen (Fig. 25-37).

Wood Lamp

• Blue-green fluorescence of scales.

• May be negative in individuals who have showered recently because the fluorescent chemical is water soluble.
• Vitiligo appears as depigmented, white, and has no scale.

Dermatopathology

• Budding yeast and hyphal forms in the most superficial layers of the stratum corneum, seen best with PAS stain.
• Variable hyperkeratosis, psoriasiform hyperplasia, chronic inflammation with blood vessel dilatation.

DIAGNOSIS

Clinical findings, confirmed by positive KOH preparation findings.

COURSE AND PROGNOSIS

Infection persists for years if predisposing conditions persist. Dyspigmentation persists for months after infection has been eradicated.

MANAGEMENT

Topical agents

Selenium sulfide (2.5%) lotion or shampoo	Apply daily to affected areas for 10–15 min, followed by shower, for 1 week
Ketoconazole shampoo	Applied same as selenium sulfide shampoo
Azole creams (ketoconazole, econazole, micronazole, clotrimazole)	Apply daily or twice daily for 2 weeks
Terbinafine 1% solution	Apply twice daily for 7 days

Systemic therapy (None of these agents is approved for use in PV in the United States)

Ketoconazole	400 mg stat (take 1 h before exercise)
Fluconazole	400 mg stat
Itraconazole	400 mg stat

Secondary prophylaxis

	Ketoconazole shampoo once or twice a week
	Selenium sulfide (2.5%) lotion or shampoo
	Salicylic acid/sulfur bar
	Pyrithione zinc (bar or shampoo)
	Ketoconazole 400 mg PO monthly

MALASSEZIA FOLLICULITIS

See "Infectious Folliculitis" Section 32.

SEBORRHEIC DERMATITIS

See "Seborrheic Dermatitis," Section 2.

FIGURE 25-36 Pityriasis versicolor: hypopigmented Multiple, small-to-medium-sized, well-demarcated hypopigmented macules on the back of a tanned individual with white skin.

FIGURE 25-37 *Malassezia furfur*: **KOH preparation** Round yeast and elongated pseudohyphal forms, so-called "spaghetti and meatballs."

TRICHOSPORON INFECTIONS

Etiology: *Trichosporon* species of yeasts
- Previously all pathogenic members of genus Trichosporon regarded as a single species, *Trichosporon beigelii.*
- Potential human pathogens: *T. asahii, T. inkin, T. asteroides, T. cutaneum, T. mucoides, T. ovoides, T. pullulans, T. loubieri.*
- Soil inhabitants.
- Common colonizers of skin, respiratory and GI tracts.

Pathogens
- Superficial infections: Piedra; infection of hair shaft
  - White piedra: *Trichosporon asahii, T. ovoides, T. inkin, T. mucoides, T. asteroides,* and *T. cutaneum*
  - Black piedra: *Piedraia hortae*
- Invasive infection in the immunocompromised host
  - *T. asahii*
  - *Blastoschizomyces capitatus,* (formerly *T. capitatus* and also known as *Geotrichum capitatum*)

Clinical findings
Piedra: asymptomatic superficial fungal infection of the hair shaft.

- *White piedra*
  - Pubic, axillary, beard, and eyebrow/eyelash hair
  - More common in temperate and semitropical regions
  - White to beige nodules on hair shaft; soft; easily removed.
- Black piedra
  - Scalp hair
  - Most common in tropical regions (high temperature, humidity)
  - Darkly pigmented, firmly attached nodules (up to a few millimeters) on the hair shaft; weakens hair shaft with hair breakage. Hard. Firmly attached.
- Disseminated trichosporonosis
  - Emerging opportunistic infection
  - Associated with neutropenia
  - Dissemination occurs to skin (erythematous or purpuric tender papules), lungs, kidneys, and spleen.
  - Differential diagnosis: disseminated candidiasis

Management: topical and/or systemic azole

TINEA NIGRA   ICD-10 : B36.1

Superficial fungal infection of the stratum corneum
Etiology: *Hortaea* (*Exophiala* or *Phaeoannellomyces*) *werneckii*
- Dematiaceous or pigmented fungus

Epideminology
- More commonly in tropical climates.
- Direct inoculation onto the skin from contact with decaying vegetation, wood, or soil seems to be the form of acquisition.

Clinical findings
- Brown to black nonscaly macule(s) with well-defined borders (Fig. 25-38) that resemble silver nitrate stains
- Distribution
  - Palm: tinea nigra palmaris
  - Sole: tinea nigra plantaris

Diagnosis: direct microscopy, visualizing abundant branching septate hyphae.
Management: topical azole.

FIGURE 25-38 Tinea nigra Uniformly tan macule on the plantar foot, present for several years. KOH preparation showed hyphae.

INVASIVE AND DISSEMINATED FUNGAL INFECTIONS

- Subcutaneous mycoses
  - Cutaneous and subcutaneous infections following local inoculation
  - Risk factors
    - Occur in otherwise healthy individuals
    - In the setting of immunocompromise, can disseminate systemically
  - Types
    - Mycetoma
    - Chromomycosis
    - Sporotrichosis

- Hematogenously disseminated infections to skin:
  - Many individuals have underlying immunocompromise.
  - Source of cutaneous inoculation
    - Primary pulmonary infection (Cryptococcosis, blastomycosis, histoplasmosis, coccidioidomycosis, penicillinosis)
    - GI tract–*Candida* spp
    - Intravascular catheters–*Candida* spp

SUBCUTANENOUS MYCOSES ICD-10: B36.1

- A heterogeneous group of fungal infections that develop at the site of transcutaneous trauma.
- Infection slowly evolves as the etiologic agent survives and adapts to the adverse host tissue environment.
- Diagnosis
  - Clinical findings

  - Histopathology
  - Fungal culture: isolation of the pathogen
- Types
  - Mycetoma
  - Chromomycosis
  - Sporotrichosis

MYCETOMA ICD-9 : 117.4 ∘ ICD-10 : B47.0 □→■* ◑

- A chronic suppurative infection originating in dermis and subcutis, extending into contiguous tissues (fascia, bone).
- Characterized by the presence of grains, which are tightly clumped colonies of the causative agent.
- Clinical findings
  - Skin findings
    - Painless swelling
    - Woody induration
    - Sinus tracts that discharge pus intermittently

- Systemic symptoms—do not develop
- Dissemination to distant sites does not occur.
- Variants and etiologic agents
  - Botryomycosis (caused by bacteria)
  - Actinomycetoma (caused by Actinomycetales organisms)
  - Eumycetoma (caused by true fungi)

Synonyms: Madura foot, maduromycetoma

*Depending on geography.

EPIDEMIOLOGY AND ETIOLOGY

Age of Onset 20–50 years
Sex 90% of patients are males
Demography

- Rural inhabitants
- Agricultural workers and laborers exposed to soil
- Tropical and subtropical regions.

Transmission

- Cutaneous inoculation of organism
  - Thorn prick
  - Wood splinter
  - Stone cut

- Contaminated with soil or plant debris
- Into foot or hand

Etiology and Epidemiology

- The predominant agent varies with the locality.
- Fungi isolated from soil except *Actinomyces israelii.*
- Tropical and subtropical climate supports growth of organisms.
- In Central/South America, 90% of cases caused by *Nocardia brasiliensis.*
- In Africa, *M. mycetomatis* is common cause.
- Most commonly seen in India, Mexico, Nigeria, Saudi Arabia, Senegal, Somalia, Sudan, Venezuela, Yemen, Zaire.
- Causative agent forms dense colonies, i.e., grains.

Risk Factors Poor hygiene, walking barefoot, necrotic injured tissue, diminished nutrition.

PATHOGENESIS

- Pathogens live in soil and enter through breaks in the skin.
- Only organisms that can survive at body temperature can produce mycetoma.
- Infection begins in skin and subcutaneous tissues, extending into fascial planes, destroying contiguous tissues.

CLINICAL MANIFESTATION

Incubation Period Lesion occurs at inoculation site weeks to years after trauma.
Duration of Lesion Lesions may continue to expand for decades.
Symptoms Relatively few, with little pain, tenderness, or fever.

Skin Lesions
Inoculation Site

- Papule/nodule at inoculation site (Fig. 25-39).
- Swelling increases slowly.
- Epidermis ulcerates and pus-containing granules (grains) drain.
- *Granules* (Fig. 25-40) are microbial colonies, small (<1–5 mm).
- Palpation: Usually not tender; pus drains on pressure.
- Distribution:
  - Unilateral on the leg, foot, hand.
  - Uncommonly: torso, arm, head, thigh, buttock.

Chronic Lesions

- Fistulae form with draining pus (Fig. 25-41).

FIGURE 25-39 Actinomycetoma A 23-year-old Hispanic female from Central America with a painful lesion for 6 months. Confluent erythematous violaceous nodules on the right prepatellar area arising in an old scar. Lesional biopsy detected *Nocardia. Nocardia brasiliensis* was isolated on culture of biopsy specimen. The lesion resolved with trimethoprim-sulfamethoxazole.

FIGURE 25-40 Mycetoma granules White granules (arrrows) in drainage from MRSA botryomycosis. (see Fig. 31-7.)

- Infection spreads to deeper tissues, into fascia, muscle, bone.
- Tissue becomes greatly distorted.
- Old mycetoma characterized by healed scars and draining sinuses.
- Central clearing gives older lesions an annular shape.

General Findings

- Fever with secondary bacterial superinfection.
- Regional lymphadenopathy occasionally.
- Osteomyelitis of contiguous bone may occur.

ETIOLOGY AND CLASSIFICATION OF MYCETOMA-LIKE CLINICAL PRESENTATION WITH GRAIN FORMATION

Type of Mycetoma	Etiologic Agents
Botryomycosis Caused by true bacteria. Not a true mycetoma.	Most common: *Staphylococcus aureus* Also: S. *epidermidis, P. aeruginosa, Escherichia coli, Bacteroides* spp., *Proteus* spp., *Streptococcus* spp.
Actinomycetoma (actinomycotic mycetoma) Caused by Actinomycetales organisms	*Actinomyces:* cause mycetoma and actinomycosis (cervical, thoracic, abdominal) *Nocardia:* cause mycetoma, lymphocutaneous infection (sporotrichoid pattern), superficial skin infections, disseminated infection with skin involvement *Actinomadura* *Streptomyces*
Eumycetoma (eumycotic mycetoma) Caused by true fungi	Most common: *Pseudallescheria boydii, Madurella grisea, M. mycetomatis* Also: *Phialophora jeanselmei, Pyrenochaeta romeroi, Leptosphaeria senegaliensis, Curvularia lunata, Neotestudina rosatti, Aspergillus nidulans* or *flavus, Acremonium* spp., *Fusarium* spp., *Cylindrocarpon* spp., *Microsporum audouinii*

DIFFERENTIAL DIAGNOSIS

Chronic Draining Subcutaneous Inflammatory Mass(es)   Osteomyelitis, botryomycosis, chromoblastomycosis, blastomycosis, bacterial pyoderma, foreign-body granuloma.

LABORATORY EXAMINATIONS

Smear of Pus from Lesion Granules   Medlar bodies (Table 25-3) visualized on KOH preparation as microbial colonies (see below).
Dermatopathology   Pseudoepitheliomatous hyperplasia of epidermis. Grains are found in purulent foci surrounded by fibrosis and mononuclear cell inflammatory cell response.
Culture   Isolate organism. Bacterial superinfection common.
Imaging   CT scan and echosonography define the extent of involvement. X-ray of bone shows multiple osteolytic lesions (cavities), periosteal new bone formation.

TABLE 25-3   Color Grains in Mycetoma and Associated Organisms

Color of Grain	Organism
Black	*Madurella mycetomatis* *M. grisea* *Leptosphaeria senegalensis*
White	*Pseudallescheria boydii* *Acremonium* spp. *Nocardia brasiliensis* *N. asteroides*
White to yellow	*N. caviae*
Pink, white, to cream	*Actinomyces israelii* *Actinomadura madurae*
Red	*A. pelletieri*

FIGURE 25-41 Eumycotic mycetoma The foot, ankle, and leg are grossly distorted with edema and confluent subcutaneous nodules, cauliflower-like tumors, and ulcerations.

DIAGNOSIS

Clinical suspicion confirmed by:

- Demonstration of grains in pus and/or
- Visualization of Medlar bodies—globular colonies of infecting organims that appear as granules or grains in pus or lesional biopsy specimen
  - ∘ White
  - ∘ Black
  - ∘ Gray
- Isolation of organism on culture.

COURSE AND PROGNOSIS

- Mycetoma runs a relentless course over many years, destroying contiguous fascia and bone.
- Actinomycetoma usually enlarges more rapidly than eumycetoma.
- Bacterial superinfections occur.
- Relapse after antifungal or antibiotic therapy common.

MANAGEMENT

Individuals are advised to seek medical attention early.

Surgery Smaller lesions can be cured by surgical excision. More extensive lesions often recur after incomplete excision. Bulk reduction surgery is performed; amputation/disarticulation avoided. Causative agent identified, and effective antimicrobial agent given.

Systemic Antimicrobial Therapy Usually continued for 10 months.

Botryomycoses Antimicrobial agents according to sensitivities of isolated organism. May be MRSA.

Actinomycotic Mycetoma May respond to prolonged chemotherapy of streptomycin combined with either dapsone or trimethoprim-sulfamethoxazole.

Eumycetoma Rarely responds to chemotherapy. Some cases caused by *M. mycetomatis* may respond to ketoconazole or itraconazole.

CHROMOMYCOSIS   ICD-9 : 117.2 ∘ ICD-10 : B43.0   ■*○

- Chronic localized invasive fungal infection of skin and subcutaneous tissues
- Etiology: pigmented (dematiaceous or dark-walled) fungi.
- Clinical findings: verrucous plaques usually occurring on the leg or foot.

Synonym: Chromoblastomycosis. One of the phaeohyphomycoses.

* Depending on geography.

EPIDEMIOLOGY AND ETIOLOGY

Age of Onset   20–60 years.
Sex   Males > females.
Etiology   Dematiaceous fungi, characterized by melanin in mycelial walls.

- *Fonsecaea pedrosoi* (most commonly)
- Also *F. compacta, Phialophora verrucosa, Cladosporium carrionii, Rhinocladiella aquaspersa, Botryomyces caespitosus.*

Risk Groups

- Living in rural areas in tropical and subtropical regions and exposed to soil while barefoot.
- Agricultural workers
- Miners
- May progress more rapidly in the immunocompromised host.

Transmission

- Cutaneous inoculation.
- Autoinoculation to other sites may occur.
- Transmission to other individuals does not occur.

Demography   Fungi isolated from soil and vegetation, preferring regions with >2.5 m (> 100 in.) of rainfall per year and mean temperatures from 12°–24°C.

CLINICAL MANIFESTATION

Duration of Lesion   Lesions may continue to expand for decades.
Symptoms   Relatively few

- Little pain, tenderness, or fever
- Usually present with
  ∘ Bacterial superinfection
  ∘ Cosmetic disfigurement
  ∘ Lymphedema.

Skin Lesions

- Inoculation site
  ∘ Single scaling nodule at site of traumatic implantation (Fig. 25-42).
- Chronic lesions (months to years)
  ∘ New crops of nodules appear.
  ∘ Expanding verrucous plaques with central clearing and islands of normal skin between verrucous macules.
  ∘ Large cauliflower-like lesions often form, which, in some cases, may become pedunculated.
  ∘ Surface of verrucous lesion: pustules, small ulcerations, "black dots" of hemopurulent material; friable granulation tissue that bleeds easily is common.
  ∘ Extension occurs via
    ▪ Lymphatic spread
    ▪ Autoinoculation
  ∘ 10–20 cm in diameter, enveloping calf or foot.
  ∘ Lymphedema of involved extremity (elephantiasis)
  ∘ Arrangement: Smaller lesions coalesce to form large verrucous masses. Central clearing gives older lesions an annular shape.
- Distribution
  ∘ Unilateral on the leg, foot
  ∘ Also, hand, thorax

DIFFERENTIAL DIAGNOSIS

Large Verrucous Plaques   Blastomycosis, tuberculosis verrucosa cutis, mycetoma, sporotrichosis, nontuberculous *Mycobacterium* infection, lepromatous leprosy, foreign-body granuloma, pyoderma gangrenosum, squamous cell carcinoma.

LABORATORY EXAMINATIONS

Smear of Pus from Lesion

- Medlar bodies (see below) visualized on 10–20% KOH preparation as black dots.
- Hyphal forms can be seen in crusts, pus, exudate.

Dermatopathology

- Warty granuloma: pseudoepitheliomatous hyperplasia, hyperkeratosis, intraepidermal abscesses containing inflammatory cells and Medlar bodies.
- Medlar bodies
  - Also known as sclerotic bodies, "copper pennies"
  - Small brown fungal forms, which are round with thick bilaminate walls
  - 4–6 μm in diameter
  - Occur singly or in clusters
- All etiologic agents appear identical in tissue.
- Older lesions show dense fibrosis in and around granulomas.

Culture   Organism in Sabouraud glucose agar shows velvety green to black, restricted, slow-growing colonies. Agents grow very slowly, requiring 4–6 weeks for identification.

DIAGNOSIS

Clinical suspicion confirmed by

- Visualization of Medlar bodies on
  - Smear of pus
  - Lesional biopsy specimen
- Isolation of organism on culture.

COURSE AND PROGNOSIS

- Bacterial superinfections.
- Recurrence after oral triazole therapy common.
- Late complication is squamous cell carcinoma arising within verrucous area.

MANAGEMENT OF CHROMOMYCOSIS

Adjunctive Therapy   Application of heat may be helpful in that lesions arise at cooler acral sites.
Surgery   Smaller lesions can be cured by surgical excision.
Parenteral Antimicrobial Chemotherapy   *Amphotericin B*: not often effective at usual dosing.
Oral Antifungal Agents   Treatment is usually continued for at least 1 year. The response is highly variable.
>   *Terbinafine,* 250 mg/d
>   *Itraconazole,* 200–600 mg/d
>   *Ketoconazole,* 400–800 mg/d

FIGURE 25-42   Chromomycosis   Hyperkeratotic and crusted plaque with old scars on the leg had been present for several decades.

SPOROTRICHOSIS   ICD-9 : 117.1 ∘ ICD-10 : B42.0   □→□ ◐ ◑

- Etiologic Agent: *Sporothrix schenckii*
- Infection occurs following accidental inoculation of skin
- Clinical findings
  - Nodule at the inoculation site; ulcerates; verrucous
  - Chronic nodular lymphangitis
  - Subcutaneous swelling

- In the immunocompromised host, disseminated infection can occur from skin or pulmonary infection.

Synonym: Rose-thorn or rose-gardener's disease

EPIDEMIOLOGY AND ETIOLOGY

Etiologic Agent   *Sporothrix schenckii*

- Dimorphic fungus
  - Tissue form is an oval, cigar-shaped yeast.
- Lives as a saprophyte on plants
- Worldwide

Sex   Males > females, especially disseminated disease.

Occupation   Occupation exposure important:

- Gardeners
- Farmers
- Florists
- Lawn laborers
- Agricultural workers
- Forestry workers
- Paper manufacturers
- Gold miners
- Laboratory workers
- In Uruguay, 80% of cases occur after a scratch by an armadillo.

Transmission

- Cutaneous local sporotrichosis
  - Commonly, subcutaneous inoculation or through small abrasion:
    - Contaminated sharp object (rose or barberry thorn, barb, wood splinter)
    - Sphagnum moss, straw, marsh hay, soils.
  - Rarely, inhalation, aspiration, or ingestion causes systemic infection.
  - Zoonosis:
    - Rarely transmitted from cats with sporotrichosis to humans.
    - Armadillos
- Lung
  - Inhalation of spores

Epidemiology

- Ubiquitous, worldwide.
- More common in temperate, tropical zones.
- Most cases isolated.
- Epidemics have occurred: exposure to cats with sporotrichosis; South African gold miners.

Risk Factors   *Cutaneous (Localized) Infection* Diabetes mellitus, alcoholism.

Disseminated Disease   HIV infection, hematologic and lymphoproliferative disease, immunosuppressive therapy.

PATHOGENESIS

- After subcutaneous inoculation, *S. schenckii* grows locally.
- Infection can be limited to the site of inoculation (*plaque sporotrichosis*).
- Infection can extend along the proximal lymphatic channels (*lymphangitic sporotrichosis*).
  - Other infections have similar lymphatic involvement, the pattern being referred to as *sporotrichoid* or resembling *lymphatic sporotrichosis*.)
- Spread beyond an extremity is rare; hematogenous dissemination from the skin remains unproven.
- The portal for extracutaneous sporotrichosis (e.g., osteoarticular) is unknown but is probably the lung.

CLINICAL MANIFESTATION

Incubation Period   3 weeks (range, 3 days to 12 weeks) after trauma or injury to site of lesion. Lesions are relatively asymptomatic, painless. Afebrile.

Skin Lesions
Fixed Cutaneous (Plaque) Sporotrichosis   Infection at inoculation site only; no lymphangiitis.

- Subcutaneous papule, pustule, or nodule appears at inoculation site several weeks after inoculation. Surrounding skin is pink to purplish. In time, skin becomes fixed to deeper tissues.
- Verrucous plaque.
- Sporotrichoid chancre; indurated ulcer may occur. Border ragged and not sharply demarcated.
- Draining lymph nodes become inflamed and enlarged.

- Crusted ulcers, ecthymatous, verrucous plaques, pyoderma gangrenosum-like, infiltrated papules and plaques may also occur.
- *Distribution:*
  ◦ Primary lesion most common on dorsum of hand or finger.
  ◦ Fixed plaque: face in children; upper extremities in adults.

Lymphangitic Sporotrichosis

- Follows lymphatic extension of local cutaneous type (Figs. 25-43, 25-44).
- Proximal to local cutaneous lesion.
- Red nodules form in intervening lymphatics; may become indurated, nodular, thickened.

FIGURE 25-43   Sporotrichosis: acute lymphangitic type   A 78-year-old gardener with tender nodules on hand and arm for 4 weeks. Erythematous nodules in a linear array in lymphatic channels on the dorsum of the hand and forearm. *S. schenckii* was isolated on culture of a lesional biopsy specimen.

FIGURE 25-44   Sporotrichosis: chronic lymphangitic type   An erythematous papule at the site of inoculation on the index finger with a linear arrangement of erythematous dermal and subcutaneous nodules extending proximally in lymphatic vessels of the dorsum of the hand and arm.

- *Distribution*: Inoculation nodule on hand/finger with chronic nodular lymphangiitis up arm.

Disseminated Sporotrichosis

- Fungus disseminates hematogenously to skin, as well as joints, eyes, and meninges.
- Cutaneous lesions
  - ◦ Crusted nodules, ulcers. May become confluent
  - ◦ Widespread
- *Distribution*: widespread lesions, usually sparing palms, soles

General examination

Lungs Pulmonary sporotrichosis presents as a single cavitary upper-lobe lesion; fibrosis.
Joints Swelling, painful joint(s) (hand, elbow, ankle, knee), often in the absence of skin lesion. Draining sinuses may occur over joints, bursae.
Hematogenous dissemination This results in skin, bone, muscle, joint, visceral, CNS (chronic meningitis) lesions.

DIFFERENTIAL DIAGNOSIS

Plaque Sporotrichosis Cutaneous tuberculosis, nontuberculous mycobacterial infection, tularemia, cat-scratch disease, primary syphilis, bacterial pyoderma, foreign-body granuloma, inflammatory dermatophytoses, blastomycosis, chromomycosis, mycetoma, leishmaniasis.
Chronic Nodular Lymphangitic Sporotrichosis
Other Infecting Agents *Mycobacterium marinum, Nocardia brasiliensis, Leishmania brasiliensis, Francisella tularensis.*

LABORATORY EXAMINATIONS

Touch Preparation In disseminated sporotrichosis (usually with advanced HIV disease), KOH solution added to smear from lesional skin biopsy specimen helps visualize multiple yeast forms.
Gram Stain In disseminated sporotrichosis (usually with advanced HIV disease), smear from crusted lesion shows multiple yeast forms.
Dermatopathology

- Granulomatous, Langerhans-type giant cells, pyogenic microabscesses.

- Organisms usually rare, difficult to visualize.
- In the immunocompromised host, yeast appear as myriads of 1- to 3-μm by 3- to 10-μm cigar shaped forms.

Culture Organism usually isolated within a few days from lesional biopsy specimen.

DIAGNOSIS

Clinical suspicion and isolation of organism on culture.

COURSE AND PROGNOSIS

- Shows little tendency to resolve spontaneously.
- Responds well to therapy, but a significant percentage relapse after completion of therapy.
- Disseminated infection in HIV-infected individuals responds poorly to all forms of therapy.

MANAGEMENT[1]

Oral Antifungal Agents

- *Itraconazole*: 200–600 mg/d. Very effective for lymphocutaneous infection; not as effective for bone/joint and pulmonary infection.
- *Fluconazole*: 200–400 mg/d reported to be effective.
- *Ketoconazole*: 400–800 mg/d reported to be effective.
- *Terbinafine*: 1000 mg/d reported to be effective.
- *Saturated solution of potassium iodide*: 4.5–9 mL/d for adults effective for lymphocutaneous infection; less effective than oral antifungal agents. Adverse events: GI disturbance, acneiform rash.

Intravenous Therapy *Amphotericin B*: For those with meningeal, pulmonary, or disseminated infection or who are unable to tolerate oral therapy for lymphocutaneous disease.

[1]Kauffman CA et al: Clin Infect Dis 30:684, 2000.

SYSTEMIC FUNGAL INFECTIONS WITH DISSEMINATION TO SKIN

Systemic fungal infections with cutaneous dissemination occur most often in the immunocompromised host.

■ Primary lung infection; can disseminate hematogenously to multiple organ systems, including the skin.
  ▪ Cryptococcosis
  ▪ Histoplasmosis

• North American blastomycosis
• Coccidioidomycosis
• Penicillinosis

■ Dissemination from GI tract or intravascular catheter; neutropenic host.
  ▪ Candidemia and disseminated candidiasis

DISSEMINATED CRYPTOCOCCOSIS   ICD-9 : 117.5 ∘ ICD-10 : B45.0

■ Cryptococcosis is a systemic mycosis
■ Primary pulmonary infection
■ Occasional hematogenous dissemination to meninges and skin

■ Dissemination occurs in advanced HIV/AIDS.
Synonyms: Torulosis

EPIDEMIOLOGY AND ETIOLOGY

• *Cryptococcus neoformans*, a yeast, serotypes A, B, C, D causing infection in humans
  ∘ Serotypes A and D designated *C. neoformans* var *neoformans*
  ∘ Serotypes B and C, *C. neoformans* var *gattii*

• In tissue, encapsulated yeastlike fungi (3.5 to 7.0 m in diameter); bud connected to parent cell by narrow pore; capsule thickness variable
• Found in soil and dried bird droppings. *C. neoformans* var. *gattii* causes localized infections (cryptococcomas) in tropical climates; associated with eucalyptus plants.
• Polysaccharide capsule is major virulence factor; basis for antigen testing.

Age of Onset   More common over the age of 40 years.
Sex   Males > females 3:1.
Incidence

• Globally, cryptococcosis (usually meningitis) is the most common invasive mycosis in HIV/AIDS, occurring in 6 to 9% of persons with advanced untreated HIV/AIDS in the United States and 20 to 30% in Africa.
• Incidence is also high in Europe and South America.
• In the industrialized nations, the incidence is much less due to immune reconstitution.

• In untreated HIV/AIDS, cutaneous dissemination occurs in 10 to 15% of cryptococcosis cases.

Risk Factors   HIV/AIDS, solid-organ transplantation, glucocorticoid therapy, sarcoidosis, lymphoma, diabetes mellitus.
Demography   Worldwide, ubiquitous. Distribution of serotype varies in geographic areas.

PATHOGENESIS

• *C. neoformans* inhaled in dust.
• Causes a primary pulmonary focus of infection that may remain localized or disseminate. Tends to resolve spontaneously.
• Progressive lung disease and dissemination occurs: in advanced untreated HIV/AIDS, hematologic malignancy, glucocorticoid therapy.
• Reactivation of latent infection in the immunocompromised host may result in hematogenous dissemination to meninges, kidneys, and skin; 10 to 15% of patients have skin lesions.

CLINICAL MANIFESTATIONS

History
Occurs in the setting of advanced HIV/AIDS

- Cutaneous lesions: usually asymptomatic
- CNS: headache most common symptom (80%), mental confusion, impaired vision for 2 to 3 months
- Lungs: pulmonary symptoms uncommon

Skin Lesions

- Papule(s) or nodule(s): with surrounding erythema that occasionally break down and exude a liquid, mucinous material. Can present as a solitary nodule in otherwise healthy individuals.
- Molluscum contagiosum-like lesions occur in HIV/AIDS-infected patients (Fig. 25-45).
- Acneiform
- Cryptococcal cellulitis: mimics bacterial cellulitis, i.e., red, hot, tender, edematous plaque on extremity; possibly multiple noncontiguous sites.
- In HIV/AIDS, lesions occur most commonly on face/scalp.

Oral Mucosa   Occur in <5% of patients, presenting as nodules/ulcers.

General Findings

- Meningoencephalitis
- In HIV/AIDS, widespread with fungemia and infection of meninges, lungs, bone marrow, genitourinary tract including prostate, and skin. Hepatomegaly and splenomegaly.

DIFFERENTIAL DIAGNOSIS

Widespread Papular Eruption in Immunocompromised Patient   Molluscum contagiosum, disseminated histoplasmosis acne, sarcoidosis, pyoderma.

LABORATORY EXAMINATIONS

Dermatopathology   Gelatinous reactions show numerous organisms in aggregates with little inflammatory response. Granulomatous reactions show tissue reaction with histiocytes, giant cells, lymphoid cells, and fibroblasts, areas of necrosis; organisms are present in smaller numbers. Capsules stain with mucicarmine stain, differentiating *C. neoformans* from *B. dermatitidis*.

Touch Preparation   Lesional skin biopsy specimen or scrapings from skin lesion smeared on microscope slide examined with KOH to identify *C. neoformans*.

CSF   With meningitis, encapsulated budding yeast is seen with India ink preparations in 40 to 60% of cases, lymphocytic pleocytosis, elevated protein, decreased glucose. Intracranial pressure may be moderately to extremely elevated.

Imaging   X-ray findings of chest variable

Culture   CSF. Lesional skin biopsy specimen. In HIV/AIDS, cryptococcosis tends to be widespread, with cultures positive in blood, sputum, bone marrow, and urine. If *C. neoformans* isolated from lesional skin biopsy specimen, extent of disease should be determined by examination of CSF, bone marrow, sputum, urine, and prostate fluid.

Cryptococcal Antigens   Sensitive and specific. Detect in CSF, serum, urine. Useful in following response to therapy and in formulating prognosis.

DIAGNOSIS

Confirmed by skin biopsy and fungal cultures.

COURSE AND PROGNOSIS

In HIV/AIDS in the absence of immune reconstitution, cryptococcal meningitis relapses in 30% of cases after amphotericin B therapy; lifelong secondary prophylaxis with fluconazole reduces relapse rate to 4 to 8%.

MANAGEMENT

Primary Prophylaxis   In some centers, fluconazole is given to HIV/AIDS-infected individuals with low CD4+ cell counts; the incidence of disseminated infection is reduced, but there is no effect on the mortality rate.

Therapy of Meningitis   Amphotericin B for 2 to 4 weeks in uncomplicated cases and for 6 weeks in complicated cases. Fluconazole (alternative).

Infection Limited to Skin   Fluconazole, 400–600 mg/d. Itraconazole (alternative), 400 mg/d.

Secondary Prophylaxis   In HIV/AIDS-disease (without immune reconstitution), lifelong secondary prophylaxis is given. Fluconazole, 200–400 mg/d; itraconazole (alternative), 200–400 mg/d.

FIGURE 25-45   Cryptococcosis: disseminated   Multiple, skin-colored papules and nodules on the face in an HIV/AIDS-infected individual represent dissemination of pulmonary cryptococcosis hematogenously to skin; meninges are also a common site of infection after fungemia. The lesions are easily mistaken for molluscum contagiosum, which occurs commonly in HIV/AIDS disease. (Courtesy of Loïc Vallant, MD.)

HISTOPLASMOSIS

- Etiologic agent: *Histoplasma capsulatum*
- Endemic areas in United States in Ohio/Mississippi river valleys
- Cutaneous lesions in histoplasmosis
  - Acute histoplasmosis: hypersensitivity reactions
    - Erythema nodosum
    - Erythema multiforme

- Progressive disseminated histoplasmosis:
  - Disseminated papules; scaling macules

Synonyms: Darling disease, cave disease, Ohio Valley disease.

ICD-9: 115.90 ∘ ICD-10: B39

EPIDEMIOLOGY AND ETIOLOGY

Etiologic Agent

- *H. capsulatum* var. *capsulatum*, an unencapsulated dimorphic fungus.
  - Mycelial (microconidia) form: naturally infectious form
  - Yeast or tissue form: Shortly after infecting host, mycelia transform to yeast, which are found within macrophages and other phagocytes.
- In Africa, *H. capsulatum* var. *duboisii*. Skin/bone lesions common.
- The fungus grows well in soil enriched with bird or bat guano.

Epidemiology

- Reported throughout the world
- Endemic areas characterized by:
  - Humidity
  - Acid soil
  - Soil enriched with bird or bat droppings promotes growth and sporulation
  - Disruption of soil leads to aerosolization of microconidia
- Activities associated with high-level exposure
  - Spelunking
  - Excavation
  - Cleaning of chicken coops
  - Demolition/remodeling of old buildings
  - Cutting dead trees
- Endemic areas
  - Americas:
    - North: Eastern and central United States, especially Ohio/Mississippi River valleys; in some areas, 80% of residents are histoplasmin-positive.
    - Central, South
  - Africa, equatorial
  - Caribbean Islands
  - Asia

Age of Onset   For disseminated infection, very old and very young.

Transmission

- Inhalation of microconidia in soil contaminated with bird or bat droppings.
- Those at risk: farmers, construction workers, children, others involved in outdoor activities (cave exploration).
- Acute pulmonary histoplasmosis may occur in outbreaks in individuals with occupational or recreational exposure.

Risk Factors for Dissemination: Immunocompromised Host

- HIV/AIDS; CD4+ T cell count <200/μL; no effective antiretroviral therapy (ART)
- Post solid organ transplant
- Lymphoma, leukemia, chemotherapy
- Advanced age.
  - Immunosuppressive drugs: prednisone, methotrexate, anti-TNF-α agents

PATHOGENESIS

- Inhalation of microconidia results in primary pulmonary infection.
- Microconidia transformed to budding yeast once engulfed by alveolar macrophages.
- Yeast grows within resting macrophages; transported to local draining lymph nodes, spreading hematogenously throughout the reticuloendothelial system.
- Granulomas form and contain organisms; fibrose and calcify.
- Severity and extent of disease depends on
  - Intensity of exposure
  - Immune status of exposed person
  - Underlying pulmonary architecture
- In HIV disease, can present as either primary histoplasmosis or reactivation of latent infection.

CLINICAL MANIFESTATION

Incubation Period

- For acute primary pulmonary infection: 5–18 days.
- For disseminated infection, 2 months.
- In severe forms of infection, presentation may be acute, resembling septicemia with associated disseminated intravascular coagulopathy.

Acute Primary Infection   90% of patients asymptomatic. If large numbers of spores inhaled, influenza-like syndrome may occur (fever 38.3°C, chills, night sweats, cough, headache, fatigue, myalgia).

Disseminated Infection

- Chronic disease syndrome.
- In HIV disease, can present as widely disseminated infection with symptoms of sepsis, adrenal insufficiency, diarrheal illness, or colonic mass.

Skin Lesions

Acute Pulmonary Histoplasmosis Cutaneous lesions represent hypersensitivity reactions to *Histoplasma* antigen(s):

- Erythema nodosum in 5–10% of persons with acute histoplasmosis. See Section 7, page 152.
- Erythema multiforme–like lesions. See Section 7.

Histoplasmosis Disseminated to Skin

- Pathogenesis:

  ○ Lesions caused by tissue infection.
  ○ Historically, lesions of mucous membranes much more common than those on skin.
  ○ HIV/AIDS: 10% of patients with disseminated histoplasmosis have cutaneous lesions.
  ○ Renal transplant patients: 4–6%.

- Lesions
  ○ Papules or nodules; erythematous, necrotic, or hyperkeratotic (Fig. 25-46)
  ○ Erythematous macules; scaling

FIGURE 25-46   Histoplasmosis, disseminated   Multiple, erythematous, scaling papules on the trunk and upper arm occurred during a 2-week period and mimicked acute guttate psoriasis in an individual with HIV/AIDS. The cutaneous lesions occurred after reactivation of pulmonary infection and fungemia. Multiple yeastlike *H. capsulatum* were demonstrated within macrophages in a lesional skin biopsy specimen. (Courtesy of JD Fallon, MD.)

- ° Folliculitis, pustules, acneiform
- ° Chronic ulcers
- ° Vegetative plaques
- ° Panniculitis
- ° Erythroderma
- ° Diffuse hyperpigmentation with Addison disease secondary to adrenal infection.

Mucous Membranes

- Oropharyngeal
  - ° Common site of involvement
  - ° Lesions: nodules, vegetations, painful ulcerations of soft palate, oropharynx, epiglottis.
- Nasal vestibule.

General Examination   Disseminated disease: hepatosplenomegaly, lymphadenopathy, meningitis.

DIFFERENTIAL DIAGNOSIS

Disseminated Disease   Miliary tuberculosis, disseminated coccidioidomycosis or cryptococcosis, leishmaniasis, lymphoma.

LABORATORY EXAMINATIONS

Dermatopathology   Identify intracellular yeast forms of *H. capsulatum* in tissue by size and staining. Differentiate from *Coccidioides immitis, Blastomyces dermatitidis,Penicillium marneffei, Leishmania donovani, Toxoplasma gondii.*
Smear   *H. capsulatum* (intracellular yeast) can be identified by smears obtained from touching lesional skin biopsy specimen to microscope slide (touch preparation); also sputum or bone marrow aspirate, stained with Giemsa stain.
Culture   Identify *H. capsulatum* from biopsy specimens of skin, oral lesions, bone marrow, sputum, lung biopsy specimen, blood, urine, lymph node, liver.
Antigen Detection   If positive, must be confirmed by culture or histopathology.

Bone Marrow Aspiration   *H. capsulatum* can be visualized in those with disseminated infection.
Imaging   Chest x-ray: interstitial infiltrates and/or hilar adenopathy (acute).

DIAGNOSIS

Clinical suspicion, confirmed by culture of organism.

COURSE AND PROGNOSIS

- Primary infection resolves spontaneously in most cases.
- Untreated chronic cavitary pulmonary infection or progressive disseminated form has a very high mortality rate, 80% of patients dying within 1 year.
- Prognosis linked to underlying condition, e.g., HIV/AIDS.
- Chronic maintenance often required. With itraconazole therapy, cure rate 80%.

MANAGEMENT

Prevention   When any material contaminated with bird or bat guano is to be disturbed in an area of endemic histoplasmosis, personal protective equipment should be used during recreational or occupational exposure.
Systemic Antimycotic Therapy   Non-life-threatening infections and for those unable to tolerate amphotericin B: Itraconazole, 400 mg twice daily PO for 12 weeks; or fluconazole, 800 mg/d PO for 12 weeks. Life-threatening and meningeal infection: Amphotericin B given IV.
Secondary Prophylaxis   In HIV disease without immune restoration, itraconazole, 200 mg/d, or fluconazole, 400 mg/d for life.

BLASTOMYCOSIS: CUTANEOUS MANIFESTATIONS ICD-9 : 116.0 ∘ ICD-10 : B40.0 □→■ ◑

- Etiologic agent: *Blastomyces dermatitidis*
- Endemic in southeastern and Great Lakes area of United States

- Primary pulmonary infection, which in some cases is followed by hematogenous dissemination to skin and other organs
Synonyms: Gilchrist disease, Chicago disease

EPIDEMIOLOGY AND ETIOLOGY

Etiologic Agent

- *Blastomyces dermatitidis,* a dimorphic fungus.
  ∘ In tissue, a yeast 10 µm in diameter with 1-µm-thick cell wall: pore of bud is wide.
  ∘ In culture, mycelial phase.
- Natural habitat: Wood debris. Lakes, river, wetlands subject to flooding.
- Zoonosis: causes blastomycosis in dogs.

Age of Onset Young, middle-aged.
Sex Males > females, 10:1.
Transmission

- Most cases are isolated.
- Occupations at risk:
  ∘ Outdoor vocation: farm workers, manual laborers
  ∘ Outdoor avocation: fishing, hunting, camping, hiking in areas of high endemicity.

Demography

- North America
  ∘ United States: Most cases occur in the southeastern, central, and Great Lakes areas.
  ∘ Canada: Toronto area
- Rarely occurs in Mexico, Central America, South America; Africa (Zimbabwe); Middle East; India.

PATHOGENESIS

- *B. dermatitidis* infection acquired from inhalation of spores (dust from soil, decomposed vegetation, or rotting wood).
- Asymptomatic primary pulmonary infection usually resolves spontaneously.
- Hematogenous dissemination may occur to skin, skeletal system, prostate, epididymis, or mucosa of nose, mouth, or larynx.
- Reactivation may occur within lung or in sites of dissemination.

- Risk factors for dissemination:
  ∘ HIV/AIDS
  ∘ Solid organ transplantation

CLINICAL MANIFESTATIONS

Incubation Period Depends on size of inoculum and immune status. Estimated median, 45 days.
Symptoms

- Primary pulmonary infection: usually asymptomatic: flulike or resembles bacterial pneumonitis.
- Chronic pulmonary infection: fever, cough, night sweats, weight loss.
- Cutaneous ulcers often painless.

Skin Lesions
Primary Pulmonary Infection Accompanied or followed by hypersensitivity reactions: erythema nodosum, erythema multiforme. See Section 7 or EN and EM.
Primary Cutaneous Blastomycosis Inoculation site infection, e.g., in laboratory workers or pathologist.
Disseminated Infection to Skin and Mucosa

- Initial lesion, inflammatory nodule that enlarges and ulcerates (Fig. 25-47); subcutaneous nodule, many small pustules on surface.
- Subsequently, verrucous and/or crusted plaque with sharply demarcated serpiginous borders.
- Peripheral border extends on one side, resembling a one-half to three-quarter moon.
- Pus exudes when crust is lifted.
- Central healing with thin geographic atrophic scar.
- Widespread lesions in HIV/AIDS
- Distribution:
  ∘ Usually symmetrically on trunk
  ∘ Also face, hands, arms, legs
  ∘ Multiple lesions in one-half of patients

- Mucous membranes:
  ◦ 25% of patients have oral or nasal lesions; one-half of those have contiguous skin lesions.
  ◦ Laryngeal infection.

General Examination *Lungs* Infiltrates, adult respiratory distress syndrome (ARDS), miliary infection, cavitary lesions.
Bones

- 50% involvement
- Osteomyelitis in thoracolumbar vertebrae, pelvis, sacrum, skull, ribs, long bones.
- May extend to form large subcutaneous abscess
  ◦ May ulcerate
  ◦ Form sinus tracts
- Septic arthritis

DIFFERENTIAL DIAGNOSIS

Verrucous Skin Lesion Squamous cell carcinoma, pyoderma gangrenosum, tumor stage of mycosis fungoides, ecthyma, tuberculosis verrucosa cutis, actinomycosis, nocardiosis, mycetoma, syphilitic gumma, granuloma inguinale, leprosy, bromoderma.

LABORATORY EXAMINATIONS

Direct Examination KOH preparation of pus or respiratory tract secretions shows large (8- to 15-μm), single, budding cells with a thick "double-contoured" wall and a wide pore of attachment.
Serology Specific diagnosis can be made with antibodies to *B. dermatitidis* antigens.
Culture Of sputum, pus from skin lesion or biopsy, prostatic secretions.
Dermatopathology Pseudoepitheliomatous hyperplasia. Budding yeast with thick walls and broad-based buds in microabscess in dermis visualized by silver stain or PAS stain. Mucicarmine stain differentiates *B. dermatitidis* from *Cryptococcus neoformans.*
Imaging Acute (primary) infection shows pneumonitis, hilar lymphadenopathy. With chronic pulmonary infection, imaging highly variable.

DIAGNOSIS

Clinical suspicion, confirmed by culture of organism from skin biopsy, sputum, pus, urine.

COURSE AND PROGNOSIS

- Most primary pulmonary blastomycosis cases are asymptomatic, self-limited.
- Cutaneous infection usually occurs months or years after primary pulmonary infection.
- Skin most common site of extrapulmonary infection, followed by bones, prostate, and meninges; rarely, adrenals and liver.
- Before amphotericin B, mortality rate in individuals with disseminated infection was 80–90%.
- Mortality rate: higher with ARDS, HIV/AIDS, solid organ transplantation.
- Cure rate with itraconazole, 95%.

MANAGEMENT

Prevention Because of the widespread extent of *B. dermatitidis* in endemic regions, avoidance is not possible.
General Care Patients with mild to moderate acute pulmonary blastomycosis can often be followed without antifungal therapy, especially if the patient is improving at time of diagnosis. Patients with meningitis or acute respiratory distress syndrome are best treated in hospital with IV amphotericin B.
Intravenous Amphotericin B In life-threatening infections: *amphotericin B*, 120–150 mg/week with a total dose of 2 g in adults. Liposomal preparations are less toxic. After initial improvement, therapy can be continued on an outpatient basis, three times weekly.
Oral Antifungal Therapy In those whose infection is non-life-threatening and/or those unable to tolerate amphotericin B: Itraconazole, 200–400 mg/d for >2 months; ketoconazole (alternative), 800 mg/d.

FIGURE 25-47 North American blastomycosis: disseminated Ulcerated, inflammatory plaque with surrounding erythema, edema, and fibrosis on the leg results from dissemination from pulmonary blastomycosis via blood to skin. The lesion must be differentiated from pyoderma gangrenosum. (Courtesy of Elizabeth M. Spiers, MD.)

DISSEMINATED COCCIDIOIDOMYCOSIS ICD-9 : 114.9 ○ ICD-10 : B38.0

- Etiologic agent: *Coccidioides*
- Endemic to desert areas of southwestern United States, northern Mexico, Central and South America
- Primary pulmonary infection, that usually resolves spontaneously
- Can disseminate hematogenously resulting in chronic, progressive, granulomatous infection in skin, lungs, bone, meninges.
- Cutaneous lesions in coccidioidomycosis

- Acute coccidioidomycosis
  - Toxic erythema (diffuse erythema, morbilliform, urticaria)
  - Erythema nodosum
  - Erythema multiforme (see Section 7, for EN, EM)
- Disseminated histoplasmosis
  - Papules, nodules, verrucous plaques

Synonyms: San Joaquin Valley fever, valley fever, desert fever

EPIDEMIOLOGY AND ETIOLOGY

Etiologic Agents

- *Coccidioides,* a dimorphic fungus. Two species: *C. immitis* and *C. posadasii.*
- On agar media and in soil: filamentous mold; form arthroconidia, which become airborne.
- In susceptible host, arthroconidia enlarge to become spherules, which contain endospores.

Race Blacks, Filipinos.
Sex Risk of dissemination greater in males, pregnant females.
Incidence Greatly increased in southern California during the past few years. Approximately 100,000 cases in the United States per year; most asymptomatic. In endemic areas: infection rates, measured by skin test reactivity, may be 16–42% or higher by early adulthood. Occurred in 25% of HIV-infected person in highly endemic regions such as Arizona or Bakersfield, CA.
Acquisition

- Exposure to dust from soil
  - Previously uncultivated desert soil.
  - Archaeologic excavations of Amerindian sites.
  - Following earthquakes in endemic areas.
- Inhalation of arthroconidia is followed by primary pulmonary infection.
- Rarely, percutaneous.

Demography

- Regions endemic for *Coccidioides* include:
  - North America
    - Southern California (San Joaquin Valley)
    - Southern Arizona, Utah, New Mexico, Nevada, southwestern Texas.
    - Mexico areas adjacent to Texas
  - Central America
  - South America (Colombia, Venezuela, northeastern Brazil, Paraguay, Bolivia, north-central Argentina).
- Primary pulmonary coccidioidomycosis occurs in individuals living in these regions (endemic) or in visitors to the regions (nonendemic).

Classification Acute self-limited pulmonary coccidioidomycosis. Disseminated coccidioidomycosis (cutaneous, osteoarticular, meningeal).

PATHOGENESIS

- Spores (microconidia) inhaled, resulting in primary pulmonary infection that is asymptomatic or accompanied by symptoms of coryza.
- Spherules contained by necrotizing granulomas.
- Failure to develop cell-mediated immunity is associated with disseminated infection and relapse after therapy.
- Dissemination outside thoracic cavitiy occurs in <1% of infections.
- Rick factors for dissemination
  - Males
  - Pregnancy: 2nd or 3rd trimester
  - African-American or Filipino ancestry
  - Advanced age
  - Persons with depressed cellular immunity
    - HIV/AIDS with CD4 T cell counts <250/μL; without adequate ART.
    - Chronic glucocorticoid therapy
    - Allogeneic solid-organ transplants
    - Treatment with TNF-α antagonists

CLINICAL MANIFESTATION

Incubation Period 1–4 weeks.
Symptoms

- About 40% of persons infected with *Coccidioides* become symptomatic. With primary pulmonary infection, influenza- or grippe-like illness with fever, chills, malaise, anorexia, myalgia, pleuritic chest pain.
- With disseminated infection, headache, bone pain.
- In HIV/AIDS, presents when CD4+ cell count is <200/μL: focal pulmonary lesions, meningitis, focal disseminated lesions, or widespread disease.

Skin Lesions
Primary Infection Manifestations of hypersensitivity: toxic erythema (diffuse erythema, morbilliform, urticaria), erythema nodosum, erythema multiforme.
Primary Cutaneous Inoculation Site (Rare)
Nodule eroding to ulcer. May have sporotrichoid lymphangitis, regional lymphadenitis.

Hematogenous Dissemination to Skin

- Initially, papule evolving with formation of pustules, plaques, nodules (Fig. 25-48).
- Abscess formation, multiple draining sinus tracts, ulcers; subcutaneous cellulitis; verrucous plaques; granulomatous nodules.
- Scars.
- Distribution: face (Fig. 25-48), especially nasolabial fold—preferential site; extremities.

General Examination *Bone* Osteomyelitis. Psoas area produces draining abscess.
CNS Signs of meningitis.

DIFFERENTIAL DIAGNOSIS

Disseminated Papules/Pustules Warts, furuncles, ecthyma, rosacea, lichen simplex chronicus, prurigo nodularis, blastomycosis, cryptococcosis, tuberculosis. In HIV-infected patient: may resemble folliculitis, molluscum contagiosum.

LABORATORY EXAMINATIONS

Dermatopathology Granulomatous inflammation; spherules in tissue.
Culture Pus, biopsy specimen grows organism on Sabouraud's medium.

DIAGNOSIS

Detection of *Coccidioides* spherules in sputum, pus, skin/tissue biopsy specimen. Isolation of *Coccidioides* on culture.

COURSE AND PROGNOSIS

- About 40% of persons infected with *Coccidioides* become symptomatic.
- Most infected residents of endemic areas heal spontaneously.
- Meningeal infection difficult to cure.
- The incidence of relapse of pulmonary or dissemiated infection is relatively high.
- In HIV/AIDS without effective ART, mortality rate is high; relapse rate very high.

MANAGEMENT

Systemic Antifungal Therapy *Non-Life-Threatening Infection* Fluconazole, 200–400 mg/d, or itraconazole.
Life-Threatening Infection Amphotericin B deoxycholate.
Secondary Prophylaxis Lifelong therapy for meningeal infection may be required and is required in HIV disease.

FIGURE 25-48 Coccidioidomycosis: disseminated Ulcerated and crusted nodules on the cheek and nose of an individual with pulmonary coccidioidomycosis with dissemination to the skin. (Courtesy of Francis Renna, MD.)

DISSEMINATED PENICILLINOSIS   ICD-9 : 117.3

- Etiologic agent: *Penicillium marneffei*, dimorphic fungus
- Disease of immunocompromised persons (HIV/AIDS) living in or traveling to Southeast Asia
- Pathogenesis
  - Primary portal of entry is the lungs
  - Hematologic dissemination may follow
- Clinical manifestations
  - Similar to those of disseminated histoplasmosis
  - Fever, chills, weight loss, anemia, generalized lymphadenopathy, and hepatomegaly

- Disseminated penicillinosis: skin lesions (Fig. 25-49)
  - Diffuse disseminated papular lesions
- Diagnosis: Small yeast cells may be seen on histopathologic examination of tissue, but definitive diagnosis depends on culture
- Management: Amphotericin B is the treatment of choice for severely ill patients. Those with less severe disease or who have responded to an initial course of amphotericin B may be treated with itraconazole

ACUTE CANDIDEMIA AND DISSEMINATED CANDIDIASIS   ICD-9 : 112.5 ○ ICD-10 : B37

- Etiologic agents: *Candida albicans* and non-*albicans* species.
- Incidence: fifth most common cause of nosocomial bloodstream infections in the United States.
- Risk factors include
  - Neutropenia
  - Immunocompromise
  - Perforation of GI tract
  - Mucosal damage due to cytotoxic agents used for cancer chemotherapy
  - Intravenous drug use
  - Third-degree burns
- High-risk patients:
  - Undergoing induction chemotherapy
  - Bone marrow transplantation
  - Liver transplantation
- Candidemia usually occurs in febrile neutropenic patients.

- Blood cultures are positive in only 50% of cases of disseminated candidiasis.
- Portal of entry: intravascular catheters, GI tract.
- Disseminated candidiasis may seed
  - Skin, presenting with small disseminated erythematous cutaneous papules (Fig. 25-50).
  - Eye
  - Liver, spleen
- On lesional skin biopsy, *Candida* yeast forms are visualized in the dermis.
- The differential diagnosis includes *Malassezia* folliculitis, which occurs on the trunk of healthy individuals.
- Candidemia has high associated morbidity and mortality.

FIGURE 25-49 Penicillinosis in HIV/AIDS: disseminated skin lesions A 27-year-old Vietnamese male with advanced untreated HIV/AIDS presented with fever, weight loss, and disseminated umbilicated skin-colored papules. Hundreds of skin-colored papules of varying sizes, many umbilicated or with central erosion and crust. (Courtesy of Hoang Van Minh.)

FIGURE 25-50 Invasive candidiasis with candidemia Multiple, erythematous papules on the hand of a febrile patient with granulo-cytopenia associated with treatment of acute myelogenous leukemia. The usual source of the infection is the gastrointestinal tract. *Candida tropicalis* was isolated on blood culture; candidal forms were seen on lesional skin biopsy.

RICKETTSIAL INFECTIONS

- Rickettsiae: small pathogens in family Ricketsiaceae (Table 26-1)
  - *Rickettsia*
  - *Orientia*
  - *Coxiella*
  - *Ehrlichia*
- Gram-negative coccobacilli/short bacilli; obligate localization/persistence within eukaryotic cells
- Transmitted to humans by arthropods: tick, mite, flea, louse; mammalian reservoirs; humans are incidental hosts
- Infections characterized by:
  - Exposure to vectors or animal reservoirs, travel to or residence in endemic locations

- Clinical findings: fever, exanthem or tâche noire (black spot or stain) (coin-like lesion with central eschar and red halo at site of vector-feeding bite site) (Table 26-1), vasculitis, hepatosplenomegaly
- Thrombocytopenia, leukopenia, elevated aminotransferase, hyponatremia
- Diagnosis: confirmed by paired serum samples after convalescence or demonstration of microbes
- Dermatopathology: microbes multiply in endothelial cells of small blood vessels and produce vasculitis with necrosis and thrombosis; disseminated intravascular coagulation (DIC) and vascular occlusion may occur
- Doxycycline is drug of choice

Rickettsiae can cause life-threatening infections. Order of decreasing case-fatality rate: *R. rickettsii* [Rocky Mountain spotted fever (RMSF)]; *R. prowazekii* (epidemic louse-borne typhus); *Orientia tsutsugamushi* (scrub typhus); *R. conorii* [Mediterranean spotted fever (MSF)]; *R. typhi* (endemic murine typhus); in rare cases, other spotted fever group organisms.

TABLE 26-1 Classification of Groups of Rickettsial Infections and Clinical Features

Groups of Rickettsial Infections	Cutaneous Findings
Tick- and gamasid mite–borne spotted fever group (SFG)	Exanthem is a major clinical and diagnostic feature
Tick-borne typhus	Tâche noire, maculopapular rash
Rickettsialpox (mite-borne)	Tâche noire, papulovesicular rash
Flea- and louse-borne typhus group rickettsial disease	Trunkal maculopapular rash
Epidemic louse-borne typhus	Generalized maculopapular rash, sparing the face, palms, and soles, possibly becoming petechial and confluent
Endemic flea-borne murine typhus	Maculopapular rash occurring on the extremities and trunk, sparing the face, palms, and soles, in 13% of patients
Chigger-borne scrub typhus	Eschar at site of chigger feeding (<50% of cases); maculopapular rash may occur, but seldom observed
Ehrlichiosis	Rash in ≤5% at onset
Q fever	Rare

TICK-BORNE SPOTTED FEVER (Table 26-2) ICD-9:066.1 ○ ICD-10:A77

ROCKY MOUNTAIN SPOTTED FEVER ICD-9:O82.0 ○ ICD-10:A77 □ ●

- Zoonosis
- Etiology: *R. rickettsii*
- Vector: various ticks
- Geography: occurs throughout Western Hemisphere (Americas)
- Most severe of rickettsial infections
- Classic triad: fever, rash, history of tick bite (not common)
- Clinical findings: sudden onset of fever, severe headache, myalgia, characteristic acral exanthem spreading centripetally

- Course: associated with significant morbidity and mortality rates
- *Synonyms*: black measles, tick typhus. Mexican spotted fever, or "fiebre manchada" (Mexico). Colombian spotted fever or "Tobia fever" (Colombia); Brazilian spotted fever, or "São Paulo fever," or "febre maculosa" (Brazil)

TABLE 26-2 Classification of Tick-Borne Rickettsial Spotted Fevers

Rickettsial group	Rickettsiae	Geographic location	Disease example
Rocky Mountain spotted fever Tick typhus	*R. rickettsii*	Western hemisphere (Americas)	Rocky Mountain spotted fever
	R. conorii	Mediterranean countries, Africa, Southeast Asia, India	Boutonneuse fever
	R. sibirica	Siberia, Mongolia, northern China	Siberian tick typhus
	R. australis	Australia	Astralian tick typhus
	R. japonica	Japan	Oriental spotted fever
	R. africae	South Africa	African tick bite fever

EPIDEMIOLOGY AND ETIOLOGY

History of RMSF   First recognized in 1896 in Snake River Valley of Idaho; originally called "black measles" because of characteristic rash.

Age   Incidence of infection highest in 5- to 9-year-old children.

Etiology   *Rickettsia rickettsii*

Transmission   Infected tick bite; inoculation through abrasions contaminated with tick feces or tissue juices. Reservoirs and vectors: wood tick *Dermacentor andersoni* in western United States; dog tick *D. variabilis* (4% infected with rickettsiae, most often with nonpathogenic species, i.e., *R. montana, R. belli*) in eastern two-thirds of United States and Canada; *Rhipicephalus sanguineus* in Mexico; and *Amblyomma cajennense* in Mexico and Central and South America. Patient either lives in or has recently visited endemic area. Only 60% have knowledge of a recent tick bite during the 2 weeks before onset of illness. 1–3% of the tick population carries pathogenic *R. rickettsii*, even in areas where majority of human cases reported.

Season   In Northern Hemisphere, cases occur mainly in spring in northern areas. In warmer southern states, most cases occur from April to end of September. The longest season and greatest number of winter-time cases occur farther south.

Demography   Americas. United States: Oklahoma, North Carolina, Virginia, Maryland, Georgia, Michigan, Alaska, Montana, South Dakota. Rarely occurs in Rocky Mountain region. Canada. Mexico. Central America (Costa Rica, Panama). South America (Colombia, Brazil, Argentina).

Incidence   In the United States, 600 cases of RMSF are reported to the Centers for Disease Control and Prevention (CDC) annually. Actual incidence is probably significantly higher. Four states (North Carolina, Oklahoma, Tennessee, South Carolina) account for 48% of U.S. cases.

PATHOGENESIS

Inoculation usually requires > 6 h feeding, after which rickettsia are released from the salivary glands. After inoculation into the dermis, initial local replication occurs in endothelial cells, followed by hematogenous and lymphatic dissemination. Organisms spread throughout body and attach to vascular endothelial cells,

the principal target. Infected foci enlarge as rickettsia spread from cell to cell, forming a network of contiguously infected endothelial cells in microcirculation of dermis, and to multiple organs and tissues. Focal infection of vascular smooth muscle causes a generalized vasculitis. Patients with severe infection of brain and lungs have high mortality rates. Increased vascular permeability results in edema, hypovolemia, hypotension, ischemia, gangrene. Rash results from extravasation of blood after vascular necrosis.

CLINICAL MANIFESTATION

Incubation Period   Range, 3–14 days (mean, 7 days) after the tick bite.

Prodrome   Fever/chills, anorexia/nausea/vomiting, irritability, malaise, severe headache, myalgia.

History of Tick Bite   60% of cases.

Symptoms   Onset is usually abrupt: fever (94%), severe headache (86%), generalized myalgia (especially the back and leg muscles, arthralgia; 83%), sudden shaking rigor, photophobia, prostration, nausea/vomiting/abdominal pain, all within the first 2 days. Symptoms are similar to those of many acute infectious diseases, making specific diagnosis difficult during the first few days. On first day of illness, only 14% of patients have characteristic rash; during first 3 days, 49% of patients have rash. In 20% of cases, rash appears only on day 6 or after. In 13% of cases, no rash is detected (spotless RMSF).

Skin Lesions

Day 1 of illness, 14% have rash; day 3, 49%. Initially, few small, pink macules. Temporal evolution of the rash is extremely helpful in the diagnosis.

Types   Tâche noire uncommon in RMSF. Early lesions, 2–6 mm, pink, blanchable macules (Figs. 26-1 and 26-2). In 1–3 days, evolve to deep red papules (Fig. 26-3). In 2–4 days, become hemorrhagic, no longer blanchable. Local edema. With DIC or prolonged hypotension, acral skin necrosis/gangrene occur, but rare.

Distribution   Characteristically, rash begins on wrists (Fig. 26-1), forearms, and ankles (Fig. 26-2) and somewhat later on palms and soles. Within 6–18 h, rash spreads centripetally to the arms, thighs, trunk (Fig. 26-3), and face. The

FIGURE 26-1 Rocky Mountain spotted fever: early Erythematous and hemorrhagic macules and papules appeared initially on the wrists of a young child.

FIGURE 26-2 Rocky Mountain spotted fever: early Erythematous and hemorrhagic macules and papules appeared initially on the ankles of an adolescent.

hemorrhagic rash involving the palms and soles occurs in 36–82% of cases and appears after the fifth day of illness in 43%. Necrosis occurs in acral extremities following hypotension.
General Findings Fever to 40°C. Hypotension, shock later in course. Hepatomegaly, splenomegaly, GI hemorrhage, encephalitis (altered consciousness, confusion, lethargy, stupor, delirium, coma), cranial nerve palsy, incontinence, renal failure, and secondary bacterial infections (lung, middle ear, parotid gland) may occur.
Variants *Spotless fever*: 13% of cases. Associated with higher mortality rate because of delay in diagnosis. *Abdominal syndrome*: Can mimic acute abdomen, acute cholecystitis, acute appendicitis. *Thrombotic thrombocytopenic purpura.*

DIFFERENTIAL DIAGNOSIS

Without Rash Influenza, enteroviral infection, infectious mononucleosis, viral hepatitis, leptospirosis, typhoid fever, gram-negative or -positive sepsis, ehrlichiosis, murine typhus, rickettsialpox.
With Rash Rubeola, rubella, meningococcemia, disseminated gonococcal infection, toxic shock syndrome, drug hypersensitivity, thrombocytopenic purpura, Kawasaki syndrome, vasculitis.

LABORATORY EXAMINATIONS

Hematology Thrombocytopenia.
Chemistry Hyponatremia, elevated aminotransferases.
Skin Biopsy Necrotizing vasculitis: rickettsia can at times be demonstrated within endothelial cells by immunofluorescence or immunoenzyme staining techniques.
Direct Immunofluorescence Specific *R. rickettsii* antigen within endothelial cells 70% sensitive; 100% specific. Treatment with antirickettsial drugs within 48 h reduces sensitivity.
Serodiagnosis Indirect immunofluorescence assay (IFA) can be used to measure both IgG and IgM anti-*R. rickettsii* antibodies. Fourfold rise in titer between acute and convalescent stages is diagnostic, with a titer of ≥64 detectable between 7 and 10 days after onset of illness.

DIAGNOSIS

Clinical and epidemiologic considerations more important than a laboratory diagnosis in early RMSF. Suspect in febrile children, adolescents, and men > 60 years of age with tick exposure in endemic areas. Diagnosis must be made clinically and confirmed later. Only 3% of patients with RMSF present with the triad of rash, fever, and history of tick bite during first 3 days of illness.

COURSE AND PROGNOSIS

Severe course is associated with older age, delay in diagnosis, delay in or no treatment, male sex, African-American race, alcoholism, G6PD deficiency. Untreated (before the availability of effective antibiotics), the fatality rate was 23%; treated, 3% (6% if >40 years of age). Fatality rate: 1.5% with known tick bite but 6.6% if no known tick exposure. Fulminant RMSF defined as a fatal disease whose course is unusually rapid (i.e., 5 days from onset to death) and usually characterized by early onset of neurologic signs and late or absent rash. In uncomplicated cases, defervescence usually occurs within 48–72 h after initiation of therapy.

MANAGEMENT

Prevention Avoid tick bites: protective clothing, tick repellants (DEET), permethrin on clothing. After possible exposure, inspect for ticks (see "Lyme Borreliosis" in Section 24).
Antirickettsial Therapy Specific antirickettsial therapy should be initiated as soon as the diagnosis is suspected clinically.
Drug of Choice Doxycycline (except for pregnant patients, history of allergy to doxycycline), 100 mg every 12 h PO or IV for adults. Tetracycline 25–50 mg/kg per day PO in four divided doses.
Alternative Chloramphenicol, 50–75 mg/kg per day in four divided doses. Ciprofloxacin reported to be effective.
Supportive Therapy For acute problems of shock, acute renal failure, respiratory failure, prolonged coma.

FIGURE 26-3 Rocky Mountain spotted fever: late Disseminated hemorrhagic macules and papules on the face, neck, trunk, and arms on the fourth day of febrile illness in an older child. The initial lesions were noted on the wrists and ankles, subsequently extending centripetally.

TICK-BORNE TYPHUS ICD-9:082.9 ∘ ICD-10:A77.0 □ ◑→●

- Occurs globally
- Vector: various ticks
- Symptomatology: ranges from mild subclinical illness to febrile life-threatening one
- Tâche noire at inoculation site
- Exanthem: macule and papules on trunk
- Treatment: doxycycline 100 mg twice daily

EPIDEMIOLOGY AND ETIOLOGY

Etiology Various rickettsiae (see Table 26-3).
Age of Onset More common in children and young adults, related to out-of-doors activities.
Sex Males > females.
Geographic Distribution See Table 26-3.
Transmission Ixodes arthropod ticks; widely distributed around the world. Bite; excoriation of feeding site inoculates rickettsiae in tick body fluid or feces.

Season Mediterranean spotted fever (MSF) occurs mainly in warmer summer months (July, August, September) when ticks are feeding.

CLINICAL MANIFESTATION

Incubation Period Range, 3–14 days (mean, 7 days) after the tick bite.
Prodrome Nonspecific.
Travel History Recent travel to or living in endemic region, e.g., recent African safari,

TABLE 26-3   Etiology and Geographic Distribution of Tick Typhus

Disease in Humans	Etiology	Distribution
Tick typhus	Similar subspecies	Primarily Mediterranean countries (southern Europe below 45th parallel), all of Africa, India, southwestern and southcentral Asia
Mediterranean spotted fever (fièvre boutonneuse, Marseilles fever), Kenya tick typhus, Israeli spotted fever, Indian tick typhus, Astrakhan spotted fever	*R. conorii,* *R. conorii israelensis,* *R. conorii caspia,* *R. aeschlimannii,* *R. slovaca,* *R. sibirica mongolitimonae,* *R. massiliae*	Mediterranean islands and surrounding lands; Africa
African tick-bite fever (tick typhus)	*R. conorii* var. *piperi* (*R. africae*)	Central, eastern, southern Africa
Siberian (North Asian) tick typhus	*R. sibirica*	Siberia, Mongolia, northern China
Queensland tick typhus	*R. australis*	Australia
Flinders Island spotted fever	*R. honei*	Flinders Island (near Tasmania)
Japanese/Oriental spotted fever	*R. japonica*	Japan

adventure travel, military service in Africa with African tick bite fever.

History of Tick Bite   Often not elicited in that rickettsiae are transmitted by tiny immature larvae and nymphs.

Symptoms   Onset is sudden in 50% of patients. Most common: headache, fever; also chills, myalgias, arthralgias, malaise, anorexia.

Skin Lesions

Tâche Noire   An inoculation eschar: papule forms at the bite site and evolves to a painless, black-crusted ulcer with red halo (resembles a cigarette burn) (Fig. 26-4) in 3–7 days. Occurs in all spotted fevers except RMSF.

Rash   About 3–4 days after appearance of tâche noire, an erythematous maculopapular eruption appears on trunk; may subsequently disseminate, involving face, extremities, palms/soles. Density of eruption heightens during next few days. In severe cases, lesions may become hemorrhagic.

Distribution   Similar pattern of spread and distribution in all spotted fevers—trunk, extremities, face (centrifugal)—*except* RMSF, which first appears at wrists and ankles and spreads centripetally.

General Findings   Conjunctivitis, pharyngitis, photophobia. Central nervous system (CNS) symptoms (confusion, stupor, delirium, seizures, coma) common in RMSF but not seen in other spotted fevers.

Lymph Nodes   Nodes proximal to tâche noire are usually enlarged and nontender.

DIFFERENTIAL DIAGNOSIS

Viral exanthems, drug eruption.

FIGURE 26-4 Tick-borne typhus; African tick bite fever: tâche noire Crusted erosion with surrounding erythema on the left hip area. The patient had just returned from a safari in South Africa. He noted onset of fever, flulike symptoms, and the hip lesion. The patient's wife photographed the tâche noire site, and emailed the image to his physician, facilitating the diagnosis. He was treated with doxycyline.

LABORATORY EXAMINATIONS

Dermatopathology *Direct Immunofluorescence* Rickettsiae can be detected in lesional biopsy specimens from site of tick bite and cutaneous lesions; also in circulating endothelial cells and various tissues obtained postmortem.
Polymerase Chain Reaction Detects rickettsial DNA in skin lesions.
Serodiagnosis Various tests are available. Antirickettsial therapy usually blunts antibody responses. Demonstration of antibodies to SFG rickettsiae by microimmunofluorescence, latex agglutination, enzyme immunoassay, Western blot, or complement fixation. Enzyme-linked immunosorbent assay (ELISA) (IgM capture assays) among the most sensitive.

DIAGNOSIS

Epidemiologic and clinical findings with identification of tâche noire confirmed by demonstration of rickettsiae by immunohistologic techniques in lesional skin biopsy specimens and/or serology. In an endemic area, patients presenting with fever, rash, and/or a skin lesion consisting of black necrotic area or a crust surrounded by erythema should be considered to have one of the rickettsial spotted fevers.

COURSE AND PROGNOSIS

In France and Spain, mortality rate similar to that of RMSF. Spotted fevers are usually milder in children. Morbidity and mortality rates are higher (up to 50%) in individuals with diabetes mellitus, cardiac insufficiency, alcoholism.

MANAGEMENT

Prevention Control host animals and vectors.
Antirickettsial Therapy Specific antirickettsial therapy abbreviates the length and severity of illness, i.e., spotted fevers, tick typhus, and rickettsialpox.
Drug of Choice Doxycycline, 100 mg PO twice daily for 7–10 days.
Alternatives Ciprofloxacin, 750 mg PO twice daily for 5 days, *or* chloramphenicol, 500 mg PO four times a days for 7–10 days, *or* josamycin (in pregnancy), PO for 5 days.

RICKETTSIALPOX   ICD-9:O83.2 ○ ICD-10:A79.1

- Etiology: *R. akari*
- Vector: mice mite (*Liponyssoides sanguineus*), other mites; transovarian transmission
- Geography: United States, Europe, Russia, South Africa, Korea, Europe
- Clinical features:
  - Tâche noire (Fig. 26-5)
  - Regional lymph nodes enlarged
  - 10–17 days after bite, nonspecific symptoms of malaise, chills/fever, headache, myalgia, nausea/vomiting/abdominal pain, cough, conjunctivitis, photophobia may occur
  - Rash: 2–6 days after onset of nonspecific symptoms, red macules and papules appear
- (Fig. 26-6); may evolve to characteristic vesicles (pox), crusted erosions occur; lesions heal without scarring
  - Fever resolves in 6–10 days without treatment with doxycycline
- Differential diagnosis: Varicella, pityriasis lichenoides et varioliformis acuta (PLEVA), viral exanthems, disseminated gonococcal infection
- Dermatopathology: Basal layer of epidermis shows vacuolar degeneration; vesiculation is subepidermal. Superficial and mid-dermal neutrophilic and mononuclear cell infiltrate are present
- Treatment: doxycline, 100 mg BID (adults)

LOUSE-BORNE TYPHUS   ICD-9:O81.0 ○ ICD-10:75.0   ☐ ◑➔●

Epidemic (Louse-Borne) Typhus (Table 26-3) *Etiology*: *R. prowazekii*. *Vector*: human louse (*Pediculus humanus corporis, Pediculus humanus capitis*); lives on clothing; microbe in louse feces inoculated by scratching. *Reservoir*: humans, flying squirrels. Epidemics associated with war/lowering of hygiene. Rickettsiae can persist for years in lymph nodes without any symptoms. *Clinical findings*: systemic infection and prostration may be severe, fever lasts for about 2 weeks; more severe and more often fatal in patients over 40 years of age. *Rash*: noted on fifth day of fever; initially on upper trunk, then disseminated; macules evolving to papules; often, no rash. During epidemics, fatality rate up to 30%. Brill-Zinsser disease is a recrudescence of a prior/-latent epidemic typhus infection.
Endemic Murine Typhus *Etiology*: *R. typhi*. *Vector*: rat flea (*Xenopsylla cheopsis*). *Reservoir*: rats, cats, opossums. *Geography*: worldwide but not reported in Britain, Scandinavia. Epidemics associated with poor hygiene as in wartime

and disaster. *Clinical findings*: resembles epidemic typhus but milder; rarely fatal. Rash in 13% of cases, noted 4 days after onset of fever; macules and papules on trunk. Latent infections in human.
Scrub Typhus *Etiology*: *Orientia* (formerly *Rickettsia*) *tsutsugamushi*. *Vector*: mites. *Reservoirs*: larval stage (chigger) of trombiculid mites (transovarian transmission), humans, rat. *Geography*: Far East, i.e., Myanmar, India, Sri Lanka, New Guinea, Japan, Taiwan. *Incidence*: high prevalence but often unrecognized. *Clinical findings*: resembles epidemic typhus; generalized lymphadenopathy. *Rash*: <50% of cases tâche noir at mite bite site or maculopapular trunkal rash after onset of fever. Pneumonitis, myocarditis and cardiac failure, encephalitis or meningitis, acute abdominal pain, granulomatous hepatitis, disseminated intravascular coagulation, or acute renal failure may develop.
Treatment: doxycycline 100 mg BID for 7 days
Synonym: Tsutsugamushi fever

FIGURE 26-5 Rickettsialpox: tâche noire A crusted, ulcerated papule (eschar) with a red halo resembling a cigarette burn at the site of a tick bite.

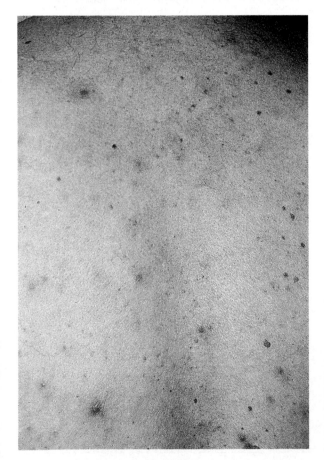

FIGURE 26-6 Rickettsialpox: exanthem Multiple but discrete erythematous papules and pustules, some with central hemorrhage and crusting, on the back after hematogenous dissemination of *R. akari* from the tick bite site.

VIRAL INFECTIONS OF SKIN AND MUCOSA

- Viral infections of skin and mucosa produce a wide spectrum of clinical manifestations.
- Viruses that cause febrile illness with exanthems are usually self-limited, with primary infection conveying lifetime immunity.
- Viruses such as human papillomavirus (HPV) and molluscum contagiosum virus (MCV) colonize the epidermis of most individuals without causing any clinical lesions.
  - Benign epithelial proliferations, i.e., warts and molluscum, occur in some colonized persons, are transient, and eventually resolve without therapy.
  - In immunocompromised individuals, however, these lesions may become extensive, persistent, and refractory to therapy.
- The eight human herpesviruses often have asymptomatic primary infection but are characterized by lifelong latent infection.
  - In the setting of immunocompromise, herpesviruses can become active and cause disease with significant morbidity and mortality rates.

POXVIRUS INFECTIONS

- The poxvirus family is a diverse group of epitheliotropic viruses that infect humans and animals.
  - The genera of poxviruses that infect humans include orthopoxvirus, parapoxvirus, molluscipoxvirus, and yatapoxvirus (Table 27–1).
  - Only smallpox virus (SPV) and molluscum contagiosum virus (MCV) cause natural disease in humans.
  - Small pox (SPV) and monkeypox virus typically cause systemic disease with rash; other poxviruses cause localized skin lesions.
  - Other poxviruses are associated with zoonotic infections.
- Poxviruses are the largest of all animal viruses and have a double-strand DNA genome.
  - They are the only DNA viruses that replicate in cytoplasm, where accumulated viral particles form eosinophilic inclusions, or Guarnieri bodies, visible by light microscopy (200–400 µm).
  - Poxviruses appear as brick-shaped or oval virus particles by electron microscopy.
  - The nucleosome contains double-strand DNA, which is surrounded by a membrane.
  - The outer surface of the lipoprotein bilayer has surface tubules that are randomly arranged and give the virion its characteristic textured appearance.
- Smallpox, or variola, has been eradicated as a naturally occurring infection.
  - Cowpox is an infection of cattle caused by cowpox virus.
  - The origins of vaccinia virus, which is used to immunize humans against smallpox, are uncertain. It may be derived from variola virus, cowpox virus, or be a hybrid of the two.
- MCV colonizes the skin of many healthy individuals, causing molluscum contagiosum, self-limited epidermal proliferations that resolve spontaneously.
- Human orf and milker's nodules are zoonotic infections that can sometimes occur in exposed humans.
- Other poxviruses that are zoonoses in animal hosts (monkeys, cows, buffalo, sheep, goats) can also infect humans.
- Poxviruses cause toxic effects on cells, which result in cell rounding and clumping, degeneration of cell architecture, and production of cytoplasmic vacuoles.
- Different poxviruses are capable of producing a localized, self-limited infection by inoculation to the skin (e.g., orf) or a fulminant systemic disease (e.g., variola).
- The same virus can affect different species in different ways.

| TABLE 27-1 Poxviruses That Infect Humans* and Cause Disease |||||

Genus and Species (Disease)	Primary Reservoir	Geographic Region	Mode of Transmission	Protection Provided by Vaccination
Orthopoxvirus				
Cowpox	Rodents	Europe, Africa, central/northern Asia	Direct contact	Yes
Monkeypox	Rodents	West/central Africa	Direct contact, respiratory droplets	Yes Yes
Vaccinia	Unknown		Direct contact	
Variola (smallpox)	Humans	U.S., Russia	Direct contact, respiratory droplets	Yes
Yatapoxvirus				
Tanapox	Nonhuman primates	Kenya, Zaire	Direct contact	No
Yatapox	Nonhuman primates	Central Africa	Direct contact	No
Parapoxvirus				
Pseudocowpox (milker's nodules and paravaccinia)	Ungulates	Worldwide	Direct contact	No
Bovine papular stomatitis (milker's nodules)	Ungulates (humans)	U.S., Canada, Africa, Australia, New Zealand, Great Britain, Europe	Direct contact	No
Orf (human orf)	Ungulates (humans)	North America, Europe, New Zealand	Direct contact	No
Sealpox	Seals	North Sea, Pacific Ocean, Atlantic Ocean	Direct contact	No
Molluscipoxvirus				
Molluscipox (molluscum contagiosum)	Humans	Worldwide	Direct contact	No

*Poxviruses that do not infect humans include camelpox and sheep and goat lumpy skin disease complex.

MOLLUSCUM CONTAGIOSUM ICD-9:078.0 ∘ ICD-10:B08.1 ■ ○→◑

- Molluscum contagiosum (MC) is a self-limited epidermal viral infection.
- Risk groups
  - Children
  - Sexually active adults
  - Immunocompromised: HIV/AIDS, organ transplant recipients
- Clinical manifestations:

- Skin-colored papules; often umbilicated
- Few to myriads of lesions
- HIV/AIDS: large nodules; confluent
- Course:
  - Healthy persons: MC resolves spontaneously
  - HIV/AIDS: if not successfully treated with antiretroviral therapy (ART), MC can become huge and confluent.

EPIDEMIOLOGY AND ETIOLOGY

Etiology

- Molluscum contagiosum virus.
- Four discrete viral subtypes, I, II, III, IV.
- 30% homology with smallpox virus.
- The virus has not been cultured.
- Not distinguishable from other poxviruses by electron microscopy.
- In many healthy adults, the epidermis and infundibulum of hair follicle are colonized by MCV.

Age, Sex   Children; sexually active adults; males > females.

Risk Factors   HIV-infected persons with low CD4+ T cell counts may have hundreds of small mollusca or giant mollusca on the face.

Transmission   Skin-to-skin contact.

Classification by Risk Groups

Children

- Mollusca commonly occur on exposed skin sites.
- Child-to-child transmission relatively low.
- Resolve spontaneously.

Sexually Active Adults

- Occur in genital region.
- Virus transmitted during sexual activity.
- Resolve spontaneously.

HIV/AIDS: Organ Transplant Recipients

- Most commonly occur on the face, spread by shaving.
- With response to ART, lesions often resolve.
- Without aggressive therapy in advanced HIV/ AIDS, mollusca enlarge; spontaneous regression does not occur.

PATHOGENESIS

- A subclinical carrier state of MCV probably exists in many adults.
- Unique among poxviruses, MCV infection results in epidermal tumor formation; other human poxviruses cause a necrotic "pox" lesion.
- Rupture and discharge of the infectious virus-packed cells occur in the umbilication/crater of the lesion.

CLINICAL MANIFESTATIONS

Duration of Lesions

- In the normal host, mollusca usually persist up to 6 months and then undergo spontaneous regression.
- In HIV/AIDS without effective ART, mollusca persist and proliferate even after aggressive local therapy.

Skin Symptoms

- Usually none.
- Cosmetic disfigurement.
- Concern about having a transmissible infection.
- Painful if superinfected.

Mucocutaneous Lesions

- Papules (1–2 mm), nodules (5–10 mm) (rarely, giant) (Fig. 27-1*A, B*). Pearly white or skin-colored. Round, oval, hemispherical, umbilicated (Fig. 27-1*B*).
- Isolated single lesion; multiple, scattered discrete lesions; or confluent mosaic plaques.
- Most larger mollusca have a central keratotic plug (Fig. 27-1*A*), which gives the lesion a central dimple or umbilication, best observed after light liquid nitrogen freeze. Gentle pressure on a molluscum causes the central plug to be extruded.
- Autoinoculation is apparent in that mollusca are clustered at a site such as the axilla (Fig. 27-2).
- Host immune response to viral antigen results in an inflammatory halo around MC (Fig. 27-2), i.e., "MC dermatitis," which usually heralds spontaneous regression; purulence may occur.
- MC can be extensive in organ transplant recipients (Fig. 27-3).
- In HIV-infected males who shave, mollusca can be confined to the beard area. Hundreds of lesions occur in HIV/AIDS patients (Fig. 27-3, 27-4; see also Fig. 31-8).
- In dark-skinned individuals, significant postinflammatory hyperpigmentation after treatment or spontaneous regression may occur. 🔳

Distribution

- Any site may be infected, especially axillae, antecubital, popliteal fossae, crural folds.
- In children: genital lesions occur via autoinoculation.
- In atopic dermatitis, MC may be widespread.
- In adults with sexually transmitted MC: groins, genitalia, thighs, lower abdomen (Fig. 27-4).
- Multiple facial MC suggest HIV infection. MC can occur in the conjunctiva, causing a unilateral conjunctivitis.

FIGURE 27-1   Molluscum contagiosum (MC): lesions   MC lesions typically are dimpled or umbilicated papules or nodules. ***A.*** Pink shiny donut-shaped papules with a depressed keratotic core on the hip of a healthy adult. ***B.*** Umbilicated papules on the moustache area and cheek of healthy teenage girl. MC commonly arise in hair follicles, the umbilication occurring at the ostium of the follicules. The keratinaceous core can be smeared on a microscope slide and stained to show intracytoplasmic molluscum bodies, viral cytoplasmic incusions.

DIFFERENTIAL DIAGNOSIS

Multiple Small Mollusca Flat warts, condylomata acuminata, syringoma, sebaceous hyperplasia.

Large Solitary Molluscum Keratoacanthoma, squamous cell carcinoma, basal cell carcinoma, epidermal inclusion cyst.

Multiple Facial Mollusca in HIV-Infected Individual Disseminated invasive fungal infection, i.e., cryptococcosis, histoplasmosis, coccidioidomycosis, penicillinosis. (See Section 25.)

LABORATORY EXAMINATIONS

Smear of Keratotic Plug Direct microscopic examination of Giemsa-stained central semisolid core reveals "molluscum bodies" (inclusion bodies).

Dermatopathology

- Epidermal cells contain large intracytoplasmic inclusion bodies, i.e., molluscum bodies, that appear as single, ovoid eosinophilic structures in lower cells of stratum malpighii.
- Molluscum bodies contain large numbers of maturing virions.
- Epidermis grows down into dermis. Infection also occurs in epithelium and follicle.

FIGURE 27-2   Molluscum contagiosum: axilla
Multiple, small pink papules in the axilla of a healthy child. The erythema surrounding the lesions represents an inflammatory response to MC and usually indicates the lesions are regressing.

FIGURE 27-3   Molluscum contagiosum in lung transplant recipient: perineum and buttocks   A 37-year-old lung transplant recipient with numerous pink papules cluster in intertriginous sites of buttocks and perineum. MC were treated with electrosurgery.

FIGURE 27-4   Molluscum contagiosum in HIV/ AIDS: confluent lesions on anogenital area   A 42-year-old male with HIV/AIDS, failing antiretroviral therapy (ART). Discrete and confluent skin-colored umbilicated papules in the anogenital area.

DIAGNOSIS

Usually made on clinical findings. Biopsy lesion in HIV-infected individual if disseminated invasive fungal infection is in the differential diagnosis.

COURSE AND PROGNOSIS

- In healthy individuals, MC resolves spontaneously without scarring, but may take up to 2 years.
- In HIV/AIDS without effective ART, mollusca often progress even with aggressive therapies, creating significant cosmetic disfigurement, especially by facial lesions. In HIV/AIDS successfully treated with ART, mollusca either do not occur or resolve after several months. Recurrence of mollusca usually indicates failure of ART.

MANAGEMENT

Prevention	Avoid skin-to-skin contact with individual having mollusca. HIV-infected individuals with mollusca in the beard area should be advised to minimize shaving facial hair or grow a beard.
Supportive therapy	In immunocompetent children and sexually active adults, mollusca regress spontaneously; painful aggressive therapy is not indicated.
Treatment of lesions	
Topical patient-directed therapy	5% imiquimod cream applied at bedtime 3–5 times per week for up to 1–3 months.
Clinician-directed therapy (office)	These procedures are painful and traumatic, especially for young children. EMLA cream applied to lesions 1 h before therapy may reduce/eliminate pain.
Curettage	Small mollusca can be removed with a small curette with little discomfort or pain.
Cryosurgery	Freezing lesions for 10–15 s is effective and minimally painful, using either a cotton-tipped applicator or liquid nitrogen spray.
Electrodesiccation	For mollusca refractory to cryosurgery, especially in HIV-infected individuals with numerous and/or large lesions, electrodesiccation or laser surgery is the treatment of choice. Large lesions usually require injected lidocaine anesthesia. Giant mollusca may require several cycles of electrodesiccation and curettage to remove the large bulk of lesions; these lesions may extend through the dermis into the subcutaneous fat.

> **HUMAN ORF**   ICD-10 : B08.0
>
> - Human orf is a parapoxvirus infection.
> - Zoonosis in ungulates
> - Occurs in humans exposed to the virus.
>
> - Clinical manifestations: Nodular lesions on exposed cutaneous sites.
>
> *Synonym*: Ecthyma contagiosum.

EPIDEMIOLOGY

Zoonosis   Sheep-pox, lip scab of sheep, scabby mouth, sore mouth, contagious pustular dermatosis, infectious pustular dermatitis.

Disease in Animals

- Ungulates (sheep, goats, yaks, deer, etc.).
- Virus survives for many months on fences, feeding basins, and surfaces in barns.
- Only newborn animals lacking viral immunity are susceptible.
  - Manifested as erythematous, exudative nodules around mouth that heal spontaneously in about a month, producing permanent immunity; lesions may become superinfected.

Transmission to Humans

- Humans are infected by
  - Inoculation of virus by direct contact with lambs (bottle feeding)
  - Indirectly via fomites (knives, shears, barbed wire, feeding troughs, barn doors, fences, etc.).
- Human-to-human infection does not occur.

Incidence   Most common in farmers, veterinarians, sheep shearers.

Season   Usually in springtime (when lambs are born) and season (Easter) of slaughter of lambs and sheep.

Demography   Occurs worldwide with epidemics in Norway and other parts of Europe, New Zealand; rare in North America.

CLINICAL MANIFESTATIONS

Skin Lesions

- Initially, one or more papule(s) to nodule(s) to plaque(s) on the hand(s) (Figs. 27-5, 27-6);

may appear very edematous to vesicular to bullous. Lesions average 1.6 cm in diameter.
- The infection goes through six clinical stages, each lasting 6 days:
  - Macule to papule, pink to red → target lesion: nodule with red center (Fig. 27-5), white middle ring, and red periphery → acute exudative nodule → regenerative dry nodule covered by a thin crust with black dots → papillomatous → regressive with dry crust (Fig. 27-6)

Distribution   Exposed sites (hands, arms, legs, face); most common site is dorsum of right index finger.

Other Findings
- Ascending lymphangitis and lymphadenopathy may occur.
- Bacterial superinfection may occur.
- More extensive infection may occur in the immunocompromised host.

DIFFERENTIAL DIAGNOSIS

Milker's nodules, anthrax, tularemia, primary inoculation tuberculosis, atypical mycobacteria infection, syphilitic chancre, sporotrichosis, pyogenic granuloma.

LABORATORY EXAMINATION

Electron Microscopy   Biopsy of lesional skin shows characteristic brick-shaped viral particles 200–380 nm in length.

DIAGNOSIS

Clinical findings with the appropriate history.

FIGURE 27-5   Human orf: multiple lesions on hands   Stage 2: Multiple blisters with target/iris patterns in lesions on the hands of a sheep herder.

COURSE

- Resolves spontaneously in 4–6 weeks, healing without scar formation.
- Erythema multiforme–like eruptions have been reported in human orf.
- Widespread lesions spread by autoinoculation may occur in atopic dermatitis.
- Lesion may be large and fail to regress in chronic lymphocytic leukemia.
- In humans, lasting immunity is conferred by infection.

MANAGEMENT

Antiviral agents are not effective. Treat bacterial superinfection.

FIGURE 27-6   Human orf: finger   A 19-year-old male of Greek heritage; lesions appeared 10 days after Greek Easter and was associated with the lamb killing for the Easter feast. Stage 6: Crusted regressing nodule on middle finger; lesion on index finger has resolved.

MILKER'S NODULES (MN)

- Cutaneous infections caused by parapoxviruses.
- Zoonosis in infected cattle
- Infection in humans is caused accidentally.

- Clincal manifestations: nodular lesions on exposed cutaneous sites.

Synonym: Milker's node.

EPIDEMIOLOGY AND ETIOLOGY

Etiology   Parapoxvirus (pseudocowpox virus), similar to that which causes orf.
Synonyms of Animal Infection   Paravaccinia, bovine papular stomatitis.
Disease in Animals   Papular lesions occur on muzzles/oral cavity of calves and on teats of cows.
Transmission to Humans   Contact with bovine lesions or teat cups of milking machines.
Incidence   Most common in dairy farmers.
Risk Factors   New milkers, young people, vacation milkers, veterinary students.
Demography   Worldwide

CLINICAL MANIFESTATIONS

Skin Lesions

- Clinical findings and course are similar to human orf.
- Lesions can present as
  - Solitary red-purple nodules (Fig. 27-7) or, less commonly, as
  - Multiple cherry-red papules and nodules, arising at site of inoculation.

Distribution   Usually on exposed sites such as hands; may occur in burn wounds. ⌫
Other Findings   Lymphadenopathy.

DIFFERENTIAL DIAGNOSIS

Human orf, smallpox vaccination site, staphylococcal abscess, herpes simplex virus infection, anthrax, tularemia, primary inoculation tuberculosis, atypical mycobacteria infection, syphilitic chancre, sporotrichosis, pyogenic granuloma.

LABORATORY EXAMINATION

See "Human Orf," above.

DIAGNOSIS

Diagnosis is usually made on history of bovine exposure and clinical findings.

COURSE

Self-limited.

MANAGEMENT

Antiviral agents are not effective. Treat bacterial superinfection.

FIGURE 27-7   Milker's nodule: finger   A single beefy eroded nodule on the finger of a dairy farmer at the site of inoculation.

SMALLPOX ICD-9:050.9 ∘ ICD-10:B03

- Etiologic agent: Poxvirus variolae
- An acute exanthematous infection.
  - Severe 3-day prodromal illness
  - Generalized rash spreading centrifugally
  - Rapidly successive papules, vesicles, pustules, umbilication, and crusting within 14 days.

- Epidemics have occurred in all populations, resulting in hundreds of millions of deaths.

Synonyms: Variola, variola major, variola minor (alastrim).

---

http://www.bt.cdc.gov/agent/smallpox/overview/disease-facts.asp
http://www.who.int/emc/diseases/smallpox/Smallpoxeradication.html

EPIDEMIOLOGY AND ETIOLOGY

- The last cases of endemic smallpox occurred in 1977.
- Eradication of the disease was declared in 1980.

Etiology

- Variola virus of the family Poxviridae, genus Orthopoxvirus (Table 27-1)
- Humans are the only host of variola.
- No longer exists naturally but is maintained in research laboratories and may be used as a bioterrorism weapon (see Appendix B).
- DNA virus that replicates in cell cytoplasm.

Occupation Laboratory workers.
Susceptibility

- Persons in the general population in the United States under age 30 have not been vaccinated.
- All such persons are susceptible to smallpox.
- Some persons born before 1972 and vaccinated may still be protected; may have milder disease if exposed and less likely to transmit infection.

Transmission

- Respiratory-droplet nuclei
  - Most likely from patients with severe disease or who are coughing
  - Contaminated clothing/bedding

- Less transmissible than measles, chickenpox, influenza.
- Secondary attack rates among unvaccinated contacts, 37–88%.
- Maximal transmissibity: from onset of enanthema through first 7–10 days of rash.

Season Winter, early spring (endemic).

Classification of Clinical Types of Variola

- *Variola major* ("ordinary")
  - 90% of cases
  - 30% mortality

- *Variola minor* (*alastrim*; modified-type)
  - 2% of cases, occurring in unvaccinated persons
  - 25% of previously vaccinated persons

- *Variola sine eruptione* occurs in:
  - Previously vaccinated contacts
  - Infants with maternal antibodies
- *Smallpox with flat lesions*
  - Case fatality 97% among unvaccinated persons
- *Hemorrhagic smallpox*
  - Near 100% case fatality rate

PATHOGENESIS

- Enters the respiratory tract, seeding mucous membranes, passing rapidly into local lymph nodes.
- After a brief period of viremia, latent period of 4–14 days occurs, during which the virus multiplies in the reticuloendothelial system.
- Another brief period of viremia precedes prodrome, during which mouth/pharynx are infected.
- Virus invades capillary endothelium of dermal layer in skin, resulting in skin lesions. Virus is abundant in skin and oropharyngeal lesions in early illness.
- Acquired immunity via cytotoxic T cells and B cells.
- Neutralizing antibodies appear during first week of illness.
- Correlation between humoral antibodies and protection from smallpox is not certain.
- Death ascribed to toxemia, associated with immune complexes, and to hypotension. Infection with smallpox confers lifelong immunity.

CLINICAL FINDINGS

Incubation Period   7–17 days (mean, 10–12).

Prodrome

- 2–3 days.
- Sudden onset of severe headache, backache, fever (±40°C); subsides over 2–3 days.
- A prodromal maculopapular or petechial rash occurring in a "swimming-trunk" distribution reported.

Mucocutaneous Lesions

- Small red macules evolve to papules (2–3 mm) over 1–2 days.
- In 1–2 more days, papules become vesicles (2–5 mm).

- Vesicles evolve to pustules (4–6 mm) 4–7 days after onset of rash (Fig. 27-8A, B), remain 5–8 days.
- Followed by umbilication and crusting (Fig. 27-8C).
- Lesions are generally all at the same stage of development.
- Palm/soles lesions persist longest.
- Pockmarks/pitted scars occur in 65–85% of severe cases, especially on the face (Fig. 27-9).
- Bacterial superinfections present as abscesses, cellulitis.
- Distribution: Initial lesions on face and extremities, then gradually become disseminated.

Mucous membrane Enanthema (tongue, mouth, oropharynx) precedes exanthem by a day. 🖉

A

B

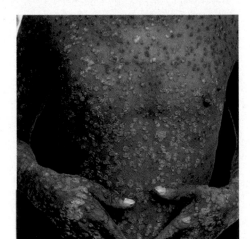

C

FIGURE 27-8   Smallpox: variola major   *A.* Multiple pustules becoming confluent on the face. ***B.*** Multiple pustules on the trunk, all in the same stage of development. ***C.*** Multiple crusted healing lesions on the trunk, arms, hands.

General Findings

- Variants: Panophthalmitis, keratitis, secondary infection of eye (1%).
- Arthritis in children (2%).
- Encephalitis (<1%)

DIFFERENTIAL DIAGNOSIS

Severe chickenpox (varicella where lesions are in different stages of development), human monkeypox (patients often have lymphadenopathy), tanapox, hand-foot-and-mouth disease (coxsackievirus A-16), insect bites, widespread molluscum contagiosum in HIV disease, adverse cutaneous drug eruption (bullous), secondary syphilis. Historically, smallpox has been confused with chickenpox, syphilis, and measles.

LABORATORY EXAMINATIONS

Specimens Skin lesions (papular, vesicular, pustular fluid; crusts); blood samples; tonsillar swabbings.

Polymerase Chain Reaction (PCR) For orthopoxvirus genes, PCR identfies variola virus.

Cultures Virus isolated on live cell cultures; DNA of orthopoxvirus identified.

Serology Does not differentiate among orthopoxvirus species. Newer methods detect IgM responses.

Dermatopathology Virus replicates in basal epithelium, causing a local cellular reaction. In papular stage, capillary dilatation and edema of papillary dermis.

Electron Microscopy Brick-shaped virus seen in negative stains.

DIAGNOSIS

An illness with acute onset of fever >38.3°C (101°F) followed by a rash characterized by firm, deep-seated vesicles or pustules in the same stage of development without other apparent cause.

Laboratory Criteria for Confirmation

- PCR identification of variola DNA in a clinical specimen, *or*
- Isolation of smallpox (variola) virus from a clinical specimen [World Health Organization (WHO) Smallpox Reference Laboratory or laboratory with appropriate reference capabilities] *plus* variola PCR confirmation.

MANAGEMENT

In the United States and most other countries possible smallpox should be reported to state health officials; diagnosis confirmed in a Biological Safety Level 4 laboratory where staff members have been vaccinated in the United States. State officials contact Centers for Disease Control and Prevention (CDC) (770–488-7100). CDC informs WHO Department of Communicable Disease Surveillance and Response Unit.

FIGURE 27-9 Smallpox: scarring on face A 50-year-old Indian male with a history of smallpox as a child has multiple depressed scars on face 40 years after smallpox infection. (Courtesy of Atul Taneja, MD.)

Immunization

- Vaccination against smallpox not performed in the United States since 1972 and in the rest of world since 1982.
- The greater majority of the global population is susceptible to smallpox.
- The U.S. military is immunized against smallpox.
- Since the threat of bioterrorism in 2001, selected health care personnel have been vaccinated in the United States.
- If an outbreak does occur, prompt recognition and vaccination would be important.
- Vaccination begun 2–3 days after exposure offers substantial protection.

Precautions

- Suspect case should be managed in negative-pressure room.
- Strict respiratory and contact isolation imperative.

Drug of Choice There is no treatment approved by the U.S. Food and Drug Administration (FDA) for orthoviruses. Cidofovir may be effective.

Bacterial Superinfection Usually *Staphylococcus aureus* or group A streptococcus.

COWPOX, MONKEYPOX, TANAPOX

- Zoonotic infections
- Accidentally transferred to humans from animal hosts.
- Rarely cause human infections in developed nations.
- When human infections do occur, the differential diagnosis includes infections associated with

bioterrorism, i.e., smallpox, anthrax, tularemia, plague.

- Identification of poxvirus can be made from skin-lesion tissue viral culture, PCR, immunohistologic analysis, or electron-microscopic methods.

COWPOX   ICD-9:051.0 ∘ ICD-10:B08.0

- Zoonosis of cats, cows, rodents, and occasionally humans.
- Jenner used cowpox isolate for vaccination.
- Reservoir:
  - Cats: most common source for human infection
  - Small rodents: voles, mice
- Source of outbreaks in cows is unknown.
- Demography: occurs in Europe and in countries of the former Soviet Union.
- Disease in cows: pustules on teats.
- Disease in cats: blisters at sites of bites/scratches.

- Disease in humans:
  - Painful papule(s), which evolve to vesicles to
  - Umbilicated pustules (surrounded by edema/erythema) to
  - Eschar or ulcer.
  - Multiple lesions occur on hands/face, which resolve in 3–4 weeks.
  - Lymphadenopathy is common.
  - Lesions may be extensive in atopic dermatitis.
  - Incidence may have increased due to discontinuation of smallpox immunization and increased numbers of immunocompromised hosts.

MONKEYPOX   ICD-9 : 057.8 ∘ ICD-10 : B04   □ ◑

- Zoonosis of captive primates and rodents
- Human cases in Africa and recently in midwestern United States.
- Transmission to:
  - Humans from pet prairie dogs via open wound or scratch or bites
  - Person-to-person transmission may occur.
- Incubation period: 4–24 days (median, 15).

- Human illness is characterized by fever, drenching sweats, and severe chills
  - Skin lesions evolve from papules to vesicopustules to serous-to-hemorrhagic crusts.
  - Lesions occur on skin, conjunctivae, and buccal mucosa.
  - Regional lymphadenopathy can occur.

TANAPOX   ICD-9 : 078.89 ∘ ICD-10 : B08.8   □ ◑

- Zoonosis of African nonhuman primates and humans.
- Transmission to humans: unknown; possibly by mosquitoes that have fed on infected monkeys.
- Disease in humans:

- Febrile illness
- 1 to 10 pruritic, indurated, ± umbilicated papules that become necrotic with red halo
  - Occur on exposed sites.
- Lymphadenopathy is common.

VACCINIA   □ ◑

- Vaccination against smallpox consists of the introduction of vaccinia virus into the outer layers of intact skin.
- Local multiplication of virus occurs
  - In some instances regional lymphadenopathy
  - Systemic symptoms ensue.
- The infection is a local one
  - Heals by scarring
  - Limited by host response.
  - Widespread and severe in atopic dermatitis

- Complications of vaccination include
  - Allergic reaction to a component of vaccine
  - Bacterial superinfection
  - Persistent/spread of local vaccinia infection.

Synonym: Cowpox.

http://www.bt.cdc.gov/training/smallpoxvaccine/reactions/sitemap.htm

EPIDEMIOLOGY AND ETIOLOGY

- Vaccinia virus, related to cowpox virus (see "Cowpox," above).
- The origin of the strains of vaccinia virus currently used for vaccination is unknown.
- Infection with cowpox virus confers immunity to smallpox.

Age, Sex Most reactions occur after first (primo) vaccination.

Season Superinfection occurs more often in warm weather.

Transmission

- Iatrogenic inoculation.
- Inadvertent transmission:
  - Autoinoculation
  - Transmission to another person
- Bioterrorism is of concern.

PATHOGENESIS

Normal Reaction (Fig. 27-10)

- Vaccinia replicates in the basal layer and disseminates from cell to cell, causing necrosis and formation of fluid-filled vesicles.
- Initial spread of virus is slowed by innate antiviral mechanisms, and, by the second week, the cell-mediated immune response begins to eliminate infected cells.
- Neutrophils, macrophages, and lymphocytes infiltrate the inoculation site, forming a confluent pustule and releasing cytokines and chemokines that cause hyperemia and edema in surrounding tissues.
  - The inflammatory process peaks 10–12 days after vaccination and begins to resolve by day 14, with shedding of the scab by day 21.
  - This sequence of events, which simulates the development of a smallpox pock, is known as a "take" reaction.
  - A successful take is required for the development of antivaccinia antibody and cell-mediated responses.

VACCINATION

Vaccine

- Inoculation against smallpox is performed using vaccinia virus.
- The vaccine currently available in the United States, Dryvax (Wyeth), is obtained from pustules on inoculated calves.
- Nearly all side effects can be predicted from the unusual nature of smallpox vaccination, which essentially employs a small circle of skin as a "culture plate" in which to grow vaccinia virus.
- Newer vaccines will be produced on cell culture.
  - Two attenuated vaccine strains have been developed and tested:
    - Modified vaccinia Ankara (MVA)
    - Japanese strain (LC16m8).

Method

- Vaccine is administered with the use of a bifurcated needle, which is dipped into reconstituted vaccine.
- 15 assertive jabs into the dermis of the upper deltoid are given in an area with a diameter of about 0.5 cm.
  - A small amount of blood should appear at the vaccination site within 20–25 s.

Contraindications   Because of adverse reactions, mandatory vaccination in the general population of the United States was discontinued in 1972 because the risk of complications outweighed the threat of endemic smallpox.

Since that time, the number of immunocompromised persons has increased markedly because of spread of HIV infection and increased numbers of patients receiving immunosuppressive medications. These persons are at risk for progressive vaccinia. (See also "Management," below.)

Vaccination contraindicated in atopic dermatitis.

CLINICAL MANIFESTATION

Mucocutaneous Lesions

Normal Vaccination Reaction

- 6–8 days after vaccination, loculated pustule (Jennerian pustule) 1–2 cm in diameter develops at site (Fig. 27-10).
- Central crusting begins and spreads peripherally over 3–5 days.
- Local edema and a dark crust remain until the third week.
- Other reactions are classified as equivocal, and another vaccination is required. 🖉
- Local "satellite" pustules may occur.

SYSTEMIC MANIFESTATIONS

- Malaise and other mild constitutional symptoms.
- Fever.
- Tender, enlarged axillary lymph nodes.

REACTIONS AND COMPLICATIONS OF VACCINIA VIRUS

Before 1972 in the United States, the risk of complication from vaccination was 1254 per 1 million vaccinations. Children under the age of 5 who were undergoing primary vaccination had the highest rates of complications. The case fatality rate was 1 per 1 million primary vaccinations; in 1968, there were nine vaccine-associated deaths.

Noninfectious Rashes

- Erythema multiforme–like
- Macular ("toxic eruption")
- Maculopapular; vesicular

- Urticarial.
- Most common 7–14 days after primovaccination or earlier after revaccination.

Noninfectious Immune-Mediated

- Encephalitis (meningoencephalitis syndrome)
- Pericarditis/myocarditis.

Bacterial Superinfection

- Presents as enlarging crusted inoculation site (impetigo or ecthyma).
- *S. aureus*, mixed; tetanus.
- GAS; Infections occur more often in persons with nasal colonization by *S. aureus* or oropharyngeal colonization with GAS.
- Contamination from soil or dung may result in tetanus.
- Other factors: trauma to site, maceration, manipulation of site.

Accidental Inoculation

- Virus usually remains localized at site of implantation but may be transposed to normal or abnormal skin/mucosa (burns, pyoderma, exanthem, eczema, other dermatitides, mucosal, corneal) elsewhere on the body or to another person.
- *Eczema vaccinatum:* inoculation on site of eczema or atopic dermatitis results in progressive and often widespread vaccinia infection.
- May occur in vaccinated or from vaccinated individual.
- Mucosal sites: conjunctiva → keratitis; mouth, airway

Congenital Vaccinia

- Vaccination during pregnancy may result in dissemination of infection to fetus.
- Infant may be stillborn or develop lesions shortly after birth.

Generalized Vaccinia

- Generalized vesicular/pustular reaction
- Self-limited, usually occurring in one crop.
- Usually occurs in a healthy individual whose antivaccinal antibody response is delayed but adequate.

Primary Vaccination Site Reaction

Day 4

Day 7

Day 14

Day 21

FIGURE 27-10 Primary smallpox vaccination site reaction Expected vaccine site reaction and progression following primary smallpox vaccination or revaccination after a prolonged period between vaccinations. Multiple pressure vaccination technique used. (Source: *http://www.bt.cdc.gov/agent/smallpox/smallpox-images/vaxsit5a.htm.*)

- Almost always benign, with normal-healing primary vaccination. May become malignant with progression (see below).

Progressive Vaccinia (Vaccinia Gangrenosa, Vaccinia Necrosa, Disseminated Vaccinia)

- Incidence during universal vaccination: 1 per million vaccines in general population.
- Vesicles fail to transform to pustules by the end of the first week. Vaccination site fails to heal and continues to enlarge forming an ulcer with raised edges. Relentless outward spread of infection from vaccination site and eventual dissemination to other areas of the body.
- Occurs only in persons with defective cellular immune function.
  - *Congenital immunodeficiency*: severe, combined immunodeficiency.
  - *Acquired immunodeficiency*: HIV disease, organ transplant recipient, chronic immunosuppression (e.g., connective tissue disorders), hypogammaglobulinemia, dysglobulinemia, malignancies (chronic lymphatic leukemia, lymphoma).

- Course is chronic and progressive, spreading deep into tissues and causing necrosis and osteomyelitis with bacterial superinfection,.
- Course: Leads to death weeks or months after vaccination.

DIFFERENTIAL DIAGNOSIS

Nonhealing/Expanding Lesion at Vaccination Site

- Abnormally large vaccination lesion: unusually strong take reaction.
- Bacterial superinfection with GAS or *S. aureus*, both of which are accompanied by an increased, rather than diminished, inflammatory response.
- Progressive vaccinia: slow pace of development, minimal inflammatory response.

LABORATORY EXAMINATIONS

Culture   Detects GAS and *S. aureus*.
Dermatopathology   Vaccinia replicates in basal epithelium, causing a local cellular reaction.

DIAGNOSIS

Clinical history, physical examination, and clinical course. Persistence of virus can be confirmed by culturing vaccinia virus from the skin lesions.

COURSE AND PROGNOSIS

Normal Vaccination Reaction

- A Jennerian pustule is classified as a major reaction, indicating successful primary vaccination; successful revaccination is indicated by palpable inflammation at 6–8 days.
- A successful vaccination confers full immunity to smallpox in >95% of persons for 5–10 years.
- Successful revaccination probably provides protection for ≥10–20 years.
- Reactions other than a Jennerian pustule are classified as equivocal, and another vaccination is required.

Progressive Vaccinia

- Lethal in infants who completely lack cellular immune function.
- Infection in adults with HIV/AIDS: may resolve if treated with vaccinia immunoglobulin (VIg).

MANAGEMENT

Contraindication to Vaccination

- If in doubt, don't vaccinate.
- Any abnormality of skin in vaccinated individual or in contacts: atopic dermatitis, eczema, burns, lichen simplex chronicus, pyodermas.
- Any immunologic defect/disorder, any hematologic disorders involving white blood cells, any inflammatory lesions of periorbital structures, GAS or *S. aureus* carrier states, any acute febrile illness, exposure to or incubation of exanthematous disease, family history of febrile convulsions or of postvaccinal encephalitis.

VIg

- Available from the CDC through state health departments for treatment of severe complications.
- May be beneficial in management of accidental inoculation, eczema vaccinatum, generalized vaccinia.

- Response of progressive vaccinia not well documented.
- Administered IM 0.6 mL/kg.

Antiviral Drug Cidofovir is protective against orthopoxvirus in animals.

Immunomodulators

- The TH1 cytokines interleukin 2 and interferon stimulate orthopoxvirus clearance.

- Local or systemic treatment with immunomodulators that potentiate a TH1 response could help suppress vaccinia infection in immunodeficient patients.

Immunosuppression Tapering or discontinuation of immunosuppressive therapies if patients are iatrogenically immunosuppressed.
Myopericarditis High-dose glucocorticoids.

HUMAN PAPILLOMAVIRUS INFECTIONS   ICD-9 : 079.4 ∘ ICD-10 : B97.7

- Human papillomaviruses (HPV) are ubiquitous in humans, causing
  - Subclinical infection
  - Wide variety of benign clinical lesions on skin and mucous membranes.
- They also have a role in the oncogenesis of cutaneous and mucosal premalignancies (Table 27-2):
  - Squamous cell carcinoma in situ (SCCIS)
  - Invasive SCC
- More than 150 types of HPV have been identified and are associated with various clinical lesions and diseases
- Cutaneous HPV infections occur commonly in the general population:
  - Common warts: Represent approximately 70% of all cutaneous warts, occurring in up to 20% of all school-age children.
    - Butcher's warts: Common in butchers, meat packers, fish handlers.
  - Plantar warts: Common in older children and young adults, accounting for 30% of cutaneous warts.

- Flat warts: Occur in children and adults, accounting for 4% of cutaneous warts.
- Oncogenic HPV can cause
  - SCCIS and invasive SCC in immunocompromised hosts, especially in those with
    - HIV/AIDS
    - Solid organ transplant recipients
    - Epidermodysplasia verruciformis (EDV).
- Mucosal warts:
  - Condyloma acuminatum (genital wart)
    - Most prevalent sexually transmitted infection (see Section 30).
  - Some HPV types have a major etiologic role in the pathogenesis of in situ as well as invasive SCC of the anogenital epithelium.
  - During delivery, maternal genital HPV infection can be transmitted to the neonate, resulting in
    - Anogenital warts
    - Respiratory papillomatosis after aspiration of the virus into the upper respiratory tract.

ETIOLOGY

- Papillomaviruses are double-strand DNA viruses of the papovavirus class, which infect most vertebrate species with exclusive host and tissue specificity.
- They infect squamous epithelia of skin and mucous membranes.
- Clinical lesions induced by HPV and its natural history are largely determined by HPV type.

- HPV are normally grouped according to their pathologic associations and tissue specificity—either cutaneous or mucosal.
- The 23 mucosal-associated HPV can be further subgrouped according to their risk of malignant transformation.
- New types of HPV are defined as possessing <90% homology to known types in six specified early and late genes.

HUMAN PAPILLOMAVIRUS: CUTANEOUS INFECTIONS ■ ○→◐

- ■ Certain human HPV types commonly infect keratinized skin.
- ■ Cutaneous warts are:
  - ▪ Discrete benign epithelial hyperplasia with varying degrees of surface hyperkeratosis
  - ▪ Manifested as minute papules to large plaques
- ■ Lesions may become confluent, forming a mosaic.
- ■ The extent of lesions is determined by the immune status of the host.

Synonym: Verruca, myrmecia.

EPIDEMIOLOGY AND ETIOLOGY

Etiology See Table 27-2.

Transmission

- • Skin-to-skin contact.
- • Minor trauma with breaks in stratum corneum facilitates epidermal infection.
- • Contagion occurs in groups—small (home) or large (school gymnasium).

Other Factors

- • Immunocompromise associated with an increased incidence of and more widespread cutaneous warts:
  - ○ HIV/AIDS
  - ○ Iatrogenic immunosuppression with solid organ transplantation.
- • Occupational risk associated with meat handling.
- • Epidermodysplasia verruciformis (EDV, see below): most commonly autosomal recessive.

▉ TABLE 27-2   Correlation of Human Papillomavirus Type with Disease

Disease	Associated HPV Types
Plantar warts	1,[*] 2, [†] 4, 63
Myrmecia	60
Common warts	1,[*] 2,[*] 4, 26, 27, 29, 41,[†] 57, 65, 77
Common warts of meat handlers	1, 2,[*] 3, 4, 7,[*] 10, 28
Flat warts	3,[*] 10,[*] 27, 38, 41,[†] 49, 75, 76
Intermediate warts	10,[*] 26, 28
Epidermodysplasia verruciformis	2,[*] 3,[*] 5,[*†] 8,[*†] 9,[*] 10,[*] 12,[*] 14,[*†] 15,[*] 17,[*†] 19, 20,[†] 21, 22, 23, 24, 25, 36, 37, 38,[†] 47, 50
Condyloma acuminatum	6,[*] 11,[*] 30,[†] 42, 43, 44, 45,[†] 51,[†] 54, 55, 70
Intraepithelial neoplasias	
Unspecified	30,[†] 34, 39,[†] 40, 53, 57, 59, 61, 62, 64, 66,[†] 67, 69, 71
Low-grade	6,[*] 11,[*] 16,[†] 18,[†] 31,[†] 33,[†] 35,[†] 42, 43, 44, 45,[†] 51,[†] 52,[†] 74
High-grade	6, 11, 16,[*†] 18,[*†] 31,[†] 33,[†] 34, 35,[†] 39,[†] 42, 44, 45,[†] 51,[†] 52,[†] 56,[†] 58,[†] 66,[†]
Cervical carcinoma	16,[*†] 18,[*†] 31,[†] 33,[†] 35,[†] 39,[†] 45,[†] 51,[†] 52,[†] 56,[†] 58,[†] 66,[†] 68, 70
Laryngeal papillomas	6,[*] 11[*]
Focal epithelial hyperplasia of Heck	13,[*] 32[*]
Conjunctival papillomas	6,[*] 11,[*] 16[*†]
Others	6, 11, 16,[†] 30,[†] 33,[†] 36, 37, 38,[†] 41,[†] 48,[†] 60, 72, 73

[*]Most common associations.
[†]High malignant potential.
NOTE: Additional information on new HPV types can be found on the HPV Sequence Data Base through the Internet (*hpv-web.lanl.gov*).
SOURCE: From RC Reichman, in E Braunwald et al (eds): *Harrison's Principles of Internal Medicine*, 15th ed. New York, McGraw-Hill, 2001.

CLINICAL MANIFESTATION

Duration of Lesions Warts often persist for several years if not treated.

Symptoms

- Cosmetic disfigurement.
- Plantar warts act as a foreign body and can be quite painful during normal daily activities, such as walking, if located over pressure points.
- More aggressive therapies such as cryosurgery often result in much more pain than that caused by the wart itself.
- Bleeding, especially after shaving.

Skin Lesions

Verruca Vulgaris (Common Wart)

- Firm papules, 1–10 mm or rarely larger (Fig. 27-11), hyperkeratotic, clefted surface, with vegetations.
- Palmar lesions disrupt the normal line of fingerprints (Fig. 27-12). Return of fingerprints is a sign of resolution of the wart.

FIGURE 27-11 Verruca vulgaris: thumb A 25-year-old male with hyperkeratotic (verrucous) papules on the dorsal thumb. The dark points represent thrombosed capillaries. The lesion resolved with electrodessication, having failed to respond to cryosurgery.

A   *B*

FIGURE 27-12 Verruca vulgaris: hands A 20-year-old immunosuppressed male with nephrotic syndrome. Multiple verrucae on the *(A)* dorsum and *(B)* palm of the hand.

- Characteristic "red or brown dots" are better seen with hand lens and are pathognomonic, representing thrombosed capillary loops.
- Isolated lesion, scattered discrete lesions.
- *Linear arrangement*: inoculation by scratching.
- *Annular warts*: at sites of prior therapy (Fig. 27-13).
- Occur at sites of trauma: hands, fingers, knees.
- *Butcher's warts*: large cauliflower-like lesions on hands of meat handlers.
- *Filiform warts* have relatively small bases, extending out with elongated cap. 🔲

Verruca Plantaris (Plantar Wart)

- Early small, shiny, sharply marginated papule (Fig. 27-14) → plaque with rough hyperkeratotic surface, studded with brown-black dots (thrombosed capillaries).
- As with palmar warts, normal dermatoglyphics are disrupted. Return of dermatoglyphics is a sign of resolution of the wart.
- Warts heal without scarring.
- Therapies such as cryosurgery and electrosurgery can result in scarring at treatment sites.

- Tenderness may be marked, especially in certain acute types and in lesions over sites of pressure (metatarsal head).
- *Mosaic warts*: Confluence of many small warts (Fig. 27-14).
- *"Kissing" warts*: lesion may occur on opposing surface of two toes (Fig. 27-15).
- Plantar foot, often solitary but may be three to six or more.
- Pressure points, heads of metatarsal, heels, toes. 🔲

Verruca Plana (Flat Wart)

- Sharply defined, flat papules (1–5 mm); "flat" surface; the thickness of the lesion is 1–2 mm (Fig. 27-16).
- Skin-colored or light brown.
- Round, oval, polygonal, linear lesions (inoculation of virus by scratching).
- Occur on face, beard area (Fig. 27-17), dorsa of hands (Fig. 27-18), shins.

Epidermodysplasia Verruciformis

- Autosomal recessive condition.
- Flat-topped papules.
- Pityriasis versicolor–like lesions, particularly on the trunk.

FIGURE 27-13   Verruca vulgaris: annular wart   A 24-year-old with an annular wart on the dorsum of the finger. The wart originally at this site was much smaller and had been treated with cryosurgery. The treated site improved but the wart expanded radially, creating the ring.

FIGURE 27-14   Verruca plantaris: plantar feet   A 71-year-old male with chronic lymphatic leukemia. Large and painful on pressure, warts are seen on the anterior feet and the toes. Multiple warts were also present on the fingers. After many failed therapeutic modalities, he was successfully treated with electron beam radiation.

FIGURE 27-15   Verruca plantaris: "kissing warts"   A 49-year-old male with HIV/AIDS has confluent warts on the hands and feet. The large warts on opposing toes are referred to as "kissing warts."

FIGURE 27-16   Verruca plana   A 12-year-old male kidney transplant recipient. Multiple brown keratotic papules are seen on the forehead and scalp.

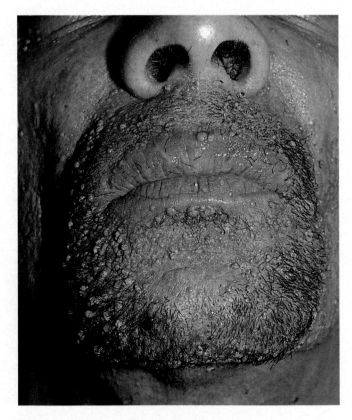

FIGURE 27-17   Verruca vulgaris   A 38-year-old male with HIV/AIDS. Confluent skin-colored papules in the beard area. Lesions resolved after successful antiretroviral therapy (ART).

- Color: skin-colored, light brown, pink, hypo-pigmented.
- Lesions may be numerous, large, and confluent.
- Seborrheic keratosis–like and actinic keratosis–like lesions.
- Linear arrangement after traumatic inoculation.
- *Distribution:* face, dorsa of hands (Fig. 27-18), arms, legs, anterior trunk.
- Premalignant and malignant lesions arise most commonly on face.
- SCC: in situ and invasive. 📖

HIV Disease, Iatrogenic Immunosuppression

- HPV-induced warts are common and may be difficult to treat successfully.

- Some have atypical histologic features and may progress to in situ and invasive SCC.

DIFFERENTIAL DIAGNOSIS

Verruca Vulgaris Molluscum contagiosum, seborrheic keratosis, actinic keratosis, kerato-acanthoma, SCCIS, invasive SCC.
Verruca Plantaris Callus, corn (keratosis), have no thrombosed capillary loops, exostosis.
Verruca Plana Syringoma (facial), molluscum contagiosum.
Epidermodysplasia Verruciformis Pityriasis versicolor, actinic keratoses, seborrheic keratoses, SCCIS, basal cell carcinoma.

FIGURE 27-18 Epidermodysplasia verruciformis-like lesions A 35-year-old female lung transplant recipient. Multiple, flat-topped, pink papules with sharp margination and minimal hyperkeratosis on the dorsa of the hands and fingers. The tape is at the site of a biopsy that showed squamous cell carcinoma in situ arising in a flat-wart lesion. Multiple lesions were also present on the legs.

LABORATORY EXAMINATION

Dermatopathology Acanthosis, papillomatosis, hyperkeratosis. Characteristic feature is foci of vacuolated cells (koilocytosis), vertical tiers of parakeratotic cells, foci of clumped keratohyaline granules.

DIAGNOSIS

- Usually made on clinical findings.
- In the immunocompromised host, HIV-induced SCC at periungual sites or anogenital region should be ruled out by lesional biopsy.

COURSE AND PROGNOSIS

- Immunocompetent individuals: Cutaneous HPV infections usually resolve spontaneously, without therapeutic intervention.
- Immunocompromised individuals: Cutaneous HPV infections may be very resistant to all modalities of therapy.
- EDV: Lesions first occur at 5–7 years of age; lesions appear progressively, becoming widespread in some. 30–50% of individuals with EDV develop malignant cutaneous lesions on areas of skin exposed to sunlight.

MANAGEMENT

Goal	Aggressive therapies, which are often quite painful and may be followed by scarring, are usually to be avoided because the natural history of cutaneous HPV infections is for spontaneous resolution in months or a few years. Plantar warts that are painful because of their location warrant more aggressive therapies.
Patient-initiated therapy	Minimal cost; no/minimal pain.
For small lesions	10–20% salicylic acid and lactic acid in collodion.
For large lesions	40% salicylic acid plaster for 1 week, then application of salicylic acid–lactic acid in collodion.
Imiquimod cream	At sites that are not thickly keratinized, apply half-strength 3 times per week. Persistent warts may require occlusion. Hyperkeratotic lesions on palms/soles should be debrided frequently; Imiquimod used alternately with a topical retinoid such as tararotene topical gel may be effective.
Hyperthermia for verruca plantaris	Hyperthermia with hot water [45°C (113°F)] immersion for 20 min two or three times weekly for up to 16 treatments is effective in some patients.
Clinician-initiated therapy	Costly, painful.
Cryosurgery	If patients have tried home therapies and liquid nitrogen is available, light cryosurgery using a cotton-tipped applicator or cryospray, freezing the wart and 1–2 mm of surrounding normal tissue for approximately 30 s, is quite effective. Freezing kills the infected tissue but not HPV.
	Cryosurgery is usually repeated about every 4 weeks until the warts have disappeared. Painful.
Electrosurgery	More effective than cryosurgery, but also associated with a greater chance of scarring. EMLA cream can be used for anesthesia for flat warts. Lidocaine injection is usually required for thicker warts, especially palmar/plantar lesions.
CO_2 laser surgery	May be effective for recalcitrant warts, but no better than cryosurgery or electrosurgery in the hands of an experienced clinician.
Surgery	Single, nonplantar verruca vulgaris:curettage after freon freezing; surgical excision of cutaneous HPV infections is not indicated in that these lesions are epidermal infections.

HUMAN PAPILLOMAVIRUS: MUCOSAL INFECTIONS

See Section 30, Sexually Transmitted Diseases

INFECTIOUS EXANTHEMS ICD-9:782.1 ○ ICD-10:B08 □→■ ○→◑

- An infectious exanthem (IE) is a generalized cutaneous eruption associated with a primary systemic infection.
  - Often accompanied by oral mucosal lesions, i.e., an enanthema.
- IEs are most commonly caused by viral agents but can also be associated with
  - Bacterial
  - Rickettsial
- Parasitic infections
- Certain IEs have fairly characteristic morphology, but in many cases an accurate diagnosis cannot be made on the basis of morphology alone.
- Historic factors may be helpful, including season, disease contacts, immunizations, previous exanthematous illnesses, and associated prodromal symptoms.

EPIDEMIOLOGY AND ETIOLOGY

Age of Onset Usually <20 years.

Etiology

RNA Viruses

- Picornaviridae
  - Poliovurus
  - Coxsackieviruses
  - Echovirus
  - Enterovirus
  - Hepatitis A virus
  - Rhinovirus
- Togaviridae
  - Rubella virus, attenuated rubella virus in vaccine
- Flaviviridae
  - Dengue
  - Hepatitis C
- Paramyxoviridae
  - Measles
  - Mumps
- Orthomyxoviridae
  - Influenza A, B, and C viruses
- Retroviridae
  - Human T-lymphotrophic virus types I and II
  - Human immunodeficiency viruses (HIV) types 1 and 2
    - Acute HIV syndrome

DNA viruses

- Parvoviridae
  - Parvovirus B19 (erythema infectiosum)
- Hepadnaviridae
  - Hepatitis B virus
- Adenoviridae

- Herpesviridae
  - Herpes simplex virus (HSV) types 1 and 2
  - Varicella zoster virus (VZV)
  - Cytomegalovirus (CMV)
  - Epstein-Barr virus (EBV)
  - Human herpesvirus (HHV) 6 and 7 (exanthem subitum, roseola infantum)
  - Kaposi sarcoma–associated virus (HHV-8)
- Poxviridae
  - Variola (smallpox) virus
  - Orf virus
  - Molluscum contagiosum virus

Bacterial

- Group A streptococcus: scarlet fever, toxic shock syndrome
- *S. aureus*: toxic shock syndrome
- *Legionella*
- *Leptospira*
- *Listeria*
- Meningococci

Mycoplasmal

- *Mycoplasma pneumoniae*

Rickettsial

- Rocky Mountain spotted fever
- Tick-borne spotted fevers
- Rickettsialpox
- Murine typhus
- Epidemic typhus

Miscellaneous

- *Strongyloides*
- *Toxoplasma*
- *Treponema pallidum*

Transmission Respiratory, food, sexual, blood.
Season Enterovirus infections: summer months.
Geography Worldwide.

PATHOGENESIS

Skin lesions may be produced by the following:

- Direct effect of microbial replication in infected cells
- Host response to the microbe
- Interaction of these two phenomena.

CLINICAL MANIFESTATION

Incubation Period Usually <3 weeks; hepatitis B virus, several months.

Prodrome Fever, malaise, coryza, sore throat, nausea, vomiting, diarrhea, abdominal pain, headache.

Mucocutaneous Lesions

- Diffuse erythema, "scarlatiniform"
- Maculopapular, "morbilliform" eruptions
- Vesicular eruptions
- Occasionally petechiae
- Mucosal: microulcerative lesions, palatal petechiae, conjunctivitis
- Confluent pink papules (morbilliform, rubeola-like, measles-like)
  - *Synonyms*: Exanthematous, maculopapular
  - Erythematous macules and/or papules (Fig. 27-19)
  - Usually central, i.e., head, neck, trunk, proximal extremities.

FIGURE 27-19 Infectious exanthem Disseminated, erythematous macules and papules, typical of the cutaneous changes with many acute infections. The eruption must be differentiated from an exanthematous (morbilliform) drug eruption. **A.** Typical distribution of lesions on the trunk and extremities. **B.** Closeup of pink macules and papules becoming confluent in some areas.

∘ Occasionally petechiae, hemorrhagic measles
• Vesicular
  ∘ Initially, vesicles with clear fluid.
  ∘ May evolve to pustules.
  ∘ In a few days to a week, roof of vesicle sloughs, resulting in erosions.
  ∘ In varicella, lesions are disseminated and may involve oropharynx.
  ∘ In hand-foot-and-mouth disease, vesicles/erosion occur in oropharynx; painful linear vesicles on palms/soles.

• Mucous membranes
  ∘ Koplik spots in measles
  ∘ Microulcerative lesions in herpangina due to coxsackievirus A (Fig. 27-20)
  ∘ Palatal petechiae in mononucleosis syndrome of EBV or CMV
  ∘ Conjunctivitis, e.g., measles

Systemic Findings

• Lymphadenopathy
• Hepatomegaly
• Splenomegaly.

DIFFERENTIAL DIAGNOSIS

Exanthematous Eruption Drug eruption, systemic lupus erythematosus, Kawasaki syndrome.

LABORATORY EXAMINATIONS

Cultures If practical.
Serology Acute and convalescent titers most helpful in specific diagnosis.

DIAGNOSIS

Usually made on history and clinical findings.

COURSE AND PROGNOSIS

Usually resolves in <10 days.

MANAGEMENT

Symptomatic.
Antimicrobial Therapy Specific antimicrobial therapy when available.

FIGURE 27-20 Infectious enanthem: herpangina Multiple, small vesicles and erosions with erythematous halos on the soft palate; some taste buds on the posterior tongue are inflamed and prominent.

RUBELLA   □ ○→●

- Etiologic agent: Rubella virus, an RNA togavirus
- A viral infection of children and adults
- Characteristic exanthem and lymphadenopathy.
- Many infections are subclinical.
- Rubella virus infecting a pregnant female, while causing a benign illness in the mother, may result

in the congenital rubella syndrome with serious chronic fetal infection and malformation.
- Childhood immunization is highly effective at preventing infection.

Synonyms: German measles, "3-day measles."

EPIDEMIOLOGY AND ETIOLOGY

Age of Onset

- Before widespread immunization, children <15 years.
- Currently, young adults.

Etiology

- *Rubella virus*, an RNA togavirus, member of *Rubivirus* genus.
- Attenuated rubella virus used in immunization can cause an illness with rubella-like rash, lymphadenopathy, and arthritis.

Occupation   Young adults in hospitals, colleges, prisons, prenatal clinics.

Transmission

- Inhalation of aerosolized respiratory droplets
- Moderately contagious
- 10–40% of cases asymptomatic
- Period of infectivity from end of incubation period to disappearance of rash.

Risk Factors

- Lack of active immunization
- Lack of natural infection.
- After immunization began in 1969, incidence has decreased by 99% in industrialized countries.

Season   Before 1969, epidemics in the United States every 6–9 years, occurring in spring.
Geography   Worldwide. Marked reduction in incidence in industrialized countries after immunization.

CLINICAL MANIFESTATION

Incubation Period   14–21 days.

Prodrome

- Usually absent, especially in young children.

- In adolescents and young adults: anorexia, malaise, conjunctivitis, headache, low-grade fever, mild upper respiratory tract symptoms.

History   Arthralgia, especially in adult women after immunization.
Immune Status   In women, rubella-like illness frequently follows administration of attenuated live rubella virus.
Mucocutaneus Lesions

- Pink macules, papules (Fig. 27-21).
- Initially on forehead, spreading inferiorly to face, trunk, and extremities during first day.
- By second day, facial exanthem fades.
- By third day, exanthem fades completely without residual pigmentary change or scaling.
- Trunkal lesions may become confluent, creating a scarlatiniform eruption.
- Mucous membranes
  ○ Petechiae on soft palate (Forchheimer sign) during prodrome (also seen in infectious mononucleosis). 🖉

General Examination

- *Lymph nodes*:
  ○ Enlarged during prodrome.
  ○ Postauricular, suboccipital, and posterior cervical lymph nodes enlarged and possibly tender.
  ○ Mild generalized lymphadenopathy may occur.
  ○ Enlargement usually persists for 1 week but may last for months.

- *Spleen*:
  ○ May be enlarged.

- *Joints*:
  ○ Arthritis in adults; possible effusion.
  ○ Arthralgia, especially in adult women after immunization.

FIGURE 27-21   Rubella
A 21-year-old male. Erythematous macules and papules appearing initially on the face and spreading inferiorly to the trunk and extremities, usually within the first 24 h. Postauricular and posterior cervical lymph nodes were enlarged. Lesions becoming confluent on the cheeks while clearing on the forehead. Truncal lesions appear 24 h after onset of facial lesions.

DIFFERENTIAL DIAGNOSIS

Exanthem   Other infectious exanthems, adverse drug eruption, scarlet fever, erythema infectiosum, enteroviral infection.
Exanthem with Arthritis   Acute rheumatic fever, rheumatoid arthritis, erythema infectiosum.

LABORATORY EXAMINATIONS

Serology   Acute and convalescent rubella antibody titers show fourfold or greater rise.
Culture   Virus can be isolated from throat, joint fluid aspirate.

DIAGNOSIS

Clinical diagnosis; can be confirmed by serology.

COURSE AND PROGNOSIS

- In most persons, rubella is a mild, inconsequential infection.

- However, when rubella occurs in a pregnant woman during the first trimester, the infection can be passed transplacentally to the developing fetus.

  - Approximately half of infants who acquire rubella during the first trimester of intrauterine life will show clinical signs of damage from the virus.
  - Manifestations of the congenital rubella syndrome are
    - Congenital heart defects
    - Cataracts
    - Microphthalmia, microcephaly, hydrocephaly, deafness

MANAGEMENT

Prevention

- Rubella is preventable by immunization.
- Previous rubella should be documented in young women: if antirubella antibody titers are negative, rubella immunization should be given.

Acute Infection   Symptomatic.

MEASLES □→■* ◑→●*

- A highly contagious childhood viral infection
- Characterized by
  - Fever, coryza, cough
  - An exanthem
  - Conjunctivitis
  - Pathognomonic enanthem (Koplik spots)
- Significant morbidity and mortality occur in acute and chronic course.

- Childhood immunization is highly effective at preventing infection.

Synonyms: Rubeola, morbilli.

* In Africa.

EPIDEMIOLOGY AND ETIOLOGY

Age of Onset

- Before measles immunization: 5–9 years of age in the United States.
- In developing countries, up to 45% of cases occur before the age of 9 months.

Etiology Measles virus, member of RNA genus *Morbillivirus* and family Paramyxoviridae.

Incidence

- United States, Europe, Canada, Japan
  - No longer endemic
  - Cases result from international importation.
- *Worldwide*: hyperendemic in many developing nations, resulting in 800,000 deaths annually.

Risk Factors

- After immunization began in 1963, incidence has decreased by 98%.
- Current outbreaks in the United States occur in inner-city unimmunized pre-school-age children, school-age persons immunized at an early age, and imported cases.
- Most outbreaks are in primary or secondary schools, colleges or universities, day-care centers.

Transmission

- Spread by respiratory droplet aerosols produced by sneezing and coughing.
- Infected persons contagious from several days before onset of rash up to 5 days after lesions appear.
- Attack rate for susceptible contacts >90–100%.
- Asymptomatic infection rare.

Season Before widespread use of vaccine, epidemics occurred every 2–3 years in late winter to early spring.

Demography

- No longer endemic in Americas and Europe.
- Hyperendemic in Africa, with 800,000 deaths annually.

PATHOGENESIS

- Virus enters cells of respiratory tract, replicates locally, spreads to local lymph nodes, and disseminates hematogenously to skin and mucous membranes.
- Viral replication also occurs on skin and mucosa.
- Modified measles, a milder form of the illness, may occur in individuals with preexisting partial immunity induced by active or passive immunization.
- Persons deficient in cellular immunity are at high risk for severe measles.

CLINICAL MANIFESTATION

Incubation Period 10–15 days.

Prodrome

- Fever
- Malaise
- Upper respiratory symptoms (coryza, hacking barklike cough)
- Photophobia, conjunctivitis with lacrimation
- Periorbital edema.
- As exanthem progresses, systemic symptoms subside.

Mucocutaneous Lesions

- Exanthem

- On the fourth febrile day, erythematous macules and papules.
- Appear on forehead at hairline, behind ears; spread centrifugally and inferiorly to involve the face, trunk (Fig. 27-22), extremities, palms/soles, reaching the feet by third day.
- Initial discrete lesions may become confluent, especially on face, neck, and shoulders.
- Lesions gradually fade in order of appearance, with subsequent residual yellow-tan stain or faint desquamation.
- Exanthem resolves in 4–6 days.
- Mucous membranes (enanthem)
  - *Oropharynx*/Koplik spots:
    - Pathognomonic.
    - Appear before exanthem.

- Cluster of tiny bluish-white spots on red background, appearing on or after second day of febrile illness, on buccal mucosa opposite premolar teeth.
- Also: entire buccal/inner labial mucosa may be inflamed; lips red.
  - *Bulbar conjunctivae*: conjunctivitis. 🔁

General Examination

- Generalized lymphadenopathy
- Diarrhea, vomiting
- Splenomegaly

Variants

Modified Measles Milder clinical findings with preexisting partial immunity.

FIGURE 27-22 Measles Erythematous flat papules, first appearing on the face and neck where they become confluent, spreading to the trunk and arms in 2 to 3 days where they remain discrete. In contrast, rubella also first appears initially on the face but spreads to the trunk in 1 day. Koplik spots on the buccal mucosa were also present. Erythematous papules have become confluent on the face on the fourth day.

Atypical Measles

- Occurs in individuals immunized with forma-lin-inactivated measles vaccine, subsequently exposed to measles virus.
- Exanthem begins peripherally and moves centrally; can be urticarial, maculopapular, hemorrhagic, and/or vesicular.
- Systemic symptoms can be severe.

Measles in Immunocompromised Host

- Rash may not occur.
- Pneumonitis, encephalitis more common.

DIFFERENTIAL DIAGNOSIS

Disseminated Maculopapular Eruption   Drug eruption, other viral exanthems (e.g., rubella), scarlet fever. Kawasaki syndrome, infectious mononucleosis, toxoplasmosis, *M. pneumoniae* infection.

LABORATORY EXAMINATIONS

Cytology   Multinucleated giant cells in secretions.
Cultures   Isolate virus from blood, urine, pharyngeal secretions.
Measles Antigen   Detect in respiratory secretions by immunofluorescent staining.
Serology   Demonstrates fourfold or greater rise in measles titer.
PCR   Detects genomic sequences of measles virus RNA in serum, throat swabs, and cerebrospinal fluid (CSF).

DIAGNOSIS

Clinical diagnosis, at times, confirmed by serology.

COURSE AND PROGNOSIS

- Self-limited infection in most patients.
- Mortality rate
  - United States: 0.3%
  - Developing countries: 1–10%.
  - Age-specific rates of complications highest among children <5 years old and adults >20 years.
- Sites of complications: respiratory tract, CNS, tract.
  - Complications more common in malnourished children, the unimmunized, and those with congenital immunodeficiency and leukemia.
  - Acute complications (9.8% of cases): otitis media, pneumonia (bacterial or measles), diarrhea, measles encephalitis (1 in 800 to 1000 cases), thrombocytopenia.
- In unimmunized HIV-infected children, fatal measles pneumonia has occurred without rash.
- Chronic complication: subacute sclerosing panencephalitis (Dawson encephalitis)

MANAGEMENT

Prevention

- Prophylactic immunization.
- The goal of eliminating indigenous measles transmission in the United States is based on four components:
  - Maintaining high coverage with a single dose of measles-mumps-rubella (MMR) vaccine among preschool-age children,
  - Achieving coverage with two doses of MMR for all school and college attendees
  - Enhancing surveillance and outbreak response
  - Increasing efforts to develop and implement strategies for global measles elimination.

Acute Infection   Symptomatic.
Secondary Bacterial Infections   Administration of appropriate antibiotics.

ENTEROVIRAL INFECTIONS

- Etiologic agent: intestinal viruses echovirus 9 and 16, coxsackie A 16 virus, enterovirus 71 (EV71)
- Enterovirus infections with rash
  - Echovirus
    - Echovirus 9 (E9): Rubelliform (discrete pink macules) rash ± fever
    - Echovirus 16: Boston exanthem, roseola-like (confluent pink papules) ± fever.

- Coxsackievirus A16, enterovirus 71
  - Hand-foot-and-mouth disease:
- A1–10, 16, 22, CB1–5; EV6, 9, 11, 16, 17, 25; EV71: Herpangina
- Other enterovirus reported to cause: erythema multiforme; vesicular, urticarial, petechial, and purpuric rashes

HAND-FOOT-AND-MOUTH DISEASE (HFMD)

- Etiologic agent: intestinal viruses, coxsackie A 16 virus, enterovirus 71
- A systemic infection

- Characterized by
  - Ulcerative oral lesions
  - Vesicular exanthem on the distal extremities
  - Mild constitutional symptoms.

EPIDEMIOLOGY AND ETIOLOGY

Age of Onset <10 years but also young and middle-age adults.

Etiology

- Enterovirus (picornavirus group, single-strand RNA, unenveloped).
- Commonly: coxsackievirus A16, enterovirus 71 (EV71).
- Also A5, 7, 9, 10; B1,2, 5.

Season Epidemic outbreaks every 3 years. In temperate climates, outbreaks during warmer months (late summer, early fall).

Transmission Highly contagious, spread from person to person by oral-oral and fecal-oral routes.

PATHOGENESIS

- Enteroviral implantation in the GI tract (buccal mucosa and ileum) leads to extension into regional lymph nodes.
- 72 h later a viremia occurs with seeding of the oral mucosa and skin of the hands and feet.

CLINICAL MANIFESTATION

Incubation Period 3–6 days.
Prodrome 12–24 h of low-grade fever, malaise, and abdominal pain or respiratory symptoms.
Symptoms Frequently 5–10 *painful* ulcerative oral lesions, leading to refusal to eat in children. Few to 100 cutaneous lesions appear together or shortly after the oral lesions and may be asymptomatic or *tender* and *painful*.

Mucocutaneous Lesions

- Lesions begin as 2- to 8-mm *macules* or *papules* that quickly evolve to *vesicles*. Early papules, pink to red.
- Vesicles have clear fluid with a watery appearance or yellowish hue.
- Characteristically, lesions arise on palms and soles, especially on sides of fingers, toes, and buttocks.
- Palms/fingers, sole/toes: vesicles
  - Characteristic "linear" shape
  - Tender, painful
  - Usually do not rupture (Fig. 27-23A).
- At other cutaneous sites, vesicles can rupture, with formation of *erosions* and *crusts*.
- Lesions heal without scarring.
- Oral lesions:
  - Macules → grayish vesicles, arising on the hard palate, tongue, buccal mucosa (Fig. 27-23B).

○ Vesicles quickly erode to 5- to 10-mm, small, punched out painful ulcers. 🔲

General Findings

- May be associated with high fever, severe malaise, diarrhea, and joint pains.
- EV17 infections may have associated CNS (aseptic meningitis, encephalitis, meningoencephalitis, flaccid paralysis), and lung involvement.
  ○ Epidemics with significant mortality in young children have occurred in China and Taiwan.

DIFFERENTIAL DIAGNOSIS

A sudden outbreak of oral and distal extremity lesions is pathognomonic for HFMD. However, if only the oral lesions are present, the differential diagnosis would include HSV infection, aphthous stomatitis, herpangina, erythema multiforme, adverse drug reaction.

LABORATORY EXAMINATIONS

Histopathology Epidermal reticular degeneration leads to an intraepidermal vesicle filled with neutrophils, mononuclear cells, and proteinaceous eosinophilic material.
Serology In acute serum, neutralizing antibodies may be detected but disappear rapidly. In convalescent serum, elevated titers of complement-fixing antibodies are found.

Tzanck Preparation Negative for both multinucleated giant cells and inclusion bodies, which are seen in HSV- and VZV-infected cells.
Viral Culture Virus may be isolated from vesicles, throat washings, and stool specimens.

DIAGNOSIS

Usually made on clinical findings.

COURSE AND PROGNOSIS

- Most commonly, HFMD is self-limited.
- Rise in serum antibodies eliminates the viremia in 7–10 days.
- A few cases have been more prolonged or recurrent.
- Serious sequelae rarely occur:
  ○ Coxsackievirus has been implicated in cases of myocarditis, meningoencephalitis, aseptic meningitis, paralytic disease, and a systemic illness resembling rubeola.
  ○ Enterovirus 71 infections have higher morbidity/mortality rates due to CNS involvement and pulmonary edema.
  ○ Infection acquired during the first trimester of pregnancy may result in spontaneous abortion.

MANAGEMENT

Symptomatic treatment, including topical application of dyclonine HC solution or lidocaine gel, may reduce oral discomfort.

HERPANGINA   🔲 ◑

- Etiologic agent: coxsackievirus A1–10, 16, 22; coxsackie B1–5; echoviruses E6, 9, 11, 16, 17, 25; enterovirus EV71
- It usually affects children <5 years and is prevalent in late summer and early fall in temperate climates.
- Clinical manifestations:
  - Sudden onset of fever, malaise, headache, anorexia, dysphagia, sore throat.
- Enanthem: 1- to 2-mm gray-white papules/vesicles that evolve to ulcers with red halos, and diffuse pharyngeal hyperemia (see Fig. 27-15).
- Distributed on the anterior tonsillar pillars, soft palate, uvula, and tonsils.
- Usually lasts 4–6 days, and its course is self-limited.

FIGURE 27-23 Hand-foot-and-mouth disease *A.* Multiple, discrete, small, vesicular lesions on the fingers and palms; similar lesions were also present on the feet. Some vesicles are typically linear. ***B.*** Multiple, superficial erosions and small, vesicular lesions surrounded by an erythematous halo on the lower labial mucosa; the gingiva is normal. In primary herpetic gingivostomatitis, which presents with similar oral vesicular lesions, a painful gingivitis usually occurs as well.

ERYTHEMA INFECTIOSUM (EI)   ICD-9 : 057.0 ○ ICD-10 : B08.3   ◨ ○➔◑

- Etiologic agent: human parvovirus B19
- Childhood exanthem associated with primary human parvovirus B19 infection.
- Characterized by
  - Edematous erythematous plaques on the cheeks ("slapped cheeks")
- Erythematous lacy eruption on the trunk and extremities.

Synonym: Fifth disease.

EPIDEMIOLOGY AND ETIOLOGY

Age of Onset

- All ages, but more common in young.
- Up to 60% of adolescents and adults are seropositive for anti-parvovirus B19 IgG.
- Symptomatic rheumatic involvement is more common in adults.

Etiology   Parvovirus, a small single-strand, unenveloped DNA virus. Human infection caused by parvovirus B19.

Sex   Symptomatic illness with arthralgias more common in adult women.

Season   Occurs year round; outbreaks in schools in late winter, early spring.

Transmission

- Virus is present in respiratory tract during the viremic stage of parvovirus B19 infection.
- Spreads via droplet aerosol.
- Secondary attack rate among close contacts, 50%.

PATHOGENESIS

- Viremia develops 6 days after intranasal inoculation of B19 into volunteers who lack serum antibodies to the virus.
- IgM and then IgG antibodies develop after a week and clear viremia.
- Significant bone marrow depression can occur at this time.
- The exanthem begins 17–18 days after inoculation and may be accompanied by arthralgia and/or arthritis; these findings are mediated by immune complexes.
- In compromised hosts, B19 can destroy erythroid precursor cells, causing severe aplastic crisis in adults and hydrops fetalis in the fetus.

CLINICAL MANIFESTATION

Incubation   4–14 days.
Contacts   Exposure to classmates or siblings with EI.
Symptoms   20–60% of individuals are symptomatic; remainder asymptomatic.

Children

- Prodrome of fever, malaise, headache, coryza 2 days before rash.
- Headache, sore throat, fever, myalgias, nausea, diarrhea, conjunctivitis, cough may coincide with rash.
- Uncommonly, arthralgias.
- Pruritus is variably present.

Adults

- Constitutional symptoms more severe, with fever, adenopathy.
- Arthritis/arthralgias involving small joints of hand, knees, wrists, ankles, feet.
- Numbness and tingling of fingers.
- Pruritus ± rash; rash usually absent in adults.

Mucocutaneous Lesions

- Edematous, confluent plaques on malar face ("slapped cheeks") (nasal bridge, periorbital regions spared) (Fig. 27-24A); lesions fade over 1–4 days.
- Nonfacial lesions, best seen on extremities, appearing after facial lesions: erythematous macules and papules that become confluent, giving a lacy or reticulated appearance (Fig. 27-24B); lesions fade in 5–9 days.
- Less commonly, morbilliform, confluent, circinate, annular.
- Rarely, purpura, vesicles, pustules, palmoplantar desquamation.
- Reticulated rash may recur. ▱

FIGURE 27-24   Erythema infectiosum   *A.* Diffuse erythema and edema of the cheeks with "slapped cheek" facies in a child. ***B.*** Discrete, erythematous macules with ring formation on the upper arm.

Distribution

- Face: "slapped cheeks". Usually absent in adults.
- Extensor surface of extremities, trunk, neck: confluent macules/papules. Adults: reticulated macules on extremities.

Other Findings Parvovirus B19 also reported to cause papular-purpuric "gloves and socks" syndrome.

Mucosal Lesions Uncommonly, enanthem with glossal and pharyngeal erythema; red macules on buccal and palatal mucosa.

General Findings

- *Adults*: More constitutional symptoms (fever, adenopathy, arthritis), especially women; often no rash.
- *Joints*: Arthralgia and/or arthritis in 10% of children; typically involving large joints.

DIFFERENTIAL DIAGNOSIS

Children with Erythema Infectiosum Childhood exanthems—rubella, measles, scarlet fever, erythema subitum, enteroviral infection, *Haemophilus influenzae* cellulitis, adverse cutaneous drug reaction.

Adults with Arthritis Lyme arthritis, rheumatoid arthritis, rubella.

LABORATORY EXAMINATIONS

Serology Demonstration of IgM anti-parvovirus B19 antibodies or IgG seroconversion. Demonstration of parvovirus B19 in serum.

Electron Microscopy Infected erythroid precursor cells show parvovirus-like particles.

Hematology During aplastic crisis: absence of reticulocytes, falling hemoglobin, hypoplasia or aplasia of erythroid series in bone marrow.

DIAGNOSIS

Usually made on clinical findings.

COURSE AND PROGNOSIS

Erythema Infectiosum "Slapped cheeks" are noted first, fading over 1–4 days. Then, reticulated rash appears on the trunk, neck, and extensor extremities. Eruption lasts 5–9 days but characteristically can recur for weeks or months, triggered by sunlight exposure, exercise, temperature change, bathing, emotional stress.

Arthralgias Self-limited, lasting 3 weeks; but may persist for several months or years.

Aplastic Crisis In patients with chronic hemolytic anemias (sickle cell anemia, hereditary spherocytosis, thalassemias, pyruvate kinase deficiency, autoimmune hemolytic anemia), transient aplastic crisis may occur, manifested by worsening anemia, fatigue, pallor.

Fetal B19 Infection Intrauterine infection may be complicated by nonimmune fetal hydrops secondary to infection of RBC precursors, hemolysis, severe anemia, tissue anoxia, high-output heart failure. Risk <10% after maternal infection.

Immunocompromised Host Prolonged chronic anemia associated with persistent lysis of RBC precursors. At risk: HIV/AIDS disease, congenital immunodeficiencies, acute leukemia, organ transplants, systemic lupus erythematosus, infants <1 year. Responds to intravenous immunoglobulin (IVIg).

MANAGEMENT

Symptomatic.

GIANOTTI-CROSTI SYNDROME (GCS)

- Etiologic agents:
  - Viruses: EBV, CMV, hepatitis B virus (ayw strain), coxsackievirus, parainfluenza virus, respiratory syncytial virus, rotavirus, adenovirus, echovirus, pox virus, poliovirus, parvovirus, HIV, hepatitis A virus, hepatitis C virus
  - Bacteria: *Mycoplasma pneumoniae, Borrelia burgdorferi, Bartonella henselae*, group A streptococcus.
  - Vaccines: influenza, diphtheria, tetanus, pertussis, BCG, *H. influenzae* type b, oral polio
- Age: children 6 months to 12 years old (See Fig. 27-25).
- Pathogenesis: immune response to transient viremia (immune complex deposition)

- Prodrome: mild, nonspecific upper respiratory infection
- Clinical manifestations: exanthem
  - Discrete, nonpruritic, erythematous, monomorphic papules (Fig. 27-25)
  - Lesions become coalescent.
  - Face, buttocks, and extensor surfaces of extremities; symmetric.
  - Typically, the trunk is spared.
- Duration is 2–8 weeks.

Synonym: Papular acrodermatitis of childhood (PAC)

FIGURE 27-25   Gianotti-Crosti syndrome   Flat papules on the cheek of a 5-year-old girl. Similar papules were also present symmetrically on forearms, elbows, and the ventral aspects of the legs.

DENGUE FEVER (DF), DENGUE HEMORRHAGIC FEVER (DHF), DENGUE SHOCK SYNDROME (DSS)   ▌→■ ❪→●

- Three clinical syndromes
  - Classic fever–arthralgia–rash syndrome, with abrupt onset of fever and muscle and joint pains, usually with retroorbital pain, photophobia, and lymphadenopathy.
  - DHF characterized by high fever, hemorrhagic phenomena, often hepatomegaly
  - DSS with circulatory failure; can be fatal
- Flavivirus infection (DEN 1–4)

- Transmitted by the bite of the *Aedes* mosquito
- Endemic to tropics in >100 countries
- Incidence: estimated 100 millions cases annually
- Rash: early flushing; later macules/papules; purpura

Synonym: Breakbone fever

EPIDEMIOLOGY AND ETIOLOGY

Etiology   Flavivirus, single-strand RNA virus. Four distinct dengue viruses (DEN-1, -2, -3, -4). Arthropod-borne virus (arbovirus). Infection confers lifelong protection against that serotype, but cross-protection between serotypes is of short duration. Infection with virus of a different serotype after the primary attack is more apt to result in severe disease, DHF, or DSS.

Vector   Transmitted by the bite of the *A. aegypti* mosquito; less commonly *A. albopictus*. Mosquito acquires virus by feeding upon viremic human; remains infective for life. These *Aedes* mosquitoes also transmit chikungunya fever. Breed near human habitation in water jars, vases, discarded containers, coconut husks, old tires. Inhabits dwellings and bites during the day. Other mosquito- and tick-borne flavivirus infections include: chikungunya fever, yellow fever, West Nile encephalitis, St Louis encephalitis, Japanese encephalitis, tick-borne encephalitis, Kyasanur Forest disease, and Omsk haemorrhagic fever

Season   Year-round transmission between latitudes 25°N and 25°S. Seasonally, *A. aegypti* as far north as Philadelphia. Global warming may be contributing to increase in number of cases of DF.

Geographic Distribution   Occurs worldwide throughout tropics. In the United States, in Texas, Puerto Rico. Most cases occurring in United States are imported in travelers returning from the tropics. Associated with human populations, urban. *Note*: chikungunya fever does not occur in the Americas and Caribbean.

Incidence   3 billion people living in areas potentially at risk; 100 million cases worldwide annually. 400,000 cases of DHF. Second most common mosquito-borne infection after

malaria. Increased incidence associated with rapid urban population growth, overcrowding, lax mosquito control.

Factors Contributing to Increase Incidence   Global warming, rapid urbanization, population growth, increase in nonbiodegradable products that can serve as sites for mosquito larvae proliferation, air travel.

Age   DHF/DSS more common in children.

PATHOGENESIS

Viremia is present at onset of fever, persisting for 3–5 days. The severe syndrome (DHF or DSS) occurs in individuals (usually children) with passively acquired (transplacental maternal antibody) or preexisting nonneutralizing heterologous dengue antibody due to previous infection with a different serotype of virus. Initial symptoms simulate usual dengue, findings abruptly worsen. DSS characterized by shock and hemoconcentration. Subsequent infection with dengue type 2 following a type 1 infection is particular risk factor for severe disease. Pathogenesis of severe syndrome involves preexisting dengue antibody. Virus-antibody complexes formed within a few days of second dengue infection; nonneutralizing enhancing antibodies promote infection of higher numbers of mononuclear cells, followed by release of cytokines, vasoactive mediators, and procoagulants, leading to the disseminated intravascular coagulation seen in DHF.

DHF   Increased vascular permeability and plasma leakage from blood vessels into tissues, thrombocytopenia, bleeding manifestations (frank hemorrhage to spontaneous petechiae or elicited by tourniquet test). Plasma leakage causes a rise in hematocrit, effusions, and edema, especially in chest, abdomen.

DSS Occurs when leakage or bleeding, or both, are sufficient to induce hypovolemic shock.

CLINICAL MANIFESTATION

Incubation Period 4–7 days after bite of infected mosquito.
Duration of Symptoms Variable; 2–5 days. Biphasic in some cases. Rash is very common in remission period or early in a second febrile phase
Symptoms *Prodrome*: Malaise, chills, headache. Rash usually asymptomatic but may be pruritic. Symptoms highly variable: subclinical to incapacitating. Sudden onset of fever, chills, malaise, nausea/vomiting, headache, photophobia, retroorbital pain, pharyngitis, back pain, severe myalgia (origin of term *break-bone fever*).

Skin Lesions
Rash estimated to occur in 50–80% of cases.

- Initial rash 1–2 days after onset of symptoms: erythema/flushing (resembles sunburn, i.e., capillary dilatation) of face, neck, chest
- Later rash 4–7 days after onset of symptoms: morbilliform eruption beginning on the trunk, spreading to extremities and face in uncomplicated dengue, lasting for 1–5 days (Fig. 27-26); petechiae; islands of sparing ("white islands in sea of red"). Correlates with immune response to virus.
- Urticaria with pruritus
- Hemorrhagic diathesis: petechiae, ecchymoses, bleeding at sites of injection or venepuncture.
- DHF
  - Islands of white in a sea of red in areas of hemorrhage and edema, especially lower legs. (Fig. 27-26)
  - Scrotal edema

Mucosal Lesions Scleral/conjunctival injection. Epistaxis. Bleeding gums, nose, GI tract.
Systemic Findings Surprisingly minimal. Adenopathy early in course. Pain on palpation

A   *B*

FIGURE 27-26 Dengue hemorrhagic fever: leg A 39-year-old developed fever and rash after a trip to Malaysia. Dermal hemorrhage, petechiae, and edema are seen on the lower leg; "white islands in a sea of red" are seen. Dengue IgG antibody was detected with borderline dengue IgM antibody. A hemorrhagic course can occur in persons who have had dengue fever previously and retain nonneutralizing heterotypic antibodies (Courtesy of C Hafner et al: Hautarzt 57:705-707, 2006.)

of muscles or epigastrium. Abdominal pain may mimic appendicitis. Encephalopathy in children. Distal sensory polyneuropathy. *DHF:* Effusions and edema in chest and abdomen. Subarachnoid hemorrhage.

DIFFERENTIAL DIAGNOSIS

Early Flushing Erythema   Chikungunya fever, sandfly fever, scarlet fever, toxic shock syndrome, Kawasaki disease, erythema infectiosum (parvovirus B19).

Morbilliform Eruption   Acute HIV syndrome, infectious mononucleosis (EBV, CMV), roseola infantum (HHV-6), measles, rubella, enterovirus, secondary syphilis, typhoid fever, chikungunya fever, West Nile virus, O'nyong-nyong fever, Myaro virus, Sindbis virus, leptospirosis, adverse cutaneous drug eruption.

LABORATORY EXAMINATIONS

Hematology   Leukopenia; thrombocytopenia. High hematocrit with DHF/DSS. Low hematocrit after hydration.

Chemistry   Aminotransferase elevations.

Dermatopathology   Nonspecific.

Reverse Transcriptase-PCR-Based Methods Rapid identification and serotyping of dengue virus in acute-phase serum, roughly during the period of fever.

Isolation of Virus   Inoculation of mosquito cell line with patient serum, coupled with nucleic acid assays to identify a recovered virus.

Serology   Viral protein-specific capture IgM or IgG enzyme-linked immunosorbent assay (ELISA) and hemagglutination inhibition test. IgM antibodies develop within a few days of illness. Neutralizing and hemagglutination-inhibiting antibodies appear within a week after onset of DF. Acute and convalescent sera show significant rise in antibody titer; most reliable evidence of active dengue infection.

CDC Dengue Branch   Both acute- and convalescent-phase serum samples sent through state/territorial health department laboratories

to CDC's Dengue Branch, Division of Vector-Borne Infectious Diseases, National Center for Infectious Diseases, 1324 Calle Cañada, San Juan, Puerto Rico 00920–3860

DIAGNOSIS

Consider diagnosis in travelers with febrile illness recently returned from endemic areas. Rapid serologic testing.

COURSE AND PROGNOSIS

Ratio of inapparent to apparent infections about 15:1 for primary infections; ratio lower in secondary infections. Temperature returns to normal after 5–6 days or may subside on about third day and rise again about 5–8 days after onset ("saddleback" form). Complete recovery is generally the outcome, although prolonged asthenia and nonspecific symptoms have been described in some cases. Death seen in cases of DF and DSS, which are leading cause of childhood death in several Asian countries. Fatality rate with DHF up to 15%; can be reduced to less than 1% with proper treatment.

MANAGEMENT

Prevention   Individuals traveling to endemic areas should be educated about preventive measures. Avoid mosquito habitat at times of peak activity; use screens/barriers and air-conditioned rooms. Apply insect repellant diethyltoluamide (DEET) to skin. Wear permethrin-impregnated clothing. Mosquito control measures in endemic areas.

Treatment   No specific antiviral therapy. Supportive measures, including analgesics (avoiding agents with platelet dysfunction) and hydration.

Vaccine   Vaccine has been developed but is not yet available commercially.

CDC Website   http://phstwlp1.partners.org:2219/ncidod/dvbid/dengue/index.htm.

HUMAN HERPESVIRUSES ICD-9:054 ○ ICD-10:B00

- Human herpesviruses (HHVs) (family Herpesviridae) are defined by the architecture of the virion, which has:
  - Core containing a linear double-strand DNA
  - Icosahedral capsid 100–110 nm in diameter composed of 162 capsomers
  - Envelope containing viral glycoprotein spikes on the surface.
- Worldwide, 60–90% of the population is infected with one or more HHVs.
- Eight HHVs have been identified:
  - Herpes simplex virus (HSV)-1 (HHV-1)
  - HSV-2 (HHV-2)
  - Varicella-zoster virus (VZV, or HHV-3)
  - Epstein-Barr virus (EBV, or HHV-4)
  - Cytomegalovirus (CMV, or HHV-5)
  - HHV-6
  - HHV-7
  - HHV-8 (Kaposi sarcoma–associated virus).
- Primary HHV infections are usually asymptomatic with the exception of VZV, which nearly always presents with symptomatic varicella.

- After primary infection, HHVs remain latent in neural or lymphoid cells and reactivate if an adequate immune response does not exist.
- HHVs are categorized into three groups: Alpha, beta, and gamma Herpesviridae (Table 27-3).
  - *Alpha Herpesviridae*: HSV-1, HSV-2, VZV are characterized by a variable host range, relatively short reproductive cycle, rapid spread in culture, rapid destruction of infected cells, and latent infection primarily, but not exclusively, of sensory ganglia.
  - *Beta Herpesviridae*: CMV has a restricted host range and spreads slowly in cultures.
  - *Gamma Herpesviridae*: EBV, HHV-6, HHV-7, HHV-8, and herpesvirus saimiri are lymphotropic, specific for either T or B lymphocytes. The HHV-8 DNA sequences are closely homologous to minor capsid and tegument protein genes of gammaherpesviridae EBV and herpesvirus saimiri.

HERPES SIMPLEX VIRUS (HSV) INFECTION

- Whether first-symptomatic or recurrent, may "typically" present clinically with grouped vesicles arising on an erythematous base on keratinized skin or mucous membrane.
- Most HSV infections are "atypical," with patch(es) of erythema, small erosions, fissures, or subclinical lesions that shed HSV.
- Once an individual is infected, HSV persists in sensory ganglia for the life of the patient, recurring with lessening in immunity.
- Clinical manifestations:

- In healthy individuals, recurrent infections are asymptomatic or minor, resolving spontaneously or with antiviral therapy.
- In the immunocompromised host, mucocutaneous lesions can be extensive, chronic, or disseminate to skin or viscera.

Synonyms: Herpes, herpes simplex, cold sore, fever blister, herpes febrilis, herpes labialis, herpes gladiatorum, scrum pox, herpetic whitlow, genital herpes, herpes progenitalis.

EPIDEMIOLOGY AND ETIOLOGY

Age of Onset Most commonly young adults; range, infancy to senescence.
Etiology HSV-1, HSV-2.

- Labialis: HSV-1 (80–90%), HSV-2 (10–20%).
- Urogenital: HSV-2 (70–90%), HSV-1 (10–30%).

- Herpetic whitlow: <20 years of age usually HSV-1; >20 years of age, usually HSV-2.
- Neonatal: HSV-2 (70%), HSV-1 (30%).

Transmission

- Most transmission occurs when persons shed virus but lack lesions.
- Usually skin-skin, skin-mucosa, mucosa-skin contact.

TABLE 27-3   Human Herpesviruses and Associated Diseases in Immunocompetent and Immunocompromised Individuals

Human Herpesvirus	Disease in Immunocompetent Individuals	Disease in Immunocompromised Individuals	Management
Herpes simplex virus-1 (HSV-1) (HHV-1)	Primary infection often asymptomatic Primary herpetic gingivostomatitis Herpes labialis Herpetic whitlow Aseptic meningitis HSV encephalitis	Widespread local infection Chronic ulcers Disseminated cutaneous infection Disseminated visceral infection	Immunization: vaccine promising Antiviral agents Acyclovir Valacyclovir Famciclovir Foscarnet
Herpes simplex virus-2 (HSV-2) (HHV-2)	Primary infection often asymptomatic Herpes genitalis, primary and recurrent Herpetic whitlow Aseptic meningitis	Widespread local infection Chronic ulcers Disseminated cutaneous infection Disseminated visceral infection	Immunization: vaccine promising Antiviral agents Acyclovir Valacyclovir Famciclovir Foscarnet
Varicella-zoster virus (VZV) (HHV-3)	Primary infection nearly always symptomatic Varicella (primary infection) Herpes zoster	Disseminated cutaneous infection Disseminated visceral infection Chronic herpes zoster Chronic ecthymatous VZV infection	Immunization: vaccine available Antiviral agents Acyclovir Valacyclovir Famciclovir Foscarnet
Epstein-Barr virus (EBV) (HHV-4)	Primary infection often asymptomatic EBV mononucleosis (primary EBV infection) Nasopharyngeal carcinoma Burkitt lymphoma Posttransplantation lymphoma T cell lymphoma, and other lymphomas Oral hairy leukoplakia	Lymphoma ???	Antiviral agents Acyclovir Ganciclovir ??? Immunization: none

TABLE 27-3 Human Herpesviruses and Associated Diseases in Immunocompetent and Immunocompromised Individuals (*Continued*)

Human Herpesvirus	Disease in Immunocompetent Individuals	Disease in Immunocompromised Individuals	Management
Cytomegalovirus (CMV) (HHV-5)	Primary infection often asymptomatic CMV mononucleosis (primary CMV infection)	Retinitis Pneumonitis Colitis	Immunization: vaccine promising Antiviral agents Ganciclovir Foscarnet Cidofovir
Human herpesvirus-6 (HHV-6)	Primary infection often asymptomatic Exanthema subitum	???	???
Human herpesvirus-7 (HHV-7)	Primary infection often asymptomatic Exanthema subitum	???	???
Human herpesvirus-8 (HHV-8)	Primary infection may present with fever and *morbilliform rash* Kaposi sarcoma	Kaposi sarcoma Body cavity lymphoma in HIV-infected individuals	

- Herpes gladiatorum transmitted by skin-to-skin contact in wrestlers.
- Increased HSV-1 transmission associated with crowded living conditions and lower socioeconomic status.

Precipitating Factors for Recurrence

- Approximately one-third of persons who develop herpes labialis will experience a recurrence; of these, one-half will experience at least two recurrences annually.
- Usual factors for herpes labialis: skin/mucosal irritation (UV radiation), altered hormonal milieu (menstruation), fever, common cold, altered immune states, site of infection (genital herpes recurs more frequently than labial).

Immunocompromising Factors Predisposing to HSV Reactivation HIV/AIDS infection, malignancy (leukemia/lymphoma), transplantation (bone marrow, solid organ), chemotherapy, systemic glucocorticoids, other immunosuppressive drugs, radiotherapy.

PATHOGENESIS

- Primary HSV infection occurs through close contact with a person shedding virus at a peripheral site, mucosal surface, or secretion.
- HSV is inactivated promptly at room temperature; aerosol or fomitic spread unlikely.
- Infection occurs via inoculation onto susceptible mucosal surface or break in skin.
- After exposure to HSV, the virus replicates in epithelial cells, causing lysis of infected cells, vesicle formation, and local inflammation.
- After primary infection at inoculation site, HSV ascends peripheral sensory nerves and enters sensory (Image 27-1) or autonomic nerve root (vagal) ganglia, where latency is established.
- Retrograde transport of HSV among nerves and establishment of latency are not dependent on viral replication in skin or neurons; neurons can be infected in the absence of symptoms.
- Latency can occur after both symptomatic and asymptomatic primary infection.

- Periodically, HSV may reactivate from its latent state and virus particles then travel along sensory neurons to skin and mucosal sites to cause recurrent disease episodes (Image 27-1).
- Recurrent mucocutaneous shedding can be associated with or without (asymptomatic shedding) lesions; virus can be transmitted to a new host when shedding occurs.
- Recurrences usually occur in the vicinity of the primary infection; may be clinically symptomatic or asymptomatic.

CLINICAL MANIFESTATION

See "Nongenital herpes simplex virus infections", below.

LABORATORY EXAMINATIONS

Direct Microscopy *Tzanck Smear* (Fig. 27-27). Optimally, fluid from intact vesicle is smeared thinly on a microscope slide, dried, and stained with either Wright or Giemsa stain. Positive, if acantholytic keratinocytes or multinucleated giant acantholytic keratinocytes are detected. Positive in 75% of early cases, either primary or recurrent.
Antigen Detection DFA Monoclonal antibodies, specific for HSV-1 and HSV-2 antigens, detect and differentiate HSV antigens on smear from lesion.
Dermatopathology Ballooning and reticular epidermal degeneration, acantholysis, and intraepidermal vesicles; intranuclear inclusion bodies, multinucleate giant keratinocytes; multilocular vesicles. Immunoperoxidase techniques can be used to identify HSV-1 and HSV-2 antigens in formalin-fixed tissue samples.
Cultures Positive HSV cultures from involved mucocutaneous site or tissue biopsy specimens.
Serology

- Antibodies to glycoprotein (g)G1 and (g)G2 detect and differentiate past HSV-1 and HSV-2 infections.
- Primary HSV infection can be documented by demonstration of seroconversion.
- Recurring herpes can be ruled out if seronegative for HSV antibodies.

Polymerase Chain Reaction To determine HSV-DNA sequences in tissue, smears, or secretion.

DIAGNOSIS

Clinical suspicion confirmed by viral culture or antigen detection. Cultures used for diagnosing first-episode infections since antibodies to (g)H1 or (g)G2 may take 2–6 weeks to develop.

MANAGEMENT

Prevention	Skin-to-skin contact should be avoided during outbreak of cutaneous HSV infection.
Topical Antiviral Therapy	Approved for herpes labialis; minimal efficacy.
Acyclovir 5% ointment	Apply q3h, 6 times daily for 7 days. Approved for initial genital herpes and limited mucocutaneous HSV infections in immunocompromised individuals.
Penciclovir 1% cream	Apply q2h while awake for recurrent orolabial infection in immunocompetent individuals.
Oral Antiviral Therapy	Currently, anti-HSV agents are approved for use in genital herpes Presumably, similar dosing regimens are effective for nongenital infections. Drugs for oral HSV therapy include acyclovir, valacyclovir, and famciclovir. Valacyclovir, the prodrug of acyclovir, has a better bioavailability and is nearly 85% absorbed after oral administration. Famciclovir is equally effective for cutaneous HSV infections.
First episode	Antiviral agents more effective in treating primary infections than recurrences.
Acyclovir	400 mg 3 times daily or 200 mg 5 times daily for 7–10 days
Valacyclovir	1 g twice daily for 7–10 days
Famciclovir	250 mg 3 times daily for 5–10 days
Recurrences	Most episodes of recurrent herpes do not benefit from pulse therapy with oral acyclovir. In severe recurrent disease, patients who start therapy at the beginning of the prodrome or within 2 days after onset of lesions may benefit from therapy by shortening and reducing severity of eruption; however, recurrences cannot be prevented.

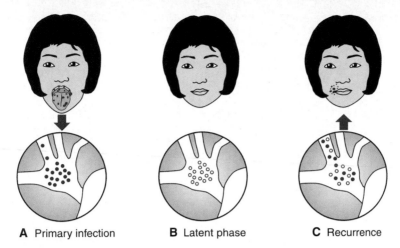

A Primary infection **B** Latent phase **C** Recurrence

IMAGE 27-1 Herpes labialis **A.** With primary HSV infection, virus replicates in the oropharyngeal epithelium, ascends peripheral sensory nerves into the trigeminal ganglion. **B.** HSV persists in a latent phase within the trigeminal ganglion for the life of the individual. **C.** Various stimuli initiate reactivation of latent virus, which then descends sensory nerves to the lips or perioral skin, resulting in recurrent herpes labialis.

FIGURE 27-27 Herpes simplex virus: positive Tzanck smear A giant, multinucleated keratinocyte on a Giemsa-stained smear obtained from a vesicle base. Compare the size of the giant cell to that of the neutrophils also seen in this preparation. An isolated acantholytic keratinocyte is also seen. Identical findings are present in lesions caused by varicella zoster virus.

Chronic suppression	Decreases frequency of symptomatic recurrences and asymptomatic HSV shedding. After 1 year of continuous daily suppressive therapy, acyclovir should be discontinued to determine the recurrence rate.
Acyclovir	400 mg twice daily
Valacyclovir	500–1000 mg per day
Famciclovir	250 mg twice daily
Mucocutaneous disease in immunocompromised individuals	Neither the need for nor the proper increased dosage of acyclovir has been established conclusively. Patients with herpes who do not respond to the recommended dose of acyclovir may require a higher oral dose of acyclovir, IV acyclovir, or be infected with an acyclovir-resistant HSV strain, requiring IV foscarnet. The roles of valacyclovir and famciclovir are not yet established.
Acyclovir	5 mg/kg IV q8h for 7–14 days, *or* 400 mg 5 times daily for 7–14 days
Oral valacyclovir *or* famciclovir	Reduces the necessity for IV acyclovir therapy.
Neonatal	
Acyclovir	20 mg/kg IV q8h for 14–21 days
Acyclovir resistance	Extremely rare in immunocompetent host. Usually occurs in immunocompromised individuals with large herpetic lesions with high HSV viral load. Resistant HSV strains are thymidine-kinase deficient. Alternative drugs: foscarnet, cidofovir. In HIV-infected patients, chronic HSV infections are mucocutaneous, rarely invasive.
Foscarnet	40 mg/kg IV q8h for 14–21 days
HIV/AIDS infections	Lesions caused by HSV are relatively common among HIV-infected persons. For severe disease, IV acyclovir therapy may be required. If lesions persist among patients undergoing acyclovir treatment, resistance to acyclovir should be suspected.
Acyclovir	Intermittent or suppressive therapy with oral acyclovir may be needed. 400 mg PO 3–5 times daily may be useful. Therapy should continue until clinical resolution is attained.
Foscarnet	For severe disease caused by proven or suspected acyclovir-resistant strains, hospitalization should be considered. Foscarnet, 40 mg/kg body weight q8h until clinical resolution is attained. Appears to be the best available treatment.

NONGENITAL HERPES SIMPLEX VIRUS INFECTION

- Nongenital HSV infection, whether primary or recurrent, is often asymptomatic.
- Lesions may present as group vesicles on an erythematous base or as a recurrent erythematous plaque ± erosions.

- *Synonyms*: Herpes, herpes simplex, cold sore, fever blister, herpes febrilis, herpes labialis, herpes gladiatorum, scrum pox, herpetic whitlow.

  For genital HSV infection, see Section 30.

CLINICAL MANIFESTATION

Incubation Period   2- to 20-day (average 6) incubation period for primary infection.
Primary Herpes

- Many individuals with primary HSV infection are either asymptomatic or have only trivial symptoms.
- Symptomatic primary herpes is uncommon.

- Characterized by vesicles at the site of inoculation (Fig. 27-28). Associated with regional lymphadenopathy
- At times accompanied by fever, headache, malaise, myalgia. It peaks within the first 3–4 days after onset of lesions, resolving during the subsequent 3–4 days.

- Primary herpetic gingivostomatitis is the most common symptom complex accompanying primary HSV infection in children.

- In young women, primary herpetic vulvovaginitis (see also Section 30).

Recurrent Herpes

- Prodrome of tingling, itching, or burning sensation usually precedes any visible skin changes by 24 h.
- Systemic symptoms are usually absent.

Mucocutanoeus Findings
Primary Herpes

- Erythema often noted initially, followed soon by grouped, often umbilicated vesicles, which may evolve to pustules (Fig. 27-28). Vesicles are often fragile, transient, not observed.
- These become eroded as the overlying epidermis sloughs.
- Erosions may enlarge to ulcerations, which may be crusted or moist.
- These epithelial defects heal in 2–4 weeks, often with resultant postinflammatory hypo- or hyperpigmentation, uncommonly with scarring.
- The area of involvement may be circumferential around the mouth.
- Regional lymphadenopathy.
- Location: oropharyngeal, labial, perioral; distal fingers; other sites. 🔋

Mucous Membranes

- Oral mucosa usually involved only in primary HSV infection with vesicles that quickly slough to form erosions (Fig. 27-29) at any site in the oropharynx, scanty to numerous; gingivitis with gingival tenderness, edema, violaceous color. Sialorrhea. Severe pain.
- Conjunctival and corneal autoinoculation may occur. 🔋

Recurrent Herpes

- Grouped vesicles on erythematous base— erosions and crusts (Fig. 27-30A–D).
- Recurrent intraoral HSV is rare. Often, only superficial erosions.

🔋

Specific Features of HSV Infections of Different Sensory Nerves: Trigeminal Nerve

- *Cold sores*: Recurrent facial herpes/cold sores (Fig. 27-30). Usually preceded by prodromal symptoms (tingling, pain, burning sensation, itching). Affect 20–40% of adults. Severe recurrences may complicate laser-resurfacing surgery.
- *Ocular HSV infections*: Recurrent keratitis is a major cause of corneal scarring and visual

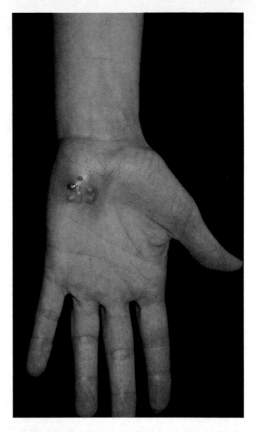

FIGURE 27-28   Herpes simplex virus infection: primary infection of the palm   A 28-year-female with a painful lesion on the palm for 3 days. A cluster of grouped pustules are seen on the palm. A red lymphangitis extends proximally on the wrist. The axillary lymph nodes were tender and enlarged. HSV-2 was detected on DFA. No antibodies to HSV-1 or -2 were detected. The infection is, thus, primary.

loss, Continuous suppression therapy is recommended.
- *Herpetic facial paralysis*: Reactivation of geniculate ganglion infection implicated in pathogenesis of idiopathic facial palsy (Bell palsy). HSV-1 shedding detected in 40% of cases. Inflammation plays a major role in pathogenesis; glucocorticoids may be effective.
- *HSV gladiatorum*: Transmission occurs during contact sports (wrestling, rugby, football). Also occurs in cervical or lumbosacral dermatomes. Prophylaxis may prevent recurrence.

Cervical and Thoracic Sensory Nerves Infections

- *Herpetic whitlow*: Prior to "Universal Precautions," occurred in health care professionals, especially dental personnel. Associated with painful neuritis in the affected finger and forearm (Fig. 27-31). May last for ≥3 weeks. ✏
- *HSV infection of the nipple*: Related to transmission of HSV from infant to mother during breast feeding.
- *HSV infections of the lumbosacral sensory nerves*: When lumbosacraal ganglia become infected subsequent to anogenital herpes, recurrent lesions can occur on genitalia as well as buttocks, thighs, perianal mucosa. Perianal herpes does not necessarily imply direct anal inoculation of HSV. Symptomatic herpes in the sacral dermatome may be accompanied by asymptomatic HSV reactivation/shedding from genital mucosa. Recurrent itching, burning, blistering, erythema below the waist should be regarded as genital HSV infection until proven otherwise.

Complications of HSV Infections of Peripheral Sensory Nervous System

- *Eczema herpeticum*: Usually follows autoinoculation of HSV (most commonly orolabial herpes) to atopic dermatitis (see "Herpes Simplex Virus: Widespread Cutaneous Infection Associated with Cutaneous Immunocompromise," below).
- *S.* aureus *superinfection*: Occurs with eczema herpeticum.
- *Erythema multiforme*: In some individuals with recurrent HSV infections, erythema multiforme may occur with each recurrence (Fig. 27-32). (See "Erythema Multiforme," Section 7.)

General Findings   Fever may be present during symptomatic primary herpetic gingivostomatitis.

Regional Lymphadenopathy   May be firm, nonfluctuant, tender; usually unilateral.

CNS   Signs of aseptic meningitis: headache, fever, nuchal rigidity, CSF pleocytosis with normal sugar content and positive HSV CSF culture.

FIGURE 27-29   Herpes simplex virus infection: primary gingivostomatitis   A 43-year-old female with history of atopic dermatitis. Multiple, very painful erosions on the lower perioral skin, lips, and tongue. Tzanck smear was positive. HSV-1 detected on DFA. Methicillin-sensitive *S. aureus* (MSSA) was isolated on bacterial culture, thus superinfecting the herpetic lesions. As in this person, primary HSV infection causes a gingivostomatitis. HSV infection recurred on the face but without oral involvement.

**FIGURE 27-30   Herpes simplex virus infection: recurrent herpes labialis   *A.* Edematous lateral upper lip 24 h after onset of tingling sensation. *B.* Grouped vesicles on moustache area 48 h after onset of symptoms. *C.* Crusted erosion on upper lip and moustache area 7 days after onset of symptoms. *D.* Painful erosion on the lower lip for 5 weeks in a 66-year-old female with severe dermatoheliosis and actinic cheilitis. The diagnosis was made on lesional biopsy.

FIGURE 27-31   Herpes simplex virus infection: herpetic whitlow   A 19-year-old male with painful finger lesions for 3 days. Painful, grouped, confluent vesicles on an erythematous edematous base of the distal finger were the first (and presumed primary) symptomatic infection.

DIFFERENTIAL DIAGNOSIS

Primary Intraoral HSV Infection   Aphthous stomatitis, hand-foot-and-mouth disease, herpangina, erythema multiforme.
Recurrent Lesion   Fixed drug eruption.

LABORATORY EXAMINATIONS

See page 816.

DIAGNOSIS

Clinical suspicion confirmed by Tzanck smear, viral culture, or antigen detection DFA.

COURSE AND PROGNOSIS

- Recurrences of HSV tend to become less frequent with the passage of time.

- Eczema herpeticum (see also page 825) may complicate various dermatoses.
- Patients with immunodeficiency may experience:
  - Cutaneous dissemination of HSV
  - Systemic dissemination of HSV
  - Chronic herpetic ulcers (see also page 828).

- Erythema multiforme may complicate each episode of recurrent herpes, occurring 1–2 weeks after an outbreak.

MANAGEMENT

See page 816.

FIGURE 27-32   Herpes simplex virus infection: recurrent erythema multiforme   A 31-year-old male with recurrent herpes labialis and disseminated lesions. Recurrent herpes labialis on the lower lip and irislike edematous papules on the dorsum of the hand.

NEONATAL HERPES SIMPLEX VIRUS INFECTION   ■ ◑ → ●

- Transmission occurs:
  - In utero
  - Intrapartum
  - Postnatal acquisition.
- The mother is the most common source of infection.
- There is usually no evidence of shedding at the time of delivery.
- Shedding also occurs from uterine cervix.
- The majority of infections are caused by HSV-2; HSV-1 is more virulent in the newborn and associated with higher morbidity and mortality rates.

- 70% of infants with neonatal HSV infection are born to mothers with asymptomatic genital herpes; 70% of cases occur in the first-born child.
- Eruption occurs on the mucous membranes (Fig. 27-33A) or on the intact skin at inoculation sites (such as monitoring sensors) (Fig. 27-33B).
- Disseminated HSV infection in neonates is difficult to diagnose in that up to 70% of infants have no mucocutaneous lesions.
- IV acyclovir therapy is mandatory in these cases.

MANAGEMENT

Prophylaxis

- Many experts recommend serotesting for HSV-1 and HSV-2 at the first prenatal visit.
- Infants born to women who asymptomatically shed HSV have reduced birth weight and increased prematurity.
- Acyclovir suppressive therapy at the end of pregnancy probably (but not documented) reduces the risk of transmission to the neonate.

Pregnancy

- The safety of systemic acyclovir for pregnant women and the fetus has not yet been established, although acyclovir appears to be completely safe in last months of pregnancy.

- Acyclovir, valacyclovir, and famciclovir are active only in cells with active viral infection.
- If HSV is acquired late in pregnancy, cesarean section is indicated.

Perinatal Infections

- Most mothers of infants who acquire neonatal herpes lack histories of clinically evident genital herpes.
- The risk for transmission to the neonate from an infected mother appears highest among women with first-episode genital herpes near the time of delivery and is low (<3%) among women with recurrent herpes.
- The results of viral cultures during pregnancy do not predict viral shedding at the time of delivery, and such cultures are not routinely indicated.

Antiviral Therapy   Acyclovir, 20 mg/kg IV q8h for 14–21 days.

FIGURE 27-33   Herpes simplex virus infection: neonatal   Neonate with fever and skin lesion. **A.** Vesicles and crusted erosions on the upper lip and large geographic ulcerations of the tongue, i.e., herpetic gingivostomatitis. **B.** Grouped and confluent vesicles with underlying erythema and edema on the shoulder, arising at the inoculation site.

HERPES SIMPLEX VIRUS: WIDESPREAD CUTANEOUS INFECTION ASSOCIATED WITH CUTANEOUS IMMUNOCOMPROMISE

- Widespread HSV cutaneous infection in underlying dermatoses occurs most commonly in atopic dermatitis (eczema herpeticum).
- Characterized by widespread vesicles and erosions.

- May occur as a primary or recurrent infection.

Synonym: Kaposi varicelliform eruption.

EPIDEMIOLOGY AND ETIOLOGY

Age of Onset Children > adults.
Etiology HSV-1 > HSV-2.
Transmission Commonly from parental herpes labialis to altered epidermis.
Risk Factors

- Most commonly, atopic dermatitis.
- More serious infections occur in erythrodermic atopic dermatitis.
- Also, Darier disease, thermal burns, pemphigus vulgaris, bullous pemphigoid, ichthyosis vulgaris, cutaneous T cell lymphoma (mycosis fungoides), Wiscott-Aldrich syndrome.

PATHOGENESIS

See "Herpes Simplex Virus Infection," page 813.

CLINICAL MANIFESTATION

- Primary eczema herpeticum may be associated with fever, malaise, irritability.
- When recurrent, history of prior similar lesions; systemic symptoms less severe.
- Primary skin disease may be pruritic; onset of eczema herpeticum associated with pain and tenderness.
- Lesions begin in abnormal skin and may extend peripherally for several weeks during the primary infection or secondary eruption.
- Superinfection with *S. aureus* is relatively common and may be painful

Mucocutaneous Lesions

- Vesicles evolving into "punched-out" erosions (Fig. 27-34).
- Vesicles are first confined to eczematous skin.
- In contrast to primary or recurrent HSV eruptions, *not* grouped but disseminated.
- May later spread to normal-appearing skin.

FIGURE 27-34 Herpes simplex virus infection: eczema herpeticum on eyelids A 36-year-old male with recurrent periorbital painful crusted erosions and atopic dermatitis. Small crusted erosion on the eyelids. DFA detected HSV-1. Bacterial culture reported MSSA and group A streptococcus (GAS). The herpetic infection had not affected the cornea.

- Erosions may become confluent, producing large denuded areas (Fig. 27-35).
- Successive crops of new vesiculation may occur.
- Common sites: face, neck, trunk.

General Examination   Primary infection may be associated with fever and lymphadenopathy.

DIFFERENTIAL DIAGNOSIS

Widespread Vesiculopustules/Erosions   Varicella, disseminated VZV infection, disseminated (systemic) HSV infection, wound infection (staphylococcal, pseudomonal, *Candida*), eczema vaccinatum.

LABORATORY EXAMINATIONS

See page 816.

DIAGNOSIS

Clinical, confirmed by detection of HSV on culture or antigen detection.

COURSE AND PROGNOSIS

- Untreated, primary episode of eczema herpeticum runs its course with resolution in 2–6 weeks.
- Recurrent episodes tend to be milder and not associated with systemic symptoms.
- Systemic dissemination can occur, especially in immunocompromised patients; reported mortality rates range from 10–50%.
- Widely distributed cutaneous HSV infection in burn patients can be difficult to detect clinically.

MANAGEMENT

Management of Underlying Dermatosis   For atopic dermatitis, see "Eczema/Dermatitis," Section 2.
Antiviral Therapy   See "Management," page 816.
Antibacterial Therapy   Treat associated bacterial superinfection. See "Bacterial Infections Involving the Skin," Section 24.

FIGURE 27-35   Herpes simplex virus infection: extensive eczema herpeticum on face   Confluent and discrete crusted erosions associated with erythema and edema of the face of a female with atopic dermatitis.

HERPES SIMPLEX VIRUS: INFECTIONS ASSOCIATED WITH SYSTEMIC IMMUNOCOMPROMISE ■ ◑ → ●

- HSV in the host with systemic immunocompromise may cause:
  - Local infection with extensive cutaneous involvement (e.g., eczema herpeticum)
  - Chronic herpetic ulcers
- Widespread systemic infection (widespread mucocutaneous lesions as well as systemic infection).

EPIDEMIOLOGY

Incidence

- Increasing due to an increasing population of immunocompromised individuals:
  - 80% in bone marrow transplant recipients
  - 65% in solid organ transplant recipients
  - 60% in those with lymphoma
  - 55% in those with leukemia
  - 25% in individuals with HIV/AIDS disease.
- Incidence of symptomatic outbreaks has decreased markedly because of the primary prophylaxis of HSV-seropositive immunocompromised individuals with oral antiviral drugs.

Risk Factors

Immunodeficiency: HIV/AIDS Infection

- Frequency and duration increase sharply as CD4+ T cell count falls to <50/μL.
  - Reduced in persons effectively treated with ART.
- In most HIV-infected individuals, frequency, duration, and severity of HSV outbreaks similar to those in immunocompetent individuals; however, asymptomatic shedding is increased.
- Disseminated cutaneous and visceral HSV infections are less common than in other immunocompromised states.
- *CDC Surveillance Case Definition for AIDS*: HSV infection for any duration in a patient older than 1 month is an AIDS-defining condition if the patient has no other cause of immunodeficiency and is without knowledge of HIV antibody status.
  - HSV infection causing a mucocutaneous ulcer that persists longer than 1 month
  - HSV infection causing bronchitis, pneumonitis, or esophagitis Immune restoration with highly active ART has markedly reduced the incidence of serious HSV infections.

Leukemia/Lymphoma HSV reactivation typically occurs during induction or reinduction within 20 days in individuals with latent HSV infection.

Bone Marrow Transplantation (BMT)

- HSV reactivation occurs within the first 5 weeks after BMT (median, day 8 posttransplantation).
- Untreated, 3% of patients die from disseminated HSV infection.

Chemotherapy

- For solid organ or BMT, congenital or acquired cellular immune defects.
- Cytotoxic cancer chemotherapy
- Glucocorticoid therapy.

Other

- Autoimmune diseases, malnutrition
- Rarely, pregnancy.
- Radiotherapy.
- Instrumentation such as nasogastric tube in debilitated patient associated with HSV esophagitis.

PATHOGENESIS

- 60–80% of HSV-seropositive transplant recipients and patients undergoing chemotherapy for hematologic malignancies will experience reactivation of HSV.
- After viremia, disseminated cutaneous or visceral HSV infection may occur.
- Factors determining whether severe localized disease, cutaneous dissemination, or visceral dissemination will occur are not well defined.

CLINICAL MANIFESTATION

Patients often hospitalized with underlying condition or disease.

Skin Symptoms Tender and painful mucocutaneous ulcers.

- *Recurrent herpetic lesion*: Mild pain in ulcers.

- *Chronic herpetic ulcers*: Mild to moderate pain.
- *Herpetic whitlow*: Severe pain.
- *Oropharyngeal ulcers*: Oral pain on eating.
- *Esophageal ulcers*: Retrosternal pain and/or painful swallowing (odynophagia) and/or dysphagia.
- *Anorectal ulcers*: Perianal/anal ulcers are usually quite painful. Anorectal ulcers are associated with pain, constipation, pain on defecation, discharge, tenesmus, and at times, sacral radiculopathy, impotence, neurogenic bladder.
- *Mucocutaneous dissemination*: Fever.

Visceral Dissemination Fever, deterioration of clinical status.

Mucocutaneous Lesions

Primary Infection

- Local infection may be widespread on the face (Fig. 27-36), oropharynx, anogenital region with initial vesiculation followed by crusted erosions.
- Without antiviral therapy, lesions may persist to become chronic herpetic ulcers.

Recurrent Herpetic Lesions

- In most immunocompromised persons, lesions appear as in the immunocompetent host.
- However, outbreaks may present with recurrent lesions (grouped crusts, erosions, ulcers) in a much larger area of involvement than usual.
- In HIV/AIDS-infected persons, large, necrotic, eroded lesions may appear over a period of a few days without apparent vesicle formation.

Chronic Herpetic Ulcers

- Recurrent lesions enlarge over weeks to months, forming large ulcers, 10–20 cm in diameter (Fig. 27-37).
- Margins may be slightly rolled, hyperplastic.
- Coalescence of ulcerations may result in linear ulcers in intergluteal cleft or inguinal fold. Base of ulcer may be crusted or moist.
- Painful on palpation. Perianal and/or rectal > genital > orofacial > digital.
- Uncommonly, ulcer on face and perineum simultaneously. 🔳

Oropharyngeal Ulcers Large ulcerations occur on the hard palate, often at the site of dental extraction. Linear ulcerations occur on the tongue.

Esophageal Ulcers

- Usually associated with oropharyngeal herpetic ulcer and swallowing HSV-infected saliva.
- Esophagoscopy: mucosal erosions/ulceration.

Genital, Perineal, Perianal, Anorectal Ulcers

- Acute ulceration of the vulva penis (Fig. 27-37), scrotum, and/or perineum may become chronic ulcers unless effectively treated.
- In individuals infected with acyclovir-resistant HSV, ulcerations do not respond to usual antiviral therapies.
- Anal ulcers usually occur via enlargement of perianal ulcers.
- Herpetic proctitis: sigmoidoscopy shows friable mucosa and ulcerations.

Mucocutaneous Dissemination

- Disseminated (nongrouped) vesicles and pustules often hemorrhagic with inflammatory halo; quickly rupture, resulting in "punched-out" erosions.

FIGURE 27-36   Herpes simplex virus infection: primary infection in HIV/AIDS   A 35-year-old male with HIV/AIDS (CD4 cell count, 400/mL). Confluent vesicles and erosions with underlying erythema and edema (5 to 6 days' duration) in the beard area. Gingivostomatitis and acute lymphadenopathy were also present, with onset 5 days after orogenital sex.

FIGURE 27-37 Herpes simplex virus infection: chronic ulcers in HIV/AIDS A 41-year-old male with HIV/AIDS with painful lesions on buttocks for 6 months. Large confluent ulcers on the buttocks and perianal area. HSV-2 was resistant to acyclovir, but resolved with IV foscarnet. Ulcers recurred during radiation to the area for metastatic squamous cell carcinoma (SCC).

FIGURE 27-38 Varicella-zoster virus infection: varicella Multiple, very pruritic, erythematous papules, vesicles ("dewdrops on a rose petal"), and crusted papules on erythematous, edematous bases on the face and neck of a young female. The spectrum of lesions, arising over 7 to 10 days, is typical of varicella.

- Lesions may be necrotic and then ulcerate (Fig. 27-38).
- Ulcers may become confluent with polycyclic well-demarcated borders; edges may be slightly raised, rolled.

Infarctive Skin Lesions   If complicated by purpura fulminans. (See Section 19)

Mucous Membranes   Oropharyngeal erosion: necrotizing gingivitis, palatal ulcers, glossitis.

General Examination

- Oropharyngeal lesions can occur in the absence of external facial lesions.
- HSV esophagitis, tracheobronchitis, and focal pneumonitis can be local infection associated with spread by aspirated or swallowed secretions.
- Diffuse interstitial pneumonitis can be a manifestation of hematogenous infection.
- HSV pneumonitis often results from endogenous reactivation.
- Widespread visceral involvement (liver, lungs, adrenals, GI tract, CNS) can occur in severely immunocompromised persons.

Variations with Specific States of Immunocompromise

Leukemia/Lymphoma

- HSV infection is often atypical, with extensive lesions on lips or nasolabial skin.
- Oropharyngeal infection manifested as necrotic gingival papillae, intraoral ulcerations that mimic thrush, or mucositis from chemotherapy or radiotherapy.

HIV/AIDS Disease

- Effective ART has dramatically reduced the occurrence of severe HSV infection in advanced HIV/AIDS.
- HSV reactivation is usually local, with chronic herpetic ulcers on the face or anogenital region.
- HSV esophagitis may coexist with candidal esophagitis.
- Persistent perianal herpes and herpetic proctitis.
- Disseminated visceral disease is uncommon.

DIFFERENTIAL DIAGNOSIS

Chronic Herpetic Ulcers   Chronic VZV infection, wound infection, ecthyma, ecthyma gangrenosum, pressure ulcer, deep mycotic (cryptococcal, histoplasmal, blastomycotic, coccidioidal) ulcer.

Oropharyngeal Ulcers   Aphthous ulcers, lymphoma, histoplasmosis with oral ulcer.

Esophageal Ulcers   CMV ulcers, aphthous (idiopathic) ulcers, *Candida* esophagitis, histoplasmosis with esophageal ulcer.

Anorectal Ulcers   HPV-induced squamous cell carcinoma, Crohn disease; amebiasis, chronic rectal abuse of ergot alkaloids.

Mucocutaneous Dissemination   VZV infection (varicella, disseminated herpes zoster), eczema herpeticum, eczema vaccinatum, disseminated vaccinia in immunosuppressed patients.

LABORATORY EXAMINATIONS

See pages 816.

Urinalysis   Hematuria due to HSV cystitis.

DIAGNOSIS

Clinical suspicion confirmed by Tzanck smear, positive HSV antigen detection DFA, or isolation of HSV on viral culture.

COURSE AND PROGNOSIS

- In most immunocompromised individuals with reactivation of HSV, clinical manifestations differ little from infections in healthy hosts.
- In renal transplant recipients, HSV is excreted in throat washings of 80% of patients shortly after grafting; two-thirds of those excreting HSV develop lesions shortly after excretion is detected.
- In some immunocompromised individuals, however, large ulcerations can persist for weeks to years.
- Herpetic ulcers facilitate superinfection with bacteria (*S. aureus* or fungi).
- HSV may disseminate to liver, lungs, adrenals, GI tract, CNS.
  - Visceral infection can be complicated by disseminated intravascular coagulation, which has a very high mortality rate.
- Factors determining whether severe localized disease, cutaneous involvement, or visceral dissemination will occur in an individual are not well defined.
- In HIV/AIDS, persons successfully treated with ART experience reduction in frequency and severity of HSV recurrences.

• Chronic herpetic ulcers that fail to respond to acyclovir should be evaluated promptly for the presence of resistant virus.
  ◦ Infection with acyclovir-resistant strains results in chronic, progressive ulcerations that persist and/or continue to enlarge despite oral and IV acyclovir treatment.
  ◦ These ulcers can enlarge to 20–30 cm in diameter and are associated with major morbidity and pain.

MANAGEMENT

Prevention *Acyclovir prophylaxis* for seropositive patients undergoing bone marrow transplantation, induction therapy for leukemia, or solid organ transplantation: acyclovir, 5 mg/kg IV q8h or 400 mg PO three times a day, from the day of conditioning, induction, or transplantation for 4–6 weeks suppresses both HSV and VZV reactivation. Also oral valacyclovir, famciclovir.
Systemic Antiviral Therapy See "Management," page 816.

VARICELLA ZOSTER VIRUS INFECTIONS

■ Varicella zoster virus (VZV) is a human herpesvirus that infects 98% of adult populations.

■ Primary VZV infection (varicella or chickenpox) is nearly always symptomatic and characterized by disseminated pruritic vesicles.

■ During primary infection, VZV establishes lifelong infection in sensory ganglia.

■ When immunity to VZV declines, VZV reactivates within the nerve cell, traveling down the neuron to the skin, where it erupts in a dermatomal pattern, i.e., herpes zoster (HZ), or shingles.

■ In the immunocompromised host, primary and reactivated VZV infection is often more severe, associated with higher morbidity rates and some mortality.

■ VZV vaccine has reduced the incidence of varicella and herpes zoster.

ICD-9:052 ◦ ICD-10:B01

EPIDEMIOLOGY AND ETIOLOGY

Age of Onset

• Without immunizaton, 90% of cases occur in children <10 years, <5% in persons older than 15 years.
• With immunization (Varivax), the incidence is markedly reduced.

Etiology

• VZV, a herpesvirus.
• Structurally similar to other herpesviruses:
  ◦ Lipid envelope surrounding nucleocapsid with icosahedral symmetry
  ◦ Total diameter of approximately 150–200 nm
  ◦ Centrally located double-strand DNA with a molecular weight of 80 million

Transmission

• Airborne droplets as well as direct contact
• Indirect contact uncommon
• Patients are contagious several days before varicella exanthem appears and until last crop of vesicles
• Crusts are not infectious.
• VZV can be aerosolized from skin of individuals with herpes zoster, which is about one-third as contagious as varicella, causing varicella in susceptible contacts.

Season In metropolitan areas in temperate climates, varicella epidemics occur in winter and spring.

PATHOGENESIS

- In varicella, VZV is thought to enter through mucosa of upper respiratory tract and oropharynx.
- Followed by local replication and primary viremia.
- VZV then replicates in cells of reticuloendothelial system with subsequent secondary viremia and dissemination to skin and mucous membranes.
- Localization of VZV in the basal cell layer is followed by virus replication, ballooning degeneration of epithelial cells, and accumulation of edema fluid.
- Second episodes of varicella have been documented but are rare.
- During the course of varicella, VZV passes from the skin lesions to the sensory nerves, travels to the sensory ganglia, and establishes latent infection.
- In herpes zoster, humoral and cellular immunity to VZV established with primary infection ebbs naturally or because of an underlying cause of immunocompromise.
- Results in VZV replication in sensory ganglia.
- VZV then travels down the sensory nerve, resulting in initial dermatomal pain, followed by skin lesions.
- Since the neuritis precedes the skin involvement, pain or itching appears before the skin lesions are visible.
- The locations of pain are varied and relate directly to the ganglion where VZV has emerged from latency to active infection.

- Prodromal symptoms may appear initially in the trigeminal, cervical, thoracic, lumbar, or sacral dermatome.
- Postherpetic neuralgia (PHN) is reflex sympathetic dystrophy (complex regional pain syndrome).

LABORATORY EXAMINATIONS

VZV Antigen Detection DFA   Smear of vesicle fluid or scraping from ulcer base/margin: Direct fluorescent antibody (DFA) test detects VZV-specific antigens. Sensitive and specific method for identifying VZV-infected lesions. Higher yield than VZV cultures.

Viral Cultures   Isolation of virus on viral culture (human fibroblast monolayers) from vesicular skin lesions, biopsy specimens, corneal scraping, and CSF is possible but more difficult than for HSV. Distinctive cytopathic effects usually appear in 3–10 days. Vesicle fluid can be cultured.

Tzanck Smear   Cytology of fluid or scraping from base of vesicle or pustule shows both giant and multinucleated acantholytic epidermal cells (as does that of HSV infections) (see Fig. 27-27).

Serology   Seroconversion documents primary VZV infection.

Dermatopathology   Lesional skin or visceral biopsy specimen shows multinucleated giant epithelial cells indicating HSV-1, HSV-2, or VZV infection. Immunoperoxidase stains specific for HSV-1, HSV-2, or VZV antigens can identify the specific herpesvirus.

VARICELLA ▪ ○

- The highly contagious primary infection caused by varicella-zoster virus.
- It is characterized by successive crops of pruritic vesicles that evolve to pustules, crusts, and at times, scars.
- This infection is often accompanied by mild constitutional symptoms

- Primary infection occurring in adulthood may be complicated by pneumonia and encephalitis.

Synonym: Chickenpox.

EPIDEMIOLOGY

Age of Onset See page 831.
Incidence

- Since introduction of varicella vaccine in 1995, incidence of varicella has decreased as vaccination coverage has increased.
- Prior to 1995, 3–4 million cases in the United States annually.

Transmission See page 831.
Season See page 831.

CLINICAL MANIFESTATION

Incubation Period 14 days (range, 10–23 days).
Prodrome

- Characteristically absent or mild.
- Uncommon in children, more common in adults: headache, general aches and pains, severe backache, malaise.
- Exanthem appears within 2–3 days.

History Exposure at day care, school, to older sibling; relative with zoster.
Skin Symptoms Exanthem usually quite pruritic.

Skin Lesions

In most children, illness begins with appearance of exanthem:

- Vesicular lesions evident in successive crops.
- Often single, discrete lesions or scanty in number in children and much more dense in adults.
- Initial lesions are *papules* (often not observed) that may appear as *wheals* and quickly evolve to *vesicles* and initially appear as small "drops of water" or "dewdrops on a rose petal" (Fig. 27-39), superficial and thin-walled with surrounding erythema.

- Vesicles become umbilicated and rapidly evolve to *pustules* and *crusts* over an 8- to 12-h period.
- With subsequent crops, all stages of evolution may be noted simultaneously, i.e., papules, vesicles, pustules, crusts, i.e., polymorphic.
- Crusts fall off in 1–3 weeks, leaving a pink, somewhat depressed base.
- Characteristic punched-out permanent scars may persist.
- Uncommonly, hemorrhage into pustular lesion occurs in otherwise healthy children, i.e., *hemorrhagic varicella.* ▰
- Complications
  - Superinfection by methicillin-sensitive *S. aureus* (MSSA), methicillin-resistant *S. aureus* (MRSA), or GAS
  - Impetigo, furuncles, cellulitis, and gangrene.

Distribution First lesions begin on face (Fig. 27-39) and scalp, spreading inferiorly to trunk and extremities.

- Most profuse in areas least exposed to pressure, i.e., back between shoulder blades, flanks, axillae, popliteal and anticubital fossae
- Density highest on trunk and face, less on extremities
- Palms and soles usually spared. ▰

Mucous Membranes Vesicles (not often observed) and subsequent shallow erosions (2–3 mm)

- Most common on palate
- Mucosa of nose, conjunctivae, pharynx, larynx, trachea, GI tract, urinary tract, vagina. ▰

General Examination Low-grade fever. Vesicopustules may occur in respiratory, GU, and GI tracts.
Pneumonitis Occurs with increased frequency in:

- Immunocompromised individuals of all ages
- Immunocompetent adolescents and adults
- More frequent/severe in pregnancy.
- 3–16% of healthy adults with varicella have radiologic evidence of VZV pneumonitis (diffuse interstitial lobular infiltrate). One-third of these will have respiratory symptoms.

Prior to antiviral therapy, morbidity/mortality was high.
CNS   Most commonly, varicella with cerebellar ataxia and encephalitis.

Variants
Bacterial Superinfection   Most commonly, *S. aureus* or GAS can cause impetigo, ecthyma, cellulitis, necrotizing fasciitis, or toxic shock syndrome in varicella lesions.
"Malignant" Varicella

- Immunosuppressed or glucocorticoid-treated individuals may develop pneumonitis, hepatitis, encephalitis, disseminated intravascular coagulation, and purpura fulminans.
- Continued VZV replication and dissemination result in prolonged high-level viremia, more extensive rash, longer period of new vesicle formation.

DIFFERENTIAL DIAGNOSIS

Widespread Vesicles/Crusts   Smallpox (all lesions are in the same stage), disseminated HSV infection, cutaneous dissemination of zoster, eczema herpeticum, eczema vaccinatum, disseminated vaccinia in immunosuppressed patients (smallpox vaccination still given in the U.S. military), rickettsialpox, enterovirus infections, bullous form of impetigo.

LABORATORY EXAMINATIONS

See "Laboratory Examinations," page 832.
Bacterial Cultures   Rule out superinfection with *S. aureus* or group A streptococcus.
Serology   Seroconversion, i.e., fourfold or greater rise in VZV titers.

DIAGNOSIS

Usually made on clinical findings alone.

COURSE AND PROGNOSIS

- In healthy children, the course is self-limited; however, a mortality rate of 1 per 50,000 cases in the United States had been reported prior to VZV immunization (100 deaths annually in the 3–4 million cases). Previously, 6500 hospitalizations annually (United States) for varicella.
- The most common complication of varicella in children <5 years is bacterial (*S. aureus*, GAS) superinfection. Bacteremia.
- In children 5–11 years of age, the most common complications are varicella encephalitis and Reye syndrome.
- In adults, prodromal symptoms are common and may be severe;
  ○ Exanthem may last for a week or more, with prolonged period of recovery.
  ○ Primary varicella pneumonia, which presents 1–6 days after appearance of rash, is relatively common in adults: 16% of adults show x-ray evidence of pneumonitis, but only 4% have clinical signs of pneumonitis. Women have a 10% risk of severe VZV pneumonitis.
  ○ VZV encephalitis may also complicate varicella in adults.
- Less common complications of varicella include viral arthritis, uveitis, conjunctivitis, carditis, inappropriate antidiuretic hormone syndrome, nephritis, and orchitis.
- The mortality rate in adults was 15 per 50,000 cases (U.S.); 25% of varicella-associated deaths did occur in adults.
- Maternal varicella during the first trimester of pregnancy:
  ○ Fetus: Fetal varicella syndrome (limb hypoplasia, eye and brain damage, skin lesions) in 2% of exposed fetuses.
  ○ Neonatal varicella has higher associated incidence of pneumonitis and encephalitis than occurs in older children.

- Immunocompromised or glucocorticoid-treated patients with varicella may manifest dissemination, hepatitis, encephalitis, and hemorrhagic complications.
- If varicella occurs at an early age when maternal antibody is still present, an individual can have a second episode of varicella.
- In HIV-infected patients, reactivation of VZV may result in chronic painful ecthymatous varicella.

In immunocompromised individuals, VZV hepatitis and pneumonitis are relatively common and are associated with significant mortality.

FIGURE 27-39 Varicella-zoster virus infection: varicella A 46-year-old female with pruritic eruption for 2 days. Multiple, pruritic, erythematous papules, vesicles on the face, neck, and chest. Several vesicles have evolved to crusted erosion. DFA detected VZV. No antibodies to VZV were detected.

FIGURE 27-40 Varicella zoster virus infection: varicella immunization varicella Asymptomatic 1-year-old male with history of varicella immunization 10 days before the onset of rash. Scattered red papules and vesicles disseminated on the chest. The vaccine contains live virus. Generalized varicella-like rash occurs in 3.8% of infants immunized, 5 to 26 days after immunization.

MANAGEMENT

Prevention

Immunization	VZV immunization is now available (Varivax) and is 80% effective in preventing symptomatic primary VZV infection. 5% of newly immunized children develop rash (Fig. 27-40). Those at high risk for varicella, who should be immunized, include: normal VZV-negative adults, children with leukemia, and immunocompromised individuals (immunosuppressive treatment, HIV infection, cancer). VZV vaccine results in both cell-mediated immunity and antibody production against the virus. Immunization with VZV vaccine may boost humoral and cell-mediated immunity and decrease the incidence of zoster in populations with declining VZV-specific immunity.

Symptomatic therapy

Lotions	Directed at reducing pruritus.
Oral antihistamines	Application gives short-term relief of pruritus.
Caution re antipyretic agents	Antipyretic administration is of concern because of a possible link between aspirin and Reye syndrome in children with varicella.

Antiviral agents

Otherwise healthy patients	If begun within 24 h after onset of varicella, decreases the severity of varicella and reduces secondary cases.
Acyclovir*	20 mg/kg (800 maximum) four times daily for 5 days
Valacyclovir	Effective but not an approved use; dosing same as for herpes zoster.
Famciclovir	Effective but not an approved use; dosing same as for herpes zoster.
VZV infection (varicella or zoster) in immunocompromised patients	
Acyclovir	10 mg/kg IV q8h for 7 days
Foscarnet (in acyclovir resistance)	40 mg/kg IV q8h for 7 days

Treatment of bacterial superinfection

Mupirocin ointment	Directed at *S. aureus* and/or group A streptococcus.
Oral antibiotics	Applied twice daily to lesions. See Table 24-1.

*In Europe, oral acyclovir is only rarely used because of better bioavailability of valacyclovir and famciclovir.

HERPES ZOSTER (HZ)   ICD-9:053 ∘ ICD-10:B02   ■ ◑

- An acute dermatomal infection associated with reactivation of VZV
- Characterized by
  - Unilateral pain
  - A vesicular or bullous eruption limited to a dermatome(s) innervated by a corresponding sensory ganglion.

- The major morbidity is postherpetic neuralgia (PHN).

Synonym: Shingles.

EPIDEMIOLOGY

Age of Onset   More than 66% are >50 years of age; 5% of cases in children <15 years.

Incidence

- In the United States, nearly 100% of adults are seropositive for anti-VZV antibodies by the third decade of life and are thus at risk for reactivation of latent VZV.
- More than 500,000 cases of HZ annually.
- Cumulative lifetime incidence: 10–20%.
- HIV/AIDS
  - In one cohort, 5% of individuals with HZ were HIV-infected and 5% had cancer.
  - Recurrent HZ < 1% of cases.
  - Occurs in 25% of HIV-infected individuals, an eight times higher incidence than the general population, ages 20–50 years;
- Renal and cardiac transplant recipients: 7–9%
- Recurrent HZ more common in immunocompromised individuals.
- Immunization to VZV in childhood will alter the epidemiology of HZ.

Risk Factors

- Most common factor is diminishing immunity to VZV with advancing age, with most cases occurring in those ≥55 years.
- However, in most cases triggering factors are not known.
- Immunocompromise:
  - Malignancy
  - Immunosuppression, especially from lymphoproliferative disorders and chemotherapy
  - Radiotherapy.
  - HIV/AIDS: eightfold increased incidence of HZ.

Pathogenesis

- In varicella VZV passes from lesions in the skin and mucosa via sensory fibers centripetally to sensory ganglia.
- In the ganglia the virus establishes lifelong latent infection.
- Reactivation occurs in those ganglia in which VZV has achieved the highest density and is triggered by immunosuppression, trauma, tumor, or irradiation (see risk factors).
- Reactivated virus can no longer be contained.
- Virus multiplies and spreads antidromically down the sensory nerve to the skin/mucosa where it produces the characteristic vesicles (Image 27-2).

Classification   HZ manifests in three distinct clinical stages: prodrome, active infection, chronic: postherpetic neuralia (PNH).

CLINICAL MANIFESTATIONS

Duration of Symptoms

- Prodromal stage: Neuritic pain or paresthesia precedes for 2–3 weeks (84% of cases).
- Acute vesiculation: 3–5 days.
- Crust formation: days to 2–3 weeks.
- PHN: months to years.
  - Chronic pain or PHN is that persisting after the lesions have healed or persisting 4 weeks after the onset of lesions, regardless of degree of healing.

Skin Symptoms
Prodromal Stage

- Pain (stabbing, pricking, sharp, boring, penetrating, lancinating, shooting), tenderness, paresthesia (itching, tingling, burning, freeze-burning) in the involved dermatome precedes the eruption.

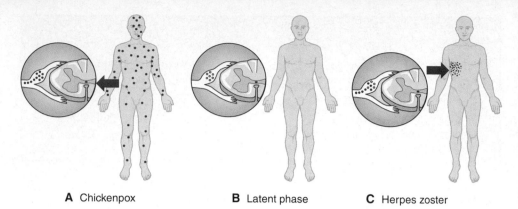

A Chickenpox **B** Latent phase **C** Herpes zoster

IMAGE 27-2 Varicella and herpes zoster A. During primary VZV infection (varicella or chickenpox), virus infects sensory ganglia. **B.** VZV persists in a latent phase within ganglia for the life of the individual. **C.** With diminished immune function, VZV reactivates within sensory ganglia, descends sensory nerves, and replicates in skin.

- Allodynia: heightened sensitivity to mild stimuli.

Active Vesiculation   Skin lesions may be pruritic but in themselves are not painful.

Zoster Sine Zoster   Nerve involvement can occur without cutaneous zoster.

Abdominal Zoster   Presents with severe abdominal (or chest pain) that may precede rash by hours to days.

Chronic Stages   PHN, described as "burning," "ice-burning," "shooting," or "lancinating," can persist for weeks, months, or years after the cutaneous involvement has resolved.

Constitutional Symptoms

- Prodromal stage and active vesiculation: flu-like symptoms such as headache, malaise, fever.
- Chronic stages: depression is very common in individuals with PHN.

Mucocutaneous Lesions

- Papules (24 h) → vesicles-bullae (Fig. 27-41 to 43) (48 h) → pustules (96 h) → crusts (7–10 days).
- New lesions continue to appear for up to 1 week.
- Erythematous, edematous base (Fig. 27-42) with superimposed clear vesicles, sometimes hemorrhagic.
- The vesicle-bulla is oval or round, may be umbilicated.
- Vesicles erode forming crusted erosions (Fig. 27-44).

- Necrotic and gangrenous lesions sometimes occur.
- Scarring is common after healing of HZ (Fig. 27-45).

Distribution

- Unilateral, dermatomal (Image 27-3).
- Two or more contiguous dermatomes may be involved (Fig. 27-41*A*, *B*).
- Noncontiguous dermatomal zoster is rare.
- Hematogenous dissemination to other skin sites in 10% of healthy individuals (Fig. 27-43*B*).

Site of Predilection   Thoracic (>50%), trigeminal (10–20%) (Figs. 27-42, 27-43, 27-45, 27-46), lumbosacral and cervical (10–20%).

Mucous Membranes   Vesicles and erosions occur in mouth, vagina, and bladder, depending on dermatome involved.

General Examination

Lymphadenopathy   Regional nodes draining the area are often enlarged and tender.

Sensory or Motor Nerve Changes   Detectable by neurologic examination. Sensory defects (temperature, pain, touch) and (mild) motor paralysis, e.g., facial palsy.

Eyes

- In ophthalmic zoster, nasociliary involvement of V-1 (ophthalmic) branch of the trigeminal nerve occurs in about one-third of cases and is heralded by vesicles on the side and tip of the nose.
- Complications include uveitis, keratitis, conjunctivitis, retinitis, optic neuritis, glaucoma,

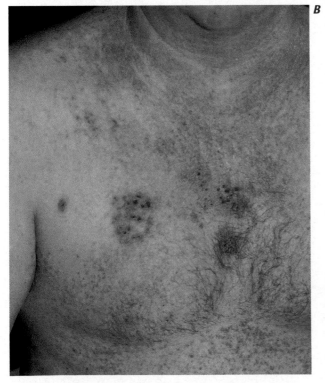

FIGURE 27-41 Varicella zoster virus infection: herpes zoster on thorax and arm A 60-year-old male being treated with prednisone for eczema has painful lesion for 3 days. Dermatomal grouped and confluent vesicles on the *(A)* right back and arm and *(B)* right pectoral area.

proptosis, cicatricial lid retraction, and extraocular muscle palsies.
- Acute retinal necrosis (rapidly progressive herpetic retinal necrosis) is more common in the immunocompromised host

Delayed Contralateral Hemiparesis

- Occurs weeks to months (mean, 7 weeks) after an episode of HZ involving the first division of the trigeminal nerve (V-1).
- Typical presentation is headache and hemiplegia occurring in a patient with recent history of HZ ophthalmicus.
- Arteriogram shows inflammation, narrowing, and thrombosis of proximal branches of anterior or middle cerebral artery.
- Pathogenesis: direct VZV invasion of cerebral arteries by extension along intracranial branches of V-1, resulting in inflammation of internal carotid artery or one of its branches on the side ipsilateral to rash.

DIFFERENTIAL DIAGNOSIS

Prodromal Stage/Localized Pain Can mimic migraine, cardiac or pleural disease, an acute abdomen, or vertebral disease.
Dermatomal Eruption Zosteriform HSV infection, phytoallergic (poison ivy, poison oak) contact dermatitis, erysipelas, bullous impetigo, necrotizing fasciitis.

LABORATORY EXAMINATIONS

See "Laboratory Exminations," page 832.

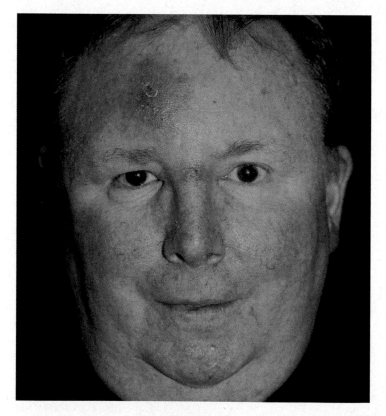

FIGURE 27-42   Varicella zoster virus infection: herpes zoster in V1 distribution   A 58-year-old male with psoriasis being treated with methotrexate and etanercept had onset of painful rash on right forehead for one day with flulike symptoms. Erythematous edematous plaques on the forehead and glabella. VZV was detected by DFA. Methotrexate and etanercept were held and valacyclovir given. He did well without complications. Etanercept was restarted in 6 weeks.

A

B

FIGURE 27-43   Varicella zoster virus infection: herpes zoster of the zygomaticotemporal nerve (branch of the V2 maxillary nerve)   A 49-year-old male with a history of left parietal glioblastoma was being treated with radiation therapy and experienced discomfort at the radiation portal site. He had been treated for bacterial infection with oral antibiotic without improvement. **A.** Clustered crusted erosions are seen on the lateral scalp; 11 disseminated vesicles were scattered on the extremities and trunk. **B.** Vesicle on the upper arm. He was treated with oral famciclovir; lesions resolved without complication.

A

B

C

Rami of the trigeminal N. {
- ■ Ophthalmic
- □ Maxillary
- ■ Mandibular

Ramus of vagus ■ Auricular

*Overlapping of greater auricular and facial nerves

Gr. occipital N. *Sm occipital N.*

Post cev. *Cervical cutaneous*

IMAGE 27-3 Dermatomes The cutaneous fields of peripheral nerves.

Electrocardiogram In prodromal stage with individuals with chest pain, rule out ischemic heart disease.

Imaging In prodromal stage, rule out organic, pleural, pulmonary, or abdominal disease.

DIAGNOSIS

Prodromal Stage Suspect HZ in older or immunocompromised individual with unilateral pain.

Active Vesiculation Clinical findings usually adequate; may be confirmed by Tzanck test and possible DFA or viral culture to rule out HSV infection.

PHN By history and clinical findings.

COURSE AND PROGNOSIS

In immunocompetent host, rash usually resolves in 2 to 3 weeks. Complications can be:

- Mucocutaneous
  - Hemorrhage, gangrene
  - Cutaneous dissemination
  - Superinfection of skin lesions

- Systemic
  - Neurologic: meningoencephalitis, cerebral vascular syndromes, cranial nerve syndromes [trigeminal (ophthalmic) branch (HZ ophthalmicus), facial and auditory nerves (Ramsay Hunt syndrome)], peripheral motor weakness, transverse myelitis
  - Visceral involvement: (pneumonitis, hepatitis, pericarditis/myocarditis, pancreatitis, esophagitis, enterocolitis, cystitis, synovitis).

- Dissemination generally occurs 6–10 days after onset of localized lesions and is most often limited to cutaneous involvement.
- Visceral dissemination can occur, involving CNS, lung, heart, and GI tract.
- Dissemination of zoster—≥ 20 lesions outside the affected or adjacent dermatomes—occurs in up to 10% of patients, usually in immunosuppressed patients. Motor paralysis occurs in 5% of patients, especially when the virus involves the cranial nerves.

The risk of PHN is 40% in patients >60 years. In one large follow-up study, PHN was present 1 month after onset of the rash in 60%; by 3 months, some pain in 24%; and by 6 months, 13% still had pain. The highest incidence of PHN is in ophthalmic zoster.

Pain with HZ is associated with neural inflammation, nerve infection during the acute reactivation, and neural inflammation and scarring with PHN.

For VZV infection in immunocompromised hosts, see page 846.

FIGURE 27-44 Varicella zoster virus infection: thoracic zoster A 39-year-old female with HIV/AIDS has had painful chest lesions for 3 weeks. Crusted and reepithelialized dermatomal erosions on the left back.

MANAGEMENT

Prevention

Immunization	Immunization with VZV vaccine may boost humoral and cell-mediated immunity and decrease the incidence of zoster in populations with declining VZV-specific immunity.
Goals of management	Relieve constitutional symptoms; minimize pain; reduce viral shedding; prevent secondary bacterial infection; speed crusting of lesions and healing; ease physical, psychological, emotional discomfort; prevent viral dissemination or other complications; prevent or minimize PHN.
Antiviral therapy	In individuals at high risk for reactivation of VZV infection, oral acyclovir can reduce the incidence of HZ. In prodromal stage: begin antiviral agent if diagnosis is considered likely; analgesics. With active vesiculation: antiviral therapy begun ≤72 h accelerates healing of skin lesions, decreases the duration of acute pain, and may decrease the frequency of PHN when given in adequate dosage.
Acyclovir	800 mg PO four times daily for 7–10 days. The 50% viral inhibitory concentration of acyclovir is three to six times higher for VZV than for HSV in vitro, and drug dose must be increased appropriately. The bioavailability of acyclovir is only 15–30% of the orally administered dose. For ophthalmic zoster and HZ in the immunocompromised host, acyclovir should be given intravenously. Acyclovir hastens healing and lessens *acute* pain if given within 48 h of the onset of the rash.*
Valacyclovir	1000 mg PO three times daily for 7 days, 70–80% bioavailable.
Famciclovir	500 mg PO three times daily for 7 days, 77% bioavailable. Reduce dose in individuals with diminished renal function.
Acyclovir-resistant VZV	Foscarnet
Immunosuppressed patients	IV acyclovir and recombinant interferon α-2a to prevent dissemination of HZ is indicated.

Supportive therapy for acute HZ

Constitutional symptoms	Bed rest, nonsteroidal anti-inflammatory drugs.
Sedation	Pain often interferes with sleep. Sleep deprivation and pain commonly result in depression. Doxepin, 10–100 mg at bed time, is an effective agent.
Oral glucocorticoids	Prednisone given early in the course of HZ relieves constitutional symptoms but has not been proven to reduce PHN.
Dressings	Application of moist dressings (water, saline, Burow solution) to the involved dermatome is soothing and alleviates pain.
Pain management	Early control of pain with narcotic analgesics is indicated; failure to manage pain can result in failure to sleep, fatigue, and depression: Best to begin with more potent analgesics and then reduce potency as pain lessens.

Chronic stages (PHN)

Pain management	Pain is that of reflex sympathetic dystrophy.
	Severe prodromal pain or severe pain on the first day of rash is predictive of severe PHN.
	Gabapentin: 300 mg three times daily. Pregabalin.
	Tricyclic antidepressants such as doxepin, 10–100 mg PO at bed time.
	Capsaicin cream every 4 h.
	Topical anesthetic such as EMLA or 5% lidocaine patch for allodynia.
	Nerve block to area of allodynia.
	Analgesics.

*In Europe, oral acyclovir is only rarely used because of greater bioavailability of valacyclovir and famciclovir.

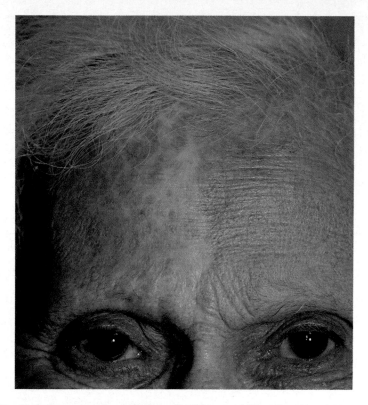

FIGURE 27-45   Varicella zoster virus infection: atrophic scar at V1 zoster site   A 90-year-old female with a history of herpes zoster 14 years previously. Hypopigmented dermatomal (V1) scar is seen on the right forehead at the site of prior zoster.

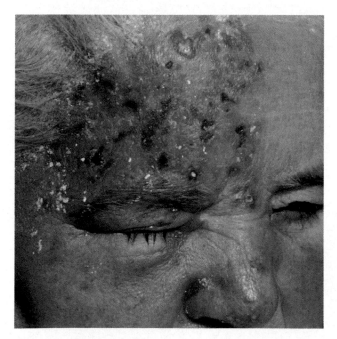

FIGURE 27-46   Varicella zoster virus infection: ophthalmic herpes zoster   Crusted ulcerations and vesicles on the right forehead and periorbital area in the ophthalmic branch of the trigeminal nerve; marked facial edema is also present. Vesicles on the tip of the nose indicate nasociliary involvement. Hutchinson rule: involvement of the nasociliary nerve suggests that eye involvement may occur.

VARICELLA ZOSTER VIRUS INFECTIONS IN THE IMMUNOCOMPROMISED HOST   ▯ ●

- In immunocompromised individuals, VZV infections can be more severe in
  - Primary infections (varicella)
  - Reactivated infections (HZ)
- Varicella cutaneous and visceral involvement can be more severe.
- Herpes zoster may

- Involve several contiguous dermatomes
- Have more extensive cutaneous necrosis
- Have wide hematogenous dissemination to
  - Mucocutaneous structures
  - Viscera (lung, liver, brain)
- Often be associated with high morbidity and mortality rates.

EPIDEMIOLOGY

Incidence The population of immunocompromised individuals is increasing, and most cases of recurrent HZ occur in immunocompromised individuals.

Risk Factors

- Immunosuppression, especially from lymphoproliferative disorders, and cancer chemotherapy.
- Herpes zoster: Often the first sign of HIV infection, preceding oral candidiasis and oral hairy leukoplakia by 1 year.
- Risk of dissemination of varicella or HZ to viscera:
  - Varicella to viscera:
    - Children undergoing cancer chemotherapy
    - Solid organ and bone marrow transplant recipients
    - HIV/AIDS infection
    - Certain cell-mediated immunodeficiency disorders of childhood.
  - Herpes zoster to viscera:
    - Hodgkin disease: 13–15% risk of HZ
    - Non-Hodgkin lymphoma: 7–9% risk for HZ
    - Solid tumors: 1–3% risk for HZ

CLINICAL MANIFESTATIONS

Skin Symptoms

- Symptoms of varicella and zoster.
- Chronic cutaneous VZV infections following hematogenous dissemination are often associated with significant lesional pain requiring narcotic analgesia for pain management.

Constitutional Symptoms Visceral dissemination usually accompanied by fever.

Mucocutaneous Lesions

Varicella and Cutaneous Dissemination of Reactivated VZV Infection (See "Varicella," page 833.) Reactivated VZV without HZ with cutaneous dissemination cannot be distinguished clinically from varicella (Fig. 27-47).

Herpes Zoster In HIV/AIDS disease and leukemia, involvement of several contiguous dermatomes is common (Fig. 27-48). (See also Section 31, Mucocutaneous Manifestations of Human Immunodeficiency Virus Disease)

Herpes Zoster with Cutaneous Dissemination

- A variable number of vesicles or bullae are seen at any mucocutaneous site, which evolve into crusted erosions.
- Lesions are disseminated and range from a few to hundreds.
- The condition thus appears clinically as zoster plus varicella. ✐

Herpes Zoster with Persistent Dermatomal Infection

- Papules and nodules, which can become hyperkeratotic or verrucous, persisting in a dermatomal pattern (single or multiple contiguous) after an outbreak of zoster (Fig. 27-49).
- Chronic ulcers can persist for months. ✐

Chronic Cutaneous VZV Infection After Hematogenous Dissemination

- Lesions on the palms or soles may present initially as bullae.
- Continual appearance of vesicles/bullae in a dermatomal or generalized distribution.
- Dissemination can occur without dermatomal HZ.
- Chronic lesions present as nodules, ulcers, crusted nodules/ulcers (ecthymatous). Postinflammatory hyper- or hypopigmentation. ✐

Systemic Findings   *Eyes*

- In HIV/AIDS disease, retinal VZV infection (acute retinal necrosis) can occur in the absence of apparent conjunctival or cutaneous involvement with subsequent loss of vision.
- Bilateral involvement in one-third of cases with subsequent loss of vision.
- VZV optic neuritis is rare.

CNS   In HIV/AIDS disease, VZV is the etiologic agent of up to 2% of CNS disease (encephalitis, polyneuritis, myelitis, vasculitis).

DIFFERENTIAL DIAGNOSIS

Primary Varicella with Visceral Dissemination
Pneumonia must be distinguished from *Pneumocystis carinii* pneumonia associated with varicella.
Herpes Zoster with Cutaneous Dissemination
Zosteriform HSV infection with dissemination.

Herpes Zoster with Visceral and Cutaneous Dissemination   Zosteriform HSV infection with dissemination. Pneumonia must be distinguished from *P. carinii* pneumonia associated with varicella.
Herpes Zoster with Persistent Dermatomal Infection   Chronic zosteriform HSV infection. Hypertrophic scars or keloids.
Chronic Cutaneous VZV Infection After Hematogenous Dissemination   Ecthyma, ecthyma gangrenosum, disseminated mycobacterial infection, deep fungal infection, syphilis.

LABORATORY EXAMINATIONS

See "Varicella Zoster Virus Infection," page 831.
Antiviral Sensitivities   When isolated, VZV from cultured lesion can be tested for sensitivity to acyclovir and other antiviral agents.
Bacterial Culture   Rule out secondary bacterial superinfection, most commonly caused by *S. aureus* (MSSA or MRSA) or group A streptococcus (GAS).

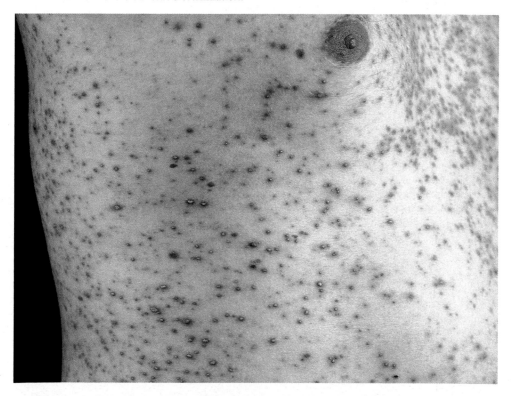

FIGURE 27-47   Varicella zoster virus infection: disseminated cutaneous, in an immunocompromised patient   Hundreds of vesicles and pustules on erythematous bases of the trunk of a patient with lymphoma. Note the absence of grouping of lesions seen in herpes simplex or herpes zoster. The eruption is indistinguishable from varicella and must be differentiated from disseminated HSV infection.

Chemistries   Abnormalities of liver function tests with VZV hepatitis.

COURSE AND PROGNOSIS

- Approximately 2–35% of children with varicella who are undergoing cancer chemotherapy experience visceral dissemination.
  - The associated mortality rate is 7–30%.
- Dissemination is more common in those with a peripheral blood lymphocyte count of <500/µL.

Children with Varicella

- Visceral involvement most commonly affects lungs; less often, liver and brain.
- Varicella pneumonia occurs 3–7 days after onset of skin lesions; can progress rapidly over a few days or remain indolent with gradual improvement over 2–4 weeks.

- Neurologic complications present 4–8 days after onset of rash; associated with poor prognosis.

Adults with HZ

- HIV/AIDS
  - Recurrent episodes occur in same or different dermatome(s)
- Hodgkin disease
  - Between 15 and 30% of patients experience significant dissemination (most often cutaneous).
- Mortality rates for disseminated zoster much lower than for children with disseminated varicella.
- PHN does not appear to be more common in immunocompromised individuals than in the general population.

MANAGEMENT

Prevention Immunization	VZV immunization is available and is 80% effective in preventing symptomatic primary VZV infection. About 5% of newly immunized children develop rash. Those at high risk for varicella who should be immunized include normal adults, children with leukemia, neonates, and immunocompromised individuals (immunosuppressive treatment, HIV infection, cancer).
Antiviral agents for VZV- and/or HSV-seropositive individuals undergoing BMT Acyclovir	Acyclovir 400 mg PO twice daily, from the day of conditioning, induction, or transplantation for 4–6 weeks, suppresses both HSV and VZV reactivation. Oral valacyclovir and famciclovir are effective.[*]
In individuals with mild to moderate immunocompromise	High-dose oral acyclovir, 800 mg five times daily for 7 days, hastens healing and lessens *acute* pain if given within 48 h of the onset of the rash. Large controlled studies in patients > 60 years have not, however, demonstrated any effect on the incidence and severity of *chronic* postherpetic neuralgia of high-dose oral acyclovir. A recent preliminary study of older patients (age 60) demonstrated a reduced frequency of persistent pain when IV acyclovir, 10 mg/kg q8h for 5 days, was given within 4 days of the onset of the pain or within 48 h after the onset of the rash. Oral valacyclovir, 1000 mg tid, famciclovir, 500 mg tid, both for 7 days.
In individuals with advanced immunocompromise	IV acyclovir or recombinant interferon α-2a to prevent dissemination of HZ is indicated.

[*]BMT, bone marrow transplantation.
[*]In Europe, oral acyclovir is rarely used because of better bioavailability of valacyclovir and famciclovir.

FIGURE 27-48 Varicella zoster virus infection: necrotizing herpes zoster Confluent, crusted ulcerations on an inflammatory base in several contiguous dermatomes in an elderly male with leukemia.

FIGURE 27-49 Varicella zoster virus infection: chronic herpes zoster in HIV disease Discrete and confluent hyperkeratotic plaques in several contiguous dermatomes persistent for 2 years in a male with advanced untreated HIV disease. The lesions were minimally symptomatic.

HHV-6 AND -7 INFECTIONS: EXANTHEMA SUBITUM (ES)   □ ◑

- Etiologic agents: primary human herpesvirus-6 (HHV-6) and HHV-7 infection
- Characterized by
  - High fever in a healthy infant (9–12 months old)

- Defervescence in 3 days followed by
- Sudden appearance of exanthem
- Complication: febrile seizure

Synonym: Roseola infantum.

EPIDEMIOLOGY AND ETIOLOGY

Age of Onset   6–24 months.
Etiology

- HHV-6 (variants -6A and -6B) and HHV-7 share genetic, biologic, and immunologic features and are T cell tropic.
- At birth, most children have passively transferred anti-HHV-6 and-7 IgG.
- Primary infection is acquired via oropharyngeal secretions.
- HHV-6 antibodies reach a nadir at 4–7 months and increase throughout infancy.
- By 12 months, two-thirds of children become infected, with peak antibody levels reached at 2–3 years of age.
- Similarly, HHV-7 antibodies reach nadir at 6 months, with level peaking at 3–4 years of age. Latent infection may persist for the lifetime of the individual.

PATHOGENESIS

Pathogenesis of ES rash is not known.

CLINICAL MANIFESTATIONS

Incubation Period   5–15 days.
Prodrome

- High fever ranging from 38.9°–40.6°C.
- Remains consistently high, with morning remission, until the fourth day, when it falls precipitously to normal, coincident with the appearance of rash.
- Infant remarkably well despite high fever.
- Asymptomatic primary HHV-6 and HHV-7 infection is common.

Symptoms   Usually absent.

Skin Lesions

- Small blanchable pink macules and papules, 1–5 mm in diameter (Fig. 27-50).

- Lesions may remain discrete or become confluent.
- Distribution: trunk and neck.

General Findings   Absent in presence of high fever. Febrile seizures are common.

DIFFERENTIAL DIAGNOSIS

Morbilliform Exanthem   See "Infectious Exanthems," page 795.

LABORATORY EXAMINATIONS

Serology   Demonstration of IgM anti-HHV-6 or anti-HHV-7 antibodies or IgG seroconversion.
Other   Viral culture and isolation from peripheral blood mononuclear cells. Demonstration of HHV-6 or HHV-7 DNA by PCR.

DIAGNOSIS

Usually made on clinical findings.

COURSE AND PROGNOSIS

- Course self-limited with rare sequelae.
- In some cases, high fever may be associated with seizures.
- Intussusception associated with hyperplasia of intestinal lymphoid tissue and hepatitis reported.
- As with other HHV infections, HHV-6 and HHV-7 persist throughout the life of the patient; Clinical manifestations associated with HHV-6 and HHV-7 reactivation have not been identified beyond doubt, but pityriasis rosea is discussed.
- An infant with HHV-6 ES may experience a second clinical syndrome, HHV-7 ES, and vice versa.

MANAGEMENT

Symptomatic.

FIGURE 27-50 Exanthema subitum Multiple, blanchable macules and papules on the back of a febrile child, which appeared as the temperature fell. (Courtesy of Karen Wiss, MD)

ARTHROPOD BITES, STINGS, AND CUTANEOUS INFECTIONS

- ■ Arthropod bites and stings:
  - • Cause a wide spectrum of reactions
  - • Transmit local and systemic infections
- ■ Superficial infestations:
  - • Epidermal: Pediculosis, scabies, tungiasis
  - • Dermal: Larva migrans, myiasis

CUTANEOUS REACTIONS TO ARTHROPOD BITES

- ■ Terrestrial arthropods that bite/sting humans: arachnids, centipedes, millipedes, insects.
- ■ Cutaneous reactions to arthropod bites (CRAB) are inflammatory and/or allergic reactions.
- ■ Characterized by an intensely pruritic eruption at the bite sites immediately to minutes to hours to days after the bite, persisting for days to weeks, manifested by solitary or grouped:
- • Urticarial papules
- • Papulovesicles
- • Bullae
- ■ Patients are often unaware of having been bitten.
- ■ In some cases, systemic symptoms may occur, ranging from mild to severe, with death occurring from anaphylactic shock.
- ■ Arthropods are vectors of many systemic infections.

EPIDEMIOLOGY

Season   Summer in temperate climates.
Etiology   5 of 9 classes of arthropods cause local and systemic reactions associated with their bites: Arachnida, Chilopoda, Diplopoda, Crustacea, Insecta.

Arthropods That Bite, Sting, or Infest

- • Arachnida (four pairs of legs): mites, ticks, spiders, scorpions
  - ○ Acarina
    - ▪ Mites: *Sarcoptes scabiei* causes scabies; *Demodex folliculorum*, human hair follicle mite; many others including food, fowl, grain, straw, harvest, animal, and house dust mites.
    - ▪ Ticks
  - ○ Araneae: spiders
  - ○ Scorpionida
- • Chilopoda and Diplopoda: centipedes, millipedes
- • Insecta (three pairs of legs)
  - ○ Anoplura: lice (*Phthirius* and *Pediculus*)

- ○ Coleoptera: beetles
- ○ Diptera: mosquitoes, black flies, midges (punkies, no seeums, sand flies), Tabandae (horseflies, deerflies, clegs, breeze flies, greenheads, mango flies); botflies, *Callitroga americana*, *Dermatobia hominis*, phlebotomid sand flies, tsetse flies
- ○ Hemiptera: bedbugs, kissing bugs
- ○ Hymenoptera: ants, bees, wasps, hornets
- ○ Lepidoptera: caterpillars, butterflies, moths
- ○ Siphonaptera: fleas, chigoe or sand flea

Arthropod-Borne Infections

- • Lyme borreliosis, tularemia, bubonic plague.
- • Scrub typhus, endemic (murine) typhus, spotted fever groups, Q fever
- • Human granulocytic anaplasmosis,
- • Tick-borne meningoencephalitis
- • Leishmaniasis, trypanosomiasis (sleeping sickness, Chagas disease).
- • Malaria, babesiosis.
- • Filariasis, onchocerciasis (river blindness), loiasis

Geographic Distribution   Worldwide.

PATHOGENESIS

Mites

- Produce pruritus and/or allergic reactions through salivary proteins deposited during feeding.
- Harvest mites (chiggers) may present as intense pruritus on the ankles, legs, belt line; mites usually fall off after feeding or may be scratched off.
- In nonsensitized individuals, 1- to 2-mm pruritic papules are seen.
- In sensitized individuals, CRAB may be papular urticaria, vesiculation, or granulomatous reaction with fever and lymphadenopathy.

Ticks (Acarina) Reactions include foreign body reactions, reactions to salivary secretions, reactions to injected toxins, and hypersensitivity reactions. *Tick paralysis* is caused by a toxin secreted in the saliva of the tick.

Spiders (Araneae)

- *Loxosceles reclusa*: Brown recluse spider bite causes reactions ranging from mild urticaria to full-thickness necrosis (*loxoscelism*).
- *Latrodectus*: "Widow" spiders inject a venom that contains a neurotoxin (α-latrotoxin) producing reactions at the bite site as well as varying degrees of systemic toxicity.
- *Tegenaria*: Hobo spider causes necrotic arachnidism in Pacific Northwest of United States.
- *Tarantula*: Mild inflammatory response to bite and from hairs shed from legs.

Scorpion (Scorpiones) Reside in tropical and arid regions. Venom also contains a neurotoxin that can cause severe local and systemic reactions.

Blister Beetles Contain the chemical cantharidin, which produces a blister when the beetle is crushed on the skin.

Black Flies Bites produce local reactions as well as black fly fever, characterized by fever, headache, nausea, generalized lymphadenitis.

Nonbiting Flies Flies commonly feed on open wounds, exudates, and skin ulcers and may deposit eggs at these sites, resulting in *wound myiasis*. Fly larvae can burrow into injured or normal skin, invading through the epidermis into the dermis, resulting in *furuncular myiasis*. In some cases, larvae move about the subcutis (*migratory myiasis*), mimicking the pattern of cutaneous larva migrans.

Bedbugs Nocturnal feedings produce a linear or grouped arrangement of papular urticaria (breakfast, lunch, and dinner).

Hymenoptera Bees, hornets, wasp bites can produce painful stings and anaphylaxis in the sensitized individual.

Caterpillars and Moths Hairs can produce local irritant and allergic reactions.

Fleas (Cat, Dog, Bird) Bites tend to cause more local reactions than human flea bites.

Chigoe or Sand Fleas (*Tunga penetrans*) Recently impregnated female flea penetrates skin of a human host, burrows into epidermis to dermal-epidermal junction, where she feeds on blood drawn from host vessels in superficial dermis (*tungiasis*). Mature eggs (150–200) are extruded singly from a terminal abdominal orifice during a period of 7–10 days. The female dies shortly after egg extrusion, and the infested tissues collapse around it.

CLINICAL MANIFESTATION

Incubation Period CRAB appears minutes to days after the bite.

Duration of Lesions Days, weeks, months.

Skin Symptoms Pruritus, pain at bite site. Systemic symptoms with systemic reaction.

Mucocutaneous Findings

Erythematous Macules Occur at bite sites and are usually transient.

Papular Urticaria

- Persistent (>48 h) urticarial papules (Figs. 28-1 to 28-5), often surmounted by a vesicle, usually <1 cm.
- Excoriations and excoriated urticarial papules, vesicles.
- Crusted painful lesions, usually purulent, may represent impetigo, ecthyma, or cutaneous diphtheria.
- Excoriated or secondarily infected lesions may heal with hyper- or hypopigmentation and/or raised or depressed scars, especially in more darkly pigmented individuals.

Bullous Lesions

- Tense bullae with clear fluid on a slightly inflamed base.
- Excoriation results in large erosion.

Tick Bites

- Attach and feed painlessly.
- Secretions can produce local reactions (Fig. 28-6), febrile illness, paralysis.

FIGURE 28-1   Papular urticaria: insect bite   A 28-year-old female with pruritic lesions on the chest. Solitary red edematous papule with early erosion on the right pectoral area. Multiple lesions were present at the site.

FIGURE 28-2   Papular urticaria: multiple insect bites   A 58-year-old male with HIV/AIDS with pruritic lesions on legs, appearing during a vacation to Puerto Rico. Multiple red papules on the lower legs. In HIV/AIDS, large reactions to insect bites can occur. In this case, the insect was not known. Papules and nodules persisted for months.

FIGURE 28-3   Papular urticaria: bedbug bites   A 77-year-old female with pruritic lesions on the neck. Excoriated papules on the posterior neck. Similar lesions were also present on the leg. Bedbugs (*Cimex lectularius*) share human domains, residing in crevices of floors and walls, in beddings, and in furniture. They usually feed only once a week and less often in cold weather. Bedbugs can travel long distances in search of a human host and can survive for 6 to 12 months without feeding. Bite reactions occur on exposed sites such as the face, neck, arms, and hands, with two to three lesions in a row ("breakfast, lunch, dinner"). In previously unexposed individuals, bite sites appear as erythematous, pruritic macules. In sensitized individuals, intensely pruritic papules, papular urticaria, or vesicles/bullae may arise at the bite sites. Changes secondary to scratching include excoriations, eczematous dermatitis, and secondary infections.

FIGURE 28-4   Papular urticaria: mites   Multiple papular urticaria at bite sites of mite *Trombicula* in the bathing trunk area. Mites fall off vegetation into clothing; multiple bites are often followed by papular urticarial reactions.

FIGURE 28-5   Insect bites: Ecchymotic lesions
A 47-year-old female with pruritic lesions on the legs. Multiple large ecchymotic lesions on the leg. The central portion appears urticarial, the peripheral area ecchymotic. Ecchymoses were not secondary to excoriation but were a manifestation of hypersensitivity.

FIGURE 28-6   Dermacentor variabilis feeding
The tick has been attached for 64 h; it is the vector of Rocky Mountain spotted fever.

- Hard *Ixodes* tick: *Erythema migrans* occurs as an enlarging plaque occurring at site of bite, characteristic of Lyme borreliosis (see Section 24); *lymphocytoma cutis* also occurs at tick bite sites.

Spiders

- *Brown recluse* and *black widow spider* bites can result in mild local urticarial reactions to full-thickness skin necrosis.
- Associated with a maculopapular exanthem, fever, headache, malaise, arthralgia, nausea/vomiting.

Diptera

- *Mosquitoes*: Bites usually present as papular urticaria on exposed sites; reactions can be urticarial, eczematous, or granulomatous.
- *Black flies*: Anesthetic is injected, resulting in painless initial bite; may subsequently become painful with itching, erythema, and edema. Black fly fever characterized by fever, nausea, generalized lymphadenitis.
- *Midges*: Bites produce immediate pain with erythema at bite site with 2- to 3-mm papulovesicles, followed by indurated nodules (up to 1 cm) persisting for many months.
- *Tabandae*: Bites painful with papular urticaria; rarely associated anaphylaxis.

- *Botfly*: Larvae penetrate skin or are deposited on open wounds producing *cutaneous myiasis*. Larvae may be fixed or migrate, resembling larva migrans. *C. americana* most common in United States.
- *D. hominis* in tropical regions causes furuncular myiasis, painful lesions that resemble pyogenic granuloma or abscess; a pruritic papule develops at the site, slowly enlarging over several weeks into a domed nodule (resembles a furuncle) with a central pore (Fig. 28-7) through which the posterior end of the larvae intermittently protrudes.
- *House flies*: Larvae deposited into any exposed skin site (ear, nose, paranasal sinuses, mouth, eye, anus, and vagina) or at any wound site (leg ulcers, ulcerated squamous and basal cell carcinomas, hematomas, umbilical stump) and grow into *maggots*, which can be seen on surface of wound (Fig. 28-8); although repulsive for the patient, maggots are very effective at debriding nonviable tissue and debris.

Hemiptera

- *Bedbug* bites produce papular urticaria that have a characteristic linear or grouped array (Fig. 28-3).
- *Reduvid (kissing bugs, assassin bugs, conenosed bugs)* bites usually present as papular urticaria;

FIGURE 28-7   Furuncular myiasis   A pruritic papule at the site of deposition of a botfly larva, slowly enlarging over several weeks into a domed nodule (resembles a furuncle). The lesion has a central pore through which the posterior end of the larva intermittently protrudes and thus respires. The larva (inset) can be induced to exit the lesion by occluding it with petrolatum or fat.

severe reactions can produce necrosis and ulceration resembling spider bites.

Fleas

• Papular pruritic urticaria at exposed bite site.
• *Tunga penetrans*: Tungiasis: Papule or vesicle
  (6–8 mm in diameter) with central black
  dot produced by posterior part of the flea's
  abdominal segments. As eggs mature and abdomen swells, papule becomes a white, pea-
  sized nodule. With intralesional hemorrhage,
  it becomes black (Fig. 28-9). With severe infestation, nodules and plaques with a honey-
  combed appearance. If lesions are squeezed,
  eggs, feces, and internal organs are extruded
  through pore. Ulceration, inflammation and

FIGURE 28-8   Wound myiasis   Multiple larvae or maggots of the housefly are seen in a chronic stasis ulcer on the ankle. The leg had been treated with Castellani paint and Unna boot for 1 week. When the dressing was removed, the maggots were visible; the base of the ulcer was red and clean, having been debrided by the maggots.

FIGURE 28-9   Tungiasis   A necrotic, periungual papule with surrounding erythema on the lateral margin of the fifth toe; the larva is visualized by removing the overlying crust.

secondary infection can occur. Sites: feet, especially under toenails, between toes, plantar aspect of the feet, sparing weight-bearing areas; in sunbathers, any area of exposed skin.

Hymenoptera

- Female bee, hornet, or wasp from modified ovipositor (stinger apparatus) sting producing immediate burning/pain, followed by intense, local, erythematous reaction with swelling and urticaria. Severe systemic reactions occur in individuals who are sensitized (0.4–0.8%), with angioedema/generalized urticaria and/or respiratory insufficiency from laryngeal edema or bronchospasm and/or shock.
- *Fire and harvester ants* produce local skin necrosis and systemic reactions to sting; bite reaction begins as an intense local inflammatory reaction that evolves to a sterile pustule.

Lepidoptera

- *Caterpillar/moth* contact can produce burning/itching sensation, papular urticaria, irritation due to histamine release, allergic contact dermatitis (Fig. 28-10), and/or systemic reactions. Wind-borne hairs can cause keratoconjunctivitis.

Systemic Findings   Systemic findings may occur associated with toxin or allergy to substance injected during bite. Many varied systemic infections can be injected during bite.

DIFFERENTIAL DIAGNOSIS

Bite Site Reactions (Erythematous Papules, Blisters)   Allergic contact dermatitis, especially to plants such as poison ivy or poison oak.
Furuncular Myiasis/Tungiasis   *Staphylococcus aureus* paronychia, *Candida* paronychia, cercarial dermatitis, scabies, fire ant bite, folliculitis.
Cutaneous Necrosis   Necrotizing soft tissue infection, vascular insufficiency, adverse cutaneous drug reaction.

LABORATORY EXAMINATIONS

Dermatopathology   *Arthropod Parts*   Arthropods such as *S. scabiei* or *T. penetrans* that burrow into the epidermis; fragments of the insect, feces, or eggs can be seen. Retained mouth parts can been seen in the skin months after the bite.
Bite Site Reactions

- In acute phase, variable epidermal necrosis, spongiosis, parakeratosis with plasma exudate; dermal inflammatory infiltrate extends into deep dermis in a wedge-shaped pattern, surrounding vessels with some extension into dermal collagen. The dermal infiltrate is mixed, composed of eosinophils, neutrophils, lymphocytes, and histiocytes. Eosinophils are usually prominent; neutrophils may predominate in reactions to fleas, mosquitoes, fire ants, and brown recluse spiders. Bullae form secondary to marked edema. Insect parts are rarely seen except in scabies and in tick bites where removal is incomplete.
- In chronic phase, lesions result from retained arthropod parts or hypersensitivity. Chronic lesions can appear as a *pseudolymphoma*.

Infection at Bite Site   The pathogen can be demonstrated in the lesional biopsy specimen by special stains.

- *Leishmania* at sandfly bite site.
- *Borrelia burgdorferi* at *Ixodes* tick bite site.

Bacterial Culture   Rule out secondary infection with *S. aureus* or GAS. Rule out systemic infection.
Serology   Rule out systemic infection.

DIAGNOSIS

Clinical diagnosis, at times confirmed by lesional biopsy.

COURSE AND PROGNOSIS

- Excoriation of CRAB commonly results in secondary infection of the eroded epidermis by GAS and/or *S. aureus* causing impetigo or ecthyma. This is especially common in humid tropical climates.
- Streptococcal skin infections are, at times, complicated by glomerulonephritis.
- Less common is secondary infection with *Corynebacterium diphtheriae*, with resultant cutaneous diphtheria (see page 637).

MANAGEMENT

Prevention

- Avoid contact with arthropods.
- Apply insect repellent such as diethyltoluamide (DEET) to skin.
- Apply permethrin spray [Permanone (United States)] to clothing.

FIGURE 28-10   Immunologic IgE-mediated contact urticaria: pine processionary caterpillar   Linear edematous papules and vesicles occurred on the exposed arm shortly after exposure to *Thaumetopoea pitycampain* in a pine forest.

- Use passive measures such as screens, nets, clothing.
- Treat flea-infested cats and dogs; spray household with insecticides (e.g., malathion, 1–4% dust) with special attention to baseboards, rugs, floors, upholstered furniture, bed frames, mattresses, and cellar.

Larvae in Skin

- *Tungiasis*: remove flea with needle, scalpel, or curette, attempting to remove all flea parts; oral thiabendazole (25 mg/kg per day) or albendazole (400 mg/d for 3 days) effective for heavy infestations.
- *Furuncular myiasis*: suffocate larvae by covering the larvae with petrolatum; remove the following day when dead.
- Oral ivermectin has been used as primary prophylaxis in animals.

Glucocorticoids

- Potent topical glucocorticoids given for a short time are helpful for intensely pruritic lesions.
- In some cases, a short tapered course of oral glucocorticoids can be given for extensive CRAB that are persistent.

Antimicrobial Agents *Secondary Infection* Antibiotic treatment with topical agents such as mupirocin ointment or antistaphylococcal/antistreptococcal agents if secondary infection is present.

Systemic Infection/Infestation Treat with appropriate antimicrobial agent.

PEDICULOSIS   ICD-9 : 132.9 ∘ ICD-10 : B85.2   ■ ○→◑

- ■ Pediculosis is an infestation of sucking lice that lay their eggs on hair shafts or in seams of clothing.
- ■ Two species of bloodsucking lice have evolved to be obligate ectoparasites of humans:
  - ▪ *Pediculus humanus*; variants of single species:
    - • *P. humanus* var. *capitis*: head louse
    - • *P. humanus* var. *humanus*: body louse
  - ▪ *Pthirius pubis*.

- ■ The two variants of *Pediculus* are similar morphologically but distinct in ecologic niches on the body and the clinical manifestations of infestation.
  - ▪ Head louse
  - ▪ Body louse (may have evolved from the head louse after humans began to wear clothes).

EPIDEMIOLOGY AND ETIOLOGY

Etiologic Agents

- Lice are 1–3 mm long, are flattened dorsoventrally, and have three pairs of legs that end in powerful claws of a diameter adapted to the region colonized.
- The female lives for 1–3 months; the head louse dies in <24 h when separated from the host.
- A female louse lays up to 300 eggs (nits) during her lifetime.
- Nits are <1 mm in diameter and, when viable, are opalescent. Nits are deposited on hair shafts emerging from the skin and hatch 6–10 days after laying, giving rise to nymphs that become adults in 10 days.
- Empty egg cases remain on the hair shaft after hatching; demonstration of empty egg cases distant from the skin is not diagnostic of active infestation.

Incidence   Hundreds of millions of cases worldwide annually.

Transmission

- Direct contact between individuals.
- Indirect contact with bedding, brushes, or clothing, according to species.
- Pediculosis and scabies may coexist in the same individual.

Secondary Infections of Excoriated Sites

- Excoriation may become secondarily infected with *S. aureus*, GAS.
- Infection can extend, resulting in cellulitis, lymphangitis, and/or bacteremia.

CLINICAL MANIFESTATIONS

Pruritus occurs in a variable proportion. Excoriations can become secondarily infected.

MANAGEMENT

Topically Applied Insecticides   Ideally, should have 100% activity against louse and egg.

- Malathion kills all lice after 5 min of exposure, and >95% of eggs fail to hatch after 10 min of exposure.
- Permethrin are synthetic pyrethoids widely used as insecticide, araricide, and insect repellant.

Lotion preparations are preferred; creams, foams, gels are also available.

Recommended Regimen

- *Permethrin*
  - ∘ *Nix*: Over-the-counter 1% product
  - ∘ *Elimite*: 5% product by prescription.
  - ∘ Product applied to infested area(s) and washed off after 10 min. Incubation period of louse eggs is 6–10 days; reapply in 7–14 days.

- *Pyrethrin* and *piperonyl butoxide* (PBO): Pyrethrins derived from extract of chrysanthemums. PBO is a synergist of pyrethrin. Kills mites louse and egg. Preparations: liquid, gels, shampoos.
- *Malathion*: 0.5% in 78% isopropyl alcohol (*Ovide*). Applied to involved site for 8–12 h; binds to hair providing residual protection. Indicated in lindane-resistant cases. Should not be used in children younger than 6 months.

Alternative Regimen

- *Pyrethrins with PBO*: Applied to scalp and washed off after 10 min.
- *Lindane 1% shampoo*: Applied for 4 min and then thoroughly washed off. (Not recommended for pregnant or lactating women.) Not totally ovicidal and lacks residual activity; in that the incubation period of louse eggs is 6–10 days, the agents should be reapplied in

7–14 days. Re-treatment may be necessary if lice are found or eggs are observed at the hair-skin junction.
- *Ivermectin*: 0.8% lotion or shampoo.

Systemic Therapy   *Oral ivermectin*: 200 μg/kg; repeat on day 10 to kill emerging nymphs.

Acquired Resistance to Insecticides   Occurs worldwide, mainly to pyrethrins and pyrethroids; also to malathion. If resistance is suspected, an alternative agent should be used. Other alternatives include newer insecticides and oral ivermectin in cases of resistance to both pyrethroids and malathion.

PEDICULOSIS CAPITIS

- An infestation of the scalp by the head louse
- Feeds on scalp and neck and deposits its eggs on hair.

- Presence of head lice is associated with few symptoms but much consternation.

EPIDEMIOLOGY AND ETIOLOGY

Etiology

- The subspecies *Pediculus humanus capitis*
- Sesame seed size, 1–2 mm.
- Feed every 4–6 h.
- Move by grasping hairs close to scalp; can crawl up to 23 cm/day.
- Lice lay nits within 1–2 mm of scalp.
- Nits are ova within chitinous case. Young lice hatch within 1 week, passing through nymphal stages, growing larger and maturing to adults over a period of 1 week.
- One female can lay 50–150 ova during a 16-day lifetime. Survive only for a few hours off scalp.

Vector of Infection   Head louse is not a vector of infectious disease.

Sex, Age of Onset   Girls > boys. 3–11 years, but all ages.

Predisposing Factors   School-age children and their mothers. More common in warmer months.

Race

- In United States, more common in whites than blacks; claws have adapted to grip cylindrical hair; hair pomade may inhibit infestation.
- In Africa, pediculosis capitis is relatively uncommon; however, lice easily grip non-cylindrical hair.

Transmission

- Head-to-head contact.
- Shared hats, caps, brushes, combs; theater seats; pillows.

- Epidemics in schools; classrooms are the main source of infestations.
- Head lice can survive off the scalp for up to 55 h.

Incidence   Most common pediculosis. Estimated that 6–12 million persons in the United States are infested annually. Bordeaux, France: up to 49% of schoolchildren. Jerusalem, Israel: 20% in 1991. Bristol, UK: 25% in 1998. Ilorin, Nigeria: 3.7% in 1987.

CLINICAL MANIFESTATION

Skin Symptoms

- Pruritus of the back and sides of scalp.
- Scratching and secondary infection associated with occipital and/or cervical lymphadenopathy.

Psychiatric Symptoms   Some individuals exhibit obsessive compulsive disorder or delusions of parasitosis after eradications of lice and nits.

Skin Findings

Infestation

- *Head lice* are identified by eye or with hand lens but are difficult to find (Fig. 28-11*A*).
- Most patients have a population of <10 head lice.
- Nits are the oval grayish-white egg capsules (1 mm long) firmly cemented to the hairs (Fig. 28-11*B*); vary in number from only a few to thousands.
- Nits are deposited by head lice on the hair shaft as it emerges from the follicle. With

recent infestation, nits are near the scalp; with infestation of long standing, nits may be 10–15 cm from the scalp.

- In that scalp hair grows 0.5 mm daily, the presence of nits 15 cm from the scalp indicates that the infestation is approximately 9 months old.
- New viable eggs have a creamy-yellow color; empty eggshells are white.
- *Sites of predilection*: Head lice nearly always confined to scalp, especially occipital and postauricular regions. Rarely, head lice infest beard or other hairy sites. Although more common with crab lice, head lice can also infest the eyelashes (*pediculosis palpebrarum*).

Skin Lesions

- *Bite reactions* at site of louse bites apparent on neck. Phases related to immune sensitivity/tolerance:
  ◦ Phase I: no clinical symptoms.
  ◦ Phase II: papular urticaria with moderate pruritus.
  ◦ Phase III: wheals immediately following bite with subsequent delayed papules/intense itching.
  ◦ Phase IV: smaller papules with mild pruritus.
- *Eczema, excoriation, lichen simplex chronicus* on occipital scalp and neck secondary to chronic scratching/rubbing.
- *Secondary impetiginization* with *S. aureus* of eczema or excoriations; may extend onto neck, forehead, face, ears.
- *Confluent, purulent mass* of matted hair, lice, nits, crusts, and purulent exudation in extreme cases.
- *Pediculid* is a hypersensitivity rash, resembling a viral exanthem.
- *Wood lamp*: Live nits fluoresce with a pearly fluorescence; dead nits do not.

Regional Lymph Nodes Postoccipital lymphadenopathy secondary to impetiginization of excoriated sites.

DIFFERENTIAL DIAGNOSIS

Small White Hair "Beads" Hair casts (inner root sheath remnants), hair lacquer, hair gels, dandruff (epidermal scales), black piedra (*Trichosporon ovoides*), white piedra (*T. inkin*)
Scalp Pruritus Impetigo, lichen simplex chronicus.
No Infestation Delusions of parasitosis.

LABORATORY EXAMINATIONS

Microscopy The louse or a nit on a hair shaft (Fig. 28-11*B*) can be examined to confirm the gross examination of the scalp and hair.
Nits 0.5-mm oval, whitish eggs. Nonviable nits show an absence of an embryo or operulum.
Louse Insect with six legs, 1–2 mm in length, wingless, translucent grayish-white body that is red when engorged with blood.
Culture If impetiginization is suspected, bacterial cultures should be obtained.

DIAGNOSIS

Clinical findings, confirmed by detection of lice. Louse comb increases chances of finding lice. Nits alone are not diagnostic of active infestation. Nits within 4 mm of scalp suggests active infestation.

MANAGEMENT

Fomite/Environmental Control

- Avoid contact with possibly contaminated items such as hats, headsets, clothing, towels, combs, hair brushes, bedding, upholstery.
- The environment should be vacuumed.
- Bedding, clothing, and head gear should be washed and dried on the hot cycle of a dryer.
- Combs and brushes should be soaked in rubbing alcohol or Lysol 2% solution for 1 h.
- Families should look for lice routinely. Many schools in the United States adhere to a "no-nit" policy before children can return after infestation.

Pediculocide Therapy See "Management," page 860.
Causes of Therapeutic Failure Misunderstanding of instructions; noncompliance; inappropriate instructions on head-lice products or from health professionals; high cost of products; misdiagnosis; psychogenic itch; incomplete ovicidal activity; inappropriate preparation (e.g., shampoo); insufficient dose-time, frequency, and/or quantity of product applied; failure to re-treat; reinfestation; live eggs not removed; acquired resistance to insecticides.
Removal of Nits After treatment and neutral shampoo, the hair is wet-combed with a fine-toothed comb to remove nits. Complete nit removal depends on comb structure, duration/technique of combing, and thoroughness.

A

FIGURE 28-11   Pediculosis capitis: multiple nits on scalp hair   _A._ Arrows: grayish-white egg capsules (nits) are firmly attached to the hair shafts, visualized with a lens. On close examination these have a bottle shape. **_B._** Under a microscope, an egg with a developing head louse, attached to a hair shaft, is seen.

B

Overnight application of petroleum jelly or HairClean 1-2-3 may facilitate removal of nits. **Pediculosis Palpebrarum** Apply petrolatum to lashes twice daily for 8 days, followed by removal of nits, _or_ physostigmine ophthalmic preparations applied twice daily for 1 or 2 days. (Eyelash infestation common with pubic lice.) **Secondary Bacterial Infection** Should be treated with appropriate doses of oral antimicrobial agent.

PEDICULOSIS CORPORIS   ⬛➔⬛ ○➔◑

- In body louse infestations, lice reside and lay eggs in clothing.
- Leave clothing to feed on human host.
- Body louse survive more than a few hours away from the human host.
- Occurs in poor socioeconomic conditions.
- Body lice are vectors of many systemic infections.

EPIDEMIOLOGY AND ETIOLOGY

Etiologic Agent

- _Pediculus humanus humanus._ Larger than head louse: 2–4 mm; otherwise indistinguishable.
- Life span 18 days. Female lays 270–300 ova. Nits: ova within chitinous case. Nits incubate for 8–10 days; nymphs mature to adults in 14 days.
- Habitat: live in seams of clothing; can survive without blood meal for up to 3 days. Grab body hairs to feed.

Risk Factors Poor socioeconomic conditions, when clothing is not changed or washed frequently: poverty, war, natural disasters, indigence, homelessness, refugee-camp populations.

Body Lice as Vectors of Disease Body lice transmit many infectious agents while feeding.

- *Bartonella quintana* causes *trench fever* (fever, myalgias, headache, meningoencephalitis, chronic lymphadenopathy, transient maculopapular eruption) and endocarditis. In United States, 15% of homeless persons tested had *B. quintana* bacteremia. *B. quintana* transmitted by fleas causes cat-scratch disease or bacillary angiomatosis.
- *Rickettsia prowazekii* causes *epidemic typhus*, characterized by fever, headache, rash, confusion. Large outbreaks (1995–1997) in Burundi, first affecting prison inmates, then >45,000 camp refugees. Small outbreak occurred in Russia in 1998. *Brill-Zinsser disease (louse-borne relapsing fever)* is recrudescence of epidemic typhus fever occurring in mild forms years after primary infection.

Skin Findings
Infestation

- Lice and nits are found in clothing seams (Fig. 28-12).
- Lice grab on to body hairs to feed.

Reactions to Bites

- Bite reactions identical to those of head lice (see page 860).
- Eczema, excoriation, lichen simplex, secondary impetiginization, postinflammatory hyperpigmentation (Fig. 28-12).
- Clothing may be stained with louse feeds, blood/serum.
- Scabies, pediculosis corporis, and *Pulex irritans* (the human flea) can coexist. 🔏

FIGURE 28-12 Pediculosis corporis   Severely malnourished, ill-kept, homeless male with multiple excoriations, erosions and crusted papules, and nodules and eczematized lesions. Lice and nits are seen in the seams of clothing (inset).

DIFFERENTIAL DIAGNOSIS

Atopic dermatitis, contact dermatitis, scabies, adverse cutaneous drug reaction.

DIAGNOSIS

Lice and eggs are found in clothing seams.

MANAGEMENT

Bedding and clothing must be systematically decontaminated.

Hygiene Measures Basic sanitation measures, and hygiene measures to assure changes of clean clothing, body washing, and sometimes shaving.

Delousing

- *Pyrethrins/pyrethroids* or *malathion* for 8–24 h is recommended in some cases.
- Outbreaks necessitate delousing of individuals with *1% permethrin dusting powder*.

Louse-Borne Infections Antibiotics are indicated if louse-borne infectious disease (trench fever, epidemic typhus) exists.

PEDICULOSIS PUBIS (PTHIRIASIS)   ■ ○→◑

- ■ Sexually transmitted disease.
- ■ Pediculosis pubis is an infestation of hair-bearing regions:
  - Most commonly the pubic area
  - Hairy parts of the chest and axillae
  - Upper eyelashes.
- ■ Manifested clinically by mild to moderate pruritus, papular urticaria, and excoriations.

Synonyms: Crabs, crab lice, pubic lice

EPIDEMIOLOGY

Age of Onset Most common in young adults; range, from childhood to senescence.
Sex More extensive infestation in males.
Etiologic Agent

- *Phthirius pubis*, the crab or pubic louse. Size 0.8–1.2 mm.
- First pair of legs vestigial; other two clawed.
- Life span 14 days.
- Female lays 25 ova. Nits incubate for 7 days; nymphs mature over 14 days.
- Mobility: adults can crawl 10 cm/day. Prefer a humid environment; tend not to wander.

Transmission

- Close physical contact: sharing bed; possibly exchange of towels.
- Sexual exposure. May coexist with another sexually transmitted infection (STI).
- Nonsexual transmission: homeless persons who have pubic lice in hair on head and back.

CLINICAL MANIFESTATION

Skin Symptoms

- Often asymptomatic.
- Mild to moderate pruritus for months.
- Patient may detect a nodularity to hairs (nits or eggs) while scratching.
- With excoriation and secondary infection, lesions may become tender and be associated with enlarged regional, e.g., inguinal, lymph node.

Skin Findings
Infestation

- *Lice* appear as 1- to 2-mm, brownish-gray specks (Figs. 28-13, 28-14) in hairy areas involved. Remain stationary for days; mouth parts embedded in skin; claws grasping a hair on either side. Usually few in number.
- *Nits* attached to hair appear as tiny white-gray specks (Fig. 28-14). Few to numerous. Eggs at hair-skin junction indicate active infestation.

Skin Lesions

- *Papular urticaria* (small erythematous papules) at sites of feeding, especially periumbilical (Fig. 28-15); blisters.
- Secondary changes of *lichenification, excoriations*.

- *Secondary infection* detected in patients with significant pruritus.
- *Maculae ceruleae* (*taches bleues*) are slate-gray or bluish-gray macules 0.5–1 cm in diameter, irregular in shape, nonblanching. Pigment thought to be breakdown product of heme affected by louse saliva.
- *Eyelash infestation*: Serous crusts may be present along with lice and nits (Fig. 29-14); occasionally, edema of eyelids with severe infestation.
- *Distribution*
  - Most common in pubic and axillary areas; also, perineum, thighs, lower legs, trunk, periumbilical (Fig. 28-15).
  - In hairy males: nipple areas, upper arms, rarely wrists; rarely, beard and moustache area.
  - In children, eyelashes (Fig. 28-14) and eyebrows may be infested without pubic involvement.
  - Maculae cerulea most common on lower abdominal wall, buttocks, upper thighs. ✏

General Findings With secondary impetiginization, regional lymphadenopathy.

DIFFERENTIAL DIAGNOSIS

Infestation Trichomycosis pubis, white piedra.
Pruritic Dermatosis Atopic dermatitis, seborrheic dermatitis, tinea cruris, folliculitis, molluscum contagiosum, scabies.

LABORATORY EXAMINATIONS

Microscopy Lice (Fig. 29-11*B*) and nits may be identified and differentiated from head/body louse with hand lens or microscope.
Cultures Bacterial cultures if excoriation impetiginized.
Serology Sexually transmitted. Testing for other STIs may be indicated in some individuals.

DIAGNOSIS

Demonstration of live adult lice, nymphs, or nits in pubic area to diagnose active infestation.

COURSE AND PROGNOSIS

- Patients should be evaluated after 1 week if symptoms persist.
- Re-treatment may be necessary if lice are found or if eggs are observed at hair-skin junction.
- Patients not responding to one regimen should be re-treated with an alternative.

MANAGEMENT

Prevention Patient and sexual partners should be treated.

A

B

**FIGURE 28-13   Pediculosis pubis: crab louse in pubis   *A.* A crab louse (arrow) on the skin in the pubic region. *B.* Adult female crab louse containing an egg suspended in mineral oil.

Screening for STIs

- 30% of persons with crab lice have another concurrent STI.
- Screen for HIV/AIDS disease, syphilis, gonorrhea, *Chlamydia* infection, herpes simplex, human papilloma virus infection, trichomoniasis, scabies.

Topical Insecticides   Hair of head/beard should be treated as well as pubic, axillary, and other body hair.

Pediculocides   See "Management," page 860.

Infestation of Eyelids   1% permethrin or vaseline if infestation is present.

Decontamination of Environment   Bedding and clothing should be decontaminated (machine-washed or machine-dried using heat cycle or dry-cleaned) or removed from body contact for at least 72 h.

Management of Sex Partner(s)   Sex partners within last month should be treated. Screening for other STIs may be indicated.

FIGURE 28-14   Pediculosis pubis: crab lice in eyelashes of a child   Crab lice (arrows) and nits on the upper eyelashes of a child; this was the only site of infestation.

FIGURE 28-15   Pediculosis pubis: papular urticaria   At this magnification only inflammatory papules (sites of crab lice bites), which are extremely pruritic, are seen on the abdomen and the inner aspects of the thighs. Closer examination reveals nits on the pubic hairs.

MITE BITES AND INFESTATIONS ■ ○

- Mites inhabit many environments including human skin.
- Environmental and animal mites can bite humans and then fall off; they do not reside or reproduce on human skin.
- Environmental mites:
  - Food mites: Cheese, grain, mold mites can cause mild contact dermatitis: baker's or grocer's itch.
  - Straw mites: Bites occur during harvest season causing dermatitis; straw itch.
  - Harvest mites: Chiggers. Bites can cause dermatitis. One species transmits *Rickettsia tsutsugamushi*, the cause of scrub typhus.
  - Dust mites: Feed on shed skin. Bodies and excreta may have a role in asthma and other allergies.
- Animal mites:
  - Fowl mites. Chicken, pigeons, etc. Bites cause papular urticaria on exposed sites.
  - Rat mites cause painful bites and dermatitis and transmit endemic/murine typhus. House mouse mite is the vector for rickettsialpox.

- *Cheyletiella* spp. (dog and cat mites) bite pet owners causing pruritic lesions on forearms, chest, abdomen.
- Canine sarcoptic mange (*Sarcoptes scabei* var. *canis*) and feline mange (*Notoedres cati*) cause a pruritic dermatosis in pet owners.
- Human mites
  - *Demodex* spp. Inhabits human hair follicle of face, scalp, upper chest. Site of habitation usually symptomatic. In some cases causes an inflammatory reaction (demodecidosis) with lesions resembling rosacea, suppurative folliculitis, or perioral dermatitis.
    - *Demodex folliculorum humanus*: Normal inhabitant of human hair follicle. Can cause rosacea-like facial lesions (demodecidosis).
    - *Demodex brevis*: Normal inhabitant of human infundibulum of sebaceous gland.
- *Sarcoptes scabiei*: causes scabies (see "Scabies," below).

SCABIES   ICD-9 : 133.0 ○ ICD-10 : B86 ■ ◑

- Scabies is a superficial epidermal infestation by the mite *Sarcoptes scabiei* var. *hominis*.
- Transmission: Usually spread by skin-to-skin contact; fomites.
- Manifestations:
  - Generalized intractable pruritus
  - Often with minimal cutaneous findings. Burrows under stratum corneum. Scabetic nodules. Eczematous dermatitis.

- The diagnosis may be easily missed and should be considered in a patient of any age with persistent generalized severe pruritus.

Synonym: Chronic undiagnosed scabies is the basis for the colloquial expression, "the 7-year itch." Hyperinfestation: crusted or hyperkeratotic or Norwegian scabies.

EPIDEMIOLOGY AND ETIOLOGY

Etiologic Agent

- *S. scabiei* var. *hominis*. Thrive and multiply only on human skin, i.e., obligate human parasite.
- Mites of all developmental stages burrow/tunnel into epidermis shortly after contact, no deeper than stratum granulosum; deposit feces in tunnels.
- Female lifespan 4–6 weeks; lays 40–50 eggs. Lays 3 eggs per day in tunnels; eggs hatch in 4 days. Burrow 2–3 mm daily, usually at night, and lay eggs during the day. Hatched larvae migrate to skin surface and mature into adults. Males and females copulate. Gravid female burrows back under stratum corneum; male falls off skin.
- Infestation;
  - Classic scabies: About a dozen females per patient are present.
  - *Hyperkeratotic* or *crusted scabies* (*Norwegian scabies*): >1 million mites may be present, or up to 4700 mites/g skin.

Incidence   Estimated at 300 million cases/year worldwide. In the past, epidemics occurred in cycles every 15 years; the latest epidemic began in the late 1960s but has continued to the present.

Age of Onset

- Children (often ≤5 years). Nodular scabies more common in children.
- Young adults (usually acquired by body contact).
- Elderly and bedridden patients; may be health care-associated in hospitals, chronic care facilities, nursing homes.

Demography

- Major public health problem in many less-developed countries.
- In some areas of South and Central America, prevalence is about 100%.
- In Bangladesh, the number of children with scabies exceeds that of children with diarrheal and upper-respiratory disease.
- In countries where human T cell leukemia/lymphoma virus (HTLV-I) infection is common, generalized crusted scabies is a marker of this infection, including cases of adult T cell leukemia/lymphoma.

Transmission

- Skin-to-skin contact: Mites transmitted by skin-to-skin contact as with sex partner, children playing, or health care workers providing care.
- Fomites: Mites can remain alive for >2 days on clothing or in bedding; hence, scabies can be acquired without skin-to-skin contact.
- Patients with crusted scabies shed many mites into their environment daily and pose a high risk of infecting those around them, including health care professionals.

Risk Factors   In nursing homes, risk factors include age of institution (>30 years), size of institution (>120 beds), ratio of beds to health care workers (>10:1).

PATHOGENESIS

- Hypersensitivity of both immediate and delayed types occurs in the development of lesions other than burrows. Infestation is usually by only approximately 10 mites.
- First infestation: For pruritus to occur, sensitization to *S. scabiei* must take place. Among

persons with their first infection, sensitization takes several weeks to develop.
- Reinfestation: After reinfestation, pruritus may occur within 24 h.
- Immunocompromised persons: Various immunocompromised states or individuals with neurologic disease predisposed to crusted or hyperkeratotic scabies. The number of infesting mites may be >1 million.

CLINICAL MANIFESTATIONS

- Patients are often aware of similar symptoms in family members or sexual partners.
- Persons with crusted scabies are often immunocompromised (HIV/AIDS, solid-organ transplant recipient) or have neurologic disorders (Down syndrome, dementia, strokes, spinal cord injury, neuropathy, leprosy).

Incubation Period   Onset of pruritus varies with immunity to the mite:

- First infestation, about 21 days
- Reinfestation, immediate, i.e., 1–3 days.

Duration of Lesions   Weeks to months unless treated. Crusted scabies may be present for years.

Skin Symptoms   *Pruritus*

- Intense, widespread, usually sparing head and neck.
- Itching often interferes with or prevents sleep.
- Often present in family members.
- One-half of patients with crusted scabies do not itch.

Rash

- Ranges from no rash to generalized erythroderma.
- Patients with atopic diathesis scratch, producing eczematous dermatitis.
- Some individuals experience pruritus for many months with no rash.
- Tenderness of lesions suggests secondary bacterial infection.

Skin Findings

- Common cutaneous findings can be classified:
  - Lesions occurring at the sites of mite infestation
  - Cutaneous manifestations of hypersensitivity to mites

- ° Lesions secondary to chronic rubbing and scratching
- ° Secondary infection.

- Variants of scabies in special hosts including those with an atopic diathesis, nodular scabies, scabies in infants/small children, scabies in the elderly, hyperkeratotic/crusted (Norwegian) scabies, scabies in HIV/AIDS disease, animal-transmitted scabies (zoonosis), scabies of the scalp, dyshidrosiform scabies, urticarial/vasculitis scabies, and bullous scabies.

Lesions at Site of Infestation
Intraepidermal Burrows

- Gray or skin-colored ridges, 0.5–1 cm in length (Figs. 28-16 to 28-18), either linear or wavy (serpiginous), with minute vesicle or papule at end of tunnel.
- Each infesting female mite produces one burrow. Mites are about 0.5 mm in length. Burrows average 5 mm in length but may be up to 10 cm.
- In persons with light colored skin, burrows have a whitish color with occasional dark specks (due to fecal scybala).
- Fountain-pen ink applied to infested skin concentrates in tunnels, highlighting and marking the burrow. Blind end of burrow where mite resides appears as a minute elevation with tiny halo of erythema or as a vesicle.
- *Distribution*: Areas with few or no hair follicles, usually where stratum corneum is thin and soft, i.e., interdigital webs of hands > wrists > shaft of penis > elbows > feet > genitalia > buttocks > axillae > elsewhere (Image 28-1). In infants, infestation may occur on head and neck. ✎

Scabietic (Scabious) Nodule

- Inflammatory papule or nodule (Fig. 28-19); burrow sometimes seen on the surface of a very early lesion.
- *Distribution*: Areola, axillae, scrotum, penis. ✎

Hyperkeratosis/Crusting Psoriasiform

- In areas of heavily infested crusted scabies, well-demarcated plaques covered by a very thick crust or scale (Figs. 29-20, 29-22).
- Warty dermatosis of hands/feet with nail bed hyperkeratosis.
- Erythematous scaling eruption on face, neck, scalp, trunk.
- *Distribution*: Most pronounced at intertriginous sites. ✎

Cutaneous Manifestations of Hypersensitivity to Mite
Pruritus   Some individuals experience only pruritus without any cutaneous findings.
"Id" or Autosensitization-Type Reactions Characterized by widespread small urticarial edematous papules mainly on anterior trunk, thighs, buttocks, and forearms.
Urticaria   Usually generalized.
Eczematous Dermatitis   At sites of heaviest infestation: hands, axillae (Figs. 28-16, 28-20).

Lesions Secondary to Chronic Rubbing and Scratching

- Excoriation, lichen simplex chronicus, prurigo nodules.
- Generalized eczematous dermatitis.
- Psoriasiform lesions. Erythroderma.

Atopy   In individuals with atopic diathesis, atopic dermatitis occurs at sites of excoriation, most commonly on the hands, webspaces of hands, wrists, axillae, areolae, waist, buttocks, penis, scrotum. In adults, the scalp, face, and upper back are usually spared; but in infants, the scalp, face, palms, and soles are involved.
Postinflammatory Hyper- and Hypopigmentation   Especially in more deeply pigmented individuals.

Secondary Infection

- Pathogens: *S. aureus*: Methicillin-sensitive *S. aureus* (MSSA) and Methicillin-resistant *S. aureus* (MRSA); GAS infection.
- Impetiginized excoriations (crusted, tender, surrounding erythema), ecthyma, folliculitis, abscess formation; lymphangitis, lymphadenitis; cellulitis; bacteremia, septicemia.
- MRSA is a major cause of secondary infection in scabies. ✎
- Acute poststreptococcal glomerulonephritis reported associated with streptococcal impetiginization.

Variants of Scabies in Special Hosts
Infants/Young Children

- Atypical lesions: vesicles, pustules, nodules; generalized; lesions concentrated on hands/feet/body folds.
- Head, palms, soles are not spared. Difficult to differentiate from infantile acropustulosis, which may be a postscabietic nonspecific reaction.

FIGURE 28-16   Scabies: webspace   Papules and burrows in typical location on the finger web. Burrows are tan or skin-colored ridges with linear configuration with a minute vesicle or papule at the end of the burrow; they are often difficult to define.

FIGURE 28-17   Scabies   Multiple, crusted, and excoriated papules and burrows on the penile shaft.

Elderly

- Altered inflammatory response may delay diagnosis.
- In bedridden patients, lesions may be concentrated on the back.
- Bullous scabies can mimic bullous pemphigoid.

Nodular Scabies

- Nodular lesions develop in 7–10% of patients with scabies.
- Nodules are 5–20 mm in diameter, red, pink, tan, or brown in color, smooth (Fig. 28-19).
- A burrow may be seen on the surface of early nodule.
- *Distribution*: Penis, scrotum, axillae, waist, buttocks, areolae (Image 28-1). Resolve with postinflammatory hyperpigmentation. May be more apparent after treatment, as eczematous eruption resolves. Upper back, lateral edge of foot (infants). Nodules are usually countable. 🔲

Crusted/Hyperkeratotic or Norwegian Scabies

- Predisposing factors: glucocorticoid therapy, Down's syndrome, HIV/AIDS disease, HTLV-I infection, organ transplant recipients, elderly.
- May begin as ordinary scabies.
- In others, clinical appearance is of chronic eczema, psoriasiform dermatitis (Fig. 28-20), seborrheic dermatitis, or erythroderma. Lesions often markedly hyperkeratotic and/or crusted.
- *Distribution*: Generalized (even involving head and neck in adults) or localized. Scale/crusts found on dorsal surface of hands, wrists, fingers, metacarpophalangeal joints, palms, extensor aspect of elbows, scalp, ears, soles, and toes. In patients with neurologic deficit, crusted scabies may occur only in affected limb. May be localized only to scalp, face, finger, toenail bed, or sole.

General Findings   Lymphadenopathy in some cases.

DIFFERENTIAL DIAGNOSIS

Pruritus, Localized or Generalized, Rash Adverse cutaneous drug reaction, atopic dermatitis, contact dermatitis, fiberglass dermatitis, dyshidrotic eczema, dermographism, physical urticaria, pityriasis rosea, dermatitis herpetiformis, animal scabies, pediculosis corporis, pediculosis pubis, lichen planus, delusions of parasitosis, metabolic pruritus.

Pyoderma   Impetigo, ecthyma, furunculosis.
Nodular Scabies   Urticaria pigmentosa (in young child), papular urticaria (insect bites), Darier disease, prurigo nodularis, secondary syphilis, pseudolymphoma, lymphomatoid papulosis, vasculitis.
Crusted Scabies   Psoriasis, eczematous dermatitis, seborrheic dermatitis, erythroderma, Langerhans cell histiocytosis.

LABORATORY EXAMINATIONS

Microscopy   *Finding the Mite*   Highest yield in identifying a mite is in typical burrows on the finger webs, flexor aspects of wrists, and penis. A drop of mineral oil is placed over a burrow, and the burrow is scraped off with a no. 15 scalpel blade and placed on a microscope slide.
Conventional Microscopy   A drop immersion of mineral oil is placed on the scraping, which is then covered by a coverslip. Three findings are diagnostic of scabies: *S. scabiei* mites, their eggs, and their fecal pellets (scybala) (Fig. 28-21).
Dermoscopy   Characteristic image of scabies, "jet-with-contrail" image.
Dermatopathology   *Scabietic burrow:* located within stratum corneum; female mite situated in blind end of burrow. Body round, 400 µm in length. Spongiosis near mite with vesicle formation common. Eggs also seen. Dermis shows infiltrate with eosinophils. *Scabietic nodules:* dense chronic inflammatory infiltrate with eosinophils. In some cases, persistent arthropod reaction resembling lymphoma with atypical mononuclear cells. *Crusted scabies:* thickened stratum corneum riddled with innumerable mites.
Hematology   Eosinophilia in crusted scabies.
Cultures   *S. aureus* and GAS cause secondary infection.

DIAGNOSIS

Clinical findings, confirmed, if possible, by microscopy (identification of mites, eggs, or mite feces). Sometimes when the mite cannot be demonstrated, a "therapeutic test" will clinch the diagnosis.

COURSE AND PROGNOSIS

Pruritus

- Often persists up to several weeks after successful eradication of mite infestation, understandable in that the pruritus is a hypersensitivity phenomenon to mite antigen(s).

FIGURE 28-18   Scabies   Papules and burrows on the lateral hand. In children, the feet and neck are often infested, sites usually spared in older individuals.

FIGURE 28-19   Scabetic nodules: penis, scrotum   Red-brown papules and nodules on the penis and scrotum; these lesions are pathognomonic for scabies, occurring at sites of infestation in some individuals.

- If reinfestation occurs, pruritus becomes symptomatic within a few days.
- Most cases resolve after recommended regimen of therapy.
- Glomerulonephritis has followed GAS secondary infection.
- Bacteremia and death have followed secondary *S. aureus* infection of crusted scabies in an HIV/AIDS-infected patient.
- Delusions of parasitosis can occur in individuals who have been successfully treated for scabies or have never had scabies.

Crusted Scabies   May be impossible to eradicate in untreated HIV/AIDS. Recurrence more likely to be relapse than reinfestation.

Nodular Scabies   In treated patients, 80% resolve in 3 months but may persist up to 1 year.

MANAGEMENT

Principles of Treatment

- Infested individuals and close physical contacts should be treated at the same time, whether or not symptoms are present.
- Topical agents are more effective after hydration of the skin, i.e., after bathing.

- Application should be to all skin sites, especially the groin, around nails, behind ears, including face and scalp.
- Sexual partners and close personal or household contacts within last month should be examined and treated prophylactically.

Scabicides

- Choice of scabicide based on effectiveness, potential toxicity, cost, extent of secondary eczematization, and age of patient.
- *Permethrin* is effective and safe but costs more than lindane.
- *Lindane* is effective in most areas of the world, but resistance has been reported. Seizures have occurred when lindane was applied after a bath or used by patients with extensive dermatitis. Aplastic anemia after lindane use was also reported.
- No controlled studies have confirmed that two applications are better than one.
- Clean clothing should be put on afterwards. Clothing and bedding are decontaminated by machine-washing at 60°C.
- Pruritus can persist for up to 1–2 weeks after the end of effective therapy. After that time, cause of persistent itching should be investigated.

Recommended Regimens

Permethrin 5% Cream Applied to all areas of the body from the neck down. Wash off 8–12 h after application. Adverse events very low.

Lindane (γ-Benzene Hexachloride) 1% Lotion or Cream Applied thinly to all areas of the body from the neck down; wash off thoroughly after 8 h. *Note*: Lindane should not be used after a bath or shower, and it should not be used by persons with extensive dermatitis, pregnant or lactating women, and children younger than 2 years. Mite resistance to lindane has developed in North, Central, and South America and Asia. Low cost makes lindane a key alternative in many countries.

Alternative Regimens

Crotamiton 10% Cream Applied thinly to the entire body from the neck down, nightly for 2 consecutive nights; wash off 24 h after second application.

Sulfur 2–10% in Petrolatum Applied to skin for 2–3 days.

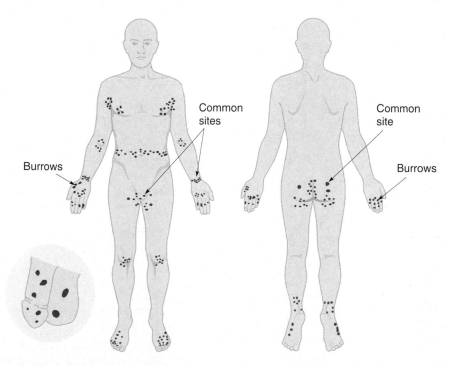

IMAGE 28-1   Scabies: Predilection sites   Burrows are most easy to identify on the webspace of the hands, wrists, lateral aspects of the palms. Scabietic nodules occur uncommonly, arising on the genitalia, especially the penis and scrotum, waist, axillae, and areolae.

FIGURE 28-20   Hyperkeratotic scabies A 79-year-old male with hyperkeratotic scabies for 4 years. The patient had been treated in his home with topical antiscabetic agents and oral ivermectin as well as extensive decontamination of his home on multiple occasions. Confluent hyperkeratotic plaques are seen on the back, buttocks, and legs. As many as five scabetic mites were seen on one microscope field (see insert).

FIGURE 28-21   Burrow with Sarcoptes scabiei (female), eggs, and feces   Female mite at the end of a burrow with eight eggs and smaller fecal particles obtained from a papule on the webspace of the hand.

Benzyl Benzoate 10% and 25% Lotions Several regimens are recommended: swabbing only once; two applications separated by 10 min, or two applications with a 24-h or 1-week interval. 24 h after application, preparation should be washed off and clothes and bedding changed. The compound is an irritant and can induce pruritic irritant dermatitis, especially on face and genitalia.

Benzyl Benzoate with Sulfiram Several regimens are recommended, swabbing only once:

Esdepallethrine 0.63%
Malathion 0.5% Lotion

Sulfiram 25% Lotion Can mimic effect of disulfiram; no alcoholic drinks should be consumed for at least 48 h.

Ivermectin 0.8% Lotion.

Systemic Ivermectin   Ivermectin, 200 μg/kg PO; single dose reported to be very effective for common as well as crusted scabies in 15–30 days. Two to three doses, separated by 1–2 weeks, usually required for heavy infestation or in immunocompromised individuals. May effectively eradicate epidemic or endemic scabies in institutions such as nursing homes, hospitals, and refugee camps. Not approved by U.S. Food and Drug Administration or European Drug Agency. Structurally similar to macrolide antibiotics.

Infants, Young Children, Pregnant/Lactating Women   Permethrin or crotamiton regimens or precipitated sulfur ointment should be used with application to all body areas. Lindane and ivermectin should not be used.

Crusted Scabies   *Scabicides*

- Lindane should be avoided because of risk of CNS toxicity.
- Multiple scabicide applications are required to all the skin.
- Treatment should also be directed at removing scale/crusts that protect mites from scabicide; nails should be trimmed.

- Oral ivermectin combined with topical therapy is most effective.
- Control of dissemination is essential and includes isolation of patient, avoidance of skin-to-skin contact, use of gloves/gowns by staff, prophylactic treatment of contacts (entire institution and visitors or family members).

Decontamination of Environment   Bedding, clothing, and towels should be decontaminated (machine washed or machine dried using heat cycle or dry-cleaned) or removed from body contact for at least 72 h. Thorough cleaning of patient's room or residence.

Treatment of Eczematous Dermatitis   *Antihistamines* Systemic sedating antihistamine such as hydroxyzine hydrochloride, doxepin, or diphenhydramine at bedtime.

Topical Glucocorticoid Ointment   Applied to areas of extensive dermatitis associated with scabies.

Systemic Glucocorticoids   Prednisone 70 mg, tapered over 1–2 weeks, gives symptomatic relief of severe hypersensitivity reaction.

Postscabietic Itching   Generalized itching that persists a week or more is probably caused by hypersensitivity to remaining dead mites and mite products. Nevertheless, a second treatment 7 days after the first is recommended by some physicians. For severe, persistent pruritus, especially in individuals with history of atopic disorders, a 14-day tapered course of prednisone (70 mg on day 1) is indicated.

Secondary Bacterial Infection   Treat with mupirocin ointment or systemic antimicrobial agent.

Scabietic Nodules

- May persist in association with pruritus for up to a year after eradication of infestation.
- Intralesional triamcinolone, 5–10 mg/mL into each lesion, is effective; repeat every 2 weeks if necessary.

CUTANEOUS LARVA MIGRANS (CLM)   ICD-9 : 126.9 ○ ICD-10 : B76

- A cutaneous infestation following percutaneous penetration and epidermal migration of larvae.
- Etiologic agent: Various nematode parasites.
- Manifestations:
  - Erythematous, serpiginous, papular, or vesicular linear lesions

- Shape of lesions indicates path of larvae in dermis.

Synonyms: Creeping eruption, creeping verminous dermatitis, sandworm eruption, plumber's itch, duckhunter's itch.

EPIDEMIOLOGY

Etiologic Agent   See Table 28-1
Cutaneous Larva Migrans

- *Ancylostoma braziliense* is most common cause in central and southeastern United States.
- Other penetrating nematode larvae: *A. caninum, Uncinaria stenocephala* (hookworm of European dogs), *Bunostomum phlebotomum* (hookworm of cattle).
- Ova of hookworms are deposited in sand and soil in warm, shady areas, hatching into larvae that penetrate human skin. Activities and occupations that pose risk include contact with sand/soil contaminated with animal feces: playing in sandbox, walking barefoot or sitting on beach, working in crawl spaces under houses, gardeners and plumbers, farmers, electricians, carpenters, pest exterminators.

Larva Currens   *Strongyloides stercoralis*: Filariform larvae can penetrate skin (usually on buttocks), producing similar lesions, i.e., *larva currens*.
Visceral Larva Migrans   Caused by *Toxocara canis, T. cati, A. lumbricoides*. Parasites enter via the GI tract and disseminate to viscera (heart and CNS) causing myocarditis and seizures; unable to reproduce in humans.
Other Migrating Cutaneous Parasitic Infestations

- Other parasites *(Gnathostoma spinigerum, Strongyloides procyonis, Dirofilaria repens, Fasciola hepatica).*
- Some forms of *myiasis* can cause migratory skin lesions.

Travel History   Most common imported ectoparasite in U.S. travelers returning to the United States after holiday.
Demographic Distribution   Endemic in deprived communities. Tropical and subtropical areas, especially southeastern United States, Caribbean, Africa, Central/South America, Southeast Asia.

PATHOGENESIS

- Humans are aberrant, dead-end hosts who acquire the parasite from environment contaminated with animal feces.
- Larvae remain viable in soil/sand for several weeks.
- Larvae penetrate human skin and migrate within the epidermis up to several centimeters a day.
- Parasite induces localized eosinophilic inflammatory reaction with edema, spongiosis, and vesicle formation.
- Most larvae are unable to develop further or invade deeper tissues and die after days or months.

TABLE 28-1   Helminthic Causes of Migratory Dermatologic Lesions

Infestation	Helminth(s)	Comments
Cutaneous larva migrans	Primarily *Ancylostoma braziliense* and *A. caninum*	Larvae of dog/cat hookworms
Dracunculiasis	*Dracunculus medinensis*	Movement of worm just below dermis before eruption
Fascioliasis	*Fasciola hepatica* and *F. gigantica*	Migratory areas of inflammation, especially with *F. gigantica*
Gnathostomiasis	*Gnathostoma spinigerum* and other *Gnathostoma* species	Migratory inflammatory lesions, 1 cm/h or faster when subcutaneous
Hookworm	*Ancylostoma duodenale, Necator americanus, A. ceylanicum*	Migratory inflammatory lesions
Loiasis	*Loa loa*	Migratory inflammatory swellings; worm may be visible crossing conjunctivae
Paragonimiasis	Primarily *Paragonimus westermani*	Subcutaneous migratory swelling or subcutaneous nodules
Spirometrosis (sparganosis)	*Spirometra erinacei, S. mansoni, S. mansonides, S. proliferum*	Subcutaneous nodules
Strongyloidiasis	*Strongyloides stercoralis*	Migratory, serpiginous lesions (larva currens), 5–10 cm/h

CLINICAL MANIFESTATIONS

Incubation Period   1–6 days from time of exposure to onset of symptoms.
Skin Symptoms   Local pruritus begins within hours after larval penetration.

Skin Lesions
Cutaneous Larva Migrans

- Serpiginous, thin, linear, raised, tunnel-like lesion 2–3 mm wide containing serous fluid (Fig. 28-22).
- Several or many lesions may be present, depending on the number of penetrating larvae.
- Larvae move a few to many millimeters daily, confined to an area several centimeters in diameter.
- *Distribution*: Exposed sites, most commonly the feet, lower legs, buttocks, hands. 🔁

Larva Currens (Cutaneous Strongyloidiasis)

- A distinctive form of larva migrans.
- Papules, urticaria, papulovesicles at the site of larval penetration (Fig. 28-23). Associated with intense pruritus.
- Occurs on skin around anus, buttocks, thighs, back, shoulders, abdomen.
- Pruritus and eruption disappear when larvae enter blood vessels and migrate to intestinal mucosa. 🔁

Systemic Findings   *Visceral Larva Migrans* Unrelated to cutaneous larva migrans. Children ingest embryonated eggs of dog or cat roundworm. Larvae disseminate to viscera with resultant seizures, myocarditis, encephalitis, and eye involvement. Characterized by persistent hypereosinophilia, hepatomegaly, and frequently pneumonitis (*Loeffler syndrome*). May be associated with urticaria.

DIFFERENTIAL DIAGNOSIS

Curvilinear Inflammatory Lesion   Larva currens, migratory lesions from other parasites, phytoallergic contact dermatitis, phytophotodermatitis, erythema migrans of Lyme borreliosis, jelly fish sting, bullous impetigo, epidermal dermatophytosis, granuloma annulare, scabies, loiasis.

LABORATORY EXAMINATIONS

Hematology   Peripheral eosinophilia.
Dermatopathology   Part of the parasite can be seen on biopsy specimens from the advancing point of the lesion(s).

DIAGNOSIS

Clinical findings.

COURSE

- Self-limited; humans are "dead-end" hosts.
- Most larvae die and the lesions resolve within 2–8 weeks; rarely, up to 2 years.

FIGURE 28-22   Cutaneous larva migrans: dorsum of foot   A 29-year-old male noted pruritic lesions on the dorsum of both feet after returning from vacation in Mexico. A serpiginous, linear, raised, tunnel-like erythematous lesion outlining the path of migration of the larva. Lesions were present bilaterally, arising in the 4–5 webspace at sites of tinea pedis. He was treated with ivermectin.

MANAGEMENT

Prevention   Avoid direct skin contact with fecally contaminated soil.

Symptomatic Therapy   Topical application of a glucocorticoid preparation under occlusion to lesion.

Anthelmintic Agents *Topical Agents* *Thiabendazole, ivermectin, albendazole* are effective topically.

Systemic Agents

- *Thiabendazole*, orally 50 mg/kg per day in two doses (maximum 3 g/d) for 2–5 days; also effective when applied topically under occlusion.
- *Ivermectin*, 6 mg twice daily.
- *Albendazole*, 400 mg/d for 3 days; highly effective.

Cryosurgery   Liquid nitrogen to advancing end of larval burrow.

Removal of Parasite   Do not attempt to extract; parasite not in visible lesion.

FIGURE 28-23   Larva currens   Multiple, pruritic, serpiginous, inflammatory lines on the buttocks at sites of penetration of *S. stercoralis* larvae.

WATER-ASSOCIATED INFECTIONS AND INFESTATIONS

- Various aquatic microorganisms can cause soft tissue infections after exposure:
  - Bacteria: *Aeromonas hydrophila, Edwardsiella tarda, Erysipelothrix rhusiopathiae, Mycobacterium marinum, Pfisteria piscicida, Pseudomonas* species, *Streptococcus iniae, Vibrio vulnificus,* other *Vibrio* species,
  - Alga: *Prototheca wickerhamii.*

- Localized cutaneous infestations, including cercarial dermatitis and seabather's eruption, can occur after exposure to microscopic marine animals (Table 28-2).
- Cnidaria (jellyfish) and Echinoderms (sea urchins, starfish) can cause envenomation.

TABLE 28-2   Comparison of Cercarial Dermatitis and Seabather's Eruption

Factor	Cercarial Dermatitis	Seabather's Eruption
Type of water	Fresh and salt	Salt
Body part involved	Uncovered	Covered and hairy areas
Geographic locale	Northern USA, Canada, Europe	Florida, Cuba
Etiology	Cercarial forms of schistosomes	Larval forms of marine coelenterates: *L. unquiculata, E. lineata*

CERCARIAL DERMATITIS   ICD-9 : 120.3 ∘ ICD-10 : B65.3

- Cercarial dermatitis (CD) is an acute pruritic papular eruption at the sites of cutaneous penetration by *Schistosoma cercariae* (larvae) of nonhuman schistosomes, whose usual hosts are birds and small mammals.

- Nonhuman schistosomes implicated: *Trichobilharzia, Gigantobilharzia, Ornithobilharzia, Microbilharzia, Schistosomatium.*

- Exposure can be to fresh, brackish, or salt water. Eggs produced by adult schistosomes living in animals are shed with animal feces into the environment; on reaching water, schistosome eggs hatch, releasing miracidia (fully developed larvae).

- Snails are the appropriate hosts for miracidia, from which they emerge as cercariae.

- These must penetrate the skin of a vertebrate host to continue development.

- Humans are dead-end hosts. Cercariae penetrate human skin, elicit an inflammatory response, and die without invading other tissues.

- CD occurs worldwide in areas with fresh and salt water inhabited by appropriate molluscan hosts.

- CD is acquired by skin exposure to fresh/salt water infested by cercariae.

- Clinical manifestations:

  - Pruritus and rash begin within hours after exposure.
  - A pruritic macular, papular, papulovesicular, and/or urticarial eruption develops at exposed sites with marked pruritus (Fig. 28-24), sparing parts of the body covered by clothing. (In contrast, seabather's eruption occurs on areas of the body covered by swimsuits.)
  - Papular urticaria occurs at each site of penetration in previously sensitized individuals.
  - In highly sensitized persons, lesions may progress to eczematous plaques, urticarial wheals, and/or vesicles, reaching a peak 2–3 days after exposure.

- Schistosomes capable of causing invasive disease in humans (*Schistosoma mansoni, S. haematobium, S. japonicum*) may cause a similar skin eruption shortly after penetration as well as late visceral complications. Lesions usually resolve within a week.

- Topical and/or systemic glucocorticoids may be indicated in more severe cases.

- CD has to be distinguished from seabather's eruption (Table 28-2).

Synonyms: Swimmer's itch, clam digger's itch, schistosome dermatitis, sedge pool itch ℮

SEABATHER'S ERUPTION   ICD-9 : 692.9

- Seabather's eruption is caused by exposure to two marine animals:
  - Larvae of the thimble jellyfish, *Linuche unquiculatum,* in waters off the coast of Florida and in the Caribbean
  - Planula larvae of the sea anemone, *E. lineata,* Long Island, NY.

- Nematocysts of coelenterate larvae sting the skin of hairy areas or under swimwear, presumably causing an allergic reaction. Some affected individuals recall a stinging or prickling sensation while in the water.

- Lesions present clinically as inflammatory papules 4–24 h after exposure. A monomorphous eruption of erythematous papules or papulovesicles

is seen most commonly: vesicles, pustules, and papular urticaria, which may progress to crusted erosions.

- In comparison with cercarial dermatitis, which occurs on exposed sites, seabather's eruption occurs at sites covered by bathing apparel (Fig. 28-25) while bathing in salt water.

- On average, lesions persist for 1–2 weeks.

- In sensitized individuals, the eruption can become progressively more severe with repeated exposures and may be associated with systemic symptoms.

- Topical or systemic glucocorticoids provide symptomatic relief. ℮

FIGURE 28-24 Cercarial dermatitis A highly pruritic papulovesicular eruption on the knees acquired after the patient waded through a slow-flowing creek.

FIGURE 28-25 Seabather's eruption This papulovesicular rash appeared on a swimmer while on vacation in the Caribbean. During swimming the patient experienced slight stinging in the regions covered by her bikini; later that evening she noticed the eruption. The rash is characteristically confined to the areas covered by the swimwear.

ENVENOMATIONS CAUSED BY CNIDARIA (JELLYFISH, PORTUGUESE MAN-OF-WAR, SEA ANEMONES, CORALS) ICD-9 : 989.5 ∘ ICD-10 : T63.6

- Cnidarian stings range from mild, self-limited irritations to extremely painful and serious injuries, depending on the:
  - Toxin of the species involved
  - Magnitude of the envenomation (Figs. 28-26, 28-27).

- Stings from box jellyfish can be fatal.
- In most cases jellyfish stings elicit toxic rather than allergic types of reactions.
- Clinical manifestations: pruritic, burning, and painful papules in linear arrangement 🔁

INJURIES CAUSED BY ECHINODERMS (SEA URCHINS, SEA STARS, AND SEA CUCUMBERS)

- *Sea urchins* have calcareous spines, which can break off in skin following a puncture wound.
- Spines are composed of calcium carbonate and a proteinaceous membrane; in certain species spines are venomous, causing excruciating pain.
- Immediate reactions are usually localized:
  - Burning pain at wound site
  - Tattooing from the spines
  - Paresthesias.

ICD-9 : E905.6

- Delayed reactions may be nodular or diffuse:
  - Foreign body reaction to spine fragments
  - Delayed-type hypersensitivity
  - Fusiform swelling of digit with pain and loss of function.
- *Sea star* injuries are similar to those caused by sea urchins.
- *Sea cucumbers* can cause a papular contact dermatitis caused by holothurin, a toxin secreted from cell walls.

FIGURE 28-26 Jellyfish envenomation Pruritic and painful papules in a linear arrangement on the leg, appearing after contact with jellyfish.

FIGURE 28-27 Fire coral envenomation A 47-year-old female with painful palms that occurred after contact with fire coral. The palms and palmar fingers are red and edematous at sites of envenomation. Fire corals are colonial marine organisms that look rather like real coral. However, they are technically not corals; they are actually more closely related to jellyfish and other stinging anemones. Fire corals are widely distributed in tropical and subtropical waters, appearing as small brushlike growths on rocks and coral. Divers often mistake fire coral for seaweed, and accidental contact is common. The very small nematocysts on fire corals contain tentacles that protrude from numerous surface pores (similar to jellyfish stings). In addition, fire corals have a sharp, calcified external skeleton that can scrape the skin.

SYSTEMIC PARASITIC INFECTIONS

CUTANEOUS AND MUCOCUTANEOUS LEISHMANIASIS ■ ◑→●

- Etiology: many species of obligate intracellular protozoa *Leishmania*; predominant species are:
  - Old World: *L. tropica, L. major, L. aethiopica*
  - New World: *L. Mexican* complex, *Viannia* subgenus
- Vector: sandflies
  - Old World: *Plebotomus*
  - New World: *Luzomyia*
- Infection of macrophages in skin (dermis), nasooropharyngeal mucosa, and the reticuloendothelial system (viscera)
- Diversity of clinical syndromes due to particular parasite, vector, and host species.
- Clinical syndromes: cutaneous, mucosal, visceral
  - Cutaneous leishmaniasis (CL) characterized by development of single or multiple cutaneous papules at the site of a sandfly bite, often evolving into nodules and ulcers,

which heal spontaneously with a depressed scar
  - Old World cutaneous leishmaniasis (OWCL) New World cutaneous leishmaniasis (NWCL)
  - Diffuse (anergic) cutaneous leishmaniasis (DCL)
  - Mucosal leishmaniasis (ML)
  - Visceral leishmaniasis (VL); kala-azar; post–kala-azar dermal leishmaniasis (PKDL)
- Management: parenteral antimonials for significant disease

Synonyms:
- OWCL: Baghdad/Delhi boil or button, oriental/Aleppo sore/evil, *bouton d'Orient.*
- NWCL: chiclero ulcer, pian bois (bush yaws), uta.
- ML: Espundia.
- VL: Kala-azar (Hindu for black fever)

ICD-9 : 085.9 ∘ ICD-10 : B55

EPIDEMIOLOGY

Etiology   Infection in humans is caused by ~20 *Leishmania* species (*Leishmania* and *Viannia* subgenera). See Table 29-1.

Stages of Parasite

- Promastrigote: flagellated form found in sandflies and culture.
- Amastigote: nonflagellated tissue form (2–4 μm in diameter); replicates in macrophage phagosomes in mammalian hosts.

Speciation   Isoenzyme patterns, kinetoplast DNA buoyant densities, specific phlebotomine vectors, monoclonal antibodies, DNA hybridization, DNA restriction endonuclease fragment analysis.

Modes of Transmission

- Vector-borne by bite of infected female phlebotomine sandflies (2–3 mm long), which become infected by taking blood meal from infected mammalian host. About 30 species of sandflies have been identified as vectors. Sandflies are weak noiseless fliers; they rest in dark, moist places, and are typically most active in evening and night-time hours.
- Other modes: congenital and parenteral (i.e., by blood transfusion, needle sharing, laboratory accident).

Reservoirs   Varies with geography and leishmanial species. Zoonosis involves rodents/canines.

- Mediterranean littoral—dogs. In endemic areas of Spain, up to 20% of dogs tested harbored parasites in skin and viscera.

TABLE 29-1 *Leishmania* Species That Cause Disease in Humans

Species[a]	Clinical Syndrome[b]	Geographic Distribution
SUBGENUS LEISHMANIA		
L. donovani complex		
L. donovani sensu strictiori	VL (PKDL, OWCL)	China, Indian subcontinent, southwestern Asia, Ethiopia,[c] Kenya, Sudan, Uganda; possibly sporadic in sub-Saharan Africa
L. infantum sensu strictiori[d]	VL (OWCL)	China, central and southwestern Asia, Middle East, southern Europe, North Africa, Ethiopia,[c] Sudan; sporadic in sub-Saharan Africa
L. chagasi[d]	VL (NWCL)	Central and South America
L. mexicana complex		
L. mexicana	NWCL (DCL)	Texas, Mexico, Central and South America
L. amazonensis	NWCL (ML, DCL, VL)	Panama and South America
L. tropica	OWCL (VL)[e]	Central Asia, India, Pakistan, southwestern Asia, Middle East, Turkey, Greece, North Africa, Ethiopia,[c] Kenya, Namibia
L. major	OWCL[f]	Central Asia, India, Pakistan, southwestern Asia, Middle East, Turkey, North Africa, Sahel region of north-central Africa, Ethiopia,[c] Sudan, Kenya
L. aethiopica	OWCL (DCL, ML)	Ethiopia,[c] Kenya Uganda
SUBGENUS VIANNIA		
L. (V.) braziliensis	NWCL (ML)	Central and South America
L. (V.) guyanensis	NWCL (ML)	South America
L. (V.) panamensis	NWCL (ML)	Central America, Venezuela, Colombia, Ecuador, Peru
L. (V.) peruviana	NWCL[g]	Peru (western slopes of Andes)

[a]Species other than those listed here have been reported to infect humans

[b]**Abbreviations:** VL, visceral leishmaniasis; PKDL, post–kala-azar dermal leishmaniasis; OWCL, Old World cutaneous leishmaniasis; NWCL, New World (American) cutaneous leishmaniasis; DCL, diffuse cutaneous leishmaniasis; ML, mucosal leishmaniasis. Clinical syndromes less frequently associated with the various species are shown in parentheses.

[c]Cutaneous and visceral leishmaniasis also are endemic in parts of Eritrea, but the causative species have not been well established.

[d]"L. infantum" and "L. chagasi" are synonymous.

[e]L. tropica also causes leishmaniasis recidivans and viscerotropic leishmaniasis.

[f]L. major–like organisms also cause New World cutaneous leishmaniasis.

[g]The cutaneous leishmaniasis syndrome caused by this species is called uta.

SOURCE: From BL Herwaldt, in AS Fauci et al (eds): *Harrison's Principles of Internal Medicine*, 17th ed, Chap. 205. New York, McGraw-Hill, 2008.

- Southern Russia—gerbils.
- For *L. major*, desert rodents.
- For *L. tropica*, rats.
- For *L. infantum*, wild canines, dogs.

Vectors Transmitted by 30 species of female sandflies of genus *Phlebotomus* (Old World) and genera *Lutzomyia* (New World). Breed in cracks in buildings, rubbish, rubble; rodent burrows, termite hills, rotting vegetation. Weak fliers; remain close to ground near breeding site. Ingest amastigotes while feeding on infected mammals (reservoir), converting to promastigotes in the gut of the sandfly; replicate in gut.

Prevalence Estimated 12 million people infected worldwide. 1.5–2 million new cases annually; 350 million individuals are at risk of infection. 50% of new cases are in children. 75,000 individuals die annually of ML.

Geography All inhabited continents except Australia; endemic in focal areas of 90 countries. Tropics, subtropics, southern Europe. >90% of cases of CL occur in Afghanistan,

Algeria, Iran, Iraq, Saudi Arabia, Syria, Brazil, Peru. Climates: Range from deserts to rain forests, rural to urban.

Iraq In 2003–2004, about 1% of U.S. soldiers who had served in Iraq developed OWCL. Sandfly season: begins in April. Long incubation period. VL also reported.

Immune status of person

- Leishmania-specific anergy: patients develop DCL.
- Poor immune response or immunosuppression (HIV/AIDS): VL
- HIV/*Leishmania* co-infection: To date, most cases of concordant infection with *Leishmania* and HIV/AIDS have been reported from Southern Europe (by 2001, 2000 cases diagnosed; 90% from Spain, Italy, France, Portugal). In the Americas, most cases reported from Brazil. Concordant infection with HIV/AIDS and *L. donovani* is associated with visceral leishmaniasis and is an emerging disease in Africa. In northwest Ethiopia, up to 30% of all visceral leishmaniasis patients are infected with HIV/AIDS. In India, co-infection increasing with highest rate of leishmaniasis and high rate of resistance to antimonial drugs.
- Hyperergic variant: Leishmaniasis recidivans caused by *L. tropica*.

PATHOGENESIS

The clinical and immunologic spectrum of leishmaniasis parallels that of leprosy. CL occurs in a host with good protective immunity. MCL occurs in those with an intense inflammatory reaction. DCL occurs with extensive and widespread proliferation of the organism in the skin but without much inflammation or tendency for visceralization. VL occurs in the host with little immune response and/or in immunosuppression. Unlike leprosy, extent and pattern are strongly influenced by the specific species of *Leishmania* involved. Additional factors that affect the clinical picture: number of parasites inoculated, site of inoculation, nutritional status of host, nature of the last nonblood meal of vector. Infection and recovery are followed by lifelong immunity to reinfection by the same species of *Leishmania*. In some cases, interspecies immunity occurs.

CLINICAL MANIFESTATION

Incubation Period Inversely proportional to size of inoculum: shorter in visitors to endemic

area. OWCL: *L. tropica major*, 1–4 weeks; *L. tropica*, 2–8 months; acute CL: 2–8 weeks or more.

Symptoms Noduloulcerative lesions usually asymptomatic. With secondary bacterial infection, may become painful.

Skin Findings

Types of Lesions Primary lesions occur at site of sandfly bite, usually on exposed site.

OWCL *L. major* Asia, Africa, Europe in tropical and subtropical zones; Middle East (Iran, Iraq, eastern Saudi Arabia, Jordan Valley of Israel and Jordan, Sinai Peninsula). More common in rural areas. Begins as small erythematous papule, which may appear immediately after sandfly bite but usually 2–4 weeks later. Papule slowly enlarges to 2 cm over a period of several weeks and assumes a dusky violaceous hue (Fig. 29-1). Eventually, lesion becomes crusted in center with a shallow ulcer and raised indurated border = volcano sign. In some cases, the center of the nodule becomes hyperkeratotic, forming a cutaneous horn. Small satellite papules may develop at periphery of lesion, and occasionally subcutaneous nodules along the course of proximal lymphatics. Rarely, lesions become locally invasive and extend into subcutaneous tissue and muscle. Peripheral extension usually stops after 2 months, and ulcerated nodule persists for another 3–6 months, or longer. The lesion then heals with a slightly depressed scar. In some cases, CL remains active with positive smears for 24 months (nonhealing chronic cutaneous leishmaniasis). The number of lesions depends on the circumstances of the exposure and extent of infection within the sandfly vector. May result in multiple lesions, up to 100 or more (Figs. 29-2 and 29-3). ▐

L. tropica Southern Europe, Iran, Iraq, Middle East, southern republics of former U.S.S.R. More common in urban areas. Clinical pattern similar to that of *L. major*, although lesions caused by *L. tropica* are more apt to be solitary, more inflammatory, last longer, and be more difficult to treat. ▐

L. infantum Countries bordering Mediterranean, including southern Europe and northern Africa. Lesions are similar to those in *L. major* form, but duration is shorter.

L. aethiopica Kenya, Sudan, Ethiopia. The common form of CL in these areas is similar to CL caused by *L. major*. In approximately 20%

FIGURE 29-1 Old World cutaneous leishmaniasis: face   A 7-year-old Jordanian female with painful lesions on the cheeks for 6 weeks. **A.** Large crusted nodules with surrounding edema on both cheeks. **B.** Three weeks after successful therapy (sodium stibo-gluconate pentostam injections; 15 mg /kg per day IM injection for 21 days), lesions have healed with minimal residual erythema and no scarring. (Courtesy of Mohammad Tawara, MD.)

of individuals, widespread skin involvement develops (DCL) that resembles lepromatous leprosy.

NWCL   *L. mexicana Complex*   Mexico, Central America, as far north as Texas, as far south as Brazil. Lesions develop in similar fashion to those caused by *L. major*. Small erythematous papule develops at sandfly bite site, evolving into ulcerated nodule (Fig. 29-4). Eventually lesion heals with a depressed scar. Enlarges 3–12 cm with raised border. Nonulcerating nodules may become verrucous. Lymphangitis, regional lymphadenopathy. Isolated lesions on hand or head usually do not ulcerate; heal spontaneously. Ear lesions may persist for years, destroying cartilage (chiclero ulcers) (Fig. 29-5).

L. braziliensis Complex   Clinical lesions similar to those of OWCL. Some strains can invade mucous membranes of mouth, nose, pharynx, larynx to cause MCL.

ML   Characterized by nasooropharyngeal mucosal involvement, a metastatic complication of CL. Caused by *Viannia* subgenus, typically *L. (V.) braziliensis*, *L. (V.) panamensis*, and *L (V.) guyanensis*. Mucosal disease usually becomes evident several years after healing of original cutaneous lesions; cutaneous and mucosal lesions can coexist or appear decades apart. Edema and inflammatory changes lead to epistaxis and coryzal symptoms. In time, nasal septum, floor of mouth, and tonsilar areas destroyed (Fig. 29-6). Results in marked disfigurement (referred to as *espundia* in South America). Death may occur due to superimposed bacterial infection, pharyngeal obstruction, or malnutrition. ✏

DCL   Resembles lepromatous leprosy; large number of parasites in macrophages in dermis; no visceral involvement. In Old World, occurs in 20% of individuals with leishmaniasis in Ethiopia and Sudan. In South America, attributed to a member of *L. braziliensis* complex. Presents as a single nodule, which then spreads locally, often through extension from satellite lesions, and eventually by metastasis. In time, lesions become widespread with nonulcerating nodules appearing diffusely over face, trunk. Responds poorly to treatment.

Leishmaniasis Recidivans (LR)   Complication of *L. tropica* infection. Dusky-red plaques with active, spreading borders and healing centers, giving rise to gyrate and annular lesions. Most commonly affects face; can cause tissue destruction and severe deformity. ✏

Post–Kala-Azar Dermal Leishmaniasis (PKDL)   Sequel to VL that has resolved spontaneously or during/after adequate treatment. Lesions appear ≥1 y after course of therapy with macular, papular, nodular lesions, and hypopigmented macules/plaques on face, trunk, extremities. Resembles lepromatous leprosy when lesions are numerous. Develops in 20% of Indian patients treated for VL caused by *L. donovani* and in a small percentage of Ethiopian patients with VL caused by *L. aethiopica.* ✏

Visceral Leishmaniasis (*VL*)   Can remain subclinical or become symptomatic, with acute, subacute, chronic course. Inapparent VL cases outnumber clinically apparent cases. Malnutrition is risk factor for clinically apparent VL. Bone marrow, liver, spleen are involved. Term *kala-azar* (Hindi for "black fever," some patients had gray color) refers to profoundly cachectic febrile patients with life-threatening disease. Occurs in China, India, former U.S.S.R., Middle East, east Africa through Sudan to west Africa, and South America. Patients present with fever, splenomegaly, pancytopenia, wasting. ✏

FIGURE 29-2   Old World cutaneous leishmaniasis
Multiple, crusted nodules on the exposed back, arising at sites of sandfly bites. Many of the lesions resemble a volcano with a central depressed center, i.e., volcano sign.

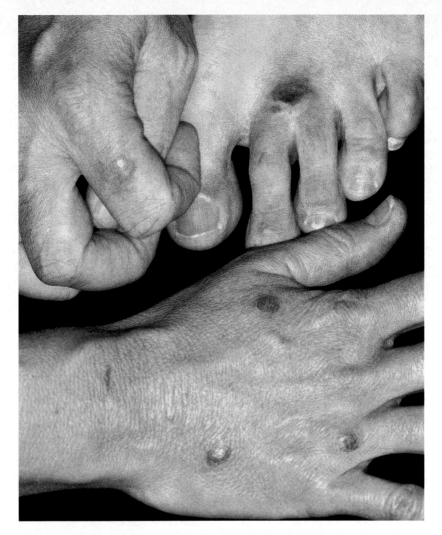

FIGURE 29-3 Old World cutaneous leishmaniasis   Multiple erythematous papules and nodules on the dorsa of hands and foot in a husband and wife who had been camping in Israel. A facial papule was present in the wife. All lesions resolved spontaneously within 2 to 3 months.

Viscerotropic Leishmaniasis Caused by *L. tropica* (typically dermotropic); recognized in U.S. soldiers who participated in Operation Desert Storm. Parasitic burdens light; non-specific manifestations of visceral infection (fatigue, fever, GI symptoms).

VL in HIV/AIDS Disease Relatively aviru-lent *Leishmania* strains can disseminate to vis-cera. Consider in HIV/AIDS-infected patient with CD4 cell count<200/μL, travel history to leishmaniasis-endemic areas, unexplained

fever, organomegaly, anemia, pancytopenia. Splenomegaly may not occur.

DIFFERENTIAL DIAGNOSIS

Acute CL Insect bite reaction, impetigo, furuncle, carbuncle, ecthyma, anthrax, orf, milker's nodule, tularemia, *M. marinum* infec-tion, tuberculosis cutis, yaws, sporotrichosis, blastomycosis, kerion, furuncular myiasis, dra-cunculosis, trypanosomal chagoma or chancre,

A   *B*

FIGURE 29-4   New World cutaneous leishmaniasis: ulcer on thigh   A 42-year-old male with HIV/AIDS
noted a painless lesion appearing on the right-medial thigh 6 weeks after returning from a vacation in Mexico.
Ulcer with rolled borders and base with granulation tissue. Leishmania were seen on lesional biopsy. *L. mexicana*
was isolated on tissue culture of lesional biopsy.

foreign-body granuloma, basal cell carcinoma, squamous cell, lymphoma.

Chronic CL and Relapsing CL   Lupus vulgaris, leprosy, sarcoidosis, granuloma faciale, Jessner lymphocytic infiltrate, lymphocytoma cutis, discoid lupus erythematosus, psoriasis, acne, rosacea, cellulitis, erysipelas, keloids, Wegener granulomatosis, syphilitic gumma.

ML   Sarcoidosis, neoplasms, midline granuloma, rhinoscleroma, paracoccidioidomycosis, histoplasmosis, leprosy, syphilis, tertiary yaws.

VL   Tropical infectious diseases that cause fever or organomegaly (typhoid fever, miliary tuberculosis, brucellosis, malaria, tropical splenomegaly syndrome, and schistosomiasis); leukemia and lymphoma.

PKDL   Syphilis, yaws, leprosy.

LABORATORY EXAMINATIONS

Serology   Lacks specificity. Cannot distinguish current from past infection.

Dermatopathology   Large macrophages filled with 2- to 4-μm amastigotes (Leishman-Donovan bodies); mixed lymphocytic, plasmacytic infiltrate. In Wright- and Giemsa-stained preparations, the amastigote cytoplasm appears blue, nucleus relatively large and red; distinctive kinetoplast is rod-shaped and stains intensely red.

Culture   Novy-MacNeal-Nicolle (NNN) medium at 22°C–28°C for 21 days grows motile promastigotes.

Touch Preparation   Macrophages containing organisms: dark, slightly flattened nucleus, and rod-shaped kinetoplast observed.

Needle Aspiration   Visualize amastigote within macrophages.

Polymerase Chain Reaction   Can detect different species of *Leishmania*. Specific and sensitive.

DIAGNOSIS

Clinical suspicion, confirmed by demonstrating:

- Intracellular nonflagellated amastigote
  - Biopsy: Giemsa-stained (skin, mucosa, liver, lymph nodes)
  - Aspirate: Splenic, bone marrow, lymph nodes

- Flagellated promastigote in culture of tissues (requires up to 21 days)

COURSE AND PROGNOSIS

CL Whether caused by *L. tropica* or *L. mexicana*, CL is self-limited. Scarring is increased by secondary bacterial infection.
MCL May extend to secondary sites. Superinfection common. Death from pneumonia.
DCL Progressive; refractory to treatment; cures rare.

MANAGEMENT

Prophylaxis No chemoprophylaxis for travelers exists. OWCL: Delay specific treatment until ulceration occurs, allowing protective immunity to develop, unless lesions are disfiguring, disabling, persist ± 6 months.
Management of Cutaneous Leishmaniasis

- Goals
  - Accelerating healing of skin lesions
  - Decreasing morbidity
  - Decreasing risk for local and mucosal dissemination and relapse
- Parasite factors
  - Tissue tropism
  - Drug sensitivities

- Extent to which lesions are of concern or bothersome because of location (facial, periarticular lesions), number, size, persistence, nodular lymphangitis.
- Parenteral Sb^v therapy recommended when optimal effectiveness is important. The first sign of a clinical response typically is decreasing induration, and relapses usually are noted first at the margins of healed lesions.

FIGURE 29-5   New World cutaneous leishmaniasis: chiclero ulcer A deep ulcer on the helix at the site of a sandfly bite. This variant typically occurs in leishmaniasis acquired in Central and South America.

FIGURE 29-6   Mucocutaneous leishmaniasis: espundia Painful, mutilating ulceration with destruction of portions of the nose. (Courtesy of Eric Kraus, MD.)

Lesional Therapy   Effective in some cases without local dissemination or risk of mucosal dissemination (e.g., for relatively benign lesions caused by *L. Mexicana* or *L. major*).

- Topical imiquimod
- Paromomycin ointments (15% paromomycin sulfate, 12% methylbenzethonium

chloride in white paraffin twice daily for 10 days)
- Cryosurgery
- Ultrasound-induced hyperthermia
- Intralesional Pentostam given weekly up to 1 mg/kg injected into borders of lesions)

Parenteral Therapy   See Table 29-2.

TABLE 29-2   Drug Regimens for Treatment of Leishmaniasis[a]

Clinical Syndrome, Drug	Route of Administration	Regimen
VISCERAL LEISHMANIASIS		
Parenteral therapy		
Pentavalent antimony[b]	IV, IM	20 mg Sb^v/kg qd for 28 days
Amphotericin B, lipid formulation[c]	IV	2–5 mg/kg qd (total: usually ~15–21 mg/kg)
Amphotericin B (deoxycholate)	IV	0.5–1 mg/kg qod or qd (total: usually ~15–20 mg/kg)
Paromomycin sulfate[d]	IV, IM	15–20 mg/kg qd for ~21 days
Pentamidine isethionate	IV, IM	4 mg/kg qod or thrice weekly for ~15–30 doses
Oral therapy		
Miltefosine[d, e]	PO	2.5 mg/kg qd for 28 days
CUTANEOUS LEISHMANIASIS		
Parenteral theraphy		
Pentavalent antimony[b]	IV, IM	20 mg Sb^v/kg qd for 20 days
Pentamidine isethionate	IV, IM	3 mg/kg qod for 4 doses or 2 mg/kg qod for 7 doses
Amphotericin B (deoxycholate)	IV	0.5–1 mg/kg qod or qd (total: up to ~20 mg/kg)
Oral therapy		
Fluconazole	PO	200 mg qd for 6 weeks[f]
Ketoconazole	PO	600 mg/d for 28 days[f]
Itraconazole	PO	200 mg bid for 28 days[f]
Miltefosine[d, e]	PO	2.5 mg/kg qd for 28 days
MUCOSAL LEISHMANIASIS		
Pentavalent antimony[b]	IV, IM	20 mg Sb^v/kg qd for 28 days
Amphotericin B (deoxycholate)	IV	1 mg/kg qod or qd (total: usually ~20–40 mg/kg)
Pentamidine isethionate	IV, IM	2–4 mg/kg qod or thrice weekly for ≥15 doses

[a]To maximize effectiveness and minimize toxicity, the listed regimens should be individualized according to the particularities of the case.

[b] The Centers for Disease Control and Prevention (CDC) provides the pentavalent antimonial (Sb^v) compound sodium stibogluconate (Pentostam; Glaxo Wellcome, PLC, United Kingdom; 100 mg Sb^v/mL) to U.S.-licensed physicians through the CDC Drug Service (404-639-3670). The other widely used pentavalent antimonial compound, meglumine antimonate (Glucantime; Rhône Poulenc, France; 85 mg Sb^v/mL), is available primarily in Spanish- and French-speaking areas of the world

[c] The lipid formulations of amphotericin B include liposomal amphotericin B, amphotericin B lipid complex, and amphotericin B cholesteryl sulfate. The U.S. Food and Drug Administration recently approved the following regimen of liposomal amphotericin B for immunocompetent patients: 3 mg/kg qd on days 1–5, 14, and 21, for a total of 21 mg/kg; for immunosuppressed patients, the approved regimen is 4 mg/kg qd on days 1–5, 10, 17, 24, 31, and 38, for a total of 40 mg/kg. Alternative regimens that have been proposed for immunocompetent patients include treatment on days 1–5 and 10 with 3–4 mg/kg qd for cases from Europe or Brazil, with 3 mg/kg qd for cases from Africa, and with 2–3 mg/kg qd for cases from India.

[d] Not commercially available as of this writing.

[e]Miltefosine, which is teratogenic in animals, should not be used to treat pregnant women. Women of child-bearing age should use effective birth control during treatment and for 2 months thereafter.

[f]Adult dosage.

SOURCE: Adapted from BL Herwaldt, in AS Fauci et al (eds): *Harrison's Principles of Internal Medicine*, 17th ed, Chap. 205. New York, McGraw-Hill, 2008.

TRYPANOSOMIASIS   ICD-9:086.9 ∘ ICD-10:B56

- Zoonosis
- Parasitic protozoan disease caused by three species of *Trypanosoma*
- Vector: reduviid bugs
- Epidemiology
  - Central and South America: *T. cruzi*
  - Africa: *T. brucei gambiense, T. brucei rhodesiense*

- Clinical findings
  - Acute: Inoculation site nodule
  - Chronic: Cardiac, gastrointestinal (GI), and central nervous system (CNS) involvment
- Course: most infected persons remain so for life. Heart, GI, and CNS involvement associated with serious morbidity and mortality

AMERICAN TRYPANOSOMIASIS (AT)   ICD-9:O86.0 ∘ ICD-10:B57

- Etiology: *T. cruzi*
- Transmission: *T. cruzi* deposited in feces of reduviid bugs onto the skin; enters host via breaks in skin, mucous membranes, or conjunctivae. Chagoma can occur at inoculation site. Can also be transmitted by transfusion of blood from infected persons, by organ transplantation, from mother to fetus, in laboratory.
- Dissemination: Via lymphatics and bloodstream to muscles.
- Geography: Central and South America
- Prevalance: 16–18 million persons infected

- Clinical findings
  - Acute infection: mild febrile illness
  - Indeterminate/asymptomatic phase: subpatent parasitemia
  - Symptomatic chronic infection:
    - Cardiac disease
    - GI disease
- Course: most infected persons remain so for life. Heart and GI involvement associated with serious morbidity and mortality

Synonym: Chagas disease.

Mucocutaneous Findings of AT
Acute AT

- *Inoculation chagoma* An indurated area of erythema and swelling (*chagoma*), at the portal of entry, occurring 7–14 days after inoculation. May be accompanied by local lymphadenopathy. Parasites located within leukocytes and cells of subcutaneous tissues. These initial local signs are followed by malaise, fever, anorexia, and edema of the face and lower extremities (Fig. 29-7).
- *Romaña sign* Unilateral painless edema of palpebrae and periocular tissues. Occurs when conjunctiva is the portal of entry. Classic finding in acute AT.
- Edema of face and lower extremities
- *Trypanosomides* Morbilliform, urticariform, or erythematopolymorphic eruptions
- *Hematogenic or metastatic chagomas* Nodule(s) caused by dissemination of infection. Hard, painful, wine-colored nodules; rarely soften or ulcerate.

Chronic AT In the immunocompromised host (HIV/AIDS disease, organ transplant recipient)

- Reactivation chagoma Nodule at inoculation site.
- *A cellulitis-mimicking plaque.*

SYSTEMIC FINDINGS OF AT

Acute AT

- Generalized lymphadenopathy
- Hepatosplenomegaly
- Severe myocarditis may occur in acute AT; most deaths are due to heart failure.

Chronic AT

- Heart (rhythm disturbances, cardiomyopathy, and thromboembolism)
- GI tract (megaesophagus, megacolon)

DIAGNOSIS

Acute AT Detect parasites in blood
Chronic AT Detect specific antibodies

HUMAN AFRICAN TRYPANOSOMIASIS (HAT)   ICD-9:O86.5 ○ ICD-10:B56   ■ ●

- Etiology: complex of *T. brucei*
  - *T. b. gambiense* causes West African sleeping sickness
  - *T. b. rhodesiense* causes East African sleeping sickness
- Transmission:
  - Vector: tsetse flies.
  - Transmission during human blood meal from infected saliva.
  - Primary reservoir
    - West African sleeping sickness: humans
    - East African sleeping sickness: Antelope and cattle
- Epidemiology

- Sub-Saharan Africa; 36 countries.
  - West Africa: Ivory Coast, Chad, Central African Republic; rural populations
  - East Africa: Sudan; workers in wild areas, rural populations, tourists in game parks
  - > 66 million persons infected
- HAT in travelers: usually East African trypanosomiasis
- Clinical findings
  - Acute
  - Chronic: Progressive neurologic impairment; death
- Course: most inexorably progressive

Synonym: Sleeping sickness

CLINICAL FINDINGS OF HAT

Acute HAT: Stage I Disease

- *Trypanosomal chancre* Appears in some patients at inoculation site (Fig. 29-7); painful; 7–14 days after tsetse-fly bite. Occurs more commonly in travelers (e.g., to game parks) than in Africans. Typically 2–5 cm, indurated; may ulcerate; resolved in few weeks. Parasites can be seen in fluid expressed from chancre and buffy coat.
- *Hemolymphatic stage* Marked by the onset of fever, arthralgias, malaise, localized facial edema, and moderate splenomegaly. Lymphadenopathy is prominent in *T. b. gambiense* trypanosomiasis.
- *Macular-papular rash* Occurs on the trunk.
- *Pruritus*
- *Winterbottom sign* Enlargement of the nodes of the posterior cervical triangle; cervical nodes also enlarged.
- *Differential diagnosis* Acute HIV/AIDS infection, malaria, typhoid fever.

FIGURE 29-7   Human East African trypanosomiasis: trypanosomal chancre   A shallow ulceration was present on the dorsum of the left foot, surrounded by a ring that contained bullae and that was, in turn, surrounded by another ring, characterized by violaceous erythema and induration; the entire lesion, which was approximately 5 cm in diameter, was painful. A macular exanthem was present on the trunk. The patient was a traveler to South Africa. *Trypanosoma brucei* was identified in an aspirate from the ulcer. (Courtesy of Edward T. Ryan, MD. N Engl J Med 346: 2069, 2002; with permission.)

- *Course* More rapid in East African type. Tourist with *T. b. rhodesiense* disease may develop systemic signs of infection (fever, malaise, headache) near the end of trip.

Chronic HAT: Stage II Disease

- *CNS invasion* Characterized by insidious development of protean neurologic symptoms. Progressive indifference and daytime somnolence develops (hence the designation "sleeping sickness").
- *Cardiac disease* East African type may develop arrhythmias and congestive heart failure before CNS disease develops.
- *Diagnosis* Detection of parasite in chancre, lymph node, blood, bone marrow.

CUTANEOUS AMEBIASIS AND ACANTHAMEBIASIS

CUTANEOUS AMEBIASIS ICD-9:006.6 ∘ ICD-10:A06.7

- Amebiasis is caused by *Entamoeba histolytica*, which infects the GI tract and rarely skin
- Incidence: 10% of world population infected with *Entamoeba*.
  - Majority of infections caused by noninvasive *E. dispar*
  - 10% of those colonized with *E. histolytica* develop amebic colitis.
- More prevalent in tropics and in rural areas; inadequate sanitation and crowding.
- Skin involvement is associated with malnutrition and immunocompromise (HIV/AIDS, solid organ transplantation)
- Clinical findings:

- CA begins as an indurated pustule that evolves to a painful ragged ulcer, foul-smelling and covered with pus or necrotic debris (Fig. 29-8).
- Usually a consequence of an underlying amebic abscess invading the skin.
- Typical sites are the perianal area (extension of sigmorectal involvement) (Fig. 29-8) or abdominal wall (draining sinus from liver or colon).
- Penis or vulva may become infected during intercourse.
- Surgical wound infections may follow removal of hepatic or abdominal abscess.
- Remote ulcers (e.g., face) may result from autoinoculation.
- Without treatment, CA progressively enlarges.

CUTANEOUS ACANTHAMEBIASIS ICD-9:006.6 ∘ ICD-10:A06.7

- Cutaneous acanthamebiasis is an infection caused by free-living *Acanthamoeba*.
- Clinical findings:
  - Primary cutaneous acanthamebiasis
    - Occurs at sites of trauma sustained in aquatic environment (streams, ponds, swimming pools).
    - Lesions begin as indurated red/violaceous deep nodules or large pustules that soon ulcerate.

- Disseminated cutaneous acanthamebiasis
  - Occurs in HIV/AIDS disease and solid organ transplant recipients
  - Disseminates from nasal/sinus colonization.
  - Presents with multiple soft red nodules that ulcerate

FIGURE 29-8   Cutaneous amebiasis: perineum   Perineal/perianal ulcer in a patient with rectal amebiasis.

SEXUALLY TRANSMITTED INFECTIONS

- Sexually transmitted infections (STIs), caused by a broad range of pathogens (Table 30-1), have a high physical and psychosocial morbidity.
- The syndromes caused by these pathogens affect both the sexually active couple and neonates born to an infected mother (Table 30-2).
- Bacterial STIs such as gonorrhea, syphilis, chancroid, donovanosis, and lymphogranuloma venereum (LGV) can easily be cured with antimicrobial therapy.
- Viral STIs, such as those caused by HIV/AIDS, human papillomavirus (HPV), and herpes simplex virus 2 (HSV-2), are chronic infections, characterized by prolonged viral shedding and opportunity for infecting a sexual partner; can only be suppressed but not cured by antiviral therapy.
- Nearly all sexually active individuals are at risk for these viral STIs. HPV persists in the anogenital mucosa for months, years, or decades after primary infection. HSV-2 infection is chronic and lifelong.

- Prevention offers the best approach to managing STIs.
- In developing nations, where STIs are more common, lack of funds for health care often limit detection and treatment of STIs as well as immunizations.
- Untreated syphilis can be a lifelong infection with long-term morbidity.
- Transmission of HIV/AIDS to neonates occurs commonly in developing nations, where the prevalence of infection is high; antiretroviral treatment of mother and neonate markedly reduces neonatal infection.
- Transmission of HSV has more immediate effects on the neonate, who is more susceptible to acute visceral infection.
- Transmission of HPV infection to the neonate can result in anogenital condyloma, and, later in life, respiratory papillomatosis.

Synonyms: Sexually transmitted diseases, genital infectious diseases, venereal disease (VD)

TABLE 30-1   Sexually Transmissible Pathogens and Associated Disease Syndromes

Pathogen	Associated Disease or Syndrome
Bacteria	
Neisseria gonorrhoeae	Urethritis, epididymitis, proctitis, cervicitis, endometritis, salpingitis, perihepatitis, bartholinitis, pharyngitis, conjunctivitis, prepubertal vaginitis, prostatitis, accessory gland infection, disseminated gonococcal infection (DGI), chorioamnionitis, premature rupture of membranes, premature delivery, amniotic infection syndrome
Chlamydia trachomatis	All of the above except DGI, plus otitis media, rhinitis, and pneumonia in infants, and reactive arthritis (Reiter) syndrome
Ureaplasma urealyticum	Nongonococcal urethritis (NGU)
Mycoplasma genitalium	(?) Nongonococcal urethritis
M. hominis	Postpartum fever, salpingitis (?)

Pathogen	Associated Disease or Syndrome
Treponema pallidum	Syphilis
Gardnerella vaginalis	Bacterial ("nonspecific") vaginosis (in conjunction with *Mycoplasma hominis* and vaginal anaerobes, such as *Mobiluncus* spp.)
Mobiluncus curtisii	Bacterial vaginosis
M. mulieris	Bacterial vaginosis
Haemophilus ducreyi	Chancroid
Calymmatobacterium granulomatis	Donovanosis (granuloma inguinale)
Shigella spp.	Shigellosis in men who have sex with men (MSM)
Campylobacter spp.	Enteritis, proctocolitis in MSM
Helicobacter cinaedi	(?) Proctocolitis; dermatitis, bacteremia in AIDS
H. fenneliae	(?) Proctocolitis; dermatitis, bacteremia in AIDS
Viruses	
HIV -1 and -2	HIV/AIDS
HSV types 1 and 2	Initial and recurrent genital herpes, aseptic meningitis, neonatal herpes
HPV	Condylomata acuminata; laryngeal papilloma; intraepithelial neoplasia and carcinoma of the cervix, vagina, vulva, anus, penis
Hepatitis A virus (HAV)	Acute hepatitis A
Hepatitis B virus (HBV)	Acute hepatitis B, chronic hepatitis B, hepatocellular carcinoma, polyarteritis nodosa, chronic membranous glomerulonephritis, mixed cryoglobulinemia (?), polymyalgia rheumatica (?)
Hepatitis C virus (HCV)	Acute hepatitis C, chronic hepatitis C, hepatocellular carcinoma, mixed cryoglobulinemia, chronic glomerulonephritis
Cytomegalovirus (CMV)	Heterophil-negative infectious mononucleosis; congenital CMV infection with gross birth defects and infant mortality, cognitive impairment (e.g., mental retardation, sensorineural deafness); protean manifestations in the immunosuppressed host
Molluscum contagiosum virus (MCV)	Genital molluscum contagiosum
Human T cell lymphotrophic virus (HTLV-I)	Human T cell leukemia or lymphoma, tropical spastic paraparesis
Human herpes virus type 8 (HHV-8)	Kaposi sarcoma, body cavity lymphoma, multicentric Castleman disease
Protozoa	
Trichomonas vaginalis	Vaginal trichomoniasis, NGU
Entamoeba histolytica	Amebiasis in MSM
Giardia lamblia	Giardiasis in MSM
Fungi	
Candida albicans	Vulvovaginitis, balanitis
Ectoparasites	
Phthirus pubis	Pubic lice infestation
Sarcoptes scabiei	Scabies

SOURCES: Adapted from W Cates, Jr, KK Holmes, in JM Last, RB Wallace (eds): *Maxcy-Rosenau-Last, Public Health and Preventive Medicine*, 14th ed. Norwalk, CT, Appleton & Lange, 1998, pp 137–155; and KK. Holmes, HH Handsfield, in AS Fauci et al (eds): *Harrison's Principles of Internal Medicine*, 14th ed. New York, McGraw-Hill, 1998.

TABLE 30-2   Selected Syndromes and Complications of Sexually Transmitted Pathogens

Syndrome or Complication	Associated Sexually Transmitted Pathogen
In men	
HIV/AIDS	HIV type 1 and 2
Urethritis	*Neisseria gonorrhoeae, Chlamydia trachomatis,* HSV, *Ureaplasma urealyticum,* (?) *Mycoplasma genitalium, T. vaginalis*
Epididymitis	*C. trachomatis, N. gonorrhoeae*
Intestinal infections	
Proctitis	*N. gonorrhoeae,* HSV, *C. trachomatis*
Proctocolitis or enterocolitis	*Campylobacter* spp., *Shigella* spp., *Entamoeba histolytica,* (?) *Helicobacter* spp.
Enteritis	*Giardia lamblia*
In women	
HIV/AIDS	HIV -1, HIV -2
Lower genitourinary tract infection	
Vulvitis	*Candida albicans,* HSV
Vaginitis	*Trichomonas vaginalis, C. albicans*
Vaginosis	*Gardnerella vaginalis, Mobiluncus* spp., other anaerobes, *Mycoplasma hominis*
Cervicitis	*N. gonorrhoeae, C. trachomatis,* HSV
Pelvic inflammatory disease	*N. gonorrhoeae, C. trachomatis, M. hominis,* anaerobes, group B streptococcus, Infertility
Postsalpingitis, postobstetrical, postabortion	*N. gonorrhoeae, C. trachomatis, M. hominis* (?)
Pregnancy morbidity	Several STIs implicated in one or more of these conditions
Chorioamnionitis, amniotic fluid infection, prematurity, premature rupture of membranes, preterm delivery, postpartum endometritis, ectopic pregnancy	
In men and women	
Rashes generalized, localized	*T. pallidum*
Neoplasm: Cervical, vulvar, vaginal, anal, and penile, intraepithelial neoplasia, carcinoma	HPV
Hepatocellular carcinoma	HBV, HCV
Kaposi sarcoma, body cavity lymphoma, Castleman disease	HHV-8
T cell lymphoma/leukemia	HTLV-I
Genital ulceration	HSV, *T. pallidum, Haemophilus ducreyi, Calymmatobacterium granulomatis, C. trachomatis* (LGV strains)
Acute arthritis with urogenital or intestinal infection	*N. gonorrhoeae, C. trachomatis, Shigella* spp., *Campylobacter* spp.
Hepatitis	HAV, HBV, HCV, CMV, *Treponema pallidum*
Anogenital warts	HPV (30 genital types)

Syndrome or Complication	Associated Sexually Transmitted Pathogen
Molluscum contagiosum	MCV
Ectoparasite infestations	*Sarcoptes scabiei, Phthirus pubis*
Mononucleosis syndrome	CMV, HIV/AIDS, Epstein-Barr Virus (EBV)
Tropical spastic paraparesis	HTLV-I
In neonates and infants	
Neonatal systemic infection, with potential cognitive impairment, deafness, death	Cytomegalovirus, HSV, *T. pallidum*, HIV/AIDS
Conjunctivitis	*C. trachomatis, N. gonorrhoeae*
Pneumonia, (?) chronic pulmonary disease	*C. trachomatis, U. urealyticum (?)*
Otitis media	*C. trachomatis*
Sepsis, meningitis	Group B streptococcus
Laryngeal papillomatosis	HPV

NOTE: For each of the above syndromes, some cases cannot yet be ascribed to any cause and must currently be considered idiopathic. "?" indicates a possible associated syndrome.

SOURCES: Adapted from W Cates, Jr, KK Holmes, in JM Last, RB Wallace (eds): *Maxcy-Rosenau-Last, Public Health and Preventive Medicine,* 14th ed. Norwalk, CT, Appleton & Lange, 1998, pp 137–155; and KK. Holmes, HH Handsfield, in AS Fauci et al (eds): *Harrison's Principles of Internal Medicine,* 17ed. New York, McGraw-Hill, 1998.

LABORATORY EXAMINATIONS

- Persons being evaluated for STIs should have a culture for gonorrhea and serotesting for HIV/AIDS and syphilis.
- Serologic testing for HPV infections is not available.
- Type-specific antibodies to glycoprotein (g)G1 and (g)G2 detect and differentiate past HSV-1 and HSV-2 infections.
- Primary HSV infection can be documented by demonstration of seroconversion.
- The development of nucleic acid amplification tests heralded a new era in sensitive and diagnostic procedures for STIs.

MANAGEMENT

The most effective way to prevent sexual transmission of STIs is to avoid sexual intercourse with an infected partner. Ideally, both new partners should get tested for STIs before initiating sexual intercourse. If a person chooses to have sexual intercourse with a partner whose infection status is unknown or who is infected with HIV/AIDS or another STI, a new condom should be used for each act of intercourse. Condom use is not completely protective against acquisition of STI because of the presence of pathogen outside the protected skin or condom breakage. HPV or HSV infections often occur at the base of the penis or pubic area, which are not protected by condoms. Chronic suppressive therapy can reduce transmission of HSV-2 (and HSV-1). Prospects for development of a vaccine for HSV-2 are excellent. An effective HPV vaccine is now available and is recommended for adolescent females to reduce the incidence of anogenital cancers. Immunization for hepatitis A and B is advised to prevent transmission of these viral infections during intercourse.

For updated information about sexually transmitted infections, see CDC website: *http://www.cdc.gov/STD/*

Management of Patients Who Have Genital Ulcers In the United States, the majority of young, sexually active patients who have genital ulcers have either genital herpes, syphilis, or chancroid. The frequency of each condition differs by geographic area and patient population; however, genital herpes is the most prevalent of these diseases. More than one of these diseases can be present in a patient who has genital ulcers. All three of these diseases have been associated with an increased risk for HIV/AIDS infection. Not all genital ulcers are caused by sexually transmitted infections.

A diagnosis based only on the patient's medical history and physical examination frequently is inaccurate. Therefore, all patients who have genital ulcers should be evaluated with a serologic test for syphilis and a diagnostic evaluation for genital herpes; in settings where chancroid is prevalent, an *H. ducreyi* infection should also be considered. Specific tests for evaluation of genital ulcers include (1) syphilis serology and either dark-field examination or direct immunofluorescence test for *T. pallidum*; (2) culture or antigen test for HSV; and (3) culture for *H. ducreyi*.

Type-specific serology for HSV-2 might be helpful in identifying persons with genital herpes (see Genital Herpes, Type-Specific Serologic Tests). Biopsy of genital ulcers might be helpful in identifying the cause of ulcers that are unusual or that do not respond to initial therapy. HIV/AIDS testing should be performed on all patients who have genital ulcers caused by *T. pallidum* or *H. ducreyi*, and should be strongly considered for those who have genital ulcers caused by HSV (see Diagnostic Considerations, sections, Syphilis, Chancroid, and Genital Herpes Simplex Virus).

Health care providers frequently must treat patients before test results are available because early treatment decreases the possibility of ongoing transmission and because successful treatment of genital herpes depends on prompt initiation of therapy. The clinician should treat for the diagnosis considered most likely, on the basis of clinical presentation and epidemiologic circumstances. In some instances, treatment must be initiated for additional conditions because of diagnostic uncertainty. Even after complete diagnostic evaluation, at least 25% of patients who have genital ulcers have no laboratory-confirmed diagnosis.

HUMAN PAPILLOMAVIRUS: MUCOSAL INFECTIONS ■ ◐

- Mucosal HPV infections are the most common STIs seen by the dermatologist.
- Only 1–2% of HPV-infected individuals have any visibly detectable clinical lesion.
- HPV present in the birth canal can be transmitted to a newborn during vaginal delivery and can cause
  - External genital warts (EGW)
  - Respiratory papillomatosis
- Warts: barely visible papules to nodules to confluent masses occurring on:
  - Anogenital: skin or mucosa
  - Oral mucosa
- HPV dysplasia of anogenital and oral skin and mucosa ranging from:
  - Mild to severe to squamous cell carcinoma (SCC) in situ (SCCIS)
  - Invasive SCC can arise within SCCIS
  - Most commonly in cervix, anal canal.

Synonyms: Condylomata acuminata, external genital warts, anogenital warts, venereal warts.

ICD-9 : 079.4 ∘ ICD-10 : B97.7

EPIDEMIOLOGY AND ETIOLOGY

Etiology

- HPV is a DNA papovavirus that multiplies in the nuclei of infected epithelial cells (see Section 27).
- More than 20 types of HPV can infect the genital tract: types 6, 11 most commonly; also types 16, 18, 31, 33 (see Table 27-2).
- Types 16, 18, 31, 33, and 35 are strongly associated with anogenital dysplasia and carcinoma.
- In individuals with multiple sexual partners, subclinical infection with multiple HPV types is common.

Age of Onset   Young, sexually active adults.

Risk Factors for Acquiring HPV Infection

- Number of sexual partners/frequency of sexual intercourse
- Sexual partner with EGW
- Sexual partner's number of sexual partners, infection with other STIs.

Transmission

- Through sexual contact: genital-genital, oral-genital, genital-anal.
- Microabrasions occur on epithelial surface allowing virions from infected partner to gain access to basal cell layer of noninfected partner.

- Digital transmission of nongenital warts probably accounts for few cases of EGW.
- During delivery, mothers with anogenital warts can transmit HPV to neonate, resulting in EGW and laryngeal papillomatosis in children.

Incidence Most sexually active individuals are subclinically infected with HPV; most HPV infections are asymptomatic, subclinical, or unrecognized. 1% of sexually active adults (15–19 years of age) develop EGW. Increased manyfold during the past two decades.

Psychosexual Impact of Genital Warts Public awareness of genital HPV infections is low. Few patients are aware of the role of HPV in anogenital cancer. Diagnosis of genital warts may result in fears about transmission and recurrence, sexual lifestyle changes (abstinence, caution, condoms), depression or low self-esteem, relationships becoming strained and/or breaking down, anxiety related to partner disclosure. Public awareness of genital HPV infection is increasing because of drug advertisements in print and television.

PATHOGENESIS

- "Low-risk" and "high-risk" HPV types both cause EGW.
- HPV infection may persist for years in a dormant state and becomes infectious intermittently.
- Exophytic warts are probably more infectious than subclinical infection.
- *Immunosuppression* may result in new extensive HPV lesions, poor response to treatment, increased multifocal intraepithelial neoplasia.
- Immunosuppressed renal transplant recipients have a 17-fold greater incidence of genital HPV infection.
- All HPV types replicate exclusively in host's cell nucleus.
- In benign HPV-associated lesions, HPV exists as a plasmid in cellular cytoplasm, replicating extrachromosomally.
- In malignant HPV-associated lesions, HPV integrates into host's chromosome, following a break in the viral genome (around E1/E2 region).

- E1 and E2 function is deregulated, resulting in cellular transformation.

EXTERNAL GENITAL WARTS

CLINICAL MANIFESTATION

Skin Symptoms

- Usually asymptomatic, except for cosmetic appearance.
- Anxiety of having STI.
- Itching, burning, bleeding, vaginal or urethral discharge, dyspareunia.
- Obstruction if large mass is uncommon.

Mucocutaneous Lesions

- Four clinical types of genital warts occur:
  - Small papular (Fig. 30-1)
  - Cauliflower-floret (acuminate or pointed) lesions (Figs. 30-2 to 30-4)
  - Keratotic warts (Fig. 30-6)
  - Flat-topped papules/plaques (most common on cervix) (Fig. 30-4).

- Color: skin-colored, pink, red, tan, brown.
- Solitary, scattered, and isolated, or form voluminous confluent masses.
- In immunocompromised individuals, lesions may be huge. (Fig. 30-6)
- Sites of predilection
  - *Male*: Frenulum, corona, glans penis, prepuce, shaft (Figs. 30-1, 30-2, 30-6), scrotum.
  - *Female*: Labia, clitoris, periurethral area, perineum, vagina, cervix (flat lesions) (Fig. 30-4).
  - *Both sexes*: Perineal, perianal (Fig. 30-5), anal canal, rectal; urethral meatus, urethra, bladder; oropharynx.

Laryngeal Papillomas

- Relatively uncommon; associated with HPV-6 and -11.
- Arise most commonly on true vocal cords of larynx.
- Age: children <5 years of age; adults >20 years of age.
- Risk of SCCIS and invasive SCC

DIFFERENTIAL DIAGNOSIS

Papular/Nodular External Genital Lesions
Normal anatomy (e.g., sebaceous glands, pearly penile papules, vestibular papillae), squamous intraepithelial lesions, SCCIS, invasive SCC, benign neoplasms (moles, seborrheic keratoses, skin tags, pilar cyst, angiokeratoma), inflammatory dermatoses (lichen nitidus, lichen planus), molluscum contagiosum, condylomata lata, folliculitis, scabietic nodules.

LABORATORY EXAMINATIONS

Pap Smear   All women should be encouraged to have an annual Pap smear since HPV is the major etiologic agent in pathogenesis for cancer of the cervix. Anal Pap test with a cervical brush and fixative solution is helpful in detecting anal dysplasia.

Dermatopathology   Biopsy is indicated if diagnosis is uncertain; the lesions do not respond to standard therapy; the lesions worsen during

FIGURE 30-1   Papular warts: penis   A 23-year-old male with penile lesions for 6 months. Multiple skin-colored papules on the penis and scrotum.

FIGURE 30-2   Condylomata acuminata: penis   A 25-year-old male with 3-month history of penile lesions. Multiple cauliflower floret-lke papules on penile shaft and foreskin.

FIGURE 30-3   Condylomata acuminata: vulva   Multiple, pink-brown, soft papules on the labia.

FIGURE 30-4   Condylomata acuminata: uterine cervix   Sharply demarcated, whitish, flat plaques becoming confluent around the cervix.

therapy; the patient is immunocompromised; warts are pigmented, indurated, fixed, and/or ulcerated; all suspect cervical lesions. Indicated in some cases to confirm diagnosis and/or rule out SCCIS or invasive SCC.

Detection of HPV DNA Presence of HPV DNA and specific HPV types can be determined on smears and lesional biopsy specimens by in situ hybridization. However, no data support the use of type-specific HPV nucleic acid tests in the routine diagnosis or management of visible genital warts.

Serology Occurrence of genital warts is a marker of unsafe sexual practices. Serologic tests for syphilis should be obtained on all patients to rule out coinfection with *T. pallidum, and all patients offered HIV/AIDS testing.*

DIAGNOSIS

Clinical diagnosis, occasionally confirmed by biopsy.

COURSE AND PROGNOSIS

- HPV is highly infectious, with an incubation period of 3 weeks to 8 months.
- Most HPV-infected individuals who develop EGW do so 2–3 months after becoming infected.
- If left untreated, genital warts may resolve on their own, remain unchanged, or grow. In placebo-treated cases, genital warts clear spontaneously in 20–30% of patients within 3 months.
- After regression, *subclinical infection may persist for life.* Recurrence may occur in individuals with normal immune function as well as with immunocompromise.
- Condylomata may recur due to persistence of latent HPV in normal-appearing perilesional skin (see "Transmission," above). Recurrences more commonly result from reactivation of subclinical infection than from reinfection by a sex partner.
- In pregnancy, genital warts may increase in size and number, show increased vaginal involvement, and have an increased rate of secondary bacterial infection of vaginal warts.
- Children delivered vaginally of mothers with genital HPV infection are at risk for developing recurrent respiratory papillomatosis in later life.

- The major significance of HPV infection is its oncogenicity.
- HPV types 16, 18, 31, and 33 are the major etiologic factors for in situ and invasive SCC:
  ○ Cervix
  ○ External genitalia: vulva and penis
  ○ Anus and perineum: homosexual/bisexual males, females

- Treatment of external genital warts is not likely to influence the development of cervical cancer. The importance of the annual Pap test should be stressed for women with genital warts.

MANAGEMENT

Prevention

- Use of condoms reduces transmission to uninfected sex partners.
- Goal of treatment is removal of exophytic warts and amelioration of signs and symptoms—not eradication of HPV.
- No therapy has been shown to eradicate HPV.
- Treatment is more successful if warts are small and have been present for <1 year.
- Risk of transmission might be reduced by "debulking" genital warts.
- Selection of treatment should be guided by preference of patient—expensive therapies, toxic therapies, and procedures that result in scarring avoided.
- A vaccine that helps protect against four types of HPV is now available for young women from ages 9 to 26 years.

Indications for Therapy

- Cosmetic
- Reduce transmissibility
- Provide relief of symptoms
- Improve self-esteem.

Primary Goal of Treating Visible Genital Warts

- Removal of symptomatic warts. Treatment can induce wart-free periods in most patients.
- Genital warts are often asymptomatic.
- No evidence indicates that currently available treatments eradicate or affect the natural history of HPV infection.
- Removal of warts may or may not decrease infectivity.
- If untreated, visible genital warts may resolve on their own, remain unchanged, or increase in size and number.

FIGURE 30-5 Condylomata acuminata: anus A 60-year-old male with Wegener granulomatosis, treated with azathioprine and prednisone with recent onset of perianal lesions. Multiple pink-tan confluent floret-like lesions surrounding the anus.

- No evidence indicates that treatment of visible warts affects the development of cervical or anal cancer.

Subclinical Genital HPV Infection (without Exophytic Warts) Subclinical genital HPV infection is much more common than exophytic warts among both men and women. Infection is often indirectly diagnosed on the cervix by Pap smear, colposcopy, or biopsy and on the penis, vulva, and other genital skin by the appearance of white areas after application of acetic acid. Treatment is not indicated.

External Genital/Perianal Warts

Patient-Applied Agents

Imiquimod, 5% cream Mechanism of action is via local cytokine release (interferon, tumor necrosis factor, interleukin). No direct antiviral activity. The cream, which is supplied in single-dose packets, is applied to the involved site by the patient, three times per week, usually at bedtime. Some patients experience local cytokine dermatitis (Fig. 30-7B). Treatment duration up to 16 weeks.

Podofilox 0.5% solution and gel. A purified and stable preparation of the active agent in podophyllin. Solution applied with a cotton swab and gel with a finger to condylomata and/or site involved (including normal-appearing skin between lesions)

FIGURE 30-6 Keratotic external genital warts (EGW): male A 46-year-old male with lesion at the base of penis for several years. A keratotic tumor at the base of the penis adjacent to the scrotum. Lesional biopsy reported EGW. Verrucous carcinoma was a concern.

twice daily for 3 days, followed by 4 days of no therapy. This cycle may be repeated as necessary for a total of four cycles. Total area of treatment should not exceed 10 cm², and total volume should not exceed 0.5 mL/d. The health care provider should apply the initial treatment to demonstrate the proper application technique and identify lesions and sites to be treated. Podofilox is contraindicated during pregnancy.

Clinician-Administered Therapy

Cryosurgery with liquid nitrogen   Apply with cotton swab or cryospray. Repeat weekly or biweekly. Relatively inexpensive, does not require anesthesia, and does not result in scarring.

Podophyllin, 10–25%   In compound tincture of benzoin. Limit the total volume of podophyllin solution applied to 0.5 mL or 10 cm² per session. Thoroughly wash off in 1–4 h. Treat <10 cm² per session. Repeat weekly if necessary. If warts persist after six applications, other therapeutic methods should be considered. Podophyllin contraindicated during pregnancy. Repeated application may cause irritation.

Trichloroacetic acid (TCA) or bichloroacetic acid bicarbonate (BCA), 80–90%   Apply only to warts: powder with talc or sodium (baking soda) to remove unreacted acid. Repeat weekly if necessary. If warts persist after six applications, other therapeutic methods should be considered.

Surgical removal   Either by tangential scissor excision, tangential shave excision, curettage, or electrosurgery.

Electrodesiccation/electrocautery   Highly effective in destruction of infected tissue and HPV. Should be attempted only by clinicians trained in the use of this modality. Electrodesiccation is contraindicated in patients with cardiac pacemakers.

Cervical Warts

For women who have exophytic cervical warts, high-grade squamous intraepithelial lesions (SIL) must be excluded before treatment is begun. Management of exophytic cervical warts should include consultation with an expert.

Vaginal Warts

Cryosurgery with liquid nitrogen   This modality is difficult due to "fog" formation, which restricts visualization of lesions.

TCA or BCA, 80–90%   Applied to warts only, powder with talc or sodium bicarbonate to remove unreacted acid if an excess amount is applied. Repeat weekly if necessary.

Podophyllin, 10–25%   In compound tincture of benzoin. Treated area must be dry before the speculum is removed. Treat with 2 cm² per session. Repeat application at weekly intervals. Systemic absorption is a concern.

Urethral Meatus Warts

Cryosurgery with liquid nitrogen   As above.
Podophyllin, 10–25%, as above.

Anal Warts

Management of warts on rectal mucosa should be referred to an expert.

Surgical removal   As above.

Oral Warts

Cryosurgery with liquid nitrogen   As above.
Surgical removal   As above.

Follow-Up

- After visible warts have cleared, a follow-up evaluation is not mandatory. Patients should be cautioned to watch for recurrences, which occur most frequently during the first 3 months.
- Because the sensitivity and specificity of self-diagnosis of genital warts are unknown, patients concerned about recurrences should be offered a follow-up evaluation 3 months after treatment. Earlier follow-up visits may also be useful to document a wart-free state, to monitor for or treat complications of therapy, and to provide the opportunity for patient education and counseling.
- Women should be counseled about the need for regular cytologic screening as recommended for women without genital warts.
- The presence of genital warts is not an indication for cervical colposcopy.

Immunocompromised Persons

- Persons who are chronically immunocompromised because of HIV/AIDS, solid organ transplantation, or other reasons may not

respond as well as immunocompetent persons to therapy for genital warts and may have more frequent recurrences after treatment.
- SCC arising in or resembling genital warts might occur more frequently among immunosuppressed persons, requiring more frequent biopsy for confirmation of diagnosis.

Management of Sex Partners

- Examination of sex partners is not necessary because role of reinfection is probably minimal.
- Most partners are probably already subclinically infected with HPV, even if no warts are visible.

A

B

FIGURE 30-7 Condylomata acuminata: anus A 45-year-old male with perianal EGW for 3 months.
A. Large perianal confluent EGW.
B. 5% imiquimod cream was applied three times weekly; cytokine dermatitis occurred after 3 weeks. EGW had completely disappeared by the 6th week of treatment.

HPV: SQUAMOUS CELL CARCINOMA IN SITU (SCCIS) AND INVASIVE SCC OF ANOGENITAL SKIN ■ ●

- HPV infection of the anogenital epithelium can result in a spectrum of changes referred to as *squamous intraepithelial lesions* (SILs), ranging from mild dysplasia to SCCIS.
- Over time, these lesions can regress, persist, progress, or recur, in some cases to invasive SCC.
- Clinically, lesions appear as multifocal macules, papules, plaques on the external anogenital region.

- Lesions involving the cervix and anus have the highest risk for transformation to invasive SCC; however, lesions can transform at any site.

Synonyms: Vulvar intraepithelial neoplasia, penile intraepithelial neoplasm, bowenoid papulosis.

EPIDEMIOLOGY AND ETIOLOGY

Terminology

- The Bethesda System (National Cancer Institute) is currently used as terminology for "dysplastic" lesions caused by HPV on anogenital sites (Table 30-3).
- The terminology applies to both cytologic (Pap test) and histologic assessments.
- Intraepithelial neoplasia are designated as cervical (CIN), vulvar (VIN), penile (PIN), and anal (AIN).
- VIN is classified as VIN1 (mild dysplasia), VIN2 (moderate dysplasia), VIN3 (severe dysplasia or carcinoma in situ), and VIN3 differentiated type, basaloid, bowenoid (warty).

Etiology HPV types 16, 18, 31, and 33 (see Table 27-2).

Transmission HPV transmitted sexually. Autoinoculation. Rarely, HPV-16 transmitted from mother to newborn with subsequent development on penis.

Incidence

- Marked increase during past two decades associated with increased sexual promiscuity.
- Cervical SCC is the second most common female malignancy worldwide, second only to breast cancer.
- It is the most frequent malignancy in developing countries—500,000 new cases and 200,000 deaths worldwide attributed to it annually.

TABLE 30-3 Bethesda System for Classification of Anogenital Dysplasia

Histologic Findings		Older Terminology/ Replaced	Still Older Terminology
Atypical proliferating suprabasal cells present in the lower one-third of the epithelium, although cytopathic changes of HPV are full thickness	Low-grade squamous intraepithelial lesion (LSIL)	Intraepithelial 1 (IN1)	Mild dysplasia
Atypical proliferating suprabasal cells present in the lower two-thirds of the epithelium, although cytopathic changes of HPV are full thickness	High-grade SIL (HSIL)	IN2 and IN3	
Atypical proliferating suprabasal cells present in the full thickness of the epithelium	Squamous cell carcinoma in situ (SCCIS)	Squamous cell carcinoma in situ (SCCIS),	Erythroplasia of Querat, Bowen disease, bowenoid papulosis
Invasive SCC present, usually arising in a field of HSIL	Invasive SCC	Invasive SCC	

Risk Factors Immunocompromised state, cigarette smoking are risk factors for more dysplastic lesions and invasive SCC.

PATHOGENESIS

- HPV-16- and -18-infected cells may not be able to differentiate fully as a result of either:
  - Functional interference of cell cycle–regulating proteins, caused by viral gene expression (e.g., interaction between HPV-16 E6 with cellular protein p53, interaction between HPV-16 E7 with cellular protein pRB); or
  - Overproduction of E5, E6, and E7.
- When this occurs, the host DNA synthesis continues unchecked and leads to rapidly dividing undifferentiated cells with morphologic characteristics of intraepithelial neoplasia.
- Accumulated chromosomal breakages, rearrangements, deletions, and other genomic mutations in these cells lead to cells with invasion capability and, ultimately, to cervical malignancy.

CLINICAL MANIFESTATION

Duration of Lesions Weeks to months to years to decades.
Incubation Period Months to years.
Systems Review Prior history of condylomata acuminata. Female partners of males may have CIN.

Mucocutaneous Lesions

- Types of lesions
  - Erythematous flat-topped papules.
  - Lichenoid (flat-topped) or pigmented papules (called *bowenoid papulosis*) (Figs. 30-8, 30-9).
  - May show confluence or form plaque(s).
  - Leukoplakia-like plaque (Fig. 30-10). Surface usually smooth, velvety.
- Colors: Tan, brown, pink, red, violaceous, white.
- Nodule or ulceration in field of SIL suggests invasive SCC (Figs. 30-11 and 30-12).
- Characteristically clusters, i.e., commonly multifocal. May be solitary.
- *Distribution*
  - Males: glans penis, prepuce (75%) (flat lichenoid papules or erythematous macules); penile shaft (25%) (pigmented papules).
  - Females: labia majora and minora, clitoris. Multicentric involvement of the cervix, vulva, perineum, and/or anus occurs not infrequently.
  - Both sexes: inguinal folds, perineal/perianal skin. Oropharyngeal mucosa.

- Sites other than external genitalia
  - May be associated with cervical dysplasia, CIN, cervical SCC.
  - Rarely, SCCIS of other sites, i.e., nail unit (periungual, nail bed); intraoral.

DIFFERENTIAL DIAGNOSIS

Multiple Skin-Colored Papules ± Hyperkeratosis
External genital warts, psoriasis vulgaris; lichen planus.
Pigmented Anogenital Macule(s)/Papule(s)
Genital lentiginosis, melanoma (in situ or invasive), pigmented basal cell carcinoma, angiokeratomas.

LABORATORY EXAMINATIONS

Dermatopathology Epidermal proliferation with numerous mitotic figures, abnormal mitoses, atypical pleomorphic cells with large hyperchromatic, often clumped nuclei, dyskeratotic cells; basal membrane intact. Koilocytosis. Recent application of podophyllin to condyloma acuminatum may cause changes similar to SCCIS.
Southern Blot Analysis Identifies HPV type.
Pap Smear Koilocytotic atypia.
Exfoliative Cytology Cervical Pap smears have been recommended annually for women ≥50 years of age. Cytology of the anal canal may also be helpful in management of individuals with a history of anal HPV infection, especially if immunocompromised (HIV/AIDS, renal transplant recipients). Anal Pap tests are obtained with a cervical brush and ThinPrep solution. By the Bethesda System, these cytologic findings are reported as atypical squamous cells of undetermined significance (ASCUS), low-grade squamous intraepithelial lesion (LSIL), high-grade (HSIL), and SCC.

DIAGNOSIS

Clinical suspicion, confirmed by biopsy of lesion.

COURSE AND PROGNOSIS

- Invasive SCC develops only through well-defined precursor lesions (Figs. 30-11, 30-12).
- Over time, these lesions can regress, persist, recur, or progress, in some cases to invasive SCC.
- Natural history of CIN is best studied: progression to invasive SCC occur in 36% of cases over a 20-year period.
- Rate of progression of AIN is not known but appears to be increasing. AIN may develop deep in glands and, although detected cytologically, can exist before visible lesions are detected with colposcopy.
- Patients with intraepithelial neoplasias, which often occur in immunocompromised individuals, should be followed indefinitely, with monitoring by exfoliative cytology and lesional biopsy specimens.

MANAGEMENT

Colposcopy   The most common indication for colposcopy is abnormal exfoliative cytology. Acetic acid, 3–5%, is applied to the cervix, which causes columnar and abnormal epithelium to become edematous. Abnormal (atypical) epithelium adopts a white or opaque appearance that can be distinguished from the normal pink epithelium. Abnormal epithelium is then biopsied. Colposcopy can also be performed on individuals with abnormal anal exfoliative cytology, and biopsy specimens obtained from abnormal site(s).

Biopsy of Lesions   In cases of documented SIL or SCCIS, biopsy specimens should be obtained from rapidly enlarging lesions, areas of ulceration or bleeding, exuberant tissue with abnormal vascularity.

Local Therapy of SIL   The only way of possibly reducing the potential risk of invasive SCC is diagnosis and eradication of intraepithelial disease. Because lesions are relatively uncommon, cases are often best managed by a dermatologist with clinical experience in the care of these patients, an oncologic gynecologist, or a colorectal surgeon. If lesion biopsy specimens do not show early invasion, lesions can be treated medically or surgically.

Medical Management   5-Fluorouracil cream has been used but is difficult to use because of erosions. Imiquimod cream 5% is also effective.

Surgical Management   Surgical excision, Mohs surgery, electrosurgery, laser vaporization, cryosurgery.

FIGURE 30-8   HPV squamous cell carcinoma in situ (SCCIS): penis   A 48-year-old male with penile lesion for 2 years. Pink-tan papules forming a 1-cm plaque on the shaft of the penis. Lesional biopsy reported SCCIS with HPV changes (koilocytosis). Electrosurgery was successful.

FIGURE 30-9 HPV squamous cell carcinoma in situ (SCCIS): vulva A 33-year-old renal transplant recipient with anogenital lesions for several years. A large pink plaque on the perineum and multiple small papules. Lesional biopsy was reported to show SCCIS with HPV changes (koilocytosis).

FIGURE 30-10 HPV squamous cell carcinoma in situ (SCCIS): vulva A 49-year-old male with HIV/AIDS noted to have anal lesion for 1 month. A white firm nodule on the rim of the anus. Biopsy reported SCCIS with HPV changes. No lesions were detected on anal colposcopy.

FIGURE 30-11   HPV-induced in situ and invasive squamous cell carcinoma: vulva   Several red nodules (invasive SCC) arising within a white plaque (SCCIS) on the left labium.

FIGURE 30-12   HPV-induced in situ and invasive squamous cell carcinoma: perineal/perianal A 38-year-old male with HIV/AIDS aware of perianal lesions for several months; he had prior history of EGW. Brown perineal and perianal macules and papules (SCCIS) with a pink nodule arising at the anal verge. The patient presented when he detected the nodule, which he thought was a hemorrhoid. Excisional biopsy of the nodule detected invasive SCC arising within SCCIS.

HERPES SIMPLEX VIRUS: GENITAL INFECTIONS   ■ ◑

- Genital herpes (GH) is a chronic sexually transmitted viral infection, characterized by symptomatic and asymptomatic viral shedding.

- In most cases, both primary infection and recurrences are asymptomatic.

- When symptomatic, primary GH may present with
  - Grouped vesicles or erosions at site of inoculation associated with significant pain
  - Regional lymphadenopathy.

- When aware of GH, individuals may notice mild symptoms, uncommonly of recurring outbreaks of vesicles at the same site.

- Most symptoms from GH relate to the psychological stigma of having a chronic incurable and transmissible STI.

- (See also "Herpes Simplex Virus Infections," Section 27.)

- Neonates are susceptible to HSV infection when exposed perinatally, with risk of significant morbidity and mortality.

Synonyms: Herpes genitalis, genital herpes simplex.

ICD-9 : 054.10 ○ ICD-10 : A60

EPIDEMIOLOGY AND ETIOLOGY

Age of Onset   Young, sexually active adults.

Etiology

- HSV-2 > HSV-1.
- Currently in the United States, 30% of new cases of GH are caused by HSV-1.
- See also Section 27.

Prevalence

- Highly variable. Depends on many factors: country, region of residence, population subgroup, sex, age. Higher among higher risk sexual behavior groups. Higher among women than men.
- Prevalence of HSV-2 seropositivity in general population: United States: 21%; Europe: 8–15%; Africa: 40–50% in 20-year-olds.
- Strongly associated with age, increasing from negligible levels in children <12 to as high as 80% among higher risk populations. In a given population, HSV-1 prevalence is almost always >HSV-2 prevalence.
- Prevalence is highest in areas of Africa and parts of the Americas. Lower in western and southern Europe than in northern Europe and North America. Lower in Asia than other areas.
- In the United States, >600,000 new infections annually; 30 million Americans are HSV-2 infected, i.e., approximately one in five adults. Older studies report the presence of antibodies to HSV-2 varies with the sexual history of the individual: nuns, 3%; middle class, 25%; heterosexuals at an STD clinic, 26%; homosexuals, 46%; lower classes, 46–60%; prostitutes, 70–80%.

Race and Sex   By HSV-2 seropositivity studies in the United States, more common in blacks: 3 in 5 men, 4 in 5 women; in whites: 1 in 5 men, 1 in 4 women. In whites, prevalence levels off after age 30 years. In blacks/Hispanics, prevalence continues to increase after age 30.

Transmission

- Usually skin-to-skin contact.
- In most cases, 70% of transmission occurs during times of asymptomatic HSV shedding, which occurs during 1% of days when no identifiable lesion is present.
- Shedding rate is higher from HSV-2 than HSV-1.
- Transmission rate in discordant couples (one partner infected, the other not) approximately 10% per year; 25% of females become infected, compared with only 4–6% of males.

- Prior HSV-1 infection is protective; in females with anti-HSV-1 antibodies, 15% become infected with HSV-2, but in those without anti-HSV-1 antibodies, 30% become infected with HSV-2.

Risk Factors for Transmission   Risk increases with number of sex partners. 40% of those with 50 different partners have genital HSV infection.

Diseases Characterized by Genital Ulcers   In the United States, most patients with genital ulcers have GH, syphilis, or chancroid. The relative frequency varies by geographic area and patient population, but in most areas GH is the most common of these diseases. More than one of these diseases may be present among at least 3–10% of patients with genital ulcers. Each disease has been associated with an increased risk for HIV/AIDS infection.

Impact of GH   The physical symptoms of GH are minor in most individuals. The major symptoms are psychological, i.e., social stigmatization and fear of harming someone through sexual intercourse.

Pregnancy and GH

- Asymptomatic HSV shedding occurs in 0.35–1.4% of women in labor in the United States.
- 32% of pregnant women have anti-HSV antibodies.
- 10% of pregnant women are at risk for primary HSV-2 infection from HSV-2 infected partners.
- Incidence of neonatal herpes: 1 in 2800 to 1 in 15,000 births.
  - 95% of newborns with HSV infection contract it during labor and delivery.
  - Transmission can occur intrauterine, perinatally, or postnatally.
  - Risk factors for neonatal HSV infection: primary GH in mother at time of delivery, absent maternal anti-HSV antibody, procedures on fetus, father with HSV infection.

- Treatment of mother with GH at time of delivery is an option for cesarean section (not approved).

PATHOGENESIS

- HSV infection is transmitted through close contact with a person shedding virus at a peripheral site, mucosal surface, or secretion.
- HSV is inactivated promptly at room temperature; aerosol or fomitic spread unlikely.

- Infection occurs via inoculation onto susceptible mucosal surface or break in skin.
- Subsequent to primary infection at inoculation site, HSV ascends peripheral sensory nerves and enters sensory or autonomic nerve root ganglia, where latency is established.
- Latency can occur after both symptomatic and asymptomatic primary infection.
- Recrudescences may be clinically symptomatic or asymptomatic.

CLINICAL MANIFESTATION

Incubation Period   2- to 20-day (average 6) incubation period.

Symptoms

- Only 10% of HSV-2 seropositive individuals are aware that symptoms are those of GH.
- 90% do not recognize symptoms of GH.

Primary GH

- Most individuals with primary infection are asymptomatic.
- Those with symptoms report fever, headache, malaise, myalgia, peaking within the first 3–4 days after onset of lesions, resolving during the subsequent 3–4 days.
- Depending on location, pain, itching, dysuria, lumbar radiculitis, vaginal or urethral discharge are common symptoms.
- Tender inguinal lymphadenopathy occurs during second and third weeks.
- Deep pelvic pain associated with pelvic lymphadenopathy.
- Some cases of first clinical episode of GH are manifested by extensive disease that requires hospitalization.

Recurrent GH

- New symptoms may result from old infections.
- Most individuals with GH do not experience "classic" findings of grouped vesicles on erythematous base.
- Common symptoms are itching, burning, fissure, redness, irritation prior to eruption of vesicles.
- Dysuria, sciatica, rectal discomfort.

Systemic Symptoms   Symptoms of aseptic HSV-2 meningitis can occur with primary or recurrent GH.

Mucocutaneous Lesions

- Most clinical lesions are minor breaks in the mucocutaneous epithelium, presenting as erosion, "abrasions," fissures.
- The "classically" described findings are *uncommon.*

Primary GH

- An erythematous plaque is often noted initially, followed soon by grouped vesicles, which may evolve to pustules; these become eroded as the overlying epidermis sloughs (Figs. 30-13, 30-14).
- Erosions are superficial; may enlarge to ulcerations; "classic" findings described below may be crusted or moist.
- These epithelial defects heal in 2–4 weeks, often with resulting postinflammatory hypo- or hyperpigmentation, uncommonly with scarring.
- The area of involvement may be circumferential around the penis, or the entire vulva may be involved.

Recurrent GH

- Lesions may be similar to primary infection but on a reduced scale. Often a 1- to 2-cm plaque of erythema surmounted with vesicles (Fig. 30-15), which rupture with formation of erosions (Fig. 30-16).
- Heals in 1–2 weeks.

Distribution   *Males*   Primary infection: glans, prepuce, shaft, sulcus, scrotum, thighs, buttocks. Recurrences: penile shaft (Figs. 30-14, 30-15), glans, buttocks.
Females   Primary infection: labia majora/minora (Fig. 30-13), perineum, inner thighs. Recurrences: labia majora / minora (Fig. 30-16), buttocks.
Anorectal Infection   Occurs following anal intercourse (often HSV-1); characterized by tenesmus, anal pain, proctitis, discharge, and ulcerations (Fig. 30-17) as far as 10 cm into anal canal.
General Findings   *Regional Lymph Nodes* Inguinal/femoral lymph nodes enlarged, firm, nonfluctuant, tender; usually unilateral.
Signs of Aseptic Meningitis   Fever, nuchal rigidity. Can occur in the absence of GH. Pain along sciatic nerve.

FIGURE 30-13   Genital herpes, primary: vulvar infection   Multiple, extremely painful, punched-out, confluent, shallow ulcers on the edematous vulva and perineum. Micturition is often very painful. Associated inguinal lymphadenopathy is common.

DIFFERENTIAL DIAGNOSIS

Anogenital Erosive(s)/Ulcer(s)   Trauma, candidiasis, syphilitic chancre, fixed-drug eruption, chancroid, gonococcal erosion.

LABORATORY STUDIES

See Section 27 "Herpes Simplex Virus Infections".

DIAGNOSIS

Because in most cases intermittent asymptomatic shedding is occurring and lesions are "atypical" (not grouped vesicles on erythematous base), GH must be confirmed by viral culture or direct fluorescent antibody (DFA) or serology.

COURSE AND PROGNOSIS

- GH may be recurrent and has no cure.
- 70% of HSV-2 infections are asymptomatic.
- HSV-2 GH recurs approximately six times per year; HSV-1 GH usually recurs, on the average, only once per year.

- Of individuals with initially symptomatic genital HSV-2 infection, almost all have symptomatic recurrences; recurrence rates are high in those with an extended first episode of infection, regardless of whether antiviral therapy is given.
- The rate of recurrence is 20% higher in men than women.
- Chronic suppressive therapy does not completely suppress viral shedding; it is reduced by 95% as detected by viral culture, and by 80% by PCR.
- Chronic suppressive therapy may reduce transmission, but this has not been documented.
- The incidence of primary infection with acyclovir-resistant HSV strains in individuals never exposed to acyclovir is 2.7% in the United States.
- Treatment of first-episode infection prevents complications such as meningitis, radiculitis.
- Erythema multiforme may complicate GH, occurring 1–2 weeks after an outbreak.

MANAGEMENT

See Table 30-5.
Website   CDC guidelines for treatment of genital ulcers:
http://www.cdc.gov/std/treatment/

FIGURE 30-14   Genital herpes, primary: penis and scrotum   A 48-year-old male with painful genital lesions for 4 days. Multiple erosions on the penis and scrotum.

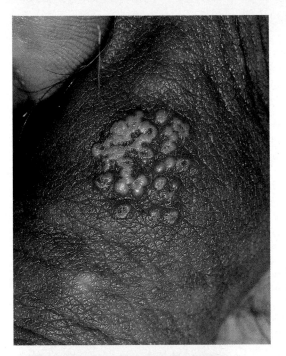

FIGURE 30-15 Genital herpes, recurrent: penis Group of vesicles with early central crusting on a red base arising on the shaft of the penis. This "textbook" presentation, however, is much less common than small asymptomatic erosions or fissures.

FIGURE 30-16 Genital herpes, recurrent: vulva Large, painful erosions on the labia. Extensive lesions such as these are uncommon in recurrent genital herpes in an otherwise healthy individual.

FIGURE 30-17 Genital herpes, recurrent: anus and perineum Multiple, painful, sharply demarcated ulcers in an HIV/AIDS male.

TABLE 30-5   Management of Genital Herpes

Prevention of GH

Sexual transmission	• Patients should be advised to abstain from sexual activity while lesions are present.
	• Use of condoms should be encouraged during all sexual exposures.
	• Efficacy of chronic suppressive therapy not proven.
	• Patients with GH should be told about the natural history of the disease, with emphasis on the potential of recurrent episodes, asymptomatic viral shedding, and sexual transmission.
	• Sexual transmission of HSV has been documented to occur during periods without evidence of lesions. In discordant couples, transmission usually occurs during period of asymptomatic shedding.
	• Risk for neonatal infection should be explained to all patients—male and female—with GH.
Perinatal transmission	Many experts recommend serotesting for HSV-1 and HSV-2 (Western blot) at the first prenatal visit. Infants born to women who asymptomatically shed HSV have reduced birth weight and increased prematurity.
Topical antiviral therapy	No significant efficacy.
Oral antiviral therapy	Antiviral agents provide partial control of symptoms and signs of herpes episodes when used to treat first clinical episode or when used as suppressive therapy. They neither eradicate latent virus nor affect subsequent risk, frequency, or severity of recurrences after drug is discontinued. Even after laboratory testing, at least a quarter of patients with GH have no laboratory-confirmed diagnosis. Many experts recommend treatment for chancroid and syphilis as well as GH if the diagnosis is unclear or if the patient resides in a community in which chancroid is present.
First clinical episode (primary or first symptomatic)	Many persons with first-episode herpes have mild clinical manifestations but later develop severe or prolonged symptoms. Therefore, patients with initial genital herpes should receive antiviral therapy.
Acyclovir	400 mg three times a day for 7–10 days, *or*
Acyclovir	200 mg five times a day for 7–10 days *or*
Valacyclovir	1 g twice a day for 7–10 days.
Famciclovir	250 mg three times a day for 7–10 days.
First clinical episode of herpes proctitis	
Acyclovir	400 mg PO 5 times daily for 10 days or until clinical resolution occurs.
Recurrent episodes	When treatment is instituted (by patient) during the prodrome or within 2 days of onset of lesions, patients with recurrent disease experience limited benefit from therapy because the severity of the eruption is reduced. If early treatment cannot be administered, most immunocompetent patients with recurrent disease do not benefit from acyclovir treatment; and for these patients it is not generally recommended.
Acyclovir	400 mg PO three times a day for 5 days, *or*
	800 mg PO twice a day for 5 days, *or*
	800 mg PO three times a day for 2 days.
Valacyclovir	500 mg PO twice a day for 3 days, *or*
	1 g PO twice a day for 3 days, *or*
Famciclovir	125 mg PO twice daily for 5 days, *or*
	1 g PO once a day for 5 days.

Oral antiviral therapy

Daily suppressive therapy	Reduces frequency of recurrences by at least 75% among patients with frequent (> 6–9 per year) recurrences. Suppressive treatment with oral acyclovir does not totally eliminate symptomatic or asymptomatic viral shedding or the potential for transmission. Safety and efficacy have been documented among persons receiving daily therapy for as long as 5 years. Acyclovir-resistant strains of HSV have been isolated from some persons receiving suppressive therapy, but these strains have not been associated with treatment failure among immunocompetent patients. *After 1 year of continuous therapy, acyclovir should be discontinued to allow assessment of the patient's rate of recurrent episodes.*
Acyclovir	400 mg PO twice a day, *or*
Valacyclovir	500 or 1000 mg PO once a day, *or*
Famciclovir	250 mg orally once a day.
Severe disease/ immuno- compromise	Patients with herpes who do not respond to the recommended dose of acyclovir may require a higher oral dose of acyclovir, IV acyclovir, or may be infected with an acyclovir-resistant HSV strain, requiring IV foscarnet. The roles of valacyclovir and famciclovir are not yet established. IV therapy should be provided for patients with severe disease or complications necessitating hospitalization (e.g., disseminated infection that includes encephalitis, pneumonitis, or hepatitis).
Acyclovir	5 mg/kg body weight IV every 8 h for 5–7 days or until clinical resolution is attained, *or* 400 mg PO 5 times a day for 7–14 days.
Oral valacyclovir *or* famciclovir	Have reduced the necessity for IV acyclovir therapy.
Neonatal	See "Neonatal HSV Infection," Section 27.
Acyclovir-resistant	See "HSV Infections," Section 27.
Foscarnet	40 mg/kg IV q8h for 14–21 days.

SYPHILIS   ICD-9:091.3 ∘ ICD-10:A50-AB

- Etiologic agent: *Treponema pallidum*
- A chronic systemic infection transmitted through skin and mucosa, with manifestations in nearly every organ system.
- Manifestations:
  - A painless ulcer or chancre on the mucocutaneous site of inoculation
  - Associated with regional lymphadenopathy (chancriform syndrome: distal ulcer associated with proximal lymphadenopathy)
  - Shortly after inoculation, syphilis becomes a systemic infection with characteristic secondary and tertiary stages (Table 30-6).

- Clinical course and response to standard therapy may be altered in HIV/AIDS.

Synonyms: Lues, the great imitator. Primary syphilis, L1; secondary syphilis, L2; tertiary syphilis, L3. The French disease, Italian disease, Spanish disease, Polish disease, Christian disease, Frank disease, British disease. Great pox (distinguishing it from smallpox). Cupid's disease. Grandgore. The Black Lion.

EPIDEMIOLOGY AND ETIOLOGY

Etiology Subspecies identified by PCR-based methods.

- Venereal syphilis: *Treponema pallidum* ssp. *pallidum* (*T. pallidum*). *T. pallidum* is a thin delicate spirochete with 6–14 spirals. Only natural host for *T. pallidum* is the human.
- Yaws: *T. pallidum* ssp. *pertenue.*
- Endemic syphilis (bejel): *T. pallidum* ssp. *endemicum.*
- Pinta: *T. carateum.*

Age of Onset In decreasing order: 20–39 years, 15–19 years, 40–49 years.

TABLE 30-6   Classification of the Clinical Stages of Syphilis (See Image 30-1)

Stage	Characterization
Primary syphilis	Localized infection at site of inoculation (chancre)
Secondary syphilis	Disseminated infection (exanthem, maculopapules, condylomata lata)
Latent syphilis	No clinical signs or symptoms of infection (seropositive)
Early	<1-year duration; any period between primary and secondary stage
Late	≥ than 1 year since patient became infected
Syphilis of unknown duration	
Late (tertiary) syphilis	Cutaneous, vascular, neurologic findings
Congenital syphilis	Acquired in utero or perinatally; early and late clinical findings

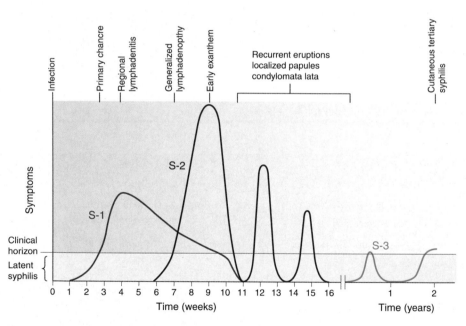

CLINICAL MANIFESTATIONS OF SYPHILIS

IMAGE 30-1   Clinical manifestations of syphilis. S-1, primary syphilis; S-2, secondary syphilis; S-3, tertiary syphilis. (From JL Bolognia, JL Jorizzo, RP Rapin, in *Dermatology.* London, New York, Philadelphia, Mosby, 2003, p. 443; with permission

Incidence   In the United States, uncommon with 36,000 cases of primary and secondary in 2006.

Race   All races; in the United States, incidence increasing in African Americans and Hispanics.

Sex   Males outnumber females 2:1 to 4:1.

Other Factors   Until recently, nearly half of all males with syphilis in the United States were male who have sex with males (MSM), but this percentage has decreased due to safer sexual practices. Incidence of syphilis, however, has markedly increased in minorities and is associated with exchange of sex for drugs. Associated with the increase in venereal syphilis is a marked increase in the number of cases of congenital syphilis.

Transmission

• *Sexual contact*: Contact with infectious lesion (chancre, mucous patch, condyloma latum,

cutaneous lesions of secondary syphilis). 60% of contacts of persons with primary and secondary syphilis become infected.
- *Congenital infection*: In utero or perinatal transmission.
- *Blood products*: One-half of cases named as contacts of infectious syphilis become infected. Refrigeration of blood kills the spirochete.

Serologic Testing Serologic testing for syphilis (STS) has declined in the United States. Currently, testing is performed in pregnant women, persons admitted to hospitals, military inductees, persons undergoing examination in physicians' offices. Premarital testing is performed in some states.

PATHOGENESIS

- The spirochetes pass through intact mucous membrane and microscopic abrasion in skin, enter lymphatics and blood within a few hours, and produce systemic infection and metastatic foci before development of a primary lesion.
- Spirochetes divide locally, with resulting host inflammatory response and chancre formation, either a single lesion or, less commonly, multiple lesions.
- Cellular immunity is of major importance in healing of early lesions and control of infection (T_H1 type).
- Primary syphilis is the most contagious stage of the disease.
- Later syphilis is essentially a vascular disease, lesions occurring secondary to obliterative endarteritis of terminal arterioles and small arteries and by the resulting inflammatory and necrotic changes.

LABORATORY EXAMINATIONS

Demonstration of the Organism *Dark-Field Microscopy* Positive in primary chancre and papular lesions of secondary syphilis, in particular condylomata lata. Unreliable in oral cavity because of the presence of saprophytic spirochetes, and negative in patients treated systemically or topically with antibiotics. Regional lymph node aspirated and aspirate examined in the dark-field microscope.
Direct Fluorescent Antibody T. pallidum (DFA-TP) Test Fluorescent antibodies are used to detect *T. pallidum* in exudate from lesion, lymph node aspirate, or tissue.

PCR Available in research laboratories.
Serologic Tests for Syphilis Positive in persons with any treponemal infection (venereal syphilis, endemic syphilis, yaws, pinta). Tests always positive in secondary syphilis.

Nontreponemal STS

- Measures IgG and IgM directed against cardiolipin-lecithin-cholesterol antigen complex.
- Rapid plasma reagin (RPR) test (automated RPR: ART).
- VDRL slide test.
  - Nonreactive in 25% of patients with primary syphilis.
- In early syphilis: either do fluorescent treponemal antibody-absorbed (FTA-ABS) test or repeat VDRL in 1–2 weeks if initial VDRL negative.
- Prozone phenomenon: if antibody titer high, test may be negative; must dilute serum.
- Becomes nonreactive or reactive in lower titers following therapy for early syphilis.

Treponemal STS

- FTA-ABS test.
  - Agglutination assays for antibodies to *T. pallidum*:
  - Microhemagglutination assay (MHA-TP; Serodia TPPA test).
  - *T. pallidum* hemagglutination test (TPHA).
- Often remain reactive after therapy; not helpful in determining infectious status of patient with past syphilis.

False-Positive STS See Table 30-7. Antigen used in nontreponemal test found in other tissues; may be positive (does not exceed 1:8 dilution).
Evaluation for Neurosyphilis Lumbar puncture indicated in following: neurologic signs or symptoms, treatment failure, serum reagin titer ≥1:32, HIV/AIDS seropositivity, other evidence of active syphilis (aortitis, gumma, visual/hearing changes), plans to administer nonpenicillin therapy. CSF examination for pleocytosis, increased protein concentration, VDRL activity. Abnormal in 40% of early syphilis and 25% of latent infection.
Evaluation for Syphilis in HIV/AIDS STS for newly diagnosed HIV/AIDS. CSF for all co-infected patients.
Dermatopathology In primary and secondary syphilis, lesional skin biopsy shows central thinning or ulceration of epidermis. Lymphocytic and plasmacytic dermal infiltrate. Proliferation of capillaries and lymphatics with endarteritis;

TABLE 30-7 Causes of False-Positive Reactions in Nontreponemal Serologic Tests for Syphilis

Cause	Rate of False-Positive Reactions,%*
ACUTE FALSE-POSITIVE REACTION (<6 MONTHS)	
Recent viral illness or immunization	1–2
Genital herpes	1–4
HIV/AIDS infection	1–4
Malaria	11
Parenteral drug use	20–25
CHRONIC FALSE-POSITIVE REACTION (≥6 MONTHS)	
Aging	9–11
Autoimmune disorders	1–20
Systemic lupus erythematosus	11–20
Rheumatoid arthritis	5
Parenteral drug use	20–25

*Data were collected from a variety of published reports.
SOURCE: SA Lukehart, in DL Kasper et al (eds): *Harrison's Principles of Internal Medicine;* 16th ed. New York, McGraw-Hill, 2005.

may have thrombosis and small areas of necrosis. Dieterle stain demonstrates spirochetes.

COURSE AND PROGNOSIS

- Even without treatment, chancre heals completely in 4–6 weeks, the infection either becoming latent or clinical manifestations of secondary syphilis appearing.
- Secondary syphilis usually manifests as macular exanthem initially; after weeks, lesions resolve spontaneously and recur as maculopapular or papular eruptions.
- In 20% of untreated cases, up to three to four such recurrences followed by periods of clinical remission may occur over a period of 1 year.
- Infection then enters a latent stage, in which there are no clinical signs or symptoms of the disease.
- After untreated syphilis has persisted for >4 years, it is rarely communicable, except in the case of pregnant women, who, if untreated, may transmit syphilis to their fetuses, regardless of the duration of their disease.
- One-third of patients with untreated latent syphilis developed clinically apparent tertiary disease.
- Gummas hardly ever heal spontaneously. Noduloulcerative syphilides undergo spontaneous partial healing, but new lesions appear at the periphery.

MANAGEMENT

See Table 30-8.

PRIMARY SYPHILIS

CLINICAL MANIFESTATIONS

Symptoms   A genital or extragenital lesion may be noted. Ulcers are usually painless unless superinfected.
Incubation Period   21 days (average); range, 10–90 days.

Skin Lesions
Chancre

- Button-like papule (Fig. 30-18) that develops at the site of inoculation into a painless erosion and then ulcerates with raised border and scanty serous exudate (Figs. 30-19 to 30-21A). Surface may be crusted. Size: few millimeters to 1 or 2 cm in diameter. Border of lesion may be raised. Palpation: most commonly, firm with indurated border; painless.
- Arrangement: single lesion; less commonly, few, multiple, or kissing lesions.
- Extragenital chancres, particularly on the fingers, may be painful.
- Atypically, genital chancres painful, especially if superinfected with *Staphylococcus aureus*.

FIGURE 30-18 Primary syphilis: penile chancre A 28-year-old male with penile lesion for 7 days. Painless ulcer on distal penile shaft with smaller erosion on the glans. The ulcer is quite firm on palpation.

FIGURE 30-19 Primary syphilis: nodule on glans A 58-year-old male with penile lesion for 10 days. Red firm nodule on the glans; the lesion resolved without therapy and did not ulcerate. Biopsy reported inflammatory changes. The diagnosis was made in retrospect when STS obtained before marriage was positive.

FIGURE 30-20 Primary syphilis: chancre on scrotum A 25-year-old male with painful lesion on scrotum for 10 days. A 1.5-cm ulcer on the scrotum, firm on palpation.

TABLE 30-8   Recommendations for the Treatment of Syphilis

Stage of Syphilis	Patients without Penicillin Allergy	Patients with Confirmed Penicillin Allergy
Primary, secondary, or early latent	Penicillin G benzathine (single dose of 2.4 million units IM, 1.2 million units in each buttock)	Tetracycline hydrochloride (500 mg PO four times a day) or doxycycline (100 mg PO twice a day) for 2 weeks
Late latent (or latent of uncertain duration), cardiovascular, or benign tertiary	Lumbar puncture CSF normal: Penicillin G benzathine (2.4 million units IM weekly for 3 weeks)	Lumbar puncture CSF normal: Tetracycline hydrochloride (500 mg PO four times a day) or doxycycline (100 mg PO Twice a day) for 4 weeks
	CSF abnormal: Treat as neurosyphilis	CSF abnormal: Treat as neurosyphilis
Neurosyphilis (asymptomatic or symptomatic)	Aqueous penicillin G (18–24 million units/d IV, given in divided doses every 4 h) for 10–14 days *or* Aqueous penicillin G procaine (2.4 million units/d IM) plus oral probenecid (500 mg four times a day), both for 10–14 days	Desensitization and treatment with penicillin if allergy is confirmed by skin testing
Syphilis in pregnancy	According to stage	Desensitization and treatment with penicillin if allergy is confirmed by skin testing

SOURCE: These recommendations are modified from those issued by the Centers for Disease Control and Prevention in 1998.

- *Sites of Predilection*: Genital sites are most common.
  - Male: inner prepuce, coronal sulcus of the glans penis, shaft, base.
  - Female: cervix, vagina, vulva, clitoris, breast; chancres observed less frequently in women because of their location within vagina or on cervix.
  - Extragenital chancres: anus or rectum, mouth, lips, tongue (Fig. 30-21*A*), tonsils, fingers (painful!), toes, breast, nipple.

General Findings   Syphilis is a systemic infection; all patients should have a thorough clinical examination. Regional lymphadenopathy appears within 7 days. Nodes are discrete, firm, rubbery, nontender, more commonly unilateral; may persist for months.

DIFFERENTIAL DIAGNOSIS

Genital Erosion/Ulcer   Genital herpes, traumatic ulcer, fixed drug eruption, chancroid, lymphogranuloma venereum.

DIAGNOSIS

Clinical suspicion, confirmed by dark-field microscopy or serologically.

SECONDARY SYPHILIS

CLINICAL MANIFESTATIONS

- Secondary syphilis appears 2–6 months after primary infection; 2–10 weeks after appearance of the primary chancre; 6–8 weeks after healing of chancre.
- Chancre may still be present when secondary lesions appear (15% of cases).

A

B

FIGURE 30-21   Primary and secondary syphilis   A 24-year-old male with painful lesion on the tongue and disseminated rash. **A.** Extragenital primary on tongue. A large ulceration on the tip of the tongue. **B.** A disseminated papulosquamous eruption, i.e., secondary syphilis, was present at the time of the examination.

- Concomitant HIV/AIDS infection may alter course of secondary syphilis.

Symptoms   Fever, sore throat, weight loss, malaise, anorexia, headache, meningismus. Mucocutaneous lesions are asymptomatic.
Duration of Lesions   Weeks.

Skin Lesions

- Macules and papules 0.5 to 1 cm, round to oval; pink brownish-red.
- *First exanthem* always macular and faint.
- *Later eruptions may be papulosquamous* (Figs. 30-21B to 30-24), pustular, or acneiform.
- Vesiculobullous lesions occur only in neonatal congenital syphilis (palms and soles).
- Uncommonly, lesions of secondary syphilis and chancre of primary syphilis occur concomitantly.
- On palpation, papules are firm; condylomata lata, soft.
- Shape of lesions may be annular or polycyclic, especially on face in dark-skinned individuals (Fig. 30-24).
- In relapsing secondary syphilis, arciform lesions.
- Always sharply defined except for macular exanthem.

- Lesions are scattered, tend to remain discrete, and usually symmetric.
- *Condylomata lata*: soft, flat-topped, moist, red-to-pale papules, nodules, or plaques (Fig. 30-25), which may become confluent.

Distribution

- Generalized eruption on the trunk (Fig. 30-21B).
- Localized eruptions most commonly are scaling and papular; localizing, especially on the head (hairline, nasolabial, scalp), neck, palms (Fig. 30-22), and soles (Fig. 30-23). Here they are often hyperkeratotic-psoriasiform.
- Condylomata lata (Fig. 30-25): most commonly in anogenital region and mouth; can be seen on any body surface where moisture can accumulate between intertriginous surfaces, i.e., axillae or toe webs.

Hair

- Diffuse hair loss, including temples and parietal scalp.
- Patchy, "moth-eaten" alopecia on the scalp and beard area.
- Loss of eyelashes, lateral third of eyebrows.

A

B

FIGURE 30-22   Secondary syphilis: disseminated papulosquamous eruption on palms   A. A solitary keratotic papule on palm of patient in Fig. 30-21; the chancre was also present on the tongue at the time of presentation of secondary syphilis. Papulosquamous lesions were also disseminated on trunk. **B.** This is the more usual appearance of secondary syphilis on the palms: multiple psoriasiform keratotic papules.

FIGURE 30-23 Secondary syphilis: annular papulosquamous eruption on soles Hyperkeratotic, scaling plaques on the plantar aspects of both feet in a 20-year-old female. Similar lesions were present on the palms but to a lesser extent. No other clinical findings were detected.

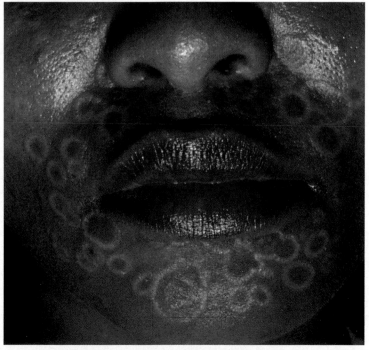

FIGURE 30-24 Secondary syphilis: annular facial lesions Annular plaques merging on the face of a South African woman. (Courtesy of Jeffrey S. Dover, MD.)

Mucous Membranes

- *Mucous patches*, i.e., small, asymptomatic, round or oval, slightly elevated, flat-topped macules and papules 0.5–1 cm in diameter, covered by hyperkeratotic white to gray membrane, occurring on the oral or genital mucosa
- *Split papules* at the angles of the mouth.

General Findings   Fever. Generalized lymphadenopathy (cervical, suboccipital, inguinal, epitrochlear, axillary) and splenomegaly.

Associated Findings

- *Musculoskeletal involvement*: periostitis of long bones, particularly tibia (nocturnal pain); arthralgia; hydrarthrosis of knees or ankles without x-ray changes. *Eyes*: acute bacterial iritis, optic neuritis, uveitis.
- *Meningovascular reaction*: CSF positive for inflammatory markers.
- *Gastrointestinal involvement*: diffuse pharyngitis, hypertrophic gastritis, hepatitis, patchy proctitis, ulcerative colitis, rectosigmoid mass).
- *Genitourinary involvement*: glomerulonephritis/nephrotic syndrome, cystitis, prostatitis.

LABORATORY EXAMINATIONS

Dermatopathology   Epidermal hyperkeratosis; capillary proliferation with endothelial swelling; perivascular infiltration by monocytes, plasma cells, lymphocytes. Spirochete is present in many tissues including skin, eye, CSF.
CSF   Abnormal in 40% of patients. Spirochetes in CSF in 30% of cases.

Liver Function   Elevated enzymes.
Renal Function   Immune complex–induced membranous glomerulonephritis.

COURSE

- In secondary syphilis there may be only one or several recurrent eruptions that appear after month-long asymptomatic intervals.
- Initial secondary syphilis eruption is a relatively faint exanthem, always macular, pink; lesions are ill-defined.
- Later lesions of early syphilis are papular, brownish, and tend to be more localized.
- Symptoms may last 2–6 weeks (4 weeks average) and may recur in untreated or inadequately treated patients.
- Secondary lesions subside within 2–6 weeks, infection entering latent stage.

DIFFERENTIAL DIAGNOSIS

Exanthem/Enanthem   Adverse cutaneous drug eruption (e.g., captopril), pityriasis rosea, viral exanthem, infectious mononucleosis, tinea corporis, tinea versicolor, scabies, "id" reaction, condylomata acuminata, acute guttate psoriasis, lichen planus.

DIAGNOSIS

Clinical suspicion confirmed by dark-field examination and/or serology. Dark-field is positive in all secondary syphilis lesions except for macular exanthem.

LATENT SYPHILIS

- No clinical signs or symptoms of infection; STS positive; CSF is normal.
- Suspected on the basis of a history of primary or secondary lesions, history of exposure to syphilis, or delivery of an infant with congenital syphilis; can occur without prior recognized primary or secondary lesions.
- A previous negative STS defines the duration of latency.
- Early latent syphilis (< 1 year) is distinguished from late latent disease (≥1 year).

- Latent disease does not preclude infectiousness or the development of gummatous skin lesions, cardiovascular lesions, or neurosyphilis.
- A pregnant woman with latent disease can infect her fetus with congenital syphilis.
- 70% of untreated patients never develop clinically evident tertiary syphilis.
- The more sensitive treponemal antibody test rarely becomes negative without treatment.

FIGURE 30-25 Secondary syphilis: condylomata lata Soft, flat-topped, moist, pink-tan papules and nodules on the perineum and perianal area. The lesions are teeming with *T. pallidum*.

FIGURE 30-26 Tertiary syphilis: noduloulcerative type Asymptomatic, red-brown, translucent, crusted, ulcerated plaque with serpiginous borders.

TERTIARY/LATE SYPHILIS

CLINICAL MANIFESTATION

Duration of Lesions

- In *untreated* syphilis, 15% of patients developed late benign syphilis, mostly skin lesions.
- Tertiary syphilis is now very rare.
- Previously, patients presenting with tertiary syphilis gave a history of lesions of 3 to 7 years' duration (range, 2–60 years); gumma develop by fifteenth year.

Gumma

- Nodular or papulosquamous plaques that may ulcerate, form circles/arc (Fig. 30-26). May expand rapidly causing destruction. May be indolent and heal with scarring. Solitary.
- Skin: any site, especially on scalp, face, chest (sternoclavicular), calf.
- Internal: skeletal system (long bones of legs), oropharynx, upper respiratory tract (perforation of nasal septum, palate), larynx, liver, stomach.

Neurosyphilis   *Asymptomatic Neurosyphilis*

- Occurs in 25% of patients with untreated late latent syphilis.
- Definition: Lack neurologic symptoms/signs and CSF abnormalities (mononuclear pleocytosis, increased protein concentrations, reactive VDRL slide test).
- 20% of patients with asymptomatic neurosyphilis progress to clinical neurosyphilis in first 10 years; risk increases with time.

Symptomatic Neurosyphilis   Meningeal, meningovascular, parenchymatous syphilis (general paresis, tabes dorsalis).

- *Meningeal syphilis*: onset of symptoms <1 year after infection; headache, nausea/vomiting, stiff neck, cranial nerve palsies, seizures, changes in mental status.
- *Meningovascular syphilis*: Onset of symptoms 5–10 years after infection; subacute encephalitis prodrome followed by stroke syndrome, progressive vascular syndrome. *General paresis*: Onset of symptoms 20 years after infection; mnemonic paresis [*p*aresis, *a*ffect, *r*eflexes (hyperactive), *e*ye (Argyll Robertson pupils), *s*ensorium (illusions, delusions, hallucinations), *i*ntellect (decrease in recent memory, orientation, calculations, judgment, insight), *s*peech].
- *Tabes dorsalis*: Onset of symptoms 25–30 years after infection; ataxic widebased gait and footslap, paresthesia, bladder disturbances, impotence, areflexia, loss of position, deep pain, temperature sensations (Charcot/neuropathic joints, foot ulcers), optic atrophy.

Cardiovascular Syphilis   Results from endarteritis obliterans of vasa vasorum. Occurs in 10% of persons with late untreated syphilis, 10–40 years after infection. Uncomplicated aortitis, aortic regurgitation, saccular aneurysm, coronary ostial stenosis.

DIFFERENTIAL DIAGNOSIS

Plaque(s) ± Ulceration ± Granulomas   Cutaneous tuberculosis, cutaneous atypical mycobacterial infection, lymphoma, invasive fungal infections.

DIAGNOSIS

Clinical findings, confirmed by STS and lesional skin biopsy; dark-field examination always negative; silver impregnation of histologic sections for demonstration of spirochetes only very rarely positive.

COURSE

- HIV/AIDS-infected individuals with neurosyphilis are more likely to present with uveitis or retinitis and have significantly higher RPR titers.
- Some, however, fail to respond immunologically to *T. pallidum* infection with antibody formation (i.e., negative STS).
- HIV/AIDS testing is advised for all patients with syphilis.
- Neurosyphilis should be considered in the differential diagnosis of neurologic disease in HIV/AIDS.
- When clinical findings suggest syphilis but STS are negative or confusing, alternative tests such as biopsy of lesions, dark-field examination, and DFA staining of lesional material should be used.

CONGENITAL SYPHILIS   □ ●

Transmission
During gestation or intrapartum. Risk of transmission: Early maternal syphilis, 75–95%; >2 years' duration, 35%.

Pathogenesis
Lesions usually develop after fourth month of gestation, associated with fetal immunologic competence. Pathogenesis depends on immune response of fetus rather than toxic effect of spirochete. Adequate treatment before sixteenth week of pregnancy prevents fetal damage. Untreated: fetal loss up to 40%.

CLINICAL MANIFESTATION

Early Manifestations   Appear before 2 years of age, often at 2–10 weeks. Infectious, resembling severe secondary syphilis in adult.

- Cutaneous: Bullae, vesicles on palms and soles, superficial desquamation, petechiae, papulosquamous lesions
- Mucosal: Rhinitis/"snuffles" (23%); mucous patches, condylomata latum.
- Bone changes: osteochondritis, osteitis, periostitis.
- Hepatosplenomegaly, jaundice, lymphadenopathy.

- Anemia, thrombocytopenia, leukocytosis.

Late Manifestations   Appear after 2 years of age. Noninfectious. Similar to late acquired syphilis in adult.

- Cardiovascular syphilis.
- Interstitial keratitis
- Eighth nerve deafness.
- Recurrent arthropathy; bilateral knee effusions (Clutton joints). Gummatous periostitis results in destructive lesions of nasal septum/palate.
- Asymptomatic neurosyphilis in 33% of patients; clinical syphilis in 25%.

Residual Stigmata

- Hutchinson teeth (centrally notched, widely spaced, pegshaped upper central incisors; "mulberry" molars (multiple poorly developed cusps).
- Abnormal facies: frontal bossing, saddle nose, poorly developed maxillae, rhagades (linear scars at angles of mouth, caused by bacterial superinfection of early facial eruption).
- Saber shins.
- Nerve deafness
- Old chorioretinitis, optic atrophy, corneal opacities due to interstitial keratitis.

HAEMOPHILUS DUCREYI: CHANCROID   □ → ■ ◑

- Chancroid is an acute STI characterized by
  - A *painful* ulcer at the site of inoculation, usually on the external genitalia
  - The development of suppurative regional lymphadenopathy.

- STI most strongly associated with increased risk for HIV/AIDS transmission.

Synonyms: Soft chancre, ulcus molle, chancre mou.

ICD-9:099.0 ○ ICD-10:A57

See CDC guidelines for treatment of genital ulcers.

ETIOLOGY AND EPIDEMIOLOGY

Etiology   *H. ducreyi*, a gram-negative streptobacillus.
Epidemiology   In the United States, chancroid usually occurs in discrete outbreaks, although the disease is endemic in some areas.
Sex   Young males. Lymphadenitis more common in males.

Risk Factors

- Transmission mainly heterosexual
- Males > females 3:1 25:1
- Prostitution significant
- Strongly associated with illicit drug use.

Transmission   Most likely during sexual intercourse with partner who has *H. ducreyi* genital ulcer. Chancroid is a cofactor for HIV/AIDS transmission; high rates of HIV/AIDS infection among those who have chancroid. 10% of individuals with chancroid have syphilis or genital herpes.

Demography Uncommon in industrialized nations. Endemic in tropical and subtropical developing countries, especially in poor, urban, and seaport populations.

PATHOGENESIS

- Primary infection develops at the site of inoculation (break in epithelium), followed by lymphadenitis.
- The genital ulcer is characterized by perivascular and interstitial infiltrates of macrophages and of CD4+ and CD8+ lymphocytes, consistent with a delayed-type hypersensitivity, cell-mediated immune response.
- CD4+ cells and macrophages in the ulcer may explain the facilitation of transmission of HIV/AIDS in patients with chancroid ulcers.

CLINICAL MANIFESTATION

Incubation period is 4–7 days.

Skin Lesions

- Primary lesion: tender papule with erythematous halo that evolves to pustule, erosion, and ulcer. Ulcer is usually quite *tender* or *painful*. Its borders are sharp, undermined, and not indurated (Figs. 30-27 and 30-28). Base is friable with granulation tissue and covered with gray to yellow exudate.
- Edema of prepuce common.
- Ulcer may be singular or multiple, merging to form large or giant ulcers (>2 cm) with serpiginous shape.

Distribution Multiple ulcers (Fig. 30-28) develop by autoinoculation.

- Male: prepuce, frenulum, coronal sulcus, glans penis, shaft.
- Female: fourchette, labia, vestibule, clitoris, vaginal wall by direct extension from introitus, cervix, perianal.
- Extragenital lesions: breast, fingers, thighs, oral mucosa. Bacterial superinfection of ulcers can occur.

General Findings
Painful inguinal lymphadenitis (usually unilateral) occurs in 50% of patients 7–21 days after primary lesion. Ulcer may heal before buboes occur. Buboes occur with overlying erythema and may drain spontaneously.

DIFFERENTIAL DIAGNOSIS

Genital Ulcer Genital herpes, primary syphilis, lymphogranuloma venereum (LGV), donovanosis, secondarily infected human bites, traumatic lesions.

Tender Inguinal Mass Genital herpes, secondary syphilis, LGV, incarcerated hernia, plague, tularemia.

LABORATORY EXAMINATIONS

Gram Stain Of scrapings from ulcer base or pus from bubo, usually not helpful.

Culture Special growth requirements; isolation difficult. Using special media, sensitivity is no higher than 80%.

Serologic Tests None available. Patients should have HIV/AIDS serology at time of diagnosis. Patients should also be tested 3 months later for both syphilis and HIV/AIDS infection if initial results are negative.

Dermatopathology May be helpful. Organism rarely demonstrated.

PCR Detects *H. ducreyi* DNA sequences.

FIGURE 30-27 Chancroid Painful ulcer with marked surrounding erythema and edema. (Courtesy of Prof. Alfred Eichmann, MD.)

DIAGNOSIS

Combination of painful ulcer with tender lymphadenopathy (one-third of patients) is suggestive of chancroid and, when accompanied by suppurative inguinal lymphadenopathy, is almost pathognomonic.

Definitive Diagnosis Made by isolation of *H. ducreyi* on special culture media (not widely available). Sensitivity 80%.

Probable Diagnosis Made if patient has following criteria:

- Painful genital ulcers
- No evidence of *T. pallidum* infection by dark-field examination of ulcer exudate or by STS performed at least 7 days after onset of ulcers
- Clinical presentation, appearance of genital ulcers, and lymphadenopathy, if present, are typical for chancroid and a test for HSV is negative.

COURSE AND PROGNOSIS

- Patients should be reexamined 3–7 days after initiation of therapy. If treatment is successful, ulcers improve symptomatically within 3 days and improve objectively within 7 days after therapy is begun.
- If no clinical improvement is evident, diagnosis may be incorrect, co-infection with another STI agent exists, the patient is HIV/AIDS-infected, treatment was not taken as instructed, or the *H. ducreyi* strain causing infection is resistant to the prescribed antimicrobial.
- The time required for complete healing is related to the size of the ulcer; large ulcers may require 14 days. Complete resolution of fluctuant lymphadenopathy is slower than that of ulcers and may require needle aspiration through adjacent intact skin—even during successful therapy.
- In HIV/AIDS, healing may be slower, and treatment failures may occur; longer treatment regimens may be advisable.

MANAGEMENT

Antimicrobial Therapy

Azithromycin	1 g PO in a single dose, *or*
Ceftriaxone	250 mg IM in a single dose, *or*
Ciprofloxacin	500 mg PO twice a day for 3 days, *or*
Erythromycin base	500 mg PO four times a day for 7 days.

Management of Sex Partners Sex partners should be referred for evaluation and treatment.

FIGURE 30-28 Chancroid Multiple, painful, punched-out ulcers with undermined borders on the vulva occurring after autoinoculation.

DONOVANOSIS   ICD-9:099.2 ∘ ICD-10:A58   ☐ ◑

- A chronic, indolent, progressive, autoinoculable, ulcerative disease, often misdiagnosed as syphilis.
- Etiologic agent: *Calymmatobacterium granulomatis*, an encapsulated intracellular gram-negative rod; closely related to *Klebsiella* spp.
- Transmission: Usually sexually. Nonsexual transmission and autoinoculation occur.
- Demography: Endemic foci in tropical and subtropical environments. Extremely rare in United States.
- Pathogenesis: Poorly understood. Mildly contagious. Repeated exposure necessary for clinical infection to occur. In most cases, lesions cannot be detected in sexual contacts.
- Clinical manifestations
  - Painless, progressive, ulcerative lesions of the genital and perianal areas. Highly vascular (i.e., a beefy red appearance) and bleed easily on contact. Spreads by continuity or by autoinoculation of approximated skin surfaces (Fig. 30-29).
  - No regional lymphadenopathy. Large subcutaneous nodule may mimic a lymph node, i.e., pseudobubo.
- Distribution of mucocutaneous lesions
  - *Males*: prepuce or glans, penile shaft, scrotum.
  - *Females*: labia minora, mons veneris, fourchette. Ulcerations then spread by direct extension or autoinoculation to inguinal and perineal skin.

- Extragenital lesions occur in mouth, lips, throat, face, GI tract, and bone.
- Variant types: Ulcerovegetative (Fig. 30-29); nodular; hypertrophic; sclerotic/cicatricial.
- Anaerobic superinfection may produce pain and foul-smelling exudate.
- Less common complications: Deep ulcerations, chronic cicatricial lesions, phimosis, lymphedema (elephantiasis of penis, scrotum, vulva), exuberant epithelial proliferation that grossly resembles carcinoma.
- Differential diagnosis in endemic area: Syphilitic chancre, chancroid, chronic herpetic ulcer, LGV, cutaneous tuberculosis, cutaneous amebiasis, filariasis, SCC.
- Diagnosis: Visualize Donovan bodies on touch or crush preparation or in lesional biopsy specimen. Rule out other or concurrent cause of genital ulcer disease.
- Course: Little tendency toward spontaneous healing. Heals with antibiotic treatment. Relapse may occur. May disseminate to spine, mimicking tuberculosis or actinomycosis.
- Recommended therapy: Trimethoprim-sulfamethoxazole (one double-strength tablet twice a day for at least 3 weeks) or doxycycline 100 mg PO twice a day for at least 3 weeks.

Synonyms: Granuloma inguinale, granuloma venereum.

FIGURE 30-29   Donovanosis: ulcerovegetative type   Extensive granulation tissue formation, ulceration, and scarring of the perineum, scrotum, and penis.

CHLAMYDIA TRACHOMATIS INFECTIONS
ICD-9:099.41 ∘ ICD-10:A56

- Etiology: *C. trachomatis*, obligate intracellular bacteria. Major outer-membrane protein delineates >20 serovars (immunotypes):
  - *Trachoma:* Serovars A, B, Ba, and C.
  - *Mucosal STIs:* Serovars D–K (most common bacterial STIs).
  - *Invasive STIs*: Serovars L_1, L_2, L_3 (in United States, L_2 most commonly)
- Incidence: Most common bacterial STI in virtually every population. 4 million cases in the United States annually.
- Prevalence in young American males: 3–5% in general medical settings or urban high schools; >10% in asymptomatic soldiers; 15–20% in heterosexual men in STI clinics.
- Chlamydial urethritis more common in heterosexual men and high socioeconomic status; gonococcal urethritis more common in homosexual men and indigent populations.

- Prevalence of cervical infection in the United States: 5% for asymptomatic college students; >10% in family planning clinics: >20% in STI clinics.
- LGV more common in homosexual men; persons returning from abroad (travelers, sailors, military personnel).
- Transmission: *Sexual: C. trachomatis* in purulent exudate is inoculated onto skin or mucosa of sexual partner and gains entry through minute lacerations and abrasions. *Perinatal.*
- Manifestations
  - Asymptomatic
  - Symptomatic mucosal infections
  - Invasive disease (LGV, hemorrhagic protocolitis).
- These infectious syndromes resemble and must be differentiated from those caused by gonococci.

SYNDROMES CAUSED BY *C. TRACHOMATIS*

Nongonococcal (NGU) and postgonococcal urethritis	20–40% of NGU in heterosexual men are chlamydial. Also caused by *U. urealyticum, T. vaginalis*, HSV.
Epididymitis	Most common cause (70%) in sexually active men <35 years.
Reactive arthritis (Reiter) syndrome	*C. trachomatis* recovered from urethra in up to 70% of men with untreated nondiarrheal reactive arthritis syndrome and associated urethritis. Chlamydial and other mucosal infections (*Salmonella, Shigella, Campylobacter*) thought to initiate aberrant, hyperactive immune response that produces inflammation at involved target organs in genetically (HA-B27 phenotype) predisposed individuals.
Proctitis	Genital immunotypes D–K (most common in the United States) or LGV immunotypes cause proctitis in homosexual men who practice receptive anorectal intercourse.
Mucopurulent cervicitis	Many women have no symptoms.
Pelvic inflammatory disease (PID)	50% of cases of PID in the United States caused by *C. trachomatis*. Intraluminal spread results in endometritis, endosalpingitis, pelvic peritonitis. Silent salpingitis causes infertility. 75% of Fitz-Hugh–Curtis syndrome caused by *C. trachomatis*.
Lymphogranuloma venereum (LGV)	See invasive infections
Perinatal infections	50–75% of newborns exposed to *C. trachomatis* at birth acquire infection. 50% of those infected develop clinical evidence of inclusion conjunctivitis; pneumonitis, otitis media also occur.
Adult inclusion conjunctivitis	Caused by exposure to infected genital secretions.
Trachoma	Responsible for 20 million cases of blindness worldwide. Transmitted from eye to eye via hands, flies, towels, other fomites. Incidence has decreased during past four decades.

PATHOGENESIS

- *C. trachomatis* preferentially infects columnar epithelium of genital tract, eye, and respiratory tract. Infection often persists for months or years in the absence of antimicrobial therapy.
- Serious sequelae often occur in association with repeated or persistent infections. Mechanism through which repeated infection elicits an inflammatory response that leads to tubal scarring and damage in the female upper genital tract unclear. Chlamydial 60-kDa heat-shock protein may induce pathologic immune response or elicit antibodies that cross-react with human heat-shock proteins.
- Chlamydial infections are often totally asymptomatic for months.
- Simultanaeous infections with gonococcus are common. Infections can persist for months or years if not treated.

LOCALIZED *C. TRACHOMATIS* INFECTION ■ ◑

SYMPTOMS

- ■ Nongonococcal Urethritis (NGU)
  - ▪ *Men:* <50% have symptoms. Urethral discharge (whitish, mucoid), dysuria, urethral itching.
  - ▪ *Women:* dysuria, frequency, pyuria.
  - ▪ Meatal erythema/tenderness; exudates.

- ■ *Proctitis* Mild rectal pain, mucous discharge, tenesmus, bleeding. On anoscopy, mild, patchy mucosa; friability, mucopurulent discharge.

- ■ *Mucopurulent Cervicitis* Many women have no symptoms or slight vaginal discharge or intermenstrual bleeding. 30-50% of asymptomatic cases have changes on speculum examination. Yellow mucopurulent discharge from endocervical columnar epithelium; friable.

- ■ *PID* Vaginal bleeding, lower abdominal pain, uterine tenderness without adnexal tenderness. Silent salpingitis results in fallopian tube scarring, ectopic pregnancy, and infertility. Endometritis, endosalpingitis, pelvic peritonitis. Symptoms of *C. trachomatis* infection are summarized in Table 30-9.

DIFFERENTIAL DIAGNOSIS

Urethritis Gonorrhea, *U. urealyticum, Mycoplasma genitalium*, trichomoniasis, herpetic urethritis.

LABORATORY EXAMINATIONS

Direct Microscopy Low sensitivity. DFA staining used for conjunctival smears.
PCR Most specific and sensitive.
Culture *C. trachomatis* can be cultured on tissue-culture cell lines in up to 60–80% of cases.
DFA Examine exudate for antigens.
Antibodies to C. trachomatis *Enzyme-Linked Immunosorbent Assay (ELISA)* 60–80% sensitive and specific; 97–99% in high-risk populations; sensitivities higher in cervical infection than urethritis in males.
DNA-RNA Hybridization As sensitive and specific as ELISA. Chlamydial DNA in urine is diagnostic.

Complement-Fixation (CF) Test Acute LGV usually has titer 1:64. Microimmunofluorescence test most sensitive and specific, identifying infecting serovar/immunotypes.

Diagnostic tests are summarized in Table 30-10.

COURSE AND PROGNOSIS

- Absence of symptoms of *C. trachomatis* infection leaves women at risk of serious chlamydia-related morbidity through the complication of PID: recurrent PID with endogenous vaginal flora, chronic pelvic pain, ectopic pregnancy, and infertility.
- PID typically affects older women, is clinically severe, and is more likely to present to hospital.
- Most common cause of epididymitis in young men.
- Other complications: conjunctivitis, reactive arthritis, pneumonitis in neonates.

TABLE 30-9   Symptoms of Sexually Transmitted *Chlamydia trachomatis* Infection

Infection	Suggestive Signs/Symptoms
NGU, PGU	Discharge, dysuria
Epididymitis	Unilateral intrascrotal swelling, pain, tenderness; fever; NGU
Cervicitis	Mucopurulent cervical discharge, bleeding and edema of the zone of cervical ectopy
Salpingitis	Lower abdominal pain, cervical motion tenderness, adnexal tenderness or masses
Urethritis	Dysuria and frequency without urgency or hematuria
Proctitis	Rectal pain, discharge, tenesmus, bleeding; history of receptive anorectal intercourse
Reactive arthritis syndrome	NGU, arthritis, conjunctivitis, typical skin lesions syndrome
LGV	Regional adenopathy, primary lesion, proctitis, systemic symptoms

TABLE 30-10   Diagnostic Tests for Sexually Transmitted *Chlamydia trachomatis* Infection

Presumptive Diagnosis*	Confirmatory Test of Choice
MEN	
Gram stain with >4 neutrophils per oil-immersion field; no gonococci	Urethral culture or nonculture test for *C. trachomatis;* urine PCR or LCR for *C. trachomatis*
Gram stain with >4 neutrophils per oil-immersion field; no gonococci; urinalysis with pyuria	Urethral culture or nonculture test for *C. trachomatis;* urine PCR or LCR for *C. trachomatis*
WOMEN	
Cervical Gram stain with ≥20 neutrophils per oil-immersion field in cervical mucus	Cervical culture or nonculture test for *C. trachomatis*; urine PCR or LCR for *C. trachomatis*
C. trachomatis always potentially present in salpingitis	Cervical culture or nonculture test for *C. trachomatis;* urine PCR or LCR for *C. trachomatis*
MPC; sterile pyuria; negative routine urine culture	Urethral and cervical cultures or nonculture test for *C. trachomatis*; urine PCR or LCR for *C. trachomatis*
ADULTS OF EITHER SEX	
Negative gonococcal culture and Gram stain; at least 1 neutrophil per oil-immersion field in rectal Gram stain	Rectal culture or direct immunofluorescence test for *C. trachomatis*
Gram stain with >4 neutrophils per oil-immersion field; lack of gonococci indicative of NGU	Urethral culture or nonculture test for *C. trachomatis*
None	Isolation of LGV strain from node or rectum, occasionally from urethra or cervix; LGV CF titer, ≥1:64; micro-IF titer, ≥1:512

*A presumptive diagnosis of chlamydial infection is often made in the syndromes listed when gonococci are not found. A positive test for *Neisseria gonorrhoeae* does not exclude the involvement of *C. trachomatis*, which often is present in patients with gonorrhea.

NOTE: CF, complement-fixing; LCR, ligase chain reaction; LGV, lymphogranuloma venereum; micro-IF, microimmunofluorescence; MPC, mucopurulent cervicitis; NGU, nongonococcal urethritis; PCR, polymerase chain reaction; PGU, post-gonococcal urethritis.

SOURCE: Adopted from WE Stamm, in AS Fauci et al (eds): *Harrison's Principles of Internal Medicine*, 17th ed. New York, McGraw-Hill, 2008.

MANAGEMENT

Screening Annually for sexually active women: adolescents, 20–25 years old, older women with risk factors (new sex partner, multiple sex partners).

Antimicrobial Therapy Cures infection and prevents ongoing tissue damage, although tissue reaction can result in scarring.

Recommended regimen		Alternative regimens	
Azithromycin	1 g PO in single dose, *or*	Erythromycin base	500 mg PO four times a day for 7 day, *or*
Doxycycline	100 mg PO twice a day for 7 day	Erythromycin ethylsuccinate	800 mg PO four times a day for 7 days, *or*
		Ofloxacin	300 mg PO twice a day for 7 days, *or*
		Levofloxacin	500 mg PO daily for 7 days.

INVASIVE *C. TRACHOMATIS* INFECTION: LYMPHOGRANULOMA VENEREUM   □ ◑

- Acute LGV in heterosexual men is characterized by a transient primary genital lesion followed by multilocular suppurative regional lymphadenopathy.
- Women, homosexual men, and–in occasional instances–heterosexual men may develop hemorrhagic proctitis with regional lymphadenitis.

- After a latent period of years, late complications include genital elephantiasis due to lymphatic involvement; strictures; and fistulas of penis, urethra, rectum.

EPIDEMIOLOGY

Sex

- *Heterosexual men*: acute infection presents as inguinal syndrome.
- *Women/homosexual men (MSM)*: Anogenitorectal syndrome most common.

Demography Sporadic/rare in North America, Europe, Australia, and most of Asia and South America. Endemic in East and West Africa, India, parts of southeast Asia, South America, and the Caribbean.

PATHOGENESIS

- Primarily an infection of lymphatics and lymph nodes.
- Lymphangitis and lymphadenitis occur in drainage field of inoculation site with subsequent perilymphangitis and periadenitis.

- Necrosis occurs; loculated abscesses, fistulas, and sinus tracts develop.
- As the infection subsides, fibrosis replaces acute inflammation with resulting obliteration of lymphatic drainage, chronic edema, and stricture.
- Inoculation site determines affected lymph nodes:

Inoculation site	Lymph node involvement
Penis, anterior urethra	Superficial, deep inguinal
Posterior urethra	Deep iliac, perirectal
Vulva	Inguinal
Vagina, cervix	Deep iliac, perirectal, retrocrural, lumbosacral
Anus	Inguinal
Rectum	Perirectal, deep iliac

CLINICAL MANIFESTATION

Incubation Period

- Primary stage: 3–12 days or longer
- Secondary stage: 10–30 days (but up to 6 months)

Acute

- Primary genital lesion noticed in fewer than one-third of men and rarely in women.
  - *In heterosexual men, women:* small painless vesicle or nonindurated ulcer/papule on penis or labia/posterior vagina/fourchette; heals in a few days.
  - *In homosexual men (MSM), women:* primary anal or rectal infection develops after receptive anal intercourse.
  - *In women:* anal/rectal infection can spread from perineum or via pelvic lymphatics.
- Infection can spread from primary site of infection to regional lymphatics.

Inguinal Syndrome

- Characterized by painful inguinal lymphadenopathy beginning 2–6 weeks after presumed exposure.
- Unilateral in two-thirds of cases; palpable iliac/femoral nodes often present on same side (Fig. 30-30).
- Initially, nodes are discrete, but progressive periadenitis results in a matted mass of nodes that may become fluctuant and suppurative.
- Overlying skin becomes fixed, inflamed, thin, and eventually develops multiple draining fistulas.
- "Groove" sign: Extensive enlargement of chains of inguinal nodes above and below the inguinal ligament; nonspecific (Fig. 30-30).

Acute LGV   Papule, shallow erosion or ulcer, grouped small erosions or ulcers (herpetiform), or nonspecific urethritis.

Heterosexual Males   Cordlike lymphangitis of dorsal penis may follow. Lymphangial nodule (bubonulus) may rupture, resulting in sinuses and fistulas of urethra and deforming scars of penis. Multilocular suppurative lymphadenopathy.

Females   Cervicitis, perimetritis, salpingitis may occur.

Female and Homosexual Males/Receptive Anal Intercourse   Primary anal rectal infection (hemorrhagic proctitis with regional lymphadenitis).

Other   Erythema nodosum in 10% of cases (see Section 7).

Secondary Stage   *Inguinal Syndrome*   Unilateral bubo in two-thirds of cases (most common presentation) (Fig. 30-30). Marked edema and erythema of skin overlying node. One-third of inguinal buboes rupture; two-thirds slowly involute. "Groove" sign: inflammatory mass of femoral and inguinal nodes separated by depression, or groove, made by Poupart ligament. 75% of cases have deep iliac node involvement with a pelvic mass that seldom suppurates.

Anogenitorectal Syndrome   Associated with receptive anal intercourse, proctocolitis, hyperplasia of intestinal and perirectal lymphatic tissue. Resultant perirectal abscesses, ischiorectal and rectovaginal fistulas, anal fistulas, rectal stricture. Overgrowth of lymphatic tissue results in lymphorrhoids (resembling hemorrhoids) or perianal condylomata.

Esthiomene   Elephantiasis of genitalia, usually females, which may ulcerate, occurring 1–20 years after primary infection.

DIFFERENTIAL DIAGNOSIS

Primary Stage   Genital herpes, primary syphilis, chancroid.

Inguinal Syndrome   Incarcerated inguinal hernia, plague, tularemia, tuberculosis, genital herpes, syphilis, chancroid, Hodgkin disease.

Anogenitorectal Syndrome   Rectal stricture caused by rectal cancer, trauma, actinomycosis, tuberculosis, schistosomiasis.

Esthiomene   Filariasis, subcutaneous mycosis.

LABORATORY EXAMINATIONS

See Table 30-10.

Imaging   MRI may show massive pelvic lymphadenopathy in women and homosexual men.

Dermatopathology   Not pathognomonic. *Primary stage*: small stellate abscesses surrounded by histiocytes, arranged in palisade pattern. *Late stage*: epidermal acanthosis/papillomatosis; dermis—edematous; lymphatics—dilated with fibrosis and lymphoplasmocytic infiltrate.

DIAGNOSIS

By DFA, culture, serologic tests, and exclusion of other causes of inguinal lymphadenopathy or genital ulcers.

COURSE AND PROGNOSIS

Highly variable. Bacterial superinfections may contribute to complications. Rectal stricture is late complication. Spontaneous remission is common.

MANAGEMENT

Antimicrobial Therapy   A 3-week course of the antimcrobial agents recommended for acute *C. trachomatis* infections is given (page 936).

FIGURE 30-30   Lymphogranuloma venereum   Striking tender lymphadenopathy occurring at the femoral and inguinal lymph nodes separated by a groove made by Poupart ligament (groove sign).

HUMAN RETROVIRAL INFECTIONS AND MUCOCUTANEOUS MANIFESTATIONS OF HIV/AIDS DISEASE

- Human retroviruses (Retroviridae) included four recognized viruses.

- Human T lymphotropic viruses (HTLV) I and HTLV-II are transforming retroviruses. HTLV-I causes adult T cell leukemia, (Section 20), anaplastic large cell lymphoma, tropical spastic paraparesis.

- Human immunodeficiency viruses, HIV/AIDS-1 and HIV/AIDS-2, are cytopathic viruses of zoonotic origins. HIV/AIDS-1 is the most common cause of HIV/AIDS disease throughout the world; it comprises several subtypes with different geographic distributions. HIV/AIDS-2 is mainly confined to West Africa.

GLOBAL HIV/AIDS PANDEMIC

AIDS was first reported by the Centers for Disease Control and Prevention (CDC) in 1981 in previously healthy men who had sex with men (MSM), who presented with *Pneumocystis carinii* pneumonia (PCP), and/or Kaposi sarcoma (KS), and/or chronic herpetic ulcers. Additional cases were soon recognized in injecting drug users (IDUs), hemophiliacs, and recipients of blood transfusions. HIV/AIDS was first isolated from an infected lymph node in 1983. The enzyme-linked immunosorbent assay (ELISA) serotest was developed in 1985 and subsequently used to determine the extent of the epidemic. Currently, sub-Saharan Africa bears the greatest burden of the epidemic worldwide. The number of new infections is escalating in countries of the former Soviet Union, India, and China. HIV/AIDS infection is manifested as opportunistic infections, aggressive cancers, and neurologic findings (dementia and neuropathy). Half of 5 million new HIV/AIDS infections occurring annually are in individuals, aged 15 to 24 years.

HIV/AIDS DISEASE AND AIDS   ICD-9:042-044 ○ ICD-10:B20-B24 ■ ●

- Originated in Africa; first recognized in the United States (1981) and shortly after in Europe.

- Transmission via sexual intercourse, exposure to blood or blood product, perinatal.

- Acute HIV/AIDS infection may be symptomatic with acute HIV/AIDS syndrome.

- Clinical findings are of opportunistic infections and neoplasms.

- Clinical course highly variable.

- Prevention: completely preventable; avoid risk-associated behaviors.

- When available, antiretroviral therapy (ART) is very effective in management of this chronic disease.

- Vaccine: none foreseeable.

EPIDEMIOLOGY AND ETIOLOGY

Age of Onset Commonly in the young, but any age.

Sex Worldwide, more common in males. In sub-Saharan Africa, equal sex distribution.

Etiology Worldwide, nearly all infections are HIV/AIDS-1. HIV/AIDS-2 causes disease in western Africa. In the United States, HIV/AIDS-1 subtype B is predominant.

Risk Factors for Transmission

- Sexual contact with an infected person. In the United States, heterosexual transmission is increasing; homosexual transmission is decreasing.
- Blood or blood products.
- Perinatal exposure (intrapartum, perinatal, breast feeding); infected mothers to infants.

Risk Factors for Acquisition Genital ulcer disease, HIV/AIDS-infected partner with high viral load (transmission more efficient), receptive anal intercourse.

Incidence Worldwide: approximately 33.2 million infections. Two-thirds of infections are in sub-Saharan Africa. United States: 56,000 new HIV/AIDS infections occurred in 2006. In 2003, 5 million new infections worldwide; 3 million deaths.

Demography Epidemic expanding in Asia, especially India and China, which have populations of >1 billion each. Rapidly expanding in Baltic States, the Russian Federation, and several Central Asian Republics.

AIDS Definition Any HIV/AIDS-infected individual with a CD4+ T cell count of <200/μL has AIDS by definition, regardless of the presence of symptoms or opportunistic diseases. See Table 31-1 for clinical categories of HIV/AIDS infection).

PATHOGENESIS

After primary HIV/AIDS infection, billions of virions are produced and destroyed each day; a concomitant daily turnover of actively infected CD4+ cells is also in the billions. HIV/AIDS infection is relatively unique among human viral infections in that, despite robust cellular and humoral immune responses that are mounted after primary infection, the virus is not cleared completely from the body (with a few exceptions). Chronic infection develops that persists with varying degrees of virus replication for a median of 10 years before an individual becomes clinically ill.

CLINICAL FINDINGS

Nearly all HIV/AIDS-infected individuals manifest some dermatologic disorder attributable to progressive immunodeficiency during the course of the infection. Some disorders are highly associated with HIV/AIDS infection, and their diagnosis often warrants HIV/AIDS serotesting (Table 31-2).

CLINICAL MANIFESTATION

For much of the course of HIV/AIDS disease, patients remain *asymptomatic*. Nonspecific complaints include: fevers, night sweats, chills, weakness, lymphadenopathy, and weight loss.

Infected individuals may appear healthy even in an advanced immunocompromised state, i.e., CD4+ cell counts approaching zero. In advanced untreated disease, wasting is common, especially in sub-Saharan Africa.

TABLE 31-1 1993 Revised Classification System for HIV/AIDS Infection and Expanded AIDS Surveillance Case Definition for Adolescents and Adults

CD4+ T Cell Categories	Clinical Categories		
	A Asymptomatic, Acute (Primary) HIV or PGL[a]	B Symptomatic, Not A or C Conditions	C AIDS-Indicator Conditions
>500/μL	A1	B1	C1
200–499/μL	A2	B2	C2
<200/μL	A3	B3	C3

[a]PGL, progressive generalized lymphadenopathy.

SOURCE: MMWR 42(No. RR-17), December 18, 1992.

TABLE 31-2   Mucocutaneous Findings Associated with HIV/AIDS Infection and Indications for HIV Serotesting

Risk for HIV Infection	Mucocutaneous Finding
High—serotesting always indicated	Acute retroviral syndrome
	Kaposi sarcoma
	Oral hairy leukoplakia
	Proximal subungual onychomycosis
	Bacillary angiomatosis
	Eosinophilic folliculitis
	Chronic herpetic ulcers (>1 month duration)
	Any sexually transmitted disease
	Skin findings of injecting drug use (IDU)
Moderate—serotesting may be indicated	Herpes zoster
	Molluscum contagiosum: multiple facial in an adult
	Candidiasis: oropharyngeal, esophageal, or recurrent vulvovaginal
Possible—serotesting may be indicated	Generalized lymphadenopathy
	Seborrheic dermatitis
	Aphthous ulcers (recurrent, refractory to therapy)

Skin Findings

In advanced untreated disease, skin findings may be common and extreme:

- Dermatologic disorders
  - Atopic dermatitis
  - Psoriasis
  - Pruritus with secondary changes of excoriation
  - Seborrheic dermatitis
  - Xerosis
  - Adverse cutaneous drug reactions
- Opportunistic infections
  - Mucosal candidiasis
  - Molluscum contagiosum
  - Herpes simplex virus (HSV); chronic herpetic ulcers
  - Varicella-zoster virus (VZV): Herpes zoster
  - Human papillomavirus (HPV) infection: skin, mucosal
- Opportunistic neoplasms
  - Kaposi sarcoma
  - Non-Hodgkin and Hodgkin lymphoma
  - Primary central nervous system (CNS) lymphoma
  - HPV-induced dysplasia and invasive squamous cell carcinoma
    - Cervix
    - Anus

- Unique to HIV/AIDS disease
  - Acute HIV/AIDS syndrome (AHS)
  - Oral hairy leukoplakia (OHL)
  - Eosinophilic folliculitis (EF)
  - Bacillary angiomatosis (BA)

Systemic Findings

Opportunistic Infections (OIs) *Myco-bacterium tuberculosis* (MTb) disease, *Myco-bacterium avium* complex (MAC) infection, bartonellosis (*Bartonella henselae, B. quintana*); syphilis; *Pneumocystis jiroveci* (previously *cari-nii*) pneumonia (PCP), candidiasis, crypto-coccosis, histoplasmosis, coccidioidomycosis, aspergillosis, penicillinosis, paracoccidioidomy-cosis; cytomegalovirus (CMV) disease, crypt-osporidiosis; HSV disease, VZV disease, human herpesvirus-8 (HHV-8), HPV, hepatitis C virus (HCV) disease, hepatitis B virus (HBV) disease; leishmaniasis.

Opportunistic Neoplasms (ONs) Kaposi sar-coma (HHV-8), non-Hodgkin lymphomas [Ep-stein-Barr virus (EBV)], cervical cancer (HPV), anal cancer (HPV).

Other AIDS dementia complex, progressive multifocal leukoencephalopathy, wasting syn-drome.

LABORATORY EXAMINATIONS

Diagnosis of HIV/AIDS Infection See Image 31-1.

CD4+ T Lymphocytes Image 31-2 illustrates the typical course of HIV/AIDS disease in the absence of any therapeutic interventions, following CD4+ T lymphocyte counts and HIV/AIDS RNA. CD4+ cell counts are used to monitor degree of immunodeficiency and response to antiretroviral therapy.

HIV/AIDS RNA HIV/AIDS RNA used to monitor response to ART.

COURSE AND PROGNOSIS

The clinical course of HIV/AIDS disease is highly variable in each individual. Some patients experience symptomatic primary infection. A prolonged asymptomatic state is common. OIs and ONs occur in advanced disease. Early in the pandemic, prophylaxis for OIs and treatment of ONs improved the prognosis. Currently, ART has been very effective in the majority of cases but may give rise to new complications such as lipodystrophy and the metabolic syndrome.

MANAGEMENT

HIV/AIDS Prevention *Sex Education* The most common mode of HIV/AIDS transmission is during sexual intercourse. Currently, in terms of numbers of new HIV/AIDS infections, female-to-male and male-to-female transmission are much more common than male-to-male. Safer sexual practices must be taught at an early age.

Transfusions and Transplantation Blood and blood by-products must be tested before administration. HIV/AIDS infection must be ruled out in donors of any transplanted organ.

Antiretroviral Therapy (ART)
Guidelines for ART evolve as new drugs become available and local resources. Websites for updated guidelines of ART are as follow:

United States:
http://www.guideline.gov/summary/summary.aspx?ss=15&doc_id=11255&nbr=5881

World Health Organization:
http://www.who.int/hiv/aids/topics/arv/en/

Immune Reconstitution Inflammatory Syndrome (IRIS) IRIS occurs in some HIV/AIDS-infected patients after initiating ART, resulting from restored immunity to specific infectious or noninfectious antigens. A paradoxical clinical worsening of a known condition or the appearance of a new condition after initiating therapy characterizes the syndrome. Potential mechanisms for the syndrome include a partial recovery of the immune system or exuberant host immunologic responses to antigenic stimuli. The overall incidence of IRIS is unknown but is dependent on the population studied and its underlying opportunistic infectious burden. The infectious pathogens most frequently implicated in the syndrome are *Mycobacteria* (MAC, MTb), VZV, HSV, CMV. Also, eosinophilic folliculitis.

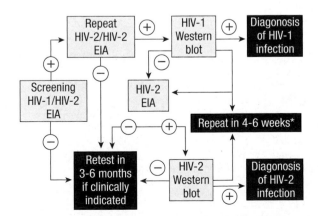

IMAGE 31-1 Algorithm of how to proceed with sero testing in case of suspected HIV/AIDS.

ACUTE HIV/AIDS SYNDROME (AHS)   ICD-10 : B23.0   ■ ●

- Primary HIV/AIDS infection
- Symptoms range from asymptomatic to severe. Symptomatic in 70% of primary infections.
- Characterized by an infectious mononucleosis-like syndrome or aseptic meningitis syndrome with fever, lymphadenopathy, and neurologic and gastrointestinal (GI) symptoms.
- Characteristic infectious exanthem, enanthem, and oral/genital ulcerations.

Incubation Period   Signs and symptoms occur within 5–30 days following HIV/AIDS exposure (most within 21–28 days).

CLINICAL MANIFESTATION

Symptoms range from asymptomatic to severe requiring hospitalization (15%). Diagnosis is often missed, considered in only 25% of cases. Between 50 and 70% of recently infected individuals experience symptomatic primary infection.

Mucocutaneous Symptoms   Cutaneous: Rash (50–60%). Exanthem usually appears 2–3 days after onset of fever, lasting 5–8 days; enanthem, asymptomatic; ulcers, painful in mouth and/or anogenital region. Pharyngitis (50–70%); oral ulcers (10–20%). Genital ulcers (5–15%).

Systemic Symptoms   Fever (>80–90%), fatigue/lethargy/malaise (>70–90%), myalgia/arthralgia (50–70%), night sweats (50%), anorexia/weight loss (25%), aseptic meningitis (24%), other neurologic symptoms (encephalitis, peripheral neuropathy, myelopathy, headache, retrobulbar pain), anorexia (21%), nausea/vomiting/diarrhea (30–60%), lymphadenopathy.

Skin Lesions
Morbilliform rash, i.e., infectious exanthem (Fig. 31-1) with pink macules, papules up to 1 cm in diameter. Ulcers occur on penis and/or scrotum. Less common: urticaria. Lesions remain discrete. Most common site of exanthem is upper thorax and collar region (100%) > face (60%) > arms (40%) > scalp, thighs (20%). Palms. ✐

Mucous Membranes   Pharyngitis. Enanthem, spotty, on hard and soft palate. Aphthous-like ulcers: 5–10 mm in diameter, round to oval, shallow with white bases surrounded by a red halo, arising on the tonsils, palate, and/or buccal mucosa; esophageal ulcers. Uncommonly, oral candidiasis.

Anogenitalia   Ulcers: prepuce of penis, scrotum, anus, anal canal. ✐

General Examination   *Lymph Nodes*   Lymphadenopathy.

Neurologic Findings   Acute meningitis; acute reversible encephalopathy with loss of memory, alteration of consciousness, and personality change.

DIFFERENTIAL DIAGNOSIS

Primary EBV infection (infectious mononucleosis) (1% of negative monospots are AHS); primary CMV infection; influenza; acute hepatitis A, B, and C infection; rubella. Syphilis: 1° and 2°. Rocky Mountain spotted fever. Adverse cutaneous drug reaction.

DIAGNOSIS

Demonstrated seroconversion of anti-HIV/AIDS antibodies by ELISA, confirmed by Western blot, confirms diagnosis of primary HIV/AIDS infection. Detection of HIV/AIDS RNA.

COURSE AND PROGNOSIS

Most individuals experience no or mild symptoms that do not prompt medical consultation. In those with symptomatic illness, the mean duration of illness in one study was 13 days (range 5–44 days). Long-term illness of >2 weeks is associated with higher risk of developing AIDS within 3 years of seroconversion.

FIGURE 31-1   Acute HIV/AIDS syndrome: exanthem   Discrete, erythematous macules and papules on the anterior trunk; associated findings were fever and lymphadenopathy. (Courtesy of Armin Rieger, MD.).

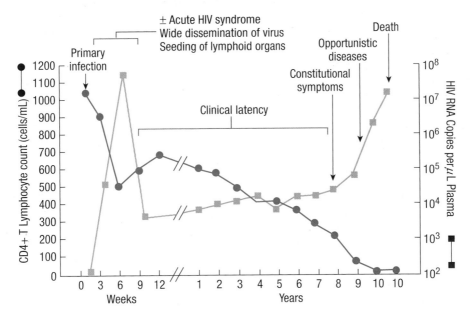

IMAGE 31-2   Typical disease course in an individual with HIV infection. (Source: AS Fauci et al: Ann Intern Med 124:654, 1996; with permission.)

EOSINOPHILIC FOLLICULITIS   ICD-9 : 704.8

- Pruritic follicular eruption of the upper trunk, face, neck, and proximal extremities
- Occurs in advanced HIV/AIDS disease and/or after initiation of ART
- Resolves with successful ART

Synonym: Eosinophilic pustular folliculitis

*Not serious itself but an indicator of serious HIV/AIDS disease.

EPIDEMIOLOGY AND PATHOGENESIS

Unknown.

CLINICAL MANIFESTATION

Moderate to intense itching unrelieved by many therapies. Pruritus may be severe, especially in those with atopic diathesis, disturbing sleep. Initially, occurred in the setting of advanced HIV/AIDS disease. Currently, occurs following initiation of ART, associated with IRIS.

Skin Lesions

Primary lesions are 3- to 5-mm erythematous, edematous, follicular papules and pustules (Fig. 31-2*A* and *B*). Dozens or hundreds of lesions may be present, in various stages of evolution. Frequently, changes secondary to scratching/rubbing are seen: excoriations/crusting of papules/pustules; atopic dermatitis, lichen simplex chronicus, prurigo nodularis.

Secondary infections of excoriated sites: impetiginization, furunculosis, cellulitis. Postinflammatory hyperpigmentation occurs in more darkly pigmented individuals and can be quite disfiguring.

Distribution   Trunk; head and neck; proximal extremities. In some individuals, lesions present only on face or on trunk. 🔲

DIFFERENTIAL DIAGNOSIS

Allergic contact dermatitis, adverse cutaneous drug reaction, atopic dermatitis, scabies, papular urticaria (insect bites), acne vulgaris, bacterial folliculitis (*Staphylococcus aureus*), *Malassezia* folliculitis.

LABORATORY EXAMINATIONS

Cultures   Negative for pathogenic organisms. Many patients with longstanding untreated EF have secondary colonization/infection with *S. aureus*.

Dermatopathology   Perifollicular and perivascular infiltrate with varying numbers of eosinophils. Epithelial spongiosis of follicular infundibulum and/or sebaceous glands associated with a mixed cellular infiltrate. Eosinophilic pustules uncommon. Special stains for bacteria, fungi, and parasites are negative.

Hematology   Eosinophilia. CD4+ cell count usually $<100/\mu L$.

DIAGNOSIS

Clinical diagnosis confirmed by biopsy of a new primary lesion (follicular papule) with cultures ruling out infectious causes.

COURSE AND PROGNOSIS

In untreated HIV/AIDS disease, the course of EF tends to be chronic and persistent. Occurring after the initiation of ART (IRIS), symptoms often persist for weeks to months if untreated.

MANAGEMENT

Pruritus is moderate to severe, significantly affecting quality of life. Changes secondary to chronic scratching such as secondary infections and lichen simplex chronicus should also be identified and treated. The most predictably effective therapy is a short tapered course of oral glucocorticoid such as prednisone. Sedating antihistamines such as hydroxyzine or doxepin are effective as antipruritics at bedtime because of sedation.

A

B

FIGURE 31-2 Eosinophilic folliculitis   Multiple, very pruritic, edematous papules with a central crust and a few pustules in a male with advanced HIV/AIDS disease (CD4+ cell count < 50/L). **A.** Distribution on the upper trunk; lesions were also present on the face and neck. **B.** Closeup showing urticarial papules, pustules, and erosion secondary to rubbing and crusts; the primary lesions resemble papular urticaria (insect bites) but are follicular.

ORAL HAIRY LEUKOPLAKIA (OHL) ICD-10 : K13.3 ■ ●*

- Benign hyperplasia of oral mucosa
- Etiology: Epstein-Barr virus (EBV)
- CD4+ cell count <300/µL
- Inferolateral surface of the tongue

- White, corrugated plaques

*Not serious itself but an indicator of serious HIV/AIDS disease.

ETIOLOGY AND PATHOGENESIS

Many adults have asymptomatic EBV infection of the oropharynx. EBV is thought to emerge from latency as HIV/AIDS-induced immuno-compromise progresses and causes the epidermal hyperplasia.

CLINICAL MANIFESTATION

Incubation Period Usually 5 to 10 years after primary HIV/AIDS infection.
Symptoms Asymptomatic, but stigmatization of HIV/AIDS disease.
Oral Mucosa White or grayish-white, well-demarcated plaque (Fig. 31-3) with corrugated texture. Most commonly on the lateral and inferior surfaces of the tongue. Often present bilaterally, but size of plaques usually not equal. Some individuals may have oropharyngeal candidiasis and/or condyloma in addition to OHL.

DIFFERENTIAL DIAGNOSIS

Thrush, condyloma acuminatum, geographic or migratory glossitis, lichen planus, tobacco-associated leukoplakia, mucous patch of secondary syphilis, squamous cell carcinoma (SCC) either in situ or invasive, occlusal trauma.

LABORATORY EXAMINATIONS

Dermatopathology Acanthotic epithelium with hyperkeratosis, hairlike projections of keratin, areas of koilocytes (ballooned cells with clear cytoplasm). *Electron microscopy*: Herpes viral structures in epithelial cells; positive for EBV markers.
Cultures Not helpful. *Candida albicans* is commonly isolated.

DIAGNOSIS

Clinical diagnosis. Does not rub off; does not clear with adequate anticandidal therapy.

COURSE AND PROGNOSIS

Usually resolves with ART.

MANAGEMENT

Reassurance that OHL is a benign viral infection is usually adequate to reduce patients' concerns, a cosmetic problem that is not precancerous.
Topical Therapy Podophyllin 25% in tincture of benzoin applied to the lesion with a cotton-tipped applicator for 5 min.
Systemic Antiviral Drugs ART indications often result in regression/clearing of OHL.

FIGURE 31-3 Oral hairy leukoplakia White plaque on the lateral tongue with corduroy-like pattern. The finding is essentially pathognomonic for HIV/AIDS infection. In this case, OHL occurred as resistance to ART evolved and CD4 count declined. OHL resolved with change in ART.

ADVERSE CUTANEOUS DRUG ERUPTIONS IN HIV/AIDS DISEASE   ICD-9 : 693.0 ∘ ICD-10 : L27.0

- Incidence of adverse cutaneous drug eruptions (ACDEs) to a variety of drugs is high in HIV/AIDS disease.
- Increases with advancing immunodeficiency.
- 95% are morbilliform

- Toxic epidermal necrolysis has high morbidity/mortality
- ART reduces the incidence of ACDE
- ART can cause a wide spectrum of ACDE

EPIDEMIOLOGY AND ETIOLOGY

Etiology   Most common drugs causing ACDE: trimethoprim-sulfamethoxazole (TMP-SMX), sulfadiazine, trimethoprim-dapsone, and aminopenicillins.

Prevalence   Drug hypersensitivity complicates 3–20% of all prescriptions in those with advanced HIV/AIDS disease, up to 100 times more common than in the general population.

PATHOGENESIS

Incidence increases with advancing immunodeficiency; may be correlated with the decline and dysregulation of immune function. After immune reconstitution by ART, some patients who had previously tolerated a drug may develop allergic cutaneous drug reactions (IRIS).

CLASSIFICATION

Drug eruptions can mimic virtually all the morphologic expressions in dermatology and must be first on the differential diagnosis in the appearance of a sudden symmetric eruption (see Section 22).

> *Exanthematous/morbilliform:* Account for 95% of ACDE in HIV/AIDS disease. Between 50 and 60% treated with TMP-SMX develop a morbilliform eruption 1–2 weeks after starting therapy.
> *Crixivan:* Retinoid dermatitis: chronic paronychia, cheilitis, pyogenic granuloma.
> *Toxic epidermal necrolysis (TEN):* The incidence of TEN caused by sulfonamides is also increased.
> *Lipodystrophy syndrome:* See below.

CLINICAL FINDINGS   See Section 22

MANAGEMENT

In most cases, the implicated or suspected drug should be discontinued. In some, such as with morbilliform eruptions, the offending drug can be continued and the eruption may resolve. In cases of urticaria/angioedema or early Stevens-Johnson syndrome (SJS)/TEN, the ACDE can be life-threatening, and the drug should be discontinued.

ACDE BY DRUG TYPE

Antiretroviral Therapy (ART)

Drug hypersensitivity commonly occurs with the nonnucleotide reverse transcriptase inhibitors (nNRTIs) nevirapine, delavirdine, and efavirenz; the nucleotide reverse transcriptase inhibitor (NRTI) abacavir; and the protease inhibitor amprenavir. ART hypersensitivity is manifested by exanthematous/morbilliform eruptions (>95%); 20% of nevirapine-treated patients experience rash, most commonly an exanthematous eruption and rarely SJS, requiring drug discontinuation. Between 18 and 50% of delavirdine-treated patients experience rash. Approximately one-half of cases of ART hypersensitivity resolve despite continuation of therapy. Drug therapy should be discontinued if the following occur: mucosal involvement, blistering, exfoliation, clinically significant hepatic dysfunction, fever >39°C, or intolerable fever or pruritus. Rechallenge with abacavir has been associated with several deaths.

Indivavir   Has a retinoid-like effect. Cheilitis (57%); diffuse dryness and pruritus; asteatotic dermatitis on the trunk, arms, and thighs; scalp defluvium; pyogenic granulomas, single or multiple.

Zidovudine (ZVD, AZT)   Longitudinal melanonychia, brown-black longitudinal streaks in the nail plate, occur in up to 40% of those treated, more commonly in blacks than in Latinos or whites. Melanonychia are usually noted in the fingers- and/or toenails within 4–8 weeks after initiation of therapy (Fig. 31-4). Pigmented macules of mucous membranes common, occurring more commonly in more heavily melanized individuals. Diffuse hyperpigmentation mimicking primary adrenal insufficiency reported. (Melanonychia and mucocutaneous pigmentation have also been reported with administration of hydroxyurea in HIV/AIDS disease.)

Enfuvirtide First of a new class of antiretroviral agents for the treatment of HIV/AIDS-1 infection, called *fusion inhibitors.* The most common type of ACDE is injection site reactions, occurring in up to 98% of patients. Many of these lesions are symptomatic. Lesional biopsy specimens show an inflammatory response consistent with a localized hypersensitivity reaction, resembling that of granuloma annulare and the recently described interstitial granulomatous drug reaction.

Other Drugs

Trimethoprim-Sulfamethoxazole Between 50 and 60% of those treated with IV TMP-SMX develop an exanthematous eruption (often associated with fever) 1 to 2 weeks after starting therapy (incidence 10 times greater than that in the general population). Successful desensitization has been accomplished in patients with prior exanthematous/morbilliform or urticarial reactions to TMP-SMX, sulfadiazine, and dapsone. Coadministration of glucocorticoids with TMP-SMX reduces incidence of ACDE. The occurrence of adverse reactions to TMP-SMX has also been noted to be associated with more rapid decline in CD4 cell counts. Sulfa drugs (sulfadiazine, TMP-SMX, sulfadoxine-pyrimethamine) can also cause severe bullous eruptions. Sulfa drugs are the most common cause of TEN, the incidence being 375 times higher than expected. TEN occurs most commonly in those with advanced HIV/AIDS disease; 21% mortality rate.

Oral Glucocorticoids Concerns: increased immunosuppression with exacerbations of opportunistic infections and neoplasms such as Kaposi sarcoma or HSV infections. Prednisone is usually well tolerated and safe, especially when given for only 1–2 weeks.

Foscarnet (Trisodium Phosphonoformate) Causes painful, penile erosions and/or ulcers in 30% of patients undergoing high-dose induction therapy for CMV retinitis, 7–24 days after starting treatment. Ulceration caused by high urinary concentration of the urinary metabolites of foscarnet. Hyperhydration reduces the risk of ulceration; in some cases, the drug must be discontinued for the ulcers to heal.

Antiretroviral Drugs
Classes of Antiretroviral Drugs

- Nucleoside and nucleotide reverse transcriptase inhibitors (NRTIs) inhibit reverse transcription by being incorporated into the newly synthesized viral DNA and preventing its further elongation.
- Nonnucleoside reverse transcriptase inhibitors (nNRTIs) inhibit reserve transcriptase directly by binding to the enzyme and interfering with its function.
- Protease inhibitors (PIs) target viral assembly by inhibiting the activity of protease, an enzyme used by HIV/AIDS to cleave nascent proteins for final assembly of new virons.
- Integrase inhibitors inhibit the enzyme integrase, which is responsible for integration of viral DNA into the DNA of the infected cell. There are several integrase inhibitors currently under clinical trial, and raltegravir became the first to receive approval by the U.S. Food and Drug Administration in October 2007.
- Entry inhibitors (or fusion inhibitors) interfere with binding, fusion, and entry of HIV/AIDS-1 to the host cell by blocking one of several targets. Maraviroc and enfuvirtide are the two currently available agents in this class.
- Maturation inhibitors inhibit the last step in gag processing in which the viral capsid polyprotein is cleaved, thereby blocking the conversion of the polyprotein into the mature capsid protein (p24). Because these viral particles have a defective core, the virions released consist mainly of noninfectious particles. There are no drugs in this class currently available, though two are under investigation, bevirimat[2] and Vivecon.

FIGURE 31-4 Adverse cutaneous drug reaction: zidovudine melanonychia A 42-year-old black female began antiretroviral therapy with zidovudine 4 months previously. Proximal nail hyperpigmentation has occurred in all fingernails and correlates with initiation of zidovudine therapy. Hyperpigmentation of skin and oral mucosa can also occur with zidovudine.

ABNORMALITIES OF FAT DISTRIBUTION (AFD)

- Associated with ART.
- Morphologic abnormalities: Varying degrees of fat redistribution, i.e., increased visceral fat; buffalo hump; decreased peripheral subcutaneous fat.
- Metabolic syndrome characterized by abdominal obesity, hypertriglyceridemia, a low high-density lipoprotein (HDL) cholesterol level, hypertension, and insulin resistance (± diabetes mellitus).

- Metabolic *changes* associated with increased risk for cardiovascular disease and diabetes.
- Morphologic abnormalities highly stigmatizing; discomfort, disability, psychological morbidity, reduce adherence to or discontinuation of effective ART.

EPIDEMIOLOGY AND ETIOLOGY

Prevalence AFD was noted in HIV/AIDS disease prior to ART; prevalence has increased drastically with widespread use of ART.
Etiology Unknown. Occurs in HIV/AIDS-infected individuals who have never been treated with ART.
Risk Factors Increasing age, current use of ART (excluding nNRTIs), longer duration of ART. Combination therapy using two NRTIs and a PI is associated with more severe disease.
  Subcutaneous lipoatrophy: Stavudine, especially when given with didanosine, zidovudine, PIs (especially indinavir), age, Caucasian, male sex.
  Visceral obesity: Age, Caucasian, male sex, restoration of health (prior wasting), effective ART.

Metabolic Abnormalities in HIV/AIDS Disease Seen most often in the context of ART (not exclusively):

- Visceral adiposity and loss of abdominal and peripheral subcutaneous fat
- Insulin resistance
- Dyslipidemia

PATHOGENESIS

Unknown. Factors in pathogenesis: (1) multiple drug-associated events in metabolic pathways and in different tissues; and (2) host predisposition: age, genetics, HIV/AIDS disease stage, inflammatory states. Metabolic changes related to direct effects of PIs on glucose, insulin, lipids, and fat, as well as effects of HIV/AIDS itself and related cytokines.

Patients with *lipoatrophy* (significantly decreased abdominal and mid-thigh subcutaneous fat) have elevated levels of plasma triglycerides. Those with obesity/mixed condition (increased intraabdominal fat) have elevated levels of plasma insulin and C-peptide. Use of stavudine correlates with fat wasting in both NRTI and PI groups. NRTI-associated mitochondrial toxicity leads to fat wasting. Stavudine-based regimens have a higher cumulative prevalence of lipoatrophy than regimens based on zidovudine, abacavir, or tenofovir. Regimens based on nelfinavir are associated with more rapid fat loss than efavirenz. In general, thymidine-based nucleoside analogues have been most associated with lipoatrophy and protease inhibitor drugs most associated with the metabolic syndrome.

CLINICAL MANIFESTATION

Cosmetic disfigurement, stigmatization. Atherosclerotic cardiovascular disease, type 2 diabetes.

Skin Findings
Loss of subcutaneous fat: First noted several months after successful ART with loss of subcutaneous fat from face (Fig. 31-5) and extremities (peripheral lipoatrophy). Results in an emaciated appearance. Face: loss of buccal fat, triangular depression below cheekbone, depression of temples, appearance of protuberant mouth because of surrounding atrophy. Rated as mild, moderate, severe. Extremities: arms, buttocks, legs; prominent veins.
   Central adiposity: Increase in subcutaneous fat in upper back and posterior neck, i.e., buffalo hump (Fig. 31-5); enlargement of breasts. Increase in visceral intraabdominal fate (protease paunch or "crix belly").
Central Adiposity/Lipohypertrophy Occurs more commonly at several anatomic locations (86%) than in one location (14%). The dorsothoracic fat pad becomes hypertrophied to a variable extent (6%) (Fig. 31-5), from mild to severe (up to 5–10 cm thick); can extend circumferentially around the neck. Breasts may become enlarged (20%) in males and females. Abdominal girth can increase due to accumulation of intraabdominal fat (60%). Lipomas.
Lipoatrophy Loss of subcutaneous fat in the face (58%) (Fig. 31-5), giving a gaunt characteristic appearance. The upper arms/shoulders (50%), buttocks/thighs (73%) also become depleted of subcutaneous fat; superficial veins are visible in these sites. There is also generalized loss of body fat. 🔲

Mixed Presentation Elements of central adiposity and lipoatrophy are present.

Systemic Findings
Coronary artery disease, peripheral artery disease. Osteonecrosis, osteopenia, osteoporosis. Hepatosteatosis. Lactic acidosis.

DIFFERENTIAL DIAGNOSIS

Fat Accumulation Cushing disease, glucocorticoid therapy, Launois-Bensaude syndrome, scleredema of diabetes mellitus.
Lipoatrophy Wasting of chronic disease, malnutrition.

LABORATORY EXAMINATIONS

Dyslipidemia: hypertriglyceridemia, hypercholesterolemia. *Insulin resistance:* glucose intolerance, diabetes mellitus. Lactic acidosis. Metabolic abnormalities associated with increased risk of cardiovascular disease.

DIAGNOSIS

Clinical diagnosis.

COURSE AND PROGNOSIS

Lipodystrophy may progress for the first 2 years of ART, then stabilize. Change in ART may result in improvement of lipodystrophy.

MANAGEMENT

For most individuals with mild to moderate lipodystrophy, changes in body habitus are not significant. However, with more severe involvement, patients may request change in ART in spite of excellent response of HIV/AIDS disease.
Metabolic Syndrome Changing NRTI may result in regression. Metabolic strategies: lipid-lowering strategies [fibric acids (clofibrate, fenofibrate, gemfibrozil)], insulin-sensitizing agents (metformin), strategies to change fat distribution (glitazones to increase subcutaneous fat, growth hormone to decrease visceral fat).
Lipoatrophy Remains the most difficult manifestation to manage. Replacing stavudine with abacavir may result in improvement in stavudine-induced lipoatrophy. For facial lipoatrophy, various filler substances have been injected into sites in the cheeks; however, the effects are evanescent and costly.

FIGURE 31-5 Fat redistribution A 51-year-old male with advanced HIV/AIDS treated for many years with ART has striking lipotrophy of the face and "buffalo hump" of the upper back and cervical neck. The facial changes are distinctive and stigmatizing.

VARIATIONS OF COMMON MUCOCUTANEOUS DISORDERS IN HIV/AIDS DISEASE

- Early in HIV/AIDS disease when immune function is relatively intact, common dermatoses, adverse cutaneous drug eruptions, and infections present as typical clinical manifestations, have the usual course, and respond to standard therapies.

- With progressive decline in immune function, each of these characteristics of a disease can be strikingly altered.

- With effective management with ART and immune reconstitution, the diseases either do not occur, resolve without specific therapy, or respond more readily to therapy.

Kaposi Sarcoma (KS)

(See also "Kaposi Sarcoma," Section 20) Early in the HIV/AIDS epidemic in the United States and Europe, 50% of homosexual men at the time of initial AIDS diagnosis had KS. In HIV/AIDS-infected individuals, the risk for KS is 20,000 times that of the general population, 300 times that of other immunosuppressed hosts. In untreated HIV/AIDS disease, KS may progress rapidly with extensive mucocutaneous and systemic involvement. KS in patients successfully treated with ART does not occur, resolves without specific therapy other than immune reconstitution, or responds better to chemotherapies.

Nonmelanoma Skin Cancers

As in solid organ transplant recipients, the incidence of ultraviolet light-induced invasive SCC is reported to be increased in HIV/AIDS of skin phototypes I to III with much UVL exposure during early decades of life. SCC can be quite aggressive, invading locally, growing rapidly, and metastasizing by lymphatics and blood, with increased morbidity and mortality.

Aphthous Stomatitis

(See also "Aphthous Ulcers," Section 34) Recurrent aphthous ulcerations may occur more frequently, become larger (often >1 cm), and/or become chronic with advanced HIV/AIDS disease. Ulcers may be quite extensive and/or multiple; commonly involving the tongue, gingiva, lips, and esophagus; at times causing severe odynophagia with rapid weight loss. Intralesional triamcinolone and/or a 1- to 2-week tapered course of prednisone (70 to 0 mg). In resistant cases, thalidomide is an effective agent.

Staphylococcus Aureus Infection

(See also "Impetigo and Ecthyma," "Abscess, Furuncle, and Carbuncle," and "Erysipelas and Cellulitis," Section 24) S. aureus is the most common cutaneous bacterial pathogen in HIV/AIDS disease. The nasal carriage rate of S. aureus is 50%, twice that of HIV/AIDS-seronegative control groups. In most instances, S. aureus infections are typical, presenting as primary infections (folliculitis, furuncles, carbuncles), secondarily impetiginized lesions (excoriations, eczema, scabies, herpetic ulcer, Kaposi sarcoma), cellulitis, or venous access device infections, all

of which can be complicated by bacteremia and disseminated infection. Methicillin-resistant S. aureus (MRSA) infections, if not diagnosed with culture and sensitives, may be more severe because of delay in initiation of effective anti-MRSA therapy (Figs. 31-6, 31-7).

Dermatophytoses

(See also "Dermatophytoses," Section 25, and "Fungal Infections: Onychomycosis," Section 33) Epidermal dermatophytosis can be extensive, recurrent, and difficult to eradicate. Proximal subungual onychomycosis occurs in advanced HIV/AIDS disease, presents as a chalky-white discoloration of the undersurface of the proximal nail plate, and is an indication for HIV/AIDS serotesting.

Mucosal Candidiasis

(See also "Candidiasis," Section 25) Mucosal candidiasis affecting the upper aerodigestive tracts and/or vulvovagina is common in HIV/AIDS disease. Oropharyngeal candidiasis, the most common presentation, is often the initial manifestation of HIV/AIDS disease and is a marker for disease progression. Esophageal and

FIGURE 31-6   Furuncle with cellulitis: MRSA   A 38-year-old male with HIV/AIDS and a painful furuncle was treated unsuccessfully with several oral antibiotics; the lesion had not been incised and drained nor cultured. When the lesion was incised and drained and culture obtained, MRSA was isolated, sensitive only to linezolid and vancomycin. The infection resolved with oral linezolid 600 mg BID for 7 days.

FIGURE 31-7   Botryomycosis: MRSA   A 35-year-old with a painful lesion on the right buttock for 10 months had been treated unsuccessfully with oral antibiotics. **A.** A large fluctuant abscess is seen on the buttock. **B.** Punch biopsies were obtained at either pole of the abscess, pus drained, and cultured. White "grains" were observed in the draining pus. The probe shows the extent of the abscess cavity. Biopsy specimen showed colonies of gram-positive cocci that were the "grains" visualized macroscopically. Culture reported MRSA, sensitive to linezolid and vancomycin. The infection resolved with oral linezolid 600 mg BID for 10 days.

tracheobronchial candidiasis occur in advanced HIV/AIDS disease and are AIDS-defining conditions. The incidence of cutaneous candidiasis may be somewhat increased; with insulin resistance associated with ART, balanoposthitis can be seen. In young children, chronic candidal paronychia and nail dystrophy are seen frequently.

Disseminated Fungal Infection

(See also "Disseminated Cryptococcosis," "Histoplasmosis," and "Disseminated Coccidioidomycosis," Section 25) Latent pulmonary fungal infections with *Cryptococcus neoformans, Coccidioides immitis, Histoplasma capsulatum,* and *Penicillium marneffei* can be reactivated in HIV/AIDS-infected individuals and disseminated to the skin and other organs. The most common cutaneous presentation of disseminated infection is molluscum contagiosum–like lesions on the face; other lesions such as nodules, pustules, ulcers, abscesses, or a papulosquamous eruption resembling guttate psoriasis (seen with histoplasmosis) also occur.

Herpes Simplex Virus Infection

(See also "Herpes Simplex Virus: Infections Associated with Systemic Immunocompromise," Section 27) Reactivated HSV-1 or HSV-2 infection is one of the most common viral OIs of HIV/AIDS disease. Most HIV/AIDS-infected persons are HSV-2 seropositive. Most reactivation is subclinical. Anogenital reactivation is particularly frequent. With increasing immunodeficiency, early lesions present with erosions or ulcerations due to epidermal necrosis without vesicle formation. Untreated, these lesions may evolve to large, painful ulcers with rolled margins in the oropharynx, esophagus, and anogenitalia. Treatment of HSV in dually infected individuals reduces genital and plasma HIV/AIDS RNA levels.

Varicella-Zoster Virus (VZV) Infection

(See also "Varicella-Zoster Virus Infections in the Immunocompromised Host," Section 27) Primary VZV infection (varicella or chickenpox) in HIV/AIDS disease can be severe, prolonged, and complicated by visceral VZV infection, bacterial superinfection, and death. Herpes zoster (HZ) occurs in 25% of HIV/AIDS-infected persons during the course of their HIV/AIDS, associated with modest decline in immune function. Cutaneous dissemination

of HZ is relatively common; however, visceral involvement is rare. With increasing immunodeficiency, VZV infection can present clinically as persistent (chronic) dermatomal verrucous lesions; one or more chronic painful ulcers or ecthymatous lesions within a dermatome; ecthymatous lesion(s), ulcer(s), or nodule(s). Untreated, these lesions persist for months. HZ can recur within the same dermatome(s) or in other dermatomes. VZV can infect the CNS causing a rapidly progressive chorioretinitis with acute retinal necrosis, chronic encephalitis, myelitis, radiculitis, or meningitis. Extensive HZ may heal with hypertrophic or keloidal scar.

Molluscum Contagiosum

(See also "Molluscum Contagiosum," Section 27) In HIV/AIDS-infected individuals, molluscum contagiosum has up to an 18% prevalence; the severity of the infection is a marker for advanced immunodeficiency. Patients may have multiple small papules or nodules or large tumors, >1 cm in diameter, most commonly arising on the face (Fig. 31-8), especially the beard area, the neck, and intertriginous sites. Shaving is a major factor in the facial spread of mollusca and should be avoided if possible. Cystlike mollusca occur on the ears. Occasionally, mollusca can arise on the non-hair-bearing skin of the palms/soles.

Human Papillomavirus (HPV) Infection

(See also "Human Papillomavirus: Mucosal Infections," Section 30) With advancing immunodeficiency, cutaneous and/or mucosal warts can become extensive and refractory to treatment. Of more concern, however, HPV-induced intraepithelial neoplasia, termed *squamous intraepithelial lesion* (SIL), is a precursor to invasive SCC (Fig. 31-9), arising most often on the cervix, vulva, penis, perineum, and anus. In HIV/AIDS-infected females, the incidence of cervical SIL is six to eight times that of controls. The current trend toward longer median survival of patients with advanced HIV/AIDS may lead to an increased incidence of HPV-associated neoplasia and invasive SCC in the future. SIL on the external genitalia, perineum, or anus is best managed with local therapies such as imiquimod cream, cryosurgery, electrosurgery, or laser surgery rather than with aggressive surgical excision.

A   *B*

FIGURE 31-8   Molluscum contagiosum, confluent: face   A 51-year-old female with **A.** extensive and confluent facial nodules. Lesions enlarged in spite of cryosurgery. **B.** All lesions resolved with electrodessication.

FIGURE 31-9   HPV infection of perineum: Condyloma acuminatum and invasive squamous cell carcinoma   A 38-year-old male with a history of perineal and perianal condylomata was poorly compliant with ART. Scissor excision of the mass was reported to show invasive SCC arising in the base of the huge condylomatous tumor. Electrodessication of the base at the time of scissor excision was curative. On reexcision, no residual SCC was detected

Syphilis (See also "Syphilis," Section 30) The clinical course of syphilis in HIV/AIDS-infected individuals is most often the same as in the normal host. However, an accelerated course with the development of neurosyphilis or tertiary syphilis has been reported within months of initial syphilitic infection.

Resources available on the World Wide Web on HIV/AIDS disease are shown in Table 31-3.

TABLE 31-3   Resources Available on the World Wide Web on HIV/AIDS

http://www.aidsinfo.nih.gov	AIDS info, a service of the U.S. Department of Health and Human Services, posts federally approved treatment guidelines for HIV and AIDS; provides information on federally funded and privately funded clinical trials and CDC publications and data
http://www.cdcnpin.org	Updates on epidemiologic data from the CDC

NOTE: CDC, Centers for Disease Control and Prevention.

PART IV

SKIN SIGNS OF HAIR, NAIL, AND MUCOSAL DISORDERS

DISORDERS OF HAIR FOLLICLES AND RELATED DISORDERS

- Hair follicles produce pigmented keratin fibers.
- Human hair has little vestigial function:
  - Contributes to a psychological perception of beauty and attractiveness.
  - Tactile sensation
  - Protects the scalp, face, and neck from UV solar radiation
  - Reduces heat loss through the scalp
- Psychology of hair: Alteration of the "normal" quantity of hair is often associated with profound psychological impact. Loss of scalp hair is considered abnormal in many societies, associating balding with old age (pattern hair loss) or impaired health (chemotherapy).
- Excess hair on the face (hirsutism, hypertrichosis) and extremities of women is often considered unattractive.
- Billions of dollars are spent annually in industrialized countries to care for hair and perceived abnormalities.

BIOLOGY OF HAIR GROWTH CYCLES

GLOSSARY OF TERMS

Hair Follicle Cycle
Life-long cyclic transformations of the hair follicle, which begins in utero (Fig. 32-1).
Anagen Growth phase; lasts variable periods of time depending on body site, e.g., scalp, eyebrows. Duration: 1–6 years; average 3 years; varies with age; determines the ultimate length of hair at a site. Scalp, beard: long anagen. Eyebrows, eyelashes, axillary/pubic hair: anagen is short; telogen prolonged. Anagen hair matrix has rapidly proliferating epithelial cells; exquisitely sensitive to drugs, growth factors, hormones, stress; immunologic and physical injury. Destruction of epithelial stem cells results in permanent hair loss.
Anagen Hairs Hairs with pigmented malleable proximal ends.
Telogen Period of relative quiescence, last variable periods of body site.
Telogen Hairs Club hairs with depigmented rounded proximal ends.

Catagen Apoptosis-driven phase between telogen and anagen phase. Duration: few weeks.
Exogen Active process of hair shaft shedding.
Effluvium Process of increased daily hair shaft shedding (normal scalp 25–100 hairs).

Hair Color
Canities Graying of hair.
Poliosis Localized white hair.

Types of Hair
Lanugo Hair Soft fine pigmented hair that covers much of fetus; usually shed before birth. Between vellus and terminal hair in length and form.
Vellus Hair Latin for "fleece." Fine, nonpigmented hair (peach fuzz) that covers the body of children and adults; growth not affected by hormones. Beard hair in women and children is vellus. Genetically determined to produce very small (but functionally fully active cycling) hair follicles located in the dermis; thin ($\leq$0.03 mm in diameter), short, often nonpigmented, usually nonmedullated hair shaft.

Intermediate Hair Shows the characteristics of vellus and terminal hairs.

Terminal Hair Thick pigmented hair found on scalp, beard, axillae, pubic area; growth is influenced by hormones. Eyebrow/eyelash hair are terminal hairs. Produced by large hair follicles located in the subcutis; hairs are generally >0.03 mm in diameter. 100,000 terminal scalp hair follicles at birth; genetically determined to produce long, thick pigmented hairs.

Hair Loss or Gain

Alopecia Hair loss, usually of the scalp.

Scarring Alopecia Cicatricial/permanent alopecia. Irreversible loss of hair follicles with disappearance of follicular orifices and skin atrophy.

Hirsutism Excessive and increased hair growth in women in locations where the occurrence of terminal hair normally is minimal or absent. It refers to a male pattern of body hair (androgenic hair) and it is therefore primarily of cosmetic and psychological concern. Hirsutism is a symptom rather than a disease and may be a sign of a more serious medical indication, especially if it develops well after puberty.

Hypertrichosis Increased growth of terminal hairs in an area where vellus hairs are normal.

ENDOCRINOLOGY OF HAIR FOLLICLES

Hair follicles can vary in size under the influence of androgens, which increase the size of hair follicles in the beard, chest, legs, and arms but decrease the size of the hair follicles in the temporal regions of the scalp; this shapes the hairline in men and many women.

The response of the hair follicle to *testosterone* and *dihydrotestosterone* (DHT) is under genetic control.

- *Dihydrotestosterone* causes growth of the prostate, growth of terminal hair, androgenetic alopecia, and acne.
- *Testosterone* causes growth of axillary hair and lower pubic hair, as well as sex drive, growth of the phallus and scrotum, and spermatogenesis.

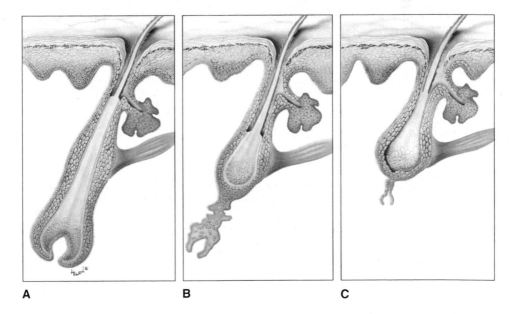

A   B   C

FIGURE 32-1 **Hair growth cycle** Diagrammatic representation of the changes that occur to the follicle and hair shaft during the hair growth cycle. **A.** Anagen (growth stage); **B.** Catagen (degenerative stage); **C.** Telogen (resting stage). (Courtesy of Lynn M. Klein, MD.)

LABORATORY EXAMINATIONS

Hair Pull   Scalp is gently pulled. Normally, three to five hairs are dislodged; shedding more hair suggests pathology.

Trichogram   Determines the number of anagen and telogen hairs and is made by epilating (plucking) 50 hairs or more from the scalp with a needleholder and counting the number of

- Anagen hairs: growing hairs with a long encircling hair sheath.
- Telogen (club) hairs: resting hairs with an inner root sheath and roots usually largest at the base.

Normally, 80–90% of hairs are in anagen phase.

Scalp Biopsy   Offers insight into pathogenesis of alopecia.

CLASSIFICATION OF ALOPECIA   ICD-9 : 704.0 ∘ ICD-10 : L63-L66

- Alopecia: diffuse (global) hair loss
- Failure of hair follicle development: e.g., hypohidrotic ectodermal dysplasia
- Hair shaft abnormalities:
  - Hair shaft abnormalities with hair breakage: trichorrhexis nodosa, trichoschisis, pili torti, trichorrhexis invaginata ("bamboo hair"), monilethrix, localized autosomal recessive hypotrichosis
  - Hair shaft abnormalities with unruly hair: Uncombable hair syndrome, woolly hair
- Abnormalities of hair follicle cycling: Short anagen syndrome, acute telogen effluvium, chronic telogen effluvium, anagen effluvium, loose anagen syndrome
- Alopecia areata
- Nonscarring hair loss, production decline: Pattern hair loss
- Traumatic hair loss: Pressure alopecia, trichotillomania, traction alopecia, tinea capitis

- Primary or acquired hair shaft abnormalities: Abnormalitiy of cycling (alopecia areata, syphilis); scalp conditions associated with focal hair loss (pityriasis amiantaea, severe scalp psoriasis or seborrheic dermatitis, scalp involvement with dermatomyositis, cutaneous T cell lymphoma, Langerhans cell histiocytosis)
- Cicatricial alopecia (destruction of the follicle) (see below):
  - Primary cicatricial alopecia [lupus erythematosus, lichen planopilaris (Graham-Little syndrome, frontal fibrosing alopecia), pseudopelade of Brocq, other [central centrifugal cicatricial alopecia (hot comb alopecia or follicular degeneration syndrome), alopecia or follicular mucinosis, folliculitis decalvans, dissecting folliculitis, acne keloidalis nuchae, acne necrotica, erosive pustular dermatosis].
  - Secondary cicatricial alopecia: hereditary or development problem.
  - Congenital cicatricial alopecia

PATHOGENESIS APPROACH TO DIAGNOSIS OF DISORDERS OF HAIR AND HAIR FOLLICLES

Pathogenetic Principle	Clinical Effect (Examples)
■ Disturbed hair follicle cycling	Effluvium (telogen effluvium, alopecia areata, androgenetic alopecia, chemotherapy-induced alopecia)
■ Unwanted hair follicle transformation	Patterned hair loss (androgenetic alopecia) Hirsutism Hypertrichosis
■ Defective hair follicle regeneration	Cicatricial alopecia (lichen planopilaris, traction alopecia, radiation-induced alopecia, folliculitis decalvans, chronic discoid lupus erythematosus)
■ Structural hair shaft defect	Hair shaft disorders (monilethrix, pili torti, trichothiodystrophy)
■ Improper/missing hair follicle development	Aplasia cutis congenita
■ Combinations of the above	Ectodermal dysplasias

Note that infectious or physical agents (e.g., staphylococci, dermatophytes, herpes–varicella zoster virus; ionizing radiation, trauma) or drugs that can lead to alopecia do so by inducing one or several of the above pathogenesis pathways (e.g., disturbed hair follicle cycling, structural hair shaft defect, defective hair follicle regeneration).

HAIR LOSS: ALOPECIA ICD-9:704.0 ∘ ICD-10:L63-L66

- Shedding of hair is termed *effluvium* or *defluvium*, and the resulting condition is called *alopecia* (Greek alópekia, "baldness").
- Individuals are often aware of and very concerned about subtle thinning of the hair.

- Alopecia classified into:
- *Noncicatricial Alopecia*: No clinical sign of tissue inflammation, scarring, or atrophy of skin.
- *Cicatricial alopecia*: Evidence of tissue destruction such as inflammation, atrophy, and scarring is apparent.

TABLE 32-1 Etiology of Hair Loss

Diffuse (global) hair loss (nonscarring)	**Focal (patchy, localized) hair loss**
Failure of follicle production	Nonscarring
Hair shaft abnormality	Production decline
Abnormality of cycling (shedding)	Triangular alopecia
Telogen effluvium	Pattern hair loss (androgenetic alopecia)
Anagen effluvium	Hair breakage
Loose anagen syndrome	Trichotillomania
Alopecia areata	Traction alopecia
	Infection (tinea capitis)
	Primary or acquired hair shaft abnormality
	Unruly hair
	Abnormality of cycling
	Alopecia areata
	Syphilis
	Scarring (cicatricial) alopecia
	(see "Scarring Alopecia," below)

NONSCARRING ALOPECIA

- Can occur globally or be focal (Table 32-1).
- Loss of scalp hair has the most cosmetic impact on individuals.

PATTERN HAIR LOSS

- Pattern hair loss is the most common type of progressive balding.
- Occurs through the combined effect of:
  - Genetic predisposition
  - Action of androgen on scalp hair follicles
- In males, pattern/extent of hair loss in males varies from bitemporal recession, to frontal and/or

vertex thinning, to loss of all hair except that along the occipital and temporal margins ("Hippocratic wreath").

Synonyms: Males: Androgenetic alopecia (AGA), male-pattern baldness, common baldness. Females: Hereditary thinning, female-pattern baldness.

ETIOLOGY AND EPIDEMIOLOGY

Etiology Combined effects of androgen on genetically predisposed hair follicles. Genetics: (1) autosomal dominant and/or polygenic; (2) inherited from either or both parents.

Age of Onset

- *Males*: May begin any time after puberty, as early as the second decade; often fully expressed in 40s.
- *Females*: Later—in about 40% occurs in the sixth decade.

Sex Males >> females.

CLASSIFICATION

Hamilton[1] classified male-pattern hair loss into stages (Fig. 32-2*A*):

Type I: Loss of hair along frontal margin.

Type II: Increasing frontal hair loss as well as onset of loss of occipital (vertex or crown).

Types III, IV, and V: Increasing hair loss in both regions with eventual confluent and complete balding of top of scalp with sparing of sides

Ludwig[2] classified hair loss in females (Fig. 32-2*B*).

PATHOGENESIS

- Testosterone is converted to (DHT) by 5α-reductase (5α-R). Two isozymes of 5α-R occur: type I and type II.
  - Type I 5α-R is localized to sebaceous glands (face, scalp), chest/back skin/liver, adrenal gland, kidney.
  - Type II 5α-R is localized to scalp hair follicle, beard, chest skin, liver, seminal vesicle, prostate, epididymis, foreskin/scrotum.
- Finasteride inhibits conversion of testosterone to DHT by type II 5α-R.
- Role of testosterone: (1) prenatal: internal sex organ development of male fetus; (2) postnatal: spermatogenesis, libido, muscle/bone mass.
- Role of DHT: (1) prenatal: external genitalia development in male fetus; (2) postnatal: scalp hair loss, prostate enlargement.
- Clinical features of type II 5α-R deficiency in men: ambiguous genitalia at birth, virilized at puberty; underdeveloped prostate, no enlargement with age; otherwise healthy (normal libido after puberty, normal bone/muscle

mass after puberty); sparse facial/body hair; no scalp hair loss with age.
- In males, testosterone produced by the testes is the major androgen. In females, androstenedione and dehydroepiandrosterone sulfate are the major peripheral androgens.
- In genetically predisposed individuals, DHT causes terminal follicles to transform into vellus-like follicles, which in turn undergo atrophy. During successive follicular cycles, hairs produced are of shorter length and of decreasing diameter.
- Conversely, androgens induce vellus-to-terminal follicle production of secondary sexual hair.

CLINICAL MANIFESTATION

Skin Symptoms Most patients present with complaints of gradually thinning hair or baldness.

- In males (Figs. 32-3, 32-4), there is a receding anterior hairline, especially in the parietal regions, which results in an M-shaped recession. Following this, a bald spot may appear on the vertex. If AGA progresses rapidly, some patients also complain of increased falling out of hair.
- In females, parietal and temporal recession is not usually a major feature, and hair loss follows a pattern depicted in Fig. 32-5; severe thinning is not common.

The cosmetic appearance of pattern hair loss is very disturbing to many persons owing to the high value that our society places on a "healthy head of hair."

Systems Review In young women, manifestations of androgen excess should be sought as significant:

- Acne
- Hirsutism
- Irregular menses
- Virilization.

However, most women with pattern hair loss are endocrinologically normal.

Skin Findings Scalp skin is normal.

- In young women, look for signs of virilization (acne, excess facial or body hair, male-pattern escutcheon).
- With advanced pattern hair loss, scalp is smooth and shiny; orifices of follicles are barely perceptible with the unaided eye.

[1] JN Hamilton: Am J Anat 71:451, 1941.

[2] E. Ludwig: Br J Dermatol 97:249, 1977.

I   II   III   IV   V

A Male

I   II   III

B Female

FIGURE 32-2 Androgenetic alopecia: patterns in males and females *A.* Hamilton classified the severity and pattern of hair loss in males into types I to V. ***B.*** Ludwig classified hair loss in females into types I to III.

Hair (Figs. 32-3 and 32-7) Hair in areas of pattern hair loss becomes finer in texture (shorter in length, reduced diameter). In time, hair becomes vellus and eventually atrophies completely.
Distribution

- Males usually exhibit patterned loss in the frontotemporal and vertex areas (Figs. 32-3, 32-4). The end result may be only a rim of residual hair on the lateral and posterior scalp (Hippocratic wreath; Fig. 32-6). In these regions hair never falls out in pattern hair loss. Paradoxically, males with extensive pattern hair loss may have excess growth of secondary sexual hair, i.e., axillae, pubic area, chest, and beard.
- Females, including those who are endocrinologically normal, also lose scalp hair according to the male pattern, but hair loss is far less pronounced. Often hair loss is more diffuse in women, following the pattern described by Ludwig (Figs. 32-2B, 32-5).

Systemic Findings In young women with AGA, look for signs of virilization (clitoral hypertrophy, acne, facial hirsutism) and, if present, rule out endocrine dysfunction.

DIFFERENTIAL DIAGNOSIS

Diffuse Nonscarring Scalp Alopecia Diffuse pattern of hair loss with alopecia areata, telogen defluvium, secondary syphilis, systemic lupus erythematosus (SLE), iron deficiency, hypothyroidism, hyperthyroidism, trichotillomania, seborrheic dermatitis.

LABORATORY EXAMINATIONS

Trichogram In pattern hair loss, the earliest changes are an increase in the percentage of telogen hairs.
Dermatopathology Abundance of telogen-stage follicles is noted, associated with hair follicles of decreasing size and eventually nearly complete atrophy.

Hormone Studies In women with hair loss and evidence of increased androgens (menstrual irregularities, infertility, hirsutism, severe cystic acne, virilization), determine:

- Testosterone: total and free
- Dehydroepiandrosterone sulfate (DHEAS)
- Prolactin

Other Studies Treatable causes of thinning hair should be excluded with measurement of thyroid-stimulating hormone (TSH), T_4, serum iron, serum ferritin, and/or total iron-binding capacity (TIBC), complete blood count (CBC), antinuclear antibodies (ANA).

DIAGNOSIS

Clinical diagnosis is made on the history, pattern of alopecia, and family incidence of AGA. Skin biopsy may be necessary in some cases.

COURSE

The progression of alopecia is usually very gradual, over years to decades.

FIGURE 32-3   Pattern hair loss: male, Hamilton type III   A 46-year-old male with bitemporal recession of hairline and frontal thinning of hair.

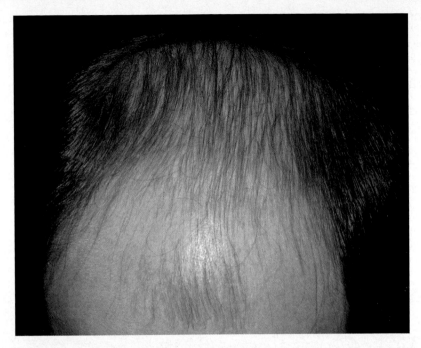

FIGURE 32-4 **Pattern hair loss: male, Hamilton types IV to V** A 37-year-old male with loss of hair in the frontotemporal and vertex areas in a male corresponding to Hamilton types IV and V.

FIGURE 32-5 **Pattern hair loss: female, Ludwig type II** A 66-year-old female with diffuse thinning of hair on the crown.

MANAGEMENT

Oral Finasteride   1 mg PO daily, competitively inhibits type II 5α-R and thus the conversion of testosterone to DHT; this results in lower serum and scalp levels of DHT. Finasteride has no affinity for androgen receptors and therefore does not block the important actions of testosterone (growth of the phallus and scrotum, spermatogenesis, libido). Most men may begin to see first benefit in slowing hair loss as early as 3 months. After 6 months, there is a regrowth of terminal hair on the vertex and anterior mid-scalp. If the drug is stopped, however, the hair that had grown will be lost within 12 months. 2% of men taking finasteride report decrease in libido and erectile function; these effects were reversible when the drug was stopped and disappeared in two-thirds of those who continued taking finasteride.

Topical Minoxidil   Topically applied minoxidil, 2% and 5% solution, may be helpful in reducing rate of hair loss or in partially restoring lost hair in both males and females.

Antiandrogens   In women with AGA who have elevated adrenal androgens, spironolactone, cyproterone acetate, flutamide, and cimetidine bind to androgen receptors and block the action of DHT. These must not be used in men.

Hairpiece   Wigs, toupees, prosthetics; hair weaves.

Surgical Treatment

Hair transplantation Grafts of one or two follicles are taken from androgen-insensitive hair sites (peripheral occipital and parietal hairy areas) to bald androgen-sensitive scalp areas.

Scalp reduction/rotation flaps

FIGURE 32-6   Pattern hair loss: male, Hamilton type V with invasive squamous cell carcinoma (SCC)   A 65-year-old white male with early onset of balding has severe dermatoheliosis with actinic keratoses, in situ SCC, invasive SCC, and multiple scars at excision sites of prior invasive SCCs. Metastatic SCC was detected in a supraclavicular lymph node, presumable from a primary scalp SCC.

FIGURE 32-7   Pattern hair loss: female, Lugwig type III with basal cell carcinoma (BCC)   A 67-year-old Greek female with advanced alopecia of the crown with BCC arising within it.

ALOPECIA AREATA ■ ◑

- A localized loss of hair in round or oval areas with no apparent inflammation of the skin. Most common on scalp.
- Nonscarring; hair follicle intact; hair can regrow.
- A cosmetic concern for the majority of patients.
- Clinical findings: Hair loss ranging from solitary patch to complete loss of all terminal hair.

- Prognosis: good for limited involvement. Poor for extensive hair loss.
- Management: intralesional triamcinolone effective for limited number of lesions.
- http://www.naaf.org

ETIOLOGY AND EPIDEMIOLOGY

Etiology   Unknown. Association with other autoimmune diseases and immunophenotyping of lymphocytic infiltrate around hair bulbs suggests an anti–hair bulb autoimmune process. 10–20% of persons with alopecia areata (AA) have a familial history of AA.

Age of Onset   Young adults (<25 years); children are affected more frequently. Can occur at any age.

Prevalence   Relatively common. 1.7% of the U.S. population experiences at least one episode of AA in a lifetime. Varies with geography and ethnicity.

PATHOGENESIS

- Chronic organ-specific autoimmune disease, mediated by autoreactive T cells affecting hair follicles and nails.
- Associated autoimmune disorders: Autoimmune thyroid disease in adults.
- Follicular damage occurs in anagen followed by rapid transformation to catagen and to telogen; then to dystrophic anagen status. While the disease is active, follicles unable to progress beyond early anagen and do not develop normal hair.

- Follicular stem cell is spared; hair follicles are not destroyed.
- White or graying hairs are frequently spared; with fulminant AA, persons may experience "going gray overnight."

CLINICAL MANIFESTATIONS

Duration of Hair Loss   Gradual over weeks to months. Patches of AA can be stable and often show spontaneous regrowth over a period of several months; new patches may appear while others resolve.

Skin Symptoms   Individuals are usually very concerned about hair loss and potential for continued, progressive balding.

Associated Findings   Autoimmune thyroiditis. Down syndrome. Autoimmune polyendocrinopathy-candidiasis–ectodermal dysplasia syndrome.

Skin Findings   Usually none. Possibly minimal erythema in area of hair loss.
Hair

- Round patches of hair loss. Single or multiple. May coalesce. Alopecia often sharply defined.
- Alopecia, normal-appearing skin with follicular openings present (Figs. 32-8 through 32-11).
- "Exclamation mark" hairs. Diagnostic broken-off stubby hairs (distal ends are broader than proximal ends) (Fig. 32-8); seen at margins of hair loss areas.
- Scattered, discrete areas of alopecia (Fig. 32-9) or confluent with total loss of scalp hair (Fig. 32-10), or generalized loss of body hair (including vellus hair).
- Diffuse AA of scalp (noncircumscribed) gives the appearance of thinned hair; can be difficult to differentiate from pattern hair loss

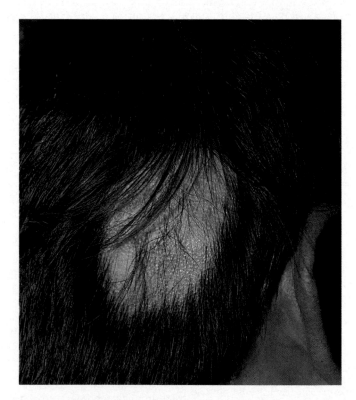

FIGURE 32-8   Alopecia areata (AA) of scalp: solitary lesion   An area of alopecia without scaling, erythema, atrophy, or scarring on the occipital scalp. The short, broken-off hair shafts (so-called exclamation point hair) appear as very short stubs emerging from the bald scalp.

of telogen effluvium, hair loss with thyroid disease.
- With regrowth of hair, new hairs are fine, often white or gray.

Sites of Predilection   Scalp most commonly. Any hair-bearing area. Beard, eyebrows, eyelashes, pubic hair.

- *Alopecia areata (AA)*: Solitary or multiple areas of hair loss. (Figs. 32-8, 32-9)
- *AA totalis (AAT)*: Total loss of terminal scalp hair. (Fig. 32-10)
- *AA universalis (AAU)*: Total loss of all terminal body and scalp hair. (Fig. 32-11)
- *Ophiasis*: Bandlike pattern of hair loss over periphery of scalp.

Nails   Fine pitting ("hammered brass") of dorsal nail plate. Also: mottled lunula, trachyonychia (rough nails), onychomadesis (separation of nail from matrix). (See also Section 33.)

DIFFERENTIAL DIAGNOSIS

Nonscarring Alopecia   White-patch tinea capitis, trichotillomania, early scarring alopecia, pattern hair loss, secondary syphilis (alopecia areolaris) ("moth-eaten" appearance in beard or scalp).

LABORATORY EXAMINATIONS

Serology   ANA (to rule out SLE); rapid plasma reagin (RPR) test (to rule out secondary syphilis).
KOH Preparation   Rule out tinea capitis.
Dermatopathology   Acute lesions show peribulbar, perivascular, and outer root sheath mononuclear cell infiltrate of T cells and macrophages; follicular dystrophy with abnormal pigmentation and matrix degeneration.

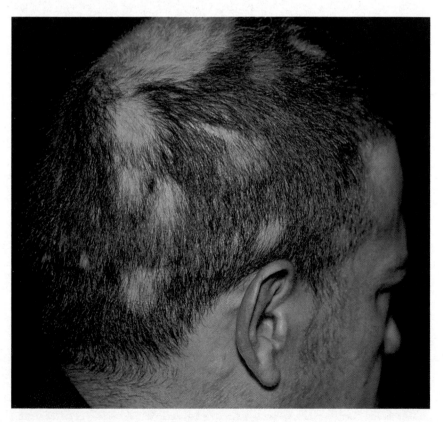

FIGURE 32-9   Alopecia areata of scalp: multiple, extensive lesions   A 46-year-old male with recent onset of alopecia areata. Multiple, confluent, involved sites on the scalp with "exclamation point hairs." Treatment with intralesional triamcinolone 3.3 mg/mL was successful.

COURSE

- Spontaneous remission is common in patchy AA but is less so with AAT or AAU.
- Poor prognosis associated with onset in childhood, loss of body hair, nail involvement, atopy, family history of AA.
- If occurring after puberty, 80% regrow hair. With extensive AA, AAT, AAU, <10% recover spontaneously.
- Recurrences of AA, however, are frequent.
- Systemic glucocorticoids or cyclosporine can induce remission of AA but do not alter the course.

MANAGEMENT

- Treatment directed at inflammatory infiltrate and growth inhibitor factors produced by inflammation. No curative treatment is currently available. Treatment for AA is unsatisfactory.
- In many cases, the most important factor in management of the patient is psychological support from the dermatologist, family, and support groups (The National Alopecia Areata Foundation, http://-www.naaf.org/).
- Persons with extensive scalp involvement such as AAT may prefer to wear a wig or hairpiece.
- Makeup applied to eyebrows is helpful. Eyebrows can be tattooed.

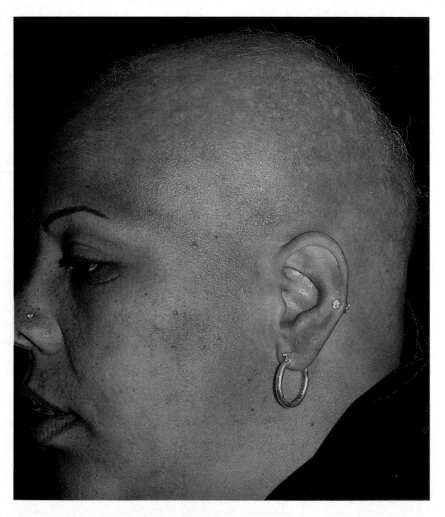

FIGURE 32-10 Alopecia areata of scalp: AA totalis *A* 41-year-old female with total loss of scalp hair, eyebrows, and eyelashes; a few, white fine regrowing hairs are seen.

FIGURE 32-11   Alopecia areata universalis (AAU)   This patient has lost all scalp hair (alopecia totalis), eyebrows, eyelashes, beard, and all body hair (alopecia universalis) and has dystrophic ("hammered brass") nails.

Glucocorticoids *Topical* Superpotent agents not usually effective.

Intralesional Injection Few and small lesions of AA can be treated with intralesional triamcinolone acetonide, 3–7 mg/mL, which can be very effective temporarily.

Systemic Glucocorticoids May induce regrowth, but AA recurs on discontinuation; risks of long-term therapy therefore preclude their use.

Systemic Cyclosporine Induces regrowth, but AA recurs when drug is discontinued.

Induction of Allergic Contact Dermatitis - Dinitrochlorobenzene, squaric acid dibutylester, or diphencyprone reported to be successful, but local discomfort due to allergic contact dermatitis and swelling of regional lymph nodes poses a problem.

Oral PUVA (Photochemotherapy) - Variably effective, as high as 30%, and worth a trial in patients who are highly distressed about the problem. Entire body must be exposed, in that the therapy is believed to be a form of systemic immune suppression.

TELOGEN EFFLUVIUM   ■ ○

- Telogen effluvium (TE) is the transient increased shedding of normal club (telogen) hairs from resting scalp follicles.
- Secondary to accelerated shift of anagen (growth phase) into catagen and telogen (resting phase)

- Results in increased daily hair loss and, if severe, diffuse thinning of scalp hair.

Synonym: Telogen deffluvium

ETIOLOGY AND EPIDEMIOLOGY

Etiology A reaction pattern to a variety of physical or mental stressors:

Endocrine: Hypo- or hyperthyroidism; postpartum; discontinuation or changing type of estrogen containing drugs

Nutritional: Deficiency: biotin, zinc, iron, essential fatty acid

Rapid weight loss, caloric or protein deprivation, chronic iron deficiency, excessive vitamin A ingestion

Physical stress: Febrile illnesses, catabolic illnesses (e.g., malignancy, chronic infection), major surgery, major trauma, acute or chronic psychological stress

Psychological stress: Anxiety, depression, bipolar disorder

Intoxication: Thallium, mercury, arsenic

Drugs: Antimitotic agents (dose dependent): cancer chemotherapy, benzimidazoles.

Antihypertensives: captopril

Anticoagulants

CNS drugs: lithium, valproic acid

Cholesterol-lowering drugs

Colchicine

Cytostatic drugs

Interferon

Penicillamine

Retinoids: vitamin A excess, retinoids (isotretinoin, acitretin, indinavir)

Selective serotonin reuptake inhibitors

Inflammatory scalp disease: Seborrheic dermatitis, erythroderma

Idiopathic: No obvious cause is apparent in a significant number of cases.

Age of Onset Any age.

Sex More common in women due to parturition, cessation of an oral contraceptive, and "crash" dieting.

Incidence Second most common cause of alopecia after androgenetic alopecia.

PATHOGENESIS

- Normal scalp: 80–90% of hairs are in anagen phase, 5% in catagen phase, and 10–15% in telogen phase; 50–100 hairs are shed as they are replaced daily.
- Telogen effluvium: many more hairs than normal are shed daily. The precipitating stimulus results in a premature shift of anagen follicles into the telogen phase. Telogen effluvium occurs in 3–4 months after the inciting event occurred. If the inciting cause is removed, shedding will resolve over the next few months as the number of hairs in telogen return to normal. Hair density may take 6–12 months to return to baseline.
- Can become chronic with decreased hair density, always has potential for reversal, does not lead to total scalp hair loss, and rarely goes beyond 50% loss.
- Chronic telogen effluvium: Persistent shedding after an acute episode suggests other pathology, e.g., early female pattern hair loss and/or thyroid malfunction.

CLINICAL MANIFESTATION

Skin Symptoms

- Patient presents with complaint of increased hair loss on the scalp that may be accompanied by varying degrees of hair thinning.
- Most individuals are anxious, fearing baldness.
- The patient often presents a plastic bag containing shed hair.
- The precipitating event precedes the telogen effluvium by 3 to 4 months.

Skin Lesions No abnormalities of the scalp are detected.

Hair (Fig. 32-12) Diffuse shedding of the scalp hair. Gentle hair pull gathers several to many club or telogen hairs.

Distribution Hair loss occurs diffusely throughout the scalp and includes the sides and back of the head. If hair loss is significant enough to result in thinning of hair, alopecia is noted diffusely throughout the scalp. Short regrowing new hairs are present close to the scalp; these hairs are finer than older hairs and have tapered ends.

Nails The precipitating stimulus for TE may also affect the growth of nails, resulting in Beau lines (see Fig. 33-23), which appear as transverse lines or grooves on the fingernail and toenail plates.

DIFFERENTIAL DIAGNOSIS

Increased Shedding of Scalp Hair ± Nonscarring Alopecia Pattern hair loss, diffuse-pattern alopecia areata, loose anagen syndrome, hyperthyroidism, hypothyroidism, SLE, secondary syphilis, drug-induced alopecia (Table 32-2).

LABORATORY EXAMINATIONS

Hair Pull Compared with the normal hair pull, in which 80–90% of hair is in the anagen phase, telogen effluvium is characterized by a reduced percentage of anagen hairs, varying with the intensity of hair shedding. See "Biology of Hair Growth Cycles" for an explanation of the hair pull.

CBC Rule out iron-deficiency anemia.

Chemistry Serum iron, iron-binding capacity.

TSH Rule out thyroid disease.

Serology ANA, RPR.

Histopathology No abnormality other than an increase in the proportion of follicles in telogen.

DIAGNOSIS

Made on history, clinical findings, hair pull, and possible biopsy, excluding other causes.

COURSE AND PROGNOSIS

Complete regrowth of hair is the rule. In postpartum TE, if hair loss is severe and recurs after successive pregnancies, regrowth may never be complete. TE may continue for up to a year after the precipitating cause.

MANAGEMENT

No intervention is needed or required. The patient should be reassured that the process is part of a normal cycle of hair growth and shedding and that full regrowth of the hair is to be expected in most cases.

FIGURE 32-12 Telogen effluvium A clump of hair in the hand, associated with striking thinning of scalp hair. The patient was HIV-infected and experienced *Pneumocystis carinii* pneumonia 10 weeks previously. Using the fingers as shown, 30 to 40 hairs could be removed with each "hair pull."

■ TABLE 32-2 Drug-Induced Alopecia*

Drugs	Features of Alopecia
ACE inhibitors	
Enalapril	Probable telogen effluvium
Anticoagulants	
Heparin	Few reports
Warfarin	Reported incidence ranges from 19 to 70% but is probably much lower; diffuse shedding with increased number of hairs in telogen phase.
Antimitotic agents	Anagen effluvium
Colchicine	Diffuse hair loss; increased number of telogen hairs
Antineoplastic agents	
Bleomycin, cyclophosphamide, cytarabine, dacarbazine, dactinomycin, daunorubicin, doxorubicin, etoposide, fluorouracil, hydroxyurea, ifosfamide, mechlorethamine, melphalan, methotrexate, mitomycin, mitoxantrone, nitrosourea, procarbazine, thiotepa, vinblastine, vincristine	
Antiparkinsonian agents	
Levodopa	Probable telogen effluvium
Antiseizure agents	
Trimethadione	Probable telogen effluvium
Beta blockers	Probable telogen effluvium
Metoprolol	
Propranolol	
Birth control agents	
Oral contraceptives	Diffuse hiar loss (telogen effluvium) 2 to 3 months after cessation of oral contraceptive
Drugs used in treatment of bipolar disorders	
Lithium	Probable telogen effluvium
Ergot derivatives (used in treatment of prolactinemia)	
Bromocriptine	Probable telogen effluvium
H₂ blockers	
Cimetidine	Onset 1 week to 11 months; probable telogen effluvium
Heavy metals (poisoning)	
Thallium	Diffuse shedding of abnormal anagen hair 10 days after ingestion; complete hair loss in 1 month; characteristic is pronounced hair loss on sides of head, also of lateral eyebrows.
Mercury and lead	Diffuse hair loss with acute and chronic exposure.
Cholesterol-lowering drugs	
Clofibrate	Occasionally associated with hair loss.
Pesticides	
Boric acid	Total scalp alopecia reported after acute intoxication; with chronic exposure hair becomes dry and falls out.
Retinoids	
Etretinate	Increased hair shedding and plucked telogen count; decreased duration of anagen phase.
Isotretinoin	Diffuse loss; probably same mechanism as above.

* Prepared by Suzanne Virnelli-Grevelink, M.D.

ANAGEN EFFLUVIUM ■ ◐

- Etiology: Radiation therapy to head; chemotherapy with alkylating agents; intoxications; protein malnutrition.
- Onset is usually rapid and extensive (Fig. 32-13).
- Pathogenesis: Occurs after any insult to hair follicle that impairs its mitotic/metabolic activity. Rapid growth arrest or damage to anagen hairs that skip catagen and telogen phases and are shed.

- More common and severe with combination chemotherapy than with the use of a single drug. Severity is generally dose dependent.
- Manifestations: *Scalp hair* loss is diffuse, extensive; also: eyebrows/lashes, beard, etc. *Nails* show transverse banding or ridging.
- Regrowth is usually rapid after discontinuation of chemotherapy.

ETIOLOGY

Anagen cycle disrupted causing varying degrees of hair follicle dystrophy:

- *Radiation therapy* to head.
- *Alkylating agents*: busulfan, carboplatin, carmustine, BCNU, chlorambucil, cisplatin, dacarbazine, estramustine, fotemustine, ifosamide, lomustine, mechlorethamine, nitrogen mustard, melphalan, oxaliplatin, procarbazine, streptozocin, temozolomide, thiotepa.
- *Intoxications*: mercury, boric acid, thallium, colchicine.
- Severe protein malnutrition.

PATHOGENESIS

- Occurs after any insult to hair follicle that impairs its mitotic/metabolic activity.
- Inhibition/arrest of cell division in hair matrix leads to thin, weakened hair shaft, susceptible to fracture with minimal trauma as well as complete failure of hair formation.
- Anagen hairs break off within the follicle or at the level of the scalp, being shed without roots, or dystrophic hairs dislodged from follicular moorings.

FIGURE 32-13   Anagen effluvium: chemotherapy   A 47-year-old male with lymphoma treated with chemotherapy. All scalp, facial, and bodily hair have fallen out. Close inspection reveals that scalp hair has begun to regrow.

- Low-dose cytostatic regimens or less cytotoxic drugs such as methotrexate cause telogen effluvium rather than anagen effluvium.
- Hair bulb itself may be damaged, and hairs may separate at the bulb and fall out.
- Rapid growth arrest or damage to anagen hairs that skip catagen and telogen phases and are shed.

CLINICAL MANIFESTATIONS

Skin   Appears normal.
Hair   Scalp hair loss is diffuse, extensive (Figs. 32-13, 32-14). Hair breaks off at the level of the scalp. Eyebrows/lashes, beard, body hair may also be lost.
Nails   Show transverse banding or ridging. Successive rounds of chemotherapy result in parallel transverse band/ridges.

COURSE

- Hair regrows after discontinuation of chemotherapy.
- Busulfan at high dose may cause permanent alopecia due to irreversible damage to hair follicle stem cell.
- Regrowth after radiation depends on type, depth, dose-fractionation; may result in irreversible hair follicle stem cell damage.

MANAGEMENT

No effective preventive measures are available. A wig is preferred by many persons.

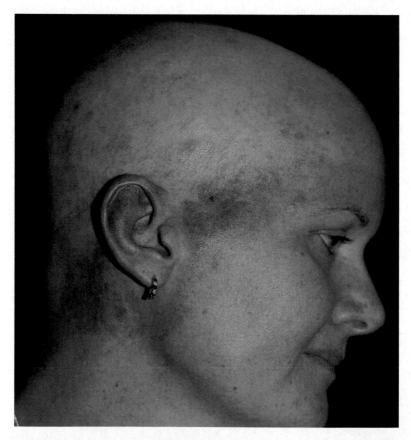

FIGURE 32-14   Anagen effluvium and acute radiation dermatitis: chemotherapy and radiation   A 43-year-old female with metastatic breast carcinoma to the brain. Chemotherapy (paclitaxel, adriamycin, cytoxan) was given with focal radiation to the brain metastasis. Loss of scalp and facial hair was seen. The angulated erythema on the neck, ear, and face demarcate the site of radiation. The patient died 3 months later of metastatic disease.

CICATRICIAL OR SCARRING ALOPECIA ☐ ◑

- Primary cicatricial (scarring) alopecia (PCA) results from damage or destruction of the hair follicles stem cells by:
  - Inflammatory (usually noninfectious) processes
  - Infection: e.g., "kerion" tinea capitis, necrotizing herpes zoster
  - Other pathologic processes: surgical scar, primary or metastatic neoplasm.

- Manifestations: Effacement of follicular orifices in a patchy or focal distribution, usually in scalp or beard.

- The end result is effacement of follicular orifices and replacement of the follicular structure by fibrous tissue (Table 32-3).

- Scarring is irreversible. Therapies are ineffective.

TABLE 32-3 Classification of Primary Cicatricial Alopecias

Lymphocytic	Chronical cutaneous (discoid) lupus erythematosus
	Lichen planopilaris (LPP)
	Classic LPP
	Frontal fibrosing alopecia
	Graham-Little syndrome
	Classic pseudopelade of Brocq
	Central centrifugal cicatricial alopecia
	Alopecia mucinosa
	Kertosis folliclaris spinulosa decalvans
Neutrophilic	Folliculitis decalvans
	Dissecting folliculitis (cellulitis)
Mixed	Folliculitis keloidalis
	Folliculitis necrotica
	Erosive pustular dermatosis
Nonspecific	

Chronic Cutaneous (Discoid) Lupus Erythematosus (CCLE) See Section 14.

- May occur without other manifestations or serologic evidence of lupus erythematosus (LE).
- Manifestations:
  - CCLE: Erythematous plaques (Figs. 32-15, 32-16, 32-17). Keratotic with follicular plugs ("carpet tacks"). Scattered. Variable in number. May become confluent. Atrophy in older patients with scarring alopecia. Postinflammatory hypopigmentation, and/or follicular plugging (Fig. 32-17).
  - SLE: diffuse scalp erythema with diffuse hair thinning (Fig. 32-16).
  - Tumid LE: violaceous dermal inflammatory plaque with overlying hair loss.

- Dermatopathology: See lupus erythermatosus, Section 14.

Lichen Planopilaris (LPP) See Lichen Planus, Section 7.

- Follicular lichen planus (LP) is associated with cicatricial scalp alopecia, resulting in permanent hair loss (Fig. 32-18).
- LPP may be or may not be associated with LP of skin or mucosa.
- Most commonly affects middle-aged women.
- Manifestations in scalp: Perifollicular erythema ± hyperkeratosis. Violaceous discoloration of scalp. Prolonged inflammation results in scarring alopecia. In some cases, follicular inflammation and scale are absent, with only areas of scarring alopecia, so-called footprints in the snow, or pseudopelade. Distribution: most common on parietal scalp; also affects other hair-bearing sites such as groin, axilla.

- Symptoms: scalp pain.
- Variants:
  - *Graham-Little syndrome*: LP-like lesions + follicular "spines"/keratosis pilaris–like lesions in areas of alopecia on scalp, eyebrows, axillary, pubic areas.
  - *Frontal fibrosing alopecia*: Frontotemporal hairline recession and eyebrow loss in postmenopausal women with perifollicular erythema (Fig. 32-19); histology shows LPP.
  - *Perifollicular erythema and follicular keratosis*: progressive scarring alopecia limited to area of pattern hair loss; overlaps with frontal fibrosing alopecia.

Pseudopelade of Brocq

- Endstage of all noninflammatory scarring alopecias and a variety of initially inflammatory disorders.

- *Pelade* is another term for alopecia areata. Pelage is the coat (hair) of an animal. Pseudopelade suggests that the clinical findings resemble those of alopecia areata.
- Manifestations:
  - Early lesions: Discrete, smooth, skin- or pink-colored irregularly shaped areas of alopecia without follicular hyperkeratosis or perifollicular inflammation (Figs. 32-19 and 32-20).
  - Pattern of alopecia: Early moth-eaten pattern with eventual coalescence into larger patches of hair loss ("footprints-in-the-snow").

- Dermatopathology: Similar to lichen planopilaris.
- Scarring alopecia is irreversible.

FIGURE 32-15   Scarring alopecia of scalp: chronic cutaneous lupus erythematosus (CCLE)   A 41-year-old white male with multiple red discoid keratotic patches on the scalp for one year. A red scaling lesion with scarring alopecia is seen on the frontal scalp. The inflammatory lesions resolved with intralesional triamcinolone and hydroxychloroquine 200 mg BID but there was no regrowth of hair.

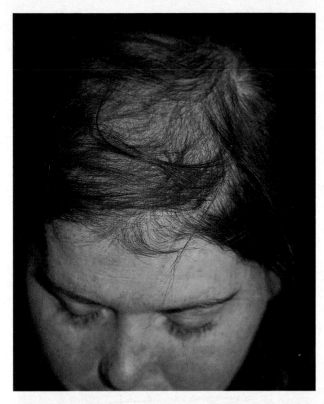

FIGURE 32-16 Diffuse and scarring alopecia of scalp: Systemic LE (SLE) and CCLE lesions A 36-year-old female with poorly controlled SLE for 3 years. Diffuse scalp alopecia is seen associated discrete discoid lesions with scarring alopecia. She has history of photosensitivity.

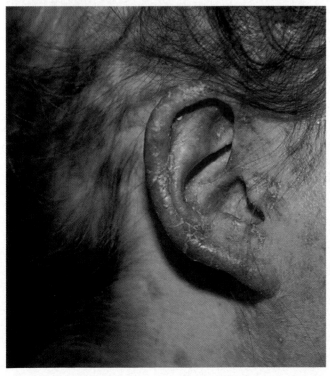

FIGURE 32-17 This is the same patient as Fig. 32-16. She has erythema of the ears and red areas of scarring alopecia on scalp.

Central Centrifugal Scarring Alopecia (CCSA)

- *Synonyms*: follicular degeneration syndrome, hot comb alopecia, pseudopelade.
- Most commonly occurs in black women. Relation to chemical processing, heat, or chronic tension on the hair is uncertain, but they are best avoided.
- Slowly progressive alopecia begins in the crown/midvertex and advances centrifugally to surrounding areas.
- Dermatopathology: Earliest most distinctive change is premature desquamation of the inner root sheath with later changes through the outer root sheath (including migration of the hair shaft), a mononuclear infiltrate primarily at the isthmus, and, finally, loss of the follicular epithelium and replacement with fibrous tissue.
- Scarring alopecia is irreversible.

Alopecia Mucinosa (Follicular Mucinosis)

- Erythematous lesions (papules, plaques, or flat patches) of alopecia, occurring mainly on scalp and/or face.

- Dermatopathology: prominent follicular, epithelial/sebaceous gland mucin, perifollicular lymphohistiocytic infiltrate without concentric lamellar fibrosis.
- May be symptom of cutaneous T cell lymphoma. (See Section 20).

Folliculitis Decalvans

- Pustular folliculitis leading to hair loss. Surviving hairs clustered, emerging from a single follicular orifice (tufted folliculitis).
- Bogginess or induration of scalp/beard with pustules, erosions, crusts (Fig. 32-21), scale.
- *Staphylococcus aureus* infection common. Whether *S. aureus* infection is the primary process or secondary is uncertain.
- Dermatopathology: acute suppurative folliculitis, early.
- Scarring alopecia is irreversible. Systemic antibiotics, rifampin, systemic and/or topical and/or intralesional glucocorticoids, and systemic retinoid have been used. *S. aureus* infection should be documented and treated with appropriate antimicrobial agent.

FIGURE 32-18   Scarring alopecia of scalp: pseudopelade of Brocq caused by lichen planus   A 66-year-old female. The scalp is smooth, shiny, devoid of hair and hair follicles in many areas; some of the remaining follicles are inflamed with perifollicular erythema and scale. Several hairs are seen emerging from a single site within the area of alopecia (arrows). The term pseudopelade implies that the lesions resemble alopecia areata.

FIGURE 32-19 Scarring alopecia of scalp: lichen planopilaris (LPP)   A 68-year-old white female with hair loss for 15 years. The frontal hairline has gradually receded; the area of alopecia lacks the pigmentation of forehead skin, which has had lifelong sun exposure. Both eyebrows have no hair; the eyebrow on the right is penciled in. The eyelashes appear normal. Biopsy was reported to show lichen planus with scarring alopecia. No other clinical findings of LP were detected. This clinical variant of LPP is called frontal fibrosing alopecia.

FIGURE 32-20 Scarring alopecia of scalp: pseudopelade of Brocq   A 38-year-old black male with progressive hair loss for 4 years. Extensive scarring alopecia with residual islands of hair follicles and hair on the vertex. Note the absence of erythema, scale, or crust.

Dissecting Folliculitis

- *Synonyms*: dissecting cellulitis, perifolliculitis abscedens et suffodiens.
- Race: most common in black men.
- Initial deep inflammatory nodules, primarily over the occiput, that progress to coalescing regions of boggy scalp (Fig. 32-22). Sinus tracts may form; purulent exudates can be expressed. *S. aureus* secondary infection common.
- Dermatopathology: early follicular plugging and suppurative follicular/perifollicular abscesses with mixed inflammatory infiltrate; later, foreign-body giant cells, granulation tissue, scarring with sinus tracts.
- Scarring alopecia is irreversible. *S. aureus* infection should be documented and treated with appropriate antimicrobial agent.

Follicultis Keloidalis Nuchae

- *Synonym*: acne keloidalis (nuchae).
- Occurs most commonly in black men.
- Usually occurs on the occipital scalp and nape of the neck, starting with a chronic papular or pustular eruption (Fig. 32-23). Results in

a spectrum of severity from small fibrotic papules to hypertrophic keloidal scar formation.
- Distribution: nape of the neck, occipital scalp.
- Early mild involvement may respond to intralesional triamcinolone. If *S. aureus* is isolated on culture, treat with appropriate antimicrobial agent.

Pseudofolliculitis Barbae

- *Synonym*: "razor bumps."
- Variant or same disease as folliculitis keloidalis.
- Occurs commonly in black males who shave.
- Related to curved hair follicles. Cut hair retracts beneath skin surface, grows, and penetrates follicular wall (transfollicular type) or surrounding skin (extrafollicular type), causing a foreign-body reaction.
- Distribution: any shaved area, i.e., beard (Fig. 32-24), scalp, pubic.
- Keloidal scarring in varying degrees occurs at involved sites.
- *S. aureus* secondary infection is common.

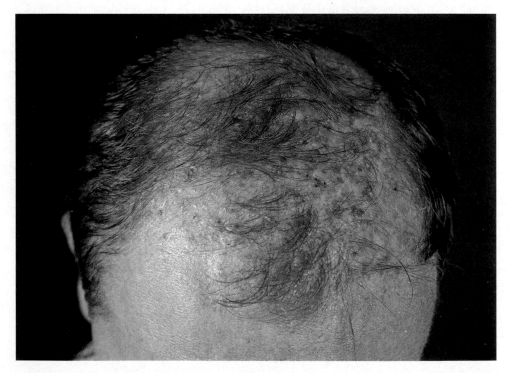

FIGURE 32-21   Scarring alopecia of scalp: folliculitis decalvans   A 50-year-old white male with hair loss for 6 years. Erythema, inflammatory papules, crusts, and scarring of the scalp. Male pattern hair loss is also present.

FIGURE 32-22 Scarring alopecia of scalp: dissecting folliculitis A 46-year-old black female with longstanding abscess formation of the scalp has resulted in very severe hypertrophic scarring. There was associated cystic acne and hidradenitis suppurativa.

FIGURE 32-23 Scarring alopecia of scalp: folliculitis keloidalis A 31-year-old black male with papular scars of 3 years' duration, becoming confluent on the occipital scalp and neck. Follicular pustules occur in the area. The condition is chronic and progressive, resulting in significant hair loss.

- Has been linked to a polymorphism of the keratin gene *KGhf*.

Acne Necrotica

- Pruritic or painful erythematous follicular-based papule with central necrosis, crusting, and healing with depressed scar.
- Lesions occur on anterior scalp, forehead, nose; at times, the trunk.
- Dermatopathology: lymphocytic necrotizing folliculitis.
- Poor response to treatment. Systemic antimicrobial agents and isotretinoin reported to be effective.

Erosive Pustular Dermatosis of Scalp

- A disease of the elderly, mainly women, although pediatric cases do occur.
- Manifestations: chronic boggy crusted plaque(s) on the scalp overlying exudative erosions and pustules, eventually leading to scarring alopecia.
- May follow trauma or treatment of actinic keratoses.

- Dermatopathology: lymphoplasmacytic infiltrate with or without foreign-body giant cells and pilosebaceous atrophy.
- Poor response to therapy. Treat documented *S. aureus* infection.

LABORATORY EXAMINATION

Scalp Biopsy   4-mm punch biopsy including subcutaneous tissue, prepared for horizontal section. A second 4-mm punch biopsy specimen for vertical sections and direct immunofluorescence.

MANAGEMENT

Glucocorticoids   Topical high-potency and intralesional glucocorticoids (e.g., triamcinolone) are the mainstay of treatment, improving symptoms and hair growth.

Antibiotics   May be effective, especially if *S. aureus* infection is documented.

FIGURE 32-24   Pseudofolliculitis barbae   A 29-year-old black male with multiple follicular papular scars in the beard; the presence of follicular pustules usually indicates secondary *Staphylococcus aureus* folliculitis. Folliculitis keloidalis is often seen on the occipital scalp and neck (see Fig. 32-23).

EXCESS HAIR GROWTH ICD-9 : 704.1 ○ ICD-10 : L68

■ Excess hair growth occurs in two patterns.
  • *Hirsutism*: occurs in women at sites where hair is under androgen control.

• *Hypertrichosis*: hair density or length beyond accepted limits of normal for age, race, sex (generalized, localized; lanugo, vellus, terminal hair).

HIRSUTISM   ■ ○

■ Excessive hair growth (women) in androgen-dependent hair patterns, secondary to increased androgenic activity.

■ Normally only postpubescent males have terminal hair in these sites.

Synonym: Unwanted hair.

ETIOLOGY AND EPIDEMIOLOGY

Definition Excessive hair growth (women) in androgen-dependent hair patterns, secondary to increased androgenic activity. However, varies with cultural and racial factors. Media heightens awareness of bodily hair, either sparse or excess. The concern of the patient might be manifestation of body dysmorphic syndrome.
Etiology See Table 32-4.
Risk Factors Familial, ethnic, and racial influences. Hirsuteness: white > black > Asian.
Prevalence in United States Survey of college-aged women: 25% had easily noticeable facial hair; 33% had hair along linea alba below umbilicus; 17% had periareolar hair. Series of

100 patients: 15% idiopathic, 3% late-onset congenital adrenal hyperplasia (CAH) (varies within ethnic group).

PATHOGENESIS

• Androgens promote conversion of vellus to terminal hairs in androgen-sensitive hair follicles: beard area, face, chest, areolae, linea alba, lower back, buttocks, abdomen, external genitalia, inner thighs.
• Dihydrotestosterone, derived from conversion of testosterone by 5α-R at the hair follicle, is the hormonal stimulus for hair growth. 50–70% of circulating testosterone in normal

---

TABLE 32-4   Etiology of Hirsutism

Androgen-secreting tumors Usually associated with irregular menses/amenorrhea.

Adrenal	Ovarian
Adenoma	Gonadal stromal tumor
Adenocarcinoma	Thecoma
Ectopic ACTH-secreting tumor	Lipoid tumor

Functional androgen excess

Adrenal enzyme deficiencies (congenital adrenal hyperplasia)	Cushing syndrome
Early onset 21-hydroxylase deficiency	Polycystic ovarian disease
Late onset 21-hydroxylase deficiency	With and without adrenal contribution
11β-hydroxylase deficiency	Hyperthecosis
3β-dehydroxylase deficiency	

"Idiopathic" hirsutism
Medication/drug-induced

women is derived from precursors, androstenedione, and DHEA; the rest is secreted directly, mostly by the ovaries. In hyperandrogenic women, a greater percentage of androgens may be secreted directly.

- In women, adrenal glands secrete androstenedione, DHEA, DHEA sulfate, and testosterone; ovaries secrete mainly androstenedione and testosterone.

CLINICAL MANIFESTATION

History

- Family history
- Drug history
- Virilization symptoms: female pattern hair loss to male pattern balding, acne, deepened voice, increased muscle mass, clitoromegaly, increased libido, personality change. Relatively recent or rapid onset of symptoms and signs *not* associated with puberty.
- Other: Amenorrhea or changes in menstruation. New-onset hypertension.

Skin Findings   Note: acne, acanthosis nigricans, striae.
Hirsutism: (1) Note amount of excess hair, (2) note all sites of hair, (3) evaluate progression and therapy.

- New growth of terminal hair (Fig. 32-25), especially on the face (Fig. 32-25A) chest (Fig. 32-25B), abdomen, upper back, shoulders.
- *Ferriman-Gallwey scale* rates hair growth in each of 11 androgen-sensitive areas (upper lip, chin, chest, upper back, lower back, upper abdomen, lower abdomen, arm, forearm, thigh, leg) from 0 (no hair growth) to 4. Score of ≥ 8 is considered hirsutism.

Cushing Syndrome   Centripetal obesity, muscle wasting (especially peripheral muscle weakness), violaceous striae.
Pelvic Examination   If polycystic ovary (PCO) syndrome is suspected.

LABORATORY EVALUATION OF HIRSUTISM

Serum Testosterone   If >200 ng/mL, exclude androgen-secreting tumor.

Serum Free Testosterone and Dehydroepiandrosterone   More sensitive; most women with moderately elevated androgen levels have polycystic ovarian syndrome.
17-Hydroxyprogesterone   Raised level suggests congenital adrenal hyperplasia; confirm diagnosis by repeat measurement after ACTH stimulation.
Serum Prolactin   Hyperprolactinemia due to macro- or microprolactinoma or treatment with neuroleptic drugs; may have associated menstrual abnormalities, infertility, or galactorrhea.
Urinary 17-Ketosteroid   Helpful in evaluating the overall amount of androgen secretion. Results checked against age-appropriate normal levels; peak levels occur at 30 years (significant decline with age thereafter).
Oligomenorrhea/Amenorrhea   Prolactin, follicle-stimulating hormone (FSH), total testosterone.
Virilization   *Serum testosterone*: 200 ng/dL in women with ovarian or adrenal tumor. *Urinary 17-ketosteroids*: elevated adrenal androgens. *Serum DHEA sulfate*: most specific to adrenals (>90% arising in adrenals); if >800 μg/d, suggestive of adrenal tumor.

MANAGEMENT

Cosmetic Treatment   Bleaching: hydrogen peroxide. Temporary removal: Shaving, waxing, chemical (Nair). Eflornithine (Vaniqua) cream. LASER epilation. Electrolysis.
Weight Loss   May be helpful in obese patients; obesity increases free testosterone levels by reducing sex hormone–biding hormone and contributes to insulin resistance.
Endocrinology Consultation   For suspected late-onset CAH, Cushing syndrome, tumor.
Systemic Antiandrogen Therapy   *Oral Antiandrogens*   Spironolactone (100–200 mg daily). Cyproterone acetate. Finasteride.
Oral Contraceptives   Inhibit androgen synthesis by inhibiting output of gonadotropins; most effective if combined with antiandrogens.
Bromocriptine   For treatment of prolactinoma.

FIGURE 32-25 Hirsutism: face and chest A 31-year-old female with hirsutism. **A.** Increased hair growth in androgen-dependent hair follicles of the sideburn area, associated with androgen excess. **B.** Increased hair growth in androgen-dependent hair follicles of the presternal and periareolar regions.

HYPERTRICHOSIS   □ ◑

- Hypertrichosis is excessive hair growth (density, length) beyond accepted limits of normal for age, race, sex in areas that are not androgen-sensitive (Fig. 32-26).

- May be generalized/universal or localized.
- May consist of lanugo, vellus, or terminal hair.

ETIOLOGY (See Table 32-5)

CLINICAL MANIFESTATION

Localized Hypertrichosis Trauma/scar/occupation-related sites of irritation. Drug-induced: topical minoxidil. Becker nevus.
Acquired Hypertrichosis Lanuginosa Production of lanugo (wasp) hair in follicles previously producing vellus hair ("malignant down"). Hair may be >10 cm in length in non-scalp areas. Can involve entire body, except for palms and soles. Fine, downy hair covers large areas of the body. In mild types, downy hair is limited to the face; hair on previously hairless areas such as the nose and eyelids is usually noticed first. Scalp, beard, and pubic hair may not be replaced.
Universal Hypertrichosis (Fig. 32-26)   Increase of lanugo, vellus, or terminal hair.

MANAGEMENT

- Find and remove the inciting cause.
- Similar to "Cosmetic Treatment" of hirsutism (see above).

TABLE 32-5   Etiology of Hypertrichosis

Universal hypertrichosis
  Congenital/hereditary generalized hypertrichosis
  Acquired generalized hypertrichosis
    Acquired hypertrichosis lanuginosa (malignancy): Usually harbinger of malignancy; of all cases of reported, 98% had malignancy of the GI tract, bronchus, breast, gallbladder, uterus, bladder; can precede neoplastic diagnosis by several years.
    Drug-induced: minoxidil (80% of those treated), diazoxide (50%), phenytoin (occurs after 2–3 months of treatment), cyclosporine (80%), PUVA, oral glucocorticoids, streptomycin, acetazolamide, oxaliazolopyrimidine, fenoterol, penicillamine
    Porphyria: porphyria cutanea tarda, hepatoerythropoietic porphyria, variegate porphyria, erythropoietic porphyria
    POEMS syndrome
    Juvenile dermatomyositis
    Hypothyroidism
    Acrodynia
    Malabsorption syndromes
    CNS-related problems of trauma: postencephalitis, multiple sclerosis, schizophrenia, head injury, hyperostosis interna, anorexia nervosa
Localized hypertrichosis
  Secondary to irritation, trauma, etc.
  Drug-induced: interferon, topical minoxidil, topical latanoprost

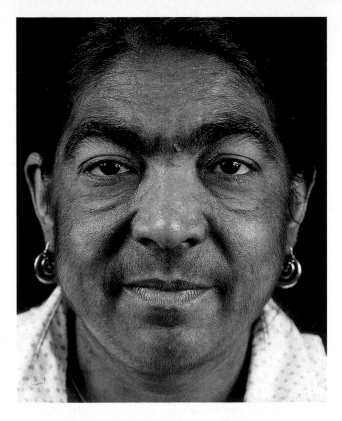

FIGURE 32-26 Hypertrichosis of face Excessive hair growth in nonandrogen-sensitive areas of the face in a female treated with cyclosporine.

INFECTIOUS FOLLICULITIS ICD-9:704.8 ○ ICD-10:L73.8

- Infectious folliculitis begins in the upper portion of the hair follicle
- Etiologic agents: Bacteria, fungi, virus, mites
- Manifestations: Follicular papule, pustule, erosion, or crust at the follicular infundibulum
- Infection can extend deeper into the entire length of the follicle (sycosis).

ETIOLOGY AND EPIDEMIOLOGY

Etiology See Table 32-6.
Predisposing Factors

- Shaving hairy regions such as the beard area, axillae, or legs facilitates follicular infection. Extraction of hair such as plucking or waxing.
- Occlusion of hair-bearing areas facilitates growth of microbes: clothing, plastic film, adhesive plaster, position (sitting occludes buttocks, lying in bed occludes back), prosthesis, natural occlusion in intertriginous sites (axillae, inframammary, anogenital). Topical climate with high temperature and relative humidity.
- Topical glucocorticoid preparations.
- Systemic antibiotic promotes growth of gram-negative bacteria; diabetes mellitus; immunosuppression.

TABLE 32-6   Classification of Infectious Folliculitis by Etiology

Infectious Agent	Organism
Bacterial	*S. aureus*: superficial (Bockhart impetigo); deep (sycosis); may progress to furuncle (boil) or carbuncle formation
	Pseudomonas aeruginosa (hot-tub) folliculitis; gram-negative folliculitis
Fungal	Dermatophytic folliculitis: tinea capitis, tinea barbae, Majocchi granuloma; *Malassezia* folliculitis; *Candida* folliculitis
Viral	Herpes simplex virus; Varicella-zoster virus; Molluscum contagiosum;
Syphilitic	Secondary syphilis: alopecia, acneiform
Infestation	Demodicidosis

CLINICAL MANIFESTATION

Symptoms   *S. aureus* and dermatophytic folliculitis can be chronic. Usually nontender or slightly tender; may be pruritic. Uncommonly, tender regional lymphadenitis.

Skin Lesions

• Papule or pustule confined to the ostium of the hair follicle, at times surrounded by an erythematous halo (Figs. 32-27, 32-28). Rupture of pustule leads to superficial erosions or crusts. Scattered discrete or more frequently grouped and clustered.
• Usually, only a small percentage of follicles in a region is infected.

• Superficial infection heals without scarring, but in darkly pigmented individuals, postinflammatory hypo- and hyperpigmentation.
• Extension of infection can progress to abscess or furuncle formation (Fig. 32-29).

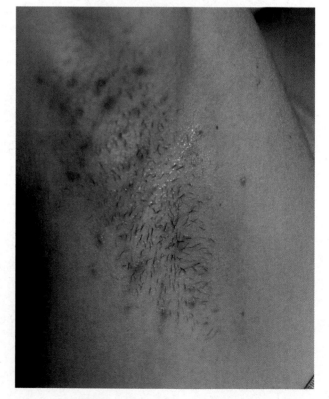

FIGURE 32-27   Infectious folliculitis, superficial in axilla: MRSA
A 25-year-old female with pruritic and tender axillary lesions for several weeks. Multiple follicular pustules and papules are seen in the vault of the shaved axilla. Shaving facilitates entry of *S. aureus* into the superficial hair follicle. The lesions resolved with minocycline.

FIGURE 32-28   Infectious folliculitis on forearm   A 44-year-old male with HIV/AIDS has had a pruritic and tender site on the forearm for several months. On examination, numerous pustules and papules are seen with mild lichen simplex chronicus. The lesions resolved with minocycline.

FIGURE 32-29   Infectious folliculitis on buttocks, deep   A 29-year-old male, with HIV/AIDS and endstage renal disease (ESRD), being treated with peritoneal dialysis has had persistent painful lesions on the buttocks for several months. Pustules and early furuncles are seen on the buttocks and perineal area.

- In chronic folliculitis, a full range of lesions is noted.
- Pseudofolliculitis barbae caused by penetration of the skin by sharp tips of shaved hairs frequently complicated by *S. aureus* secondary infection (see Fig. 32-24).

Distribution *Face* *S. aureus.* Gram-negative folliculitis: resembles or may coexist with acne vulgaris. Molluscum contagiosum. Demodicidosis resembles rosacea.
Beard Area *S. aureus* folliculitis: folliculitis (sycosis) barbae, most commonly of shaved beard area Dermatophytic folliculitis: tinea barbae; papulopustules may coalesce to deeply infiltrated kerion. Herpes simplex virus. Molluscum contagiosum. Demodicidosis resembles rosacea.
Scalp *S. aureus.* Dermatophytic.
Neck *S. aureus* in shaved area and nape of neck, occipital scalp, especially in diabetics. Pseudofolliculitis in shaved area. Keloidal folliculitis in nape of neck; follicular keloids to large nodular–tumorous keloidal masses. (see page 986)
Legs Occurs in women who shave legs. In India, a chronic folliculitis occurs in young men, lasting for years. Pustular dermatitis atrophicans of the legs reported commonly from West Africa, usually affecting the shins, sometimes the thighs and forearms.
Trunk *S. aureus* in axillae, especially in those who shave. *Pseudomonas aeruginosa* ("hot tub") folliculitis (Fig. 32-30). *Malassezia* folliculitis. *Candida* folliculitis on the back of hospitalized patients with fever who lie in supine position.
Buttocks Common site for *S. aureus* folliculitis. Dermatophytic.

Variants
S. aureus Folliculitis Can be either superficial folliculitis (infundibular) (Fig. 32-27) or deep (sycosis) (extension beneath infundibulum) with abscess formation (Figs. 32-28, 32-29). In the shaved beard area, also known as sycosis vulgaris, or barber's itch. In severe cases (lupoid sycosis), the pilosebaceous units may be destroyed and replaced by fibrous scar tissue.

Gram-Negative Folliculitis Occurs in individuals with acne vulgaris treated with oral antibiotics. "Acne" typically worsens, having been in good control. Characterized by small follicular pustules and/or larger abscesses on the cheeks.
Hot Tub Folliculitis Occurs on the trunk following immersion in spa water (Fig. 32-30).
Dermatophytic Folliculitis Infection begins in the perifollicular stratum corneum and spreads into follicular ostia and hair shafts (see Section 25). (Fig. 32-31)
Tinea Capitis   (see Section 25)

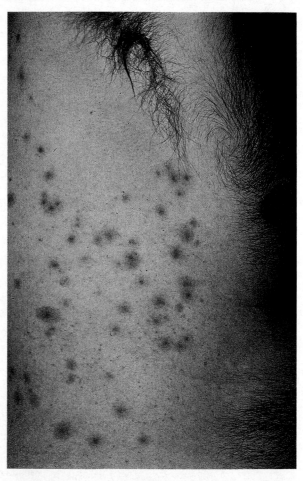

FIGURE 32-30   Infectious folliculitis ("hot tub"): *P. aeruginosa*   A 31-year-old male with painful lesions on the trunk. Multiple follicular pustules are seen, having appeared 3 days after bathing in a hot tub. *P. aeruginosa* was isolated on culture from a lesion. The lesions resolved spontaneously within a week. If symptomatic, ciprofloxacin 500 mg BID can be given.

FIGURE 32-31 Dermatophytic folliculitis: *Trichophyton rubrum* A 32-year-old male with HIV/AIDS had a pruritic rash on the buttocks for one year; topical glucocorticoids and antifungal agents had not been effective. Multiple follicular papules and scaling erythema are seen on the sacral area; tinea cruris and pedis were also present. KOH preparation showed septated hyphae. The lesions resolved with oral terbinafine.

In dermatophytic Majocchi granuloma, scattered papules, pustules and nodules, usually associated with tinea cruris or tinea corporis.

Malassezia Folliculitis More common in subtropical and tropical climates. Pruritic, monomorphic eruption characterized by follicular papules and pustules on the trunk, most often on the back (Fig. 32-32), upper arms, and less often on the neck and face; excoriated papules. Absence of comedones differentiates it from acne vulgaris (see Section 25). *Synonym*: Pityrosporum folliculitis.

Candida albicans Occurs in sites of occluded skin such as the back of a hospitalized febrile patient or under plastic dressing, especially if topical glucocorticoid preparations are used. Large follicular pustules (see Section 25).

Herpetic Folliculitis Occurs predominantly in the beard area (viral sycosis) in men. Characterized by follicular vesicles and later crusts (Fig. 32-33).

Molluscum Folliculitis Presents as umbilicated skin-colored papules in a follicular and perifollicular distribution over the beard area.

Syphilitic (Luetic) Folliculitis: Secondary Nonscarring alopecia of the scalp and beard (alopecia areolaris); "moth-eaten" appearance. *Synonym*: Alopecia syphilitica.

Demodicidosis Clinical presentation: perifollicular scaling (pityriasis folliculorum or rosacea-like erythematous follicular papules and pustules with a background of erythema on the face. Etiology: *Demodex folliculorum*.

DIFFERENTIAL DIAGNOSIS

Follicular Inflammatory Disorders Acneiform disorders (acne vulgaris, rosacea, perioral dermatitis), HIV-associated eosinophilic folliculitis, chemical irritants (chloracne), acneiform adverse cutaneous drug reactions [epidermal growth factor receptor inhibitors (e.g., erlotinib), halogens, glucocorticoids, lithium], keloidal folliculitis, pseudofolliculitis barbae.

Regional Differential Diagnosis *Face*: acne, rosacea, perioral dermatitis, keratosis pilaris, pseudofolliculitis barbae (ingrowing hairs). *Scalp*: folliculitis necrotica. *Trunk*: acne vulgaris, pustular miliaria, transient acantholytic disease (Grover disease). *Axillae and groins*: hidradenitis suppurativa.

LABORATORY FINDINGS

Direct Microscopy *Gram Stain* S. *aureus:* gram-positive cocci. Also visualizes fungi.
KOH Preparation Dermatophytes: hyphae, spores. *M. furfur:* multiple yeast forms; *Candida:* mycelial forms.
Culture *Bacterial* S. *aureus, P. aeruginosa;* gram-negative folliculitis: *Proteus, Klebsiella, Escherichia coli.* In cases of chronic relapsing folliculitis, culture nares and perianal region for S. *aureus* carriage.
Fungal Dermatophytes; *C. albicans.*
Viral Herpes simplex virus (HSV).
Dermatopathology The following features should be evaluated: Are microorganisms present? Is the inflammatory infiltrate predominantly follicular or perifollicular? What region of the pilosebaceous structure is involved? Is the inflammatory process acute suppurative (neutrophilic), chronic lymphocytic, or granulomatous (foreign-body response to keratin subsequent to rupture of follicle)? Is any portion of the pilosebaceous structure destroyed?

DIAGNOSIS

Clinical findings confirmed by laboratory findings.

COURSE AND PROGNOSIS

- S. *aureus* folliculitis can progress to deeper follicular and perifollicular infection with abscess (furuncle, carbuncle) or cellulitis.

- Infection of multiple contiguous follicles results in a carbuncle.
- Many types of infectious folliculitis tend to recur or become chronic unless the predisposing conditions are corrected.

MANAGEMENT

Prophylaxis *Correct underlying predisposing condition.* Washing with antibacterial soap or benzoyl peroxide preparation or isopropyl/ethanol gel.
Antimicrobial Therapy *Bacterial Folliculitis* See Table 24-2.
Gram-negative Folliculitis Associated with systemic antibiotic therapy of acne vulgaris. Discontinue current antibiotics. Wash with benzoyl peroxide. In some cases, ampicillin (250 mg four times daily) or trimethoprim-sulfamethoxazole four times daily. Isotretinoin.
Fungal Folliculitis Various topical antifungal agents. For dermatophytic folliculitis: terbinafine, 250 mg PO for 14 days, or itraconazole, 100 mg twice daily for 14 days. For *Candida* folliculitis: fluconazole or itraconazole, 100 mg twice daily for 14 days.
Herpetic Folliculitis See "Herpes Simplex Virus Infections" (Section 27).
Demodicidosis Permethrin cream. Ivermectin, 200 μg/kg (usual range, 12–18 mg) stat.
Pseudofolliculitis Barbae Rule out secondary S. *aureus* infection. Discontinue shaving. Use beard clipper instead of safety razor. Destruction of hair follicle: electrolysis; laser hair removal.

FIGURE 32-32   Infectious folliculitis: *Malassezia furfur*   A 41-year-old Hispanic male with trunkal rash for 2 months. Multiple, discrete, follicular papulopustules on the chest. Lesional biopsy showed yeast forms of *Malassezia furfur*. The lesions resolved after treatment with oral itraconazole.

FIGURE 32-33   Infectious folliculitis: herpes simplex virus   A 40-year-old healthy male with discrete and grouped pustules and erosions in the beard area for 3 weeks. HSV was isolated on culture. No pathogens were isolated on bacterial culture. Lesions resolved with oral acyclovir.

DISORDERS OF THE NAIL APPARATUS

- The nail apparatus is made up of:
  - Nail plate, the horny "dead" product
  - Four specialized epithelia: proximal nail fold; nail matrix; nail bed; hyponychium
- Fingernails add function to multiple uses of the hands, protect the terminal digits; add to esthetics of the fingers.

- Toenails protect the distal toes and contribute to pedal biomechanics.
- Nail apparatus disorders can be traumatic, structural, primary, manifestations of cutaneous disease (e.g., psoriasis), neoplastic, infectious, or manifestations of systemic diseases (e.g., lupus erythematosus).

COMPONENTS OF THE NORMAL NAIL APPARATUS (See Image 33-1)

Nail Plate   The hard protective tool, the product of the nail apparatus. Rests on and is firmly attached to nail bed, which is attached to underlying bone. Surrounded on three sides by nail folds. Made of three horizontal layers: thin dorsal lamina, thicker intermediate lamina, ventral layer from nail bed. Hardness of nail plate due to high sulfur matrix protein. Nail plate shape relates to shape of underlying phalangeal bone. Longitudinal ridging increases with aging.

Proximal Nail Fold (PNF)   Covers proximal one-quarter of the nail plate. Has two epithelial surfaces, dorsal and ventral.

Dorsal PNF   Similar to skin; thinner; devoid of pilosebaceous units. Devoid of dermatoglyphic markings.

Ventral PNF   Covers ¾ of nail plate. Closely adherent to nail plate surface; keratinizes with a granular layer.

Dermis of PNF   Contains numerous capillaries that run parallel to skin surface. Can be visualized with dermoscope: permits observation of arterial and venous limbs of capillaries, which are arranged in parallel rows and appear as fine regular loops with a small space between afferent and efferent vessels. Morphology altered in collagen vascular disease.

Cuticle   Junction of two epithelial surfaces of PNF, projects distally onto nail surface, sealing PNF and nail. Protects structures at base of nail

(germinative matrix) from irritants, allergens, bacterial/fungal pathogens. Loss of cuticle produces potential space or pocket: inflammation of this pocket results in chronic paronychia.

Lateral Folds   Usually cover lateral edges of plate.

Lunula   Underlies proximal fold. Normally is white. Represents most distal region of the matrix.

Free Margin   Distal nail. Natural shape same as contour of distal lunula.

Nail Matrix   Proximal matrix underlies nail plate to distal border of lunula. Distal matrix is that portion distal to distal border of lunula. Produces the major part of nail plate. As in epidermis, possesses a dividing basal cell layer producing keratinocytes, which differentiate, harden, die, and contribute to nail plate—analogous to epidermal stratum corneum. Keratinocytes mature and keratinize without keratohyalin (granular layer) formation. Melanocytes are present in lower layers and produce melanin. Linear longitudinal pigmented bands may be seen in persons of darker skin phototypes.

Nail Bed   Consists of epidermal part (ventral matrix) (no more than two to three cells thick) and underlying dermis closely apposed to periosteum of distal phalanx. Within connective tissue network lie blood vessels, lymphatics, a fine network of elastic fibers, and scattered fat cells. Subcutaneous fat layer is absent. Normally pink due to vasculature as seen through the translucent nail plate.

Onychocorneal Band Thin distal transverse white band, which marks the most distal portion of attachment of the nail plate to nail bed. Disruption causes onycholysis.

Onychodermal Band Area from onychocorneal band to nail plate free edge.

Hyponychium Space under free margin of nail plate, from point of separation of nail plate from nail bed to the distal end of the nail plate. Extension of hyponychium proximally is onycholysis.

GLOSSARY OF ABNORMALITIES OF THE NAIL APPARATUS

Beau Lines Transverse depression in nail plate. Single nail involvement is usually traumatic. Multiple nail involvement indicates systemic cause. Etiology: Trauma (manicure, onychotillomania); dermatologic disease (eczema, erythroderma, paronychia); systemic disorders (drugs, pyrexia, viral infection (hand-foot-and-mouth disease, measles); Kawasaki syndrome; peripheral ischemia.

Onychomadesis Periodic separation of the proximal portions of the nail plate from the matrix and bed with subsequent shedding of the nails. Single nail: usually traumatic. Multiple nails: systemic cause. *Etiology*: same as Beau lines.

Koilonychia Spoon nails; thinned concave nails. Physiologic in children; in adults, most commonly occupational or iron deficiency.

True Leukonychia White opaque discoloration of the nail plate associated with distal nail matrix damage; may be punctate, striate, or diffuse. *Single nail*: traumatic, psoriasis. *Punctate leukonychia*: small white opaque spots; commonly seen following trauma or as the only finding in psoriasis. *Transverse leukonychia*: multiple transverse opaque parallel bands; commonly associated with matrix trauma of manicure or tight shoes. *Diffuse leukonychia*: nail plate completely opaque and white. Fungal infections cause superficial white onychomycosis and proximal subungual onychomycosis.

Apparent Leukonychia White discoloration that fades with pressure; abnormalities of color of nailbed; nail transparency maintained. Occurs with chemotherapeutic drugs and systemic disease.

Melanonychia Caused by activation or proliferation of nail matrix melanocytes. Melanin hyperpigmentation of the nail, either partial (longitudinal) or complete. *Etiology*: race, HIV/AIDS, inflammatory nail disorders, drugs (AZT), Addison disease, pregnancy, Laugier-Huntziker syndrome, trauma. Single band may represent nail matrix nevus or melanoma.

Longitudinal Erythronychia Nail bed disorder. Red band extending from proximal nail fold to

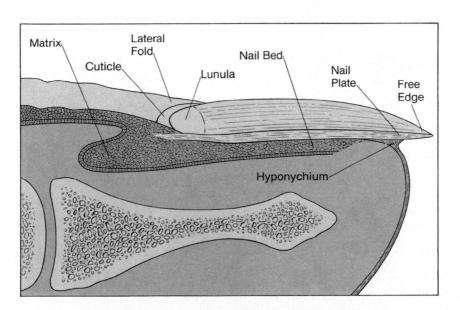

IMAGE 33-1 Schematic drawing of normal nail.

distal edge. *Etiology*: solitary caused by onycho-papilloma or other benign subungual tumor; multiple seen in Darier disease.

Onychauxis   Nail plate appears to be thickened due to subungual hyperkeratosis of nailbed. Common in psoriasis, eczema, distal subungual onychomycosis.

Onychia   Inflammation of the matrix of the nail resulting in shedding of nail.

Onychoclasis   Breaking of the nail.

Onychocryptosis   Ingrowing nail.

Onychogryphosis   Hypertrophy of the nail(s), producing a hooked or incurved clawlike deformity.

Onycholysis   Separation of the nail plate from the nail bed, usually beginning at the free margin and progressing proximally. Common in psoriasis, trauma, distal subungual onychomycosis.

Onychomalacia   Softening of the nail(s).

Onychomycosis   Tinea unguium. Fungal infection of periungual and nail bed skin with gradual involvement of the surface of the nail plate.

Onychorrhexis   Longitudinal ridging and fissuring of the nail plate with brittleness and breakage. Common with aging. Occurs in lichen planus.

Longitudinal Grooves   Usually single. Caused by tumors (digital myxoid cyst) of the proximal nail fold.

Onychoschizia   Splitting or lamination of the nail plate, usually in the horizontal plane at the free edge.

Onychotillomania   Compulsive picking or tearing at the nails.

Pitting of Nail Plate   Results from small areas of abnormal keratinization of proximal nail matrix. Punctate depressions of the nail plate surface. Common in psoriasis; also atopic dermatitis. Geometric and superficial pits seen in alopecia areata (hammered brass nails).

Longitudinal Ridging   Increases normally with aging.

Trachonychia   Nails rough due to excessive longitudinal ridging, often thinned. Twenty-nail dystrophy or sandpaper nails associated with proximal nail matrix damage: alopecia areata, lichen planus, psoriasis, dermatitis. May regress spontaneously.

Thinning of Nail Plate   Sign of matrix disorder.

Thickening of Nail Plate   Consequence of nail bed disorders.

LOCAL DISORDERS OF NAIL APPARATUS

Local disorders affecting the nail apparatus can result in a spectrum of chronic nail diseases.

CHRONIC PARONYCHIA   ICD-9 : 681.02 ○ ICD-10 : L03.0   ■ ◑

- Associated with damage to cuticle: mechanical or chemical.
- At risk: adult women; food handlers, housecleaners.
- Chronic dermatitis of proximal nail fold and matrix: chronic inflammation (eczema, psoriasis) with loss of cuticle, separation of nail plate from proximal nail fold (Fig. 33-1).
- Predisposing factors:
  - Dermatosis: psoriasis, dermatitis [atopic, irritant (occupational), allergic contact], lichen planus
  - Drugs: oral retinoids (isotretinoin, acitretin), indinavir
  - Foreign body: hair, bristle, wood splinters.
- Manifestations: first, second, and third fingers of dominant hand; proximal and lateral nail folds erythematous and swollen; cuticle absent.

- Intermittently, persistent low-grade inflammation may flare into subacute painful exacerbations, resulting in discolored transverse ridging of lateral edges.
- Secondary infection/colonization: *Candida* spp., *Pseudomonas aeruginosa*, or *Staphylococcus aureus*. Nail plate may become discolored; green undersurface with *Pseudomonas*. Infection associated with painful acute inflammation.
- *Management*:
  - Protection
  - Treat the dermatitis with glucocorticoid: topical, intralesional triamcinolone, short course of prednisone
  - Treat secondary infection.

FIGURE 33-1 Chronic paronychia A 64-year-old female who works as a cleaner has had hand "dermatitis" for many years. The distal fingers and periungual skin are red and scaling. The cuticle is absent; a pocket is present, formed as the proximal nail folds separate from the nail plate. The nail plates show trachonychia (rough surface with longitudinal ridging) and onychauxis (apparent nail plate thickening due to subungual hyperkeratosis of nailbed). The underlying problem is psoriasis. *Candida albicans* or *S. aureus* can cause space infection in the "pocket" with intermittent erythema and tenderness of the nail fold.

ONYCHOLYSIS   ICD-9:703.8 ∘ ICD-10:L60.1   ■ ◐

- Detachment of nail from its bed at distal and/or lateral attachments (Fig. 33-2).
- Onycholysis creates a subungual space that collects dirt and keratinous debris; grayish-white color due to presence of air under nail, but color varies from yellow to brown; area may be malodorous when the overlying nail plate is removed.
- Etiology:
  - Primary: Idiopathic (fingernails in women; mechanical or chemical damage to the onychodermal band); trauma (fingernails, occupational injury; toenails, podiatric abnormalities, poorly fitting shoes).
  - Secondary: Vesiculobullous disorders (contact dermatitis, dyshidrotic eczema, herpes simplex); nail bed hyperkeratosis (onychomycosis, psoriasis, chronic contact dermatitis); nail bed tumors; drugs.
- In psoriasis, yellowish-brown margin is visible between pink normal nail and white separated areas. In "oil spot" or "salmon-patch" variety (Fig. 33-2),

nail plate–nail bed separation may start in middle of nail.
- Colonization with *P. aeruginosa* results in a biofilm on the undersurface of the onycholytic nail plate, causing a brown or greenish discoloration (Fig. 33-3).
- Other secondary pathogens that can colonize/infect the space are *Candida* spp., dermatophytes, and numerous environmental fungi.
- Underlying disorders in fingernail onycholysis: trauma (e.g., splinter), psoriasis, photoonycholysis (e.g., doxycycline), dermatosis adjacent to nail bed (e.g., psoriasis, dermatitis, chemical exposure), congenital/hereditary.
- Underlying toenail onycholysis: additional factors of onychomycosis (*Trichophyton rubrum*), shoe trauma.
- *Management*: debride all nail separated from nail bed (patient should continue weekly debridement); remove debris on nail bed; treat underlying disorders.

GREEN NAIL SYNDROME   □ ◐

- Usually associated with onycholysis (see above). *P. aeruginosa*, the most common cause, produces the green pigment pyocyanin (Fig. 33-3).

- *Management*: debride "lytic" nail. See above.

FIGURE 33-2   Onycholysis   A 60-year-old female with fingernail problems for 10 years. Distal onycholysis of fingernails with little subungual debridement. Mild chronic paronychia is present with loss of cuticle. Psoriasis is the likely underlying problem.

FIGURE 33-3   Onycholysis with *Pseudomonas* colonization   Psoriasis has resulted in distal onycholysis of the thumbnail. A biofilm of *Pseudomonas aeruginosa* has produced the green-black discoloration of the undersurface of the onycholytic nail. Onycholysis resolved following the debridement and treatment of the nailbed with glucocorticoid cream.

ONYCHAUXIS AND ONYCHOGRYPHOSIS   ■ ○

- *Onychauxis*: Thickening of entire nail plate, seen in elderly (Fig. 33-4).
- *Onychogryphosis*: Onychauxis with ram's hornlike deformity, most commonly of great toe (Fig. 33-4).
  - Nail is severely distorted, thickened, brownish, ±spiraled, without attachment to nail bed.

- *Etiology*: pressure from footware in elderly; also, inherited autosomal dominant.
- Keratin produced by matrix at uneven rates, with faster-growing site determining direction of deformity.

FIGURE 33-4 Onychauxis A 73-year-old male with nail dystrophy for decades. The great toenails appear grossly thickened with transverse ridging (onychauxis) with some medial deviation (onychogryphosis or ram's horn deformity). The lateral view shows the thickness of the nail plate, separation from the nailbed (onycholysis), and the small area of attachment to the nail matrix.

PSYCHIATRIC DISORDERS

Repeated manipulation of the nail apparatus can result in changes of the paronychial skin and the nail plate.

Habit-tic Deformity *Synonyms:* central longitudinal grooved dystrophy, onychodystrophia mediana canaliformis. Washboard nail plate (Fig. 33-5). Caused by chronic, mechanical injury. Cuticle is pushed back with inflammation and thickening of proximal nail fold. Occurs most commonly on thumbnail(s), as compulsive disorders (tic habit), caused by the index finger repeatedly picking at cuticle of thumbnail.

Obsessive Compulsive Disorder Repeat picking at the paronychia skin can result in lichen simplex chronicus. *S. aureus* secondary infection is a common complication. In extreme cases, the nail plate can be destroyed (Fig. 33-6); nail biting.

FIGURE 33-5 Habit-tic deformity A 58-year-old male with thumbnail deformity for decades. The nail plates of both thumbs are dystrophic with transverse ridging and discoloration. The cuticle is absent and the proximal nail folds excoriated. When the proximal nails and nail fold with covered with tape continually, normal nails regrew in 5 months.

FIGURE 33-6 Compulsive nail picking A 56-year-old male with nail dystrophy for decades. The cuticles are not formed, the proximal nail folds inflamed and excoriated. The patient has been manipulating the fingernail apparatus for decades. The breaks in the integrity provide a portal of entry for *S. aureus* and acute paronychia.

NAIL APPARATUS INVOLVEMENT OF CUTANEOUS DISEASES

PSORIASIS ■ ◐

- Most common dermatosis affecting the nail apparatus
- >50% of persons with psoriasis have nail involvement at one point in time, with lifetime involvement up to 80–90%

- See also "Psoriasis," Section 3

LABORATORY EXAMINATION

KOH preparation and/or nail clipping to pathology for PAS stain to rule out fungal colonization/infection. Onychomycosis more common in nails with onycholysis.

CLINICAL FINDINGS

Skin Typical psoriatic lesion on nail folds (Fig. 33-7).

Matrix

- *Pitting or elkonyxis*: Punctate depressions; small, shallow; vary in size, depth, shape (Fig. 33-7A). Characteristically, isolated, deep. May occur as regular lines (transverse; long axis) or grid-like pattern. Uncommon on toenails.

- *Trachyonychia*: Nail dull, rough, fragile (Fig. 33-7B).
- *Serial transverse depressions*: May mimic "washboard" nails of tic habit (pushing back cuticle).
- *Longitudinal ridging*: Resembles melted wax.
- *Punctate leukonychia*: 1- to 2-mm white spots in nail plate. (mistakenly attributed to trauma) (Fig. 33-7C).
- *Leukonychia*: Proximal matrix involvement: surface rough and nail coarse (Fig. 33-7C).

Nail Bed

- *"Oil" spots*: Oval, salmon-colored nail beds (Fig. 33-7A, D).
- *Onycholysis*: Secondary to "oil" spots affecting hyponychium medially or laterally (Fig. 33-7A).

FIGURE 33-7 Psoriasis vulgaris ***A.*** Multiple nail pits on the dorsal nail plate, "oil staining" of the nail bed, and distal onycholysis. ***B.*** Trachonychia (rough surface) with oil staining, and distal onycholysis. ***C.*** Punctate leukonychia is pathognomonic for psoriasis and may be the only finger. As can be seen in the nail below with traumatic subungual hemorrhage, punctate leukonychia did not occur at this site of trauma. ***D.*** Oil staining, distal onycholysis, longitudinal ridging, adherence of the cuticle to the distal nail plate.

- *Colonization of onycholytic nail:* May affect nail bed or undersurface of nail (biofilm). *Candida,* environmental fungi (e.g., *Aspergillus*), *Pseudomonas.* Predisposes to distal/lateral onychomycosis in toenail. Up to 21% of psoriatic nails have secondary onychomycosis.
- *Subungual hyperkeratosis:* Nail plate becomes raised off hyponychium.
- *Splinter hemorrhages.*

Variant Acrodermatitis continua of Hallopeau: relapsing periungual and subungual pustules with onycholysis (see Section 3). Acute episodes with onycholysis with nail bed erythema and scaling. Often misdiagnosed as bacterial or fungal infection.

DIFFERENTIAL DIAGNOSIS

Onycholysis, onychomycosis, trauma (toenails), eczema, alopecia areata.

MANAGEMENT

- Often unsatisfactory. See "Psoriasis," Section 3.
- For matrix involvement, intralesional triamcinolone 3–5 mg/mL may be effective.
- For nail bed psoriasis, topical steroid (occluded) reduces hyperkeratosis.
- Systemic therapy such as methotrexate or "biologics" often improves nail apparatus psoriasis.

LICHEN PLANUS (LP)   □ ◑

- Nail involvement occurs in 10% of individuals with disseminated LP.
- Nail apparatus involvement may be the only manifestation.
- One, several, or all 20 nails may be involved ("twenty-nail syndrome," where there is loss of all 20 nails without any other evidence of lichen planus elsewhere on the body).
- Similar changes are seen in lichenoid graft-versus-host disease
- Course: May destroy nails.
- See also "Lichen Planus," Section 7.

CLINICAL MANIFESTATONS

Skin   Dorsum of PNF: swelling with blue/red discoloration of PNF.
Matrix

- *Small focus in matrix*: Bulge under proximal nail fold (Fig. 33-8A).
- *Subsequent longitudinal red line*: Thinned nail plate evolving into distal split nail (onychorrhexis) (Fig. 33-8B).
- *Diffuse matrix involvement*: Selective atrophy of nail plate with onychorrhexis and/or transverse splitting.
- *Red lunula*: Focal or disseminated.
- *Melanonychia, longitudinal*: Transitory.
- *Complete nail split.*
- *Pterygium formation (scar, matrix destroyed)*: Partial loss of the central nail plate presents as a V-shaped extension of skin of proximal nail fold adherent to nail bed (Fig. 33-8A, B).
- *"Idiopathic atrophy of nails"*: Acute progressive nail destruction leading to diffuse nail atrophy with and without pterygium; complete loss of nail (anonychia) (Fig. 33-8B, C, D).
- *Ulcerative LP*: Bulla formation, erosion, hemorrhage, scarring; cutaneous lesions usually present on palms/soles.

Nail Bed   Onycholysis, distal subungual hyperkeratosis, bulla formation, permanent anonychia.
Variants

- *20-nail dystrophy of childhood*: Resolves spontaneously.
- *LP-like eruptions following bone marrow transplant*: Graft-versus-host disease.
- *Drug-induced LP-like reaction.*
- *Permanent anonychia*: May be only manifestation of LP.

MANAGEMENT

- See "Lichen Planus," Section 7.
- Intralesional triamcinolone
- Systemic glucocorticoids

ALOPECIA AREATA (AA)   □ ○

- See "Nonscarring Alopecia," Section 32.
- Manifestations:
  - Geometric pitting (Fig. 33-9) (small, superficial, regularly distributed in geometric pattern)
- Hammered brass appearance
- Mottled erythema of lunulae
- Trachonychia (roughness caused by excessive longitudinal striations)

A

B

C

D

FIGURE 33-8   Lichen planus   A. Middle finger: Involvement of the proximal fold and matrix has caused trachonychia, longitudinal ridging, and pterygium formation. Index finger: destruction of the matrix and nail plate is complete with anonychia. Seven of ten fingernails are involved; the others are normal. **B.** Involvement of the nail matrix with scarring or pterygium formation proximally dividing the nail plate in two. The patient has hepatitis C virus infection and oral involvement with erosive lichen planus. **C.** Early involvement of the matrix with thinning of the thumbnail plates. **D.** Same patient as Fig. 33-10C two years later, the nail plate is completely destroyed, i.e., anonychia.

FIGURE 33-9   Alopecia areata: trachonychia   The nail plate is rough with a "hammered brass" appearance.

DARIER DISEASE (DARIER-WHITE DISEASE, KERATOSIS FOLLICULARIS)   □ ○

Nail changes are pathognomonic: longitudinal streaks (red and white); distal subungual hyperkeratotic papules with distal V- or wedge-shaped fissuring of nail plate (Fig. 33-10).

FIGURE 33-10   Darier disease   A 65-year-old female with pruritic rash on trunk for decades. Erythematous excoriated papules on the trunk with red and white longitudinal streaks on the fingernails.

CHEMICAL IRRITANT OR ALLERGIC DAMAGE OR DERMATITIS   ◧ ○

Chemicals in nail polish and adhesive for paste-on nails can cause damage to the nail plate, i.e., discoloration, onychoschizia. Irritant or allergic contact dermatitis can also occur on the paronychial skin.

FIGURE 33-11   Chemically damaged nail   False nail glued to the fingernail has chemically damaged the nail plate with leukonychia and onychoschizia.

NEOPLASMS OF THE NAIL APPARATUS   ICD-9 : 703.8

■ Benign tumors: Fibroma/fibrokeratoma, subungual exostosis, myxoid cyst, glomus tumor (painful red nail bed patch), onychomatrixoma, nail matrix nevi.

■ Malignant tumors: Squamous cell carcinoma, melanoma, Merkel cell tumor.

MYXOID CYSTS OF DIGITS

(See "Digital Myxoid Cyst," Section 9)

■ Pseudocyst or ganglion originates in distal interphalangeal joint, associated with osteoarthritis (Herberden nodes).

■ Lesions can present on the proximal nail fold (Fig. 33-12), above and compressing the matrix,

resulting in a longitudinal depressed groove in the nail plate.

■ When cysts expand between the periosteum and matrix, nail becomes dystrophic with a dusky red lunula.

LONGITUDINAL MELANONYCHIA

■ *Manifestations*: Tan, brown, or black longitudinal streak within nail plate (Fig. 33-13).

■ *Pathogenesis*: (1) Increased melanin synthesis in normally nonfunctional matrix melanocytes, (2) increase in total number of melanocytes synthesizing melanin, (3) nevomelanocytic nevus (junctional, Fig. 33-13).

■ *Onset*: Congenital or acquired. Most originate in distal matrix.

■ *Differential diagnosis*: Focal activation of nail matrix (e.g., trauma), hyperplasia of nail matrix melanocytes, nevomelanocytic nevus (junctional), drug-induced [e.g., zidovudine (AZT)] hydroxychloroquine, or melanoma of nail matrix.

FIGURE 33-12   Myxoid cysts A 62-year-old male with nail deformity of one year's duration. Dermal erythema and swelling of the proximal nail folds with associated longitudinal groove of the nail plate. Clear gelatinous fluid has drained from the index finger on the right (crusted site). Degenerative joint disease is present in both distal interphalangeal joints.

FIGURE 33-13   Junctional nevomelanocytic nevus of the nail matrix A junctional nevus is present in the nail matrix resulting in a longitudinal brown stripe in the nail bed. The proximal nail fold/ cuticle are not pigmented.

NAIL MATRIX NEVI

- Appear as longitudinal melanonychia (Fig. 33-13).
- Onset: childhood.

- Course: color and width change with aging.

ACROLENTIGINOUS MELANOMA (ALM) (See Section 12)

- *Mean age*: 55–60 years. *Incidence*: 2–3% of melanomas in whites; 15–20% in blacks, Asian, Native Americans. Usually asymptomatic; most patients notice pigmented lesion, especially after trauma.
- *Dermatopathology*: In situ or invasive.
- *Findings*: Arises subungually or periungually, presenting with longitudinal melanonychia and/or nail plate dystrophy (Fig. 33-14). Matrix lesions usually present as ALM in whites or broadening of an existing ALM in blacks.
- *Hutchinson sign*: Periungual extension of brown-black pigmentation onto proximal and lateral nail folds (Fig. 33-14).

- 25% of ALM may be amelanotic (pigmentation not obvious or prominent).
- *Distribution*: Thumbs, great toes (hallux).
- *Differential diagnosis*: Subungual hemorrhage.
- *Indications for biopsy*: Periungual pigmentation, adult age, change in color/width of band, hyperpigmented lines with the band, proximal portion of band wider than distal; thumb, index finger, or toe involvement; blurred margins, history of trauma.
- *Prognosis*: 5-year survival rates from 35–50%.

SQUAMOUS CELL CARCINOMA (See Section 11)

- SCC in situ (SCCIS) occurring periungually is usually caused by the oncogenic human papillomavirus (HPV) types 16 and 18.
  - *Findings*: Skin-colored or hyperpigmented, keratotic, hyperkeratotic, or warty papules/plaques; onycholysis; failure of nail formation.
  - *Distribution*: Proximal and lateral nails, matrix, hyponychium (Fig. 33-15).
- *Invasive SCC* arises within SCCIS.
  - *Symptoms*: Pain if periosteal invasion has occurred.

- *Findings*: Solitary nodule is most common, often destroying the nail.
- *Distribution*: Much more common on fingers (thumb and index finger most often) than toes; multiple fingers may be involved in the immunocompromised host.
- *Management*: Mohs surgery or amputation of digit for more deeply invasive lesions involving periosteum.

FIGURE 33-14   Acrolentiginous melanoma   The melanoma arose in the nail matrix of the thumb with resultant nail plate dystrophy, subungual melanosis, and extension into the proximal nail fold and beyond it (Hutchinson sign). (See also Fig. 12-12.)

FIGURE 33-15   HPV-induced in situ squamous cell carcinoma in HIV/AIDS: nail bed and glans penis
A 51-year-old male with HIV/AIDS and fingernail dystrophy. SCCIS had been excised by Mohs micrographic surgery 5 years previously. The right index fingernail bed with hyperkeratotic failure of nail plate formation. Pink papules are seen on the glans penis. Biopsy of the nailbed and penile papules reported SCCIS with HPV-induced changes (koilocytosis).

INFECTIONS OF THE NAIL APPARATUS   ICD-9:681.9

- Dermatophytes are the most common pathogens infecting the nail apparatus.
- *S. aureus* and group A streptococcus cause acute soft tissue infection of the nail fold.

- *Candida* and *S. aureus* can cause secondary infection of chronic paronychia.
- Recurrent herpes simplex virus infection.

BACTERIAL INFECTIONS

- *S. aureus* is the most common cause of acute paronychia.

- Felon is an acute infection of the finger tip.
- *Management*: See "Antimicrobial Therapy," Section 24.

ACUTE PARONYCHIA   ICD-10 ∘ L03.0

- Acute infection of lateral or proximal nail fold.
- Usually associated with break in integrity of epidermis (e.g., hang nail), trauma.

- *Findings*: Throbbing pain, erythema, swelling, pain, ± abscess formation (Fig. 33-16).
- Infection may extend deeper, forming a felon.

FELON   ICD-9:681.01 ∘ ICD-10:L03.0

- Soft tissue infection of pulp space of distal phalanx (Fig. 33-17); closed space infection of multiple compartments created by fibrous septa passing between the skin and periosteum.
- *History*: Penetrating injury, splint, paronychia.
- *Findings*: Pain, erythema, swelling, abscess (Fig. 33-17); abscess may break in center of pulp space and decompress spontaneously, with slough of necrotic skin over pulp space.
- *Distribution*: Thumb, index finger.

- *Complications*: Osteitis, osteomyelitis of distal phalanx, sequestration of diaphysis of the phalanx; rupture into distal interphalangeal joint with septic arthritis; extension into distal end of flexor tendon sheath, producing tenosynovitis.
- *Course*: May be rapid and severe; contained by unyielding skin of fingertip, infection creates tension with microvascular compromise, necrosis, and abscess formation.

FUNGAL INFECTIONS AND ONYCHOMYCOSIS

- *Candida* spp. usually cause "space" infections of chronic paronychia or onycholytic nail and can cause destruction of the nail in the immunocompromised host.
- Dermatophytes infect the skin around the nail apparatus and cause superficial destruction of nail.
- Environment fungi cause secondary colonization of diseased nail and are rarely primary pathogens.

- *Onychomycosis*: Chronic progressive fungal infection of nail apparatus, most commonly caused by dermatophytes, less often by *Candida* spp.; molds can be cultured from diseased nails but are not primary pathogens.
- *Candida onychia*: Onychomycosis caused by *Candida* spp.
- *Tinea unguium*: Onychomycosis caused by dermatophytes.

FIGURE 33-16 Acute paronychia A 40-year-old healthy male with painful swelling of right-index finger. The proximal nail fold red and edematous (cellulitis) with pus formation.

FIGURE 33-17 Felon A 60-year-old female with painful finger for 3 days. An abscess is seen on the fingertip with surrounding erythema and swelling. Methicillin-sensitive *S. aureus* (MSSA) was isolated on culture of the pus.

CANDIDA ONYCHIA

- *Candida albicans* infections of the nail apparatus occur most often on fingers, most commonly as secondary infection of chronic paronychia.
- *Candida* can cause distal and lateral onycholysis, especially in diabetics.

- Invasion of nail plate usually occurs only in the immunocompromised host, i.e., chronic mucocutaneous candidiasis (CMC) or HIV/AIDS disease.

ETIOLOGY AND EPIDEMIOLOGY

Etiology *C. albicans* and other species. Normal flora, which causes infection if local ecology is changed in favor of yeast or in association with altered immune status. See "Candidiasis," Section 25.

Classification

- Subungual infection associated with onycholysis
- Intermittent flares of chronic paronychia
- Colonization in tinea unguium

- Total nail dystrophy (TND) (Fig. 33-18): CMC and HIV/AIDS disease.

Chronic Mucocutaneous Candidiasis See "Candidiasis," Section 25.

CLINICAL FINDINGS

See "Candidiasis," Section 25.
HIV/AIDS Candidal onychia and paronychia are common in children with HIV/AIDS, often associated with mucosal candidiasis.

Nail Apparatus *Chronic Paronychia with Acute Candidal Flare* *Candida* spp. can cause intermittent painful infection of chronic paronychia with pain, tenderness, erythema, ± pus. Nail may become dystrophic with areas of opacification; white, yellow, green, or black discoloration; with transverse furrowing.
Subungual Candidiasis ± Abscess These occur in onycholytic space. Risk factor: diabetes.
Colonization in Tinea Unguium Secondary pathogen in distal/lateral onychomycosis.
Total Nail Dystrophy Proximal/lateral nail folds are inflamed and thickened. Fingertips appear bulbous. Nail is invaded and may eventually become totally dystrophic (Fig. 33-18). Nail apparatus thickens due to nail dystrophy and subungual hyperkeratosis. HIV/AIDS: one nail may be involved. CMC: 20 nails may be involved in time.
Other Findings   See "Candidiasis," Section 25.

DIFFERENTIAL DIAGNOSIS

Tinea unguium, psoriasis, eczema, chronic paronychia, lichen planus.

MANAGEMENT

See "Candidiasis," Section 25.

FIGURE 33-18   *Candida* onychomycosis: total dystrophic type   The entire fingernail plate is thickened and dystrophic and is associated with a paronychial infection; both findings were caused by *C. albicans* in an individual with advanced HIV/AIDS disease.

TINEA UNGUIUM/ONYCHOMYCOSIS   ■ ◑

- Symptoms: unsightly; nails lose protective and manipulative function;
- Complications:
  - Pain in toenail with pressure from shoes
  - Predispose to secondary bacterial infections
  - Ulcerations of the underling nail bed
- Complications occur more commonly in the growing population of immunocompromised individuals and diabetics
- See also Section 25

CLASSIFICATION BY ANATOMIC SITE INVOLVED

Distal and Lateral Subungual Onychomycosis (DLSO)   (Figs. 33-19 and 33-20) Infection begins in stratum corneum of hyponychial area or nail fold, extending subungually, and progressively involves the nail centripetally and medially. May be either primary, i.e., involving a healthy nail apparatus, or secondary (e.g., psoriasis) associated with onycholysis. *Findings:* Onycholysis, subungual hyperkeratosis, yellow-brown discoloration of keratinaceous debris. Always associated with tinea pedis.
Superficial White Onychomycosis (SWO) Pathogen invades surface of dorsal nail (Fig. 33-21). *Etiology:* *Trichophyton mentagrophytes* or *T. rubrum* (children). Much less commonly, mold: *Acremonium, Fusarium, Aspergillus terreus.*
Proximal Subungual Onychomycosis (PSO) Pathogen enters by way of the posterior nail fold–cuticle area and then migrates along the

proximal nail groove to involve the underlying matrix, proximal to the nail bed, and finally the underlying nail (Fig. 33-22). *Etiology*: *T. rubrum*. *Findings*: Leukonychia that extends distally from under proximal nail fold. Usually one or two nails involved. Always associated with immunocompromised states.

ETIOLOGY AND EPIDEMIOLOGY

Age of Onset Children or adults. Once acquired, usually does not remit spontaneously. Therefore, the incidence increases with advancing age; 1% of individuals <18 years affected; almost 50% of those >70 years.

Sex Somewhat more common in men.

Etiologic Agents Between 95 and 97% caused by *T. rubrum* and *T. mentagrophytes*. Much less common: *Epidermophyton floccosum*, *T. violaceum*, *T. schoenleinii*, *T. verrucosum* (usually infects only fingernails).

Molds Rarely, primary pathogens in onychomycosis, but rather secondarily colonize already dystrophic nails/nail apparatus. *Acremonium*, *Fusarium*, and *Aspergillus* spp. can rarely cause SWO. Dermatosis such as psoriasis, which results in onycholysis and subungual hyperkeratosis, or dermatophytic onychomycosis can be secondarily colonized/infected by molds. More than 40 mold species have been reported

FIGURE 33-19 Onychomycosis of toenails: distal and lateral subungual type (DLSO) A 4-year-old female with toenail dystrophy for 2 years and atopic dermatitis. The toenails are white, caused by onycholysis and subungual hyperkeratosis. The dorsum of the feet show erythema and scaling, i.e., tinea pedis. PAS stain of nail clipping shows septate hyphae. *T. rubrum* was detected on culture.

FIGURE 33-20 Onychomycosis of toenails: distal and lateral subungual type (DLSO) A 69-year-old male with toenail dystrophy for decades. The toenails show advanced dystrophy. Distal onycholysis and subungual hyperkeratosis cause apparent discoloration of the nails. The nail plate itself is not thickened. Colonization of the hyperkeratotic nailbed with environmental mold or *Pseudomonas* increases the discoloration.

to be isolated from dystrophic nails, including *Scopulariopsis brevicaulis, Aspergillus* spp., *Alternaria* spp., *Acremonium* spp., *Fusarium* spp., *Scytalidium dimidiatum (Hendersonula toruloidea), S. hyalinum.*

Etiology of Anatomic Types of Onychomycosis DLSO: *T. rubrum, T. mentagrophytes.* PSO: *T. rubrum.* SWO: *T. mentagrophytes.*

Geographic Distribution Worldwide. Etiologic agent varies in different geographic areas. More common in urban than in rural areas (associated with wearing occulsive footwear).

Prevalence Incidence varies in different geographic regions. In the United States and Europe, up to 10% of adult population affected (related to occlusive footwear). In developing nations where open footwear is worn, uncommon.

Transmission *Dermatophytes* Anthropophilic dermatophyte infections are transmitted from one individual to another, by fomite or direct contact, commonly among family members. Some spore forms (arthroconidia) remain viable and infective in the environment for up to 5 years.

Molds Ubiquitous in environment; not transmitted between humans.

Risk Factors Atopics are at increased risk for *T. rubrum* infections. Diabetes mellitus, treatment with immunosuppressive drugs, HIV/AIDS. For toenail onychomycosis, most important factor is wearing of occlusive footwear.

PATHOGENESIS

Primary Onychomycosis/Tinea Unguium Invasion occurs in an otherwise healthy nail. The probability of nail invasion by fungi increases with defective vascular supply (i.e., with increasing age, chronic venous insufficiency, peripheral arterial disease), in posttraumatic states (lower leg fractures), or disturbance of innervation (e.g., injury to brachial plexus, trauma of spine).

Secondary Onychomycosis Infection occurs in already altered nail apparatus, such as psoriatic or traumatized nail. Toenail onychomycosis usually occurs after tinea pedis; fingernail involvement associated with tinea manuum, tinea corporis, or tinea capitis. Infection of first and fifth toenails probably occurs secondary to damage to these nails by footwear.

DLSO (Figs. 33-19 and 33-20) Nail bed produces soft keratin stimulated by fungal infection that accumulates under the nail plate, thereby raising it, a change that clinically gives involved nail an altered cream color rather than normal transparent appearance. Dense keratin of nail plate is not involved primarily. Accumulated subungual keratin promotes further fungal growth and keratin production. Matrix is usually not invaded, and production of normal nail plate remains unimpaired despite fungal infection. In time, dermatophytes create air-containing tunnels within the nail plate; where the network is sufficiently dense, nail is opaque. Often invasion follows longitudinal ridges of nail bed. Subungual location of infection prevents effective topical antifungal agents.

CLINICAL MANIFESTATION

Approximately 80% of onychomycosis occurs on the feet, especially on the big toes; simultaneous occurrence on toe- and fingernails is not common.

DLSO White patch is noted on the distal or lateral undersurface of the nail and nail bed, usually with sharply demarcated borders. In time, whitish color can become discolored to a brown or black hue. Progressive involvement of nail can occur in a matter of weeks, as in HIV/AIDS, or more slowly over a period of months or years. With progressive infection, the nail becomes opaque, thickened, cracked, friable, raised by underlying hyperkeratotic debris in hyponychium (Figs. 33-19 and 33-20). Sharply marginated white streaks beginning at the distal nail margin and extending proximally are filled with keratinaceous debris and air. Toenails are involved much more commonly than fingernails. First and fifth toenails are infected most frequently. Involvement of the fingernails is usually unilateral. When fingernails are involved, pattern is usually two feet and one hand.

SWO A white chalky plaque is seen on the proximal nail plate, which may become eroded with loss of the nail plate (Fig. 33-21). Diagnostically, the involved nail can be removed easily with a curette in comparison with a traumatized nail, which has white, air-containing areas. In some cases, the entire superficial nail plate may become involved. SWO may coexist with DLSO. Occurs almost exclusively on the toenails, rarely on the fingernails.

PSO (Fig. 33-22) A white spot appears from beneath proximal nail fold. In time, white discoloration fills lunula, eventually moving distally to involve much of undersurface of the nail. Patients treated with oral azoles show interruption of involved nail. Occurs more commonly on toenails.

DIFFERENTIAL DIAGNOSIS

DLSO Psoriatic nails ("oil drop" staining of the distal nail bed and nail pits is seen in psoriasis but not onychomycosis), paronychial psoriasis or eczema. Reiter syndrome and keratoderma blennorrhagicum, onychogryphosis, pincer nails, congenital nail dystrophies.
SWO Traumatic or chemical injury to nail, psoriasis with leukonychia.

LABORATORY EXAMINATIONS

All clinical diagnoses of onychomycosis should be confirmed by laboratory testing (see "Dermatophytoses," Section 25).
Nail Samples For DLSO: distal portion of involved nail bed; SWO: involved nail surface; PSO: punch biopsy through nail plate to involved nail bed.
Direct Microscopy Direct microscopic examination of nail samples is used to confirm the clinical diagnosis. Keratinaceous material from involved nail scrapings is placed on glass slide, covered with glass coverslip, suspended in a solution of potassium hydroxide (KOH), and gently heated. Specific identification of pathogen is usually not possible by microscopy, but, in most cases, yeasts can be differentiated from dermatophytes by morphology.
Fungal Culture Isolation of the pathogen permits better use of oral antifungal agents. Samples of infected nail are inoculated onto Sabouraud agar with or without cycloheximide. Isolation of mold from psoriatic nail or tinea unguium is mostly colonizer and not primary pathogen.
Histology of Nail Clipping Indicated if clinical findings suggest onychomycosis after negative KOH wet mounts. PAS stain is used to detect fungal elements in the nail. *Most reliable technique for diagnosing onychomycosis.*

DIAGNOSIS

Clinical diagnosis is never adequate. Clinical findings confirmed by finding fungal forms in KOH preparation, nail clipping, and/or isolation of pathogenic fungus on culture.

COURSE AND PROGNOSIS

Without effective therapy, onychomycosis does not resolve spontaneously; progressive involvement of multiple toenails is the rule. DLSO

FIGURE 33-21   Onychomycosis of toenails: superficial white type (SWO) The dorsal nail plate is chalky white. White nail dystrophy can easily be treated by curettage; KOH preparation of the curetting shows hyphae.

FIGURE 33-22   *Tinea unguium*: proximal subungual onychomycosis type (PSO) The proximal nail plate is a chalky white color due to invasion from the undersurface of the nail matrix. The patient had advanced HIV/AIDS disease.

persists after topical treatment of tinea pedis and often results in repeated episodes of epidermal dermatophytosis of feet, groin, and other sites. Tinea pedis and/or DLSO provide portal of entry for recurrent bacterial infections (*S. aureus*, group A streptococcus), especially cellulitis of lower leg after venous harvesting. Prevalence in diabetics estimated to be 33%; DLSO contributes to severity of foot problems: superficial bacterial infection, ulceration, cellulitis, osteomyelitis, necrosis, amputation. *Diabetics need early intervention and should be screened regularly by a dermatologist and/or podiatrist.* Untreated HIV/AIDS is associated with increased prevalence of dermatophytoses.

Long-term relapse rate with newer oral agents such as terbinafine or itraconazole reported to be 15–21% 2 years after successful therapy; long-term follow-up studies not yet reported. Causes of relapse/reinfection uncertain: reinfection, immunologic incompetence, persistent trauma, unknown causes. Mycologic cultures may be positive without any clinically apparent disease. Nail/foot hygiene is important: benzoyl peroxide soap in shower or antifungal preparation or ethanol/isopropyl gel.

MANAGEMENT

See Section 25 and Table 33-1.

TABLE 33-1 Management of Tinea Unguium	
Debridement	Debride dystrophic nails; patients should debride weekly. In DLSO, nail and hyperkeratotic nail bed should be removed. In SWO, abnormal nail can be debrided with curette.
Topical agents	Available as lotions and lacquer. *Usually not effective* except for SWO.
	Ciclopirox (Penlac) nail lacquer: monthly professional nail debridement recommended.
Systemic agents	*Note:* In systemic treatment of onychomycosis, nails usually do not appear normal after the treatment times recommended because of slow growth of nail. If cultures and KOH preparations are negative after these time periods, medication can nonetheless be stopped and nails will usually regrow normally.
Allylamines	Most effective against dermatophyte infections; also efficacious against selected other fungi.
Terbinafine	250 mg/d for 6 weeks for fingernails and 12–16 weeks for toenails.
Azoles	Drugs in this category are usually effective in treatment of nail infections caused by dermatophytes, yeasts, and molds.
Itraconazole: approved (USA) for onychomycosis. Effective in dermatophytes and *Candida* only.	200 mg/d for 6 weeks (fingernails), 12 weeks (toenails) (continuous therapy). 200 mg twice daily for first 7 days of each month for 2 months (fingernails) (pulse dosing). Although not approved for toenail onychomycosis, pulse dosing is used, given for 3–4 months.
Fluconazole: not approved (USA) for onychomycosis. Effective in dermatophytes and *Candida*.	Reported effective at dosing of 150–400 mg 1 day per week or 100–200 mg/d until the nails grow back normally. Effective in yeasts and less so in dermatophytes.
Ketoconazole: not approved for onychomycosis.	Prolonged therapy as for onychomycosis has highest incidence of liver function abnormalities.
	Effective at 200 mg/d; more effective for *Candida* than dermatophytes; however, infrequently hepatotoxicity and antiandrogen effect have limited its long-term use for onychomycosis.
Secondary prophylaxis	Recommended for all patients. The entirety of both feet should be treated. Prophylaxis should be simple to use and inexpensive:
	Antifungal cream, lotion, or powder daily.
	Antiseptic gels: ethanol or isopropyl alcohol.
	Pedicures/manicures: make sure instruments are sterilized or individuals have their own.

Indications for Systemic Therapy Fingernail involvement, limitation of function, pain (thickened great toenails with pressure on nail bed, ingrowing toe nails), physical disability, potential for secondary bacterial infection, source of recurrent epidermal dermatophytosis, quality-of-life issues (poorer perceptions of general and mental health, social functioning, physical ap-pearance, difficulty in trimming nails, discomfort in wearing shoes). Early onychomycosis easier to cure in younger, healthier individuals than in older individuals with more extensive involvement and associated medical conditions. *It is essential to prove (fungal) infection before starting systemic treatment; differentiate onychomycosis from other nail dystrophies.*

NAIL SIGNS OF MULTISYSTEM DISEASES ICD-9 : 703.8

A wide spectrum of systemic disorders can affect the nail apparatus.

TRANSVERSE OR BEAU LINES: 20 NAILS

Systemic disease implicated if all 20 nails involved. *Pathogenesis*: Occur after any severe, sudden, acute, particularly febrile illness; damage to matrix. *Etiology*: High fever, postnatal, cytotoxic drugs, severe adverse cutaneous drug reaction. *Findings*: Transverse, bandlike depressions in nail, extending from one lateral edge to the other, affecting all nails at corresponding levels (Fig. 33-23). If duration of disease completely inhibits matrix activity for 7–14 days, transverse depression results in total division of nail plate (onychomadesis). Multiple parallel lines with chemotherapy. *Duration*: Thumbnails (lines present for 6–9 months) and large nails (lines present for up to 2 years) are most reliable markers.

LEUKONYCHIA

True Leukonychia Attributable to matrix dysfunction:

- *Total leukonychia*: Usually inherited
- *Subtotal leukonychia*: Distal nail pink
- *Transverse leukonychia*: 1- to 2-mm wide arcuate bands
- *Punctate leukonychia*: Psoriasis, trauma
- *Longitudinal leukonychia*: Darier disease (Fig. 33-10)

Pseudoleukonychia Superficial white onychomycosis (Fig. 33-21), chemical damage to nail keratin.
Apparent Leukonychia Due to alteration of matrix and/or nail bed (e.g., apparent macrolunula); may involve all fingernails:

- *Terry-type leukonychia*
  - *Association*: Hepatic disorders.

- *Findings*: Opaque white plate obscuring lunula and extending to within 1–2 mm from distal edge of nail (Fig. 33-24). Involves all nails evenly.
- *Uremic Half-and-Half Nail of Lindsay*
  - *Association*: Renal disorders.
  - *Findings*: Proximal nail dull white obscuring lunula (20–60% of nail); distal nail pink/reddish.
- *Banded nails (Muehrcke lines)* (Fig. 33-35)
  - Paired, narrow, white transverse bands.
  - *Association*: Cancer antineoplastic chemotherapy, hypoalbuminemia; unilateral following trauma.
  - *Findings*: Bands are parallel to lunula, separated from one another, and from lunula, by strips of pink nail.

FIGURE 33-23   Cancer chemotherapy: Beau lines   Multiple transverse ridging of multiple fingernails was associated with chemotherapy for breast cancer.

FIGURE 33-24   Apparent leukonychia: Terrytype nails   The proximal two-thirds of the nail plate is white, whereas the distal third shows the red color of the nailbed.

YELLOW NAIL SYNDROME   □ ◑

Symptoms: Nails stop growing. *Association*: Lymphedema, respiratory tract disease (bronchiectasis, chronic bronchitis, malignant neoplasms), rheumatoid arthritis, internal malignancies. *Pathogenesis*: Arrest in nail growth. *Findings*: Nails hard, excessively curved from side to side; diffuse pale yellow to dark yellow-green discoloration (Fig. 33-25). Cuticles absent. Secondary onycholysis common. *Distribution*: 20 nails.

PERIUNGUAL FIBROMA   □ ○

Synonym: Koenen tumors. *Association*: Tuberous sclerosis (see "Tuberous Sclerosis," Section 15); occur in 50% of individuals. *Onset*: Puberty. *Findings*: Usually multiple, small to large, elongated to nodular tumors; produce a longitudinal groove in nail plate due to matrix compression (Fig. 33-26).

FIGURE 33-25 Yellow nail syndrome Diffuse yellow-to-green color of the fingernails, nail thickening, slowed growth, and excessive curvature from side to side of all ten fingernails.

FIGURE 33-26 Tuberous sclerosis: periungual fibroma A 42-year-old female with tuberous sclerosis. A skin-colored tumor is seen emerging from beneath the proximal nail fold associated with a longitudinal groove in the nail plate.

SPLINTER HEMORRHAGES   □→■ ○

Subungual epidermal ridges extend from lunula distally to hyponychium, fitting in a "tongue-and-groove" fashion between similarly arranged dermal ridges (Fig. 33-27). Rupture of fine capillaries along these longitudinal dermal ridges results in splinter hemorrhages. *Distal splinter hemorrhages* seen with minor trauma (most common cause, occurring in up to 20% of normal population); psoriasis, atopic der-

matitis. *Proximal splinter hemorrhages*: sideropenic anemia, bacterial endocarditis (Fig. 33-28), trichinosis, antiphospholipid antibody syndrome, altitude sickness. *Findings*: Fingernails. Tiny linear structures, usually 2–3 mm long, arranged in the long axis of nail; plum-colored when formed, darkening to brown or black within 1–2 days; they subsequently move superficially and distally with nail growth.

NAIL FOLD/PERIUNGUAL ERYTHEMA AND TELANGIECTASIA   □ ○

Associated with connective tissue (collagen-vascular) disease.
Periungual Erythema   *Association*: Systemic lupus erythematosus (SLE), dermatomyositis (DM). HIV/AIDS or hepatitis C virus infection. *Findings*: Periungual erythema, edema, alterations of cuticle, secondary nail changes.
Telangiectasia   *Association*: Scleroderma, SLE, DM; rheumatoid arthritis. *Findings*: Linear wiry

vessels perpendicular to nail base overlie proximal nail folds (Fig. 33-29); usually bright red; may be black if thrombosed. SLE and DM: arise within erythema. Scleroderma and DM: enlarged capillary loops with *reduced* capillary density and avascular areas.
Cuticle Hyperkeratosis and Hemorrhages   SLE and DM.
Discoid LE   Figure 33-30

PTERYGIUM INVERSUM UNGUIUM

Nail plate adheres to fingertip skin in scleroderma.

FIGURE 33-27   Trauma: subungual hemorrhage   Trauma to the proximal nail resulted in hemorrhage and a tranverse depression across the nail plate. Hemorrhage extends to the longitudinal dermal ridges.

SYSTEMIC AMYLOIDOSIS

Nail dystrophy resembling lichen planus with severe onychodystrophy (nail plate thinned, longitudinally fissured with subungual hemorrhages) can precede diagnosis of primary systemic amyloidosis. Biopsy of nail apparatus confirms the diagnosis of amyloidosis with amyloid deposits in the superficial dermis of the nail matrix (Fig. 33-31).

FIGURE 33-28   Infective endocarditis: splinter hemorrhage   Subungual hemorrhage in the midportion of the fingernail bed in a 60-year-old female with enterococcal endocarditis; subconjunctival hemorrhage was also present.

FIGURE 33-29   Systemic lupus erythematosus: nail fold erythema and telangiectasis   A 64-year-old female with systemic LE with arthritis, fatigue, and photosensitivity for decades. Proximal nail folds are enlarged with erythema, telangiectasis, and thromboses. The cuticle is elongated.

FIGURE 33-30   Discoid lupus erythematosus: Nail fold and matrix involvement and nail dystrophy   A 46-year-old female with chronic cutaneous LE for several decades. Proximal nail folds show erythema, scarring, and depigmentation associated with nail matrix inflammation.

FIGURE 33-31   Systemic amyloidosis   A 52-year-old male with systemic amyloidosis; nail findings preceded the diagnosis of systemic amyloidosis. The nail findings resemble those seen in lichen planus. The matrix is inflamed with resultant thinning of the proximal nail plaque and disintegration of the plate distally.

KOILONYCHIA   □ ○

Spoon-shaped nails (Fig. 33-32). *Etiology* (more often due to local rather than systemic factors): physiologic (early childhood); thin nails (old age, peripheral vascular disease); soft nails (mainly occupational); hereditary and congenital; Plummer-Vinson syndrome (iron-deficiency anemia, dysphagia, glossitis). *Findings*: In early stages, nail plate becomes flattened; later, edges become everted upwards and nail appears concave.

CLUBBED NAILS   ■ ○

Angle between proximal nail fold and nail plate is >180°. May occur with or without cyanosis. *Pathogenesis*: Hypertrophy of soft tissue components of digital pulp; hyperplasia of fibrovascular tissue at base of nail (nail can be "rocked"); local cyanosis. *Etiology*:

- Cardiovascular disorders: Aortic aneurysm, congenital and acquired cardiovascular disease
- Bronchopulmonary disorders: Intrathoracic neoplasms, chronic intrathoracic suppurative disorders

- Gastrointestinal disorders: Inflammatory bowel disease, GI neoplasms, hepatic disorders, multiple polyposis, bacillary dysentery, amoebic dysentery
- Chronic methemoglobinemia

Findings: Digit is bulbous; nail plate enlarged and excessively curved (Fig. 33-33). Increased curvature usually affects all 20 nails.

FIGURE 33-32   Koilonychia   The fingernail plate is concave; no other nails were involved. There were no associated systemic factors.

FIGURE 33-33   Lung cancer: clubbed fingers   Bulbous enlargement and broadening of the fingertips in a smoker with lung cancer. The tissue between the nail and underlying bone has a spongy quality giving a "floating" sensation when pressure is applied downward and forward at the junction between the plate and proximal fold. Cigarette smoke has stained the left middle finger.

DRUG-INDUCED NAIL CHANGES ■ ○

See Table 33-2.
Drugs causing adverse nail changes are similar to those causing adverse changes in cutaneous and mucosal sites.

- Chemotherapy: Beau lines (Fig. 33-23), onychomadesis, Muehrcke lines, hemorrhagic onycholysis, pyogenic granulomas (Fig. 33-35), melanonychia

- Antiretrovirals: Melanonychia [zidovudine (AZT)]; pyogenic granuloma (indinavir)
- Beta-blockers: Digital ischemia
- Bleomycin: Digital ischemia
- PUVA: Photo-onycholysis, melanonychia
- Retinoids: Nail fragility, pyogenic granuloma, paronychia

TABLE 33-2 Drug-Induced Nail Changes

Nail findings	Causative drug
Discoloration (non-melanin) (Fig. 33–34)	Antimalarials: chloroquine, hydroxychloroquine, quinacrine
	Minocycline
	Gold, Silver
Melanonychia (Fig. 33-35)	Zidovudine (AZT)
	Psoralens
	Chemotherapeutic drugs: 5-fluorouracil (Fig. 33–35), daunorubicin, doxorubicin
Leukonychia: true	Chemotherapeutic drugs
Leukonychia: apparent	Chemotherapeutic drugs
	Polypharmacy: anthracyclines, vincristine
Beau lines, onychomadesis (Fig. 33–23)	Chemotherapeutic drugs
Paronychia; paronychial pyogenic granuloma (Fig. 33–16)	Retinoids: isotretinoin, acitretin
	Indinavir
	Methotrexate
	EGFR antagonists
Ischemic changes	β-Blockers

FIGURE 33-34 Nail discoloration: quinacrine Bluish discoloration of the nail in a patient with SLE treated with quinacrine.

FIGURE 33-35 Nail discoloration and transverse bands (Muehrcke lines): chemotherapy Period transverse bands on the fingernail in a patient with breast cancer being treated with chemotherapy (5-fluorouracil).

SECTION 34

DISORDERS OF
THE MOUTH

- Oral mucosa covers and protects tissues beneath it and conveys sensory information from the surface.
- Normal function is required for mastication, deglutition, chemosensory function, phonation.

- Structures of mouth: lips, oral mucosa, gingivae, tongue, palate, teeth.
- Impaired oral mucosal health causes pain, malnutrition, infection, compromised immune function, and exacerbations of medical disorders.

DISEASES OF THE LIPS ICD-9:528.5 ○ ICD-10:K13.0

ANGULAR CHEILITIS (PERLÈCHE) ■ ◑

- Intertrigo. Associated with increased moisture at commissures.
- *Predisposing factors*: thumbsucking in children; sagging face and loss of teeth in older persons; candidiasis in immunocompromised persons; *S. aureus* in atopic dermatitis and isotretinoin treatment.

- *Findings*: erythema and maceration at commissures (see Fig. 25-29); white candidal colony.
- *Diagnosis*: KOH for candidiasis; culture for *S. aureus, Candida*.
- *Management*: Identify and treat causes.

ACTINIC CHEILITIS ■ ◑

Actinic/solar keratoses, usually of the lower lip. Rule out squamous cell carcinoma in situ or invasive if pa-

pule or nodule or ulcer occur. (See "Solar Keratosis," Section 10.)

CONDITIONS OF THE TONGUE ICD-9:528.6, 528.7, 529 ○ ICD-10:K14

FISSURED TONGUE ■ ○

- Normal variant in up to 11% of population. Asymptomatic.
- *Findings*: Multiple folds with anterior-posterior orientation on the dorsal surface of the tongue (Figs. 34-1, 34-2).

- *Associated disorders*: Psoriasis, Down syndrome, acromegaly, Sjögren syndrome.

Synonyms: Lingua fissurata, lingua plicata, scrotal tongue, grooved tongue, furrowed tongue.

BLACK OR WHITE HAIRY TONGUE

- *Pathogenesis*: Defective desquamation of filiform papillae resulting in hair-like projections on the dorsum of the tongue.

- *Associations*: Heavy tobacco use, mouth breathing, systemic antibiotic therapy, poor oral hygiene, general debilitation, radiation therapy, chronic use of bismuth-containing antacids, lack of dietary roughage.

- *Symptoms*: Gagging sensation, altered taste, halitosis, cosmetic disfigurement.

- *Findings*: Furry plaques on dorsal tongue (Fig. 34-2). Chromogenic bacteria or exogenous pigment stain tongue: white, yellow, green, brown, black. Candidiasis may occur secondarily.

- *Management*: Eliminate predisposing factors; good oral hygiene.

Synonym: Lingua villosa (nigra)

FIGURE 34-1   Fissured tongue   Deep furrows on the dorsum of the tongue are asymptomatic.

FIGURE 34-2   Hairy and fissured tongue   A 57-year-old healthy male. Tongue has a white surface due to retained keratin. A midline fissure is also present.

ORAL HAIRY LEUKOPLAKIA (See Section 31)

- *Pathogenesis*: Epstein-Barr virus infection; low CD4 cell counts.

- *Findings*: White corrugated plaques on lateral aspects of tongue (see Fig. 31-3). Does not occur in successfully treated HIV/AIDS.

MIGRATORY GLOSSITIS ICD-9:529.1 ∘ ICD-10:K14.1

Irregular areas of dekeratinized and desquamated filiform papillae (red in color) are surrounded by elevated whitish or yellow margins (Fig. 34-3).

Etiology: unknown; possible link with psoriasis Incidence: common; usually asymptomatic
Synonym: Geographic tongue

FIGURE 34-3 Migratory glossitis Areas of hyperkeratosis alternate with areas of normal pink epithelium, creating a geographic pattern in a female with psoriasis.

DISEASES OF THE GINGIVA, PERIODONTIUM, AND MUCOUS MEMBRANES ICD-9:523 ∘ ICD-10:K06

GINGIVITIS AND PERIODONTITIS

- *Gingivitis*: Erythema, edema, blunting of interdental papillae without bone loss. Predisposing factors: poor oral hygiene, tobacco use, diabetes.
- *Periodontitis*: Chronic infection of connective tissue, periodontal ligament, and alveolar bone; most common cause of tooth loss in adults.
- *Course*: Accumulation of subgingival calculus (calcified plaque) and *Actinobacillus actinomyc-* *etemcomitans* infection results in painless soft-tissue edema, insidious alveolar bone resorption, deepening periodontal pockets, and tooth loss.
- Predisposing factors for periodontitis: Malocclusion, oral contraception, diabetes, glucocorticoids; HIV/AIDS.

Synonym: Periodontal disease

EROSIVE GINGIVOSTOMATITIS

Reaction pattern associated with viral infection, autoimmunity, lichen planus, erythema multiforme, pemphigus, cicatricial pemphigoid.

Findings: Erythema and edema of gingivae. Other mucocutaneous sites may be affected.

LICHENOID MUCOSITIS

Findings: Reticulated white plaques and painful erosions on mucosal surfaces.

Etiology: Lichen planus (LP), drugs (NSAIDs, antihypertensive agents), allergic contact dermatitis, graft-versus-host disease.

Synonym: Periodontal disease.

LICHEN PLANUS (See Section 7)

- *Incidence*: 40–60% of inividuals with LP have oropharyngeal involvement. Erosive ulcerative LP is painful.
- *Findings:*
  - Milky-white papules
  - Reticulate (netlike) patterns of lacy-white hyperkeratosis [buccal mucosa (Fig. 34-4), lips (see Fig. 7-7), tongue, and gingivae]
  - Hypertrophic LP—leukoplakia with Wickham, striae usually on the buccal mucosa
- Atrophic LP—shiny plaque often with Wickham striae in surrounding mucosa
- Erosive/ulcerative LP—superficial erosions with overlying fibrin clots that are seen on the tongue and buccal mucosa (Fig. 34-4)
- Bullous LP—intact blisters (rupture and result in erosive LP)
- Desquamative gingivitis—bright red gingiva (Fig. 34-5).

FIGURE 34-4 Lichen planus: Wickham striae Poorly defined violaceous plaque with lacy, white pattern on the buccal mucosa.

FIGURE 34-5   Lichen planus: desquamative gingivitis   The gingival margins are erythematous, edematous, and retracted in a 72-year-old female. The lesions were painful, making dental hygiene difficult, resulting in plaque formation on the teeth.

ACUTE NECROTIZING ULCERATIVE GINGIVITIS (ANUG)   □ ◑

- *Precipitating factors*: Poor oral hygiene, HIV/AIDS, immunosuppression, alcohol and tobacco use, nutritional deficiency.
- *Findings* (Fig. 34-6): Punched-out ulcers of the interdental papillae. Gingival hemorrhage, severe pain, foul odor/halitosis, fever, lymphadenopathy; alveolar bone destruction.

- *Etiologic agents*: *Bacteroides fusiformis, Prevotella intermedia, Borrelia vincentii, Treponema, Selenomonas.*
- *Management*: Systemic antibiotics such as clindamycin, metronidazole, amoxicillin. Dental hygiene.

Synonyms: Trench mouth, Vincent disease.

GINGIVAL HYPERPLASIA   ◧ ○

- *Findings*: Hypertrophy of both the free and attached gingivae, particularly the interdental papillae (Fig. 34-7).
- *Inflammatory enlargement*: Most common cause of gingival enlargement. Caused by edema and infective cellular infiltration caused by prolonged exposure to bacterial plaque; fibrosis occurs if untreated.
- *Drug-induced fibrous hyperplasia of gingivae*: May cover the teeth and is associated with:
  - Anticonvulsants: phenytoin, succinimides, valproic acid
  - Calcium channel blockers: nifedipine, verapamil
  - Cyclosporine
- *Systemic conditions/disorders*
  - Pregnancy, puberty, vitamin C deficiency, glycogen storage disease
  - Chronic myelomonocytic leukemia (Fig 34-7)

Synonyms: Gingival enlargement, hypertrophic gingivitis

FIGURE 34-6   Acute necrotizing ulcerative gingivitis (ANUG)   Very painful gingivitis with necrosis on marginal gingiva, edema, purulence, and halitosis in a 35-year-old female with advanced HIV disease. ANUG resolved with oral clindamycin.

FIGURE 34-7   Gingival hyperplasia: acute monocytic leukemia   A 37-year-old female with recent diagnosis of AML. The gingivae show hyperplasia due to infiltration with leukemic monocytes.

APHTHOUS ULCERATION ICD-9:528.2 ∘ ICD-10:K12.0

- Recurrent painful mucosal lesions.
- Most common cause of oral ulcerations; incidence up to 30% of otherwise healthy persons.
- May be associated with systemic diseases such as HIV/AIDS and Behçet disease.

Synonyms: Aphthae, canker sore, aphthous (ancient Greek word for "ulcer") stomatitis.

EPIDEMIOLOGY

Etiology Idiopathic. Can arise at site of minor mucosal injury, e.g., bite.
Pathogenesis Cell-mediated immune reaction pattern.
Age at Onset Any age; often during second decade, persisting into adulthood, and becoming less frequent with advancing age.
Classification

- Simple versus complex aphthosis based on clinical course.
  ∘ Simple: 1–3 oral ulcers that recur 1–3 times per year.
  ∘ Complex: Continuous ulcers and associated with systemic disease or genital ulcers.
- Major aphthous ulcers (AU) may persist for ≥6 weeks, healing with scarring.
- Behçet disease should be considered in patients with persistent oropharyngeal AU, with or without anogenital AU, associated with systemic findings (eye, nervous system). See Section 14.

CLINICAL MANIFESTATION

Symptoms Even though small, AU can be quite painful, which may impair nutrition. A burning or tingling sensation may be felt before ulceration. In persons with severe AU, malaise: weight loss associated with persistent, painful AU.
Mucosal Findings

- At times, small, painful red macule or papule before ulceration
- More commonly, ulcer(s) <1 cm (Figs. 34-8 and 34-9), covered with fibrin (gray-white), with sharp, discrete, and at times edematous borders. White-gray base with an erythematous rim.
- Most commonly single; at times, multiple or numerous small, shallow, grouped—i.e., herpetiform AU (HAU). Major AU (MaAU)may heal with white, depressed scars.

- Number of ulcers: Minor AU (MiAU), 1–5; MaAU, 1–10: HAU, up to 100.
- *Distribution*: Oropharyngeal, anogenital, any site in the GI tract. Oral lesions most commonly on the buccal and labial mucosa, less commonly on tongue, sulci, floor of mouth. MiAU rarely occur on the palate or gums. MaAU often occur on soft palate and pharynx. Also, esophagus, upper and lower GI tract, and anogenital epithelium.

General Findings With MaAU, occasionally tender cervical lymphadenopathy.
Associated Disorders Behçet disease (see Section 14), cyclic neutropenia, HIV/AIDS [acute HIV/AIDS syndrome, AIDS (large chronic AU)], reactive arthritis; periodic fever, aphthous stomatitis, Crohn disease, pharyngitis and adenitis (PFAPA; occurs in young children with associated high fever occurring periodically every 3–5 weeks with AU, pharyngitis, and/or lymphadenitis).

DIFFERENTIAL DIAGNOSIS

Primary herpetic gingivostomatitis, hand-foot-and-mouth disease, herpangina, primary HIV/AIDS infection, Behçet disease, squamous cell carcinoma (SCC), bullous disease, lichen planus, Reiter syndrome, adverse drug reaction.

LABORATORY

Dermatopathology Nondiagnostic. Rule out specific cause of ulcer, i.e., infection (syphilitic chancre, histoplasmosis), inflammatory disorders (lichen planus), or cancers (SCC).

DIAGNOSIS

Usually made on clinical findings, ruling out other causes.

FIGURE 34-8 Aphthous ulcers: minor   Multiple, very painful, gray-based ulcers with erythematous halos on the labial mucosa.

COURSE

Tend to recur during adulthood. Uncommonly, may be almost constant in the oropharynx or anogenitalia, referred to as *complex aphthosis*.

MANAGEMENT

Intralesional Triamcinolone   3–10 mg/mL in lidocaine very effective for immediate relief of pain and resolution of ulcers.

Systemic Therapy

- *Prednisone*: In persons with large, persistent, painful AU interfering with nutrition, a brief course of prednisone is effective (70 mg, tapered by 10 or 5 mg/d).
- *Thalidomide*: Effective in HIV/AIDS, Behçet disease, large painful AU. Adverse effects: peripheral sensory neuropathy. Teratogenesis. *Tumor necrosis factor* (TNF) α *inhibitor*: Adalimumab and Infliximab reported to be effective.

FIGURE 34-9 Aphthous ulcers: major   A 52-year-old female with advanced HIV/AIDS with a 5-month history of painful lesions on the tongue. Two huge painful deep ulcers on the lateral tongue. Ulcers resolved with intralesional triamcinolone injection.

LEUKOPLAKIA   ICD-9:528.6 ∘ ICD-10:K13.2   □ ○→●

- Leukoplakia is a chronic white plaque/lesion in the oropharynx.
- Premalignant leukoplakia has histologic atypia.
- Leukoplakia is descriptive clinical term regarding morphology: *squamous cell carcinoma, in situ and invasive, must be ruled out.*
- *Findings:* a white plaque that cannot be wiped off and cannot be diagnosed as any other distinct lesion.

- Leukoplakia may be premalignant or malignant.
- Definitive diagnosis should be made on clinical findings and/or histology.
- When diagnosis is definitive histologically, "leukoplakia" is no longer appropriate.

The differential diagnosis of leukoplakia is shown in Table 34-1.

TABLE 34-1   Differential Diagnosis of Leukoplakia

Lesion/Disorder	Characteristics
Leukoedema	Grayish-white opalescence of buccal mucosa; variant of normal. Histology: acanthosis.
Frictional keratosis	Keratosis secondary to friction (e.g., sharp tooth, rough or overextended denture border).
Chronic chewing: lip, tongue, cheek	Form of frictional keratosis. Surface white, rough. On buccal mucosa, wedge-shaped.
Linea alba	Occurs on buccal mucosa at edge of teeth (occlusal plane). Occurs normally or with teeth-clenching.
Nicotine stomatitis	Chemical irritation from smoking pipe, cigar, cigarette. Occurs on hard palate; obstructs minor salivary glands on palate; ducts become inflamed. Ducts appear raised, erythematous dots on posterior hard palate and soft palate. White appearance resolves with cessation of smoking. Not considered premalignant.
Tobacco chewer's white lesion	Develops where chewing tobacco is held. Mucosa granular or wrinkled. *Location:* mucobuccal fold. Lesion is premalignant. Usually resolves with discontinuation of tobacco.
Hairy tongue (Fig. 34-2)	Elongation of filiform papillae of dorsal tongue; color white, brown, or black. See above.
Aspirin/chemical burn	Occurs following placement of aspirin tablet on mucosal surface. Mucosal surface becomes necrotic; white/painful lesion loosely adherent, easily sloughs off.
Oral hairy leukoplakia (see Fig. 31-3)	See above and HIV disease (Section 31). White corduroy appearance on inferolateral aspect of tongue.
Premalignant leukoplakia	Severity linked to duration and quantitiy of tobacco and alcohol use. Location: lip, tongue, floor of mouth. Erythroleukoplakia (speckled leukoplakia) has the highest rate of malignant transformation).
HPV: condyloma acuminatum, verruca vulgaris (Fig. 34-18), squamous papilloma	*Findings:* white papules, plaques; small, sessile, papillated, exophytic. Solitary, multiple, mosaic.
Verrucous carcinoma	See below.
Other white lesions	Keratoacanthoma, squamous acanthoma, submucous fibrosis (betel nut chewing), white sponge nevus

ERYTHEMATOUS LESIONS AND/OR LEUKOPLAKIA ◘ ◑→●

- Erythematous lesions ± leukoplakia appear red because of inflammation, hemorrhage, increased angiogenesis, epithelial atrophy, acantholysis, ulceration.

- The differential diagnosis is shown in Table 34-2.

TABLE 34-2 Differential Diagnosis of Erythematous Lesion and/or Leukopkakia

Lesion/Disorder	Characteristics
Dysplasia, squamous cell carcinoma in situ (SCCIS) (Fig. 34-10)	Findings: white (leukoplakic, red/white; erythroleukoplakic), or red (erythroplakic). Suspicious lesions have erythroplakic components with poorly defined borders, nonhomogeneous colorations, ulcerations.
Invasive SCC (Figs. 34-11, and 34-12)	See below.
Candidiasis: erythematous	See Section 25, "Candidiasis."
Migratory glossitis (geographic tongue)	Findings: mixed red/white areas on dorsal tongue, depapillation, sharply marginated by whitish rim; maplike or "geographic" appearance. Course: intermittently remits and recurs, creating the appearance of migration lesions (Fig. 34-3) over days to weeks. Etiology: idiopathic; may be associated with psoriasis. About 40% of patients also have a fissured tongue.
Radiotherapy (XRT)-induced mucositis	Onset after XRT: 1–2 weeks. Findings: mucosal painful erythema, necrosis, ulceration. Salivary dysfunction. Stomatodynia, dysphagia. Dessicated lips and oral mucosa, dental caries, candidiasis, poorly fitting dentures. Healing begins after completion of XRT.
Chemotherapy-induced mucositis	Similar to those of XRT-induced mucositis.
Oral lichen planus (Fig. 34-4)	See "Lichen Planus," above. Lichenoid form: lacelike pattern on buccal mucosa, gingiva. Erosive, ulcerative form: buccal, labial, gingival, glossal mucosa. Lichenoid lesions occur as adverse mucosal drug reactions, graft-versus-host disease.
Lupus erythematosus (Fig. 34-17)	See "Lupus Erythematosus," Section 14.

PREMALIGNANT AND MALIGNANT NEOPLASMS   ICD-10:C14

DYSPLASIA AND SQUAMOUS CELL CARCINOMA IN SITU (SCCIS)

- *Etiology*: Tobacco-related habits [smoking moist snuff, pan (betel nut)]; human papillomavirus (HPV).
- *Risk factors*: Tobacco use, alcohol use, oral lichen planus.
- *Oncogenesis*: Complex, multifocal process, multiclonal field carcinogenesis, and intraepithelial clonal spread; multifocal nature of early process reduces efficacy of local treatment.
- *Findings*: Chronic, ± solitary patch/plaque on oropharyngeal mucosa. ± Reddish velvety appearance with either stippled or patchy regions of leukoplakia (Fig. 34-10). ± Smooth patch with minimal or no leukoplakia.
- *Size*: Usually <2 cm. *Location*: Floor of mouth (men); tongue and buccal surface (women).
- *Course*: Most dysplasia do not progress to invasive SCC; some do.
- Biopsy all lesions that persist for >3 weeks without definitive diagnosis.

FIGURE 34-10   Squamous cell carcinoma in situ: inferolateral tongue   A 72-year-old male with an asymptomatic lesion on the tongue noticed by his dentist. A 6-mm white plaque (leukoplakia) on the tongue. Biopsy reported SCCIS. The lesion was excised.

ORAL INVASIVE SQUAMOUS CELL CARCINOMA (See also Section 11)

- High associated morbidity and mortality, accounting for about 5% of all neoplasms in men and 2% of those in women.
- *Findings*: Usually appears as a granulating, velvety plaque or nodule with stippled hyperkeratosis ± ulceration (Fig. 34-11) (lips, floor of the mouth, central and lateral sides of the tongue).
- Biopsy all lesions that persist for >3 weeks without definitive diagnosis.
- *Management*: Aggressive surgical intervention.

FIGURE 34-11 Invasive squamous cell carcinoma: palate An advanced leukoplakic tumor on the hard palate of a cigarette smoker.

ORAL VERRUCOUS CARCINOMA

- *Etiology*: Oncogenic HPV types 16, 18.
- *Findings*: Extensive hyperkeratotic white leukoplakia (Fig. 34-12).

- *Course*: Metastasizes late. Biopsy all lesions that persist for >3 weeks without definitive diagnosis.
- *Management*: Aggressive surgical intervention.

FIGURE 34-12 Verrucous carcinoma: buccal mucosa Extensive thick plaque arising on the buccal mucosa.

OROPHARYNGEAL MELANOMA (See also Section 12) □ ●

- *Incidence*: 4% of primary oral malignancies.
- For the most part, lesions are asymptomatic; often advanced when first detected.
- *Findings*: Presents as pigmented lesion (Fig. 34-13), with variegation of color and irregular borders; rarely amelanotic. In situ lesions are macular; sites of invasion are usually raised within the in situ lesion.

- *Distribution*: 80% arise on pigmented mucosa of the palate and gingiva.
- *Risk factors*: More deeply pigmented individuals (Africans) have higher proportional incidence rates of mucosal melanoma than whites (because of the lower incidence of cutaneous melanoma).

FIGURE 34-13 Melanoma: hard palate A large, highly variegated pigmented lesion in a 63-year-old male. Lesional biopsy of a raised part showed invasive acrolentiginous melanoma.

SUBMUCOSAL NODULES

MUCOCELE ICD-9:527.6 ∘ ICD-10:K11.6 ◧ ○

- These arise following rupture of minor salivary gland.
- *Findings*: Nodule with mucus-filled cavity, with a thick roof (Fig. 34-14). Chronic lesions are firm, inflamed, poorly circumscribed nodules; bluish, translucent; fluctuant.

- *Location*: Develops at sites where minor salivary glands are easily traumatized: mucous membranes of the lip and floor of the mouth.
- *Course*: Chronic, recurrent, and then it presents as a firm, inflamed nodule.

Synonym: Ranula

FIGURE 34-14 **Mucocele** A well-defined, soft bluish submucosal fluctuant nodule on the lip. Thick clear mucus drained when the lesion was incised.

IRRITATION FIBROMA ICD-10 : M8810/0

- This is a submucosal nodular scar, occurring at a site of recurrent trauma (Fig. 34-15).
- *Findings*: Sessile or pedunculated, well-demarcated nodule, usually 2 cm in diameter (may be large if neglected). Normal color of the mucous membrane to pink-red; firm to hard.

- *Location*: Buccal mucosa along bite line; tongue, gingiva, labial mucosa.

Synonym: Bite fibroma

FIGURE 34-15 **Irritation fibroma: lower lip** A 58-year-old female with a lesion on the lip for 10 years. She frequently bites it when chewing. There is a rubbery pink nodule at the reflection of the labial mucosa.

CUTANEOUS ODONTOGENIC (DENTAL) ABSCESS   □ ◑

- A periapical dental abscess can extend into the overlying soft tissues, tracking and draining on the face. (Fig. 34-16).

FIGURE 34-16   Cutaneous odontogenic absces: cheek   A 23-year-old healthy female notes a lesion on the cheek for 6 months. **A.** Nodule on the lower left cheek near the jawline with surrounding erythema and scar-like depression. **B.** Molar with advanced caries and underlying dental abscess.

CUTANEOUS DISORDERS INVOLVING THE MOUTH

Cutaneous disorders may present in oral mucosa; may be confined to this site for months before cutaneous involvement occurs.

PEMPHIGUS VULGARIS (PV) (See also Section 6)   ICD-9:694.4 ∘ ICD-10:L10.0

- Often presents in oral mucosa; may be confined to this site for months before cutaneous bullae occur.
- *Findings*: Blisters are very fragile, rupture easily, rarely seen. Sharply marginated erosions of the mouth (buccal mucosa, hard and soft palate, and gingiva) are presenting symptoms. Erosions are extremely painful, interfering with nutrition.
- Biopsy confirms diagnosis (see "Pemphigus Vulgaris," Section 6).

PARANEOPLASTIC PEMPHIGUS (See also Section 18)   ICD-9:694.4

- Painful mucosal erosions. Cutaneous blisters and erosions. (See Fig. 18-19).
- Confirmed or occult malignancy.
- Acantholysis, keratinocyte necrosis, interface dermatitis. IgG and complement (C3) within the epidermal intercellular spaces and basement membrane. Circulating antibodies specific for stratified or transitional epithelium.

BULLOUS PEMPHIGOID (See also Section 6)   ICD-9:694.5 ∘ ICD-10:L12.0

- In contrast to pemphigus vulgaris, bullous pemphigoid uncommonly affects the oropharynx.
- *Findings*: Blisters, which initally are tense, erupt on the buccal mucosa and the palate, rupture, and leave sharply defined erosions that are practically indistinguishable from those of PV.
- However, erosions less painful and less extensive than in PV, where lesions occur only in the oropharynx.
- Diagnosis, see "Bullous Pemphigoid," Section 6.

CICATRICIAL PEMPHIGOID (See Section 6)   ICD-9 : 694.6 ∘ ICD-10 : L12.1   ☐ ●

- Autoimmune mucosal blistering disease that heals with scarring.
- Clinical manifestations dependent on sites involved. Persistent painful erosions on mucous membranes. Desquamative gingivitis with painful

erosions on tongue, buccal, and palatal mucosa. Ocular synblepharon.
- Sequelae: decreased vision/blindness; hoarseness, upper airway compromise, esophageal stenosis.

SYSTEMIC DISEASES INVOLVING THE MOUTH

LUPUS ERYTHEMATOSUS (See also Section 14)   ICD-9 : 710.0 ∘ ICD-10 : L93

- Mucosal involvement occurs in approximately 25% of those with chronic cutaneous lupus erythematosus (CCLE).
- *Findings*: Lesions: painless erythematous patches to chronic plaques, sharply marginated, irregularly scalloped white borders, radiating white striae, and telangiectasia. In older lesions: central depression, painful ulceration.

- *Distribution*: buccal mucosa; palate (Fig. 34-17), alveolar process, tongue. Chronic plaques may also appear on the vermilion border of the lips (Fig. 34-18).
- In acute systemic lupus erythematosus (SLE), ulcers arise in purpuric necrotic lesions of the palate (80%), buccal mucosa, or gums.

BEHÇET DISEASE See above and Section 14

STEVENS-JOHNSON SYNDROME / TOXIC EPIDERMONECROLYSIS See Section 8

ADVERSE DRUG REACTIONS See Section 22
ACTINIC CHEILITIS ■ ◑

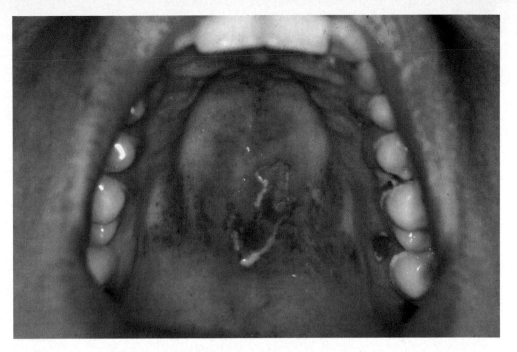

FIGURE 34-17 Lupus erythematosus: hard palate Erythematous eroded plaques were associated with chronic cutaneous LE.

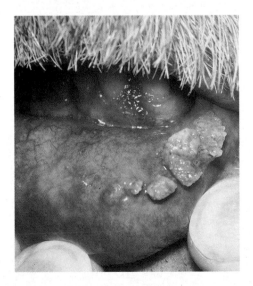

FIGURE 34-18 Condyloma acuminatum: mucosal lip A 35-year-old male with advanced HIV/AIDS has had oral lesions for 6 months. Cluster of white cauli-flower-floret-like lesions on the mucosa of the lower lip.

DISORDERS OF THE GENITALIA, PERINEUM, AND ANUS

- Anogenital skin and mucosa are subject to unique disorders because of their special anatomy.
- Dermatologic and systemic disorders occur in the anogenital region.
- Primary neoplasms arise in these areas, most commonly associated with chronic human papillomavirus (HPV) infection.
- Sexually transmitted as well as other infections also occur commonly in these sites.

VARIANTS OF GENITAL ANATOMY

These normal structures, newly observed, give rise to great concerns about sexual transmitted infections such as anogenital warts and molluscum contagiosum.

PEARLY PENILE PAPULES

- Normal anatomic structures. *Incidence*: Up to 19%.
- *Symptoms*: Asymptomatic; may arouse some anxiety when first noted.
- *Clinical findings*: Skin-colored 1- to 2-mm, discrete, domed papules evenly distributed circumferentially around the corona (Fig. 35-1), giving a cobblestone pattern.
- *Differential diagnosis*: Condylomata acuminatum, molluscum contagiosum
- *Histology*: Angiofibromas.
- *Management*: Reassurance: normal anatomic structures.

Synonym: Angiofibromas

SEBACEOUS GLAND PROMINENCE

- Normal sebaceous glands. Analogous to sebaceous gland on mucosa of mouth.
- *Locations*: Penis, vulva.
- *Manifestation*: 2-mm dermal papule; cream colored. May be arranged in rows.

Synonyms: Tyson glands, sebaceous hyperplasia, "ectopic" sebaceous glands, Fordyce condition

FIGURE 35-1   Pearly penile papules   Pink (skin-colored), 1- to 2-mm papules are seen regularly spaced along the corona of the glans penis. These structures, which are part of the normal anatomy of the glans, are commonly mistaken for condylomata or molluscum contagiosum.

ANGIOKERATOMA   ■ ○

- Ectatic thin-walled blood vessels in the superficial dermis with overlying epidermal hyperplasia.
- Increasingly common with aging.
- Multiple purple, smooth, 2- to 5-mm papules. Bleed with trauma. (See Section 9, Fig. 9-27).
- *Location*: Scrotum, glans penis, penile shaft. Labia, vulva

- Differentiate from angiokeratomas of Fabry disease (usually pinhead size, found on bathing trunk area and upper thighs), Kaposi sarcoma.
- *Management*: Reassurance. electrosurgery

Synonym: Angiokeratomas of Fordyce

CHRONIC PAIN SYNDROME   ◧ ○

- *Pathogenesis*: Unknown.
- *Symptoms*: Itching, burning, redness, pain on vulva, penis/scrotum, or perineum.
- *Manifestations*: Absence of mucocutaneous findings.

- Differentiate from dysmorphophobia, depression, psychosis.

Synonyms: Penodynia, scrotodynia, red or burning scrotum syndrome, vulvodynia, perineal pain.

DISORDERS SPECIFIC TO GENITAL ANATOMY

SCLEROSING LYMPHANGITIS OF PENIS

- *Etiology*: Trauma associated with vigorous sexual activity.
- *Pathogenesis*: Lymphatic stasis may result in thrombosed lymphatic vessels. Subsequent recanalization and fibrosis of walls of lymphatic vessels.
- *Clinical findings*: Painless, firm, at times nodular, translucent serpiginous cord appears suddenly, usually parallel to corona; not attached to overlying epidermis (Fig. 35-2).
- *Course*: Resolves spontaneously in weeks to months.

Synonyms: Nonvenereal sclerosing lymphangitis, penile venereal edema, Mondor phlebitis

CHRONIC LYMPHEDEMA OF THE GENITALIA

- Acute idiopathic scrotal edema. Occurs in young boys. Resolves spontaneously in 1–4 days. Differentiate from acute scrotum. Also reported in adults with dengue hemorrhagic fever, Henoch-Schönlein purpura.
- Lymphogranuloma venereum (see Section 30). Occurs in chronic undiagnosed infection. Both sexes. Referred to as *esthiomene*: elephantiasis due to lymphatic obstruction. Chronic. Deformitiy of penis referred to as "saxaphone penis."
- Chronic recurrent bacterial infection (Fig. 35-3).
- Kaposi sarcoma.
- Filarial or lymphatic elephantiasis. Caused by parasitic worms such as *Wuchereria bancroftii, Brugia malayi, B. timori*. Associated with elephantiasis of legs.

Synonym: Lymphangiofibrosis thrombotica occlusiva

PLASMA CELL BALANITIS AND VULVITIS

- Asymptomatic red glistening plaque(s) on glans penis (Fig. 35-4) or vulva.
- Differentiate from squamous cell carcinoma in situ.
- *Management*: Circumcision is curative.

Synonym: Zoon balanitis

*In uncircumcised males

FIGURE 35-3   Chronic lymphedema: scrotum   A 29-year-old male with history of recurrent scrotal infections and scrotal swelling. The scrotum is huge with noncompressible lymphedema and the penis is retracted. Recurrent bacterial infections have destroyed lymphatic channels.

FIGURE 35-2   Sclerosing lymphangitis: penis   A dermal cord on the distal shaft parallel to the corona.

FIGURE 35-4   Plasma cell balanitis   A 65-year-old male with penile lesion for 10 years. Solitary red glistening plaque in an uncircumcised male. Biopsy confirmed the diagnosis.

PHIMOSIS, PARAPHIMOSIS, BALANITIS XEROTICA OBLITERANS   ICD-9:605 ○ ICD-10:N47

- *Phimosis*: nonretractable foreskin. *Etiology*: Lichen sclerosus, nonspecific balanoposthitis (posthitis is inflammation of foreskin or prepuce), lichen planus, cicatricial pemphigoid, chronic lymphedema, Kaposi sarcoma. Precludes examination of glans for precancerous changes (Fig. 35-5).

- *Balanitis xerotica obliterans*: End stage of chronic phimosis. Foreskin fibrotic, contracted, fixed over

  glans and cannot be retracted over glans. Most often end-stage lichen sclerosus, which is commonly referred to as BXO (see Section 7, lichen sclorosus).

- *Paraphimosis*: Foreskin fixed in retraction. *Etiology*: vigorous sexual activity, acute contact urticaria, acute allergic contact dermatitis, lichen sclerosus (Fig. 35-6).

FIGURE 35-5   Phimosis   The prepuce or foreskin has been chronically inflamed with scarring andis no longer retractable over the glans penis

FIGURE 35-6   Paraphimosis   The prepuce or foreskin has been retracted proximally over the glans and cannot be replaced to the normal position covering the glans. The shaft is edematous.

MUCOCUTANEOUS DISORDERS

GENITAL (PENILE/VULVAR/ANAL) LENTIGINOSES   ■ ○

- *Onset*: Adulthood.
- *Clinical findings*: Tan, brown, intense blue-black; usually variegated, 5- to 15-mm macules
- *Sites*: In clusters on vulva (labia minora, Fig. 35-7), penis (glans, shaft) (Fig. 35-8), and perianal areas.
- *Course*: Persist for years without change in size.
- *Histology*: No significant melanocytic hyperplasia; nevus cells are not present; pigmentation due to increased melanin in basal cell layer.

- *Differential diagnosis*: Melanoma in situ, PUVA lentigo, fixed drug reaction, blue nevus, HPV-induced intraepithelial neoplasia (IN).
- *Diagnosis*: Dermoscopy rules out in situ melanoma; histology confirms diagnosis.
- Extensive lesions that cannot be easily removed should be followed photographically; areas that show significant change should be biopsied.

Synonyms: Penile lentigo, vulvar melanosis

FIGURE 35-7   Genital lentiginoses: vulva   Multiple, variegated dark brown macules, bilateral on the labia minora. Lesions had been present for >5 years and are multifocal in origin. Acrolentiginous melanoma in situ must be ruled out.

FIGURE 35-8   Genital lentiginoses: penis   A 42-year-old male with pigmentation of penis for 20 years. Variegated macular pigmentation of the glans and foreskin. Biopsy confirms the diagnosis, ruling out melanoma and HVP-infection (SCCIS).

VITILIGO AND LEUKODERMA (See also Section 13)

- *Etiology*: Loss of melanocytes results in depigmentation. Vitiligo. Chemically induced leukoderma.

- *Isomorphic* or *Koebner phenomenon*: Depigmentation at sites of injury: genital herpes, cryosurgery, imiquimod therapy.

- Wood lamp examination: Differentiates depigmentation from hypopigmentation.

- *Clinical findings*: Sharply dermarcated, depigmented, white macules (Fig. 35-9); examine skin for other depigmented areas.

- *Differential diagnosis*: Lichen sclerosus, site of genital herpes; iatrogenic after cryo-, electro-, or laser surgery.

FIGURE 35-9   Vitiligo: penis   Depigmentation of the proximal penile shaft. Multiple macules have become confluent. The lesions were an isolated finding.

PSORIASIS VULGARIS (See also Section 3)

- *Incidence*: Most common noninfectious dermatosis occurring on the glans penis and vulva.

- *Onset*: May be initial presentation of psoriasis.

- *Clinical findings*: (1) Erythematous scaling plaques on nonoccluded skin (Fig.35-10); (2) intertriginous psoriasis, well-dermarcated erythematous plaques without scale in naturally occluded skin (Fig. 35-11).

- *Distribution [intertriginous (inverse) psoriasis]*: Penis, vulva, intergluteal cleft, inguinal folds.

- *Differential diagnosis*: Lichen planus (LP), fixed drug eruption, condyloma acuminata, HPV-induced intraepithelial neoplasia, squamous cell carcinoma (SCC) in situ, invasive SCC.

FIGURE 35-10   Psoriasis vulgaris: shaft of penis   Well-demarcated scaling plaques on the penile shaft of a 25-year-old male. "Pinking" of the intergluteal cleft and nail findings of psoriasis were also present. The patient presented to a clinic for sexually transmitted disease.

FIGURE 35-11   Psoriasis vulgaris: intertriginous   A 75-year-old male with inguinal rash for decades, unresponsive to topical antifungal agents. An erythematous plaque is seen in the left inguinal area. Biopsy confirmed psoriasis, excluding extramammary Paget disease.

LICHEN PLANUS (See also Section 7)

- Commonly associated with LP at other sites: however, may occur as initial or sole manifestation.
- *Symptoms*: Not pruritic; pain in eroded lesions, anxiety about sexually transmitted disease (STD).
- *Clinical findings*: Violaceous flat-topped papules, discrete or confluent. Lacy white surface pattern most commonly on glans. Older lesions may have grayish hue with melanin incontinence. Annular lesions occur on glans and shaft (Fig. 35-12). Bullous and/or erosive LP (Fig. 35-13) on glans, vulva.
- *Distribution*: Glans, penile shaft (Fig. 35-12), vulva.
- *Course*: Spontaneous remission; erosive LP may persist for decades; SCC rarely. ⚡

FIGURE 35-12   Lichen planus, annular: penis   Violaceous annular plaques on the distal shaft and glans of a 26-year-old patient, present for >1 year. White lacelike plaques were also present on the buccal mucosa.

FIGURE 35-13   Lichen planus, erosive: penis
A 36-year-old male with painful erosions on penis for 6 months. He had previously been diagnosed and treated for herpes genitalis without improvement. Erythematous lesions on the glans and foreskin with erosions. Biopsy confirmed the diagnosis. Lesions resolved with intralesional triamcinolone injections.

LICHEN NITIDUS

- Probably micropapular variant of lichen planus.
- 1- to 2-mm papules on shaft of penis (Fig. 35-14).

FIGURE 35-14 Lichen nitidus: penis
Flat-topped papules on the shaft of the penis.

LICHEN SCLEROSUS (See also Section 7)

- *Symptoms*: Pruritus, burning; pain with ulceration.
- *Clinical findings*: Early: erythema ± hypopigmentation. Later: typical ivory- or porcelain-white macules and plaques; white due to loss of dermal vasculature (Fig. 35-15). Ecchymosis (Figs. 35-15, 35-16, 35-17), bullae, and/or erosions may occur in involved sites. May obstruct urethral orifice.
- *Demography*: Ten times move common in female. Causes of phimosis (Fig. 35-15) in boys.

- *End stage*: Balanitis xerotica obliterans (BXO). Effacement of normal architectural features: labia minora and clitoral hood may be reabsorbed (Fig. 35-16).
- *Course*: Invasive SCC can arise in this site of chronic inflammation.
- *Management*: Clobetasol ointment; monitor for steroid-induced atrophy pimecrolimus, tacrolimus.

Synonym: Lichen sclerosus et atrophicus

FIGURE 35-15   Lichen sclerosus: penis   A 17-year-old male with phimosis (inability to retract foreskin) for 6 months. White plaques on the periurethral glans and on the reflection of the foreskin. Lesions resolved with topical clobetasol ointment.

FIGURE 35-16   Lichen sclerosus: vulva and perineum   A large white sclerotic plaque extensively involving the anogenital region. The clitoral and labia minora region is completely atrophic (agglutination). Ecchymoses are noted in association with atrophy. Ulcerations can occur and are painful. Sclerosis was improved with clobetasol ointment therapy.

FIGURE 35-17 Lichen sclerosus: penis A 67-year-old male with lesions on the penis for 10 years. **A.** Whitish plaques on glans with typical ecchymoses; the urethral orifice was constricted. **B.** Five years later, the penis had become atrophic and submerged within the pubic fat, making urination difficult. A white sclerotic plaque with ecchymoses is seen on the stretched skin of the ventral penile shaft.

MIGRATORY NECROLYTIC ERYTHEMA (See also Section 18) □ ●

- Manifestation of glucagonoma syndrome.

- Painful erythematous plaques, glistening surface, serpiginous border surrounded by scaling. (See Fig. 18-14).

GENITAL APHTHOUS ULCERATIONS (See Section 34) ◧ ◖

- Idiopathic ulcers on scrotum or vulva. May be associated with oral aphthous ulcerations. May occur as a manifestation of primary HIV/AIDS.

- Occur as part of the syndrome complex of Behçet disease (Fig. 35-18). (See also Figs. 14-14 and 14-15).

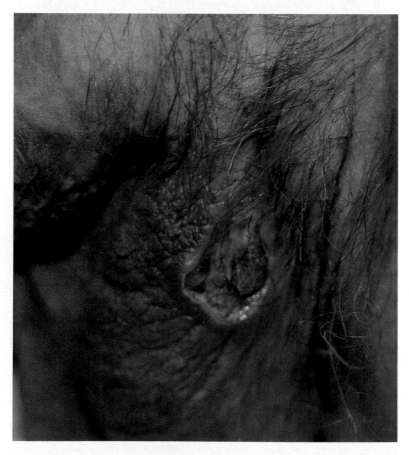

FIGURE 35-18 Aphthous ucler, Behçet disease: scrotum A 42-year-old male with recurrent scrotal ulcerations, treated with azathioprine. A large ulcer with gray base and elevated margins is seen on the scrotum. The ulcer healed with thalidomide 50 mg BID.

ECZEMATOUS DERMATITIS

ALLERGIC CONTACT DERMATITIS (See also Section 2)   ■ ◑

- On genitalia is often more florid and symptomatic than at other sites.
- *Allergens*: Topically applied agents (medications, lubricants); haptens blotted onto genitals by hands (e.g., poison ivy sap).
- *Symptoms*: Intense pruritus, burning sensation; edema.

- *Clinical findings*: Erythema, microvesicles; edema; exudation of genitals (Fig. 35-19). With phytodermatitis (e.g., poison ivy or oak), lesions are usually present at other sites.
- *Differential diagnosis*: Genital herpes, atopic dermatitis, irritant dermatitis

FIGURE 35-19   Allergic contact dermatitis: penis Striking edema of the distal penile shaft associated with severe pruritus in a 21-year-old patient. He had touched poison ivy with his hands, transferring the resin to his penis while urinating; pruritus and then edema occurred within 24 h of exposure. The magenta-colored pigment is Castellani paint. The patient was initially seen in an urgent care unit where a diagnosis of cellulitis was made. Pruritus is the distinguishing feature of allergic contact dermatitis.

ATOPIC DERMATITIS, LICHEN SIMPLEX CHRONICUS (LSC), PRURITUS ANI   ■ ◑

- Atopic dermatitis: Usually associated with more widespread involvement but can be isolated to genitalia.
- Lichen simplex chronicus: Chronic rubbing/scratching result in a single plaque on scrotum (Fig. 35-20) vulva or anus (Fig. 35-21), persisting for years or decades. In dark skin, hypo- and hyperpigmentation occur (see Section 2).

- Pruritus ani: Can occur in the absence of any identifiable dermatologic disorder. Chronic pruritus and rubbing often produce some lichenification (Fig. 35-17). *Risk factors*: Atopic diathesis; multifactorial. *Secondary infection*: *Staphylococcus aureus,* group A and B streptococci, *Candida albicans,* and herpes simplex virus. *Management*: Discontinue compulsive rubbing/scratching; maintenance of perianal hygiene.

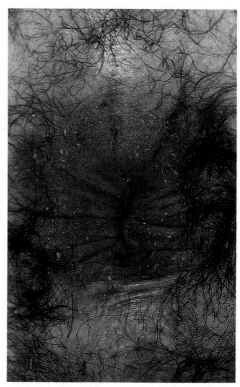

FIGURE 35-20   Lichen simplex chronicus: scrotum   Pruritic bilateral erythematous hyperpigmented plaques in a 46-year-old Hispanic male. Lesions had been present for >20 years. Lesions resolved following an injection of intralesional triamcinolone (3 mg/mL).

FIGURE 35-21   Lichen simplex chronicus: pruritus ani   The patient had experienced intense anal pruritus for many years. Perianal erythema with mild lichen simplex chronicus and fissure is associated with chronic rubbing of the skin.

FIXED DRUG ERUPTION (See also Section 22)

- Large blisters occur on the male genitalia commonly; evolve to painful erosion (Fig. 35-22).

- With repeated drug exposure, blisters/erosions recur at the same site.

FIGURE 35-22   Fixed drug eruption: trimethoprim-sulfamethoxazole   Violaceous bullae that had ruptured, occurring on the dorsum of the penis (glans and shaft), recurring after treatment with trimethoprim-sulfamethoxazole in a male with HIV/AIDS.

PREMALIGNANT AND MALIGNANT LESIONS

SQUAMOUS CELL CARCINOMA IN SITU

- *Terminology*: Squamous cell carcinoma in situ (SCCIS) is generic; intraepithelial neoplasia (IN) is HPV-induced SCCIS.
- *Etiology*: HPV infection, chronic low-grade balanoposthitis (poor hygiene, LS) in older individuals; chronic dermatoses (ulcerative lichen planus, lichen sclerosus).
- *Clinical findings*: Solitary, well-defined, irregularly bordered, red patch with a glazed-to-velvety surface hyperkeratosis on the penis (Fig. 30-8) or vulva; associated dermatoses. HPV-associated lesions are usually multifocal, occurring at any sites of the anogenital region (Fig. 35-23).

- *Diagnosis*: Lesional biopsy.
- *Course*: Appearance of a nodule or ulcer suggests progression to invasive SCC (Fig. 35-24). In HPV-associated SCCIS, rate of transformation to invasive SCC is relatively low; rate is higher for vulvar SCCIS: Rate of invasiveness and metastasis higher when associated with poor hygiene/chronic balanoposthitis. (See also Sections 11 and 30.)

Synonyms: Erythroplasia of Queyrat; Bowen disease, bowenoid papulosis.

FIGURE 35-23   HPV-induced squamous cell carcinoma in situ: perianal   A 35-year-old male with HIV/AIDS with asymptomatic anal lesion for several years. A well-demarcated pink perianal plaque. Anal Pap test showed low-grade squamous intraepithelial lesion (LSIL). All clinical findings resolved with 5% imiquimod cream and effective antiretroviral therapy. He has remained lesion-free for 6 years.

HPV-INDUCED INTRAEPITHELIAL NEOPLASIA (IN) AND SQUAMOUS CELL CARCINOMA IN SITU (See also Section 30)

- *Etiology*: HPV types 16, 18, 31, 33.
- *Risk factors*: Immunosuppression, occurring in HIV/AIDS disease, iatrogenically induced immunosuppression in solid organ transplantation.
- *Clinical findings*: Erythematous patches and papules (flat-topped), (Figs. 30-8, 35-23, 35-25); pigmented papules. *Arrangement*: Solitary, clustering, confluence, plaque(s) formation. *Distribution*: Mucosa and anogenital and inguinocrural skin.

- *Course*: Spontaneous resolution; persist for years; multiple new lesions appear; progress to invasive SCC. Progression to invasive SCC highest in cervix, anus. Monitor cervix/anus by periodic Pap testing (cytology) to detect dysplastic changes.
  - IN I: mild dysplasia
  - IN II: moderate dysplasia
  - IN III: neoplastic cells penetrate into upper third of epithelial layers; SCCIS
  - Invasive SCC: neoplastic cells penetrate stromal layer of epithelium

FIGURE 35-24 Squamous cell carcinoma in situ arising in lichen sclerosus: vulva A 60-year-old patient with longstanding genital lichen sclerosus. Erythema and erosions with marked atrophy of the labia minora and clitoris. Lesional biopsy of a white hyperkeratotic area shows associated SCC in situ arising in lichen sclerosus.

FIGURE 35-25 HPV-induced invasive squamous cell carcinoma: perineum A 35-year-old HIV/AIDS-infected male presented with a perineal tumor of several months duration. Histology of the excised specimen showed invasive SCC.

INVASIVE ANOGENITAL SQUAMOUS CELL CARCINOMA

INVASIVE SCC OF PENIS

- *Risk factors*: Lack of circumcision, poor penile hygiene, phimosis (25–75%), low socioeconomic status, HPV infection (15–80%), UV-radiation exposure, tobacco use.
- *Demography*: More common in developing nations (up to 10% of cancers in men; rare in industrialized nations).
- *Precancerous lesion/disorders*: Phimosis, chronic balanoposthitis, pseudoepitheliomatous keratotic and micaceous balanitis, lichen planus, lichen sclerosus, giant condyloma, HPV-induced IN.
- *Symptoms*: Precursor lesion, itching/burning under foreskin, ulceration of glans or prepuce.
- *Clinical findings*: Subtle induration; small excrescence; small papule; warty growth to an obvious extensive carcinoma with sloughing. Necrosis and/or secondary infection in phimotic foreskin. Extends along the penile shaft and involves corpora cavernosa. Rarely, bleeding, urinary fistula, and urinary retention occur.
- *Distribution*: Glans (48%), prepuce (21%), glans and prepuce (9%), prepuce glans and shaft (14%), coronal sulcus (6%), shaft (<2%).
- *Metastasis*: Inguinal lymph node metastases; distant sites rare. ⚡

INVASIVE SCC OF VULVA

- *Risk factors*: HPV infection, abnormal cervical Pap test, immunosuppression, HIV/AIDS disease, advanced age, increased number of sexual partners, younger age at first episode of intercourse, tobacco use, lichen planus, lichen sclerosus (Fig. 35-24).
- *Symptoms*: Vulvar pruritus, localized pain, discharge, dysuria, bleeding, ulceration.
- *Clinical findings*: IN, bulky whitish or pigmented lesion of thickened or hard skin; verrucoid, polypoid, papular. *Location*: 65% arise on labia majora.

INVASIVE SCC OF CUTANEOUS ANUS

- *Etiology*: Oncogenic HPV infection. *Risk factors*: Chronic immunosuppression, HIV/AIDS disease. *Location*: (1) Cutaneous, (2) junction of columnar and squamous epithelium.
- *Precursor lesion*: Anal IN. *Clinical findings*: Papule, nodule, ulcerated nodule (Fig. 35-25).

GENITAL VERRUCOUS CARCINOMA

- *Etiology*: HPV infection.
- *Clinical findings*: Large, cauliflower-like, warty tumors (Fig. 35-26).
- *Distribution*: Vulva, penis, anus.
- *Course*: Slow-growing; rarely metastasize. ⚡

MALIGNANT MELANOMA OF THE ANOGENITAL REGION (See also Section 12)   ☐ ●

- Incidence: Rare.

- *Precursor lesions*: Preexisting pigmented lesion or de novo from epidermal melanocytes.

- *Clinical findings*: Macules or papules with variegation of brown-black color, irregular borders, and often with papular elevation (Fig. 35–26) or ulceration.

- *Distribution*: Males: glans (67%), prepuce (13%), urethral meatus (10%), penile shaft (7%), and coronal sulcus (3%) (Fig. 35-26); females: labia minora, clitoris (Fig. 35-27).

- *Differential diagnosis*: Genital lentiginosis, old fixed drug eruption, SCC, hemangioma, intraepithelial neoplasia (Bowenoid papulosis).

- *Histologic types*: Acral lentiginous melanoma; rarely, desmoplastic melanoma.

- *Prognosis*: Poor because of early metastases via lymphatic vessels; most patients die within 1–3 years. 🖉

FFIGURE 35-26   Melanoma, invasive: penis   A violaceous nodule arising in an area of macular variegated hyperpigmentation in a 60-year-old male. The macular lesions had been present for 5 years and resembled genital lentiginosis. The most common histologic type of genital melanoma is the acrolentiginous melanoma.

FIGURE 35-27   Melanoma, invasive: vulva   A violaceous nodule in a black plaque in a 52-year-old female.

EXTRAMAMMARY PAGET DISEASE (See also Section 18)   □ ●

- Often undiagnosed for years or decades; treated as intertrigo.
- Well-demarcated plaques in underpants area (Fig. 35-28). ⟳

KAPOSI SARCOMA (See Section 20)   □ → ■ ◑

- Common in advanced untreated HIV/AIDS.
- *Location*: Penis and scrotum.
- *Manifestations*: Violaceous papules, nodules, plaques; become confluent. Edema of penis and scrotum (Fig. 35-29). ⟳

ANOGENITAL INFECTIONS

- Bacterial infections, see Section 24
- Mucocutaneous anogenital fungal infections, see Section 25
  - Dermatophytosis and tinea versicolor occur on keratinizing skin only. Rarely occur on shaft of penis
- Candidiasis is common on naturally occluded sites on the penis, vulva, vagina
- STI, see Section 29

FIGURE 35-28 **Extramammary Paget disease (EMP): penis, scrotum, inguinal area** A 94-year-old male with recurrent red plaques for several years. EMP had been excised by Mohs micrographic surgery twice previously but recurred. Well-demarcated bright red plaques are seen. Biopsy confirmed the diagnosis. The lesions were effectively treated with electron beam radiotherapy.

FIGURE 35-29 **Kaposi sarcoma: penis** A 46-year-old male with HIV/AIDS has swelling of penis and legs for 8 months. Multiple nodules are seen on the glans and shaft of the penis. Massive swelling of the penis was caused by tumor infiltration and lymphatic obstruction, resulting in urinary obstruction. Similar obstruction caused edema of both legs. The patient was noncompliant with antiretroviral therapy and treatment of Kaposi sarcoma

GENERALIZED PRURITUS WITHOUT SKIN LESIONS (PRURITUS SINE MATERIA)

- Persistent severe pruritus, like pain, is a dominating factor in existence; from day to day it takes over one's life. Intense pruritus may, in fact, be more maddening for the patient than pain.

- The physician, therefore, often feels somewhat helpless in the management of these unfortunate patients.

- Pruritus leads to sleepless nights; a state of permanent fatigue ensues that precludes work and confounds family relationships. Most skin eruptions and rashes are more or less pruritic, but there are states where there is severe pruritus in the absence of skin lesions, except for scratch marks (Fig. 36-1). This is called *pruritus sine materia* (from Latin, "itch without physical substrate").

- The diagnostic approach to the patient with generalized pruritus without identifiable skin lesions is a *diagnosis of exclusion*.

- This pruritus may be intrinsic to the skin but not due to a skin disease with specific lesions.

- It may be a symptom of a skin disease that at the time of examination does not manifest with specific lesions.

- It may be due to an internal organ disease, metabolic and endocrine conditions, or hematologic disease.

- It may be a manifestation of malignant tumors, psychogenic states, or HIV-1 infection; or it may be related to injected or ingested drugs.

- The various causes of pruritus sine materia are listed in Table 36-1, and an algorithm of how to approach a patient with pruritus sine materia is shown in Table 36-2.

- A careful history and physical examination are essential and should take into account the different types of itching and their duration, the quality of itching, and its distribution and timing.

- It is understood that any patient referred with generalized pruritus without skin lesions should be assumed to have minimal or latent disease of the skin until proven otherwise.

- Skin signs may be clinically inapparent, perhaps confined to only circumscribed areas, and this is particularly important with regard to the exclusion of scabies, pediculosis, or conditions such as urticaria factitia.

MOST IMPORTANT CAUSES

Chronic renal disease: Pruritus is one of the most important and distressing problems of chronic renal failure, affecting up to 50% of patients. Secondary skin lesions may develop due to intense scratching, such as nummular eczema, prurigo nodularis, or lichenified plaques.

Cholestasis: Distressing persistent pruritus accompanying biliary obstruction starts with an acral distribution and becomes generalized. It may be due to both bile salts in the skin and elevated levels of opioid peptides.

Endocrine disease: Intractable itching occurs in thyrotoxicosis, probably due to increased blood flow, and in hypothyroidism, where it is probably due to excessive skin dryness. In contrast to previous beliefs, pruritus is not a feature of diabetes mellitus but can be a manifestation of diabetic neuropathy.

Hematologic disease: Pruritus occurs in about 50% of patients with polycythemia vera, often after contact with water ("bath itch"), and may be associated with raised blood histamine levels. In Hodgkin disease it is a presenting symptom, and it occurs in leukemias; in cutaneous mastocytosis (without visible skin lesions), it usually occurs locally following rubbing the skin.

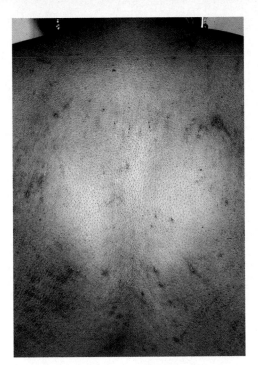

FIGURE 36-1 Pruritus without diagnostic skin lesions This patient had multiple scratch marks due to compulsive scratching because of severe pruritus. There were no other, and in particular, diagnostic lesions. Workup revealed biliary cirrhosis without jaundice.

HIV infection: Pruritus may occur as a primary symptom of HIV infection and may be pruritus sine materia or be associated with infestations; xerosis; or hepatic disease, renal disease, lymphoma, or adverse drug reactions.

Senile pruritus: This is common in persons aged ≥70 years and in many patients. No causes found. Desiccation of the skin may be one reason, but sometimes pruritus may also be provoked by water contact mimicking aquagenic pruritus (see below).

Psychiatric disease: Localized pruritus is often a common manifestation of chronic anxiety, and persistent rubbing of the localized area will result in lichenification. Parasitophobia is a more serious problem (see Section 23).

Aquagenic pruritus: This pruritus, usually in the middle aged and elderly, is provoked

TABLE 36-1 Causes of Pruritus Sine Materia

Metabolic, endocrine conditions
Hyperthyroidism
Hypothyroidism
Pregnancy related

Malignant neoplasms
Lymphoma, myeloid and lymphatic leukemia, myelodysplasia
Multiple myeloma
Hodgkin disease
Other cancer (rare)

Drug ingestion
Subclinical drug sensitivities
Aspirin, alcohol, dextran, polymyxin B, morphine, codeine, scopolamine, D-tubocurarine, IV hydroxyethyl starch

Infestations
Scabies*
Pediculosis corporis, capitis, pubis
Hookworm (ancylostomiasis)
Onchocerciasis
Ascariasis

Renal disease
Renal failure

Hematologic disease
Polycythemia vera
Paraproteinemia, iron deficiency

Hepatic disease
Obstructive biliary disease
Pregnancy (intrahepatic cholestasis) (see Section 15)

Psychogenic states
Transitory:
Periods of emotional stress
Persistent:
Delusions of parasitosis
Psychogenic pruritus
Neurotic excoriations
Anorexia nervosa

Latent dermatoses and miscellaneous conditions
Xerosis (dry skin, "winter itch")
Senile pruritus
Bullous pemphigoid (without skin lesions)
Dermatitis herpetiformis (without skin lesions)
Atopic dermatitis (without skin lesions)
Factitious urticaria (dermographism)
Fiber glass exposure
Aquagenic pruritus
Notalgia paresthetica
Brachioradial pruritus

*Diagnostic lesions may or may not be present.

TABLE 36-2 Approach to the Diagnosis of Generalized Pruritus Without Diagnostic Skin Lesions

It is critical to recognize that nonspecific skin changes can be induced by rubbing and scratching. The false conclusion that a dermatologic cause for itching is necessarily present just because a rash can be seen is a trap that must be avoided. The approach to the patient with persistent generalized pruritus begins with careful history and meticulous examination of the (entire) skin, followed by additional attention to the general history, review of systems, general physical examination, and investigations as outlined below.

Initial Visit

1. Detailed history of pruritus:
   - Are there any skin lesions that precede the itching?
   - Is the itching continuous or does it occur in waves?
   - Is the itching related to certain times of the day, does it occur at night, and does it keep the patient awake?
   - Is the itching related to environmental conditions (heat, cold); is it related to emotional stress, physical exertion, sweating; contact with water?
2. Examine carefully for subtle primary skin disorders as a cause of the pruritus; xerosis or asteatosis, scabies, pediculosis (nits?). Discrete papules on elbows, scalp (dermatitis herpetiformis), on scrotum or shaft of penis (scabies).
3. Check for dermographism, rub skin for Darier sign (see "Mastocytosis Syndromes," Section 19).
4. Repeat history related to pruritus. Obtain history of constitutional symptoms, weight loss, fatigue, fever, malaise. History of oral or parenteral medication that can be a cause of generalized pruritus without a rash.
5. General physical examination including *all* the lymph nodes; rectal examination and stool guaiac in adult patients.
6. If dry skin or winter itch is a reasonable possible explanation, give the patient bath oil, followed by an emollient ointment. No soap; the bath is therapeutic, not for cleansing the skin; shower to clean.
7. Follow-up appointment in 2 weeks.

Subsequent Visit(s)

If no relief from symptomatic treatment given on the first visit, proceed as follows:

1. Detailed review of systems.
2. Laboratory tests: complete blood tests including erythrocyte sedimentation rate, fasting blood sugar, renal function tests, liver function tests, hepatitis antigens, thyroid tests, stool and serologic examination for parasites.
3. If the diagnosis has not been established at this point, the patient should be referred for complete workup including pelvic examination and Pap smear.

SOURCE: Adapted from JD Bernhard (ed): *Itch Mechanisms and Management of Pruritus.* New York, McGraw-Hill, 1994, pp. 211–215.

by contact with water of any temperature; it lasts up to 1 h, and there are no visible signs on the skin. Elevated levels of histamine have been found in the blood and skin of such patients, and this condition must be distinguished from "bath-itch" in polycythemia vera or water-induced senile pruritus. The causes are unknown; since no lesions can be found, such patients are often labeled as neurotic.

Notalgia paresthetica: This is a common localized itch usually in the interscapular area, sometimes more widespread (Fig. 36-2). The sensations are part itch/part paresthesia. It is probably a neuropathic itch due to the entrapment of spinal nerves as they emerge through the muscle fascias of the back.

Brachioradial pruritus: This is a localized pruritus on the outer surface of the upper arm, elbow, and forearm, often associated with clinical evidence of chronic sun damage and xerosis (hence "golfer's itch").

MANAGEMENT

1. Identify and treat underlying disease.
2. Treat xerosis with baths and emollients.
3. UVB and narrow-band (311 nm) phototherapy or PUVA (in renal-, biliary-, aquagenic-, and polycythemia vera–related pruritus).
4. Nolaxone, naltrexone, or odansetron; cholestyramine in cholestatic itch (but ineffective in total biliary obstruction).

FIGURE 36-2 Notalgia paresthetica This condition in the interscapular region is characterized by intense pruritus without skin lesions. The erythema seen here is due to rubbing and scratching.

PRURITUS ANI   ICD-9:698.0 ◦ ICD-10:L29.0

- Many patients, in desperation, become resigned to accepting pruritus ani as part of their lives and endure the embarrassment and the sleepless nights.

- *Pruritus ani* is pruritus of the anal skin without evidence of a primary dermatologic disorder sometimes seen in this region, e.g., dermatophytosis, candidiasis, psoriasis, or seborrheic dermatitis, or of hemorrhoidal nodes.

- Pinworms are a rare cause and are seen usually only in children.

- The major factor in the pathogenesis of pruritus ani is irritation from the presence of fecal soiling on the anal skin; this is most often the result of incomplete cleansing of the area after defecation but also results in some persons from the weakness of the anal sphincter, which allows for fecal soiling when the rectum is distended by the arrival of feces or with flatus.

- The vicious cycle is irritation → itching → rubbing with the development of lichenification → more pruritus.

- When lichenification is present, control begins with a *very limited* course of potent topical glucocorticoids to reduce lichenification. The main thrust of management, however, must be directed at provoking factors:
  - *Paroxysmal compulsive rubbing and scratching of the anal sphincter and skin around it.* Anxiety and stress appear to contribute to the itching. The "fits" of rubbing or scratching occur most often after defecation and at night, when the patient is often awakened by the itching. These bouts of pruritus can be somewhat relieved by menthol-camphor lotions.
  - *Poor anal hygiene.* Strict, "squeaky" cleansing with cotton pledgets soaked in water is ideal. "Baby wipes" available in any supermarket/drugstore will also do the job. Whenever possible, a shower or tub bath is the best method of cleansing; a more convenient method is with a bidet. After cleansing the area, liberal application of talcum powder helps absorb the fecal soiling that can occur during the day; ointments and oily lotions may actually aggravate the pruritus.

APPENDICES

APPENDIX A: "TRAVEL" DERMATOLOGY

With the marked increase in international travel in the past decades among persons of all walks of life and all ages, it is necessary to ask patients with skin lesions where they have lived and traveled. This is particularly true for infectious skin disease or infectious systemic disease with skin manifestations. Website *http://www.cdc.gov/travel/index.com* gives information on diseases endemic in different parts of the world and on modes of acquisition. Links provide updated information relevant to diagnosis and thus appropriate treatment.

It is important to keep in mind that a patient with an infection acquired in one geographic location may undergo medical evaluation in another location where the infection is not endemic. Also, many infections may be rare or sporadically acquired in regions outside of endemic areas. An example is anthrax. Sporadic infection may be acquired in any geographic location by way of contact with imported contaminated animal products.

Equally important to note is that infections that require a specific vector for transmission have a distribution limited by the vector distribution. However, presence of the vector is not sufficient for disease to occur. For example, a mosquito competent to transmit dengue is found in many states in the southern United States. However, in recent years, transmission of dengue has been documented only rarely within the United States (Texas). Dengue, of course, is common in Asia and in other parts of the world.

APPENDIX B: DERMATOLOGIC MANIFESTATIONS OF DISEASES INFLICTED BY BIOLOGIC WARFARE/BIOTERRORISM

The use of microbial pathogens as potential or actual weapons of terrorism and warfare dates from antiquity. In 2001, the anthrax attacks via the U.S. postal system resulted in 12 cutaneous and 10 inhalational cases of anthrax with 4 deaths. These caused a tremendous amount of anxiety, had an impact on the U.S. postal system, and led to a functional interruption of the activities of the legislative branch of the U.S. government. The Working Group for Civilian Biodefense has compiled a list of characteristics of biologic agents that can be used as bioweapons (Table B-1), and the U.S. Centers for Disease Control and Prevention (CDC) has classified potential biologic agents into three categories: A, B, and C (Table B-2). Category A agents are the priority pathogens requiring special attention for public health preparedness. Many of these lead to skin signs and symptoms and are therefore of major concern to dermatologists. The potential bioterrorism diseases with dermatologic manifestations are

- Anthrax
- Plague
- Smallpox
- Smallpox vaccine (vaccinia)
- Tularemia
- Viral hemorrhagic fevers

Full information on plague and the viral hemorrhagic fevers as well as infections with anthrax by inhalation can be obtained at the CDC website *http://www.bt.cdc.gov/agent/agentlist.asp.*

Also, information on all of these agents and related links can be obtained at the following web-sites:

- *www.bt.cdc.gov/agent/smallpox/diagnosis/pdf/spox-poster-full.pdf*

- *http://www.cdc.gov/ncidod/dvrd/spb/mnpages/disinfo.htm*
- *http://jama.ama-assn.org/cgi/content/full/287/18/2391*

TABLE B-1   Key Features of Biologic Agents Used as Bioweapons

1. High morbidity and mortality	6. Potential to cause anxiety
2. Potential for person-to-person spread	7. Availability of pathogen and feasibility of production
3. Low infective dose and highly infectious by aerosol	8. Environmental stability
4. Lack of rapid diagnostic capability	9. Database of prior research and development
5. Lack of universally available effective vaccine	10. Potential to be "weaponized"

SOURCE: From L Borio et al: JAMA 287:2391, 2002, with permission.

TABLE B-2   CDC Category A, B, and C Agents

Category A
Anthrax (*Bacillus anthracis*)
Botulism (*Clostridium botulinum toxin*)
Plague (*Yersinia pestis*)
Smallpox (*Variola major*)
Tularemia (*Francisella tularensis*)
Viral hemorrhagic fevers
    Arenaviruses: Lassa, New World (Machupo, Junin, Guanarito, and Sabia)
    Bunyaviridae: Crimean, Congo, Rift Valley
    Filoviridae: Ebola, Marburg
    Flaviviridae: Yellow fever, Omsk fever, Kyasanur Forest

Category B
Brucellosis (*Brucella* spp.)
Epsilon toxin of *Clostridium perfringens*
Food safety threats (e.g., *Salmonella* spp., *Escherichia coli* 0157:H7, *Shigella*)
Glanders (*Burkholderia mallei*)
Melioidosis (*B. pseudomallei*)
Psittacosis (*Chlamydia psittaci*)
Q fever (*Coxiella burnettii*)
Ricin toxin from *Ricinus communis* (castor beans)
Staphylococcal enterotoxin B
Typhus fever (*Rickettsia prowazekii*)
Viral encephalitis [alphaviruses (e.g., Venezuelan, eastern, and western equine encephalitis)]
Water safety threats (e.g., *Vibrio cholerae, Cryptosporidium parvum*)

Category C
Emerging infectious disease threats such as Nipah, hantavirus, and SARS coronavirus.

SOURCE: Centers for Disease Control and Prevention and the National Institute of Allergy and Infectious Diseases.

APPENDIX C: CHEMICAL BIOTERRORISM AND INDUSTRIAL ACCIDENTS

Chemical agents have been used as weapons on a large scale in World War I, in the Iraq-Iran War, by Iraq against Kurdish civilians, and in the Sarin attacks in Japan. Industrial hazardous materials (HAZMATs), produced in chemical plants, could also be used as weapons in chemical terrorism.

Table C-1 lists potential agents for such attacks and the symptoms they elicit. Of these, the blistering agent sulfur mustard is one of the

TABLE C-1   Recognizing and Diagnosing Health Effects of Chemical Terrorism

Agent	Agent Name	Unique Characteristics	Initial Effects
Nerve	Cyclohexyl sarin (GF)	Miosis (pinpoint pupils)	Miosis (pinpoint pupils)
	Sarin (GB)	Copious secretions	Blurred/dim vision
	Soman (GD)	Muscle twitching/ fasciculations	Headache
	Tabun (GA)		Nausea, vomiting, diarrhea
	VX		Copious secretions/sweating
			Muscle twitching/fasciculations
			Breathing difficulty
			Seizures
Asphyxiant/blood	Arsine	Possible cherry red skin	Confusion
	Cyanogen chloride	Possible cyanosis	Nausea
	Hydrogen cyanide	Possible frostbite*	Patients may gasp for air, similar to asphyxiation but more abrupt onset
			Seizures prior to death
Choking/pulmonary damage	Chlorine	Chlorine is a greenish	Eye and skin irritation
	Hydrogen chloride	yellow gas with	Airway irritation
	Nitrogen oxides	pungent odor	Dyspnea, cough
	Phosgene	Phosgene gas smells like newly mown hay or grass	Sore throat
			Chest tightness
		Possible frostbite*	
Blistering/vesicant	Mustard/Sulfur mustard (HD, H)	Mustard (HD) has an odor like burning garlic or horseradish	Severe irritation
	Mustard gas (H)		Redness and blisters of the skin
	Nitrogen mustard (HN-1, HN-2, HN-3)		Tearing, conjunctivitis, corneal damages
	Lewisite (L)	Lewisite (L) has an odor like penetrating geranium	Mild respiratory distress to marked airway damage
	Phosgene oxime (CX)	Phosgene oxime (CX) has a pepperish or pungent odor	May cause death
			Dry mouth and skin
Incapacitating/ behavior-altering	Agent 15/BZ	May appear as mass drug intoxication with erratic behaviors, shared realistic and distinct hallucinations, disrobing and confusion	Initial tachycardia
			Altered consciousness, delusions, denial of illness, belligerence
		Hyperthermia	Hyperthermia
		Mydriasis (dilated pupils)	Ataxia (lack of coordination)
			Hallucinations
			Mydriasis (dilated pupils)

* Frostbite may occur from skin contact with liquid arsine, cyanogen chloride, or phosgene.
SOURCE: State of New York, Department of Health.

most likely agents to be used in a terrorist attack scenario, and it also induces skin lesions (see website *http://www.bt.cdc.gov/agent/agentlist.asp*).

Following exposure and an asymptomatic latent period, erythema, pruritus, burning, and pain may present; initial blistering of the skin will start on the second day after exposure and will progress for up to 2 weeks. Vesicles coalesce, forming large blisters, and wound healing is considerably slower than for a comparable thermal burn. Differential diagnoses are thermal burn or scalding, toxic epidermal necrolysis, and staphylococcal scalded skin syndrome. (See also W R Heymann: Threats of biological and chemical warfare on civilian populations. J Am Acad Dermatol 2004, 51:452.)

APPENDIX D: DRUG USE IN PREGNANCY[1]

The developing fetus can potentially be affected by any medication given to the mother. The disastrous effects of thalidomide and stilbestrol on the exposed offspring led to the development of the U.S. Food and Drug Administration (FDA) categories that are now assigned before a drug is released (Table D-1).

Table D-2 lists safe treatments for dermatologic diseases in pregnancy, and the common dermatologic diseases, the drugs used for them, and the drugs' pregnancy categories are listed in Table D-3.

TABLE D-1   FDA Pregnancy Categories for Drugs

A   No fetal risk in controlled studies.
B   No risk to human fetus despite possible animal risk or no risk in animal studies but human studies lacking.
C   Human risk cannot be ruled out. Animal studies may or may not show risk.
D   Evidence of risk to human fetus.
X   Contraindicated in pregnancy.

TABLE D-2   Safe Treatments for Dermatologic Disorders During Pregnancy

Disease	Medication Name
Acne	Topical clindamycin, erythromycin, benzoyl peroxide
Rosacea	Topical metronidazole, azelaic acid
Psoriasis	Topical glucocorticoids, calcipotriol, broad band UVB
Dermatitis	Topical glucocorticoids, chlorpheniramine or diphenhydramine
Genital human papillomavirus infection	Liquid nitrogen, trichloracetic acid
Herpes simplex virus infection	Acyclovir
Fungal infections	Topical antifungals
Bacterial infections	Penicillins, cephalosporins after first trimester, azithromycin

[1] Source: Skin Therapy Letter. S.Maddin ed. Vol 11, No 4, May 2006

TABLE D-3 Common Dermatologic Diseases, Drugs Used and Their Pregnancy Categories

Disease	Drug	FDA Pregnancy Category
Acne and rosacea	Topical erythromycin	B
	Topical clindamycin	B
	Topical benzoyl peroxide	C
	Topical tretinoin	C, but not advised
	Topical adaptalene	C, but not advised
	Topical tazarotene	X
	Topical metronidazole	B
	Topical azelaic acid	B
	Systemic tetracyclines	D
	Systemic erythromycin	B
	Systemic isotretinoin	X
Psoriasis	Topical glucocorticoids	C
	Topical calcipotriene	C
	UVB phototherapy	Considered safe
	PUVA	Considered potential teratogen, but adverse outcomes not reported
	Systemic methotrexate	X
	Systemic acitretin	X
	Alefacept	B
	Efalizumab	B
	Etanercept	B
Dermatitis	Systemic glucocorticoids	C
	Topical tacrolimus	C
	Topical pimecrolimus	C
	Systemic chlorpheniramine	B
	Systemic diphenyldramine	B
Viral infection	Imiquimod	B
	Podophyllin	C, not recommended
	Podophyllinotoxin	C, not recommended
	Acyclovir	B
	Famciclovir	B
	Valacyclovir	B
Fungal infection	Topical antifungals	considered safe
	Systemic terbinafine	B
	Systemic fluconazole	C, not recommended
	Topical fluconazole	C, considered safe
	Systemic itraconazole	C, avoidance suggested in first trimester
Bacterial infection	Systemic penicillin	B
	Systemic cephalosporin	B; possible association between certain cephalopsorins and congenital malformations in first trimester
	Systemic azitromycin	C

INDEX

Page numbers followed by an "f" indicate figures and images; page numbers followed by "t" indicate tables.